Management of Acute Coronary Syndromes

CONTEMPORARY ◊ CARDIOLOGY
Christopher P. Cannon, Series Editor

MANAGEMENT OF ACUTE CORONARY SYNDROMES

Second Edition

Edited by

CHRISTOPHER P. CANNON, MD

Brigham and Women's Hospital, Boston, MA

Foreword by

EUGENE BRAUNWALD, MD

Brigham and Women's Hospital, Boston, MA

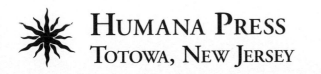

HUMANA PRESS
TOTOWA, NEW JERSEY

For additional copies, pricing for bulk purchases, and/or information about other Humana titles, contact Humana at the above address or at any of the following numbers: Tel.: 973-256-1699; Fax: 973-256-8341, E-mail: humana@humanapr.com; or visit our Website: http://humanapress.com

Due diligence has been taken by the publishers, editors, and authors of this book to assure the accuracy of the information published and to describe generally accepted practices. The contributors herein have carefully checked to ensure that the drug selections and dosages set forth in this text are accurate and in accord with the standards accepted at the time of publication. Notwithstanding, as new research, changes in government regulations, and knowledge from clinical experience relating to drug therapy and drug reactions constantly occurs, the reader is advised to check the product information provided by the manufacturer of each drug for any change in dosages or for additional warnings and contraindications. This is of utmost importance when the recommended drug herein is a new or infrequently used drug. It is the responsibility of the treating physician to determine dosages and treatment strategies for individual patients. Further it is the responsibility of the health care provider to ascertain the Food and Drug Administration status of each drug or device used in their clinical practice. The publisher, editors, and authors are not responsible for errors or omissions or for any consequences from the application of the information presented in this book and make no warranty, express or implied, with respect to the contents in this publication.

Cover design by Patricia F. Cleary.

This publication is printed on acid-free paper. ∞
ANSI Z39.48-1984 (American National Standards Institute) Permanence of Paper for Printed Library Materials.

Printed in the United States of America.   10 9 8 7 6 5 4 3 2 1

Library of Congress Cataloging-in-Publication Data

Management of acute coronary syndromes / edited by Christopher P. Cannon; foreword by Eugene Braunwald.--2nd ed.
             p.;cm.–(Contemporary cardiology)
      ISBN 1-58829-130-8 (alk. paper) (hb); 1-58829-309-2 (pb)
      Includes bibliographical references and index.
        1. Coronary heart disease. 2. Myocardial infarction. I. Cannon, Christopher P. II. Contemporary cardiology (Totowa, N.J.: unnumbered)
      [DNLM: 1. Coronary Disease–therapy, 2. Acute Disease–therapy. WG 300 M2656 2003]
      RC685.C6 M33 2003
      616.1'23–dc21   2002068765

FOREWORD

Coronary artery disease, the great scourge of our times, may express itself in two major clinicopathologic forms. The chronic form is caused by progressive atherosclerotic narrowing of the coronary arterial bed and usually presents as angina secondary to ischemia precipitated by increased myocardial oxygen demand, i.e., "demand ischemia." Treatment consists of pharmacological agents and other measures to reduce oxygen demand, and when this approach is inadequate, surgical or catheter-based revascularization. The acute form, on the other hand, results form a sudden reduction in myocardial oxygen supply caused, most commonly, by a thrombus on a fissured or eroded coronary atherosclerotic plaque that previously had not caused critical obstruction. This causes "supply ischemia," which may result in a variety of clinical syndromes, including unstable angina, non-Q-wave myocardial infarction, and Q-wave myocardial infarction. These acute coronary syndromes are responsible for more than half a million deaths and a million hospitalizations each year in the United States. The incidence is similar in other developed nations and it is rising at an alarming rate in portions of the world.

The management of patients with acute coronary syndromes represents one of the critical challenges to contemporary cardiology. This field has been the subject of intensive investigation that has led to major advances in our understanding of the pathophysiology, as well as in the diagnosis and management, of patients with these conditions.

Management of Acute Coronary Syndromes, Second Edition captures the many important recent developments in this rapidly moving area of cardiology. Dr. Cannon deserves thanks and congratulations for having organized a group of experienced clinicians and clinical investigators who present a comprehensive, up-to-date, and eminently readable picture of the field. This book is certain to aid cardiologists, internists, and emergency physicians in their management of patients with acute coronary syndromes.

Eugene Braunwald, MD

PREFACE

Over the past decade, there has been a revolution in our understanding of both the pathophysiology and the management of acute coronary syndromes (ACS). The conversion of a stable atherosclerotic lesion to a ruptured plaque with thrombosis has provided a unifying hypothesis for the etiology of acute coronary syndromes. From this, the concept of a "spectrum" of myocardial ischemia has provided a framework for understanding the pathogenesis, clinical feature, treatment, and outcome of patients across the spectrum of myocardial ischemia.

Furthermore, a new paradigm for acute coronary syndromes has emerged with the results of the Thrombolysis in Myocardial Ischemia (TIMI) IIIB trial: Though thrombolytic therapy has proven clearly beneficial in patients with ST segment elevation, no benefit has been observed in patients with unstable angina or non-ST elevation MI. Angiographic studies, including TIMI I and TIMI IIIA, have shown that this difference in outcome results from the initial status of the infarct-related artery, which usually demonstrates 100% coronary occlusion in ST elevation MI, in contrast to a patent, but stenotic coronary lesion in unstable angina and not-ST elevation MI. Thus, a classification of ST elevation MI vs non ST segment elevation ACS provides the critical information regarding the pathophysiology and acute management of the patient.

Accordingly, *Management of Acute Coronary Syndromes,* now in its *Second Edition,* is the first book to approach the management of acute coronary syndromes based on this new paradigm. The initial sections are devoted to understanding the pathophysiology of ACS, as well as the diagnostic tools for assessing patients. There are then two separate sections, one for ST elevation MI and the other for non-ST elevation ACS, which discuss the state-of-the-art management of these two groups of patients. I have felt privileged to have colleagues who are each world-renowned experts in their fields to provide concise, evidence-based recommendations on the optimal management of patients. The latest clinical trial data with numerous figures and tables are provided so that the reader will be able to have quickly available the key information that supports the recommended therapies. It is hoped that this compilation of the latest information will facilitate improvement in the management of patients with acute coronary syndromes.

On a personal level, my interest in acute coronary syndromes grew from many sources. First and foremost in guiding me has been my father, Paul Cannon, whose dedication to medicine and science has been a strong role model for me. His initial work in the measurement of coronary blood flow with radionuclide imaging two decades ago helped define the very basic pathophysiology of angina pectoris. He has also been one of my clinical teachers, as he has for many others at Columbia University College of Physicians and Surgeons over the past 30 years, teaching the students, housestaff, and fellows about the clinical presentation of angina to the acute management of myocardial infarction in the coronary care unit. The second major influence came from the writings of Fuster, Willerson, Braunwald, and others, on the emerging understanding of plaque rupture and coronary thrombosis in the pathophysiology of unstable angina. The new and rapidly emerging field sparked both my interest and enthusiasm to focus on acute coronary syndromes where new treatments might be of benefit to patients. Next, beginning with my fellowship at the Brigham, it has been my privilege to work with Eugene Braunwald, for nearly a decade in conducting the Thrombosis in Myocardial Infarction (TIMI) trials. His expertise, insight, innovation, and judgment have been the greatest example any student of medicine could hope for. His support and teaching throughout has fueled my enthusiasm for design and participation in clinical trials and scientific research studies, with the goal of improving patient care. Finally, my numerous other colleagues in the TIMI Group, notably Carolyn McCabe, Michael Gibson, and Elliott Antman, and in the entire cardiology community have been a constant inspiration to delve deeper into trying to understand and improve the management of patients with acute coronary syndromes.

Christopher P. Cannon, MD

CONTENTS

Part III   ST-Segment Elevation Myocardial Infarction

Part IV   Non-ST-Segment Elevation Myocardial Infarction

Part V   Special Aspects of Acute Coronary Syndromes

CONTRIBUTORS

H. VERNON ANDERSON, MD • *Professor of Medicine, Texas Heart Institute and the University of Texas at Houston, Houston, TX*

JEFFREY L. ANDERSON, MD • *Professor of Medicine, University of Utah School of Medicine, and Associate Chief of Cardiology, LDS Hospital, Salt Lake City, UT*

ANNEMARIE ARMANI, MD • *University of Massachusetts Medical School, Worcester, MA*

BRUCE BECKER, MD, MPH • *Centers for Behavioral and Preventive Medicine, The Miriam Hospital, Providence, RI*

RICHARD C. BECKER, MD • *Professor of Medicine, University of Massachusetts Medical School, and Director, Coronary Care Unit, Anticoagulation Services and Cardiovascular Thrombosis Research Center, UMass-Memorial Medical Center, Worcester, MA*

ROGER S. BLUMENTHAL, MD, FACC • *Director, the Johns Hopkins Ciccarone Center for the Prevention of Heart Disease, and Associate Professor of Medicine, Johns Hopkins University School of Medicine, Baltimore, MD*

BETH C. BOCK, PhD • *Centers for Behavioral and Preventive Medicine, The Miriam Hospital, Providence, RI*

EUGENE BRAUNWALD, MD • *Distinguished Hersey Professor of Medicine, Faculty Dean for Academic Programs, Brigham and Women's Hospital and Massachusetts General Hospital, Harvard Medical School, and Chief Academic Officer, Partners HealthCare System, Boston, MA*

SORIN J. BRENER, MD • *Department of Cardiovascular Medicine, The Cleveland Clinic Foundation, Cleveland, OH*

CHRISTOPHER P. CANNON, MD • *Associate Professor of Medicine, Cardiovascular Division, Brigham and Women's Hospital and Harvard Medical School, Boston, MA*

RODOLFO CARRILLO-JIMENEZ, MD • *Cardiology Fellow, Mount Sinai Medical Center, Miami Beach, FL*

BERNARD R. CHAITMAN, MD, FACC • *Division of Cardiology, Department of Internal Medicine, St. Louis University School of Medicine, St. Louis, MO*

ROBERT H. CHRISTENSON, PhD • *Pathology Department, University of Maryland Medical Center, Baltimore, MD*

MARC COHEN, MD • *Division of Cardiology, MCP Hahnemann University, Philadelphia, PA*

IAN CONDE-POZZI, MD • *Baylor College of Medicine and The Methodist Hospital, Houston, TX*

JAMES C. FANG, MD • *Cardiovascular Division, Brigham and Women's Hospital, Boston, MA*

W. BRIAN GIBLER, MD • *Department of Emergency Medicine, University of Cincinnati Medical Center, Cincinnati, OH*

C. MICHAEL GIBSON, MS, MD • *Harvard Clinical Research Institute, Harvard Medical School, Boston, MA*

MARY M. HAND, MSPH, RN • *National Heart, Lung, and Blood Institute, National Institutes of Health, Bethesda, MD*

CHARLES H. HENNEKENS, MD, DrPH • *Visiting Professor of Medicine and Epidemiology and Public Health, University of Miami School of Medicine, and Associate Director for Cardiovascular Research, Mount Sinai Medical Center, Miami Beach, FL*

DAVID R. HOLMES, JR., MD • *Internal Medicine and Cardiovascular Diseases, Mayo Clinic Rochester, Rochester, MN*

ALICE K. JACOBS, MD • *Cardiology Division, Boston Medical Center, Boston, MA*

IK-KYUNG JANG, MD • *Cardiology Division, Massachusetts General Hospital, Harvard Medical School, Boston, MA*

NEAL S. KLEIMAN, MD, FACC • *Section of Cardiology, Department of Medicine, Baylor College of Medicine and The Methodist Hospital, Houston, TX*

GERVASIO A. LAMAS, MD • *Director for Cardiovascular Research and Academic Affairs, Mount Sinai Medical Center, Miami Beach, FL*

COSTAS T. LAMBREW, MD • *Division of Cardiology, Maine Medical Center, Portland, ME*

GARY E. LANE, MD • *Department of Cardiovascular Diseases, Mayo Clinic Jacksonville, Jacksonville, FL*

JOSEPH LAU, MD • *Division of Clinical Care Research, New England Medical Center, Boston, MA*

JANE A. LEOPOLD, MD • *Boston Medical Center, Boston, MA*

NANCY SINCLAIR MCNAMARA, RN, BSN • *Cardiology Resource/Research Nurse-Coordinator, Exeter Hospital, Exeter, NH*

ALI MOUSTAPHA, MD • *Assistant Professor of Medicine, Louisiana State University School of Medicine in Shreveport, Shreveport, LA*

JAMES E. MULLER, MD • *Director of Clinical Research in Cardiology, Harvard Medical School, Massachusetts General Hospital, Boston, MA*

SABINA A. MURPHY, MPH • *Harvard Clinical Research Institute, Boston, MA*

L. KRISTIN NEWBY, MD • *Duke Clinical Research Institute, Durham, NC*

PATRICK T. O'GARA, MD • *Associate Professor of Medicine, Cardiovascular Division, Brigham and Women's Hospital and Harvard Medical School, Boston, MA*

E. MAGNUS OHMAN, MD • *The University of North Carolina–Chapel Hill, Chapel Hill, NC*

TERJE R. PEDERSEN, MD, PhD • *Head, Cardiology Department, Medical Clinic, Aker Hospital, University of Oslo, Oslo, Norway*

JORGE PLUTZKY, MD, FACC • *Cardiovascular Division, Brigham and Women's Hospital, Boston, MA*

J. HECTOR POPE, MD • *Assistant Professor of Emergency Medicine, Tufts University School of Medicine, Boston and Springfield, MA*

JEFFREY J. POPMA, MD • *Associate Professor of Medicine, Cardiovascular Division, Brigham and Women's Hospital and Harvard Medical School, Boston, MA*

SANJEEV PURI, MD • *Division of Cardiology, Department of Internal Medicine, St. Louis University School of Medicine, St. Louis, MO*

HANI A. RAZEK, MD • *Division of Cardiology, Department of Internal Medicine, University of Arkansas, Little Rock, AR*

MARC S. SABATINE, MD, MPH • *Cardiology Division, Department of Medicine, Massachusetts General Hospital, Boston, MA*

PETER M. SAPIN, MD, FACC • *Department of Internal Medicine, Alaska Native Medical Center, Anchorage, AK*

HARRY P. SELKER, MD, MSPH • *Professor of Medicine, Tufts University School of Medicine, Boston, MA*

KANWAR P. SINGH, MD • *Brigham and Women's Hospital and Harvard Clinical Research Institute, Harvard Medical School, Boston, MA*

PETER H. STONE, MD • *Associate Professor of Medicine, Cardiovascular Division, Brigham and Women's Hospital and Harvard Medical School, Boston, MA*

SERENA TONSTAD, MD, PhD • *Consultant, Preventive Cardiology, Medical Clinic, Ulleval University Hospital, Oslo, Norway*

ERIC J. TOPOL, MD • *Department of Cardiovascular Medicine, The Cleveland Clinic Foundation, Cleveland, OH*

WILLIAM S. WEINTRAUB, MD • *Division of Cardiology, Emory School of Medicine, Atlanta, GA*

THOMAS P. WHARTON, JR., MD, FACC • *Medical Director, Cardiology Section and Cardiac Catheterization Laboratory, Exeter Hospital, Exeter, NH*

YEREM YEGHIAZARIANS, MD • *Cardiovascular Division, Brigham and Women's Hospital, Boston, MA*

ROBERT J. ZALENSKI, MD, MA • *Department of Emergency Medicine, Wayne State University School of Medicine, and John D. Dingel Veterans Hospital, Detroit, MI*

JAMES S. ZEBRACK, MD • *University of Utah School of Medicine, Salt Lake City, UT*

I PATHOPHYSIOLOGY

1

The Spectrum of Myocardial Ischemia

The Paradigm of Acute Coronary Syndromes

Christopher P. Cannon, MD *and*
Eugene Braunwald, MD

CONTENTS

INTRODUCTION

Traditionally, ischemic heart disease has been divided into several separate syndromes: stable coronary artery disease, unstable angina (UA)*(1,2)*, non-Q wave myocardial infarction (MI), and Q wave MI. However, the understanding of the conversion of a stable atherosclerotic lesion to a ruptured plaque with thrombosis has provided a unifying hypothesis for the etiology of acute coronary syndromes (ACS)*(3–7)*. The concept of myocardial ischemia as a spectrum provides a framework for understanding the pathogenesis, clinical features, treatment and outcome of patients across the nexus of myocardial ischemia (Fig. 1).

However, a new paradigm for ACS emerged with the results of the Thrombolysis in Myocardial Ischemia (TIMI) IIIB trial: while fibrinolytic therapy is clearly beneficial in patients with ST segment elevation (STE) *(8)*, no benefit was observed in patients without STE *(9)*. Thus, it was observed that pharmacologic reperfusion therapy applies only to patients with STEMI, and is not indicated for patients without STEMI *(8–10)* Angio-

From: *Contemporary Cardiology: Management of Acute Coronary Syndromes, Second Edition*
Edited by: C. P. Cannon © Humana Press Inc., Totowa, NJ

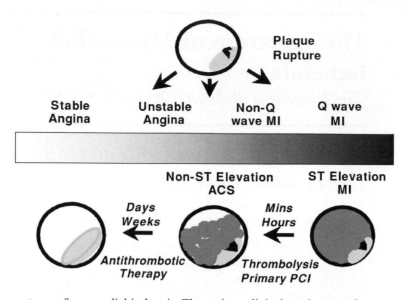

Fig. 1. The spectrum of myocardial ischemia. The various clinical syndromes of coronary artery disease can be viewed as a spectrum, ranging from patients with stable angina to those with acute Q wave MI. Across the spectrum of the ACS, atherosclerotic plaque rupture leads to coronary artery thrombosis: in acute Q wave MI, which usually presents with STE on the electrocardiogram, complete coronary occlusion is present. In those with UA or non-Q wave MI, a flow-limiting thrombus is usually present. In patients with stable angina, thrombus is rarely seen. The overall treatment objective is to move the patients back to a stable lesion. In acute STEMI, the objective over the first minutes to hours is to open the artery and achieve reperfusion. In patients with UA and non-STEMI, the goal is to stabilize or passivate the active thrombotic lesion over a period of hours to days. Then, over a period of months to years, the goal is to try to heal the lesion with risk-factor reduction with treatment of hypercholesterolemia, hypertension, diabetes, and smoking cessation, in an attempt to reduce the likelihood of subsequent rupture of the coronary plaques. Adapted with permission from ref. *135*.

graphic studies have shown that this difference in outcome is due to the initial status of the infarct-related artery, which usually exhibits 100% occlusion in STEMI (11,12), in contrast to a patent, but severely stenotic coronary lesion in non-STE ACS *(13,14)* (Fig. 1).

Thus, because of the advent of acute reperfusion therapy, the old distinction of Q wave vs non-Q wave MI (usually made days following MI) is no longer as useful for acute management. Instead, a classification of STEMI vs non-STE ACS provides the critical information regarding the pathophysiology and acute management of the patient. Patients with UA and non-STEMI share a similar pathophysiology, although the non-STEMI patients are at higher risk of subsequent events and appear to benefit more from more aggressive antithrombotic and interventional therapies.

Accordingly, in this book, separate sections are devoted to the management of these two broad types of patients with ACS, those with STEMI and those with non-STE ACS. It should be noted that STE is not a perfectly sensitive marker of acute occlusion *(15)*, and thus new technologies for proper identification and triage of patients with ACS are being evaluated extensively, as reviewed in Chapters 7 and 8. There are more than 1.8 million patients admitted every year to hospitals in the United States, with approx 1.42 million patients with UA/non-STEMI as compared with approx 400,000 patients with acute STEMI *(16)*.

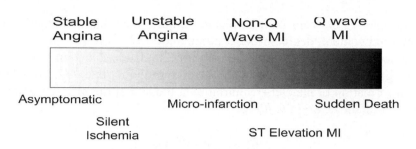

| Stable Angina | Unstable Angina | Non-Q Wave MI | Q wave MI |

Asymptomatic   Micro-infarction   Sudden Death

Silent Ischemia   ST Elevation MI

Fig. 2. The complete clinical spectrum of myocardial ischemic syndromes.

CLINICAL SPECTRUM OF ACS

It is useful to note that there are several other groups of patients who fall on this spectrum of myocardial ischemia (Fig. 2) Among patients with stable coronary artery disease, many apparently stable patients have active lesions, which are prone to rupture over the subsequent months and years *(17)*. Although most patients remain clinically stable *(18)*, it is estimated that nearly all of these patients with "stable" coronary artery disease have subclinical plaque rupture events *(19,20)*.

Between patients with stable angina and those with UA are a high-risk group with clinically stable symptoms, yet significant ambulatory ischemia that can be detected by ambulatory Holter monitoring *(21,22)*. Similarly, between patients with UA and non-STEMI, a patient may have what has been called a microinfarction *(23)* or infarctlet with a very small elevation of cardiac markers such as troponin T or I *(24–26)*.

At the extreme right of the spectrum of ischemic heart disease (Fig. 2) are patients with sudden cardiac death. Many patients have an acute coronary occlusion as the etiology of the cardiac arrest. However, with aggressive emergency medical services which respond rapidly and treat with advanced cardiac life support (ACLS) procedures, more patients are presenting with resuscitated "sudden cardiac death" *(27)*. Indeed, the National Heart Attack Alert Program (NHAAP) has as one of its major goals the improvement of emergency medical systems and early identification and treatment of acute MI patients as a means to reduce the overall mortality from MI *(28–31)*. If more patients with cardiac arrest can be successfully resuscitated in the pre-hospital setting, they may become candidates for reperfusion and other therapies for ACS.

PLAQUE RUPTURE

Atherothrombosis is a silent process that usually commences 20–30 yr prior a patient's presentation with a clinical syndrome *(3,4)*. Hypercholesterolemia, hypertension, diabetes, smoking and other coronary risk factors damage the endothelium which initiates the atherosclerotic process *(3,4,32)*, When the endothelium is dysfunctional, macrophages bind to endothelial adhesion molecules and can infiltrate the endothelial cell. Low density lipoprotein (LDL) molecules are able to penetrate into the vessel wall, the macrophages digest the LDL, becoming foam cells, which thereby create a lipid-filled atherosclerotic plaque *(4,33)*. Oxidized LDL may also have a direct toxic affect on the endothelium and smooth muscle cells, which contribute to the instability of the atherosclerotic plaque.

Then, multiple factors contribute to plaque rupture, including endothelial dysfunction, plaque lipid content, degree of local inflamation *(34),* coronary artery tone at the site of irregular plaques, and local shear stress forces, platelet function *(35,36),* the status of the coagulation system (i.e., a potentially prothombotic state) *(37,38),* all of which culminate in formation of platelet-rich thrombi at the site of the plaque rupture or erosion and the resultant ACS *(5,39,40).*

INFLAMMATION

A large body of evidence now points to a role for inflammation, which appears to play a key role in the development of atherosclerosis *(41)* and the development of ACS *(42–46).* Infectious agents, e.g., *Chlamydia pneumoniae,* may be one of the underlying causes of diffuse inflammation in the pathogenesis of coronary artery disease *(47–52).* Evidence from histologic studies *(47–52)* and several initial *(53–55)* (but not all) *(56)* treatment trials suggests *C. pneumoniae* may be an important and potentially treatable cause of ACS.

THROMBOSIS

The central role of coronary artery thrombosis in the pathogenesis of ACS is supported by a substantial body of evidence *(4,5,14,39,40,57–61).* Six sets of observations contribute to this concept: (*i*) at autopsy, thrombi can usually be identified at the site of a ruptured plaque*(5,39);* (*ii*) coronary atherectemy specimens obtained from patients with acute MI or UA demonstrate a high incidence of acute thrombotic lesions *(61);* (*iii*) coronary angioscopic observations indicate that thrombus is frequently present *(57,59,60);* (*iii*) coronary angiography has demonstrated ulceration or irregularities suggesting a ruptured plaque *(62,63)* and/or thrombus in many patients *(14,58);* in the TIMI III A trial, coronary angiograms in 306 patients with non-STE ACS revealed an apparent thrombus (globular intraluminal radiololucency) in 35% of all primary culprit lesions and a possible thrombus (adherent, flat intraluminal mass) in an additional 40% *(14);* (*v*) evidence of ongoing thrombosis has been noted with elevation of several markers of platelet activity and fibrin formation *(3,6,64–70);* and (*vi*) the improvement in the clinical outcome of patients with ACS by antithrombotic therapy with aspirin *(71–74),* heparin *(73–77),* low-molecular-weight heparin *(78–80),* clopidogrel *(81),* and platelet glycoprotein IIb/IIIa inhibitors *(82,83).*

PATHOPHYSIOLOGIC SPECTRUM

Across the spectrum of myocardial ischemia, markers of inflammation, thrombosis, and platelet activation increase in frequency in parallel with the clinical severity of the ACS (Fig. 3). Markers of inflammation, such as C-reactive protein (CRP), are found in 13% of patients with stable coronary artery disease vs 65% of patients with UA and 76% of patients with acute MI *(43).* Similarly, antibodies to *C. pneumoniae* are found in a higher percentage of patients with ACS than non-ACS patients *(84).* Activated platelets and markers of ongoing thrombosis, such as fibrinopeptide A, are also found more often in patients with ACS *(36,38,70,85–88).*

Coronary angiographic and angioscopic findings follow the same pattern across the spectrum of myocardial ischemia (Fig. 4). Angiographic studies have documented

	Stable Angina	Unstable Angina	Non-Q Wave MI	Q wave MI

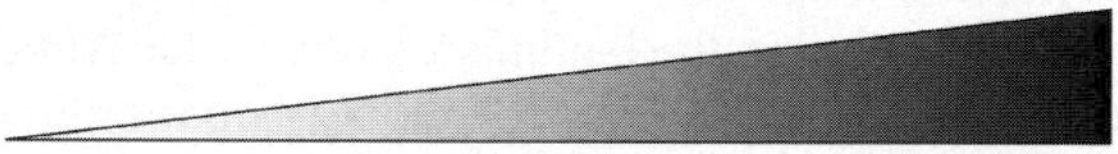

		Non-ST Elevation ACS	ST Elevation MI
↑ CRP	13%	65%	76%
Chlamydia	25%	75%	90%
Increased FPA / TAT	0-5%	60-80%	80-90%
Activated Platelets	0-5%	70-80%	80-90%

Fig. 3. The pathophysiology of acute ischemic syndromes. Atherosclerotic plaque rupture leads to coronary artery thrombosis, as indicated by angiographic evidence of thrombus or biochemical markers of increased fibrinopeptide A (FPA), thrombin–antithrombin complexes (TAT), or activated platelets. In acute Q wave MI, which usually presents with STE on the electrocardiogram, complete coronary occlusion is present. In those with unstable angina or non-Q wave MI, a flow-limiting thrombus is usually present, but complete occlusion of the artery is uncommon. In patients with stable angina, thrombus is rarely seen. Mortality increases with the severity of the acute ischemic syndrome. Data from Becker et al. *(38,70)*, Merlini et al. *(37)*, Trip et al. *(87)*, Liuzzo et al. *(43)*, Kruskal et al. *(136)*, and Mazzoli et al. *(84)*.

	Stable Angina	Unstable Angina	Non-Q Wave MI	Q wave MI

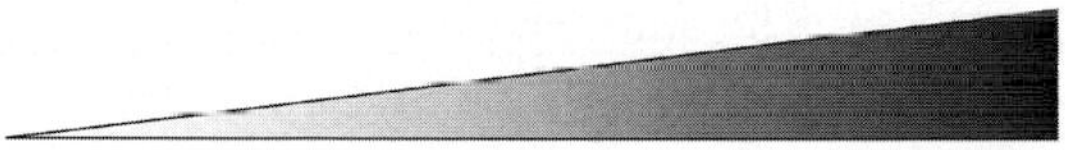

		Non-ST Elevation ACS	ST Elevation MI
Angiographic Thrombus	0-1%	40-75%	>90%
Morphology	Smooth	Ulcerated	Occluded
Acute Coronary Occlusion	0-1%	10-25%	>90%
Angioscopy	No clot	"White clot"	"Red clot"

Fig. 4. Angiographic findings across the spectrum of ACS. Data from the TIMI Investigators *(12,14)*, Van Belle et al. *(89)*, DeWood et al. *(11,13)*, Sacks et al. *(137)*, Mizuno et al. *(60)*, and Sherman et al. *(57)*.

"white" thrombi, predominantly platelet-rich thrombi, in patients with UA and non-STEMI, as compared with "red" thrombi in patients with acute STEMI *(57,89,90)*. This distinction was also noted in the landmark study by DeWood, in which coronary thrombi were aspirated with Fogarty catheters from patients with acute STEMI *(11)*. Coronary angiography in patients with STEMI usually documents total occlusion of the infarct-related artery *(11,12)*. In patients with ACS without STE, active lesions are frequently observed, with irregular borders, associated intraluminal lucencies (which may represent thrombus), and ulcerated or eccentrically localized obstructions *(14,62,63)*. Such lesions are more likely to be associated with the pathologic features of plaque rupture, hemorrhage, and superimposed thrombus *(5,39)*. In addition, activated macrophages can frequently be identifed in the hinge-point of the plaques, which may contribute to plaque rupture *(40)*. In patients with stable angina, nonactive lesions (which have symmetric, concentric, and with smooth borders) are usually observed *(14,62,63)*. The typical deformities are smooth with an hourglass configuration and absence of intraluminal lucencies on coronary angiography. The presence of angiographic thrombus thus shows a gradient across the spectrum of ACS.

NEW PARADIGM OF CLINICAL SYNDROMES

The extent of local thrombosis at the site of coronary plaque rupture is largely responsible for the severity of the clinical syndrome (Fig. 1). If the thrombosis causes total occlusion of the coronary artery, persistent ischemic pain and STE develop, which usually evolves into a Q-wave MI *(11,12)*. In some patients, the amount of local thrombosis is extensive, but the obstruction is subtotal, resulting in a flow-limiting coronary stenosis and myocardial ischemia (e.g., UA) sometimes associated with myocardial necrosis (NSTEMI) *(13,14)*. Plaque rupture plays a major role even in patients with stable angina: large numbers of plaques are found to have undergone rupture and healing in the past *(5,17,61)*. Indeed, it is estimated that up to 99% of all plaque ruptures are clinically silent events *(19)*. This highlights the importance of continued antithrombotic therapy for all patients with coronary artery disease.

STEMI: THE OPEN ARTERY THEORY

The "open artery theory" explains the beneficial effects of fibrinolytic therapy and catheter-based revascularization in acute STEMI: early achievement of an open infarct-related artery is associated with improved outcome *(91)*. If occlusion persists for more than 30 min, myocardial necrosis develops in the territory at risk (Fig. 5). If the area at risk is large and the artery remains occluded, left ventricular function is impaired. Fibrinolytic therapy acts to interrupt this cascade of events. By lysing the coronary thrombus, reperfusion of the infarct-related artery is achieved. This leads to a limitation of infarct size and decreases the extent of left ventricular dysfunction *(92)*. The most important result of thrombolysis is improved survival *(93,94)*.

Beginning with animal studies *(95)*, the initial angiographic studies in patients using intracoronary streptokinase *(96,97)* and numerous other angiographic studies over the subsequent 20 yr have all lent strong support to this theory *(91,98)*. An overview of all the angiographic studies that used the TIMI flow grading system *(12)*, comprising over 4200 patients, found that patients who achieved complete and normal coronary perfusion,

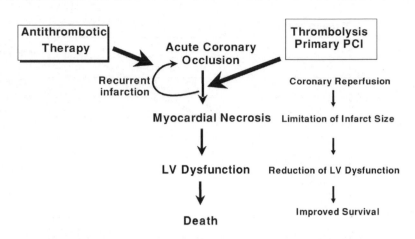

Fig. 5. The pathophysiology of acute STEMI and the paradigm of thrombolytic therapy.

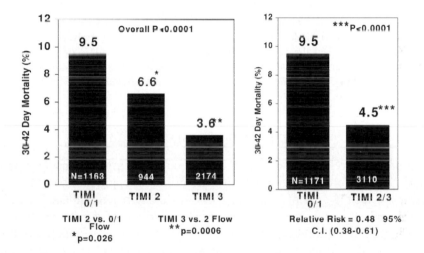

Fig. 6. The relationship between TIMI flow grade at 90 min following fibrinolytic therapy and subsequent mortality. Adapted with permission from ref. *98*.

graded TIMI grade 3 flow, at 90 min had the lowest mortality, 3.6%, compared with 9.5% with patients with TIMI grade 0 or 1 flow ($p < 0.00001$) (Fig. 6) *(98)*. Patients with slowed or delayed coronary flow in the infarct-related artery compared to the uninvolved artery, graded as TIMI grade 2 flow, had an intermediate mortality of 6.6% and a relative risk of mortality that was significantly better than an occluded artery *(98)* These findings have also been confirmed in the Global Use of Strategies to Open Occluded Arteries (GUSTO) angiographic substudy, in which the mortality rates of patients with TIMI flow grades 2 and 3 were adjusted for differences in baseline characteristics *(99)*. A direct relationship between full reperfusion and lower mortality also is also seen in an overview of trials of primary angioplasty and fibrinolytic therapy (Fig. 7) *(100)*. When plotting the percentage of patients in various trials vs the corresponding mortality, a strong correlation between increasing rates of early TIMI grade 3 flow and lower mortality is observed *(100)*.

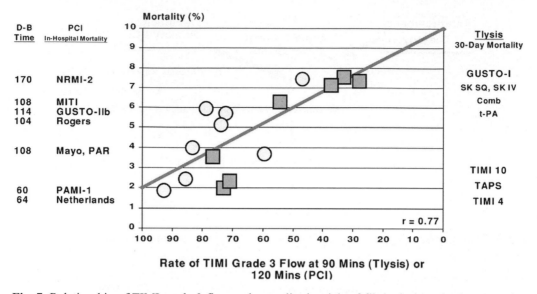

Fig. 7. Relationship of TIMI grade 3 flow and mortality in trials of fibrinolysis and primary angioplasty. For each trial listed in the left and right columns, the rate of TIMI grade 3 flow is plotted against the mortality observed in that group in the trial. Circles indicate the trials of primary angioplasty and squares indicate fibrinolysis trials. Adapted with permission from Cannon CP, Braunwald E. *J Thromb Thrombolysis* 1996;3:109–117

PARADIGM FOR NON-STE ACS

Among patients presenting without STE, the coronary artery is usually patent (i.e., TIMI grade 2 or 3 flow). In these patients, the principal approach is to use antithrombotic therapy, with the goal of preventing thrombus extension, enhancing endogenous fibrinolysis, and ultimately allowing healing (passivation) of the disrupted plaque. As shown in Fig. 8, if antithrombotic therapy is present at the time of plaque rupture, it can limit the degree of thrombosis and subsequent lesion stenosis. A corresponding reduction in the severity of the ACS episode has been seen in several trials comparing patients who were receiving aspirin vs not *(101,102)*. Another goal of antithrombotic therapy is to prevent the coronary thrombus from progressing to a complete occlusion. Over a period of days to weeks, antithrombotic therapy acts to passivate the lesion and allow endogenous fibrinolysis to dissolve the acute thrombosis and restore the acute lesion to a stable plaque.

MEDICAL TREATMENT

An overview of the medical treatment of ACS is shown in Fig. 9. As discussed, aspirin has been shown in numerous studies to be beneficial across the entire spectrum of myocardial ischemia, from primary prevention of MI *(103,104)* to prevention of death or MI in all ACS *(71–74,94,105)*. Aspirin is also a very effective agent for secondary prevention of events *(106,107)*.

Heparin has also been shown to be beneficial in reducing death or MI in non-STE ACS *(73,75–77)*. Low-molecular-weight heparin also significantly reduces death or MI com-

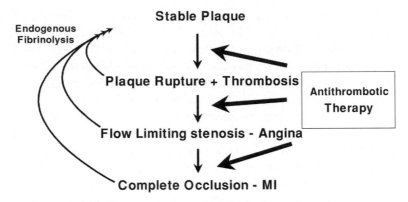

Fig. 8. The paradigm of antithrombotic therapy for non-STE ACS: antithrombotic therapy plays a major role in the treatment and prevention of ACS. If present at the time of plaque rupture (or administered acutely at the time of a clinical event), antithrombotic therapy can limit the development of thrombosis or the degree of thrombosis and subsequent lesion stenosis, which causes clinical ischemia (e.g., UA). Antithrombotic therapy could also prevent the local thrombosis from progressing to a complete occlusion (i.e., an MI). Over a period of days to weeks, antithrombotic therapy acts to passivate the lesion and allow endogenous fibrinolysis to dissolve the acute thrombosis and restore the acute lesion to a stable plaque. Adapted with permission from ref. *135*.

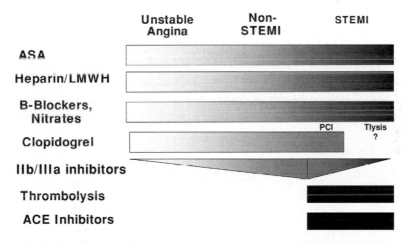

Fig. 9. Medical treatments across the spectrum of myocardial ischemia. Aspirin, heparin, beta-blockers, and nitrates are all uniformly beneficial across the spectrum; fibrinolytic therapy and the acute use of angiotensin converting enzyme inhibitors is only beneficial in patients presenting with acute MI with STE (or new left bundle branch block). Glycoprotein IIb/IIIa inhibitors are more beneficial in patients with non-STEMI (i.e., positive troponin) and in those undergoing primary percutaneous coronary intervention (PCI), and of some benefit in conjunction with reduced-dose fibrinolytic therapy. Clopidogrel has been shown to be beneficial in patients with UA/non-STEMI, and in those undergoing PCI, but trials are still ongoing in patients with fibrinolytic therapy.

pared with aspirin alone *(78)*, and one agent, enoxaparin, has been shown to be superior to heparin in patients with non-STE ACS *(79,80)* In STEMI, heparin improves infarct-related artery patency following tissue plasminogen activator *(108–110)*. The low-molecular-weight heparin enoxaparin has also recently been shown to reduce the incidence of death, MI, or recurrent ischemia following thrombolytic therapy *(111–113)*.

Beta-blockers, nitrates, and calcium antagonists are useful in the majority of patients with ACS (10,114). Angiotensin converting enzyme (ACE) inhibitors have been shown to be beneficial in patients post-MI (115,116) and, more recently, in acute STEMI in the Gruppo Italiano per lo Studio della Sopravvivenza nell'Infarto Miocardico (GISSI)-3, International Study of Infarct Survival (ISIS)-4, and Chinese trials (117–119).

Most recently, inhibition of the platelet glycoprotein IIb/IIIa receptor has been shown to be beneficial in patients with non-STE ACS *(82,83)*, especially those who have a positive troponin *(120,121)*. In STEMI, promising results with IIb/IIIa inhibitors have been observed with primary angioplasty *(122–124)*, and reduction in recurrent ischemic events (but not mortality) has been seen when used in conjunction with reduced-dose firbinotlytic therapy *(113,125,126)*.

CLINICAL COURSE

Mortality following ACS is influenced by the patients' baseline characteristics, the severity of the initial and recurrent event(s), and the extent of coronary artery disease and left ventricular dysfunction *(18,127–130)*. Following any of the ACS, patients remain at risk for recurrent events with approx 15–25% of patients developing recurrent ischemia or infarction by 1 yr *(131,132)*. If such recurrent events occur, subsequent mortality is higher *(133,134)*. Thus, early identification and treatment of the patient to prevent recurrent ischemic complications is important and is described in detail in this book.

REFERENCES

1. Braunwald E. Unstable angina: a classification. Circulation 1989;80:410–414.
2. Conti CR, Brawley RK, Griffith LSC, et al. Unstable angina pectoris: morbidity and mortality in 57 consecutive patients evaluated angiographically. Am J Cardiol 1973;32:745–750.
3. Fuster V, Badimon L, Cohen M, Ambrose JA, Badimon JJ, Chesebro J. Insights into the pathogenesis of acute ischemic syndromes. Circulation 1988;77:1213–1220.
4. Fuster V, Badimon L, Badimon JJ, Chesebro JH. The pathophysiology of coronary artery disease and the acute coronary syndromes. N Engl J Med 1992;326:242–50,310–318.
5. Falk E. Unstable angina with fatal outcome: dynamic coronary thrombosis leading to infarction and/or sudden death. Circulation 1985;71:699–708.
6. Willerson JT, Golino P, Eidt J, Campbell WB, Buja M. Specific platelet mediators and unstable coronary artery lesions. Experimental evidence and potential clinical implications. Circulation 1989;80: 198–205.
7. Falk E, Shah PK, Fuster V. Coronary plaque disruption. Circulation 1995;92:657–671.
8. Fibrinolytic Therapy Trialists' (FTT) Collaborative Group. Indications for fibrinolytic therapy in suspected acute myocardial infarction: collaborative overview of early mortality and major morbidity results from all randomised trials of more than 1000 patients. Lancet 1994;343:311–322.
9. The TIMI IIIB Investigators. Effects of tissue plasminogen activator and a comparison of early invasive and conservative strategies in unstable angina and non-Q-wave myocardial infarction: results of the TIMI IIIB Trial. Circulation 1994;89:1545–1556.

10. Braunwald E, Mark DB, Jones RH, et al. Unstable Angina: Diagnosis and Management. Clinical Practice Guideline Number 10. Agency for Health Care Policy and Research and the National Heart, Lung, and Blood Institute, Public Health Service, U.S. Department of Health and Human Services, Rockville, MD, 1994.

11. DeWood MA, Spores J, Notske R, et al. Prevalence of total coronary occlusion during the early hours of transmural myocardial infarction. N Engl J Med 1980;303:897–902.

12. TIMI Study Group. The Thrombolysis in Myocardial Infarction (TIMI) Trial: phase I findings. N Engl J Med 1985;312:932–936.

13. DeWood MA, Stifter WF, Simpson CS, et al. Coronary arteriographic findings soon after non-Q wave myocardial infarction. N Engl J Med 1986;315:417–423.

14. The TIMI IIIA Investigators. Early effects of tissue-type plasminogen activator added to conventional therapy on the culprit lesion in patients presenting with ischemic cardiac pain at rest. Results of the Thrombolysis in Myocardial Ischemia (TIMI IIIA) Trial. Circulation 1993;87:38–52.

15. Gibbons RJ, Christian TF, Hopfenspirger M, Hodge DO, Bailey KR. Myocardium at risk and infarct size after thrombolytic therapy for acute myocardial infarction: implications for the design of randomized trials of acute interventions. J Am Coll Cardiol 1994;24:616–623.

16. Braunwald E, Antman EM, Beasley JW, et al. ACC/AHA guidelines for the management of patients with unstable angina and non ST segment elevation myocardial infarction: a report of the American College of Cardiology/American Heart Association Task Force on Practice Guidelines (Committee on the Management of Unstable Angina and Non-ST Segment Elevation Myocardial Infarction). J Am Coll Cardiol 2000;36:970–1056.

17. Chester MR, Chen L, Kaski JC. Angiographic evidence for frequent "silent" plaque disruption in patients with stable angina. J Am Coll Cardiol 1995;Special Issue:428A.

18. Mark DB, Nelson CL, Califf RM, et al. Continuing evolution of therapy for coronary artery disease. Initial results from the era of coronary angioplasty. Circulation 1994;89:2015–2025.

19. Webster MWI, Chesebro JH, Smith HC, et al. Myocardial infarction and coronary artery occlusion: a prospective 5-year angiographic study. J Am Coll Cardiol 1990;15:218A.

20. Davies MJ. The composition of coronary-artery plaques. N Engl J Med 1997;336:1312–1314.

21. Gottlieb SO, Weisfeldt ML, Ouyang P, Mellits ED, Gertenblith G. Silent ischemia as a marker for early unfavorable outcomes in patients with unstable angina. N Engl J Med 1986;1986:1214–1219.

22. Rocco MB, Nabel EG, Campbell S, et al. Prognostic importance of myocardial ischemia detected by ambulatory monitoring in patients with coronary artery disease. Circulation 1988;78:877 884.

23. Fung AY, Jue J, Thompson CR, Davies C, Schreiber WE. Diagnosis of microinfarction in acute ischemic syndromes is of prognostic value. J Am Coll Cardiol 1994;Special Issue:316A.

24. Hamm CW, Ravkilde J, Gerhardt W, et al. The prognostic value of troponin T in unstable angina. N Engl J Med 1992;327:146–150.

25. Antman EM, Tanasijevic MJ, Thompson B, et al. Cardiac-specific troponin I levels to predict the risk of mortality in patients with acute coronary syndromes. N Engl J Med 1996;335:1342–1349.

26. Morrow DA, Cannon CP, Rifai N, et al. Ability of minor elevations of troponin I and T to predict benefit from an early invasive strategy in patients with unstable angina and non-ST elevation myocardial infarction: results from a randomized trial. JAMA 2001;286:2405–2412.

27. Eisenberg MS, Horwood BT, Cummins RO, Reynolds-Haertle R, Hearne TR. Cardiac arrest and resuscitation: a tale of 29 cities. Ann Emerg Med 1990;19:179–186.

28. National Heart Attack Alert Program Coordinating Committee—60 Minutes to Treatment Working Group. Emergency department: rapid identification and treatment of patients with acute myocardial infarction. Ann Emerg Med 1994;23:311–329.

29. National Heart Attack Alert Program Coordinating Committee Access to Care Subcommittee. 9-1-1: rapid identification and treatment of acute myocardial infarction. Am J Emerg Med 1995;13:188–195.

30. National Heart Attack Alert Program Coordinating Committee Access to Care Subcommittee. Staffing and equipping emergency medical services systems: rapid identification and treatment of acute myocardial infarction. Am J Emerg Med 1995;13:58–65.

31. National Heart Attack Alert Program Coordinating Committee Access to Care Subcommittee. Emergency medical dispatching: rapid identification and treatment of acute myocardial infarction. Am J Emerg Med 1995;13:67–73.

32. Vita JA, Treasure CB, Nabel EG, et al. Coronary vasomotor response to acetylcholine relates to risk factors for coronary artery disease. Circulation 1990;81:491–497.

33. Libby P. Molecular bases of the acute coronary syndromes. Circulation 1995;91:2844–2850.

34. Moreno PR, Bernardi VH, Lopez-Cuellar J, et al. Macrophages, smooth muscle cells, and tissue factor in unstable angina. Implications for cell-mediated thrombogenicity in acute coronary syndromes. Circulation 1996;94:3090–3097.

35. Weiss EJ, Bray PF, Tayback M, et al. A polymorphism of a platelet glycoprotein receptor as an inherited risk factor for coronary thrombosis. N Engl J Med 1996;334:1090–1094.

36. Ault K, Cannon CP, Mitchell J, et al. Platelet activation in patients after an acute coronary: results from the TIMI 12 trial. J Am Coll Cardiol 1999;33:634–639.

37. Merlini PA, Bauer KA, Oltrona L, et al. Persistent activation of coagulation mechanism in unstable angina and myocardial infarction. Circulation 1994;90:61–68.

38. Becker RC, Tracy RP, Bovill EG, et al. Surface 12-lead electrocardiogram findings and plasma markers of thrombin activity and generation in patients with myocardial ischemia at rest. J Thromb Thrombolysis 1994;1:101–107.

39. Davies MJ, Thomas A. Plaque fissuring—the cause of acute myocardial infarction, sudden ischemic death, and crescendo angina. Br Heart J 1985;53:363–373.

40. Shah PK, Falk E, Badimon JJ, et al. Human monocyte-derived macrophages induce collagen breakdown in fibrous caps of atherosclerotic plaques. Potential role of matrix-degrading metalloproteinases and implications for plaque rupture. Circulation 1998;92:1565–1569.

41. Ridker PM, Cushman M, Stampfer MJ, Tracy RP, Hennekens CH. Inflammation, aspirin, and the risk of cardiovascular disease in apparently healthy men. N Engl J Med 1997;336:973–979 [published erratum appears in N Engl J Med 1997;337:356].

42. Berk BC, Weintraub WS, Alexander RW. Elevation of C-reative protein in "active" coronary artery disease. Am J Cardiol 1990;65:168–172.

43. Liuzzo G, Biasucci LM, Gallimore JR, et al. The prognostic value of C-reactive protein and serum amyloid A protein in severe unstable angina. N Engl J Med 1994;331:417–424.

44. Haverkate F, Thompson SG, Pyke SDM, Gallimore JR, Pepys MB, for the European Concerted Action on Thrombosis and Disabilities Angina Pectoris Study Group. Production of C-reactive protein and risk of coronary events in stable and unstable angina. Lancet 1997;349:462–466.

45. Morrow DA, Rifai N, Antman EM, et al. C-reactive protein is a potent predictor of mortality independently and in combination with troponin T in acute coronary syndromes: a TIMI 11A substudy. J Am Coll Cardiol 1998;31:1460–1465.

46. Cannon CP, Weintraub WS, Demopoulos L, et al. High-sensitivity C-reactive protein (hs-CRP) to predict 6 month mortality and relative benefit of invasive vs. conservative strategy in patients with unstable angina: primary results of the TACTICS-TIMI 18 C-Reactive Protein substudy. J Am Coll Cardiol 2001;37(Suppl. A):315A.

47. Linnanmaki E, Leinonen M, Mattila K, Nieminen MS, Valtonen V, Saikku P. *Chlamydia pneumoniae*-specific circulating immune complexes in patients with chronic coronary heart disease. Circulation 1993;87:1130–1134.

48. Saikku P, Leinonen M, Mattila K, et al. Serological evidence of an association of a novel *Chlamydia*, TWAR, with chronic coronary heart disease and acute myocardial infarction. Lancet 1988;2:983–986.

49. Thom DH, Grayston JT, Siscovick DS, Wang SP, Weiss NS, Daling JR. Association of prior infection with *Chlamydia pneumoniae* and angiographically demonstrated coronary artery disease. JAMA 1992; 268:68–72.

50. Blasi F, Cosentini R, Raccanelli R, et al. A possible association of *Chlamydia pneumoniae* infection and acute myocardial infarction in patients younger than 65 years of age. Chest 1997;112:309–312.

51. Danesh J, Collins R, Peto R. Chronic infection and coronary heart disease: is there a link? Lancet 1997; 350:430–436.

52. Libby P, Egan D, Skarlatos S. Roles of infectious agents in atherosclerosis and restenosis. An assessment of the evidence and need for future research. Circulation 1997;96:4095–4103.

53. Gurfinkel E, Bozovich G, Daroca A, Beck E, Mautner B, for the ROXIS Study Group. Randomised trial of roxithromycin in non-Q wave coronary syndromes: ROXIS pilot study. Lancet 1997;350: 404–407.

54. Gupta S, Leathan EW, Carrington D, Mendall MA, Kaski JC, Camm AJ. Elevated *Chlamydia pneumoniae* antibodies, cardiovascular events, and azithromycin in male survivors of myocardial infarction. Circulation 1997;96:404–407.

55. Sinisalo J, Mattila K, Valtonen V, et al. Effect of 3 months of antimicrobial treatment with clarithromycin in acute non-q-wave coronary syndrome. Circulation 2002;105:1555–1560.

56. Dunne MW. Rationale and design of a secondary prevention trial of antibiotic use in patients after myocardial infarction: the WIZARD (weekly intervention with zithromax [azithromycin] for atherosclerosis and its related disorders) trial. J Infect Dis 2000;181(Suppl. 3):S572–S578.
57. Sherman CT, Litvack F, Grundfest W, et al. Coronary angioscopy in patients with unstable angina pectoris. N Engl J Med 1986;315:913–919.
58. Brunelli C, Spallarossa P, Ghigliotta G, Ianetti M, Caponnetto S. Thrombosis in refractory unstable angina. Am J Cardiol 1991;68:110B–118B.
59. Uchida Y, Fujimori Y, Hirose J, Oshima T. Percutaneous coronary angioscopy. Jpn Heart J 1992;33: 271–294.
60. Mizuno K, Satumo K, Miyamoto A, et al. Angioscopic evaluation of coronary artery thrombi in acute coronary syndromes. N Engl J Med 1992;326:287–291.
61. Sullivan E, Kearney M, Isner JM, Topol EJ, Losordo DW. Pathology of unstable angina: analysis of biopsies obtained by directional coronary atherectomy. J Thromb Thrombolysis 1994;1:63–71.
62. Ambrose JA, Winters SL, Arora RR, et al. Angiographic evolution of coronary artery morphology in unstable angina. J Am Coll Cardiol 1986;7:472–478.
63. Ambrose JA, Hjemdahl-Monsen CE, Borrico S, Gorlin R, Fuster V. Angiographic demonstration of a common link between unstable angina and non-Q-wave myocardial infarction. Am J Cardiol 1988,61. 244–247
64. Fitzgerald DJ, Roy L, Catella F, Fitzgerald GA. Platelet activation in unstable coronary disease. N Engl J Med 1986;315:983–989.
65. Theroux P, Latour JG, Leger-Gautier C, Delaria J. Fibrinopeptide A and platelet factor four levels in unstable angina. Circulation 1987;75:156–162.
66. Robertson RM, Robertson D, Roberts LJ, et al. Thromboxane A_2 in vasotonic angina pectoris. N Engl J Med 1981;304:998–1003.
67. Alexopoloulos D, Ambrose JA, Stump D, et al. Thrombosis-related markers in unstable angina. J Am Coll Cardiol 1991;17:866–871.
68. Hirsch PD, Hillis LD, Campbell WB, Firth BG, Willerson JT. Release of prostaglandins and thromboxane into the coronary circulation in patients with ischemic heart disease. N Engl J Med 1981;304: 685–691.
69. van der Berg EK, Schmitz JM, Benedict CR, Malloy CR, Willerson JT, Dehmer GJ. Transcardiac serotonin concentration is increased in selected patients with limiting angina complex coronary lesion morphology. Circulation 1989;79:116–124.
70. Becker RC, Tracy RP, Bovill EG, Mann KG, Ault K, for the TIMI-III Thrombosis and Anticoagulation Study Group. The clinical use of flow cytometry for assessing platelet activation in acute coronary syndromes. Coron Artery Dis 1994;5:339–345.
71. Lewis HD, Davis JW, Archibald DG, et al. Protective effects of aspirin against acute myocardial infarction and death in men with unstable angina. N Engl J Med 1983;309:396–403.
72. Cairns JA, Gent M, Singer J, et al. Aspirin, sulfinpyrazone, or both in unstable angina. N Engl J Med 1985;313:1369–1375.
73. Theroux P, Ouimet H, McCans J, et al. Aspirin, heparin or both to treat unstable angina. N Engl J Med 1988;319:1105–1111.
74. The RISC Group. Risk of myocardial infarction and death during treatment with low dose aspirin and intravenous heparin in men with unstable coronary artery disease. Lancet 1990;336:827–830.
75. Theroux P, Waters D, Qiu S, McCans J, de Guise P, Juneau M. Aspirin versus heparin to prevent myocardial infarction during the acute phase of unstable angina. Circulation 1993;88:2045–2048.
76. Cohen M, Adams PC, Parry G, et al. Combination antithrombotic therapy in unstable rest angina and non-Q-wave infarction in nonprior aspirin users. Primary end points analysis from the ATACS trial. Circulation 1994;89:81–88.
77. Oler A, Whooley MA, Oler J, Grady D. Adding heparin to aspirin reduces the incidence of myocardial infarction and death in patients with unstable angina. A meta-analysis. JAMA 1996;276: 811–815.
78. Fragmin during Instability in Coronary Artery Disease (FRISC) Study Group. Low-molecular-weight heparin during instability in coronary artery disease. Lancet 1996;347:561–568.
79. Cohen M, Demers C, Gurfinkel EP, et al. A comparison of low-molecular-weight heparin with unfractionated heparin for unstable coronary artery disease. N Engl J Med 1997;337:447–452.
80. Antman EM, McCabe CH, Gurfinkel EP, et al. Enoxaparin prevents death and cardiac ischemic events in unstable Angina/Non-Q-wave myocardial infarction: results of the Thrombolysis In Myocardial Infarction (TIMI) 11B trial. Circulation 1999;100:1593–1601.

81. Clopidogrel in Unstable Angina to Prevent Recurrent Events Trial Investigators. Effects of clopidogrel in addition to aspirin in patients with acute coronary syndromes without ST-segment elevation. N Engl J Med 2001;345:494–502.

82. The Platelet Receptor Inhibition for Ischemic Syndrome Management in Patients Limited by Unstable Signs and Symptoms (PRISM-PLUS) Trial Investigators. Inhibition of the platelet glycoprotein IIb/IIIa receptor with tirofiban in unstable angina and non-Q-wave myocardial infarction. N Engl J Med 1998;338:1488–1497.

83. The PURSUIT Trial Investigators. Inhibition of platelet glycoprotein IIb/IIIa with eptifibatide in patients with acute coronary syndromes. N Engl J Med 1998;339:436–443.

84. Mazzoli S, Tofani N, Fantini A, et al. *Chlamydia pnermoniae* antibody response in patients with acute myocardial infarction and their follow-up. Am Heart J 1998;135:15–20.

85. Becker RC, Bovill EG, Corrao JM, et al. Platelet activation determined by flow cytometry persists despite antithrombotic therapy in patients with unstable angina and non-Q wave myocardial infarction. J Thromb Thrombolysis 1994;1:95–100.

86. Becker RC, Bovill EG, Corrao JM, et al. Dynamic nature of thrombin generation, fibrin formation, and platelet activation in unstable angina and non-Q-wave myocardial infarction. J Thromb Thrombolysis 1995;2:57–64.

87. Trip MD, Manger Cats V, can Capelle FJL, Vreeken J. Platelet hyperreactivity and prognosis in survivors of myocardial infarction. N Engl J Med 1990;322:1549–1554.

88. Tofler GH, Brezinski D, Schafer AI, et al. Concurrent morning increase in platelet aggregability and the risk of myocardial infarction and sudden cardiac death. N Engl J Med 1987;316:1514–1518.

89. Van Belle E, Lablanche J-M, Bauters C, Renaud N, McFadden EP, Bertrand ME. Coronary angioscopic findings in the infarct-related vessel within 1 month of acute myocardial infarction. Natural history and the effect of thrombolysis. Circulation 1998;97:26–33.

90. Inoue K, Ochiai H, Kuwaki K. The mechanism of reocclusion after successful coronary thrombolysis as validated by percutansous angioscopy. J Am Coll Cardiol 1994;13A.

91. Braunwald E. The open-artery theory is alive and well—again. N Engl J Med 1993;329:1650–1652.

92. Braunwald E. Myocardial reperfusion, limitation of infarct size, reduction of left ventricular dysfunction, and improved survival: Should the paradigm be expanded? Circulation 1989;79:441–444.

93. Gruppo Italiano per lo Studio della Streptochinasi nell'Infarto Miocardico (GISSI). Effectiveness of intravenous thrombolytic treatment in acute myocardial infarction. Lancet 1986;1:397–402.

94. ISIS-2 (Second International Study of Infarct Survival) Collaborative Group. Randomised trial of intravenous streptokinase, oral aspirin, both, or neither among 17,187 cases of suspected acute myocardial infarction: ISIS-2. Lancet 1988;2:349–360.

95. Reimer KA, Lowe JE, Rasmussen MM, Jennings RB. The wavefront phenomenon of ischemic cell death. 1. Myocardial infarct size vs duration of coronary occlusion in dogs. Circulation 1977;56:786–794.

96. Rentrop KP, Blanke H, Karsch KR, Kreuzer H. Initial experience with transluminal recanalization of the recently occluded infarct-related coronary artery in acute myocardial infarction. Comparison with conventionally treated patients. Clin Cardiol 1979;2:92–105.

97. Ganz W, Buchbinder N, Marcus H, et al. Intracoronary thrombolysis in evolving myocardial infarction. Am Heart J 1981;101:4–13.

98. Cannon CP, Braunwald E. GUSTO, TIMI and the case for rapid reperfusion. Acta Cardiol 1994;49: 1–8.

99. Simes RJ, Topol EJ, Holmes DR, et al. Link between the angiographic substudy and mortality outcomes in a large randomized trial of myocardial reperfusion. Importance of early and complete infarct artery reperfusion. Circulation 1995;91:1923–1928.

100. Cannon CP, Braunwald E. Time to reperfusion: the critical modulator in thrombolysis and primary angioplasty. J Thromb Thrombolysis 1996;3:117–125.

101. Garcia-Dorado D, Theroux P, Tornos P, et al. Previous aspirin use may attenuate the severity of the manifestation of acute ischemic syndromes. Circulation 1995;92:1743–1748.

102. Borzak S, Cannon CP, Kraft PL, et al. Effects of prior aspirin and anti-ischemic therapy on outcome of patients with unstable angina. Am J Cardiol 1998;81:678–681.

103. Willard JE, Lange RA, Hillis LD. The use of aspirin in ischemic heart disease. N Engl J Med 1992; 327:175–81.

104. Steering Committee of the Physicians' Health Study Research Group. Final report on the aspirin component of the ongoing Physicians' Health Study. N Engl J Med 1989;321:129–135.

105. Roux S, Christeller S, Ludin E. Effects of aspirin on coronary reocclusion and recurrent ischemia after thrombolysis: a meta-analysis. J Am Coll Cardiol 1992;19:671–677.
106. Klimt CR, Knatterud GL, Stamler J, Meier P, for the PARIS II Investigator Group. Persantine-Aspirin Reinfarction Study. Part II. Secondary coronary prevention with persantine and aspirin. J Am Coll Cardiol 1986;7:251–269.
107. Antiplatelet Trialist' Collaboration. Collaborative overview of randomised trials of antiplatelet therapy—I: prevention of death myocardial infarction and stroke by prolongued antiplatelet therapy in various categories of patients. BMJ 1994;308:81–106.
108. Bleich SD, Nichols T, Schumacher RR, Cooke DH, Tate DA, Teichman SL. Effect of heparin on coronary patency after thrombolysis with tissue plasminogen activator in acute myocardial infarction. Am J Cardiol 1990;66:1412–1417.
109. Hsia J, Hamilton WP, Kleiman N, Roberts R, Chaitman BR, Ross AM, et al. A comparison between heparin and low-dose aspirin as adjunctive therapy with tissue plasminogen activator for acute myocardial infarction. N Engl J Med 1990;323:1433–1437.
110. de Bono DP, Simoons MI, Tijssen J, et al. Effect of early intravenous heparin on coronary patency, infarct size, and bleeding complications after alteplase thrombolysis: results of a randomized double blind European Cooperative Study Group trial. Br Heart J 1992;67:122–128.
111. Baird SH, McBride SI, Trouton TG, Wilson C. Low molecular weight heparin versus unfractionated heparin following thrombolysis in myocardial infarction. J Am Coll Cardiol 1998;31(Suppl. A):191A.
112. Antman EM, Louwerenburg HW, Baars HF, et al. Enoxaparin as adjunctive antithrombin therapy for ST-elevation myocardial infarction: results of the ENTIRE-Thrombolysis in Myocardial Infarction (TIMI) 23 Trial. Circulation 2002;105:1642–1649.
113. The Assessment of the Safety and Efficacy of a New Thrombolytic Regimen (ASSENT)-3 Investigators. Efficacy and safety of tenecteplase in combination with enoxaparin, abciximab, or unfractionated heparin: the ASSENT-3 randomised trial in acute myocardial infarction. Lancet 2001;358:605–613.
114. Ryan TJ, Anderson JL, Antman EM, et al. ACC/AHA guidelines for the management of patients with acute myocardial infarction: a report of the American College of Cardiology/American Heart Association Task Force on Practice Guidelines (Committee on Management of Acute Myocardial Infarction). J Am Coll Cardiol 1996;28;1328–1428.
115. Pfeffer MA, Braunwald E, Moye LA, et al. Effect of captopril on mortality and morbidity in patients with left ventricular dysfunction after myocardial infarction. N Engl J Med 1992;327:669–677.
116. The Acute Infarction Ramipril Efficacy (AIRE) Study Investigators. Effect of ramipril on mortality and morbidity of survivors of acute myocardial infarction with clinical evidence of heart failure. Lancet 1993;342:821–828.
117. Gruppo Italiano per lo Studio della Sopravvivenza nell'Infarto Miocardico. GISSI-3: effect of lisinopril and trasdermal glyceryl trinitrate sinly and together on 6-week mortality and ventricular function after acute myocardial infarction. Lancet 1994;343:1115–1122.
118. ISIS-4 Collaborative Group. ISIS-4: randomized factorial trial assessing early oral captopril, oral mononitrate, and intravenous magnesium sulphate in 58,050 patients with suspected acute myocardial infarction. Lancet 1995;345:669–685.
119. Chinese Cardiac Study Collaborative Group. Oral captopril versus placebo among 13,634 patients with suspected myocardial infarction: interim report from the Chinese Cardiac Study(CCS-1). Lancet 1995;345:686–687.
120. Hamm CW, Heeschen C, Goldmann B, et al. Benefit of abciximab in patients with refractory unstable angina in relation to serum troponin T levels. N Engl J Med 1999;340:1623–1629.
121. Heeschen C, Hamm CW, Goldmann B, et al. Troponin concentrations for stratification of patients with acute coronary syndromes in relation to therapeutic efficacy of tirofiban. Lancet 1999;354:1757–1762.
122. Lefkovits J, Ivanhoe RJ, Califf RM, et al. Effects of platelet glycoprotein IIb/IIIa receptor blockade by a chimeric monoclonal antibody (abciximab) on acute and six-month outcomes after percutaneous transluminal coronary agioplasty for acute myocardial infarction. Am J Cardiol 1996;77:1045–1051.
123. Montalescot G, Barragan P, Wittenberg O, et al. Platelet glycoprotein IIb/IIIa inhibition with coronary stenting for acute myocardial infarction. N Engl J Med 2001;344:1895–1903.
124. Stone GW, Grines CL, Cox DA, et al. Comparison of angioplasty with stenting, with or without abciximab, in acute myocardial infarction. N Engl J Med 2002;346:957–966.
125. Antman EM, Giugliano RP, Gibson CM, et al. Abciximab facilitates the rate and extent of thrombolysis: results of TIMI 14 trial. Circulation 1999;99:2720–2732.

126. The GUSTO V Investigators. Reperfusion therapy for acute myocardial infarction with fibrinolytic therapy or combination reduced fibrinolytic therapy and platelet glycoprotein IIb/IIIa inhibition: the GUSTO V randomised trial. Lancet 2001;357:1905–1914.
127. DeBusk RF, Blomqvist CG, Kouchoukos NT, et al. Identification and treatment of low-risk patients after acute myocardial infarction and coronary bypass surgery. N Engl J Med 1986;314:161–166.
128. Morrow DA, Antman EM, Charlesworth A, et al. TIMI risk score for ST-elevation myocardial infarction: a convenient, bedside, clinical score for risk assessment at presentation: an intravenous nPA for treatment of infarcting myocardium early II trial substudy. Circulation 2000;102:2031–2037.
129. Antman EM, Cohen M, Bernink PJ, et al. The TIMI risk score for unstable Angina/Non-ST elevation MI: A method for prognostication and therapeutic decision making. JAMA 2000;284:835–842.
130. Boersma E, Pieper KS, Steyerberg EW, et al. Predictors of outcome in patients with acute coronary syndromes without persistent ST-segment elevation. Results from an international trial of 9461 patients. Circulation 2000;101:2557–2567.
131. Anderson HV, Cannon CP, Stone PH, et al. One-year results of the Thrombolysis in Myocardial Infarction (TIMI) IIIB clinical trial. A randomized comparison of tissue-type plasminogen activator versus placebo and early invasive versus early conservative strategies in unstable angina and non-Q-wave myocardial infarction. J Am Coll Cardiol 1995;26:1643–1650.
132. Cannon CP, McCabe CH, Stone PH, et al. The electrocardiogram predicts one-year outcome of patients with unstable angina and non-Q wave myocardial infarction: results of the TIMI III Registry ECG Ancillary Study. J Am Coll Cardiol 1997;30:133–140.
133. Cannon CP, Sharis PJ, Schweiger MJ, et al. Prospective validation of a composite end point in thrombolytic trial of acute myocardial infarction (TIMI 4 and 5). Am J Cardiol 1997;80:696–699.
134. Mueller HS, Forman SA, Manegus MA, et al. Prognostic significance of nonfatal reinfarction during 3-year follow-up: results of the Thrombolysis in Myocardial Infarction (TIMI) Phase II Clinical Trial. J Am Coll Cardiol 1995;26:900–907.
135. Cannon CP. Optimizing the treatment of unstable angina. J Thromb Thrombolysis 1995;2:205–218.
136. Kruskal JB, Commerford PJ, Franks JJ, Kirsch RE. Fibrin and fibrinogen-related antigens in patients with stable and unstable coronary artery disease. N Engl J Med 1987;317:1361–1365.
137. Sacks FM, Pasternak RC, Gibson CM, Rosner B, Stone P. Effect on coronary atherosclerosis of decrease in plasma cholesterol concentrations in normocholesterolemic patients. Harvard Atherosclerosis Reversibility Project (HARP) Group. Lancet 1994;344:1182–1186.

2

Linking Biochemistry, Vascular Biology, and Clinical Events in Acute Coronary Syndromes

Richard C. Becker, MD *and*
Annemarie Armani, MD

CONTENTS

INTRODUCTION

The clinical expression of disease recognized as acute coronary syndromes represents the culmination of many diverse and complex cellular, biochemical, and biologic processes within the coronary arterial vasculature. Although unique in their own right, atherosclerosis and thrombosis share common origins and are intimately linked by a common denominator, inflammation. An increasing knowledge base and in-depth understanding of vascular biology has provided a clearer view of atherothrombosis and, with it, the platform for targeted therapies and management.

VASCULAR ENDOTHELIUM

The vascular endothelium is responsible for vessel responsiveness and thromboresistance. It is a multifunctional organ system composed of metabolically active and physiologically responsive component cells that meticulously regulate blood flow and myocardial perfusion.

From: *Contemporary Cardiology: Management of Acute Coronary Syndromes, Second Edition*
Edited by: C. P. Cannon © Humana Press Inc., Totowa, NJ

Basic Anatomy

Vascular endothelial cells form a single layer of simple squamous lining cells. The cells themselves are polygonal in shape, varying between 10 and 50 μm in diameter, and elongated in the long axis, orienting the cellular longitudinal dimension in the direction of blood flow. The endothelial cell has three surfaces: nonthrombogenic (luminal), adhesive (subluminal), and cohesive. The luminal surface is smooth and devoid of electron-dense connective tissue. Its luminal membrane or glycocalyx adds significantly to the vessels' thromboresistant properties, carrying a negative charge that repels similarly charged circulating blood cells. The subluminal (abluminal) surface adheres to connective tissue within the subendothelial zone. Small processes penetrate a series of internal layers to form myoendothelial junctions with subjacent smooth muscle cells. The cohesive surface of the vascular endothelium joins adjacent cells to one another by cell junctions of two basic types, occluding (tight) and communicating (gap).

Intrinsic Thromboresistance

As an active site of protein synthesis, endothelial cells synthesize, secrete, modify, and regulate connective tissue components, vasodilators, vasoconstrictors, anticoagulants, procoagulants, fibrinolytic proteins, and prostanoids. The intrinsic thromboresistant properties of a normally functioning vascular endothelium include three distinct yet integrated systems that entenuate platelets, fibrin and coagulation factor- mediated thrombotic processes.

Platelet-Directed Cell Surface Proteins

PROSTACYCLIN

Prostacyclin (PGI_2) is a potent vasodilating substance released locally in response to biochemical and mechanical mediators. PGI_2, by increasing intracellular cyclic adenosine monophosphate, also inhibits platelet aggregation.

NITRIC OXIDE

Furchgott and Zawadski [1] first discovered that acetylcholine-mediated vasodilation requires an intact vascular endothelium (i.e., it is endothelium-dependent). Nitric oxide is an L-arginine derivative that relaxes smooth muscles by increasing intracellular cyclic guanosine monophosphate. It is released locally in response to a number of biochemical mediators, including thrombin, bradykinin, thromboxane A_2, histamine, adenine nucleotides, shear stress, and aggregating platelets. In addition to vasoactive properties, nitric oxide is also a potent inhibitor of platelet adhesion and aggregation. Moreover, nitric oxide and PGI_2 appear to have synergistic antiaggregatory properties (Fig. 1).

Fibrin-Directed Cell Surface Proteins

PLASMINOGEN ACTIVATORS

Vascular endothelial cells synthesize and release activators that are capable of converting plasminogen to the serine protease plasmin, an enzyme that proteolytically degrades fibrin (and fibrinogen). Tissue plasminogen activator (tPA) and urokinase-type plasminogen activator generate plasmin locally; therefore, fibrinolysis is limited to the immediate environment. Stimuli for the release of vascular plasminogen activators include epinephrine, thrombin, heparin, interleukin-1 (IL-1), venous occlusion, aggre-

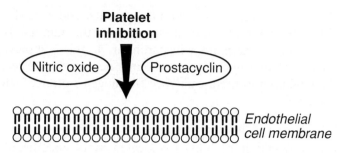

Fig. 1. The attenuation of platelet aggregation is a vital component of natural vascular thromboresistance. Nitric oxide and PGI_2 are particularly important.

gating platelets, and desamino-8-D-arginine vasopressin. (Plasminogen activators and their role in atherosclerosis and thrombosis will be discussed in a section to follow.)

Coagulation Factor-Directed Cell Surface Proteins

HEPARIN-LIKE MOLECULES

Endothelial cells are capable of synthesizing heparin-like molecules with anticoagulant properties *(2)*. Thus, vascular thromboresistance is mediated, at least in part, through the interaction of heparin-like substances with antithrombin and heparin cofactor II (both located on the endothelial surface), thus accelerating the neutralization of hemostatic (procoagulant) proteins.

Heparin cofactor II, a potent inhibitor of thrombin, is secreted by the liver into circulating blood, where it is present at a concentration of 1.0–2.0 μm/L. Unlike antithrombin, heparin cofactor II is activated predominantly by dermatan sulfate; however, under high-shear stress conditions, heparan sulfate can stimulate its inhibiting action as well. In vivo, thrombin inhibition by heparin cofactor II appears to be mediated by the interaction of dermatan sulfate with the vessel wall, predominantly in the extracellular matrix *(3,4)*. At least four distinct subspecies have been identified in endothelial cells: two high-molecular-weight complexes, a heterodimeric form bound to fibronectin, and two small molecules referred to as decorin and biglycan *(5)*.

ANTITHROMBIN

Antithrombin is a 58,000-Dalton plasma glycoprotein that circulates at a concentration of 2.3 mmol/L and is capable of neutralizing the coagulation proteins thrombin and factors IXa, Xa, XIa, and XIIa by covalent binding at their active sites.

PROTEIN C AND PROTEIN S

Protein C is synthesized in the liver and is secreted into plasma as a two-chain disulfide-bonded glycoprotein. It acts as an important anticoagulant (activated protein C [APC]) by selectively deactivating the activated forms of factor V and factor VIII (principally by cleaving their heavy chains). Protein S facilitates the anticoagulant function of APC by promoting its interaction with factors Va and VIIIa. Because protein S enhances APC-mediated factor Va inactivation by only twofold, the existence of an APC-independent anticoagulant effect has been suggested *(6)*. Indeed, protein S is able to inhibit both the prothrombinase complex and the intrinsic tenase complex. Protein S can also interact directly with factor Va and factor VIIIa.

Both protein C and protein S are found on the vascular endothelial surface. Thrombomodulin, an integral membrane protein located on the luminal surface of most endothelial cells, forms a 1:1 complex with thrombin. In this complex, thrombin activates protein C (while at the same time thrombin is neutralized). Accordingly, thrombomodulin is able to inhibit thrombin-catalyzed fibrinogen clotting, factor V activation, and platelet activation.

TISSUE FACTOR PATHWAY INHIBITOR-1

Tissue factor pathway inhibitor (TFPI)-1 is located on the endothelial surface. It acts against the combined action of tissue factor and factor VII in the presence of factor Xa. The proposed mechanism for inhibition involves the formation of a quaternary complex with TFPI and factor X in a two-step reaction: factor Xa generated by tissue factor–factor VIIa complex binds reversibly with TFPI, and the binary complex formed binds, in a calcium-dependent manner, to membrane-bound tissue factor–factor VIIa *(7)*. In essence, TFPI prevents the extrinsic coagulation cascade from activating the prothrombinase complex; however, it has also been recognized that TFPI inhibits the intrinsic coagulation cascade, supporting the role of tissue factor on factor VIIIa and factor IX-mediated clotting *(8)*. The presence of factor IX also impairs TFPI-mediated inhibition of tissue factor VIIa.

In the presence of glycosaminoglycans, including heparin, heparan sulfate, and dextran sulfate, the release of TFPI from endothelial cell storage sites is increased by several fold *(9)*.

TISSUE FACTOR PATHWAY INHIBITOR-2

TFPI-2 is found within human umbilical vein endothelial cells, the liver, and the placenta and has been shown to inhibit tissue factor VIIa, kallikrein, factor XIa, and factor X activation by factor IXa *(10,11)*. It does not independently (in the absence of heparan sulfate) inactivate factor Xa or thrombin.

ANNEXIN V

The annexins are unique family of nonglycosylated proteins that bind to negatively charged phospholipids, including phosphatidylserine and phosphatidylethanolamine *(12)*. One of the 13 recognized annexins, annexin V, is a potent endothelial surface-based anticoagulant, which can displace phospholipid-dependent coagulation factors. It also impairs platelet adhesion Fig. 2.

ATHEROSCLEROSIS
Endothelial Cell Performance

Coronary atherosclerosis is diffuse in nature, primarily involving the vessel intima (composed of the endothelium, the underlying basement membrane, and a layer of myointimal cells). A structurally and functionally normal coronary artery vasodilates in response to acetylcholine, physical exercise, or mechanical provocation. In contrast, an atherosclerotic coronary artery undergoes paradoxic vasoconstriction when exposed to acetylcholine, and a progressive decrease in cross-sectional luminal area follows rapid ventricular pacing. The failure to vasodilate prevents an increase in physiologic blood flow and, in addition, subjects the endothelial surface to excessive shear stress and injury.

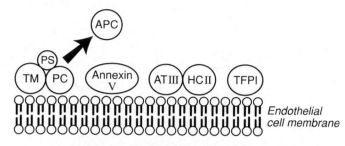

Fig. 2. The modulation of coagulation is a vital component of natural vascular thromboresistance. Protein C (PC) binds to surface thrombomodulin (TM) and, in the presence of protein S (PS), forms C APC, which then neutralizes two coagulation proteases—factor V and factor VIII. TFPI, antithrombin (AT), heparin cofactor II (HCII), and annexin V are also important components of thromboresistance.

It has become apparent that hypercholesterolemia adversely effects endothelial cell function (even before the development of atherosclerosis), and although morphologically intact, the vascular endothelium in regions of atherosclerosis fails to release nitric oxide *(13)*. Hypercholesterolemia has been shown to impair endothelium-dependent vascular relaxation in coronary resistance vessels—the vascular bed responsible for regulating myocardial tissue perfusion *(14)*.

Vascular endothelial cells are strategically positioned to play an important role in the regulation of local clotting processes. The cells are also ideally positioned to promote thrombosis, when needed, following vascular injury. Damaged and dysfunctional endothelial cells, however, quickly lose their ability to maintain thromboresistance and can, in fact, promote pathologic thrombosis. Indeed, assembly of the prothrombinase complex can take place on the endothelial surface of atherosclerotic vessels. Moreover, impaired local fibrinolytic activity attenuates clot dissolution.

Even the earliest stages of coronary atherosclerosis are associated with decreased endothelium-dependent dilation of the microvasculature, which may impair epicardial blood flow and increase cell–vessel wall interactions *(15)*.

In addition to losing its thromboresistant capabilities, the dysfunctional vascular endothelium can become, in essence, prothrombotic. Following vascular injury, endothelial cells amplify the coagulant response through the synthesis and expression of factors VIII, IX, and X *(16,17)*. Moreover, an abnormal endothelium can produce tissue factor, impair fibrinolytic activity, and decrease the effectiveness of the APC-mediated anticoagulant pathway (by impairing thrombomodulin–thrombin interactions on the endothelial surface) *(18)*.

Endothelial Cell Responses to Thrombotic Stimuli

Comprehensive thromboresistance includes an appropriate response to thrombotic stimuli, preventing thrombus growth. Unfortunately, dysfunctional endothelial cells lose their ability to synthesize and secrete proteins capable of inhibiting platelets and coagulation proteins. A prime example is the response to thrombin. Under normal circumstances thrombin stimulates platelet-mediated vasoconstriction (caused by thromboxane A_2 release), which is prevented by the simultaneous thrombin-induced release of prosta-

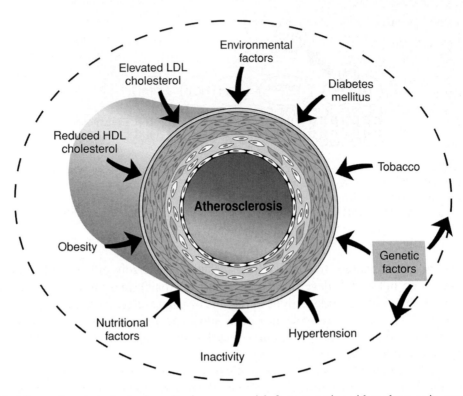

Fig. 3. Atherosclerosis is the end result of numerous risk factors, acting either alone or in combination. The overall impact of any given risk factor(s) is likely determined by genetic regulatory mechanisms.

cyclin and nitric oxide from endothelial cells. In atherosclerotic vessels, the response to thrombin is almost entirely vasoconstrictive (and prothrombotic) *(19)*.

Atherogenesis

Macroscopic Pathology

Coronary atherosclerosis, the most common underlying condition among patients with acute coronary syndromes, has been described macroscopically over the past century and a half by removed pathologists and clinicians ranging from Von Rokitansky and Virchow to Osler. The pathologic sequence of events includes an initiating step, defined as the fatty streak, followed by plaque maturation and transition, setting the stage for intravascular thrombosis. The progression of coronary atherosclerosis varies widely among individuals, as does the time course and influence of recognized risk factors (Fig. 3).

Microscopic Pathology

Observations at the microscopic and cellular levels have contributed substantially to unraveling several of the mysteries that surround human atherosclerosis and have fostered clear view of the mechanisms leading to intravascular thrombosis. It is now evident that the atherosclerotic plaque and its cellular components represent an ideal substrate for thrombus formation. Thus, the term "atherothrombosis" appears fitting.

DEVELOPMENTAL ANATOMY AND CELLULAR BIOLOGY

In experimental animals, focal sites of predilection for either spontaneous or dietary-induced atherosclerosis can be determined reliably prior to plaque development. These areas are delineated by their in vivo uptake of the protein-binding azo dye Evans blue. Salient features of these lesion-prone areas include increased endothelial permeability to an intimal accumulation of plasma proteins, including albumin, fibrinogen, and low-density lipoproteins (LDL). There is also increased endothelial cell turnover. Overall, the prelesion area within endothelial cells takes on a unique appearance, and the surface glycocalyx is two- to fivefold thinner than normal endothelial cells *(20)*.

Lesion-prone areas within blood vessel walls exhibit a unique property of blood monocyte recruitment, followed by accumulation of these cells in the subendothelial space, a process that is accelerated in the presence of hyperlipidemia. Based on the available information, it appears that at least two processes are pivotal in the initiation of atherosclerosis: (*i*) an enhanced focal endothelial transcytosis of plasma proteins, including LDL, which accumulate in the widened proteoglycan-rich subendothelial space, and (*ii*) the preferential recruitment of blood monocytes to the intima, a process that is markedly augmented by even a short period of hyperlipidemia. Thus, the lesion-prone subendothelial space has two key participants in atherosclerosis, namely, the monocyte (macrophage) and LDL.

Monocyte recruitment in the intimal space of lesion-prone areas is thought to be mediated by an enhanced generation of chemoattractants of which monocyte chemoattractant protein-1 (MCP-1), a cationic peptide synthesized and secreted by both arterial smooth muscle cells and endothelial cells, is of particular importance. It is also recognized that the production of MCP-1 is stimulated by minimally modified (oxidized) LDL, whereas oxidized LDL itself is chemotactic *(21)*.

ATHEROMATOUS PLAQUE GROWTH, EVOLUTION, AND ULTRASTRUCTURE

After monocytes attach to the morphologically intact but dysfunctional endothelium (receptive stage), there is a net directed migration of monocytes through the endothelium to the subendothelial space, where they undergo differentiation. The phenomenon of monocyte activation–differentiation plays an important role in atherosclerosis, particularly with regard to plaque remodeling and lesion progression. This complex process proceeds by means of at least two mechanisms: (*i*) the generation of reactive oxygen species (free radicals); and (*ii*) the phenotypic modulation of expression of the scavenger receptor or family of receptors. The chemical modification of LDL results in its avid uptake by monocytes (now considered macrophages), and the subsequent transformation to foam cells follows. The specific receptor responsible for the uptake of modified LDL fails to down-regulate; as a result, a substantial amount of intracellular LDL cholesterol accumulates. When the influx of LDL particles exceeds the capacity of the macrophage scavenger receptors to remove them from the intracellular space, oxidized LDL particles accumulate within the arterial intima (Fig. 4A). These particles are cytotoxic, causing both injury and death to endothelial cells, smooth muscle cells, and macrophages. The net result is disruption of the relatively fragile macrophage-derived foam cells, leading to release of their intracellular lipid into the extracellular compartment of the intima; this sequence of events gives rise to the origin of the pultaceous cholesteryl ester-rich core of the atherosclerotic plaque (Fig. 4B) *(22–25)*.

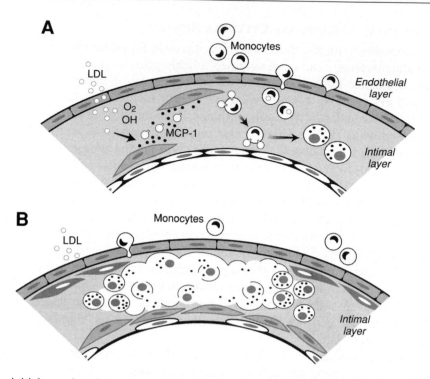

Fig. 4. The initial step in atherosclerosis involves monocyte and LDL binding to a dysfunctional endothelial surface (receptive stage). Monocyte activation and chemical modulation (oxidation) of LDL (modified LDL) results in avid uptake and transformation to macrophages (foam cells). Transformed smooth muscle cells synthesize and secrete MCPs that participate in monocyte recruitment and migration within the intimal layer. The influx of modified LDL exceeds the capacity of macrophage surface receptors (impaired down-regulation), allowing accumulation of potentially cytotoxic LDL particulars in the extracellular space. This step is a pivotal step in the development of a lipid core.

LIPID (NECROTIC) CORE

The release of copious foam cell lipids to the extracellular compartment induces a second cascade of inflammatory responses within the vascular intimal layer. In particular, granulomatous foci involving macrophages, lymphocytes, and multinucleate giant cells surround and invade the extracellular lipid.

Besides foam cell death, what other mechanisms can account for the formation of extracellular lipid deposits? New lines of evidence suggest that lipoproteins, particularly LDL, aggregate and then fuse with one another in the extracellular space to form microscopically evident lipid deposits *(26–32)*. Structures resembling lipoprotein aggregates have been visualized in human atherosclerosis by electron microscopy, and lipid aggregates containing apolipoprotein B (apo B) have also been isolated.

A number of proteins and peptides have been detected in relative abundance within or near the atherosclerotic core. Many of the proteins found in this region are relatively hydrophobic, including the apolipoproteins, C-reactive protein (CRP), and the 70- and 60-kDa heat shock proteins. A list of proteins and peptides detected by immunologic methods in the atherosclerotic lipid core is given in (Table 1).

Cells that border and penetrate the atherosclerotic core not only participate in the deposition (or removal) of core lipids but can also be influenced by the accumulating lipids

Table 1
Proteins and Peptides Found in the Lipid Core of Atheromatous Plaques

Myeloperoxides	Heat-shock protein 60
Hyaluronectin	Heat-shock protein 70
Albumin	Fibrinogen
CRP	Tissue factor
Complement factor C3	Apolipoproteins
C56-9 neoantigen	Apo B
	Apo A
	Apo E

and proteins. Complement components have been found in relative abundance in the core, and both toxic and chemotactic responses may be generated via activation of complement. Antigenic markers of complement activation, including C3D and the terminal C5B-9 neoantigen, have been found in the atherosclerotic core, and terminal C5B-9 has been detected coincident with the cholesterol-rich vesicles in the subendothelium *(33–38)*.

INFECTION AND ATHEROGENESIS

The link between infection and atherosclerosis has been investigated with great enthusiasm given the potential for widely implementable therapies (Table 2).

Chlamydia pneumonia titers are increased among some patients with atherosclerosis, and the organism has been isolated from atheromatous plaques *(39,40)*. Although the pathobiologic relationships have not been elucidated fully, *C. pneumoniae* accelerates LDL uptake in monocytes and facilitates their transition to foam cells. Infected endothelial cells also become prothrombotic with decreased synthesis of tissue factor pathway inhibitor, plasminogen activator, and increased tissue factor expression *(41)*.

Cytomegalovirus (CMV) exhibits atherogenic effects through the synthesis of one of more proteins that stimulate smooth muscle cell proliferation *(42)* and LDL uptake within monocytes. CMV also impairs fibrinolysis, increases production of lipoprotein-a (Lpa), and increases platelet adhesion.

The available evidence supports chronic rather than acute infection as a potential pro-atherogenic factor in genetically susceptible individuals. Infection has been linked to hypertriglyceridemia, hyperfibrinogenemia, reduced high-density lipoprotein levels, anticardiolipin antibodies, and elevated CRP levels, suggesting both direct and indirect effects on both atherogenesis and thrombogenesis.

Thrombogenesis

PLAQUE RUPTURE

The clinical expression of atherosclerotic disease activity is determined by pathologic events leading to coronary thrombosis. In this regard, there are two key factors: (*i*) the propensity of plaques to rupture, and (*ii*) the thrombogenicity of exposed plaque components.

The morphologic characteristics of plaques that determine their propensity to rupture have been determined. Pathology based-studies using necropsy and atherectomy tissue samples have shown convincingly that plaques associated with intraluminal thrombosis

Table 2

The Potential Link Between Infectious Agents and Atherosclerotic Vascular Disease

Infectious agent	Association suggested in animal models	Comments	Association suggested in humans	Comments
Cytomegalovirus	0		+++	• Detected in atheromatous tissue. • Serologic evidence for link with atherosclerosis. • Associated with allograft disease. • Potential role in restenosis. • Alters cellular function.
Chlamydia pneumonia	+++	• Developed de novo atherosclerotic changes with infection in rabbits. • Azithromycin treatment shown to prevent atherosclerosis.	+++	• Often subclinical infection • Detected in atheroma. • Serologic evidence for link with atherosclerosis. • Detected in asymptomatic atherosclerosis. atherosclerotic disease.
Helicobacter pylori	0		+	• Alters cellular function. • Associated with elevated inflammatory markers. • Limited serologic data. • No evidence for detection in atheromatous plaques.
Herpes Simplex Virus	+++	• Marek's disease (herpes virus in chickens) associated with atherosclerosis.	+	• Detected in atheroma. • Serologic data lacking.

Table 2 (*continued*)
The Potential Link Between Infectious Agents and Atherosclerotic Vascular Disease

Infectious agent	Association suggested in animal models	Comments	Association suggested in humans	Comments
Coxsackie B Virus	++	• Acute coronary arteritis in mice.	0	• No serologic data. • Not detected in atheroma.
Pasteurellamulticoda	++	• Shown to enhance atherosclerotic changes in rabbits on high cholesterol diets.	0	
Periodontal disease: *Porphyromonas* Streptococcus viridans Streptococcus anguis	0		++	• Epidemiological associations observed. • *S. viridans* detected in atheroma.
Hepatitis A	0		+/0	• Seropositivity which may or may not be of pathological significance.

are rich in extracellular lipid and that the lipid core of these vulnerable or rupture-prone plaques occupies a large proportion of the overall plaque volume. The degree of cross-sectional stenosis involving the vessel lumen is typically <50% *(43)*. In addition to the predominant lipid core, vulnerable plaques are characterized by a thin fibrous cap and high macrophage density *(44)*. Whereas most individuals with atherosclerotic coronary artery disease exhibit a diversity of plaque types, most have a preponderance of one specific type (vulnerable or nonvulnerable) (Fig. 5). The genetic and acquired determinants of plaque type are subjects of intense investigation.

The lipid core of an advanced atherosclerotic plaque is bordered at its luminal aspect by a fibrous cap, at its edges by the shoulder region, and on its abluminal side by the plaque base. Because the lipid core contains a substantial amount of prothrombotic substrate (to be discussed in a subsequent section), the fibrous cap, separating the core from circulating blood components within the vessel's lumen, determines the overall stability of the plaque. In turn, the extracellular matrix of the fibrous cap, consisting of several proteinaceous macromolecules, including collagen (types I and III) and elastin secreted by transformed smooth muscle cells, determines its integrity.

The point should once again be made that core size and fibrous cap thickness are not related to absolute plaque size nor to the degree of luminal stenosis. The determinants of core size have not been fully elucidated, although death of lipid-filling macrophages by apoptosis (programmed cell death) is a possibility. Fibrous cap thickness appears to be related to macrophage and smooth muscle cell activity, particularly their production of metalloproteinases that degrade connective tissue.

Matrix metalloproteinases, part of a superfamily of enzymes that include collagenases, gelatinases, and elastases, require activation from proenzyme precursors to attain enzymatic activity. Under normal circumstances, tissue inhibitors hold these enzymes in check; however, exposure of smooth muscle cells to the cytokines IL-1 and tumor necrosis factor-α (TNF-α) causes induction of interstitial collagenase and stromelysin. Macrophages exposed to inflammatory cytokines also stimulate the production of matrix-degrading enzymes *(45–47)*.

Coronary atherectomy specimens from patients with acute coronary syndromes contain a 92-kDa gelatinase that is produced predominantly by macrophages and smooth muscle cells *(48)*. Within atherosclerotic plaques, the highest stress regions have a twofold greater matrix metalloproteinase (MMP-1) expression than the lowest stress regions. Overexpression of MMP-1 in vulnerable plaques is associated with a substantial increase in circumferential stress. Degradation and weakening of the collagenous extracellular matrix at critical points of high shear stress may play an important role in the pathogenesis of plaque rupture.

Fibrous cap thickness can be maintained by smooth muscle cell-mediated collagen synthesis (local repair); however, interferon-γ (IFN-γ), an inflammatory cytokine found within atherosclerotic plaques, decreases the ability of smooth muscle cells to express the collagen gene. Because only T-lymphocytes can elaborate IFN-γ *(49,50)*, it has been suggested that chronic immune stimulation within atherosclerotic plaques leads to the production of IFN-α from T cells that subsequently inhibits collagen synthesis in vulnerable regions of the fibrous cap. IFN-γ can also contribute to apoptosis and, therefore, may be a key biochemical determinant of plaque vulnerability (Fig. 6).

Human mast cells contain proteoglycans and proteolytic enzymes, including chymase and tryptase. In normal coronary arteries, mast cells amount to 0.1% of all nucleated

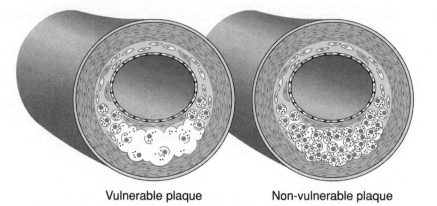

Vulnerable plaque   Non-vulnerable plaque

Fig. 5. Vulnerable plaques are typified by (*i*) a prominent lipid core; (*ii*) a thin fibrous cap; and, (*iii*) high inflammatory cell density located at the plaque shoulders. By contrast, nonvulnerable plaques contain few extracellular lipid particles and are fibrotic, making disruption a less common event.

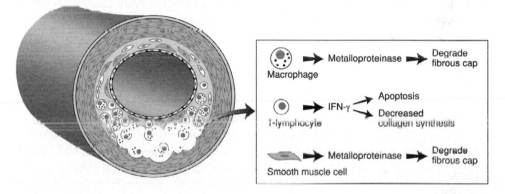

Fig. 6. Plaque vulnerability is determined by both structure and intrinsic activity. Macrophages and smooth muscle cells synthesize and secrete matrix metalloproteinases that can degrade the fibrous cap. IFN-γ, an inflammatory cytokine secreted by T lymphocytes, participates in programmed cell death (apoptosis) and inhibits collagen synthesis, thereby weakening the plaque's supporting framework.

cells; however, within the fibrous cap, lipid core, and shoulder regions of atheromatous lesions, there are 5-, 5-, and 10-fold increased densities, respectively *(51)*. Electron and light microscopic studies of mast cells in the plaque shoulder region have revealed evidence of degradation, a sign of activation that may contribute to matrix degradation and plaque rupture in acute coronary syndromes *(52)*.

Models of Plaque Rupture

Shear stress

The coronary arterial intimal surface is constantly exposed to the dynamic influences of circulating blood that creates shear stress. Assuming a constant viscosity, shear stress is described by the following formula: $T = Udv/dr$, where U is viscosity, V is velocity, and r is the radius of the vessel. Within arterial segments containing laminar flow, shear stress (τ) = $4 \mu Q/pr^3$. Therefore, shear stress is directly proportional to flow (Q) and inversely proportional to the cube of the vessel's radius. In coronary atherosclerosis, the lumen is reduced in size and there is increased flow velocity, ultimately leading to increased shear stress.

There is evidence *(53)* that atherosclerosis typically develops in low-flow/low-shear stress segments of the coronary arterial tree. Low-shear stress may also contribute, at least initially, to impaired vasoreactivity and thromboresistance by reducing the local stimulus to both prostaglandin and nitric oxide synthesis and release. It appears that unsteady (turbulent) flow is particularly detrimental to endothelial cell function *(54)*.

In contrast to plaque development, plaque disruption occurs most often in regions of high shear stress.

WALL STRESS

Plaque rupture occurs when the forces acting directly on the plaque exceed its tensile strength. Pressure generated within the arterial lumen exerts both radial and circumferential force, which must be countered by radial and circumferential wall tension. According to the law of Laplace, T (circumferential wall tension) $= pr/h$, where p is the intraluminal pressure, r is the vessel radius, and h is the wall thickness. Thus, atherosclerotic vessels with a thickened intima and small internal diameter maintain relatively low wall tension. This may explain why plaque rupture is more likely to occur in vessels with less severe stenosis.

STRESS DISTRIBUTION

Computer models have been developed to study the relative stress distribution within atherosclerotic coronary arteries *(55)*. Overall, the circumferential stress is greatest at the intimal layer. In plaques that contain a large lipid pool, most of the stress is localized to the overlying fibrous cap. As the stiffness of the cap increases, the maximal circumferential stress shifts from the center of the cap to the lateral edges or "shoulder" region.

The thickness of the fibrous cap is a major determinant of circumferential stress and the plaque's predisposition to rupture. In the presence of a constant luminal dimension, there is increasing stress with enlargement of the lipid core. With increasing fibrous cap thickness, even in the presence of decreasing luminal area, circumferential stress decreases. Another important feature is the lipid core itself, which, because of its semi-fluid nature, bears very little circumferential stress. Instead, stress is displaced to the fibrous cap.

FREQUENCY OF STRESS

Much like fatigue fractures occurring in metal, the frequency, extent, and localization of stress play important roles in plaque rupture. Atherosclerotic plaques, particularly fibrous caps overlying large lipid cores, become progressively more stiff with increasing stress and frequency of stress. Elevations in heart rate have been slow to increase stiffness and circumferential stress at the plaque's shoulder regions *(56)*.

TRIGGERS FOR PLAQUE RUPTURE

Triggering events for plaque rupture are among the most contemplated and investigated areas in cardiovascular medicine. It has become clear, however, that triggers have less impact when they occur in the absence of a vulnerable plaque. This important feature allows for the development of several lines of prevention. Potential triggers include plasma catecholamine surges and increased sympathetic activity, blood pressure surges, exercise, emotional stress, changes in heart rate and myocardial contraction (angulation of coronary arteries), coronary vasospasm, and hemodynamic forces *(57–63)*. This subject is discussed in chapter 3.

Prevention of Plaque Rupture

Plaque rupture is the end result of a dynamic interplay between factors intrinsic to the plaque itself and extrinsic factors. The intrinsic factors primarily relate to rupture vulnerability; the extrinsic forces deliver the final blow. Each can be addressed when contemplating options for prevention.

Lipid-lowering strategies, antioxidants, anti-inflammatory agents, inhibitors of macrophages and their secreted proteins, and gene therapy can be used individually or concomitantly to change the plaque's composition, making it less prone to rupture. β-Adrenergic blockers *(64)* and angiotensin-converting enzyme inhibitors *(65)* can reduce extrinsic forces capable of causing damage. The future in both basic and clinical research undoubtedly will devote considerable time, effort, and resources to these areas.

Cellular Plaque Components: Intrinsic Thrombogenicity

Pathologic studies performed on patients who died suddenly or who recently experienced an episode of unstable angina or myocardial infarction (MI) often reveal intraluminal thrombus anchored to a ruptured atherosclerotic plaque. Primarily based on the results of in vitro experiments and studies conducted in static systems, the thrombogenic capacity of atherosclerotic plaques has been attributed to collagen, fatty acids, and phospholipids. Fuster and colleagues *(66)* have investigated dynamic thrombus formation using an ex vivo perfusion chamber and reported that the greatest stimulus was, in fact, the atheromatous core, yielding a sixfold greater degree of platelet deposition and thrombus production than other substrates, including foam cell rich matrix, collagen-rich matrix, collagen-poor matrix without cholesterol crystals, and segments of normal intima. There is mounting evidence that tissue factor is the predominant thrombogenic mediator found within the atheromatous core. This substrate will be discussed in a section to follow.

Cholesterol sulfate, present within human atherosclerotic plaques and plasma, is a substrate for platelet adhesion through a specific, but not yet defined, receptor. It, in all likelihood, plays a role in both atherosclerosis and prothrombotic potential of disrupted plaques *(67)*.

VASCULAR THROMBOSIS

In most instances, thrombosis occurring in the arterial system is composed of platelets and fibrin in a tightly packed network (white thrombus). By contrast, venous thrombi consist of a tightly packed network of erythrocytes, leukocytes, and fibrin (red thrombus).

The process of vascular thrombosis, particularly in the arterial system, is dynamic, with clot formation and dissolution occurring almost simultaneously. The overall extent of thrombosis and ensuing circulatory compromise is therefore determined by the predominant force that shifts the delicate balance. If local stimuli exceed the vessel's own thromboresistant mechanisms, thrombosis will occur. If, on the other hand, the stimulus toward thrombosis is not particularly strong and the intrinsic defenses are intact, clot formation of clinical importance is unlikely. In some circumstances, systemic factors contribute to or magnify local prothrombotic factors, shifting the balance toward thrombosis *(68)*.

Overall, the site, size, and composition of thrombi forming within the arterial circulatory system is determined by: (*i*) alterations in blood flow; (*ii*) thrombogenicity of cardiovascular surfaces; (*iii*) concentration and reactivity of plasma cellular components; and (*iv*) effectiveness of physiologic protective mechanisms.

Defining Steps

PLATELET DEPOSITION

Platelets attaching to nonendothelialized or disrupted surfaces undergo adherence by activation and distribution along the involved area and subsequent recruitment to form a rapidly enlarging platelet mass.

The process of platelet deposition involves: (*i*) platelet attachment to collagen or exposed surface adhesive proteins; (*ii*) platelet activation and intracellular signaling; (*iii*) the expression of platelet receptors for adhesive proteins; (*iv*) platelet aggregation; and (*v*) platelet recruitment mediated by thrombin, thromboxane A_2, and adenosine diphosphate.

COAGULATION FACTOR ACTIVATION

Thrombin is rapidly generated in response to vascular injury. It also plays a central role in platelet recruitment and the formation of an insoluble fibrin network. The thrombotic process is localized, amplified, and modulated by a series of biochemical reactions driven by the reversible binding of circulating proteins (coagulation factors) to damaged vascular cells, elements of exposed subendothelial connective tissue (especially collagen), platelets (which also express receptor sites for coagulation factors), and macrophages. These events lead to an assembly of enzyme complexes that increases local concentrations of procoagulant material; in this way, a relatively minor initiating stimulus can be amplified greatly to yield a thrombus.

FIBRIN FORMATION

The final phase in thrombus formation involves the generation of a stable fibrin network that provides the structural support for the circulating blood's cellular elements and the scaffolding for vascular remodeling. In this pivotal process, thrombin cleaves two small peptides, fibrinopeptide A and fibrinopeptide B, to form fibrin monomers, which in turn polymerize to form soluble fibrin strands. An orderly assembly, branching, and lateral association of fibrillar strands follows, terminating with factor XIII-mediated covalent crosslinking to form a mature fibrin network (mature thrombus).

PATHOLOGY OF THROMBOTIC EVENTS

There is evidence that the growth of atheromatous plaques occurs in a stepwise yet dynamic fashion in response to vascular injury. The clinical expression of a broad potential of pathobiologic events ranges from asymptomatic plaque growth to complete coronary arterial occlusion with a fatal outcome (Fig. 7).

James Herrick (1912) *(69)* is credited with describing the association between acute coronary thrombosis and acute MI, paving the way toward a greater understanding of acute coronary syndromes. Support for the disrupted plaque theory as a precipitant or nidus for coronary thrombosis can be traced to the work of Saphir et al. (1735) *(70)*, followed by the observations of Chapman (1965) *(71)*, Constantinides (1966) *(72)*, Bouch and Montgomery (1970) *(73)*, Ridolfi and Hutchins (1977) *(74)*, Falk (1983) *(75)*, and

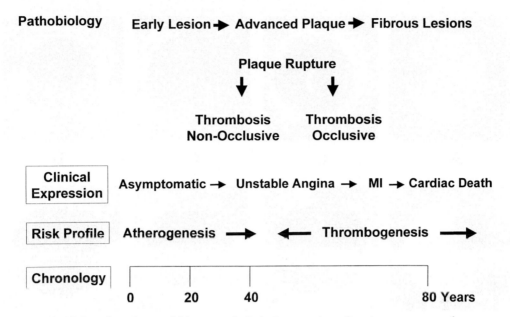

Fig. 7. Pathobiology-based natural history and clinical expression of acute coronary syndromes.

Davies and Thomas (1985) *(76)*. Additional support for the role of thrombosis-mediated processes in clinical events can be found in autopsy-based series that have revealed coronary microthrombi among patients with sudden cardiac death *(75,76)*.

THEORY OF DYNAMIC PLAQUE DISRUPTION AND ARTERIAL THROMBOSIS

Despite early views, the evidence suggests that plaque disruption and coronary arterial thrombosis are not random events in atherosclerosis, rather the process is sudden and dynamic. In a series of 42 patients undergoing coronary angiography before and after MI, Little and colleagues (1988) *(43)* found that most had a stenosis of <50% of the infarct-related vessel prior to the event. Similar findings were reported by Taeymans. Computer-based modeling also supports the dynamic nature of coronary occlusion *(77)*. Comparing a rigid stenosis and a dynamic stenosis in which proximal vessel constriction and distal collapse were simulated, the latter model (with an added potential for vasoconstriction and passive collapse) required a much smaller thrombus burden for complete occlusion.

ATHEROSCLEROTIC PLAQUE IMAGING

The fine structure and composition of an atherosclerotic plaque rather than the degree of stenosis determines the likelihood of future clinical events. As a result, imaging modalities capable of characterizing the plaques internal environment have strong appeal. Having information on both plaque composition and luminal features may also be useful during atherosclerosis coronary interventions.

A majority of imaging modalities are catheter-based; however, more generalizable techniques are being developed and studied. High frequency intravascular ultrasound (20–40 MHz) provides tomographic images of the arterial wall and is able to quantitate luminal and plaque area as well as morphologic features including calcification and inti-

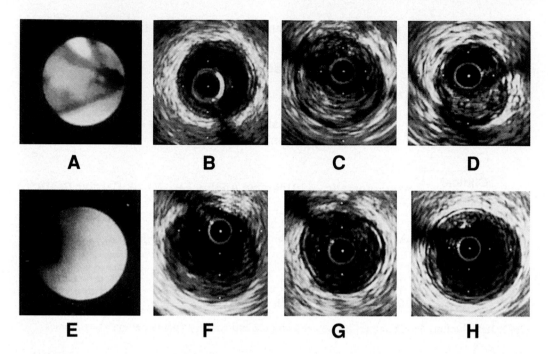

Fig. 8. (**A**) Angioscopic image of the left anterior descending artery in a patient with acute MI demonstrating yellow plaque. (**B,C,D**) Intravascular ultrasound images as depicted in lesion A demonstrating compensatory enlargement. (**B**) At the defined proximal reference site the external elastic membrane (EEM) cross-sectional area (CSA) was 11.8 mm². (**C**) At the culprit lesion, EEM CSA was 13.5 mm². (**D**) At the distal reference site, EEM CSA was 9.6 mm². The remodeling ratio (RR) was 1.26. (**E**) Angioscopic image of the left anterior descending artery in a patient with stable angina demonstrating white plaque. (**F,G,H**) Intravascular ultrasound images at the same lesion as E demonstrating paradoxical shrinkage. (**F**) At the proximal reference site, EEM CSA was 17.1 mm². (**G**) At the culprit lesion EEM CSA was 10.1 mm². (**H**) At the distal reference site, EEM CSA was 15.3 mm². The RR was 0.62 *(79)*.

mal dissection *(78)*. Axial resolution to approximately 150 mHz is possible, permitting identification of lipid-rich regions and features of the plaques' fibrous cap.

Intervascular ultrasound with elastography is a unique method which allows both visual characterization of the plaque and its mechanical properties. Tissue components compare differently in response to applied pressure allowing determination of mechanical and structural integrity *(79)* (Fig. 8).

Coronary angioscopy, although not used frequently in North American catheterization laboratories, is a sensitive means to detect atherosclerotic plaques, grossly approximate their lipid composition, determine the presence of fibrous cap disruption and identify associated thrombosis formation *(80)*.

Magnetic resonance imaging (MRI) (high resolution fast spin echo) represents a promising tool for studying the progression and regression of atherosclerosis over time. In addition, recently developed intravascular techniques can accurately assess plaque size and vulnerability (for rupture) *(81)*.

A variety of innovative imaging modalities under development include optical coherence tomography, nuclear scintigraphy, thermometry, and Raman spectroscopy *(82)*.

CLINICAL EXPRESSION OF PATHOBIOLOGICAL EVENTS

Acute MI

Occurring in upwards of one million individuals yearly in the United States, ST-segment elevation MI represents the most commonly observed arterial thrombotic event in clinical practice. In the vast majority of cases, fissuring or rupture of an atherosclerotic plaque within a major epicardial coronary artery is followed by occlusive thrombosis, typically anchored to the damaged vascular surface and exposed plaque components.

It is of interest and of clinical importance that plaque rupture does not occur randomly throughout the coronary tree. Instead, there are vulnerable sites located in:

- the proximal portion of the left anterior descending coronary artery;
- the right coronary artery near the origin of its marginal branch; and
- the left circumflex coronary artery at the origin of the first obtuse marginal branch.

In general terms, the severity of vessel wall injury determines the extent of thrombosis. Mild injury (type I) is typically associated with the deposition of platelets in a single (nonocclusive) layer. Moderate injury (type II) provokes a loosely adherent platelet mass that can quickly be dispersed by normal blood flow. Severe injury (type III) leads to platelet adherence, activation, and stimulation of the coagulation cascade, producing an occlusive thrombus. Type III injury is present in most of patients with MI.

Unstable Angina/Non-ST-Segment Elevation MI

Angiographic, angioscopic, and pathologic studies have shown that atherosclerotic plaque disruption accompanied by varying degrees of intraluminal thrombosis is the primary pathologic event in unstable angina/non-ST segment elevation MI (non-ST segment elevation acute coronary syndromes). Mounting evidence suggests that chronic recurrent plaque rupture of mild to moderate severity may contribute to plaque development and its natural history. Thrombosis occurs with each episode, but may not be of sufficient mass (clot burden) to compromise coronary arterial blood flow. Over time, however, plaque growth occurs, obstructing the coronary lumen. Thus, the obstructive lesion is a combination of mature plaque and layers of aged thrombus, consisting primarily of platelets in a tightly packed fibrin network.

In some patients, non-ST-segment elevation MI has clinical features reminiscent of ST-segment elevation MI, progressing suddenly, because of plaque rupture and occlusive intracoronary thrombosis. Experience has shown that these patients frequently have multivessel coronary artery disease and, therefore, represent a high-risk group.

Most patients with unstable angina/non-ST-segment elevation MI have advanced underlying atherosclerotic coronary artery disease with nearly uniform distribution of single, double, and triple vessel involvement. The available evidence suggests that the clinical conversion from asymptomatic or stable angina to unstable angina is a direct result of pathologic changes within the atheromatous plaque, specifically plaque fissuring, disruption, and intraluminal thrombosis. Angiographic studies have revealed a high prevalence of eccentric irregular narrow-necked stenoses with overhanging edges (type II lesion) and reduced thrombolysis in myocardial infarction (TIMI) flow (83). In contrast, patients with stable angina most often exhibit concentric symmetric stenoses or eccentric broad-necked stenoses (type I lesion).

The presence of intracoronary thrombosis and the overall thrombus burden has varied greatly in studies of patients within unstable angina/non-ST-segment elevation MI. On average, thrombus has been reported in 40–50% of patients. The variability can be traced to differences in clinical presentation (accelerated angina, angina at rest, postinfarction angina), variability in electrocardiographic features (T-wave inversion, ST-segment shifts), the time frame of clinical assessment (early, late), and the method of imaging.

Coronary angioscopy has proved to be a useful tool in the evaluation of coronary arterial morphology. In a landmark study by Forrester and colleagues (84), angioscopy was performed at the time of bypass grafting in 20 patients, 10 with unstable angina and 10 with advanced but clinically stable coronary artery disease. All patients with accelerated angina exhibited complex-appearing plaques (Fig. 9A), and all patients with angina at rest had thrombus (Fig. 9B). In contrast, patients with stable coronary disease had neither of these features. These observations, representing a pathobiology–clinical correlation "snapshot," suggest strongly that plaque morphology, in general, and intracoronary thrombosis, in particular, are major determinants of disease expression.

Unique Characteristics of Acute Coronary Syndromes

Although plaque disruption with thrombus formation has been associated with acute coronary syndromes, including unstable angina and MI, determinants of which particular entity within the spectrum of possibilities a patient will develop have not been fully elucidated. The challenge becomes greater when one considers that plaque disruption is not an uncommon event, yet only certain individuals experience symptoms, as a clinical expression of mechanical and biochemical events, which characterize acute coronary syndromes.

The available evidence suggests that although plaque rupture is a common theme in acute coronary syndromes, the degree and composition of the associated thrombus burden differs. Percutaneous angioscopy performed in patients with unstable angina frequently reveals gray-white nonocclusive thrombi; reddish occlusive thrombi are seen in patients with acute MI. These characteristics suggest that unstable angina is a platelet-mediated phenomenon and, by contrast, acute MI is predominantly fibrin-mediated. Autopsy-based studies have drawn similar conclusions. In a study of 14 patients with unstable angina and 32 patients with a fatal first MI, Kragel et al. (85) observed a predominance of platelets within nonocclusive thrombi in those with a diagnosis of unstable angina, whereas thrombi in patients with acute MI consisted almost entirely of fibrin and were occlusive. The investigators also found that the extent or depth of plaque rupture, approximated by the presence of hemorrhage, was less in patients with unstable angina when compared with those with acute MI.

The question then remains: what are the determinants of disease progression (or suppression) and clinical expression in acute coronary syndromes? Our group has shown that patients with unstable angina and non-ST-segment elevation MI exhibit varying degrees of platelet activation and thrombin generation, suggesting that not only the thrombotic stimulus may differ, but that regulation of thrombus growth may differ as well (Table 3).

Microvascular Disease

The supply–demand paradigm of myocardial ischemia, when considered comprehensively, takes both epicardial and microvascular conditions into consideration. Because tissue perfusion is regulated at the microvascular level and downstream resistance to flow has

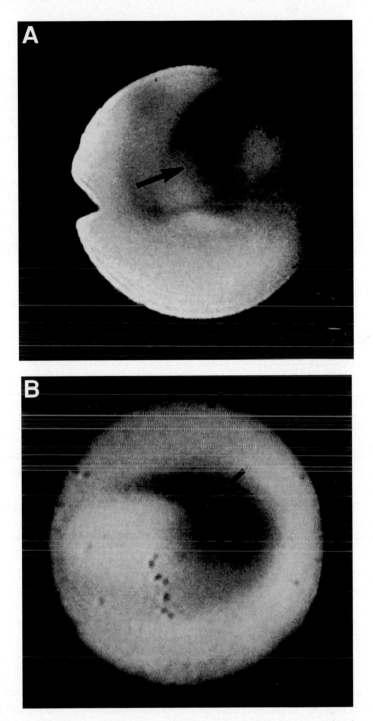

Fig. 9. (**A**) Coronary angioscopy in a patient with unstable angina. An eccentric plaque with disruption is evident (arrow). Reprinted with permission from ref. *84.* (**B**) Coronary angioscopy in a patient with unstable angina at rest. Intraluminal thrombus (nonocclusive) is visualized (arrow). Reprinted with permission from ref. *48.*

Table 3
Multidimensional Determinants of Clinical Expression and
Cardiac Events in Coronary Atherosclerosis

Vascular endothelium	Atherosclerotic plaque	Coronary artery	Systemic factors
Vasoreactivity	Composition Thrombogenicity	Degree of stenosis Site and flow characteristics of stenosis	Platelets Activatability
Thromboresistance	Depth of rupture	Extent of disease	Coagulation factors Prothrombotic state

Regeneration capacity	Inflammatory response	Collateral circulation	Neuroendocrine status
			  Sympathetic tone
			  Renin–angiotensin
			  Tone

Prothrombotic potential	Redox state Diet Gender	Preconditioning	Age
Preconditioning	Passivatibility Genetic regulation		

a strong influence on epicardial hemodynamics, it is important to understand microvascular disorders that characterize coronary artery disease in its most active phases.

One of the earliest events in acute myocardial ischemia is microvascular damage and dysfunction *(86)*. Although injury may be the direct result of diminished nutritive blood flow, evidence also suggests that platelet micro-embolism, platelet–leukocyte aggregates, and inflammatory cytokines play important roles. The restoration of epicardial blood flow following fibrinolytic therapy or percutaneous intervention may also contribute by supplying oxygen-derived free radicals and neutrophils, leading to complement activation and expression of adhesion molecules that incite a vicious cycle of inflammation, injury, reduced tissue perfusion, and myocardial ischemia (Fig. 10). Accordingly, the management of acute coronary syndromes, particularly ST-segment elevation MI, must consider therapies that address the macrovascular and microvascular circulatory systems *(87)*.

VASCULAR BIOLOGY, BIOCHEMISTRY, AND EMERGING CONCEPTS IN ATHEROTHROMBOSIS

C-Reactive Protein

The link between inflammation and thrombosis in atherosclerotic vascular disease is complex; however, CRP may represent an important mediator given its association with both atherogenesis and thrombogenesis. In the Speedwell study *(88)*, CRP correlated strongly with D-dimer levels, which is a marker of fibrin formation (and subsequent degradation). This observation is particularly relevant when one considers the ability of D-dimer (and other fibrin-related products) to activate neutrophils and monocytes, increase secretion of cytokines (IL-1, IL-6), and stimulate the hepatic synthesis of acute-phase proteins including CRP *(89)*.

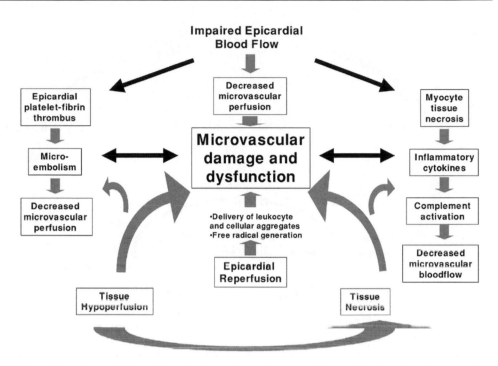

Fig. 10. Impaired myocardial perfusion in the setting of acute MI is a multidimensional process that is mediated by microcirculatory dysfunction. Impaired epicardial coronary blood flow impairs microvascular perfusion either directly or indirectly through myocardial necrosis-mediated inflammatory responses, which are either cytotoxic or compromise microvascular responsiveness. Epicardial to microcirculatory vessel platelet-fibrin microemboli also contribute to impaired distal flow and perfusion. Lastly, the restoration of blood flow may have either a transient or prolonged impact on microvascular performance by delivering leukocytes, platelet–leukocyte aggregates, and oxygen-derived free radicals.

CRP can be found within macrophages of atheromatous plaques where it interacts with a specific cell surface receptor CD 32. The co-localization of CRP and LDL cholesterol suggest that it plays a major role in transport and atherosclerotic plaque development (Fig. 11). Once present, CRP up-regulates adhesion molecule expression, activates complement, and induces monocyte tissue factor expression (88–90).

The strong correlation between elevated CRP concentrations (measured by a high sensitivity assay) and vascular thrombotic events, while not proving cause and effect provides, at the very least, a readily attainable prognostic marker (Table 4) (91). The potential relevance both pathologically and clinically is further underscored by the ability of therapeutic agents, including "statins" and aspirin, to reduce CRP (and predict treatment response) (92,93).

Tissue Factor

Shortly after tissue injury, including even superficial trauma to the endothelium, thrombin-like activity can be detected that persists for weeks thereafter (94,95). The expression of tissue factor mRNA and antigen within atherosclerotic plaques has been characterized by in situ hybridization and immunohistochemistry (96). In atherectomy specimens obtained from human carotid arteries, tissue factor mRNA and antigen can be detected in macrophages, mesenchymal intimal cells, and extracellular matrix (97).

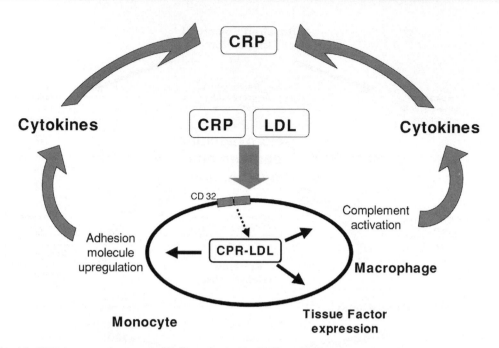

Fig. 11. CRP is more than an "epi phenomenon" of atherosclerotic vascular disease. In response to cytokine stimulation, it co-localizes with LDL-cholesterol, facilitating monocyte entry via CD32, a cell surface receptor. Once internalized, the CRP-LDL-cholesterol complex incites complement activation, tissue factor expression, and surface adhesion molecule "up-regulation."

Table 4
High Sensitivity (HS) CRP and Its Correlation with Atherothrombotic Events

	Endpoint				
	Coronary heart disease (CHD)-death	*MI*	*Stroke*	*Peripheral vascular disease (PVD)*	*Cardiovascular death*
Relative risk for future cardiovascular events					
5.0					
4.0	X				X
3.0		X		X	
2.0			X		
1.0					

Adapted with permission from Ridker PM. Circulation 2001;103:1813–1818.

Patients with unstable angina demonstrate high concentrations of tissue factor antigen and activity within coronary atherectomy specimens *(98)*, and it has been suggested that this potent procoagulant protein found within the lipid core may be released from macrophages during cell death or in the form of shed vesicles *(99)* (Fig. 12).

The impact of therapies designed to reduce myocardial ischemia or attenuate thrombotic potential on endothelial performance must be considered. One frequently used agent, unfractionated heparin, exerts prothrombotic effects by adversely affecting

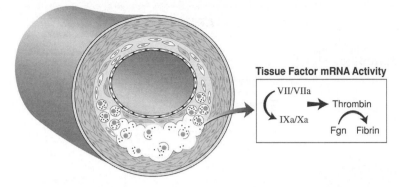

Fig. 12. Tissue factor is a strong stimulus for intravascular coagulation, particularly after plaque disruption. In addition to activating factor X directly (extrinsic coagulation cascade) the TF-VII$_a$ complex generates thrombin (and the conversion of fibrinogen [FgN] to fibrin) via the extrinsic coagulation cascade by factor IX activation (cascade cross-talk).

endothelial-mediated thromboresistance to tissue factor, which is an important trigger for thrombosis in atherosclerotic coronary artery disease. Under normal circumstances, TFPI is released from endothelial cells, neutralizing the tissue factor, VIIa complex and factor Xa. Unfractionated heparin causes a release of TFPI (*100*), contributing to its overall anticoagulant effects; however, prolonged administration depletes intracellular storage pools, compromising both anticoagulant potency and thromboresistance capacity. This phenomenon may help explain the limitations of unfractionated heparin in acute coronary syndromes and the clustering of thrombotic events that follow its abrupt discontinuation (*101*).

Thrombin

Thrombin, a multifunctional serine protease generated at sites of vascular injury, is a potent platelet activator and possesses a variety of actions on inflammatory cells, the vascular endothelium, and smooth muscle cells. Arterial wall-associated thrombin activity is expressed following coronary angioplasty (*102*), and thrombin bound to the subendothelial extracellular matrix is functionally active, localized, and protected from inactivation by circulating inhibitors (*103*).

The multiple cell-activating functions of thrombin contribute to hemostatic, inflammatory, proliferative, and reparative responses of injured vessel walls (Fig. 13). In human atheroma, a functional thrombin receptor is expressed in regions rich in macrophages and smooth muscle cells. Local thrombin generation in areas of dysfunctional endothelium and either fissured or ruptured atherosclerotic plaques activates surrounding cells, thereby contributing to plaque growth, inflammation, and thrombosis (*104*).

Monocytes

Cultured endothelial cells exposed to monocytes release less nitric oxide, and the monocyte-derived cytokines, IL-1, and TNF-α, down-regulate nitric oxide synthase (*105*). Overall, the adhesion of monocytes to endothelial cells, as well as their secretory products, diminishes the steady-state levels of nitric oxide synthase, an event associated with an attenuated release of biologically active nitric oxide. The observed suppression is both monocyte concentration and time-dependent (*106*).

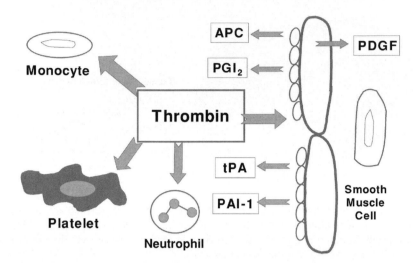

Fig. 13. Beyond serving as the pivotal enzyme for all coagulation processes, thrombin exhibits a broad range of direct cellular activating (and inhibiting) properties as well. Platelet, monocyte, and neutrophil activation (and interactions) may be particularly important in the determination of an inflammatory-pro-thrombotic environment. Thrombin's effect on dysfunctional endothelial cells includes increased PAI-1 secretion and decreased APC secretion. Thrombin-mediated platelet-derived growth factor (PDGF) synthesis participates in smooth muscle cell migration and plaque growth. PGI_2 and tPA secretion are decreased as well. The latter may also be functionally defective (impaired fibrinolytic potential).

Nitric oxide is generated under basal conditions by vascular endothelial cells, and several lines of evidence suggest that the continuous tonic release of nitric oxide is important in maintaining normal vasoreactivity and thromboresistance by means of its potent vasodilating and platelet-inhibiting potential, respectively.

Monocytes and macrophages from atheromatous plaques exhibit a coagulant response to a variety of stimuli, including IL-1 and products of activated lymphocytes *(107)*. Monocytes from patients with unstable angina express significant procoagulant activity; however, they must first bind to lymphocytes *(108)*. In addition, only activated lymphocytes can stimulate monocyte procoagulant activity.

The impact of T lymphocytes on atherosclerotic disease progression and expression is supported by studies showing a relationship between immune-mediated IFN-γ signaling and acute coronary syndromes. Monocytes from patients with acute coronary syndromes exhibit a molecular fingerprint of recent activation (transcription of STAT [transcription-1 proteins], up-regulation of inducible genes (D64 and IP-10) *(109)*, and monoclonal T cell populations have been detected in atherosclerotic plaques obtained from patients with fatal MI *(110)*. Although there is little question that antigen-specific stimulation is of paramount relevance in atherogenesis, an alternate pathway of T cell activation, independent of antigen presentation, might involve IL-15-A, a macrophage-released cytokine that shares biologic similarities with IL-2 and induces proliferation of mature T cells, generation of cytotoxic T cells, induction of CD 40 ligand expression, and release of proinflammatory cytokines *(111)*.

Smooth Muscle Cells

The smooth muscle cell is ubiquitous in its role as both a pro-atherosclerotic and pro-thrombotic mediator. Similar to endothelial cells and monocytes, smooth muscle cells

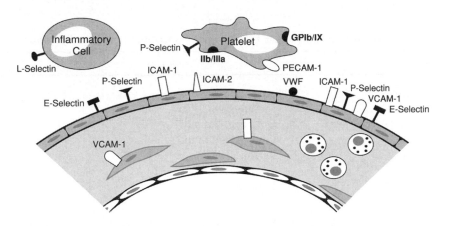

Fig. 14. The dysfunctional vascular endothelium, transformed intima, and modified cellular components of the developing plaque are a virtual warehouse of inflammatory proteins and expressed receptors that mediate the adhesion of cells to one another and to structural components of the cell surface matrix. ICAM, intercellular adhesion molecule; VCAM, vascular cell adhesion molecule; PECAM, platelet endothelial cell adhesion molecule; vWF, von Willebrand factor; GP, glycoprotein.

express tissue factor *(112)*. In addition, they can release inflammatory cytokines in response to thrombotic activation that activate platelets and/or monocytes *(113)*.

Cell Adhesion Molecules

In both physiologic and pathologic states, cell surface receptors mediate the adhesion of cells (endothelial cells, monocytes, lymphocytes, neutrophils, smooth muscle cells, platelets) to one another and to structural components of the extracellular matrix. To date, six families of cell adhesion molecules have been described—integrins, selectins, immunoglobulins, adhesion molecules, proteoglycans, and mucins (Fig. 14).

Integrins comprise a superfamily of heterodimeric transmembrane proteins composed of noncovalently associated α- and β-subunits (Table 5). To date, 8 β-subunits and 12 α-subunits have been identified *(114,115)*. Integrins have been grouped according to their composition, which typically includes various combinations of α-subunits joined with a common β-subunit. Most integrins that bind matrix molecules recognize the tripeptide Arg-Gly-Asp (RGD) that can be found in fibrinogen, fibronectin, fibronectin, vitronectin, laminin, and type 1 collagen. Not all cellular interactions with matrix proteins are mediated by their RGD sequence.

Selectins are composed of a lectin domain, an epithelial growth factor domain, and complement regulatory-like molecules. P- and E-selectins bind to common sites of carbohydrates, and C-selectin binds to mucin-like endothelial cell glycoproteins. P-selectin (CD62, granule membrane protein, platelet activation-dependent granule external membrane protein) can be found within platelet α-granules and endothelial cells (Weibel-Palade bodies). Because P-selectin binds to monocytes and neutrophils, it is felt to play an important role in platelet–leukocyte and endothelial cell–leukocyte interactions. The interaction of fibrinogen and P-selectin may have a particularly important role in regulating inflammatory and thrombotic responses (Table 6).

Members of the immunoglobulin superfamily, including intercellular adhesion molecules (ICAM-1, ICAM-2) and vascular cell adhesion molecules (VCAM) play an

Table 5
Major Integrins and Their Ligands that Contribute to Atherothrombosis

Integrin	Ligands
VLA integrins	
α, β_1 (VLA-1)	Laminin, collagen
α_2, β_1 (VLA-2)	Collagen, laminin
α_3, β_1 (VLA-3)	Fibronectin, laminin, collagen
α_4, β_1 (VLA-4)	Fibronectin, VCAM-1
α_5, β_1 (VLA-5)	Fibronectin
α_6, β_1 (VLA-6)	Laminin
Leukocyte integrins	
α_2, β_2	ICAM-1, ICAM-2
$\alpha m, \beta_2$	ICAM-1, fibrinogen, factor X
$\alpha x, \beta_2$	Fibrinogen
Cytoadhesions	
AIIb, β_3	Fibrinogen, fibronectin, vitronectin
$\alpha IV, \beta_3$	Vitronectin, fibrinogen, thrombospondin

VLA, very late antigens; ICAM, intercellular adhesion molecule; VCAM, vascular cell adhesion molecule.

important role in the transmigration of leukocytes. The cytokines TNF-α, IL-1, and IFN-γ stimulate the expression of ICAM on the vascular endothelial surface. Endothelial VCAM-1 supports the adhesion of lymphocytes, monocytes, eosinophils, and basophils. Platelet endothelial cell adhesion molecule (PECAM-1) exists on platelets, T lymphocytes, and monocytes, suggesting that it contributes to leukocyte migration and thrombosis (Table 7).

Cadhesions represent a group of proteins whose major function is the maintenance of tight gap junctions and intercellular spacing within the vascular endothelium.

Proteoglycans constitute a large protein family with glycoaminoglycan side chains that mediate lymphocyte binding and epithelial cell binding to collagen, fibronectin, and thrombospondin. The glycoprotein Ib/IX complex is the most well-known cell adhesion molecule of the mucin family. It contains a thrombin binding site and a von Willebrand factor binding site.

Cytokines and Provoked Inflammatory Responses

Histologic studies have shown that atherosclerotic plaques contain foci of monocytes, macrophages, and activated lymphocytes. The cytokine secretory capacity of monocytes expressing TNF, IL-1, IL-6, and IFN-λ is also increased. The acute-phase reactants CRP and amyloid A protein are elevated in a majority of patients with unstable angina and identify those patients who were more likely to suffer an in-hospital ischemic–thrombotic event (116). The prognostic value of fibrinogen, an acute phase protein directly involved with the cascade of events leading to thrombosis, has also been determined in patients with unstable angina and non-ST-segment elevation MI in whom elevations identify increased risk of spontaneous ischemia, MI, and death (117) (Table 8).

Table 6
Selectins: Cellular Distribution and Interactions

Cell	Distribution	Binding site
L-Selectin	All leukocytes	Endothelial cells
E-Selectin	Activated endothelial cells	Neutrophils, monocytes, T lymphocytes
P-Selectin	Platelets, endothelial cells (Weibel-Palade)	Neutrophils, monocytes, T lymphocytes

Table 7
Adhesion Molecules

Glycoprotein	Distribution
ICAM-1	Endothelial cells, fibroblasts, hematopoietic cells
ICAM-2	Endothelial cells, fibroblasts, hematopoietic cells
VCAM-1	Endothelial cells, smooth muscle cells
PECAM-1	Platelets, endothelial cells

ICAM, intercellular adhesion molecule; VCAM, vascular cell adhesion molecule; PECAM, platelet-endothelial cell adhesion molecule.

Patients with accelerated atherosclerosis and MI at a young age (<45 yr) frequently have detectable circulating immune complexes (118). Similarly, patients with acute MI have increased plasma concentrations of IL-1, IL-6, IL-8, and TNF-α, and the intensity of the acute inflammatory response after infarction is associated with short-term mortality (119). The inflammatory state also may determine the overall response to treatment (120).

Plasminogen Activator Inhibitor-1

Plasminogen activator inhibitor (PAI)-1 is a globular glycoprotein with a molecular weight of 50,000 and comprised of 379 amino acids in a single chain. The primary structure of PAI-1 designates it as a member of the superfamily of serine protease inhibitors (serpins), and it is structurally similar to other serpins, including angiotensinogen, antithrombin III, and α-2-antiplasmin. PAI-1 was first isolated by Van Mourik et al. (121) and has been cloned by several investigative groups (122,123).

At least three distinct conformations of the intact PAI-1 molecule have been identified. In its latent form, PAI-1 is not susceptible to cleavage by tPA nor does it form complexes with tPA. However, in its active form, it is both susceptible to cleavage and does form complexes with the tPA molecule. The active form of PAI-1 is the inhibitory form of the molecule. In its conformation, the reactive site of PAI-1 is readily accessible to cleavage by plasminogen activators; once this peptide bond is cleaved, a complex is formed between plasminogen activators and PAI-1. Thus, the active form of PAI has been appropriately termed a suicide substrate. It has a circulating half-life of approx 60 min (124).

Latent PAI-1 has been crystallized, and its structure determined; it is inactive because part of its reactive centers is inaccessible to binding. Latent conformation of PAI appears to be a preferred state, and spontaneous reversions of latent PAI to an active state have not been described. However, if latent PAI is chemically denatured and allowed to refold,

Table 8
Major inflammatory Cytokines

Cytokine	Predominant cell of origin	Biologic activity
IL-1	Endothelial cells Activated macrophages	T cell activation; cytokine production
IL-2	Activated T cell	Activated natural killer cells stimulate IL-2, TNF-α
IL-6	Monocytes, macrophages, T cells, endothelial cells	Differentiatial of B cells; stimulate production of acute phase proteins and cytokines
INF-γ	Activated T cells	Oxygen-derived free radical production expression of MHC I and II; monocyte and macrophage activation
TNF-α	Monocytes, macrophages	Cytokine production; endothelial cell injury; pro-thrombotic effects, cellular proliferation

IL, interleukin; TNF-γ, tumor necrosis factor α; INF-γ, interferon γ; and MHC, major histocompatibility complex.

a fraction of the material will resume the active conformation *(125)*. It has been determined that most PAI-1 secreted into the blood is in the active state, although some of the PAI stored within platelets is inactive. The mechanisms responsible for activating latent PAI have not been fully described, but negatively charged phospholipids have been reported to activate the latent form of PAI in vitro *(126)*.

The primary source of PAI-1 in the circulation is thought to be the endothelium *(127);* however, this is not the only synthetic site. Other sites of synthesis include the liver and vascular smooth muscle cells. Platelets store large quantities of PAI-1, which can be secreted following aggregation. Endothelial cells also have the capacity to secrete PAI-1 abluminally *(128)*. The relative abundance of vitronectin in the subendothelial matrix provides a mechanism for preserving PAI-1 activity. The PAI-1-vitronectin complex may represent the physiologically relevant form of the inhibitor in the extracellular matrix.

A wide array of compounds has been found to stimulate endothelial PAI-1 production. Inflammatory cytokines, including IL-1 and TNF, can induce PAI-1 synthesis. Transforming growth factor-β, epidermal growth factor, and insulin can also stimulate PAI-1 production. Thrombin is a potent stimulus for PAI-1 in cultured endothelial cells *(129)*.

An excess of PAI-1 reduces the efficiency of the fibrinolytic system, creating a permissive environment toward vascular thrombosis. There is compelling evidence that PAI-1 exists in excess quantities within human atherosclerotic vessels *(130)*. Elevated levels of PAI-1 are a risk factor for both venous and arterial thrombolic events. PAI-1 excess has been identified in young survivors of acute MI *(131)*. It has also found in excess among survivors of MI who subsequently experienced a second event *(132)* (Fig. 15).

Plasma Fibrinolytic Factors

Lipoprotein (A) is composed of an LDL particle linked to a unique glycoprotein, apo A, which exhibits marked structural similarities to the plasma zymogen plasminogen. Experimental evidence suggests that increased levels of lipoprotein (A) impair fibrinolysis through binding to plasminogen receptors on fibrin, endothelial cells, mononuclear cells, and platelets.

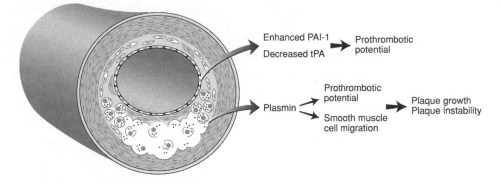

Fig. 15. Vascular plasminogen activators and their inhibitors play an important role in both plaque activity (predisposing to disruption) and thrombosis. TPA, tissue plasminogen activator; (PAI-1), plasminogen activator inhibitor.

Renin–Angiotensin System

Angiotensin II has been shown to promote the growth of vascular smooth muscle cells *(133,134)*, and it has been suggested that angiotensin-converting enzyme (ACE) inhibitors can reduce neointimal proliferation. Activity of the endogenous fibrinolytic system is regulated, in large part, by two proteins secreted by the vascular endothelium, tPA and its primary inhibitor PAI-1. Both endogenous tPA and PAI-1 have been implemented in the pathogenesis of thromboembolic disorders. Infusion of angiotensin II in low physiologic doses results in a rapid and significant increase in circulating levels of PAI-1 antigen *(135)*. Effects are apparent within 45 min of initiating the infusion; moreover, the effect of angiotensin II on PAI-1 production appears to be a simple dose-response relationship. Angiotensin II preferentially induces the synthesis of PAI-1 I in both cultured endothelial cells and murine astrocytes *(136)*. In cultured endothelial cells, angiotensin II induces a dose-dependent increase in PAI-1 messenger RNA and in the concentrations of secreted PAI-1 in the media. Platelets express receptors for angiotensin II, and while angiotensin II is not a direct platelet agonist, it does sensitize platelets to the effects of other known agonists. As a result, angiotensin-treated platelets are more sensitive to the aggregating effects of epinephrine, adenosine diphosphate, and collagen. Work by Vaughn and colleagues *(137)* suggests that angiotensins, including angiotensin III and angiotensin IV (particularly the latter), has a direct effect on endothelial cell and smooth muscle cell PAI-1. The findings of at least one clinical trial suggest that ACE inhibitor therapy in survivors of anterior MI results in a marked depression of PAI-1 concentrations in plasma within 2 wk of treatment initiation *(137)*.

ACE is found in high concentrations within hypercellular plaques and bordering areas of clustered macrophages and T lymphocytes. Additionally, angiotenic II receptors exist in close proximity to sites of plaque rupture among patients with unstable angina *(138)*.

Plasma Coagulation Factors and Cardiac Events

Epidemiologic studies have examined factor VII and fibrinogen, two components of the natural hemostatic mechanism. In the Northwick Park Study *(139)*, factor VII coagulant activity was shown to correlate with cardiovascular mortality. Fibrinogen also correlated strongly, as did factor VIII, although less strongly than other hemostatic markers. The potential importance of factor VIII, however, is strengthened by the low incidence of atherosclerotic coronary artery disease in hemophiliacs. In the Atherosclerosis Risk Communities study, which included 15,800 individuals from four diverse areas in the United States *(140)*, baseline measurements of factor VIII and von Willebrand factor were performed to determine their relationship to the development of coronary atherosclerosis. In a univariate analysis, both factors were positively associated with plasma triglycerides and negatively associated with high-density lipoprotein cholesterol.

As in the Northwick Park Study, several large-scale epidemiologic studies have identified an association between both factor VIII activity and fibrinogen and the incidence of atherosclerotic coronary artery disease. In the Framingham Study *(141)*, fibrinogen and coronary disease were strongly correlated, and the association was stronger than was the association between cholesterol (and other standard risk factors) and coronary disease.

Involvement of the fibrinolytic system in the development of acute coronary syndromes has recently led investigative groups to explore several markers as predictors of thrombotic cardiovascular events. In a study of 213 consecutive patients with angina pectoris and angiographically confirmed coronary artery disease, tPA mass concentration was the only laboratory marker significantly associated with mortality at a mean follow-up of 7 yr *(142)*.

Diabetes Mellitus

Diabetes mellitus, increasing rapidly on a world-wide basis, is linked strongly to atherothrombosis *(143,144)*. The linkage of glucose (glycosylation) to proteins produces an insoluble product known as advanced glycation end-products (AGEs) *(145)*, which promote atherosclerosis through several unique mechanisms. AGE has been shown to deplete nitric oxide, thereby impairing endothelium-dependent dilation. It also binds specific macrophage receptors, stimulating cytokine release and smooth muscle cell proliferation. AGE increases the secretion of platelet-derived growth factor and enhances chemotaxis of blood monocytes *(146)*.

Glycosylation of lipoproteins contributes to atherosclerosis through the following sequence of events. Glycosylated LDL, not being recognizing by LDL receptors, increases cholesteryl ester synthesis and accumulation in macrophages. In addition, glycosylation of LDL impairs its own degradation and permits more LDL to be bound by local matrix proteins, where oxidation can take place *(147)* (Fig. 16).

The glycosylation of HDL increases its clearance and decreases the physiologic HDL receptor-mediated cholesterol removal process *(148)*.

Hyperinsulinemia is recognized as an important contributor to atherogenesis in the sitting of Type II diabetes. High fasting insulin concentrations are an independent predictor of ischemic heart disease-related events in men *(149)*.

TNF-α is increased in the insulin-resistant state *(150)* and decreases the expression of nitric oxide synthase and increases the expression of ICAM-1 *(151)*.

Diabetes is associated with a heightened thrombotic capacity that is multifactorial in origin. Endothelial dysfunction with impaired thromboresistance, increased sympathetic tone, reduced fibrinolytic potential, elevated coagulation factor concentrations (VII, IX, X, XII, fibrinogen), and enhanced platelet aggregation in response to a variety of biochemical mediators contribute collectively *(152)*.

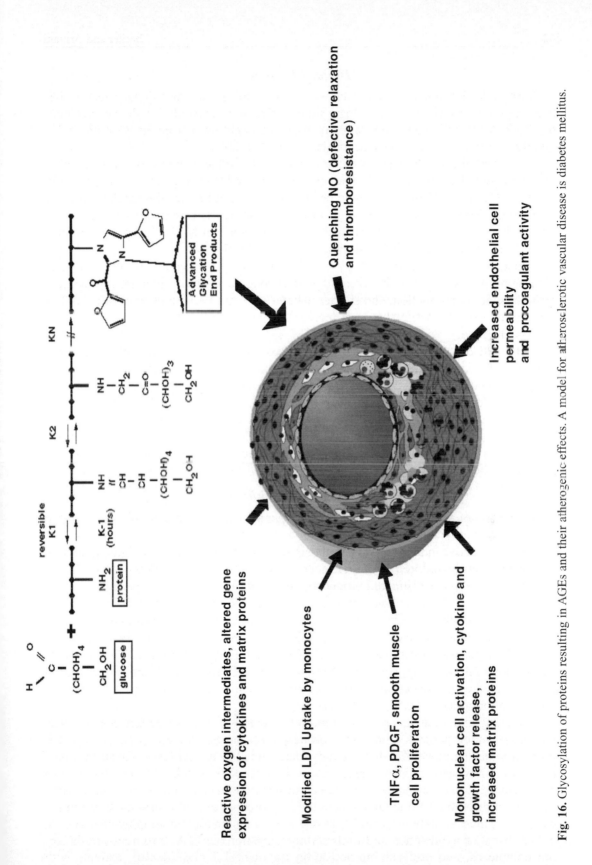

Fig. 16. Glycosylation of proteins resulting in AGEs and their atherogenic effects. A model for atherosclerotic vascular disease is diabetes mellitus.

51

Dietary Factors

A possible link among atherosclerosis, thrombotic events, and dietary factors has been explored in several epidemiologic studies. The first, referred to as the Seven Country Study *(153)*, observed a correlation between total calories consumed as saturated fats and the occurrence of coronary heart disease-related death.

The potential direct impact of dietary factors on cardiac events was investigated in the Lyon Diet Heart Study *(154)*. Patients with a prior MI were given a diet previously shown in the Seven Country Study to be associated with a low cardiovascular mortality (the Cretan Mediterranean Diet, high in α-linolenic acid). Compared with a control group, dietary intervention patients had a lower incidence of MI and cardiac death during a 27-mo follow-up period (risk ratio 0.27; $p = 0.001$).

Hypercholesterolemia, induced by a high dietary intake of saturated fatty acids and cholesterol, is associated with increased platelet coagulant activity, platelet aggregation, thromboxane A_2 production, and shorter platelet survival. Elevations in plasma cholesterol have also been associated with increases in prothrombin and coagulation factors VII and X *(155)*.

Factor VII coagulant activity (VIIc) increases with rising plasma triglycerides and dietary fat intake. It has been proposed that the association between fat consumption and VIIc is related to increased concentrations of triglyceride-rich lipoprotein particles on the intrinsic coagulation pathway. The metabolism of triglyceride-rich lipoproteins may generate a negatively charged surface, which then activates the contact system of coagulation (factor XII, factor XI, prekallikrein, high molecular weight kininogen). Support for this hypothesis is derived from studies showing reduced prothrombin activation fragment 1.2 concentrations with triglyceride-reducing therapies *(156)*.

Markers of Thrombosis

In clinical practice, limited means exist to assess the physiologically relevant balance between in vivo anticoagulation and thrombosis. Ideally, if tests were readily available that reflected active intravascular thrombosis, clot dissolution, and thrombotic potential, treatment could be tailored more precisely. Conceptually, these markers could also be used to provide mechanistic and prognostic information.

Thrombin, a 308-amino acid serine protease, plays a central role in the natural history of ruptured atherosclerotic plaques. Thrombin, in essence, determines the extent of thrombus formation at sites of vascular injury. Thrombin activity can be assessed in plasma by measuring fibrinopeptide A (FPA) concentrations. Actually, FPA represents fibrin formation resulting from thrombin's activity on fibrinogen. Thrombin generation is represented by plasma concentrations of prothrombin activation fragment 1.2, thrombin-antithrombin complexes, and APC (Fig. 17).

Eisenberg and colleagues *(157)* reported previously that thrombin activity was increased among patients with acute coronary thrombosis. Our group has shown that both thrombin activity and platelet activity (determined by the expression of surface proteins using flow cytometry) are increased in acute coronary syndromes and that heightened activity persists even after the acute clinical symptoms have resolved *(158)*. Plasma markers of thrombin activity and generation may provide useful information during the early assessment of patients with MI at rest in whom electrocardiographic changes are either absent or nondiagnostic. In this setting, elevations in FPA, thrombin–antithrombin complexes, and prothrombin activation fragment 1.2 may identify patients with

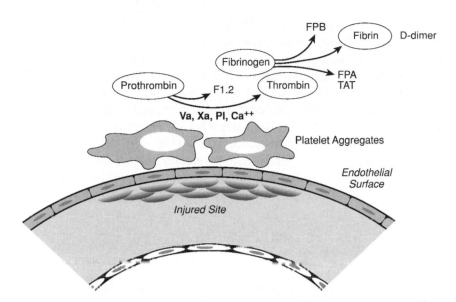

Fig. 17. The conversion of prothrombin to thrombin is mediated by the prothrombinase complex (coagulation factors Va and Xa, phospholipid, and calcium [Ca^{2+}]). This enzymatic reaction typically takes place on existing platelet aggregates; however, it can also occur on a dysfunctional endothelial surface. During the generation of thrombin, which can be neutralized to some degree through binding to antithrombin (thrombin–antithrombin duplex [TAT]), a peptide fragment (prothrombin activation peptide F1.2) appeared in plasma where it can be measured. The thrombin-medicated conversion of fibrinogen to fibrin yields two peptides, fibrinpeptide A (FPA) and fibronopeptide B (FPB). Newly generated thrombin can either be complexed to antithrombin (TAT) or participate in the conversion of fibrinogen to fibrin. D-Dimer is a breakdown product of fibrin.

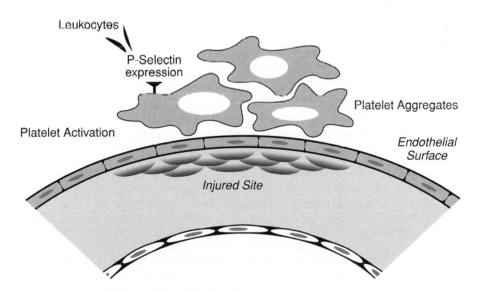

Fig. 18. Activated platelets undergo numerous structural and functional changes. Surface markers of activation, including P-selectin, can be measured using flow cytometry as can platelet–leukocyte heterotypic aggregates.

active coronary artery disease *(159)*. D-Dimer, a breakdown product of fibrin, has shown promise as a diagnostic marker among patients with venous thromboembolic disease and is currently being evaluated in the setting of acute coronary syndromes. Rapid bedside tests are available that may be useful in the early management of these patients. The combined measurement of several biochemical markers that reflect decreased myocardial perfusion (troponin), inflammation (fibrinogen, CRP, amyloid A protein, leukocyte activation) and thrombosis (platelet activation, thrombin generation, fibrin formation, thrombin-mediated platelet activation) (Fig. 18) or combination markers (platelet–leukocyte aggregates, fibrinogen–P-selectin interaction) could potentially offer the greatest wealth of information on the pathobiology, prevention, and treatment of acute coronary syndromes *(160)*.

REFERENCES

1. Furchgott RF, Zawadski JV. The obligatory role of endothelial cells in the relaxation of arterial smooth muscle cells by acetycholine. Nature 1980;288:373–376.
2. Marcum JA, Rosenberg RD. Heparin-like molecules with anticoagulant activity are synthesized by cultured endothelial cells. Biochem Biophys Res Commun 1985;126:365–372.
3. Vogel KG, Peterson DW. Extracellular, surface and intracellular proteglycans produced by human embryo lung fibroblasts in culture. J Biol Chem 1981;256:13235–13240.
4. Jarvelainen HT, Kinsella MG, Wight TN, Sandell LJ. Differential expression of small chondroitin/dermatan sulfate proteoglycans, PG-I/biglycan and PG-II/decorin, by vascular smooth muscle and endothelial cells in culture. J Biol Chem 1991;266:23274–23279.
5. Kresse H, Hausser H, Schonherr E, Bittner K. Biosynthesis and interactions of small chondroitin/dermatan sulfate proteoglycans. Eur J Clin Chem Clin Biochem 1994;32:259–266.
6. Heeb MJ, Mesters RM, Tans G, Rosing J, Griffin JH. Binding of protein S to factor Va associated with inhibition of prothrombinase that is independent of activated protein C. J Biol Chem 1993;268:2872–2877.
7. Broze GJ Jr, Warren LA, Novotny WF, Higuchi DA, Girard TJ, Miletich JP. The lipoprotein-associated coagulation inhibitor that inhibits factor VII-tissue factor complex also inhibits factor Xa: insight into its possible mechanism of action. Blood 1988;71:335–343.
8. van't Veer C, Hackeng TM, Delahaye C, Sixma JJ, Bouma BN. Activated factor X and thrombin formation triggered by tissue factor on endothelial cell matrix in a flow model: effect of the tissue factor pathway inhibitor. Blood 1994;84:1132–1139.
9. Kaiser B, Hoppensteadt DA, Jeske W, Wun TC, Fareed J. Inhibitory effects of TFPI of thrombin and factor Xa generation in vitro—modulatory action of glycosaminoglycans. Thromb Res 1994;75:609–619.
10. Sprecher CA, Kisiel W, Mathewes S, Foster DC. Molecular cloning, expression, and partial characterization of a second human tissue-factor-pathway inhibitor. Proc Natl Acad Sci USA 1994;91:3353–3357.
11. Petersen LC, Sprecher CA, Foster DC, Blumberg H, Hamamoto T, Kisiel W. Inhibitory properties of a novel human Kunitz-type protease inhibitor homologous to tissue factor pathway inhibitor. Biochemistry 1996;35:266–272.
12. Tait JF, Gibson D, Fujikawa K. Phospholipid binding properties of human placental anticoagulant protein-I, a member of the lipocortin family. J Biol Chem 1989;264:7944–7951.
13. Yamamoto H, Bossaller C, Cartwright J Jr, Henry PD. Videomicroscopic demonstration of defective cholinergic arteriolar vasodilation in atherosclerotic rabbit. J Clin Invest 1988;81:1752–1758.
14. Sellke FW, Armstrong ML, Harrison DG. Endothelium-dependent vascular relaxation is abnormal in the coronary microcirculation of atherosclerotic primates. Circulation 1990;81:1585–1593.
15. Zeiher AM, Drexler H, Wollschlager H, Just H. Endothelial dysfunction of the coronary microvasculature is associated with impaired coronary blood flow regulation in patients with early atherosclerosis. Circulation 1991;84:1984–1992.
16. Stern DM, Drillings M, Nossel HL, Harlet-Jensen A, LaGamma KS, Owen J. Binding of factors IX and Ixa to cultured endothelial cells. Proc Natl Acad Sci USA 1983;80:4119–4123.
17. Stern DM, Nawroth PP, Kisiel W, Vehar G, Esmon CT. The binding of factor Ixa to cultured bovine aortic endothelial cells. J Biol Chem 1985;260:6717–6722.

18. Colucci M, Balconi G, Lorenzet R, Pietra A, Locati D, Donati MB, et al. Cultured human endothelial cells generate tissue factor in response to endotoxin. J Clin Invest 1983;71:1893–1896.

19. Yang Z, Arnet U, Bauer E, et al. Thrombin-induced endothelium-dependent inhibition and direct activation of platelet-vessel wall interaction: role of prostacyclin, nitric oxide, and thromboxane A2. Circulation 1994;86:2266–2272.

20. Caplan BA, Gerrity RG, Schwartz CJ. Endothelial cell morphology in focal areas of in vivo Evans Blue uptake in the young pig aorta. I. Quantitative light microscopic findings. Exp Mol Pathol 1974; 21:102–117.

21. Jauchem JR, Lopez M, Sprague EA, Schwartz CJ. Mononuclear cell chemoattractant activity from cultured arterial smooth muscle cells. Exp Mol Pathol 1982;37:166–174.

22. Schwartz CJ, Valente AJ, Sprague EA, Kelley JL, Suenram CA, Rozek MM. Atherosclerosis as an inflammatory process: the roles of the monocyte-macrophage. Ann NY Acad Sci 1985;454:115–120.

23. Schwartz CJ, Valente AJ, Sprague EA, Kelley JL, Suenram CA, Graves DT, et al. Monocyte-macrophage participation in atherogenesis: inflammatory components of pathogenesis. Semin Thromb Hemost 1986;12:79–86.

24. Goldstein JL, Ho YK, Basu SK, Brown MS. Binding site on macrophages that mediates uptake and degradation of acetylated low density lipoprotein, producing massive cholesterol deposition. Proc Natl Acad Sci USA 1979;76:333–337.

25. Brown MS, Basu SK, Falck JR, Ho YK, Goldstein JL. The scavenger cell pathway for lipoprotein degradation: specificity of the binding site that mediates the uptake of negatively charged LDL by macrophages. J Supramol Str 1980;13:67–81.

26. Khoo JC, Miller E, McLoughlin P, Steinberg D. Enhanced macrophage uptake of low density lipoprotein after self-aggregation. Arteriosclerosis 1988;8:348–358.

27. Frank JS, Fogelman AM. Ultrastructure of the intima in WHHL and cholesterol-fed rabbit aortas prepared by ultra-rapid freezing and freeze-etching. J Lipid Res 1989;30:34967–34978.

28. Guyton JR, Klemp KF, Mims MP. Altered ultrastructural morphology of self-aggregated low density lipoproteins: coalescence of lipid domains forming droplets and vesicles. J Lipid Res 1991;32: 953–962.

29. Lovanen PT, Kokkonen JO. Modification of low density lipoproteins by secretory granules of rat serosal mast cells. J Biol Chem 1991;266:4430–4436.

30. Steinbrecher UP, Lougheed M. Scavenger receptor-independent stimulation of cholesterol esterification in macrophages by low density lipoproteins extracted from human aortic intima. Arterioscler Thromb 1992;12:608–625.

31. Xu XX, Tabas I. Sphingomyelinase enhances low density lipoprotein uptake and ability to induce cholesterl ester accumulation in macrophages. J Biol Chem 1991;266:24849–24858.

32. Tirzui D, Bobrian A, Tasca C, Simionescu M, Simionescu N. Intimal thickenings of human aorta contain modified reassembled lipoproteins. Atherosclerosis 1995;112:101–114.

33. Hollander W, Colombo MA, Kirkpatrick B, Paddock J. Soluble proteins in the human atherosclerotic plague: with special reference to immunoglobulins, C3-complement component, alpha I-antitrypsin and alpha 2-macroglobulin. Atherosclerosis 1979;34:391–405.

34. Rus HG, Niculescu F, Constantinescu E, Cristea A, Vlaicu R. Immunoelectron-microscopic localization of the terminal C5b-9 complement complex in human atherosclerotic fibrous plaque. Atherosclerosis 1986;61:35–42.

35. Reynolds GD, Vance RP. C-reactive protein immunohistochemical localization in normal and atherosclerotic human aortas. Arch Pathol Lab Med 1987;111:265–269.

36. Hoff HF, Heideman CL, Gaubatz JW, Scott DW, Titus JL, Gotto AM Jr. Correlation of apolipoprotein B retention with the structure of atherosclerotic plaques from human aortas. Lab Invest 1978;38:560–567.

37. Hansson GK, Seifert PS. Complement receptors and regulatory proteins in human atherosclerotic lesions. Arteriosclerosis 1989;9:802–811.

38. Seifert PS, Hugo F, Hansson GK, Bhakdi S. Prelesional complement activation in experimental atherosclerosis. Lab Invest 1989;60:747–754.

39. Saikku P, Mattila K, Nieminen MS, et al. Serological evidence of an association of a novel *Chlamydia*, TWAR, with chronic coronary heart disease and acute myocardial infarction. Lancet 1988;2: 983–986.

40. Gupta S, Leathrm EW, Carrington D, et al. Elevated *Chlamydia pneumoniae* antibodies, cardiovascular events, and azithromycin in male survivors of myocardial infarction. Circulation 1997;96:404–407.

41. Gaydos CA, Summersgil JT, Sahney NN, et al. Replication of *Chlamydia pneumoniae* in vitro in human macrophages, endothelial cells, and aortic artery smooth muscle cells. Infect Immun 1996;64: 1614–1620.
42. Speir E, Huang ES, Modali R, et al. Interaction of human cytomegalovirus with p53: possible role in coronary restenosis. Scand J Infect Dis Suppl 1995;99:78–81.
43. Little WC, Constantinescu M, Applegate RJ, et al. Can coronary angiography predict the site of a subsequent myocardial infarction in patients with mild-to-moderate coronary artery disease? Circulation 1988;78:1157–1166.
44. Davies MJ, Thomas AC. Plaque fissuring—the cause of acute myocardial infarction, sudden ischemic death and crescendo angina. Br Heart J 1985;53:363–373.
45. Davies MJ, Richardson PD, Woolf N, Katz DR, Mann J. Risk of thrombosis in human atherosclerotic plaques: role of extracellular lipid, macrophage, and smooth muscle cell content. Br Heart J 1993;69: 377–381.
46. Moreno PR, Falk E, Palacios IF, Newell JB, Fuster V, Fallon JT. Macrophage infiltration in acute coronary syndromes: implications for plaque rupture. Circulation 1994;90:775–778.
47. Galis Z, Sukhova G, Kranzhofer R, Clark S, Libby P. Macrophage foam cells from experimental atheroma constitutively produce matrix-degrading proteinases. Proc Natl Acad Sci USA 1995;92: 402–406.
48. Brown DL, Hibbs MS, Kearney M, Loushin C, Isner JM. Identification of 92-kD gelatinase in human coronary atherosclerotic lesions. Association of active enzyme synthesis with unstable angina. Circulation 1995;91:2125–2131.
49. Amento EP, Ehsani N, Palmer H, Libby P. Cytokines positively and negatively regulate interstitial collagen gene expression in human vascular smooth muscle cells. Arterioscler Thromb 1991;11: 1223–1230.
50. Hansson GK, Holm J, Jonasson L. Detection of activated T lymphocytes in the human atherosclerotic plaque. Am J Pathol 1989;135:169–175.
51. Kaartinen M, Penttila A, Kovanen PT. Accumulation of activated mast cells in the shoulder region of human coronary atheroma, the predilection site of atheromatous rupture. Circulation 1994;90: 1669–1678.
52. Constantinides P. Infiltrates of activated mast cells at the site of coronary atheromatous erosion or rupture in myocardial infarction. Circulation 1995;92:1084–1088.
53. Enos WF, Holmes RH, Beyer J. Coronary disease among United States soldiers killed in action in Korea. JAMA 1953;152:1090.
54. Davies PF, Remuzzi A, Gordon EJ, Dewey CF Jr, Gimbrone MA Jr. Turbulent fluid shear stress induces vascular endothelial cell turnover in vitro. Proc Natl Acad Sci USA 1986;83:2114–2117.
55. Loree HM, Kamm RD, Stringfellow RG, Lee RT. Effects of fibrous cap thickness on peak circumferential stress in model atherosclerotic vessels. Circ Res 1992;71:850–858.
56. Lee RT, Grodzinsky AJ, Frank EH, Kamm RD, Schoen FJ. Structure dependent dynamic mechanical behavior of fibrous caps from human atherosclerotic plaques. Circulation 1991;83:1764–1770.
57. Tofler GH, Stone PH, Maclure M, et al. Analysis of possible triggers of acute myocardial infarction (The MILIS Study). Am J Cardiol 1990;66:22–27.
58. Behar S, Halabi M, Reicher-Reiss H, et al. Circadian variation and possible external triggers of onset of myocardial infarction. Am J Med 1993;94:395–400.
59. Tofler GH, Muller JE, Stone PH, Forman S, Solomon RE, Knatterud GL, Braunwald E. Modifiers of timing and possible triggers of acute myocardial infarction in the TIMI II population. J Am Coll Cardiol 1992;20:1049–1055.
60. Mittleman MA, Maclure M, Tofler GH, Sherwood JB, Goldberg RJ, Muller JE. Triggering of acute myocardial infarction by heavy exertion: protection against triggering by regular exertion. N Engl J Med 1993;329:1677–1683.
61. Willich SN, Lewis M, Lowel H, Arntz HR, Schubert F, Schroder R. Physical exertion as a trigger of acute myocardial infarction. N Engl J Med 1993;329:1684–1690.
62. Williams RB. Psychological factors in coronary artery disease: epidemiological evidence. Circulation 1987;76(Suppl. I):I-117–I-123.
63. Jern C, Eriksson E, Tengborn L, Risberg B, Wadenvik H, Jern S. Changes of plasma coagulation and fibrinolysis in response to mental stress. Thromb Hemost 1989;62:767–771.
64. Yusuf S, Peto J, Lewis J, Collins R, Sleight P. Beta blockade during and after myocardial infarction: an overview of the randomized trials. Prog Cardiovasc Dis 1985;27:335–371.

65. The SOLVD Investigators. Effects of enalapril on mortality and the development of heart failure in asymptomatic patients with reduced left ventricular ejection fractions. N Engl J Med 1992;327: 685–691.

66. Fernandez-Ortiz A, Badimon JJ, Falk E, et al. Characterization of the relative thrombogenicity of atherosclerotic plaque components: implications for consequences of plaque rupture. J Am Coll Cardiol 1994;23:1562–1569.

67. Merten M, Dong JF, Lopez JA, Thiagarajan P. Cholesterol sulfate: a new adhesive molecule for platelets. Circulation 2001;103:2032–2034.

68. Burke AP, Farb A, Malcom GT, Liang YH, Smialek J, Virmani R. Coronary risk factors and plaque morphology in men with coronary disease who died suddenly. N Engl J Med 1997;336:1276–1282.

69. Herrick JB. Clinical features of sudden obstruction of the coronary arteries. JAMA 1912;59: 2015–2020.

70. Saphir O, Priest WS, Hamburger WW, Katz LN. Coronary arteriosclerosis, coronary thrombosis, and the resulting myocardial changes. An evaluation of their respective clinical pictures including the electrocardiographic records, based on the anatomical findings. Am Heart J 1935;10:567–595.

71 Chapman I. Morphogenesis of occluding coronary artery thrombosis. Arch Pathol 1965;80:256–261.

72. Constantinides P. Plaque fissures in human coronary thrombosis. J Atheroscler Res 1966;6:1 17.

73. Douch DC, Montgomery GL. Cardiac lesions in fatal cases of recent myocardial ischaemia from a coronary care unit. Br Heart J 1970;32:795–803.

74. Ridolfi RL, Hutchins GM. The relationship between coronary artery lesions and myocardial infarcts: ulceration of atherosclerotic plaques precipitating coronary thrombosis. Am Heart J 1977;93: 468 486.

75. Falk E. Unstable angina with fatal outcome: dynamic coronary thrombosis leading to infarction and/or sudden death. Circulation 1985;71:699–708.

76. Davies MJ, Thomas A. Thrombosis and acute coronary-artery lesions in sudden cardiac ischemic death. N Engl J Med 1984;310:1137–1140.

77. Santamore WP, Yelton Jr BW, Ogilby JD. Dynamics of coronary occlusion in the pathogenesis of myocardial infarction. J Am Coll Cardiol 1991;18:1397–1405.

78. Losordo DW, Rosenfeld K, Kaufman J, Pieczek A, Isner JM. Focal compensatory enlargement of human arteries in response to progressive atherosclerosis. Circulation 1994;89:2570–2577.

79. Takano M, Mizuno K, Okamatsu K, et al. Mechanical and structural characteristics of vulnerable plaques-assembly coronary angioscopy and intravascular ultrasound. J Am Coll Cardiol 2001;38: 99–104.

80. Thieme T, Wernecke KD, Meyer R, et al. Angioscopic evaluation of atherosclerotic plaques: validation by histomorphologic analysis and association with stable and unstable coronary syndromes. J Am Coll Cardiol 1996;28:1–6.

81. Toussanint JF, Lamuraglia GM, Southern JF, Fuster V, Kantor HL. Magnetic resonance images lipid, fibrous, calcified, hemorrhagic and thrombotic components of human atherosclerosis in vivo. Circulation 1996;94:932–938.

82. Pasterkamp G, Falk E, Woutman H, Borst C. Techniques characterizing the coronary atherosclerotic plaque: influence on clinical decision making? J Am Coll Cardiol 2000;36:13–21.

83. Dangas G, Mehran R, Wallenstein S, et al. Correlation of angiographic morphology and clinical presentation in unstable angina. J Am Coll Cardiol 1997;29:519–525.

84. Sherman CT, Litvack F, Grundfest W, et al. Coronary angioscopy in patients with unstable angina pectoris. N Engl J Med 1986;315:913–919.

85. Kragel AH, Gertz SD, Roberts WC. Morphologic comparison of frequency and types of acute lesions in the major epicardial coronary arteries in unstable angina pectoris, sudden coronary death and acute myocardial infarction. J Am Coll Cardiol 1991;18:801–808.

86. Kloner RA, Rude RE, Carlson N, et al. Ultrastructural evidence of microvascular damage and myocardial cell injury after coronary artery occlusion: which comes first? Circulation 1980;62:945–952.

87. Roe MT, Ohman EM, Mass ACP, et al. Shifting the open-artery hypopiesis downstream: the quest for optimal reperfusion. J Am Coll Cardiol 2001;37:9–18.

88. Rus HG, Vlaicu R, Miculescu F. Interleukin-6 and interleukin-8 protein and gene expression in human arterial atherosclerotic wall. Atherosclerosis 1996;127:263–271.

89. Sukovich DA, Kauser K, Shirley FS, et al. Expression of interleukin-6 in atherosclerotic lesions of male ApoE-knockout mice: inhibition by 17beta-estradiol. Arterioscler Thromb Vasc Biol 1998;18: 1498–1505.

90. Cermak J, Key NS, Bach RR, Balla J, Jacobs HS, Vercellotti GM. C-reactive protein induces human peripheral blood monocytes to synthesize tissue factor. Blood 1993;82:513–520.
91. Ridker PM. High sensitivity C-reactive protein. Circulation 2001;103:1813–1818
92. Crisby M, Nordin-Fredriksson G, Shah PK, et al. Pravastatin treatment increases collagen content and decreases lipid content, inflammation, metalloproteinases, and cell death in human carotid plaques. Circulation 2001;103:926–933.
93. Ridker PM, Rifai N, Lowenthal SP. Rapid reduction in C-reactive protein with cerviastatin among 785 patients with primary hypercholesterolemia. Circulation 2001;103:1191–1193.
94. Hatton MWC, Moar SL, Richardson M. Deendothelialization *in vivo* initiates a thrombogenic reaction at the rabbit aorta surface. Correlation of uptake of fibrinogen and antithrombin III with thrombin generation by the exposed subendothelium. Am J Pathol 1989;135:499–508.
95. Hatton MWC, Southward SMR, Ross-Ouellet B, DeReske M, Blajchman MA, Richardson M. An increased uptake of prothrombin, antithrombin, and fibrinogen by the rabbit balloon-deendothelialized aorta surface in vivo is maintained until reendothelialization is complete. Arterioscler Thromb Vasc Biol 1996;16:1147–1155.
96. Marmur JD, Thiruvikraman SV, Fyfe BS, et al. Identification of active tissue factor in human coronary atheroma. Circulation 1996;94:1226–1232.
97. Wilcox JN, Smith KM, Schwartz SM, Gordon D. Localization of tissue factor in the normal vessel wall and in the atherosclerotic plaque. Proc Natl Acad Sci USA 1989;86:2839–2843.
98. Annex BH, Denning SM, Channon KM, et al. Differential expression of tissue factor protein in directional atherectomy specimens from patients with stable and unstable coronary syndromes. Circulation 1995;91:619–622.
99. Toschi V, Gallo R, Lettino M, et al. Tissue factor modulates the thrombogenicity of human atherosclerotic plaques. Circulation 1997;95:594–599.
100. Sandset PM, Abildgaard V, Larson ML. Heparin induces release of extrinsic coagulation pathway inhibitor. Thromb Res 1988;50:803–813.
101. Becker RC, Spencer FA, Li YouFu, et al. Thrombin conversion after the abrupt cessation of intravenous unfractionated heparin among patients with acute coronay syndromes. J Am Coll Cardiol 1999;34:1020–1027.
102. Barry WL, Gimple LW, Humphries JE, et al. Arterial thrombin activity after angioplasty in an atherosclerotic rabbit model. Time course and effect of hirudin. Circulation 1996;94:88–93.
103. Bar-Shavit R, Eldor A, Vlodavsky I. Binding of thrombin to subendothelial extracellular matrix. Protection and expression of functional properties. J Clin Invest 1989;84:1096–1104.
104. Nelken NA, Soifer SJ, O'Keefe J, Vu T-KH, Charo IF, Coughlin SR. Thrombin receptor expression in normal and atheroosclerotic human arteries. J Clin Invest 1992;90:1614–1621.
105. Lundgren CH, Sawa H, Sobel BE, Fujii S. Modulation of expression of monocyte/macrophage plasminogen activator activity and its implications for attenuation of vasculopathy. Circulation 1994;90:1927–1934.
106. Marczin N, Antonov A, Papapetropoulos A, et al. Monocyte-induced downregulation of nitric oxide synthase in cultured aortic endothelial cells. Arterioscler Thromb Vasc Biol 1996;16:1095–1103.
107. Gupta M, Doellgast GJ, Cheng T, Lewis JC. Expression and localization of tissue factor-based procoagulant activity (PCA) in pigeon monocyte-derived macrophages. Thromb Haemost 1993;70:963–969.
108. Serneri GG, Abbate R, Gori AM, et al. Transient intermittent lymphocyte activation is responsible for the instability of angina. Circulation 1992;86:790–797.
109. Liuzzo G, Vallejo AN, Kopecky SL, et al. Molecular fingerprint of interferon-γ signaling in unstable angina. Circulation 2001;103:1509–1514.
110. Liuzzo G, Goronzy JJ, Yang H, et al. Monoclonal T-cell proliferation and plaque instability in acute coronary syndromes. Circulation 2000;102:2883–2888.
111. Houtkamp MA, van der Wal AC, deBoar OJ, et al. Interleukin-15 expression in atherosclerotic plaques: an alternative pathway for T cell activation in atherosclerosis? Arterioscler Thromb Vasc Biol 2001;21:1208–1213.
112. Schonbeck U, Mach F, sukhova GK, et al. CD 40 ligation induces tissue factor expression in human vascular smooth muscle cells. Am J Pathol 2000;156:7–14.
113. Loppnow H, Libbey P. Proliferating or interleukin activated human vascular smooth muscle secrete copious interleukin 6. J Clin Invest 1990;85:731–738.
114. Hynes RO. Integrins: a family of cell surface receptors. Cell 1987;48:549–554.

115. Plow EF, Ginsberg MH. Cellular adhesion: GPIIb/IIIa as a prototypic adhesion receptor. Prog Hemost Thromb 1989;9:117–156.
116. Liuzzo G, Biasucci LM, Gallimore JR, et al. The prognostic value of C-reactive protein and serum amyloid A protein in severe unstable angina. N Engl J Med 1994;331:417–424.
117. Becker R, Cannon C, Bovill E, et al. Prognostic value of plasma fibrinogen concentration in patients with unstable angina and non-Q-wave myocardial infarction (TIMI IIIB Trial). Am J Cardiol 1996;78: 142–147.
118. Lefvert A, Hamsten A, Holm G. Association between circulating immune complexes, complement C4 null alleles, and myocardial infarction before age 45 years. Arterioscler Thromb Vasc Biol 1995;15: 665–668.
119. Neumann FJ, Ott I, Gawaz M, et al. Cardiac release of cytokines and inflammatory responses in acute myocardial infarction. Circulation 1995;92:748–755
120. Furman M, Becker R, Yarzebski J, Savegeau J, Gore J, Goldberg R. Effect of elevated leukocyte count on in-hospital mortality following acute myocardial infarction. Am J Cardiol 1996;78:945–948.
121. Van Mourik JA, Lawrence PA, Loskutoff DJ. Purification of an inhibitor of plasminogen activator (antiactivator) synthesized by endothelail cells. J Biol Chem 1984; 259:14914–14921.
122. Ginsburg D, Zcheb R, Yang AY, ct al. cDNA cloning of human plasminogen activator-inhibitor from endothelial cells. J Clin Invest 1986;78:1673–1680.
123. Ny T, Sawdey M, Lawrence D, Millan JL, Loskutoff DJ. Cloning and sequence of cDNA coding for the human β-migrating endothelial-cell-type plasminogen activator inhibitor. Proc Natl Acad Sci USA 1986;83:6776–6780.
124. Declerck PJ, DeMol M, Alessi MC, et al. Purification and characterization of a plasminogen activator inhibitor 1 binding protein from human plasma. J Biol Chem 1988;263:15454–15461.
125. Vaughan DE, Declerck PJ, Reilly TM, Park K, Collen D, Fasman GD. Dynamic structural and functional relationships in recombinant plasminogen activator inhibitor-1 (rPAI-1). Biochim Biophys Acta 1993;1202:221–229.
126. Lambers JW, Cammenga M, Konig BW, Mertens K, Pannekoek H, van Mourik JA. Activation of human endothelial cell-type plasminogen activator inhibitor (PAI-1) by negatively charged phospholipids. J Biol Chem 1987;262:17492–17496.
127. Sprengers ED, Kluft C. Plasminogen activator inhibitors. Blood 1987;69:381 387.
128. Sprengers ED, Princen HM, Kooistra T, van Hinsbergh VW. Inhibition of plasminogen activators by conditioned medium of human hepatocytes and hepatoma cell line Hep G2. J Lab Clin Med 1985;105: 751–758.
129. Dichek D, Quertermous T. Thrombin regulation of mRNA levels of tissue plasminogen activator and plasminogen activator inhibitor-1 in cultured human umbilical vein endothelial cells. Blood 1989; 74:222 228.
130. Schneiderman J, Sawdey MS, Keeton MR, et al. Increased type 1 plasminogen activator inhibitor gene expression in atherosclerotic human arteries. Proc Natl Acad Sci USA 1992;89:6998–7002.
131. Hamsten A, Wiman B, Faire UD, de Faire U, Blomback M. Increased plasma levels of a rapid inhibitor of tissue plasminogen activator in young survivors of myocardial infarction. N Engl J Med 1985;313: 1557–1563.
132. Hamsten A, de Faire U, Walldius G, et al. Plasminogen activator inhibitor in plasma: risk factor for recurrent myocardial infarction. Lancet 1987;2:3–9.
133. Berk BC, Vekshtein V, Gordon HM, Tsuda T. Angiotensin II-stimulated protein synthesis in cultured vascular smooth muscle cells. Hypertension 1989;13:305–314.
134. Katz AM. Angiotensin-II: hemodynamic regulator or growth factor? J Mol Cell Cardiol 1990;22: 739–747.
135. Ridker PM, Gaboury CL, Conlin PR, Seely EW, Williams GH, Vaughan DE. Stimulation of plasminogen activator inhibitor in vivo by infusion of angiotensin II: evidence of a potential interaction between the renin angiotensin system and firinolytic function. Circulation 1993;87:1969–1973.
136. Olson JA Jr, Shiverick KT, Ogilvie S, Buhi WC, Raizade MK. Angiotensin II induces secretion of plasminogen activator inhibitor-I and a tissue metalloprotease inhibitor-related protein from rat brain astrocytes. Neurobiology 1991;88:1928–1932.
137. Vaughan DE, Rouleau J-L, Ridker PM, Arnold JMO, Menapace FJ, Pfeffer MA. Effects of ramipril on plasma fibrinolytic balance in patients with acute anterior myocardial infarction. Circulation 1997;96: 442–447.

138. Neri Serneri GG, Boddi M, Poggesi L, et al. Activation of cardioa resin-angiotension system in unstable angina. J Am Coll Cardiol 2001;38:49-55.
139. Brozovic M, Stirling Y, Harricks C. Factor VII in an industrial population. Br J Haematol 1974;28:381–391.
140. Conlan MG, Folsom AR, Finch A, et al. Associations of factor VII and von Willebrand factor with age, race, sex and risk factors for atherosclerosis. Thromb Haemost 1993;3:380–385.
141. Kannel WB, Wolf PA, Castelli WP, D'Agostino RB. Fibrinogen and risk of cardiovascular disease. JAMA 1987;258:1183–1186.
142. Jansson JH, Olofsson BO, Nilsson TK. Predictive value of tissue plasminogen activator mass concentration on long term mortality in patients with coronary artery disease: a 7-year follow up. Circulation 1993;88:2030–2034.
143. American Diabetes Association. Consensus statement: detection and management of lipid disorders in diabetes. Diabetes Care 1996:19(Suppl. 1):S96–S102.
144. Krolewski AS, Kosinski EJ, Warram HJ, et al. Magnitude and determinants of coronary artery disease in juvenile-onset, insulin-dependent diabetes mellitus. Am J Cardiol 1987;59:750–755.
145. Schwartz CJ, Valente AJ, Sprague EA, et al. Pathogenesis of the atherosclerotic lesion: implications for diabetes mellitus. Diabetes Care 1992;15:1156–1157.
146. Bierman EL. Atherogenesis in diabetes. Arterioscler Thromb 1992;12:647–656.
147. Lyon TJ. Lipoprotein glycation and its metabolic consequences. Diabetes 1992;41(Suppl. 2;67–73.
148. Raman M, Nesto RW. Heart disease in diabetes mellitus. Endocrinol Metab Clin North Am 1996;25:425–438.
149. Pyorala K, Savolainedn E, Kaukola S, et al. Plasma insulin as a coronary heart disease risk factor: Relationship to other risk factors and predictive value during 9 1/2 year follow-up of the Helsinki Policemen Study. Acta Med Scand 1985;701(Suppl.)38–52.
150. Kern PA, Saghizadeh M, Ong JM, Bosch RJ, Deem R, Simsolo RB. The expression of tumor necrosis factor in human adipose tissue. Regulation by obesity, weight loss, and relationship to lipoprotein lipase. J Clin Invest 1995;95:2111–2119.
151. Haraldsen G, Kvale D, Lien B, Farstad IN. Brandtzaeg P. Cytokine-regulated expression of E-selectin, intercellular adhesion molecule-1 (CAM-1), and vascular cell adhesion molecule-1 (VCAM-1) in human microvascular endothelial cells. J Immunol 1996;156:2558–2565.
152. Festa A, D'Agostino R Jr, Mykkanen L, et al. Relative contributionof insulin and its precursors to fibrinogen and PAI-1 in a large population with different states of glucose tolerance. The Insulin Resistance Atherosclerosis Study (IRAS). Arterioscler Thromb Vasc Biol 1999;19:562–568.
153. Keys A. Coronary heart disease in seven countries. Circulation 1970;41:1–211.
154. Walker ID, Davidson JF, Hutton I. Disordered fibrinolytic potential in coronary heart disease. Thromb Res 1977;15:114A.
155. Tremoll E, Maderna P, Calil S, et al. Increased platelet sensitivity and thromboxane B2 formation in type-II hyperlipoproteinemic patients. Eur J Clin Invest 1984;14:329–333.
156. Wilkes HC, Meade TW, Barzegar S, et al. Gemfibrozil reduces plasma prothrombin fragment F1+2 concentration, a marker of coagulability, in patients with coronary heart disease. Thromb Haemost 1992;67:503–506.
157. Eisenberg PR, Sherman LA, Schectman K, Perez J, Sobel BE, Jaffe AS. Fibrionopeptide A: a marker of acute coronary thrombosis. Circulation 1985;71:912–918.
158. Becker RC, Bovill E, Corrao JM, et al. Platelet activity persists among patients with unstable angina and non-Q wave myocardial infarction. J Thromb Thrombolysis 1994;1:95–100.
159. Becker RC, Tracy RP, Bovill EG, et al. Surface 12-lead electrocardiographic findings and plasma markers of thrombin activity and generation in patients with myocardial ischemia at rest. J Thromb Thrombolysis 1994;1:101–107.
160. Furman MI, Bernard MR, Krueger LA, et al. Circulating monocyte-platelet aggregates are an early marker of acute myocardial infarction. J Am Coll Cardiol, 2001;4:1002–1006.

3

Triggers of Acute Coronary Syndromes

Peter M. Sapin, MD and James E. Muller, MD

CONTENTS

INTRODUCTION

The likelihood that acute myocardial infarction is triggered by a specific event has been a subject of debate since the earliest description of this disorder, which incorporated the belief that specific physical or mental events precipitated the attack *(1)*. Controversy concerning the events precipitating acute myocardial infarction continued for decades *(2,3)*, until 1960 when Master published a retrospective study of over 2600 patients with acute myocardial infarction *(4)*. This study was the largest to that date addressing the triggering of myocardial infarction. While no formal statistical analysis was applied, it was concluded from the data that the onset of myocardial infarction was unrelated to physical effort, to time of day, to day of the week, or to the occupation of the patient. In the last 15 yr, as knowledge of the pathological processes underlying acute coronary syndromes has advanced, the possibility of the existence of specific triggers of the onset of acute myocardial infarction and related syndromes has been reconsidered.

The current concept holds that acute coronary syndromes result from a breach in the surface of an atherosclerotic plaque, either by frank rupture of the fibrous cap overlying the plaque or, less commonly, by endothelial denudation of the cap *(5–12)*. This event exposes collagen, tissue factor, and the lipid material underlying the luminal surface of the plaque to blood. The interaction between the inner constituents of the plaque and its cap and blood where platelets and clotting factor proteins are available for activation, initiates

From: *Contemporary Cardiology: Management of Acute Coronary Syndromes, Second Edition*
Edited by: C. P. Cannon © Humana Press Inc., Totowa, NJ

the formation of intracoronary thrombus. The competition between thrombosis and intrinsic fibrinolytic processes determines the natural history of the plaque rupture. One possible outcome is a voluminous thrombus little diminished by fibrinolysis, causing total coronary occlusion, extensive myocardial ischemia with electrocardiographic ST segment elevation, and myocardial infarction. A different clinical syndrome might be expected to result from a smaller thrombus mass that is spontaneously lysed—transient symptoms, with or without ischemic electrocardiographic changes, and without myocardial infarction. Another acute presentation of coronary artery disease is sudden cardiac death. There is evidence that acute changes in plaque morphology can be found in a majority of such cases *(13)*, and mechanisms, including ischemia and reperfusion, hemodynamic factors, metabolic alterations, and autonomic influences, are implicated *(14)*.

The triggering of acute coronary syndromes requires two elements: a substrate and the triggering events or circumstances. The substrate is an atherosclerotic plaque with features predisposing it to superficial erosion or rupture. The plaque exists in a microenvironment which includes the physical forces that stress or deform the plaque, coronary vasomotor tone and endothelial function, circulating catecholamines and other vasoactive substances, and the state of the intracoronary hemostatic environment. The activities and circumstances that may be recognized as triggering events for acute coronary syndromes produce their effects through alterations in the microenvironment, which favor plaque erosion or rupture and intracoronary thrombus formation (Fig. 1).

TRANSFORMATION FROM STABLE TO VULNERABLE ATHEROSCLEROTIC PLAQUE

There is considerable heterogeneity in the structure of atherosclerotic plaques, and numerous investigations have attempted to identify special features of plaques that are involved in acute ischemic syndromes *(5–12)*. It has been observed in patients experiencing acute myocardial infarction, who have coincidentally undergone coronary arteriography at some point prior to the acute event, that the site of coronary occlusion is often not the site of the most stenotic lesion in the coronary tree *(15,16)*. It is now recognized that acute ischemic syndromes are often precipitated at atherosclerotic sites that are only minimally obstructive, suggesting that features other than plaque bulk contribute to the risk of a given plaque acting as the site of an acute coronary occlusion *(15,16)*. Detailed anatomic studies of plaque structure at the site of rupture and thrombosis in patients who have died from acute myocardial infarction have identified a variety of morphologic features that are more likely to be found in these plaques compared to plaques at other, presumably more stable, sites *(5–12)*. These features include a relatively large physically soft lipid pool and a fibrous cap overlying the plaque, which is relatively thin *(5–12)*. There is evidence that plaques with a thinner cap and larger underlying lipid pool may be more susceptible to physical forces that cause the cap to fissure, usually at the edge of the plaque, thus setting in motion the thrombogenic cascade leading to an occlusive clot *(5–12)*. The fibrous cap, separating the thrombogenic core material from the blood, is figuratively the "no-man's land" between stable and unstable coronary artery disease. It appears to be a site of intense biologic activity and is a dynamic structure *(11,12)*.

Two important findings in the caps of vulnerable plaques are a reduced smooth muscle cell content and increased numbers of inflammatory cells, such as activated macrophages,

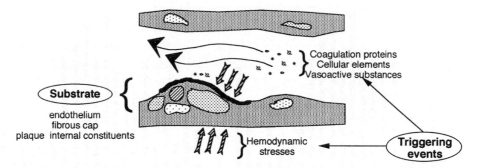

Fig. 1. Substrate, triggering events, and the physiologic processes linking the two. Atherosclerotic plaques with varying structural, cellular, and biochemical characteristics form the substrate for acute coronary events. The plaque is in contact with circulating cellular elements, coagulation proteins, and vasoactive substances produced locally in the endothelium and circulating systemically. The plaque also is acted upon by physical forces related to systemic hemodynamics and coronary blood flow. Triggering events exert their effects by modifying local physiologic processes to promote plaque disruption and intracoronary thrombosis.

T cells, and mast cells. Smooth muscle cells produce collagen and other proteins, which thicken and strengthen the cap. The inflammatory cells produce a variety of substances which inhibit collagen formation or degrade that which exists. Substances produced by inflammatory cells can also induce smooth muscle cell apoptosis (programmed cell death). These changes in the composition of the cap reduce its strength, favoring rupture or erosion. Recent studies in patients have shown that higher serum levels of systemic markers of inflammation predict a higher risk of acute coronary disease (17 19). The spe cific mechanisms by which these proinflammatory modulators become augmented in the vessel wall are as yet unknown. The possibility that infectious agents, either within the vascular wall or at remote sites, might constitute this link is under investigation, but conclusions are still controversial (20,21).

The susceptability of an individual to plaque disruption and resulting coronary disease events may also depend on the presence of specific inherited polymorphisms of genes controlling proteins involved in the development of atherosclerotic plaque and in thrombosis. For example, in a prospective study of 3052 men in the Northwick Park Heart Study, initially free of coronary heart disease, cigarette smokers who were carriers of the E4 allele of apolipoprotein E had a significantly increased risk (2.79-fold, 95% confidence interval 1.59–4.91) of myocardial infarction or coronary artery surgery, with no increased risk imparted by this allele in exsmokers (22). In another study of 444 patients with angiographically severe severe coronary disease, those with certain alleles of the Factor VII gene were significantly less likely to have experienced a myocardial infarction (23).

EVIDENCE FOR TRIGGERING
Periodicity in the Onset of Acute Cardiac Events
MORNING INCREASE IN ACUTE CARDIOVASCULAR DISEASE ONSET

The frequency of acute myocardial infarction onset over the 24-h period has been reexamined since the work of Master (4). Muller and others in 1985 examined data from the Multicenter Investigation of the Limitation of Infarct Size (MILIS) trial, involving

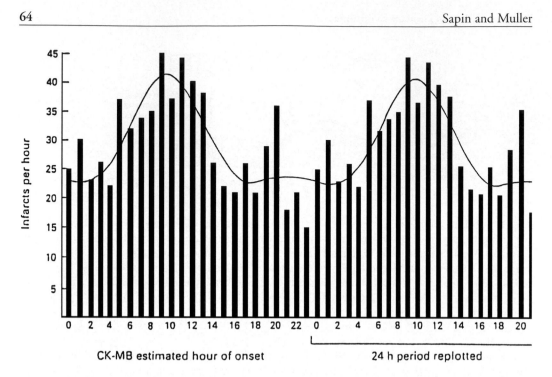

Fig. 2. Circadian variation in myocardial infarction onset. The number of infarctions/h is plotted on the Y-axis vs the time of onset on the X-axis (24-h clock) for 849 patients experiencing acute myocardial infarction. The hour of onset of infarction is determined from extrapolated from creatine phosphokinase MB fraction levels. There is a significant excess of infarctions between the hours of 6 AM and noon, with a small secondary peak at 7 to 8 PM. Reprinted with permission from ref. *24.*

849 patients *(24).* Serial cardiac muscle enzyme levels were used to estimate the time of the onset of infarction. These investigators identified a prominent morning increase in the incidence of infarction onset, peaking from 9 AM to noon, with a smaller peak in the early evening. A nadir in the incidence of infarction onset was observed at night (Fig. 2). Similar findings were reported from the Intravenous Streptokinase in Acute Myocardial Infarction (ISAM) trial of 1741 patients, with infarction occurring 1.8× more frequently between 6 AM and noon, compared to the other quarters of the day *(25).* This pattern, with a predominance of infarctions beginning in the morning hours, and a relative paucity beginning during what would be considered hours of sleep (midnight to 6 AM), has been confirmed in many other studies *(26–35).* Some but not all investigators have also reported a second, smaller peak in the incidence of infarction onset during the late afternoon or evening hours. A meta-analysis of 30 studies encompassing 66,635 patients found a relative risk for myocardial onset between 6 AM and noon of 1.38 (95% confidence interval 1.37–1.40) *(36).* This study calculated that 27.7% of morning non-fatal infarctions and 8.8% (95% confidence interval 8.5–9.0%) of all nonfatal myocardial infarctions could be attributed to the excess morning risk of acute myocardial infarction (Fig. 3).

A similar pattern of circadian variation occurs in acute coronary and vascular events other than nonfatal myocardial infarction. The onset of chest pain at rest in patients hospitalized with unstable angina pectoris also shows a statistically significant morning peak *(37–41).* In the Thrombolysis in Myocardial Infarction (TIMI) III study of unstable angina and non-Q wave myocardial infarction, 31.4% of 7730 patients entered into

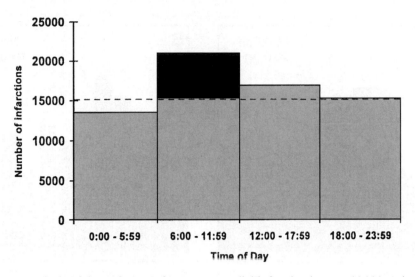

Fig. 3. Meta-analysis of time of onset of acute myocardial infarction in over 66,000 patients. In these studies the 24-h period is divided into 6-h segments, beginning at midnight. The dotted line shows the expected number of infarctions for each 6-h time period, and the black shaded area shows the excess incidence of infarctions occurring during the 6 AM to noon segment. Reprinted with permission from ref. *36*.

the registry roster had onset of pain between 6 AM and noon *(37)* (Fig. 4). One study of 1167 patients with non-Q wave myocardial infarction failed to show a significant diurnal variation in time of onset of symptoms *(41)*. However, the larger TIMI III study demonstrated a significant morning excess of events in both the unstable angina and non-Q wave myocardial infarction subgroups *(37)*.

Ambulatory monitoring of patients with stable coronary artery disease and myocardial ischemia also demonstrates an increase in the number of episodes of transient myocardial ischemia occurring during the morning hours, between 6 AM and noon, again sometimes with a secondary peak in the late afternoon *(42–47)* (Fig. 5). A multicenter European study of over 1087 stable angina patients found both early morning (9 AM to noon) and afternoon (3 PM to 6 PM) peaks in anginal attack frequency *(48)*. Another study of transient myocardial ischemia in the early posthospital phase of acute myocardial infarction demonstrated the peak incidence of ischemic episodes to be in the early evening hours rather than in the morning *(49)*. This suggests that circadian patterns may be altered transiently by an event such as acute myocardial infarction.

Ischemic stroke represents another vascular catastrophe with pathogenesis similar to that of myocardial ischemic events. A significant variation in the time of onset of stroke symptoms, with a dominant peak in the 6 AM to noon time frame, has been demonstrated *(50,51)*. Even when accounting for stroke patients awakening with symptoms, when the time of onset may not be known, over 50% of strokes in one study *(50)* and 38% in another *(51)* were thought to have had their onset between 6 AM and noon.

The timing of sudden cardiac death also appears to have a similar circadian variation, demonstrated in two studies of the Massachusetts population *(52,53)*, a group of patients with advanced heart failure dying suddenly *(54)*, and in patients receiving antiarrhythmic agents during the Cardiac Arrhythmia Supression Trial (CAST) *(55)*. A meta-analysis also reviewed 19 published studies of the time of onset of sudden cardiac death (5834

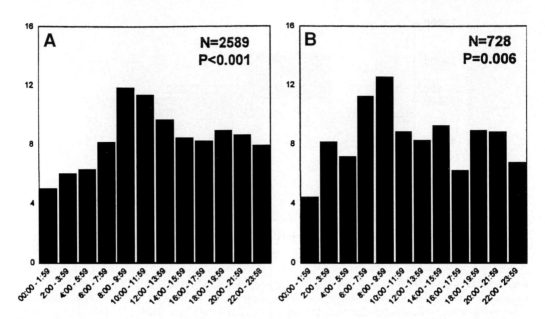

Fig. 4. The circadian variation in the timing of the onset of unstable angina pectoris and non-Q wave myocardial infarction, from the TIMI III Registry. The percent of patients with onset of symptoms in each 2-h time period (X-axis) is shown. The *p*-values are the result of the chi-square goodness-of-fit test for a uniform distribution, indicating a highly significant nonuniformity. Reprinted with permission from ref. *37*.

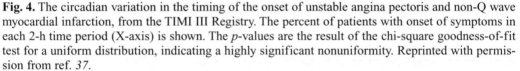

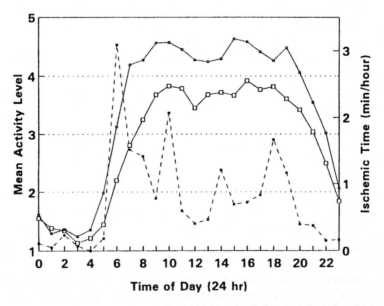

Fig. 5. Circadian variation in myocardial ischemic burden in patients undergoing 24-hourly ambulatory monitoring. The solid lines indicate the level of physical and mental activity (Y-axis on left) throughout the 24-h cycle (X-axis). These levels increase in the morning, remain elevated throughout the day, and decrease at night. The dotted line plots the total duration of myocardial ischemia per hour (Y-axis on right). There is a prominent morning peak in ischemic time, paralleling the rise in the level of physical and mental activity. However, ischemic time decreases after the morning hours despite maintenance of high physical and mental activity levels. Reprinted with permission from ref. *42*.

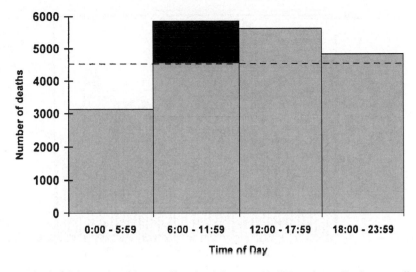

Fig. 6. Meta-analysis of time of sudden cardiac death in over 19,000 patients. In these studies, the 24-h period is divided into 6-h segments, beginning at midnight. The dotted line shows the expected number of infarctions for each 6-h time period, and the black shaded area the excess incidence of sudden deaths occurring during the 6 AM to noon segment. Reprinted with permission from ref. *36*.

events) *(36)*. The relative risk of sudden cardiac death was 1.29× greater (95% confidence interval 1.26–1.32) in the morning period compared to the rest of the day. The morning excess of sudden cardiac deaths accounted for 22.5% of morning sudden deaths and 6.8% (95% confidence interval 6.4–7.1%) of all sudden deaths (Fig. 6). Ventricular tachycardia and ventricular fibrillation are the most frequent arrhythmias causing sudden cardiac death. Several studies of patients with automatic implantible cardioverter-defibrillators (AICD) capable of documenting the time of arrhythmias *(56–61)* and a study of the arrival time in the emergency room of patients with ventricular fibrillation *(62)*, demonstrated a morning peak and a nighttime nadir of the frequency of these events (Fig. 7).

The relationship between morning and myocardial infarction has prompted consideration that the time of awakening, rather than the time of day *per se*, may better explain the variation in the time of onset of acute coronary syndromes. In one study of 224 patients, the relative risk of acute myocardial infarction onset between 6 and 9 AM was 1.8 (95% confidence interval 1.3–2.4) *(63)*. After adjustment for individual wake times, the relative risk of infarction onset in the first 3 h after awakening increased to 2.4 (95% confidence interval 1.8–3.1). Another study of 137 patients found 23% of patients to report the onset of symptoms of myocardial infarction within 1 h of awakening *(64)*. In the CAST experience of 3309 patients with a history of myocardial infarction, 24% experienced symptom onset within 4 h of awakening *(65)*. In patients with sudden cardiac death, the relative risk for the first 3 h after awakening was 2.6 (95% confidence interval 1.6–4.2) compared to other times of the day *(66)*. Studies of ambulatory patients undergoing Holter monitoring to detect myocardial ischemic episodes found that ischemic time increased significantly for the 2 h after awakening *(42,46)*. This increase was observed even after correction for the greater level of physical and mental activity, which independently influenced ambulatory ischemia *(42)*. The multicenter European

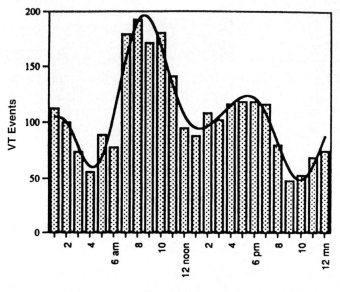

Fig. 7. Circadian variation in frequency of ventricular tachyarrhythmic events in 32 patients with automatic implantable defibrillators capable of recording the time of occurrence of arrhythmias. The Y-axis represents the number of events vs time of day. The predominance of events during the 6 AM to noon time period is statistically significant by analysis of variance (ANOVA) ($p = 0.007$). The curve is a fourth-order harmonic regression curve, demonstrating a significant periodicity in the frequency of events over time ($R^2 = 0.91$, $p < 0.001$). Reprinted with permission from ref. *57.*

angina study cited above found 50% of anginal attacks to occur within 6 h of awakening *(48)*. While the hours of sleep (generally midnight to 6 AM) have been shown to encompass the lowest frequency of the onset of acute coronary syndromes, one study found that in patients with stable coronary disease, arising at night was strongly associated with the occurrence of transient myocardial ischemia detectable by ambulatory monitoring *(67)*.

OTHER PATTERNS IN THE TIMING OF ACUTE CARDIAC EVENTS

In addition to variation in frequency of acute cardiac events over the course of a typical 24-h sleep–wake cycle, other temporal and environmental cycles have been shown to affect the timing of these events. Several studies have shown that myocardial infarctions are more likely to occur on Monday *(26,68–70)*. One group demonstrated that this pattern was present only in a working, as opposed to a nonworking, population *(68)*, although this was not confirmed in another study *(34)*. One interesting observation has been made concerning 148 sudden cardiac deaths over a 10-yr period on the Hawaiian Island of Kauai *(71)*. While the occurrence of sudden death in local residents demonstrated the typical 6 AM to noon peak, sudden death in visitors coming from 2500 to 5400 miles distant (3–6 time zones) showed a peak in the 6 PM to midnight time period. This may reflect altered sleep–wake cycles induced by "jet lag."

A seasonal variation, with a peak in wintertime admissions for acute myocardial infarction and a summertime trough, has also been reported *(28,34,69)*. One group studied the daily frequency of myocardial infarction over a 10-yr period and found correlations to varying weather patterns from year-to-year; higher incidence correlated with lower temperature and higher humidity *(72)*. A study of vital statistics from five Minneapolis–St. Paul winters found no statistical relation between air temperature and cardiovascular mortality *(73)*. However, this study found that snowfall influenced mortality on the day of occurrence and for 2 d following snowfall. The combination of rain and snow was found to produce a dramatic increase in mortality from acute myocardial infarction. Similar observations were made in Toronto, Ontario, Canada *(74)*. On the other hand, a large multicenter study did find a significant increase in cardiovascular disease event rates with decreasing air temperatures *(75)*. A recent study in patients with event-recording implantable cardioverter-defibrillators (ICD) found that the frequency of ventricular tachyarrhythmias correlated with the temperature calculated to be "felt" by the individual. "Felt-temperatures" in the range considered to represent thermal stress were associated with higher frequencies of arrhythmia *(76)*. The role that climate, as opposed to nonmeteorological features of seasonal transitions, may play as a modifier of susceptibility to acute coronary disease onset is unclear. While the seasonal distribution of myocardial infarction existed without regard to climate in a multicenter, 259,891-patient U.S. study *(77)*, a study of 540 acute MI patients in Taiwan, a country with a year-round uniform subtropical climate found no such seasonal variation *(78)*.·

Many of the studies examining the circadian variation of acute myocardial infarction have performed analyses in subgroups of patients, with the goal of gaining insights into triggering mechanisms by identifying differences in circadian rhythms between groups with different characteristics. In most studies, age, sex, cigarette smoking, prior myocardial infarction, or angina pectoris have not affected circadian patterns. The findings for diabetic patients have been less consistent, with some studies showing attenuation of circadian variation of myocardial infarction onset in diabetics *(26,27,69,79)*, and others showing preserved circadian variation *(24,31,80)*. One study found circadian variation to be present in treated diabetic subjects, and abolished in untreated patients *(81)*.

Specific Activities as Potential Triggers of Acute Myocardial Infarction

Morning and awakening appears to trigger acute coronary syndromes. Other environmental changes, such as the transition from weekend to work week and changes in weather cycles, may also function as triggers. Many investigators have sought specific events identifiable by patients as triggers. Studies using interview techniques to determine the fraction of patients reporting a suspected "triggering activity" in the time period immediately preceding the onset of symptoms have found that 25 to >50% of patients describe moderate to heavy physical exertion, unusual emotional stress, lack of sleep, overeating or use of alcohol, noncardiac illness or surgery, or some other activity as ongoing at the time of, or in the 24 h preceding, the onset of infarction *(82–85)*. However, these data are limited by recall bias and by the difficulty of obtaining appropriate control data, i.e., the frequency with which the activity occurs without an acute event following.

New epidemiological techniques have allowed a more sophisticated study of the relationship between specific patient activities and the onset of acute cardiac events. One such approach is the case-crossover method, which uses the patient as his or her own control to calculate the relative risk of a rare acute event such as a myocardial infarction following an intermittently performed activity suspected of being a trigger *(86)*. This method reduces some of the bias inherent in this type of study.

Table 1
Relative Risk of Myocardial Infarction Following Triggering Events, Including the Effect of Exercise Frequency on Risk

Trigger (reference)	Duration of risk increase	Overall RR MI of triggering MI	RR of triggering MI stratified by exercise frequency	
			<1/wk	3 to 4/wk
Exercise (88)	1 h	5.9 (4.6–7.7)	107 (67–171)	8.6 (3.6–20.5)
Sexual intercourse (94)	2 h	2.5 (1.7–3.7)	3.0 (2.0–4.5)	1.2 (0.4–3.7)
Anger (103)	2 h	2.3 (1.7–3.2)	*	*
Morning (36)	*	1.38 (1.37–1.40)	*	*
Cocaine use (105)	1 h	23.8 (8.3–66.3)	*	*
Marijuana use (106)	1 h	4.8 (2.4–9.5)	*	*

RR, relative risk (95% confidence intervals); MI, myocardial infarction.
Duration, time period after trigger for which relative risk of infarction remained >1.0.
Anger, "very angry, furious, or enraged".
Exercise frequency, sessions of ≥6 METS of effort (vigorous exertion with panting, overheating).
*, not reported.

PHYSICAL EXERTION

The role of physical exertion as a trigger of myocardial infarction has been a subject of controversy, since most infarctions occur at rest or with mild activity (Table 1). One study of 1194 German patients reported 7.1% of infarct patients to have engaged in ≥ 6 metabolic equivalents (METS) of exertion at the onset of infarction vs 3.9% of a control group (87). From case-crossover analysis, the relative risk of having engaged in this level of activity within 1 h of the onset of infarction was 2.1 (95% confidence interval 1.1–3.6). This increased risk was modified by the frequency with which the patient engaged in physical exercise on a routine basis. Exercise ≥4×/wk was associated with a relative risk of only 1.3 (95% confidence interval 0.8–2.2), whereas exercise <4×/wk imparted a relative risk of 6.9 (95% confidence interval 4.1–12.2). Similar findings emerged from the Myocardial Infarction Onset Study of 1228 patients, which also used the case-crossover method (88). Although only 4.4% of patients reported heavy physical exertion within 1 h of the onset of myocardial infarction, the relative risk of infarction within 1 h of heavy exertion (≥ 6 METS) was 5.9 (95% confidence interval 4.6–7.7). This risk increase persisted for 1 h after exercise (Fig. 8). These investigators also found that regular exercise lowered the risk of exertion-related infarction. The relative risks of infarction following exertion among individuals who exercised 1, 1 to 2, 3 to 4, and ≥5×/wk were 107, 19.4, 8.6, and 2.4, respectively (Fig. 9) (Table 1). Known coronary artery disease, age, sex, and a variety of other clinical variables did not influence the increased relative risk of myocardial infarction imparted by exercise, with the exception of diabetes mellitus, where the relative risk was significantly higher (18.9 vs 5.4 for nondiabetics).

Similar results concerning the incidence of sudden cardiac death during exercise and the protective effect of regular exercise, were reported by Siscovick et al. (89) In a group of men who spent less than 20 min/wk engaged in vigorous exercise, the risk of sudden death during exercise was increased 56-fold, as compared to a five-fold increase in risk seen in men exercising more than 20 min/d. The absolute risk of sudden death was very

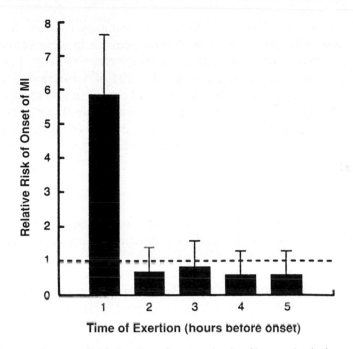

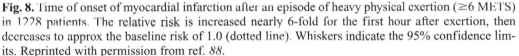

Fig. 8. Time of onset of myocardial infarction after an episode of heavy physical exertion (≥6 METS) in 1228 patients. The relative risk is increased nearly 6-fold for the first hour after exertion, then decreases to approx the baseline risk of 1.0 (dotted line). Whiskers indicate the 95% confidence limits. Reprinted with permission from ref. *88.*

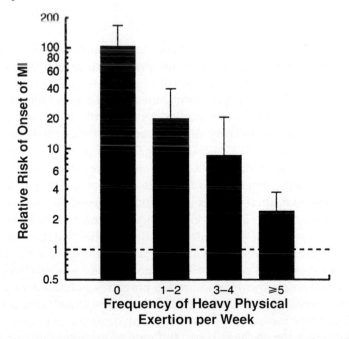

Fig. 9. Relation between risk of exertion triggered myocardial infarction and weekly frequency of heavy exertion. The relative risk of myocardial infarction (Y-axis) following heavy exertion is approx 100-fold in individuals who perform no heavy exertion during the week and falls to approx 2.4-fold for individuals with >5 sessions of heavy exertion per week. Whiskers indicate the 95% confidence limits. The dotted line indicates the baseline risk. Reprinted with permission from ref. *88.*

low, 1 cardiac death per 20,000 joggers per year. In marathon runners, the sudden death incidence was lower still: among over 200,000 participants in separate marathon races, 3 such deaths occurred during or immediately after the race *(90)*. The Physician's Health Study, involving 21,481 male physicians initially free of self-reported cardiovascular disease, identified 122 cases of sudden death over 12 yr of follow-up. The relative risk of sudden death during and up to 30 min after exercise was 16.9 (95% confidence interval 10.5–27.0). This study also identified a protective effect of habitual exercise, with a gradient of relative risk from 74.1 for individuals exercising $<1\times$/wk to 10.9 for those exercising $\geq5\times$/wk *(91)*.

SEXUAL ACTIVITY

Anecdotal reports have related sexual intercourse to the onset of myocardial infarction *(92,93)*, but there are little systematic data addressing this question. The Myocardial Infarction Onset Study interviewed 858 patients who were sexually active in the year prior to their myocardial infarction: 9% reported sexual activity within 24 h and 3% reported sexual activity within 2 h of the index acute myocardial infarction *(94)*. From case-crossover analysis, the relative risk of myocardial infarction following intercourse was 2.5 (95% confidence interval 1.7–3.7). In contrast to the data for physical exertion, where the period of increased risk persisted for 1 h, the post-coital risk remained elevated for 2 h. There was no difference between patients with and without a history of angina pectoris; however, it was observed that regular exercise at ≥6 METs $\geq3\times$/wk decreased the relative risk to a nonsignificant 1.2 (95% confidence interval 0.4–3.7) (Table 1).

MENTAL STRESS AND ANGER

Several studies have suggested that psychologically stressful life events, such as the death of a spouse, are potential triggers for myocardial infarction and sudden death *(95,96)*. Other data have shown that periods of general calamity increase the frequency of myocardial infarction. For example, during the 1991 Persian Gulf War, Iraqi missile attacks on Israel nearly doubled the relative frequency of cardiovascular deaths in that country on the day of attack *(97)* (Fig. 10). Immediately following severe earthquakes in Athens *(98)*, Hyogo, Japan *(99)*, and Los Angeles *(100)*, researchers documented an increase in cardiovascular mortality. In Los Angeles, there were 24 sudden cardiac deaths on the day of the quake, compared to an average of 5 such deaths per day the preceding week. Only 3 of the 24 deaths occurred in relation to unusual physical exertion *(100)*.

Events such as the death of a loved one, earthquake, and war occur rarely and thus are of lesser importance when one is considering daily activities that may function as triggers of acute cardiovascular disease onset. The relation between acute cardiac events and more commonly experienced periods of high emotion, such as anger, has been suggested by work examining post-myocardial infarction prognosis in relation to personality characteristics. For example, one study addressing the controversial subject of the "Type A" personality found that increased first year post-myocardial infarction mortality correlated not with "global Type A" test scores, but with scores reflecting the subcomponents of anger expression, cynicism, and irritability *(101)*. A relation between mental stress and cardiac prognosis is suggested by another study of 126 patients, over half of whom demonstrated a mental stress-induced fall in left ventricular ejection fraction *(102)*. The relative risk of cardiac death, nonfatal myocardial infarction, or coronary revasculariza-

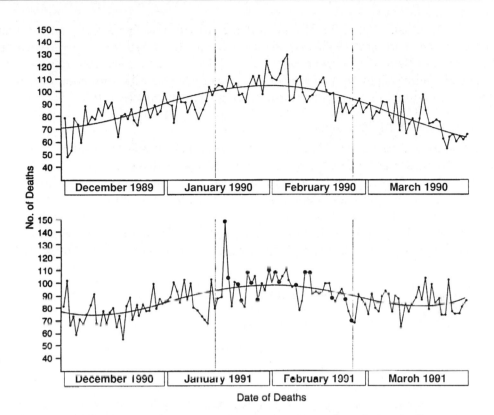

Fig. 10. The daily frequency of deaths in Israeli citizens >24 yr of age during the Persian Gulf War (bottom plot) compared to the same time period the year before (top plot) On January 18, 1991 (left vertical line) missiles launched from Iraq exploded in the Tel Aviv and Haifa areas. Daily warnings and attacks followed (larger filled points) until February 25 (right vertical line). The chi-square good-ness-of-fit test demonstrated significant inhomogeneity for the daily mortality during the 5-wk peri-od, almost entirely due to the excess of cardiovascular deaths during the 24-h period of January 18. Reprinted with permission from ref. *97.*

tion in that group was 2.4× (95% confidence interval 1.13–5.14) that of the patients who had no mental stress-induced change in left ventricular ejection fraction.

A more precise relation between anger and acute myocardial infarction was eluci-dated by the Myocardial Infarction Onset Study, again using the case-crossover design *(103).* The relative risk of onset of myocardial infarction following an episode of anger was 2.3 (95% confidence interval 1.7–3.2), and remained at this level for 2 h (Table 1). Further analysis of these data found that the relative risk increase was influenced by the socioeconomic status of the individual subject *(104).* In patients with less than a high school education, the risk increase was greater (relative risk 3.3), and the risk increase was least in patients with some college education (relative risk 1.6).

EXPOSURE TO SPECIFIC SUBSTANCES

Further analysis of the data from the Myocardial Infarction Onset Study has identified an increased risk of myocardial infarction following exposure to specific substances. One such analysis identified a nearly 24-fold increase in the risk of myocardial infarction in the 60 min following cocaine use (95% confidence interval 8.5–66.3) *(105).* Another report from the same group found a 4.8-fold increase in risk of infarction in the 60 min after smoking marijuana (95% confidence interval 2.4–9.5) *(106)*. The Myocardial Infarction Onset Study, which was conducted in the Boston area, also identified small but statistically significant risk increases (1.48–1.69) for myocardial infarction on days of higher concentrations of particulate airborne pollutants in that city *(107)*.

SUPERIMPOSITION OF TRIGGERS

One study compared the change in acute myocardial infarction incidence immediately following an earthquake between two intense quakes that occurred in Los Angeles in 1994 and San Francisco in 1989 *(108)*. Interestingly, there was no statistically significant increase in hospital admission for acute myocardial infarction for the San Francisco quake, which occurred at 5:04 PM, compared to the Los Angeles quake which occurred at 4:31 AM and was followed by a highly significant increase in myocardial infarction admission rate for that day. This suggests that in some circumstances, specific triggers may need to act in concert with circadian variations in cardiac vulnerability to produce their effect.

LINKING TRIGGERS AND ACUTE CORONARY EVENTS
Circadian Changes in Physiologic Variables

Daily activities and experiences, which act as triggers of acute coronary syndromes, must act through the perturbation of the physiologic milieu in which a vulnerable atherosclerotic plaque exists (Fig. 11). Circadian variation in hemodynamic variables has been studied to explain the circadian variation of acute cardiac events. The morning hours are associated with a rise in arterial blood pressure and an increase in heart rate, both of which are reduced during sleep *(109,110)*. This hemodynamic surge appears to be related to assumption of the upright posture *(111)*. Most studies have shown that episodes of ambulatory ischemia are related to an increase in rate–pressure product *(111)*, and that ambulatory myocardial ischemia is more frequent and more prolonged in the morning *(42–47)*. Angina patients and normal subjects have a significantly greater blood pressure and heart rate response during an exercise test in the morning compared to the response during an afternoon exercise test *(112)*.

In another study, the rate–pressure product at which ischemia was induced was lower in the morning, in parallel with an increase in postischemic forearm vascular resistance *(113)*. A study of forearm blood flow found vasodilatory responses to acetylcholine to be greater in normal subjects in the morning compared to afternoon; however, no such morning increase in endothelium-dependent vasodilation was found in subjects with coronary artery disease *(114)*. One study directly examined circadian variation in coronary artery tone. Segments of artery with dysfunctional endothelium showed exaggerated constrictor responses to acetylcholine and also greater dilator responses to nitroglycerin at 6 AM as compared to 1 PM, whereas segments with normal endothelium showed no diurnal variations *(115)*. These data suggest that, in addition to the morning increase in myocardial oxygen demand, coronary disease patients may have increased coronary vascular resistance plus a morning blunting of compensatory vasodilatory responses.

A number of hemostatic variables follow a circadian rhythm paralleling that of cardiac events *(116)*. The morning hours are associated with an increase in platelet aggregability, which occurs with the assumption of the upright posture *(117–119)*. Plasma

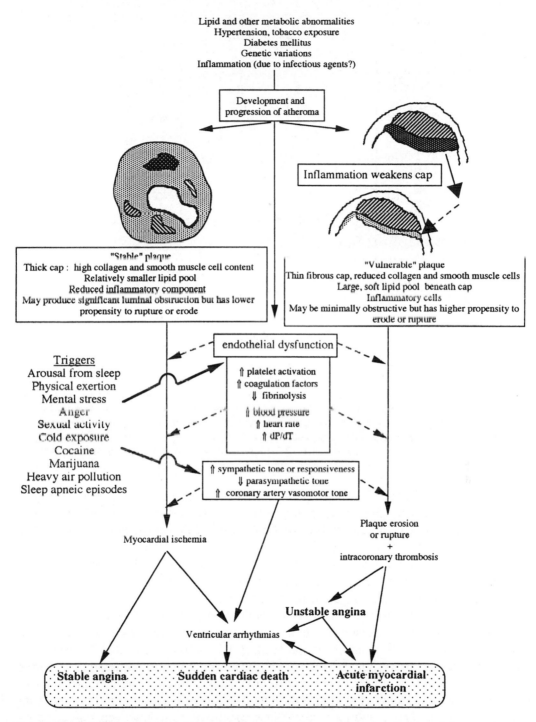

Fig. 11. Potential mechanisms linking atherogenic risk factors, plaque evolution and the transformation from stable to vulnerable plaque, and the means by which external triggers produce various acute coronary syndromes.

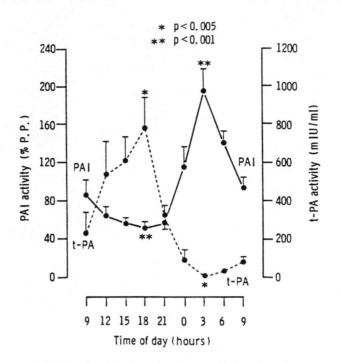

Fig. 12. Circadian variation in physiologic processes mediating the triggering of acute coronary events. The level of plasminogen activator inhibitor (higher levels favor thrombosis) in 6 healthy volunteers undergoing sampling every 3 h (including during sleep from midnight to 8 AM) is shown by the dotted line. The level of tissue-type plasminogen activator (higher levels favor fibrinolysis) is shown by the solid line. Whiskers indicate standard error of the mean. Asterisks indicate significant difference between peak and nadir values. The balance of factors in the morning favors thrombosis, and in the evening, the balance of factors favors fibrinolysis. Reprinted with permission from ref. *126.*

viscosity *(120)*, fibrinogen levels *(121)*,white blood cell aggregation *(122),* and lipoprotein (a) levels *(123)* increase in the morning. These changes favor thrombosis. The morning hours bring a decrease in resting tissue-type plasminogen activator (tPA) levels *(124–127)* and an increase in tPA inhibitor, PAI-1 *(124–128),* which reduces the activity of the intrinsic fibrinolytic system (Fig. 12). Recent studies of other markers of coagulability and fibrinolysis have further strengthened the appreciation of the morning hours as a period of relative hypercoagulability *(129,130).*

The activity of the autonomic nervous system has been studied to elucidate circadian patterns. Plasma norepinephrine falls to a nadir at night and increases in the morning in association with awakening and resumption of upright activty *(131,132).* Forearm vascular resistance has been shown to increase in the morning in normal subjects, a change attenuated by phentolamine but not nitroprusside, suggesting that the increase in vasomotor tone in the morning is mediated through α-adrenergic activity *(133).* A morning withdrawal of vagal tone and an increase in sympathetic tone has been suggested by spectral analysis of heart rate variability *(134–139).* Autonomic nervous system dysfunction in diabetic patients with coronary artery disease was shown to be associated with a blunted circadian pattern of myocardial ischemia *(140).*

Circadian variation has been shown for electrophysiologic variables such as the length of the refractory period *(141)* and the QT interval *(142).* Increased QT interval

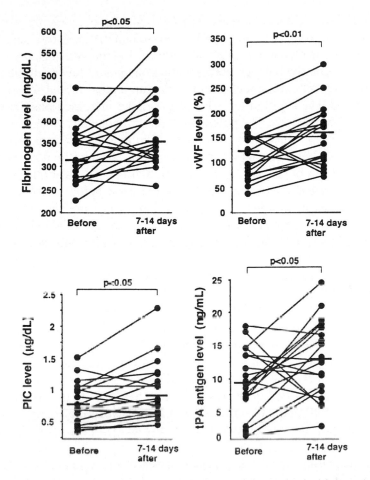

Fig. 13. In 42 elderly patients who experienced "high stress" but no physical injury during a major earthquake in Japan, levels of coagulation and fibrinolyis-related proteins increased significantly following the quake. Blood samples from within the 60 d preceeding the quake were available for analysis (X-axis, before) and were matched with samples 7–14 d after the quake. In addition to fibrinogen levels, results are reported for plasmin-α2-plasmin inhibitor complex (PIC, a fibrinolytic factor), von Willebrand factor (vWF, an endothelial cell derived factor), and tissue-type plasminogen (tPA antigen, also a fibrinolytic factor). Reprinted with permission from ref. *99.*

dispersion (difference between the longest and shortest QT interval in a given patient) has been considered to represent inhomogeneous ventricular repolarization and is thought to be a risk factor for malignant ventricular arrhythmias *(143,144)*. Variations in QT interval dispersion throughout the day support the concept of the morning hours as a period of heightened sympathetic tone, and that autonomic imbalance, with increased sympathetic nervous system output or sensitivity, may be a risk factor for malignant ventricular arrhythmias and sudden cardiac death *(143,144)*.

Physical Exertion and Mental Stress

Various forms of physical exertion have been shown to be triggers of acute myocardial infarction, and investigators have found marked changes in hemodynamic variables associated with exertion. Both dynamic and static forms of exercise increase blood pressure, heart rate, and plasma catecholamines *(145,146)*. Similar changes are seen with mental stress and cold exposure *(145,146)*. While exercise and mental stress have been demonstrated to increase platelet activity, they also appear to increase fibrinolytic activity, and it is not clear whether the balance in these situations would favor thrombosis or thrombolysis *(145)*. A recent experimental study using an animal model found that surges in epinephrine blood levels within the physiologic range increased platelet deposition on damaged arterial walls *(147)*. The potential effect of mental stress on hemodynamic and hemostatic variables is illustrated by a study of individuals who experienced a major earthquake in Japan, but escaped physical injury *(99)*. The investigators compared a variety of measures of hemodynamic and hemostatic status 7–14 d after the quake with samples that were coincidentally obtained during the 60 d before the quake. There were significant increases in systolic and diastolic blood pressure, hematocrit, fibrinogen level, and von Willebrand factor level (which reflects endothelial cell dysfunction), D-dimer (which reflects the formation and degradation of fibrin—its elevation is an indicator of activation of the hemostatic system), and two fibrinolytic factors. All values decreased to prequake levels after 4–6 mo (Fig. 13).

Obstructive Sleep Apnea

It is increasingly recognized that many adults have sleep disordered breathing patterns characterized as obstructive sleep apnea and hypopnea. There appears to be a high prevalence of these abnormalities in patients with cardiovascular disease, in the range of 30–50% *(148)*. There is evidence that the disorder may increase the relative risks of myocardial infarction *(149,150)*, sudden death *(151)*, and cardiovascular death *(152)*. One small study of 40 patients admitted with acute myocardial infarction found a significantly higher prevalence of sleep apnea in patients with myocardial infarction onset in the morning *(153)*.

Apneic events during sleep result in acute increases in blood pressure, vascular resistance, and sympathetic nervous system activity, and some events may be associated with hypoxemia *(148)*. In 17 patients with moderate and severe obstructive sleep apnea, platelet aggregation induced by epinephrine was increased at midnight and 6 AM (compared to 8 PM), in contrast to an overnight decrease in this variable in 15 age-matched controls *(154)*. A similarly small study found an overnight increase in whole blood viscosity in obstructive sleep apnea patients compared to controls *(155)*. Therefore, it is not surprising that studies have identified myocardial ischemic episodes in association with obstructive sleep apnea *(156,157)*. Despite these suggestive data, one recent review identified methodologic difficulties in a number of the epidemiologic studies prior to 1996 and cast doubt on the significance of obstructive sleep apnea as an independent risk factor for acute cardiac events *(158)*.

THERAPEUTIC CONSIDERATIONS
β-*Adrenergic Blocking Drugs*

Given the pivotal role of the sympathetic nervous system as a mediator of the triggering process, close attention has been paid to the effects of β-adrenergic blocking agents on the onset of acute coronary syndromes. Several studies of the circadian variation of the time of onset of acute myocardial infarction reported that the morning excess of events was attenuated in patients taking β-blockers compared to patients not taking these

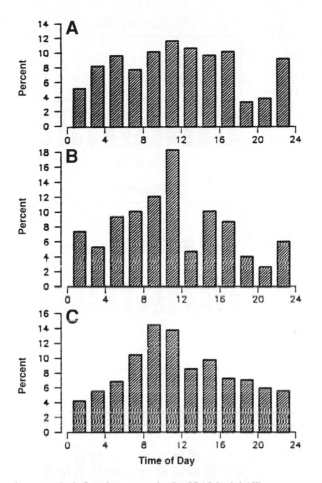

Fig. 14. The morning increase in infarctions seen in the ISAM trial (**C**) was preserved in patients taking calcium channel blocking agents (**B**) but was attenuated in patients taking β-blocking drugs (**A**). Reprinted with permission from ref. 25.

agents at the time of the acute event *(24,25,27,35,69,159)* (Fig. 14). β-Blocking agents also have been shown to reduce the morning increase in frequency of ventricular tachyarrhythmias in patients with AICDs *(160)* and to attenuate the morning increase in sudden cardiac deaths in postmyocardial infarction patients *(161)*. Studies of unstable angina and non-Q wave myocardial infarction have not demonstrated this beneficial effect of β-blockade on the circadian variation of these events *(37,41)*. However, this finding is still consistent with a beneficial effect of β-blockers on triggering mechanisms, in that it may represent a β-blocker therapy-related shift in morning events from acute myocardial infarction to less serious acute ischemic syndromes *(37)*. Several randomized prospective studies of β-blocker therapy in patients with ambulatory ischemia have also shown a beneficial effect of these drugs on the frequency of acute ischemic events *(162,163)*.

Calcium Channel Blocking Agents and Nitrates

The ability of other anti-ischemic drugs such as calcium channel blocking agents and nitrates to blunt potential triggering mechanisms is less clear. Two large studies

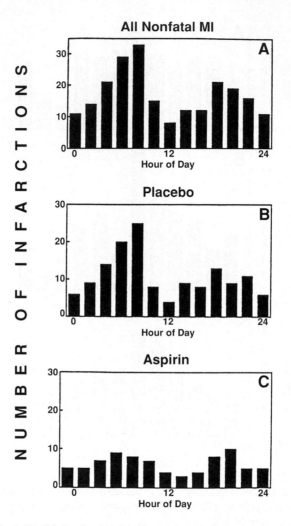

Fig. 15. In the Physician's Health Study, the significant ($p < 0.001$) morning increase among 211 non-fatal myocardial infarctions (top panel) was preserved in patients randomized to placebo ($p < 0.001$) (middle panel) and attenuated ($p = 0.16$) in patients randomized to aspirin, 325 mg every other day (bottom panel). Reprinted with permission from ref. *169*.

of the circadian variation in the time of onset of acute myocardial infarction identified a subset of patients taking calcium channel blockers and found a persistent morning increase in infarctions in these patients *(27,35)* (Fig. 14). On the other hand, some smaller trials reported the absence of a morning increase in infarction *(159)* and sudden cardiac death *(164)* in patients taking calcium channel blocking agents. Two subset analyses from trials reporting nitrate usage described no beneficial effect of this agent on the circadian variation of myocardial infarction onset *(35,139)*. However, one study found that the lack of use of nitrates or calcium channel blockers in the 24 h prior to the onset of infarction was associated with a higher frequency of infarction during physical exertion *(35)*.

Angiotensin-Converting Enzyme Inhibitors and Angiotensin II Type 1 Receptor Antagonists

These agents have effects beyond their simple hemodynamic benefits. Angiotensin-converting enzyme inhibitors influence the intravascular hemostatic environment to favor fibrinolysis *(165)* and improve endothelial function *(166)*. The recent Heart Outcomes Prevention Evaluation (HOPE) study *(167)* found that treatment with ramipril significantly reduced the rates of acute myocardial infarction, stroke, and cardiac arrest in over 9000 patients with coronary and other vascular disease. A recent clinical study found that irbesartan, an antagonist of the angiotensin II type 1 receptor, significantly reduced levels of several substances recognized as markers of inflammation, which are elevated in patients with coronary artery disease *(168)*. Thus, angiotensin-converting enzyme inhibitors and related agents may also be considered as having a role in preventing the triggering of acute coronary disease.

Antithrombotic Agents

The effect of aspirin on the circadian pattern of myocardial infarction is also uncertain. In the TIMI Phase II and the International Study of Infarct Survival (ISIS) 2 patient populations, a history of aspirin use or nonuse at the time of infarction did not affect the morning increase in infarction incidence *(27,35)*. In contrast, the Physician's Health Study followed 22,071 healthy middle-aged men randomized to aspirin or placebo over 5 yr *(169)*. The aspirin group had a 44.8% reduction in the incidence of nonfatal infarction, with an additional 25.2% reduction between 4 AM and 10 AM (Fig. 15). One other study of consecutive myocardial infarction admissions reported a beneficial effect of aspirin similar to that in the Physician's Health Study *(69)*. The Myocardial Infarction Onset Study also found that regular users of aspirin had a reduction in the relative risk of myocardial infarction induced by episodes of anger *(103)*.

The efficacy of thrombolytic agents also appears to have a circadian variation. In one study of 692 patients undergoing coronary arteriography 90 min after receiving intravenous tissue-type plasminogen activator, complete patency was observed in 42% of patients given the drug between noon and midnight, compared to 29% of patients given the drug between midnight and noon ($p < 0.001$) *(170)*. Two smaller studies demonstrated similar effects *(171,172)*.

Treatment of Myocardial Ischemia and Triggering

Episodes of myocardial ischemia may presage the onset of acute coronary events and may trigger malignant ventricular arrhythmias. Studies of β-blocking agents *(44, 173,174)*, calcium channel blocking agents *(175,176)*, and their combination *(173,176)* have shown that both agents alone or in combination can reduce the total number of ischemic episodes in a 24-h period, and that β-blocking drugs are particularly effective at attenuating the well-documented morning increase in ischemia *(44,173,174)*. The effect of β-blockers may be mediated by the reduction of heart rate, as heart rate increases precede most episodes of ambulatory ischemia *(111,173,174)*. Long-acting calcium channel blocking agents may not have the same effect on the circadian variation of ischemic episodes *(44,175)*. Calcium channel blocking agents such as nifedipine appear to prevent ischemic episodes that are unrelated to heart rate increases, suggesting that their effect may be mediated by increasing myocardial oxygen supply rather than by decreasing myocardial oxygen demand *(174)*. One randomized crossover study comparing atenolol, amlodipine, and placebo found that atenolol was more effective at suppressing episodes of ambulatory ischemia, whereas amlodipine was more effective at suppressing exercise-induced ischemia *(177)*.

β-Blocking agents have been shown to blunt the heart rate and blood pressure increases that occur in association with mental stress and with handgrip *(178)*, but do not appear to affect indices of hemostatic function *(178,179)*. This further supports the role of β-blockade as primarily a modifier of the hemodynamic factors thought to play a role in the triggering of acute coronary events.

The link between ischemia suppression and cardiac prognosis is supported by at least two randomized studies. The Atenolol Silent Ischemia Study randomized 306 patients to atenolol or placebo *(162)*. The group treated with the β-blocker had significantly fewer episodes of ischemia on ambulatory monitoring, and after 1 yr of follow-up had significantly fewer cardiac events (relative risk 0.44 [95% confidence interval 0.26–0.75]). The Total Ischemic Burden Bisoprolol Study followed 520 patients for 1 yr, with a similar result: patients randomly assigned to the β-blocking agent bisoprolol had significantly fewer cardiac events *(163)*.

HMG CoA Reductase Inhibitors and Plaque Stabilization

An emerging concept, which is relevant to the issue of triggering of acute coronary disease, is that of plaque stabilization *(11,12)*. An atherosclerotic lesion, which is more resistant to rupture, will be less likely to do so when exposed to a trigger that can induce plaque disruption. Angiographic studies of aggressive lipid-lowering therapy identified a disproportionately dramatic reduction in cardiac events compared to tiny changes in the arteriographic appearance of the coronary arteries. Large clinical studies demonstrating the success of both primary *(180)* and secondary *(181)* coronary event prevention strategies, using β-hydroxy-β-methylglutaryl (HMG) CoA reductase inhibitors (statins), have supported the concept that these drugs have their beneficial effects on coronary events by altering the composition and milieu of the plaque rather than by reducing plaque bulk and coronary stenosis severity. There are a variety of mechanisms by which the most prominent effect of statins, lipid lowering, may improve plaque stability. These include increases in collagen content, decreases in macropahges, and decreases in the expression of metalloproteinases and proinflammatory substances *(11,12)*. Dietary factors *(182)* and other drugs, such as fibrates, which do not lower low-density lipoprotein (LDL) but have statin-like effects on cardiac event rates *(183)*, can affect the function of receptors that limit the activation of vascular inflammatory responses *(11,12)*. These represent changes that favor plaque stability and, thus, reduced susceptability to triggering of acute coronary disease.

OTHER IMPLICATIONS FOR PATIENT MANAGEMENT

A number of practical clinical considerations emerge from the current state of knowledge of the triggering of acute cardiovascular events. One of these is information given to patients concerning the role of activities as precipitants of past or future acute events. A number of specific triggers—awakening, heavy physical exertion, sexual activity, anger, cocaine and marijuana use, and heavy air pollution—have been linked by sophisticated epidemiological studies to the onset of acute myocardial infarction.

Data concerning triggering of acute cardiac disease onset are of value when a physician is involved in a legal debate over the role of a given event in precipitating acute cardiovascular disease.

It is important to specify the difference between the absolute and relative risk of cardiac events in relation to specific triggers when advising patients concerning activities. The baseline risk of myocardial infarction in a sedentary but otherwise healthy middle aged man is estimated at 1%/yr, or an hourly risk (8760 h/yr) of slightly greater than 1/1 million *(184,185)*. The Physician's Health Study involving maddle aged male physicians found an absolute risk of sudden death during or immediately after exertion to be 1/1.5 million episodes of exertion *(91)*. As an example, consider this individual engaging in sexual activity, which triples the risk of myocardial infarction onset during the 2 post-coital hours *(94)*. Sexual activity 2×/wk would be predicted to increase the annual mortality from 1 to only 1.06%. These statistics should be reassuring to individuals concerned about the possibility of intercourse-induced myocardial infarction. On the other hand, heavy physical exertion in a sedentary patient increases relative risk of myocardial infarction 100-fold *(86)*. For a hypothetical post-infarction patient with an annual myocardial infarction risk of 4%, 1 h of active singles tennis 1×/wk as his or her sole form of exercise, increases the annual myocardial infarction risk from 4 to 6% *(86)*.

Regular physical exercise has beneficial effects on a variety of health-related parameters, including cardiovascular disease and mortality *(186–188)*. These benefits include reducing the increased risk of acute myocardial infarction immediately following heavy exertion and intercourse. Healthy individuals at risk for coronary artery disease, as well as patients with known cardiovascular disease should be encouraged to begin and maintain a program of regular exercise after appropriate medical screening *(188)*. Given the well-documented morning increase in the risk of myocardial infarction and sudden cardiac death, a prudent recommendation concerning the timing of exercise sessions might be that patients, with a higher baseline risk of events, who are sedentary, and beginning a regular exercise program, perform exercise at times other than in the morning. After the patient has become conditioned to a schedule of regular moderate to heavy exercise, and the relative risk of an exercise-related event decreases, morning exercise times can be included.

β-Blocking drugs are ideal agents for modulating the surges in sympathetic nervous system activity that appear to be associated with myocardial ischemia and acute cardiac events. This class of drugs should be the first choice for the treatment of patients with coronary artery disease and myocardial ischemia and for post-myocardial infarction patients. The ability of β-blockers to blunt the morning increase in infarctions suggests that these agents may be beneficial in some patients without clinically manifest coronary disease, and thus, β-blocker therapy could reasonably be considered as the first line agent for treatment of hypertension in patients who are considered to be at high risk for the presence of underlying atherosclerotic coronary artery disease. There are no data concerning the effect of β-blocker therapy on prognosis in patients with atherosclerotic coronary artery disease, no prior infarction, and no demonstrable ischemia. The role of calcium channel blocking drugs in the management of patients with coronary disease is controversial *(189,190)*. The data on the ability of calcium channel blockers, as monotherapy, to blunt the morning increase in infarctions and ambulatory ischemic episodes are conflicting, although these drugs reduce the total burden of ambulatory ischemic episodes. Given the early morning increase in cardiac events, it may be preferable to select drug formulations with long half-lives to provide a pharmacological effect over the entire 24-h period *(191,192)*. The Controlled-Onset Verapamil Investigation of Cardiovascular Endpoints (CONVICE) study, utilizing a new controlled-onset extended release verapamil formulation, was a randomized trial designed to compare this agent to either atenolol or hydrochlorothiazide, as a test of the "chronotherapuetic" hypothesis. While the new agent was highly effective at controlling blood pressure, the trial was terminated prematurely by the industry sponsor *(193)*. Thus, there is, at present, little data addressing the efficacy of a chronotherapuetic approach to cardiovascular phamacology *(194)*.

The evidence of a morning procoagulant state and the possible reduction in morning cardiac event rate with aspirin provides further strength to the recommendation for indefinite use of this drug for patients with proven or suspected coronary atherosclerosis. The demonstration of morning resistance to thrombolysis could conceivably influence clinical decision making concerning management of patients presenting with acute myocardial infarction at different times of the day. Although there are, as yet, no data to support a change in current thrombolytic drug dosing strategies, some authors have suggested a possible need for varying drug dosages for patients presenting at different times of the day *(195,196)*.

The data tying states of high emotional and mental stress to myocardial ischemia and acute cardiac events also have potential implications regarding therapy. Individuals with coronary artery disease who suffer frequent periods of emotional stress or outbursts of anger might be considered for pharmacotherapy or counseling to attempt to reduce the frequency and severity of these experiences. However, studies to date have not clearly shown that such therapy reduces the incidence of acute cardiac events in patients *(197)*. In addition, heightened preparations by emergency service personnel for dealing with victims of acute cardiac disease can be considered during periods of general calamity such as natural disasters.

FUTURE DIRECTIONS

Further investigations into the mechanisms by which the atherosclerotic plaque and its hemostatic milieu undergoes transformation from a stable to a vulnerable configuration will identify new targets for pharmacologic and other manipulations to reduce the ability of a given trigger or combination of triggers to induce plaque rupture and intracoronary thrombosis. Certain genetic variants may confer particular susceptability to various triggers, allowing more targeted recommendations for primary and secondary prevention. The use of serum markers of inflammation to predict cardiac events may evolve such that risk increases over shorter time periods may be appreciable; i.e., a heightened risk for the next month as opposed to the next 6–12 mo. If this could be accomplished, it might facilitate adjustments of lifestyle and therapy during relatively short periods of significantly increased susceptibility to external triggers.

In addition to improving the understanding of plaque biology, clinically applicable methods will need to be developed to detect vulnerable plaques in patients *(198)*. Contrast arteriography, currently the most widely used technique to visualize the coronary arteries, visualizes the degree to which plaques obstruct the arterial lumen and can determine gross features of plaque such as large ulcerations *(16)*. Arteriography has limited ability to identify obstructive plaques that are likely to produce acute coronary

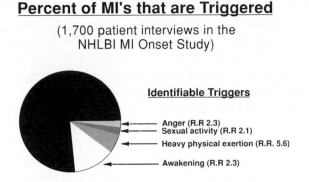

Percent of MI's that are Triggered

(1,700 patient interviews in the
NHLBI MI Onset Study)

Identifiable Triggers

Anger (R.R 2.3)
Sexual activity (R.R 2.1)
Heavy physical exertion (R.R. 5.6)
Awakening (R.R 2.3)

At least 245,000 MI's per year are triggered.

Fig. 16. Percent of myocardial infarctions that are triggered. Reprinted with permission from ref. *209*.

syndromes and cannot identify the minimal nonobstructive lesions that are often the culprits in acute syndromes *(16)*. Intravascular ultrasound, a clinically available imaging modality, has greatly improved the ability to visualize the structure of the coronary artery, albeit with limited resolution *(199)*. Emerging new technologies, such as optical coherence tomography *(200,201)*, magnetic resonance imaging of the coronary arteries *(202)*, thermal detection techniques *(203,204)*, intravascular electrical impedance imaging *(205)*, and various forms of spectroscopy may provide a superior means of imaging vulnerable plaques. Near infrared spectroscopy *(206–208)* has the potential to image both the architecture as well as the biochemical composition of atherosclerotic material.

Current data suggest that the well-characterized triggers of infarction account for 15–20% of all infarctions *(209)* (Fig. 16). It is likely that further epidemiological studies will identify additional triggers, particularly the less well studied issues related to mental stress, and to the onset of events occurring during sleep. It is not possible to free human beings from the circumstances that appear to trigger the onset of acute cardiovascular disease. The goals of future research will be to elucidate further the mechanisms connecting human circumstances to plaque rupture and intracoronary thrombosis and to develop therapy to weaken or sever these links.

SUMMARY: KEY POINTS

- Current data suggest at least 15–20% of acute myocardial infarctions may be triggered.
- All acute cardiovascular events studied have displayed a circadian variation, with a morning (6 AM to noon) excess (relative risk almost 1.4) and a nighttime nadir. The risk is further increased with adjustment for time of awakening.
- Besides awakening, other triggers of acute myocardial infarction identified in carefully controlled epidemiologic studies include, heavy physical exertion, sexual intercourse, and outbursts of anger. Exposure to substances such as marijuana, cocaine, and heavy air pollution have also been shown to be triggers.

- Despite the excess of relative risk of infarction (risk increases of 1.5- to 100-fold) imparted by these activities, the low risk of myocardial infarction, on an hourly basis, keeps the absolute risk increase imparted by these activities quite small in most cases.
- The relative risk of physical exertion or sexual activity triggering infarction can be reduced by vigorous exercise several times weekly.
- Most physiologic processes thought to be implicated in the genesis of acute coronary syndromes display a similar circadian pattern. The morning hours are characterized by an increase in blood pressure, heart rate, sympathetic nervous system activity, and by a relatively prothrombotic, hypofibrinolytic state.
- β-Blockers and aspirin have been demonstrated to attenuate the morning increase in infarction incidence.

REFERENCES

1. Obraztsov VP, Strazhesko ND. The symptomatology and diagnosis of coronary thrombosis. In: Vorobeva VA, Konchalovski MP, eds. Works of First Congress of Russian Therapists. Comradeship Typography of A.E. Mamontov, Moscow, 1910, pp. 26–43.
2. Sproul J. A general practitioner's views on the treatment of angina pectoris. N Engl J Med 1936;215: 443–452.
3. Phipps C. Contributory causes of coronary thrombosis. JAMA 1936;106:761–762.
4. Master AM. The role of effort and occupation (including physicians) in coronary occlusion. JAMA 1960;174:942–948.
5. Davies MJ. Stability and instability: two faces of coronary atherosclerosis. Circulation 1996;94: 2013–2020.
6. Fuster V. Mechanisms leading to myocardial infarction: insights from studies of vascular biology. Circulation 1994;90:2126–2146.
7. Falk E, Shah PK, Fuster V. Coronary plaque disruption. Circulation 1995;92:657–671.
8. Libby P. Molecular basis of the acute coronary syndromes. Circulation 1995;91:2844–2850.
9. Falk E. Why do plaques rupture? Circulation 1992;86(Suppl. III):III-30–III-42.
10. Schroeder AP, Falk E. Pathophysiology and inflammatory aspects of plaque rupture. Cardiol Clin 1996;14:211–220.
11. Shah PK. Plaque disruption and thrombosis. Cardiol Rev 2000;8:31–39.
12. Libby P. Current concepts of the pathogenesis of the acute coronary syndromes. Circulation 2001;104: 365–372.
13. Davies MJ, Thomas A. Thrombosis and acute coronary artery lesions in sudden cardiac ischemic death. N Engl J Med 1984;310:1137–1140.
14. Myerburg RJ, Kessler KM, Castellanos A. Pathophysiology of sudden cardiac death. Pacing Clin Electrophysiol 1991;14:935–943.
15. Little WL, Constantinescu M, Applegate RJ, et al. Can coronary angiography predict the site of a subsequent myocardial infarction in patients with mild-to-moderate coronary artery disease? Circulation 1988;78:1157–1166.
16. Little WL, Applegate RJ. The role of plaque size and degree of stenosis in acute myocardial infarction. Cardiol Clin 1996;14:221–228.
17. Ridker PM, Rifai N, Pfeffer M, Sacks F, Lepage S, Braunwald E. Elevation of tumor necrosis factor-alpha and increased risk of recurrent coronary events after myocardial infarction. Circulation 2000; 101:2149–2153.
18. Ridker PM, Rifai N, Stampfer MJ, Hennekens CH. Plasma concentration of interleukin-6 and the risk of future myocardial infarction among apparently healthy men. Circulation 2000;101:1767–1772.
19. Ridker PM, Hennekens CH, Buring JE, Rifai N. C-reactive protein and other markers of inflammation in the prediction of cardiovascular disease in women. N Engl J Med 2000;342:836–843.
20. Libby P, Egan D, Skarlatos S. Roles of infectious agents in atherosclerosis and restenosis: an assessment of the evidence and need for future research. Circulation 1997;96:4095–4103.

21. Danesh J, Whincup P, Walker M, et al. *Chlamydia pneumoniae* IgG titres and coronary heart disease: prospective study and meta-analysis. BMJ 2000;321:208–213.
22. Humphries SE, Talmud PJ, Hawe E, Bolla M, Day INM, Miller GJ. Apolipoprotein E4 and coronary heart disease in middle-aged men who smoke: a prospective study. Lancet 2001;358:115–119.
23. Girelli D, Russo C, Ferraresi P, et al. Polymorphisms in the Factor VII gene and the risk of myocardial infarction in patients with coronary artery disease. N Engl J Med 2000;343:774–780.
24. Muller JE, Stone PH, Turi ZG, et al. Circadian variation in the frequency of onset of acute myocardial infarction. N Engl J Med 1985;313:1315–1322.
25. Willich SN, Linderer T, Wegschieder K, Leizorovicz A, Alamercery I, Schroeder R. Increased morning incidence of myocardial infarction in the ISAM study: absence with prior beta-adrenergic blockade. Circulation 1989;80:853–858.
26. Gnecchi-Ruscone T, Piccaluga E, Guzetti S, Contini M, Montano N, Nicolis E. Morning and Monday: critical periods for the onset of acute myocardial infarction. The GISSI 2 study experience. Eur Heart J 1994;15:882–887.
27. ISIS-2 (Second International Study of Infarct Survival) Collaborative Group. Morning peak in the incidence of myoardial infarction: experience in the ISIS-2 trial. Eur Heart J 1992;13:594–598.
28. Marchant B, Ranjadayalan K, Stevenson R, Wilkinson P, Timmis AD. Circadian and seasonal factors in the pathogenesis of acute myocardial infarction: the influence of environmental temperature. Br Heart J 1993;69:385–387.
29. Thompson DR, Sutton TW, Jowett NI, Pohl JE. Circadian variation in the onset of chest pain in acute myocardial infarction. Br Heart J 1991;65:177–178.
30. Zornosa J, Smith M, Little W. Effect of activity on circadian variation in time of onset of acute myocardial infarction. Am J Cardiol 1992;69:1089–1090.
31. Hansen O, Johansson BW, Gullberg B. Circadian distribution of onset of acute myocardial infarction in subgroups from analysis of 10,791 patient treated in a single center. Am J Cardiol 1992;69:1003–1008.
32. Behar S, Halabi M, Reicher-Reiss H, et al. Circadian variation and possible external triggers of onset of myocardial infarction. SPRINT Study Group. Am J Med 1993;94:395–400.
33. Van der Palen J, Doggen CJ, Beaglehole R. Variation in the time and day of onset of myocardial infarction and sudden death. N Z Med J 1995;108:332–334.
34. Spielberg C, Falkenhahn D, Willich SN, Wegscheider K, Voller H. Circadian, day-of-week, and seasonal variability in myocardial infarction: comparison between working and retired patients. Am Heart J 1996;132:579–585.
35. Tofler GH, Muller JE, Stone PH, et al. Modifiers of timing and possible triggers of acute myocardial infarction in the Thrombolysis in Myocardial Infarction Phase II (TIMI II) Study Group. J Am Coll Cardiol 1992;20:1049–1055.
36. Cohen MC, Rohtla KM, Lavery CE, Muller JE, Mittleman MA. Meta-analysis of the morning excess of acute myocardial infarction and sudden cardiac death. Am J Cardiol 1997;79:1512–1516.
37. Cannon CP, McCabe CH, Stone PH, et al. Circadian variation in the onset of unstable angina and non-Q-wave acute myocardial infarction (the TIMI III Registry and TIMI IIIB). Am J Cardiol 1997;79: 253–258.
38. Behar S, Reicher-Reiss H, Goldbourt U, Kaplinsky E. Circadian variation in pain onset in unstable angina pectoris. Am J Cardiol 1991;67:91–93.
39. Beamer AD, Lee TH, Cook EF, et al. Diagnostic implications for myocardial ischemia of the circadian variation of the onset of chest pain. Am J Cardiol 1987;60:998–1002.
40. Figueras J, Lidon RM. Circadian rhythm of angina in patients with unstable angina: relationship with extent of coronary artery disease, coronary reserve, and ECG changes during pain. Eur Heart J 1994; 15:753–760.
41. Kleiman NS, Schechtman KB, Young PB, et al. Lack of diurnal variation in the onset of non-Q wave infarction. Circulation 1990;81:548–555.
42. Krantz DS, Kop WJ, Gabbay FH, et al. Circadian variation of ambulatory myocardial ischemia. Triggering by daily activities and evidence for an endogenous circadian component. Circulation 1996;93: 1364–1371.
43. Mulcahy D, Dakak N, Zalos G, et al. Patterns and behavior of transient myocardial ischemia in stable coronary disease are the same in both men and women. A comparative study. J Am Coll Cardiol 1996;27:1629–1636.
44. Mulcahy D, Keegan J, Cunningham D, et al. Circadian variation of total ischemic burden and its alteration with anti-anginal agents. Lancet 1988;2:755–759.

45. Taylor CR, Hodge EM, White DA. Circadian rhythm of angina: similarity to circadian rhythms of myocardial infarction, ischemic ST segment depression, and sudden cardiac death. The Amlodipine Angina Study Group. Am Heart J 1989;118:1098–1099.

46. Rocco MB, Barry J, Campbell S, et al. Circadian variation of transient myocardial ischemia in patients with coronary artery disease. Circulation 1987;75:395–400.

47. Hausmann D, Nikutta P, Trappe HJ, Daniel WG, Wenzlaff P, Lichtlen PR. Circadian distribution of the characteristics of ischemic episodes in patients with stable coronary artery disease. Am J Cardiol 1990; 66:668–672.

48. Willich SN. European survey on circadian variation of angina pectoris (ESCVA): design and preliminary results. J Cardiovasc Pharmacol 1999;34(Suppl. 2):S9–S13.

49. Mickley H, Pless P, Nielsen JR, Moller M. Circadian variation of transient myocardial ischemia in the early out-of-hospital period after first acute myocardial infarction. Am J Cardiol 1991;67: 927–932.

50. Argentino C, Toni D, Rasura M, et al. Circadian variation in the frequency of ischemic stroke. Stroke 1990;21:387–389.

51. Marler JR, Price TR, Clark GL, et al. Morning increase in the onset of ischemic stroke. Stroke 1989; 20:473–476.

52. Willich SN, Levy D, Rocco MB, Tofler GH, Stone PH, Muller JE. Circadian variation in the incidence of sudden cardiac death in the Framingham Heart Study. Am J Cardiol 1987;60:801–806.

53. Muller JE, Ludmer PL, Willich SN, et al. Circadian variation in the frequency of sudden cardiac death. Circulation 1987;75:131–138.

54. Moser DK, Stevenson WG, Woo MA, Stevenson LW. Timing of sudden death in patients with heart failure. J Am Coll Cardiol 1994;24:963–967.

55. Peters RW, Mitchell LB, Brooks MM, et al. Circadian pattern of arrhythmic death in patients receiving encainide, flecainide, or moricizine in the Cardiac Arrhythmia Supression Trial (CAST). J Am Coll Cardiol 1994;23:283–289.

56. Mallavarapu C, Pancholy S, Schwartzman D, et al. Circadian variation of ventricular arrhythmia recurrences after cardioverter-defibrillator implantation in patients with healed myocardial infarcts. Am J Cardiol 1995;75:1140–1144.

57. Lampert R, Rosenfeld L, Batsford W, Lee F, McPherson C. Circadian variation of sustained ventricular tachycardia in patients with coronary artery disease and implantable cardioverter-defibrillators. Circulation 1994;90:241–247.

58. Behrens S, Galecka M, Bruggemann T, et al. Circadian variation of sustained ventricular tachyarrhythmias terminated by appropriate shocks in patients with an implantable cardioverter defibrillator. Am Heart J 1995;130:79–84.

59. Auricchio A, Klein H. Circadian variations of ventricular tachyarrhythmias detected by the implantable cardioverter-defibrillator. G Ital Cardiol 1997;27:113–122.

60. Englund A, Behrens S, Wegscheider, Rowland E. Circadian variation of malignant ventricular arrhythmias in patients with ischemic and nonischemic heart disease after cardioverter-defibrillator implantation. J Am Coll Cardiol 1999;34:1560–1568.

61. Grimm W, Menz WM, Hoffman J, Maisch B. Circadian variation and onset mechanisms of ventricular tachyarrhythmias in patients with coronary disease versus idiopathic dilated cardiomyopathy. Pacing Clin Electrophysiol 2000;23:1939–1943.

62. Arntz HR, Willich SN, Oeff M, et al. Circadian variation of sudden cardiac death reflects age related variability in ventricular fibrillation. Circulation 1993;88:2284–2289.

63. Willich SN, Lowel H, Lewis M, et al. Association of wake time and the onset of myocardial infarction. Triggers and mechanisms of myocardial infarction (TRIMM) pilot study. Circulation 1991;84 (Suppl. 6):V162–V167.

64. Goldberg RJ, Brady P, Muller JE, et al. Time of onset of symptoms of acute myocardial infarction. Am J Cardiol 1990;60:140–144.

65. Peters RW, Zoble RG, Liebson PR, Pawitan Y, Brooks MM, Proschan M. Identification of a secondary peak in myocardial infarction onset 11 to 12 hours after awakening: the Cardiac Arrhythmia Supression Trial (CAST) experience. J Am Coll Cardiol 1993;22:998–1003.

66. Willich SN, Goldberg RJ, Maclure M, Perriello L, Muller JE. Increased onset of sudden cardiac death in the first three hours after awakening. Am J Cardiol 1992;70:65–68.

67. Barry J, Campbell S, Yeung AC, Raby KE, Selwyn AP. Waking and rising at night as a trigger of myocardial ischemia. Am J Cardiol 1991;67:1067–1072.

68. Willich SN, Lowel H, Lewis M, Hormann A, Anrtz HR, Keil U. Weekly variation of acute myocardial infarction. Increased Monday risk in the working population. Circulation 1994;90:87–93.
69. Sayer JW, Wilkinson P, Ranjadalayan K, Ray S, Marchant B, Timmis AD. Attenuation or absence of circadian and seasonal rhythm of acute myocardial infarction. Heart 1997;77:325–329.
70. Thompson DR, Pohl JE, Tse YY, Hiorns RW. Meteorological factors and the time of onset of chest pain in acute myocardial infarction. Int J Biometeorol 1996 39:116–120.
71. Couch RD. Travel, time zones, and sudden cardiac death. Am J Forensic Med 1990;11:106–111.
72. Hirasawa K, Tateda K, Shibata J, Yokoyama K. Multivariate analysis of meteorological factors and evaluation of circadian rhythm: their relation to the occurrence of acute myocardial infarction. J Cardiol 1990;20:797–805.
73. Baker-Blocker A. Winter weather and cardiovascular mortality in Minneapolis-St. Paul, Am J Public Health 1982;72:261–265.
74. Anderson TW, Rochard C. Cold snaps, snowfall, and sudden death from ischemic heart disease. Can Med Assoc J 1979;121:1580–1583.
75. Danet S, Richard F, Montaye M, et al. Unhealthy effects of atmospheric temperature and pressure on the occurrence of myocardial infarction and coronary deaths. A 10-year survey: the Lille-World Health Organization MONICA project (Monitoring trends and determinants in cardiovascular disease). Circulation 1999;100:E1 E7.
76. Fries RP, Heisel AG, Jung JK, Schieffer HJ. Circannual variation of malignant ventricular tachyarrhythmias in patients with implantable cardioverter-defibrillators and either coronary artery disease or idiopathic dilated cardiomyopathy. Am J Cardiol 1997;79:1194–1197.
77. Spencer FA, Goldberg RJ, Becker RC, Gore JM. Seasonal distribution of acute myocardial infarction in the Second National Registry of Myocardial Infarction. J Am Coll Cardiol 1998;31:1226–1233.
78. Ku CS, Yang CY, Lee WJ, Chiang HT, Liu CP, Lin SL. Absence of a seasonal variation in myocardial infarction onset in a region without temperature extremes. Cardiology 1998;89:277–282.
79. Fava S, Azzopardi J, Muscat IIA, Fenech FF. Absence of circadian variation in the onset of acute myocardial infarction in diabetic subjects. Br Heart J 1995;74:370–372.
80. Hjalmarson A, Gilpin EA, Nicod P, et al. Differing circadian patterns of symptom onset in subgroups of patients with acute myocardial infarction. Circulation 1989;80:267–275.
81. Tanaka T, Fujita M, Fudo T, Tamaki S, Nohara R, Sasayama S. Modification of the circadian variation of symptom onset of acute myocardial infarction in diabetes mellitus. Coron Artery Dis 1995;6: 241–244.
82. Tofler GH, Stone PH, Maclure M, et al. Analysis of possible triggers of acute myocardial infarction (the MILIS study). Am J Cardiol 1990;66:22–27.
83. Sumiyoshi T, Haze K, Saito M, Fukami K, Goto Y, Hiramori K. Evaluation of clinical factors involved in onset of myocardial infarction. Jpn Circ J (Japan) 1986;50:164–173.
84. Smith M, Little WC. Potential precipitating factors of the onset of myocardial infarction, Am J Med Sci 1992;303:141–144.
85. Stewart RA, Robertson MC, Wilkins GT, Low CJ, Restieaux NJ. Association between activity at onset of symptoms and outcome of acute myocardial infarction. J Am Coll Cardiol 1997;29:250–253.
86. Maclure M. The case-crossover design: a method for studying transient effects on the risk of acute events. Am J Epidemiol 1991;133:144–153.
87. Willich SN, Lewis M, Lowel H, Arntz R, Schubert F, Schroeder R. Physical exertion as a trigger of acute myocardial infarction. Triggers and Mechanisms of Myocardial Infarction Study Group. N Engl J Med 1993;329:1684–1690.
88. Mittleman A, Maclure M, Tofler GH, Sherwood JB, Goldberg RJ, Muller JE . Triggering of myocardial infarction by heavy physical exertion. Protection against triggering by regular exertion. Determinants of Myocardial Infarction Onset Study Investigators. N Engl J Med 1993;329:1677–1683.
89. Siscovick DS, Weiss NS, Fletcher RH, Lasky T. The incidence of primary cardiac arrest during vigorous exercise. N Engl J Med 1984;311:874–877.
90. Maron BJ, Poliac LC, Roberts WO. Risk for sudden cardiac death associated with marathon running. J Am Coll Cardiol 1996;28:428–431.
91. Albert CM, Mittleman MA, Chae CU, Min-Lee I, Hennekens CH, Manson JoAnn E. Triggering of sudden death from cardiac causes by vigorous exertion. N Engl J Med 2000;343:1355–1361.
92. Nalbangtil I, Yigthbasi O, Kiliccioglu B. Sudden death in sexual activity. Am Heart J 1976;91: 405–406.
93. Ueno M. The so-called coition death. Jpn J Leg Med 1963;17:330–340.

94. Muller JE, Mittleman MA, Maclure M, Sherwood JB, Tofler GH, for the Determinants of Myocardial Infarction Onset Study Investigators. Triggering of myocardial infarction by sexual activity. Low absolute risk and prevention by regular physical exertion. JAMA 1996;275:1405–1409.
95. Cottington EM Matthews KA, Talbott EM, Kuller LH. Environmental events preceeding sudden death in women. Psychosom Med 1980;42:567–575.
96. Parkes CM, Benjamin B, Fitzgerald RG. Broken heart: a statistical study of increased mortality among widowers. Br Med J 1969;1:740–743.
97. Kark JD, Goldman S, Epstein L. Iraqi missle attacks on Israel. The association of mortality with a threatening stressor. JAMA 1995; 273:1208–1210.
98. Trichopoulos D, Katsouyanni K, Zavitsanos X, Tzonou A, Dalla-Vorgia P. Psychological stress and fatal heart attack: the Athens (1981) earthquake natural experiment. Lancet 1983;1:441–444.
99. Kario K, Matsuo T, Kobayashi H, Yamamoto K, Shimada K. Earthquake-induced potentiation of acute risk factors in hypertensive elderly patients: possible triggering of cardiovascular events after a major earthquake. J Am Coll Cardiol 1997;29:926–933.
100. Leor J, Poole WK, Kloner RA. Sudden cardiac death triggered by an earthquake. N Engl J Med 1996; 334:413–419.
101. Julkunen J, Idanpaan-Heikkila U, Saarinen T. Components of Type A behavior and the first year prognosis of a myocardial infarction. J Psychosom Res 1993;37:11–18.
102. Jiang W, Babyak M, Krantz DS, et al. Mental stress induced myocardial ischemia and cardiac events. JAMA 1996;275:1651–1656.
103. Mittleman MA, Maclure M, Sherwood JB, et al. Triggering of acute myocardial infarction onset by episodes of anger. Determinants of Myocardial Infarction Onset Study Investigators. Circulation 1995; 92:1720–1725.
104. Mittleman MA, Maclure M, Nachnani M, Sherwood JB, Muller JE. Educational attainment, anger, and the risk of triggering myocardial infarction onset. The Determinants of Myocardial Infarction Onset Study Investigators. Arch Intern Med 1997;157:769–775.
105. Mittleman MA, Mintzer D, Maclure M, Tofler GH, Sherwood J, Muller JE. Triggering myocardial infarction by cocaine. Circulation 1999;99:2737–2741.
106. Mittleman MA, Lewis RA, Maclure M, Sherwood J, Muller JE. Triggering myocardial infarction by marijuana. Circulation 2001;103:2305–2309.
107. Peters A, Dockery DW, Muller JE, Mittleman MA. Increased particulate air pollution and the triggering of myocardial infarction. Circulation 2001;103:2810–2815.
108. Brown DL. Disparate effects of the 1989 Loma Prieta and 1994 Northridge earthquakes on hospital admissions for acute myocardial infarction: importance of superimposition of triggers. Am Heart J 1999;137:830–836.
109. Tsuda M, Hayashi H, Kanematsu K, Yoshikane M, Saito H, Comparison between diurnal distribution of onset of infarction in patients with acute myocardial infarction and circadian variation of blood presure in patients with coronary artery disease. Clin Cardiol 1993;16:543–547.
110. Kawano Y, Tochikubo O, Minamisawa K, Miyajima E, Ishii M. Circadian variation of hemodynamics in patients with essential hypertension: comparison between early morning and evening. J Hypertens 1994;12:1405–1412.
111. Deedwania PC. Hemodynamic changes as triggers of cardiovascular events. Cardiol Clin 1996;14: 229–238.
112. Saito D, Matsubara K, Yamanari H, et al. Morning increase in hemodynamic response to exercise in patients with angina pectoris. Heart Vessels 1993;8:149–154.
113. Quyyumi AA, Panza JA, Diodati JG, Lakatos E, Epstein SE. Circadian variation in ischemic threshold. A mechanism underlying the circadian variation in ischemic events. Circulation 1992;86:22–28.
114. Shaw JA, Chin-Dusting JPF, Kingwell BA, Dart AM. Diurnal variation in endothelium-dependent vasodilatation is not apparent in coronary artery disease. Circulation 2001;103:806–812.
115. El-Tamimi H, Mansour M, Pepine CJ, Wargovich TJ, Chen H. Circadian variation in coronary tone in patients with stable angina. Circulation 1995;92:3201–3205.
116. Aranha Rosito GB, Tofler GH. Hemostatic factors as triggers of cardiovascular events. Cardiol Clin 1996;14:239–250.
117. Brezinski DA, Tofler GH, Muller JE, et al. Morning increase in platelet aggregability: association with assumption of the upright posture. Circulation 1988;78:35–40.
118. Tofler GH, Brezinski DA, Schaefer AI, et al. Concurrent morning increase in platelet aggregability and the risk of myocardial infarction and sudden death. N Engl J Med 1987;316:1514–1518.

119. Willich SN, Arntz HR, Lowel H, Lewis M, Schroeder R. Wake up time, thrombocyte aggregation, and the risk of acute coronary heart disease. The TRIMM (Trigger and Mechanisms of Myocardial Infarct) Study Group. Z Kardiol 1992;81(Suppl. 2):95–99.

120. Ehrly AM, Jung G. Circadian rhythm of human blood viscosity. Biorheology 1973;10:577–583.

121. Petralito A, Mangiafico RA, Gibilino S, Cuffari MA, Miano MF, Fiore CP. Daily modifications of plasma fibrinogen, platelet aggregation, Howell's time, PTT, TT, and antithrombin III in normal subjects and in patients with vascular disease. Chronobiologica 1982;9:195–201.

122. Bridges AB, Scott NA, McNeill GP, Pringle TH, Belch JJF. Circadian variation of white blood cell aggregation and free radical indices in men with ischemic heart disease. Eur Heart J 1992;13:1632–1636.

123. Bremner WF, Sothern RB, Kanabrocki EL, et al. Relation between circadian patterns in levels of circulating lipoprotein (a), fibrinogen, platelets, and lipid variables in men. Am Heart J 2000;139:164–173.

124. Angleton P, Chandler WL, Schmer G. Diurnal variation of tissue-type plasminogen activator and its rapid inhibitor (PAI-1). Circulation 1989;79:101–106.

125. Bridges AB, McLaren M, Saniabadi A, Fisher TC, Belch JJF. Circadian variation of endothelial cell function, red blood cell deformity, and dehydrothromboxane B2 in healthy volunteers. Blood Coagul Fibrinolysis 1991;2:447–452.

126. Andreotti F, Davies GJ, Hackett DR, et al. Major circadian fluctuations in fibrinolytic factors and possible relevance to time of onset of myocardial infarction, sudden cardiac death, and stroke. Am J Cardiol 1988;62:635–637.

127. Bridges AB, McLaren M, Scott NA, Pringle TH, McNeill GP, Belch JJ. Circadian variation of tissue plasminogen activator and its inhibitor, von Willebrand factor antigen, and prostacyclin stimulating factor in men with ischemic heart disease. Br Heart J 1993;69:121–124.

128. Sayer JW, Gutteridge C, Syndercombe-Court D, Wilkinson P, Timmis AD. Circadian activity of the endogenous fibrinolytic system in stable coronary artery disease: effects of beta-adrenoreceptor blockers and angiotensin-converting enzyme inhibitors. J Am Coll Cardiol 1998;32:1962–1968.

129. Kapiotis S, Jilma B, Quehenberger P, Ruzicka K, Handler S, Speiser W. Morning hypercoagulability and hypofibrinolysis. Diurnal variations in circulating activated factor VII, prothrombin fragment F1 + 2, and plasmin-plasmin inhibitor complex. Circulation 1997;96:19–21.

130. Fujino T, Katou J, Fujita M, et al. Relationship between serum lipoprotein(a) level and thrombin generation to the circadian variation in the onset of acute myocardial infarction. Atherosclerosis 2001,155. 171–178.

131. Linsell CR, Lightman SL, Mullen PE, Brown MJ, Causon RC. Circadian rhythms of epinephrine and norepinephrine in man. J Clin Endocrin Metab 1985;60:1210–1215.

132. Stene M, Panagiotis N, Tuck MI, Sowers JR, Mayes D, Berg G. Plasma norepinephrine levels are influenced by sodium intake, glucocorticoid administration, and circadian changes in normal man. J Clin Endocrin Metab 1980;51:1340–1345.

133. Panza JA, Epstein SE, Quyyumi AA. Circadian variation in vascular tone and its relation to alpha-sympathetic vasoconstrictor activity. N Engl J Med 1991;325:986–990.

134. Furlan R, Guzzetti S, Crivellaro W, et al. Continuous 24 hour assessment of the neural regulation of systemic arterial pressure and RR variabilities in ambulant subjects. Circulation 1990;81:537–547.

135. Burr R, Hamilton P, Cowan M, et al. Nycthemeral profile of nonspectral heart rate variability measures in women and men. Description of a normal sample and two sudden cardiac arrest subsamples. J Electrocardiol 1994;27(Suppl.):54–62.

136. Marchant B, Stevenson R, Vaishnav S, Wilkinson P, Ranjadayalan K, Timmis AD. Influence of the autonomic nervous system on circadian patterns of myocardial ischemia: comparison of stable angina with the early post infarction period. Br Heart J 1994;71:329–333.

137. Klingenheben T, Rapp U, Hohnloser SH. Circadian variation of heart rate variability in postinfarction patients with and without life-threatening ventricular tachyarrhythmias. J Cardiovasc Electrophysiol 1995;6:357–364.

138. Lombardi F, Sandrone G, Mortara A, et al. Circadian variation of spectral indices of heart rate variability after myocardial infarction. Am Heart J 1992;123:1521–1529.

139. Malik M, Farrell T, Camm AJ. Circadian rhythm of heart rate variability after acute myocardial infarction and its influence on the prognostic value of heart rate variability. Am J Cardiol 1990;66:1049–1054.

140. Zarich S, Waxman S, Freeman RT, Mittleman M, Hegarty P, Nesto RW. Effect of autonomic nervous system dysfunction on the circadian pattern of myocardial ischemia in diabetes mellitus. J Am Coll Cardiol 1994;24:956–960.

141. Kong TQ Jr, Goldberger JJ, Parker M, Wang T, Kadish AH. Circadian variation in human ventricular refractoriness. Circulation 1995;92:1507–1516.
142. Ong JJC, Sarma JSM, Venkataraman K, Levin SK, Singh BN. Circadian rhythmicity of heart rate and QTc interval in diabetic autonomic neuropathy: implications for the mechanism of sudden death. Am Heart J 1993;125:744–752.
143. Ishida S, Nakagawa M, Fujino T, Yonemochi H, Saikawa T, Ito M. Circadian variation of QT interval dispersion: correlation with heart rate variability. J Electrocardiol 1997;30:205–210.
144. Molnar J, Rosenthal JE, Weiss JS, Somberg JC. QT interval dispersion in healthy subjects and survivors of sudden cardiac death: circadian variation in twenty-four hour assessment. Am J Cardiol 1997;79:1190–1193.
145. Muller JE, Tofler GH, Stone PH. Circadian variation and triggers of onset of acute cardiovascular disease. Circulation 1989;79:733–743.
146. Mittleman MA, Sisovick DS. Physical exertion as a trigger of myocardial infarction and sudden cardiac death. Cardiol Clin 1996;14:263–270.
147. Badimon I, Martinez-Gonzalez J, Royo T, Lassila R, Badimon JJ. A sudden increase in plasma epinephrine levels transiently enhances platelet deposition of severely damaged arterial wall-studies in a porcine model. Thromb Hemost 1999;82:1736–1742.
148. Roux F, D'Ambrosio C, Mohsenin V. Sleep-related breathing disorders and cardiovascular disease. Am J Med 2000;108:396–402.
149. Partinen M, Guilleminault C. Daytime sleepiness and vascular morbidity at seven-year followup in obstructive sleep apnea patients. Chest 1990;97:27–32.
150. Schafer H, Koehler U, Ewig S, Hasper E, Tasci S, Luderitz B. Obstructive sleep apnea as a risk marker in coronary artery disease. Cardiology 1999;92:79–84.
151. Seppala T, Partinen M, Penttila A, Aspholm R, Tiainen E, Kaukianen A. Sudden death and sleeping history among Finnish men. J Intern Med 1991;229:23–38.
152. Peker Y, Hedner J, Kraiczi H, Loth S. Respiratory disturbance index: an independent predictor of mortality in coronary artery disease. Am J Resp Crit Care Med 2000;162:81–86.
153. Aboyans V, Cassat C, Lacroix P, et al. Is the morning peak of acute myocardial infarction's onset due to sleep related breathing disorders? A prospective study. Cardiology 2000;94:188–192.
154. Sanner BM, Konermann M, Tepel M, Groetz J, Mummenhoff C, Zidek W. Platelet function in pateints with obstructive sleep apnoea syndrome. Eur Respir J 2000;16:648–652.
155. Nobili L, Schiavi G, Bozano E, De Carli F, Ferrillo F, Nobili F. Morning increase of whole blood viscosity in obstructive sleep apnea syndrome. Clin Hemorheol Microcirc 2000;22:21–27.
156. Schefer H, Koehler U, Ploch T, Peter JH. Sleep-related myocardial ischemia and sleep structure in patients with obstructive sleep apnea and coronary heart disease. Chest 1997;111:387–393.
157. Franklin KA, Nilsson JB, Sahlin C, Naslund U. Sleep apnoea and nocturnal angina. Lancet 1995;345:1085–1087.
158. Wright J, Johns R, Watt I, Melville A, Sheldon T. Health effects of obstructive sleep apnea and the effectiveness of continuous positive airway pressure: a systematic review of the reserach evidence. BMJ 1997;314:851–860.
159. Woods KL, Fletcher S, Jagger C. Modification of the circadian rhythm of onset of acute myocardial infarction by long term antianginal treatment. Br Heart J 1992;68:458–461.
160. Behrens S, Ehlers C, Bruggeman T, et al. Modification of the circadian pattern of ventricular tachyarrhythmias by beta-blocker therapy. Clin Cardiol 1997;20:253–257.
161. Peters RW, Muller JE, Goldstein S, Byington R, Friedman LM. Propanolol and the morning increase in the frequency of sudden cardiac death (BHAT study). Am J Cardiol 1989;63:1518–1520.
162. Pepine CJ, Cohn PF, Deedwania PC, et al. Effects of treatment on outcome in mildly symptomatic patients with ischemia during daily life. The Atenolol Silent Ischemia Study. Circulation 1994;90:762–768.
163. Von Arnim T. Prognostic significance of transient ischemic episodes: response to treatment shows improved prognosis Results of the Total Ischemic Burden Bisoprolol Study (TIBBS) follow-up. J Am Coll Cardiol 1996;28:20–24.
164. Andersen L, Sigurd B, Hansen J. Verapamil and circadian variation of sudden cardiac death. Am Heart J 1996;131:409–410.
165. Vaughn D, Jean-Lucien R, Ridker P, et al. Effects of ramipril on plasma fibrinolytic balance in patients with acute anterior infarction. Circulation 1997;96:442–448.

166. Mancini GB, Henry GC, Macaya C, et al. Angiotensin converting enzyme inhibition with quinapril improves endothelial vasomotor dysfunction in patients with coronary artery disease. The TREND (Trial on Revensing Endothelial Dysfunction) Study. Circulation 1996;94:258–265.

167. Yusuf S, Sleight P, Pogue J, Bosch J, Davies R, Dagenais G. Effects of an angiotensin-converting-enzyme inhibitor, ramipril, on cardiovascular events in high-risk patients. The Heart Outcomes Prevention Evaluation Study Investigators. N Engl J Med 2000;342:145–153.

168. Navalkar S, Parthasarathy S, Santanam N, Khan BV. Irbesartan, an angiotensin type 1 receptor inhibitor, regulates markers of inflammation in patients with premature atherosclerosis. J Am Coll Cardiol 2001;37:440–444.

169. Ridker P, Manson JE, Buring J, Muller JE, Hennekens CH. Circadian variation of acute myocardial infarction and the effect of low dose aspirin in a randomized trial of physicians. Circulation 1990;82: 897–902.

170. Kurnik PB. Circadian variation in the efficacy of tissue-type plasminogen activator. Circulation 1995; 91:1341–1346.

171. Kono T, Morita H, Nishina T, et al. Circadian variations of onset of acute myocardial infarction and efficacy of thrombolytic therapy. J Am Coll Cardiol 1996;27:774–778.

172. Fujita M, Araie E, Yamanishi K, Miwa K, Kida M, Nakajima H. Circadian variation in the success rate of intracoronary thrombolysis for acute myocardial infarction. Am J Cardiol 1993;71:1369–1371.

173. Egstrup K. Attenuation of circadian variation by combined antianginal therapy with supression of morning and evening increases in transient myocardial ischemia. Am Heart J 1991;122:648–655.

174. Andrews TC, Fenton T, Toyosaki N, et al. Subsets of ambulatory myocardial ischemia based on heart rate activity: circadian distribution and response to anti-ischemic medication. Circulation 1993;88:92–100.

175. Deanfield JE, Detry JM, Lichtlen PR, Magnani B, Sellier P, Thaulow E. Amlodipine reduces transient myocardial ischemia in patients with coronary artery disease: double blind Circadian Anti Ischemia Program in Europe (CAPE Trial). J Am Coll Cardiol 1994;24:1460–1467.

176. Parmley WW, Nesto RW, Singh BN, Deanfield J, Gottlieb SO. Attenuation of the circadian patterns of myocardial ischemia with nifedipine GITS in patients with chronic stable angina. J Am Coll Cardiol 1992;19:1380–1386.

177. Davies RF, Habibi H, Klinke WP, et al. Effect of amlodipine, atenolol, and their combination on myocardial ischemia during treadmill exercise and ambulatory monitoring. Canadian Amlodipine/Atenolol in Silent Ischemia Study (CASIS) Investigators. J Am Coll Cardiol 1995;25:619–625.

178. Jimenez AH, Tofler GH, Chen X, Stubbs ME, Solomon HS, Muller JE. Effects of nadolol on hemodynamic and hemostatic responses to potential mental and physical triggers of myocardial infarction in subjects with mild systemic hypertension. Am J Cardiol 1993;72:47–52.

179. Andreotti F, Kluft C, Davies GJ, Huisman LG, deBart AC, Maseri A. Effect of propanolol (long acting) on the circadian fluctuation of tissue-plasminogen activator and plasminogen activator inhibitor-1. Am J Cardiol 1991;68:1295–1299.

180. Shepherd JS, Cobbe SM, Ford I, et al. Prevention of coronary heart disease with pravastatin in men with hypercholesterolemia. N Engl J Med 1995;333:1301–1307.

181. Randomized trial of cholesterol lowering in 4444 patients with coronary artery disease: the Scandinavian Simvastatin Survival Study (4S). Lancet 1994;344:1383–1389.

182. de Lorgeril M, Salen P, Martin JL, Monjaud I, Delaye J, Mamelle N. Mediterranean diet, traditional risk factors, and the rate of cardiovascular complications after myocardial infarction: final report of the Lyon Diet Heart Study. Circulation 1999;99:779–785.

183. Rubins HB, Robins SJ, Collins D, et al. Gemfibrazol for the secondary prevention of coronary heart disease in the with low levels of high-density lipoprotein cholesterol: Veterans Affairs High-Density Lipoprotein Cholesterol Intervention Trail Study Group. N Engl J Med 1999;341:410–418.

184. Anderson KM, Wilson PW, Odell PM, Kannel WB. An updated coronary risk profile: a statement for health professionals. Circulation 1991;83:356–362.

185. Anderson KM, Odell PM, Wilson PW, Kannel WB. Cardiovascular disease risk profiles. Am Heart J 1993;121:293–298.

186 Berlin JA, Colditz GA. A meta-analysis of physical activity in the prevention of coronary heart disease. Am J Epidemiol 1990;132:612–628.

187. Blair SN, Kohl HW 3rd, Barlow CE, Paffenbarger RS Jr, Gibbons LW, Macera CA. Change in physical fitness and all-cause mortality: a prospective study of healthy and unhealthy men and women. JAMA 1995;273:1093–1098.

188. Fletcher GF, Balady G, Blair SN, et al. Benefits and recommendations for physical activity programs for all Americans: a statement for health professionals by the committee on exercise and cardiac rehabilitation of the council on clincial cardiology, American Heart Association. Circulation 1996;94: 857–862.

189. Yusuf S. Calcium antagonists in coronary artery disease and hypertension. Time for reevaluation? Circulation 1995;92:1079–1082.

190. Buring JE, Glynn RJ, Hennekens CH. Calcium channel blockers and myocardial infarction. A hypothesis formulated but not yet tested. JAMA 1995;274:654–655.

191. Bertolet BD, Hill JA, Pepine CJ. Treatment strategies for daily life silent myocardial ischemia: a correlation with potential pathogenetic mechanisms. Prog Cardiovasc Dis 1992;35:97–118.

192. Flack JM, Yunis C. Therapeutic implications of the epidemiology and timing of myocardial infarction and other cardiovascular diseases. J Hum Hypertens 1997;11:23–28.

193. Sica D. Lessons learned from prematurely terminated clinical trials. Curr Hypertension Reports 2001; 3:360–366.

194. Munger MA, Kenney JK. A chronobiologic approach to the pharmacotherapy of hypertension and angina. Ann Pharmacother 2000;34:1313–1319.

195. Kurnik PB. Practical implications of circadian variations in thrombolytic and thrombotic activities. Cardiol Clin 1996;14:251–262.

196. Braunwald E. Morning resistance to thrombolytic therapy. Circulation 1995;91:1604.

197. Frasure-Smith N, Lesperance F, Prince RH, et al. Randomised trial of home-based psychosocial nursing intervention for patients recovering from myocardial infarction. Lancet 1007;350:473–479.

198. Naghavi M, Madjid M, Khan MR, Mohammadi RM, Willerson JT, Casscells SW. New developments in the detection of vulnerable plaque. Curr Atheroscler Rep 2001;3:125–135.

199. Nissen S. Coronary angiography and intravascular ultrasound. Am J Cardiol 2001;87:15A–20A.

200. Brezinski ME, Tearney GJ, Bouma BE, et al. Optical coherence tomography for optical biopsy. Properties and demonstration of vascular pathology. Circulation 1996;93:1206–1213.

201. Jang IK, Bouma BE, Kang DH, et al. Visualization of coronary atherosclerotic plaques in patients using optical coherence tomography: comparison with intravascular ultrasound. J Am Coll Cardiol 2002;39:604–609.

202. Toussaint JF, LaMuraglia GM, Southern JF, Fuster V, Kantor HL. Magnetic resonance images fibrous, calcified, hemorrhagic, and thrombotic components of human atherosclerosis in vivo. Circulation 1996;94:932–938.

203. Casscells W, Hathorn B, David M, et al. Thermal detection of cellular infiltrates in living atherosclerotic plaques: possible implications for plaque rupture and thrombosis. Lancet 1996;347:1447–1451.

204. Stefanadis C, Diamantoupoulos L, Vlachopoulos C, et al. Thermal heterogeneity within human atherosclerotic coronary arteries detected invivo: a new method of detection by application of a special thermography catheter. Circulation 1999;99:1965–1971.

205. Konings MK, Mali WP, Viergever MA. Develoment of an intravascular impedance catheter for detection of fatty lesions in arteries. IEEE Trans Med Imaging 1997;16:439–446.

206. Cassis LA, Lodder RA. Near-IR imaging of atheromas in living arterial tissue. Anal Chem 1993;65: 1247–1256.

207. Dempsey RJ, Cassis LA, Davis DG, Lodder RA. Near-infrared imaging and spectroscopy in stroke research: lipoprotein distribution and disease. Ann NY Acad Sci 1997;820:149–169.

208. Jaross W, Neumeister V, Lattke P, Schuh D. Determination of cholesterol in atherosclerotic plaques using near infrared diffuse reflection spectroscopy. Atherosclerosis 1999;147:327–337.

209. Cohen MC, Muller JE. Triggers of acute myocardial infarction. In: Gersh BJ, Rahimtoola SH, eds. Acute Myocardial Infarction. Elsevier, New York, 1996, pp. 91–105.

4

Insights into the Pathophysiology of Acute Ischemic Syndromes Using the TIMI Flow Grade, TIMI Frame Count, and TIMI Myocardial Perfusion Grade

C. Michael Gibson, MS, MD,
Sabina A. Murphy, MPH,
and Jeffrey J. Popma, MD

INTRODUCTION

For over a decade now, the Thrombolysis in Myocardial Infarction (TIMI) flow grade classification scheme has been successfully used to assess coronary blood flow in acute coronary syndromes (1). Although this scheme has been a valuable tool for comparing the efficacy of reperfusion strategies and in identifying patients at higher risk for adverse

From: *Contemporary Cardiology: Management of Acute Coronary Syndromes, Second Edition*
Edited by: C. P. Cannon © Humana Press Inc., Totowa, NJ

outcomes in acute coronary syndromes, there are limitations to this classification scheme *(2,3)*. To overcome these limitations, the TIMI Angiographic Core Laboratory developed a new index of coronary blood flow called the TIMI frame count *(2)*. In contrast to the TIMI flow grades (TFGs), which are subjective categorical variables, the TIMI frame count is an objective continuous variable of epicardial flow *(2)*. There has also been a recent shift toward focus on microvascular perfusion. One method developed to assess tissue level perfusion is the TIMI myocardial perfusion grade (TMPG) *(4)*. The goal of this chapter is to review these three methods and to discuss the insights into the pathophysiology of acute coronary syndromes provided by these indexes of coronary blood flow and myocardial perfusion.

TFG CLASSIFICATION SCHEME

The original definition of the TFGs from the TIMI 1 study in 1986 are as follows *(1)*:

Grade 0:   No perfusion. No antegrade flow beyond the point of occlusion.
Grade 1:   Penetration without perfusion. Contrast material passes beyond the area of obstruction but fails to opacify the entire coronary bed distal to the obstruction for the duration of the cineangiographic filming sequence.
Grade 2:   Partial perfusion. Contrast material passes across the obstruction and opacifies the coronary distal to the obstruction. However, the rate of entry of contrast material into the vessel distal to the obstruction or its rate of clearance from the distal bed (or both) are perceptibly slower than its flow into or clearance from comparable areas not perfused by the previously occluded vessel.
Grade 3:   Complete perfusion. Antegrade flow into the bed distal to the obstruction occurs as promptly as antegrade flow into the bed proximal to the obstruction, and clearance of contrast material from the involved bed is as rapid as clearance from an uninvolved bed in the same vessel or the opposite artery.

Recently, several groups have begun to define "TIMI grade 3 flow" as opacification of the coronary artery within three cardiac cycles *(5,6)*. As the definition above shows, this is not how TIMI grade 3 flow was originally defined *(1)*. This substantial departure from the original definition of TIMI grade 3 flow will result in much higher rates of TIMI grade 3 flow. In the majority of patients with TIMI grade 3 flow in thrombolytic trials (TIMI 4, 10A, and 10B) *(7–9)*, it requires just under 1 s (26.8 ± 9.1 frames or 0.9 s, $n = 693$) or one cardiac cycle to traverse the length of the artery. Obviously, increasing the time for dye to go down the artery by a factor of three (i.e., from one to three cardiac cycles) that is permissible to qualify for TIMI grade 3 flow greatly increases the rate of TIMI grade 3 flow. Data from the TIMI Angiographic Core Laboratory suggests that the "three cardiac cycle" definition of TIMI 3 flow, results in an approx 10% increase over the original definition of TIMI grade 3 flow *(10)*.

It is possible that TIMI grade 1 flow may sometimes be classified as TIMI grade 2 flow. In the TIMI Angiographic Core Laboratory, we follow the original definition in classifying TIMI grade 2 flow: the dye must reach the apex of the heart during the duration of filming. It is our experience that TIMI grade 1 flow comes in two varieties: one in which the dye barely penetrates the lesion and the other in which dye penetrates the lesion fairly well but the dye moves down the artery so slowly that the operator stops filming before it reaches the apex. We interpret the original definition of TIMI grade 1 flow very literally, and if the dye is not filmed as it reaches the apex, we classify this as TIMI grade 1 flow. It is unclear if other angiographic core laboratories would classify dye that may reach the apex, but is not filmed reaching the apex, as TIMI grade 2 flow. If they do classify flow in this fashion, then this may account for the higher rates of mortality that have been reported by other angiographic core laboratories for TIMI grade 2 flow.

LIMITATIONS OF THE TFG CLASSIFICATION SCHEME

One limitation of the TFG classification scheme is a high rate of interobserver variability in the assessment of TFGs. The rate of agreement between an angiographic core laboratory and clinical centers is best when determining if a culprit artery is either open or closed (κ value = 0.84 $\pm$ 0.05, which indicates good agreement) *(2)*. In contrast, the rate of agreement is only moderate when assessing TIMI grade 3 flow (κ value = 0.55 $\pm$ 0.05) and is actually poor in the assessment of TIMI grade 2 flow (κ value = 0.38 $\pm$ 0.05) *(2)*. Even between experienced angiographic core laboratories, there can be a frequent lack of concordance. In a recent study, the rate of agreement between two core laboratories in the assessment of TIMI grades 2 and 3 flows was only 83%, and three experienced angiographic core laboratories achieved complete agreement in only 71% of the cases *(3)*.

For many years it has been assumed that there are distinct categories of coronary blood flow. However, we have shown that coronary blood flow is unimodally distributed as a continuous variable *(2)*. It has also been assumed that the flow in the nonculprit artery (the flow used as the "gold standard" for assessing TIMI grade flow in the infarct related artery) is truly "normal". As will be discussed below, this assumption is not well justified. Finally, as newer reperfusion strategies achieve a higher rate of TIMI grade 3 flow, this categorical method may have limited statistical power and sensitivity in distinguishing the efficacy of different reperfusion strategies, as there may be a range of velocities associated with TIMI grade 3 flow *(2)*.

TIMI FRAME COUNT

To overcome the above limitations associated with the TIMI flow grade classification scheme, we have recently described a more objective and precise method of estimating coronary blood flow, in which the number of cineframes required for dye to reach standardized distal landmarks are counted, called the TIMI frame count *(2)*. In the first frame used for TIMI frame counting, a column of dye touches both borders of the coronary artery and moves forward (Fig. 1). In the last frame, dye begins to enter (but does not necessarily fill) a standard distal landmark in the artery (Fig. 1). These standard distal landmarks are as follows: in the right coronary artery the first branch of the posterolateral artery; in the circumflex system the most distal branch of the obtuse marginal branch, which includes the culprit lesion in the dye path; and in the left anterior descending (LAD) artery the distal bifurcation which is also known as the "moustache," "pitch fork," or "whales tail" (Fig. 1). These frame counts are corrected for the longer length of the LAD by dividing by 1.7 to arrive at the corrected TIMI frame count (CTFC) *(2)*.

In contrast to the conventional TIMI flow grade classification scheme, the CTFC is quantitative rather than qualitative, it is objective rather than subjective, it is a continuous rather than a categorical variable, and it is reproducible *(2)*. Indeed, with respect to

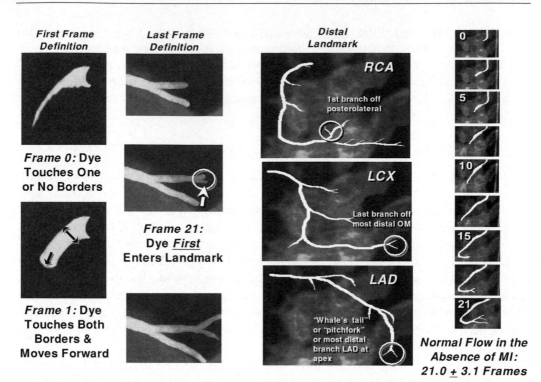

Fig. 1. The TIMI frame counting method. In the first frame (lower left panel), a column of near or fully concentrated dye touches both borders of the coronary artery and moves forward. In the last frame (second column), dye begins to enter (but does not necessarily fill) a standard distal landmark in the artery. These standard distal landmarks are as follows: the first branch of the posterolateral artery in the right coronary artery (upper panel, third column); in the circumflex system the most distal branch of the obtuse marginal branch which includes the culprit lesion in the dye path (mid panel, third column); and in the left anterior descending artery the distal bifurcation which is also known as the "moustache", "pitch fork" or "whales tail" (lower panel, third column).

variability, the mean absolute value of the difference between two consecutive hand injections of the infarct-related artery was only 4.7 ± 3.9 frames ($n = 85$) *(2)*. Other groups, such as Ivanc and Ellis et al., have shown even better measures of reproducibility *(11)*. These authors examined angiograms on two separate occasions separated in time by 6 mos, and found a correlation of 0.97 in their readings over time and a correlation of 0.99 among three different observers *(11)*. There was a 0.7–2.0 frame difference between observers *(11)*. In a recent study where two experienced angiographic core laboratories (Global Use of Strategies to Open Occluded Coronary Arteries [GUSTO] and TIMI) analyzed the same films for a fibrinolytic trial, there were discrepancies in 21% of TFG readings (41 out of 194, $\kappa = 0.76$); however, excellent concordance in trial results were seen using the CTFC (overall median difference = 0 frames) with no significant difference being observed between the two core laboratories *(12)*.

Normal flow in normal arteries in the absence of acute myocardial infarction (MI) has been found to be 21.0 ± 3.1 frames ($n = 78$)*(2)*, with the 95% confidence interval for normal flow extending from >14 frames to <28 frames. Despite differences in the length of the coronary arteries, the force of injections, the diameter of the arteries, heart rates, cardiac output, and catheter engagement, we have found that the standard

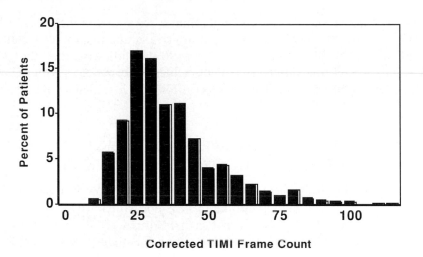

Fig. 2. Shown here is a histogram displaying the percent of patients with a given CTFC (grouped by bins of 5 frames) following thrombolysis in the TIMI 4, TIMI 10A, and TIMI 10B trials. Note that very few patients have a CTFC > 100.

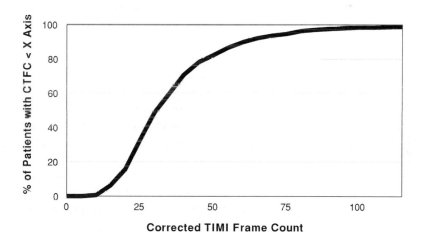

Fig. 3. Cumulative distribution function of corrected TIMI frame counts in 960 patients from the TIMI 4, 10A, and 10B studies. Any CTFC can be chosen on the X-axis as a definition of thrombolytic success. The corresponding value on the Y-axis displays the percent of patients that satisfy that definition of success. Only approx one quarter of patients have normal flow (i.e., a CTFC < 28) following thrombolysis.

deviation among 78 arteries with normal flow was only 3.1 frames, a coefficient of variation of approx 14% *(2)*. We have recently studied the impact of the force of injection and shown that the CTFC following power injections performed at the 10th and 90th percentile of human injection rates differ from each other by only 2 frames *(13,14)*.

Using the CTFC, coronary blood flow appears to be unimodally distributed as a continuous variable *(2)* (Figs. 2 and 3). Thus, any division of flow into normal and abnormal categories is arbitrary. Although we do not use the CTFC to determine the TFGs, in a retrospective analysis, the TIMI Angiographic Core Laboratory tended to classify flow as TIMI grade 2 flow if the CTFC was >40 (approx 1.3 s) *(2)*. In the TIMI 4, 10A and 10B trials *(7–9)*, the 90-min CTFC in culprit arteries is unimodally distributed with a mean CTFC of 35.6 ± 20.8 frames ($n = 960$) at 90 min following thrombolysis (Figs. 2 and 3). Approximately one quarter of patients achieved normal flow with a CTFC <28 frames, (i.e., within the 95% confidence interval for flow in patients without acute MI) (Fig. 3).

NONCULPRIT FLOW AS A FLAWED GOLD STANDARD AGAINST WHICH TO GAUGE FLOW IN ACUTE MI

Traditionally, it has always been assumed that the basal flow in nonculprit arteries in the setting of acute MI following thrombolysis is normal. However, using the CTFC, basal flow in the uninvolved artery is in fact not normal *(2)*. In the setting of acute MI, the mean CTFC at 90 min following thrombolysis among the nonculprit arteries (30.9 ± 15.0, $n = 1,817$) *(15)* was 45% higher than minimally diseased arteries with normal flow in the absence of acute MI (21.0 ± 3.1, $p < 0.001$), but returned to that of normal arteries by 18–36 hours following thrombolysis (21.3 ± 7.1, $n = 76$, $p = NS$) *(2)*.

This problem is further complicated by the fact that nonculprit arteries may not all be slowed to the same degree depending upon their location. We have shown that flow in nonculprit LAD arteries was disproportionately slowed by 36% when compared to that in uninvolved circumflex arteries which confounds the classification of conventional TFGs *(2)*. While our original study showed that the CTFC in LAD culprits is on the whole higher (reflecting slower flow) than that in other locations at 90 min following successful thrombolysis, the CTFC for TIMI grade 3 flow was actually 32% lower for LAD culprits when compared to the circumflex artery (25.7 vs 34.0 frames) *(2)*. This paradox was explained by the fact TIMI grade 3 flow in culprit LAD arteries was gauged against faster flow in nonculprit circumflex arteries (22.5 frames), and consequently, few LAD culprits (26.2%) achieved a rapid enough velocity to be classified as achieving TIMI grade 3 flow. In contrast, flow in circumflex culprits was graded against the 36% slower flow in nonculprit LADs (30.5 frames), and therefore, most circumflex arteries (92%) were classified as achieving TIMI grade 3 flow *(2)*. Thus, the conventional notion that flow in uninvolved arteries is normal may be erroneous and may lead to the misclassification of TFGs. In the right coronary artery (RCA), no other normal artery is even present for comparison. The complexity of visual flow grade assessment is further compounded by the fact that international cinefilms are filmed at a wide but subtle variety of speeds (12.5, 15, 25, 30, 50, 60 frames/s).

In addition to these reductions in basal nonculprit flow, Uren et al. have shown in position emission tomography (PET) scanning experiments that the coronary vasodilatory response (the ratio of myocardial blood flow after the administration of dipyridamole to the basal myocardial blood flow) in angiographically normal nonculprit arteries remains reduced at 1 wk following acute MI as compared with control patients without acute MI (1.53 ± 0.36 vs 3.17 ± 0.72, $p = 0.009$) *(16)*. Similarly, in a study by Marjorie et al. in isolated perfused rat hearts, basal coronary blood flow in acute MI hearts was completely normalized within 1 wk, whereas maximal coronary blood flow was not normalized until 5 wk after acute MI *(17)*. Thus, acute MI impairs both basal and maximal flow in nonculprit territories. In addition, Wyatt and Corday have shed some light on the pathophysiology of delayed flow in remote areas of the heart by demonstrating that focal necrosis (micro-infarcts) and regional lactate derangements occur in the nonoccluded (remote) posterior segments of the left and right ventricles after occlusion of the proximal LAD in closed chest dogs *(18,19)*.

We have reported that the predictors of delayed flow in the nonculprit artery include slower flow in the culprit artery, a longer length of culprit vessel distal to the stenosis (i.e., a bigger infarct), a tighter stenosis in the nonculprit artery, and pulsatile flow in the culprit artery *(15)*. The observation relating pulsatile culprit flow to delayed nonculprit flow sheds light on the potential mechanism of global flow delays. Doppler velocity wire studies have shown that a pulsatile pattern of flow with systolic flow reversal is observed in the setting of the no reflow phenomenon and that this flow pattern reflects heightened downstream microvascular resistance.

We have recently reported that flow improves in the nonculprit artery as flow improves in the culprit artery in the setting of acute MI *(15)*. The CTFC in nonculprit arteries improved by 3.3 frames between 60 and 90 min following thrombolysis ($p <$ 0.0001) *(15)*. When flow improved in the associated culprit artery between 60 and 90 min, nonculprit artery flow improved by 7.4 frames ($p = 0.0003$) *(15)*. In contrast, when flow did not improve in the associated culprit artery, there was no significant improvement in the nonculprit artery flow (1.0 frame, $p = $ NS) *(15)*. Similarly, in the setting of percutaneous transluminal coronary angioplasty (PTCA) for unstable angina syndromes, we have shown that PTCA of the culprit lesion was associated with a 3-frame improvement in the nonculprit artery after the intervention *(20)*. Again, if abnormal flow was present in the nonculprit artery at baseline (i.e., CTFC > 28), then the improvements in nonculprit flow were more dramatic (10 frames) *(20)*. It could be speculated that the delayed flow in nonculprit arteries may be the result of more extensive necrosis in shared microvasculature, or a result of vasoconstriction mediated through either a local neurohumoral or paracrine mechanism. Further studies are needed, however, to determine the cause of delayed flow in the nonculprit arteries.

TIMI MYOCARDIAL PERFUSION GRADE

It has recently become apparent that epicardial flow does not necessarily imply tissue level or microvascular perfusion *(21,22)*. This led to the recent development of a new angiographic measure of tissue level perfusion, the TIMI myocardial perfusion grade (TMPG) *(4)*, as follows:

TMPG 3:   Normal entry and exit of dye from the microvasculature. There is the ground glass appearance (blush) or opacification of the myocardium in the distribution of the culprit lesion that clears normally, and is either gone or only mildly/moderately persistent at the end of the washout phase (i.e., dye is gone or is mildly/moderately persistent after 3 cardiac cycles of the washout phase and noticeably diminishes in intensity during the washout phase), similar to that in an uninvolved artery. Blush that is of only mild intensity throughout the washout phase, but fades minimally, is also classified as grade 3.

TMPG 2:   Delayed entry and exit of dye from the microvasculature. There is the ground glass appearance (blush) or opacification of the myocardium in the distribution of the culprit lesion that is strongly persistent at the end of the washout phase (i.e., dye is strongly persistent after three cardiac cycles of the washout phase and either does not or only minimally diminishes in intensity during washout).

TMPG 1:   Dye slowly enters but fails to exit the microvasculature. There is the ground glass appearance (blush) or opacification of the myocardium in the distribution of the culprit lesion that fails to clear from the microvasculature, and dye staining is present on the next injection (approx 30 s between injections).

TMPG 0:   Dye fails to enter the microvasculature. There is either minimal or no ground glass appearance (blush) or opacification of the myocardium in the distribution of the culprit artery indicating lack of tissue level perfusion.

The TMPG has been shown to be a multivariate predictor of mortality in acute MI (Fig. 4) *(4)*. The TMPG permits risk stratification even within epicardial TIMI grade 3 flow. Despite achieving epicardial patency with normal TIMI grade 3 flow, those patients whose microvasculature fails to open (TIMI myocardial perfusion grade 0/1) have a persistently elevated mortality of 5.4%. In contrast, those patients with both TIMI grade 3 flow in the epicardial artery and TIMI myocardial perfusion grade 3 have a mortality under 1% *(4)*.

The TIMI flow grades and the TIMI myocardial perfusion grades can be combined to identify a group of patients at very low risk and alternatively very high risk for mortality. Those patients with both TIMI grade 3 flow and TIMI myocardial perfusion grade 3 flow had a mortality of 0.7% while those patients with both TIMI grade 0/1 and TIMI myocardial perfusion grade 0/1 flow had a mortality of 10.9% *(4)*.

In order to quantitatively characterize the kinetics of dye entering the myocardium using the angiogram, digital subtraction angiography (DSA) was developed. DSA is performed at end diastole by aligning cineframes images before dye fills the myocardium with those at the peak of myocardial filling to subtract spine, ribs, diaphragm, and the epicardial artery (Fig. 5). A representative region of the myocardium is sampled that is free of overlap by epicardial arterial branches to determine the increase in the Gray scale brightness of the myocardium when it first reached its peak intensity. The circumference of the myocardial blush is measured using a handheld planimeter. The number of frames required for the myocardium to first reach its peak brightness is converted into time (s) by dividing the frame count by 30. In this way, the rate of rise in brightness (Gray/s) and the rate of growth of blush (cm/s) can be calculated.

Compared to normal patients, microvascular perfusion was reduced in acute MI patients on DSA as demonstrated by a reduction in peak Gray (brightness) (10.9 ± 5.7 vs $7.8 \pm 8.9, p < 0.0001$), the rate of rise in Gray/s (2.8 ± 1.4 vs $2.1 \pm 2.5, p < 0.0001$), the blush circumference (19.4 ± 5.4 vs $13.6 \pm 10.7, p < 0.0001$), and the rate of growth in circumference (cm/s)(5.2 ± 2.0 vs $3.7 \pm 3.1, p < 0.0001$) *(23)*. However, while DSA perfusion was impaired overall in the setting of acute MI, TMPG grade 3 in the setting of acute MI did not differ from that in normal patients when studied quantitatively as shown by similar peak Gray (10.9 ± 5.7 vs 10.6 ± 6.1), rate of growth in Gray/s (2.8 ± 1.4 vs 3.1 ± 2.1), the blush circumference (19.4 ± 5.4 vs 18.0 ± 10.3), and the rate of growth in circumference (5.2 ± 2.0 vs 4.9 ± 2.4) ($p = $ NS for all) *(23)*.

In myocardial contrast echocardiography (MCE) studies by Ito et al. *(21,22)*, the culprit artery was patent after angioplasty or thrombolysis within 24 h of symptom onset in 126 patients with anterior MI. However, despite epicardial patency, one-fourth of

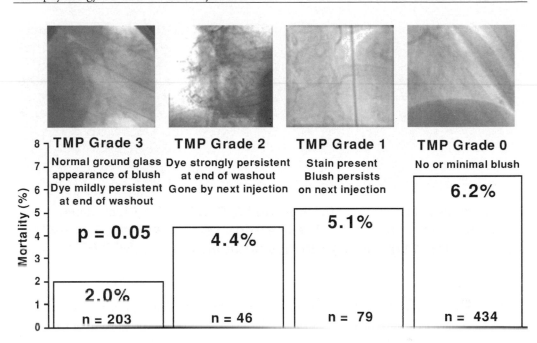

Fig. 4. The TMPG assesses tissue level perfusion using the angiogram and is a multivariate predictor of mortality in acute MI. The TMPG permits risk stratification even within epicardial TIMI grade 3 flow. Despite achieving epicardial patency with normal TIMI grade 3 flow, those patients whose microvasculature fails to open (TMPG 0/1) have a persistently elevated mortality of 5.4%. In contrast, those patients with both TIMI grade 3 flow in the epicardial artery and TMPG 3 have a mortality under 1%.

patients had a lack of tissue level perfusion and the no reflow phenomenon, and these patients had a higher rate of adverse outcomes (sustained arrhythmias, pericardial effusion, cardiac tamponade, congestive heart failure, or death), and a lower rate of improvement in global (5 vs 11%) as well as regional left ventricle (LV) contractile function (standard deviations [SD]/chord) (-0.4 vs -0.9) (21,22).

Several mechanisms have been postulated in the development of the no reflow phenomenon following acute MI, such as a loss of microvasculature integrity and profound spasm of microvasculature, caused by the release of potent vasoconstrictors from activated platelets (e.g., serotonin) or neutrophil infiltration and platelet fibrin clots in the microvasculature (24–30). Adjunctive therapies such as superoxide dismutase, catalase, adenosine, verapamil, papaverine, ketanserine (a serotonin inhibitor), and other new therapies targeted at the microvasculature may warrant further investigations (31–33).

Unlike the epicardial artery, the microvasculature responds poorly to nitroglycerine due to impaired synthesis of endothelium-derived relaxing factor (EDRF) (27). Calcium channel blockers act directly on vascular smooth muscle rather than EDRF and may be of benefit in minimizing microvascular spasm. Indeed, in a prospective trial by Taniyama et al. (34), MCE has been used after primary angioplasty to demonstrate that the low reflow ratio (ratio of no flow zone plus low reflow zone to the risk area) decreased by 45% after the administration of 0.5 mg of intracoronary verapamil (from 0.39 ± 0.23 to 0.29 ± 0.17, $p < 0.05$) (34). Of note, the improvement in the regional

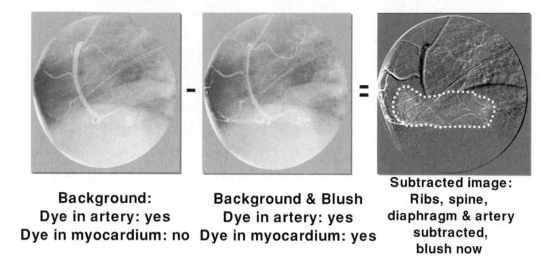

Background:
Dye in artery: yes
Dye in myocardium: no

Background & Blush
Dye in artery: yes
Dye in myocardium: yes

Subtracted image:
Ribs, spine,
diaphragm & artery
subtracted,
blush now
apparent

Fig. 5. Digital subtraction angiography (DSA) was developed in order to quantitatively characterize the kinetics of dye entering the myocardium using the angiogram. DSA is performed at end diastole by aligning cineframes images before dye fills the myocardium with those at the peak of myocardial filling to subtract spine, ribs, diaphragm, and the epicardial artery. A representative region of the myocardium is sampled that is free of overlap by epicardial arterial branches to determine the increase in the Gray scale brightness of the myocardium when it first reached its peak intensity. The circumference of the myocardial blush is measured using a handheld planimeter. The number of frames required for the myocardium to first reach its peak brightness is converted into time (s) by dividing the frame count by 30. In this way the rate of rise in brightness (Gray/s) and the rate of growth of blush (cm/s) can be calculated.

wall motion score index from baseline to follow-up study at 24 d was higher in the verapamil-treated group than in the control group (0.7 ± 0.8 vs $0.2 \pm 1.3, p < 0.05$) *(34)*. A major question has been whether microvascular spasm is an epiphenomenon in acute MI and if improving microvascular spasm will lead to improved clinical outcomes. This small preliminary study suggests that intracoronary verapamil can attenuate microvascular spasm and that it can in turn augment basal tissue level perfusion. It provides a critical link in relating these improvements in tissue perfusion to improved wall motion in patients with acute MI *(34)*.

RELATIVE CONTRIBUTION OF THE EPICARDIAL STENOSIS AND MICROVASCULAR RESISTANCE TO FLOW DELAYS IN ACUTE MI

While the no reflow phenomenon exists in many patients with acute MI, the magnitude of its contribution to flow delays following thrombolysis is unclear and may be relatively small. For instance, verapamil administration in the previous study reduced the CTFC by only 9 frames (from 50 ± 15 to 41 ± 14, $n = 40$; $p < 0.01$) *(34)*. The relief of the residual stenosis by conventional PTCA and the scaffolding provided by intracoronary stent placement present unique opportunities to examine the potential role of both the residual stenosis and intraluminal obstruction to flow delays following thrombolysis *(35)*. Unlike conventional PTCA, intracoronary stenting relieves any residual intraluminal obstruction caused by dissection planes that may cause baffling and non-laminar flow. Any persistent delay in flow following adjunctive stenting is unlikely to be due to the residual stenosis or intraluminal obstruction and most likely represents the contribution of downstream microvasculature resistance. Both rescue and adjunctive PTCA of the residual stenosis at 90–120 min largely normalized discrepancies in pre-PTCA frame counts between the TFGs *(35)*. Adjunctive and rescue angioplasty also restored flow in culprit vessels that were nearly identical to that of nonculprit arteries in the setting of acute MI (30.5 vs 30.5 frames, p = NS) *(35)*. These observations should not, however, be misinterpreted as demonstrating that PTCA restores completely "normal" flow. It is important to note that post-PTCA CTFCs and nonculprit CTFCs of 30 are both in actuality abnormally slowed, and they are nearly 45% slower (p < 0.001) than the CTFC of 21 previously reported in patients without acute MI and normal flow *(2)*. Despite a 13% residual diameter stenosis and the relief of intraluminal obstruction that would be anticipated following stent placement, flow was persistently delayed to 26 frames, and likewise, 34% of stented vessels had abnormal flow with a CTFC $\geq$ 28 (the 95th percentile of the upper limit of normal) *(35)*. This persistent delay is unlikely to be due to either the residual stenosis or intraluminal obstruction and most likely represents the contribution of downstream microvascular resistance. To summarize the magnitude of flow delays attributable to microvascular resistance, nonculprit and culprit artery flow following relief of the stenosis by PTCA/stenting is delayed by approx 5 to 10 frames and likewise, treatment of heightened microvascular resistance with verapamil improves flow by approx 9 frames.

Recently, we have reported the multivariable determinants of coronary blood flow at 90 min following thrombolysis, and a map of the multiple colinearities that we have observed is shown in Fig. 6 *(35)*. Obviously, the residual percent stenosis plays a critical role, with the average 70% stenosis increasing the CTFC by approx 17 frames *(35)*. The presence of residual thrombus adds approx 4 frames *(35)*. Thus, superior revascularization strategies will reduce the residual stenosis and eliminate thrombus. There were also some unanticipated contributors to delayed to flow, such as the timing of reperfusion; i.e., those patients who were patent at 60 min had 15 frames faster flow than those patients who achieved flow between 60 and 90 min. LAD infarcts had slower flow by 8 frames than infarcts in other locations. It could be speculated that left system infarcts have slower flow due to the fact that they have lesions that are located more proximally, they subtend the thicker LV wall, and there is higher wall stress in the LV than in the right ventricle (RV) *(35)*.

RANGE OF VELOCITIES THAT CONSTITUTES TIMI GRADE 3 FLOW

As newer reperfusion strategies are reported to achieve a higher incidence of TIMI grade 3 flow, a categorical scale may fail to distinguish their efficacies because there is a range of dye velocities that constitute TIMI grade 3 flow *(2,36–38)*. Even if two reperfusion strategies result in the same proportion of TIMI grade 3 flow, the TIMI grade 3 flow of one strategy may be faster than the TIMI grade 3 flow of another strategy, and there may be a difference in the dye velocity between the two strategies when analyzed as a continuous variable using the CTFC. This range of velocities that constitutes TIMI grade 3 flow can be demonstrated by the following example *(37)*. We have developed a new method of measuring absolute velocity called the PTCA guidewire velocity *(37)*.

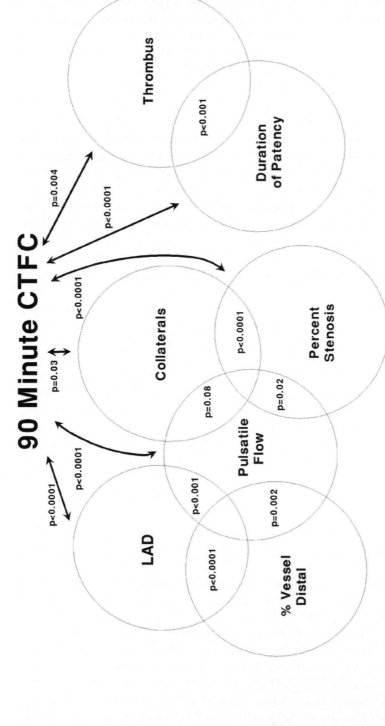

Fig. 6. Multiple variables determine flow at 90 min, and they are often related to each other. For instance, LAD location, the percent of the vessel distal to the stenosis, and the presence of a pulsatile flow pattern were all related to each other as well as the 90-min CTFC. In particular, there was a greater percent of the culprit vessel distal to the stenosis in patients with an LAD lesion (76.6 ± 11.1% [n = 252] vs 61.4 ± 22.9% [n = 422], p < 0.0001); LAD lesions predominated in patients with pulsatile flow (61.1% LAD [n = 66 out of 108] vs 38.9% non-LAD [n = 42 out of 108], p < 0.001); and finally patients with a pulsatile flow pattern also had a greater percent of the vessel distal to the stenosis (72.9 ± 16.2% [n = 97] vs 65.8 ± 21.3% [n = 548], p = 0.002). Patients with pulsatile flow had less severe percent stenoses (68.6 ± 18.8% [n = 106] vs 73.0 ± 18.9% [n = 733], p = 0.02), and pulsatile lesions tended to be collateralized less frequently (pulsatile lesions collateralized in 9.5% [n = 10 out of 105] of cases, and nonpulsatile lesions collateralized in 16% [n = 116 out of 723] of cases, p = 0.08). Patients who were patent for less than 30 min also had a higher incidence of thrombus (50.0% [n = 24 out of 48] vs 21.4% [n = 119 out of 555], p < 0.001).

106

After PTCA, the guidewire tip is placed at the coronary landmark, and a Kelly clamp is placed on the guidewire where it exits the Y-Adapter. The guidewire tip is then withdrawn to the catheter tip, and a second Kelly clamp is placed on the wire where it exits the Y-Adapter. The distance between the 2 Kelly clamps outside the body is the distance between the catheter tip and the anatomic landmark inside the body. Velocity (cm/s) may be calculated as this distance [(cm) ÷ TFC (frames)] × film frame speed (frames/s). Flow (cm³/s) may be calculated by multiplying this velocity (cm/s) and the mean cross-sectional lumen area (cm²) along the length of the artery to the TIMI landmark *(37)*. In 30 patients, velocity increased from 13.9 ± 8.5 cm/s pre-PTCA to 22.8 ± 9.3 cm/s post-PTCA ($p < 0.001$). Despite TIMI grade 3 flow, both before and after PTCA in 18 patients, velocity actually increased 38% from 17.0 ± 5.4 cm/s to 23.5 ± 9.0 cm/sec ($p = 0.01$). For all 30 patients, flow doubled from 0.6 ± 0.4 cm³/s pre-PTCA to 1.2 ± 0.6 cm³/s post-PTCA ($p < 0.001$). In the 18 patients with TIMI grade 3 glow both before and after PTCA, flow increased 86% from 0.7 ± 0.3 cm³/s to 1.3 ± 0.6 cm³/s ($p = 0.001$) *(37)*. These data illustrate the wide range of velocities associated with TIMI grade 3 flow and the potential that TIMI grade 3 flow can be improved upon and made faster. A range of velocities that constitutes different TFGs has also been described using the Doppler velocity wires *(39–41)*. We have also planimetered the length of arteries from the angiogram and combined this with the frame count to calculate what is called the quantitative coronary angiography (QCA) velocity, and we have shown that the QCA velocity proximal and distal to the lesion is almost identical to that reported using Doppler velocity wires *(42,43)*.

CORONARY BLOOD FLOW IN THE ASSESSMENT OF THROMBOLYTIC AGENTS

A variety of thrombolytic agents have been developed over the past two decades with the hope of improving coronary blood flow and, hence, mortality in acute MI. Initial efforts to restore antegrade flow to occluded vessels began with the administration of intracoronary thrombolytic agents in the late 1970s and the early 1980s *(44–47)*. These recanalization trials and the intracoronary route of thrombolytic administration were logistically demanding, and they were soon replaced by trials involving the simpler and the more rapid intravenous route of thrombolytic administration in 90-min patency trials in the mid 1980s *(47,48)*. The original open artery hypothesis, namely that early and full reperfusion would lead to improved clinical outcomes, was subsequently confirmed by large-scale megatrials with angiographic substudies that linked improved 90-min patency profiles of front-loaded recombinant tissue plasminogen activator (rtPA) to improved left ventricular function and, in turn, to improved mortality *(49,50)*.

The interobserver variability inherent in the TFG classification scheme is reflected in the wide range of rates of TIMI grade 3 flow reported for a single drug, front-loaded tissue-type plasminogen activator (tPA). A pooled analysis involving 1492 patients from all large angiographic thrombolytic trials of front-loaded tPA to date, reveals a 90-min patency rate of 82% (60% rate of TIMI 3 flow and 22% rate of TIMI 2 flow) *(50–57)* (Fig. 7). As shown in Fig. 7, the rates of TIMI grade 3 flow vary tremendously from a high of 71% in the initial report of Neuhaus et al. *(51)* to a low of 45% in the RAPID 2 trial *(57)*. The overall rate of TIMI grade 3 flow in the TIMI Angiographic Core Laboratory over the years has been 60%, which is the same as the rate reported across all

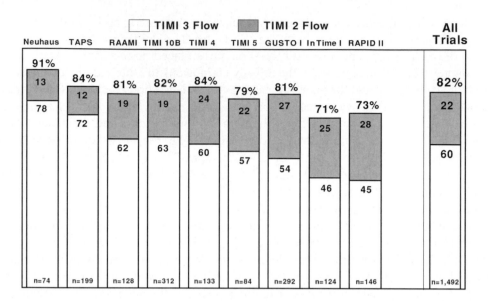

Fig. 7. The interobserver variability in the assessment of TIMI grade 3 flow for a single drug (tPA) is shown here. The rate of TIMI grade 3 flow following front-loaded tPA administration extends from a high value of 71% to a low value of 45%. Overall, the rate of TIMI grade 3 flow is 60%, the same as that reported over the years by the TIMI Angiographic Core Laboratory.

trials to date. Thus, the TIMI Angiographic Core Laboratory reflects the central tendency of how TIMI grade 3 flow is read in a variety of angiographic core laboratories from around the world.

In an effort to improve upon this 60% rate of TIMI grade 3 flow, variants of tPA have been developed such as recombinant plasminogen activator (rPA) *(57)*, which is a nonglycosylated deletion mutant of wild-type tPA, novel plasminogen activator (NPA), and a genetically engineered mutant of tPA (TNK) *(54)*. The Reteplase vs Alteplase Patency Investigation during Myocardial Infarction (RAPID-2) trial was a small angiographic patency study which demonstrated a higher 90-min rate of TIMI grade 3 flow for rPA compared to tPA (60 vs 45%, $p = 0.01$). It should be noted that this 45% rate of TIMI grade 3 flow for front-loaded tPA was significantly lower than the rates reported in many of the trials in Fig. 7. Consistent with the 60% rate of TIMI grade 3 flow observed for rPA, the results of the Global Use of Strategies to Open Occluded Coronary Arteries (GUSTO) III trial demonstrated no significant difference in mortality at 30 d (7.47% for rPA vs 7.24% for tPA, $p = 0.54$) or the combined endpoint of death/disabling stroke (7.89% for rPA vs 7.91% for tPA, $p = 0.97$) *(58)*. Both TNK and NPA have also achieved approx 60% rates of TIMI grade 3 flow at the doses studied *(54)*.

ADJUNCTIVE MECHANICAL INTERVENTION TO FURTHER IMPROVE FLOW

As the previous section indicates, stand alone thrombolytic therapy faces a formidable challenge in increasing the rate of TIMI grade 3 flow beyond 60%. While there are clear angiographic benefits to rescue (opening a closed artery) and adjunctive PTCA (further dilating an open artery with TIMI grade 2 or 3 flow) as discussed above, the clinical benefits are less clear. Previously the routine use of immediate adjunctive conventional angioplasty to supplement the results of thrombolysis has not been shown to be any more efficacious than a conservative approach of deferred angioplasty (59–61). PTCA/stenting in the subgroup of patients with suboptimal TIMI 2 flow has not been fully assessed. Preliminary results from the TIMI study group have shown that in the 38 patients in which TIMI grade 2 flow was dilated, TIMI grade 3 flow was restored in 34 patients (89.5%), and the mean post-intervention CTFC was 30.8 6 26.8 frames (62). The 30-d risk of death or recurrent MI was 11.2% in patients who were medically managed for TIMI grade 2 flow (12 out of 107) and was 10.0% in those patients who were treated with PTCA/stenting for TIMI grade 2 flow (4 out of 40) (p 5 NS) (62). Thus, PTCA/stenting may not offer a major advantage in clinical outcomes over medical management. Larger randomized trials are obviously needed to ascertain the clinical benefit (if any) of mechanical intervention over medical management for TIMI grade 2 flow following thrombolysis.

If thrombolytic therapy is not effective in opening the infarct related artery, a "rescue" or "salvage" PTCA may be performed. Experience with rescue angioplasty sheds important light on the relative importance of coronary blood flow and the timing with which that flow is achieved. In the TIMI 4 trial, although successful rescue angioplasty for an occluded artery at 90 min resulted in a much higher rate of TIMI 3 flow than successful thrombolysis (86.5 vs 64.8%, $p = 0.002$), this higher rate of grade 3 flow was achieved later, at over 120 min after thrombolysis, and this time, delay may explain in part the higher rate of mortality (9.6%) for this strategy than successful thrombolysis (3.3%) (Fig. 8) *(63)*.

Direct or primary angioplasty in acute MI has been demonstrated to achieve high rates of patency and TIMI grade 3 flow in several small angiographic trials *(63–71)*. In the initial study in this area, the Primary Angioplasty in Myocardial Infarction (PAMI) investigators reported a success rate of 97.1% for primary angioplasty *(64)*. There was a trend for patients treated with primary angioplasty to have a lower mortality rate than patients treated with thrombolysis alone (2.6 vs 6.5%, respectively, $p = 0.06$) in this trial. However, other randomized trials of primary angioplasty at the time, each involving less than 100 patients per treatment arm, revealed no significant difference in mortality between the two strategies *(65–67)*.

These early comparisons of primary angioplasty with thrombolysis, however, were limited by the use of either older dosing regimens of tPA or streptokinase (SK), rather than utilizing the more efficacious regimen of front-loaded tPA. Fortunately, the most recent randomized trial in this field (the GUSTO IIb trial) overcomes many of these limitations in its comparison of direct angioplasty to front-loaded tPA in a large series of 1138 patients *(68)*. The composite endpoint of the trial (death, reinfarction or stroke) was lower in the primary angioplasty group than the front-loaded tPA group (9.6 vs 13.7%, $p = 0.03$), and there was a trend for the 30-d mortality rate to also be slightly lower (5.7 vs 7.0%, $p = $ NS) with this strategy *(68)*. In contrast to the 90–99% success rate previously reported by primary angioplasty operators and the 84% rate reported in the GUSTO IIb trial, only 73% of patients achieved TIMI grade 3 flow following angioplasty in this trial when the TFGs were evaluated by an independent angiographic core laboratory. Although this core laboratory rate of TIMI grade 3 flow is lower than the rate assessed by the primary PTCA operators themselves, this 73% rate of TIMI grade 3 flow following primary PTCA still compares favorably with the 60% rate reported

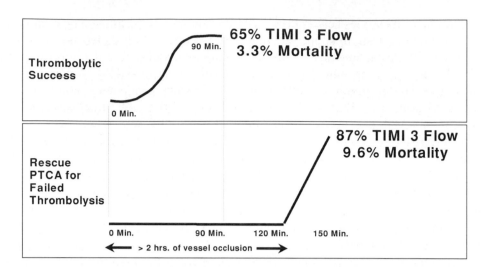

Fig. 8. Data from the TIMI 4 rescue PTCA experience, which shows that TIMI grade 3 flow is not always associated with improved outcomes if it is achieved too late. In the TIMI 4 trial, although successful rescue angioplasty for an occluded artery at 90 min resulted in a much higher rate of TIMI 3 flow than successful thrombolysis (86.5 vs 64.8%, $p = 0.002$), this higher rate of grade 3 flow was achieved later, at over 120 min after thrombolysis, and this time delay may explain in part the higher rate of mortality (9.6%) for this strategy than successful thrombolysis (3.3%).

for all trials of front-loaded tPA to date. It is also notable that the survival curves did not diverge early (i.e., within 24 h), but rather they began to diverge at 1 to 2 wk in this trial, indicating that the occurrence of reinfarction, rather than early flow, may be driving the force in the mortality differential between the strategies.

While individual trials, including the relatively large GUSTO IIb trial, were unable to show significant difference in mortality between the two strategies, a meta-analysis of all ten randomized trials of primary angioplasty to date, involving 2066 patients (large enough to detect clinically relevant differences), reveals lower rates of mortality at 30 d (4.4 vs 6.5%, $p = 0.02$), death/reinfarction (7.2 vs 11.9%, $p < 0.001$), and stroke (0.7 vs 2.0%, $p = 0.007$) when primary angioplasty is compared with thrombolysis *(72)*.

While primary angioplasty may restore a high rate of TIMI 3 flow, stenting may further improve upon lumen dimensions and may relieve intraluminal obstruction due to dissection planes and thrombus. In a pooled analysis of 20 nonrandomized trials of primary stenting within 24 h of acute MI involving 1357 patients, the incidence of mortality was 2.4%, the incidence of stent thrombosis was 1.5%, and the incidence of emergency coronary artery bypass graft (CABG) was 1.3% *(73)*. Even if stenting was the ideal treatment modality for acute MI, it is unclear how many patients would have vessels ideally suited in size for stent placement. In a pooled analysis of quantitative angiographic data from the TIMI 4, 10A and 10B trials, only 69% of patients had a proximal reference segment diameter (PRSD) > 2.75 mm, and only 56% of patients had a PRSD > 3.0 mm *(73)*. Given these restraints regarding the adequacy of vessel size, randomized trials of intracoronary stenting may facilitate the enrollment of patients with right coronary artery lesions, and this may result in favorable clinical outcomes in these trials. Thus, adequate reporting of the outcomes in smaller vessels and the number of patients excluded on the basis of reference segment diameter is needed to further evaluate the generalizability of the primary stenting technique.

As stated previously, the rate of agreement between an angiographic core laboratory and clinical centers is only moderate in assessing TIMI grade 3 flow, and it is poor in the assessment of TIMI grade 2 flow (2). Indeed, while the PAMI investigators have reported a 96% rate of TIMI grade 3 flow following stent placement in acute MI (6), the TIMI study group has reported a much lower 83% rate of TIMI grade 3 flow following adjunctive stent placement following thrombolysis (35). As discussed previously, the 3 cardiac cycle definition used by the PAMI group may increase the rates of TIMI grade 3 flow by 10% (10). As suggested by Drs. Topol, Ellis and Califf, the disparity in the rate of TIMI grade 3 flow following primary angioplasty in the PAMI and GUSTO trials may be overstated, and a more objective method of assessing coronary blood flow such as the TIMI frame count may be the preferred method in the assessment of TIMI grade 3 flow in these interventional trials (69). As discussed previously, the TIMI frame count method indicates that stenting does not restore a CTFC of 21 to infarct arteries, highlighting the fact that downstream microvascular resistance remains elevated despite relief of the epicardial stenosis.

When comparing thrombolytic and interventional strategies, it must be kept in mind that a successful revascularization strategy is one that opens arteries both fully and quickly. Fig. 9 shows the relationship between vessel patency and the time after a patient comes to the emergency room. As shown in Fig. 9, the advantage of a thrombolytic regimen is speed, and the advantage of an interventional strategy is a higher rate of full reperfusion. The data for thrombolytic agents is taken from Kawai et al. (74), in which they performed cardiac catheterization at 15, 30, 45, 60, 75, and 90 min after the administration of a thrombolytic agent that is a variant of tPA. By 15 min after thrombolytic administration, 37% of culprit arteries were patent, and by 45 min after thrombolytic administration, 74% were patent (74). This 74% rate of patency is 90% of the treatment effect that is achieved by 90 min (84% patency). If the patient undergoes primary PTCA with a door to balloon time of 120 min (shown by the light grey line in Fig. 9), the GUSTO IIb trial has shown that there will be a 25% spontaneous rate of vessel opening. As shown by the blocked area in Fig. 9, there will be a significant amount of time during which the patency rates for a thrombolytic will exceed that of primary angioplasty. This is what we have termed the early PTCA "flow debt". At 120 min, however, the patency for PTCA will exceed that of thrombolysis. If the primary PTCA is performed quicker, with a door to balloon time of 75 min as shown by the dark grey line in Fig. 9, then by 75 min, the patency rate for the interventional strategy will exceed that for lysis. This is what we would term the late "flow debt" for thrombolysis. Despite the superior patency of the interventional strategy at 75 min, it appears that thrombolytics may open a substantial number of vessels more quickly prior to the performance of the intervention. Thus, while interventional strategies may achieve a higher rate of patency, it appears that thrombolytics have an advantage of opening arteries very quickly in a substantial number of patients. Thus, the challenge for interventional strategies is to achieve even earlier opening than is currently the case, and the challenge for thrombolytic agents remains to achieve higher rates of patency.

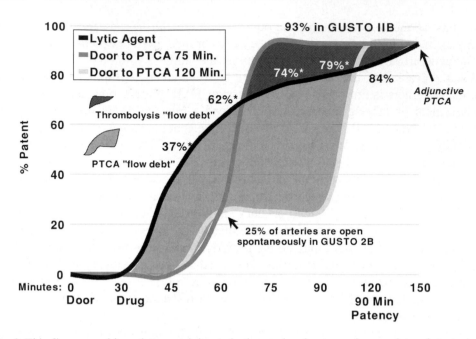

Fig. 9. This figure combines data pertaining to both speed and patency for a variety of strategies. If a patient enters the door at time 0, 30 min later they will be given a thrombolytic (as signified by "drug"). From the data of Kawai et al. *(74)* (shown by the dark black line), 15 min after lytic administration (45 min after presentation) there will be a 37% patency rate, at 30 min after lytic administration a patency rate of 62%, at 45 min a patency rate of 74%, and at 90 min a patency rate of 84%. Thus, speed of reperfusion is the advantage of a thrombolytic agent. If the patient undergoes primary PTCA with a door to balloon time of 120 min (shown by the light grey line), the GUSTO IIb trial has shown that there will be a 25% spontaneous rate of vessel opening, however, as shown by the blocked area, there will be a significant amount of time during which the patency rates for a thrombolytic will exceed that of primary angioplasty. This is what we have termed the early PTCA "flow debt". At 120 min, however, the patency for PTCA will exceed that of thrombolysis. If the primary PTCA is performed more quickly, with a door to balloon time of 75 min as shown by the dark grey line, then by 75 min, the patency rate for the interventional strategy will exceed that for lysis. This is what we would term the late flow debt for thrombolysis. Despite the superior patency of the interventional strategy at 75 min, it appears that thrombolytics may open a substantial number of vessels more quickly prior to the performance of the intervention.

RELATIONSHIP OF CORONARY BLOOD FLOW
TO CLINICAL OUTCOMES

Several thrombolytic trials have demonstrated an important relationship between the different TFGs at 90 min after thrombolysis and clinical outcomes *(50,75–78)*. The GUSTO angiographic substudy involving 1431 patients provided important insight into the mechanism linking TIMI 3 flow with reduced mortality *(50)*. While the rate of TIMI grade 2 flow did not differ significantly among the thrombolytic regimens (25% with SK and subcutaneous heparin regimen, 28% with SK and intravenous [IV] heparin regimen, 27% with tPA and IV heparin regimen, 35% with tPA and SK combination regimen, p = NS), the rate of TIMI 3 flow was highest for the tPA with IV heparin regimen (54% compared to 29% for SK with subcutaneous heparin regimen, 32% for SK with IV heparin regimen, 38% for the tPA and SK combination regimen) *(50)*.

The mortality rate of 7.4% for patients with TIMI 2 flow approximated that of TIMI 0 or 1 flow (mortality 8.9%) (50). In contrast, TIMI 3 flow was associated with nearly half this mortality (4.4%) *(50)*. This trial also linked improved TIMI flow grades with improved LV ejection fractions *(50)*. Thus, it appears that the survival benefit of front-loaded tPA (6.3% mortality as compared with 1% higher mortality with the other regimens in GUSTO) was due, at least in part, to the improved coronary blood flow (both higher patency and TIMI 3 flow rates) in the infarct-related artery with this regimen *(50)*.

The results of GUSTO 1 raise important questions as to the potential mortality benefits that could be accrued by improved flow at 90 min following thrombolysis. An increase in the rate of TIMI 3 flow by 22% (from 32% with SK and IV heparin to 54% with front-loaded tPA) reduced the mortality by 1% (from 7.4% with SK and IV heparin to 6.3% with front-loaded tPA) in this trial *(50)*. If there is a linear relationship, to improve mortality by yet another 1%, the rate of TIMI grade 3 flow in the infarct-related artery would need to improve by another 20% from the current mean value of 60% in all thrombolytic trials to approx 80%. The achievement of 80% rates of TIMI grade 3 flow appears to be a formidable challenge given the previous observation that there was only a 73% rate of TIMI grade 3 flow following primary angioplasty in GUSTO IIb *(68)*.

To further evaluate the relationship between TFGs at 90 min after thrombolysis and clinical outcome, a pooled analysis of all angiographic thrombolytic trials performed to date, involving 5498 patients, is presented in Fig. 10. The 30- to 42-d mortality rate was lowest (3.7%) in patients with TIMI 3 flow at 90 min following thrombolysis and was significantly lower than that in patients with TIMI grade 2 flow (6.1%, $p < 0.0001$) or TIMI grade 0/1 flow (9.3%, $p < 0.0001$) flow (Fig. 10) The mortality rate difference between patients with TIMI 2 and 0/1 flows was also significant ($p = 0.003$) (Fig. 10). It is only with the larger sample size of this pooled data does the distinction between TIMI 0/1 and TIMI 2 flows become apparent. This pooled data analysis reconfirms the superiority of achieving complete reperfusion (i.e., TIMI 3 flow) after thrombolysis. Although TIMI grade 2 flow (partial perfusion) is not equivalent to TIMI 3 flow, it nevertheless confers a significant survival advantage compared with TIMI 0/1 flow and, therefore, should not be regarded as a failure of reperfusion, but rather as intermediate in benefit between TIMI grades 0/1 and 3 flows.

The assessment of the clinical significance of TIMI grade 2 flow has, however, been confounded by the tremendous interobserver variability in the visual assessment of coronary blood flow *(2)*. In addition, TIMI grade 2 flow encompasses a wide spectrum of flows from markedly delayed to near normal flows *(2)*. Finally, the analysis of the relationship between TIMI grade 2 flow to clinical outcomes is confounded by the observation that most of TIMI grade 2 flow is observed in LAD arteries (63%), and most of TIMI grade 3 flow has been observed in right coronary arteries (approx 75%). This statistical colinearity in infarct artery location and coronary blood flow could explain, at least in part, the significant differences in clinical outcomes *(2)*.

The more objective CTFC is also related to clinical outcomes *(79–83)*. In the TIMI 4, 10A and 10B trials, the flow in the infarct-related artery in survivors was significantly faster than in patients who died (CTFCs of $49.5 \pm 32.3, n = 1195$ vs $69.6 \pm 35.4, n = 53$, respectively; $p = 0.0003$) *(79)*. In this data set, mortality increases by 0.7% for every 10-frame rise in CTFC ($p < 0.001$) *(79)*. Thus, the CTFC at 90 min following thrombolysis

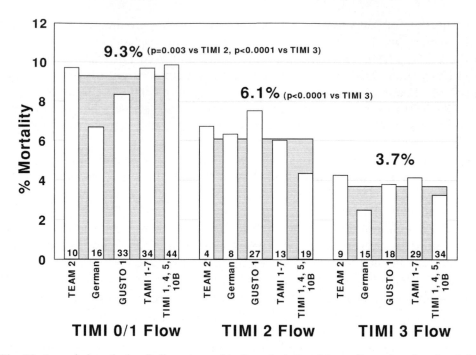

Fig. 10. A pooled analysis of all angiographic thrombolytic trials performed to date involving 5498 patients. The 30- to 42-day mortality rate was lowest (3.7%) in patients with TIMI grade 3 flow at 90 min following thrombolysis, which was significantly lower than that in patients with either TIMI grade 2 flow (6.1%, $p < 0.0001$) or TIMI grade 0/1 flow (9.3%, $p < 0.0001$).

would be required to increase from its current value of 35 frames to approx 21 frames (normal flow) to improve mortality by 1% *(79)*. This is a formidable challenge given that flow in nonculprit arteries at 90 min is approx 30 frames and that culprit CTFCs following adjunctive PTCA are also approx 30 frames.

None of the patients in the TIMI studies who have had a CTFC < 14 (hyperemic or TIMI grade 4 flow) died by 30 d *(79)*. Likewise, in the Randomized Efficacy Study of Tirofibon for Outcomes and Restenosis (RESTORE) trial (tirofiban plus heparin vs heparin alone in patients undergoing angioplasty for acute ischemic syndromes), the postangioplasty culprit flow in survivors was significantly faster than in those patients who died (CTFCs 20.4 ± 16.7, n=1073 vs 33.4 ± 27.1, $n = 10$ respectively; $p = 0.017$) *(80)*. Again, none of the 376 patients with a CTFC < 14 following angioplasty died in this trial, underscoring the fact that within the subgroup of patients with normal flow, there may be further subgroups with even better flow *(80)*. The CTFC in this trial was also related to a lower rate of restenosis, even when post-procedure diameters were corrected for *(81)*. Thus, not only is bigger better, but faster is better also *(81)*.

We have also shown recently that slower flow distal and not proximal to the lesion is related to adverse outcomes following thrombolysis *(79)*. Higher CTFCs are also related to increased myoglobin release *(82)*. We have also shown that other more refined measures of coronary blood flow, such as the QCA velocity, are also related to clinical outcomes *(83)*.

REFERENCES

1. The TIMI Study Group. The Thrombolysis in Myocardial Infarction (TIMI) trial. Phase I findings. N Engl J Med 1985;312:932–936.
2. Gibson CM, Cannon CP, Daley WL, et al. The TIMI frame count: a quantitative method of assessing coronary artery flow. Circulation 1996;93:879–888.
3. Ross AM, Neuhaus KL, Ellis SG. Frequent lack of concordance among core laboratories in assessing TIMI flow grade after reperfusion therapy. Circulation 1995; 92:I-345.
4. Gibson CM, Cannon CP, Murphy SA, et al. Relationship of TIMI myocardial perfusion grade to mortality following thrombolytic administration. Circulation 2000;101:125–130.
5. Gulba DC, Tanswell P, Dechend R, et al. Sixty minute alteplase protocol: a new accelerated recombinant tissue type plasminogen activator regimen for thrombolysis in acute myocardial infarction. J Am Coll Cardiol 1997;30:1611–1617.
6. Stone GW, Brodie BR, Griffin JJ, et al. Prospective, multicenter study of the safety and feasibility of primary stenting in acute myocardial infarction: in-hospital and 30-day results of the PAMI stent pilot trial. J Am Coll Cardiol 1998;31:23–30.
7. Cannon CP, McCabe CII, Diver DJ, et al. Comparison of front-loaded recombinant tissue-type plasminogen activator, anistreplase and combination thrombolytic therapy for acute myocardial infarction: results of the Thrombolysis in Myocardial Infarction (TIMI) 4 trial. J Am Coll Cardiol 1994;24:1602–1610.
8. Cannon CP, McCabe CH, Gibson CM, Ghali M, et al. TNK-tissue plasminogen activator in acute myocardial infarction: results of the thrombolysis in myocardial infarction (TIMI) 10A dose-ranging trial. Circulation 1997;95:351–356.
9. Cannon CP, Gibson CM, McCabe CH, et al. TNK-tissue plasminogen activator compared with front-loaded alteplase in acute myocardial infarction: results of the TIMI 10B trial. Circulation 1998;98:2805–2814.
10. Gibson CM, Ryan K, Sparano A, et al. Methodologic drift in the assessment of TIMI grade 3 flow and its implications with respect to the reporting of angiographic trial results. Am Heart J 1999;137:1179–1184.
11. Ivanc TB, Crowe TD, Balazs EM, Debowey DL, Ellis SG. Reproducibility of the corrected TIMI frame count in angiograms of MI patients receiving thrombolysis. J Am Coll Cardiol 1998; 31:11A.
12. Moliterno D, Antman EM, Ohman M, et al. Concordance between core labs in trial results using TIMI flow grades and frame counts. Circulation 2000;102:II-590.
13. Dodge JT, Nykiel M, Altman J, Hobkirk K, Brennan M, Gibson CM. Coronary artery injection technique: a quantitative in vivo investigation using modern catheters. Cardiac Catheterization Diag, 1998; 44:34–39.
14. Dodge JT, Rizzo M, Nykiel M, et al. Impact of injection rate on the TIMI Frame Count. Am J Cardiol 1998;81:1268–1270.
15. Gibson CM, Ryan KA, Murphy SA, et al. Impaired coronary blood flow in non-culprit arteries in the setting of acute myocardial infarction. J Am Coll Cardiol 1999;34:974–982.
16. Uren NG, Crake T, Lefroy DC, DeSilva R, Davies GJ, Maseri A. Reduced coronary vasodilator function in infarcted and normal myocardium after myocardial infarction. N Engl J Med 1994;331:222–227.
17. Marjorie HJ, Debets JM, Snoeckx LH, Daeman MJ, Smits JF. Time related normalization of maximal coronary flow in isolated perfused hearts of rats with myocardial infarction. Circulation 1996;93:349–355.
18. Wyatt HL, Forrester JS, Luz PL, Diamond GA, Chagrasulis R, Swan HJC. Functional abnormalities in non-occluded regions of myocardium after experimental coronary occlusion. Am J Cardiol 1976; 37:366–372.
19. Corday E, Kaplan L, Brasch J, et al. Consequences of coronary arterial occlusion on remote myocardium: effects of occlusion and reperfusion. Am J Cardiol 1975;36:385–392.
20. Gibson CM, Goel M, Murphy SA, et al. Global impairment of coronary blood flow in the setting of acute coronary syndromes: a RESTORE substudy. Am J Cardiol 2000;86:1375–1377.
21. Ito H, Tomooka T, Sakai N, et al. Lack of myocardial perfusion immediately after successful thrombolysis. A predictor of poor recovery of left ventricular function in anterior myocardial infarction. Circulation 1992;85:1699–1705.

22. Ito H, Maruyama A, Iwakura K, et al. Clinical implications of the no reflow phenomenon. A predictor of complications and left ventricular remodeling in reperfused anterior wall myocardial infarction. Circulation 1996;93:223–228.

23. Gibson CM, Luu L, Kermgard SR, et al. Validation of myocardial perfusion grades using digital subtraction angiography (DSA). Am J Coll Cardiol 2001;37:333A

24. Kloner RA, Ganote CE, Jennings RB. The "no reflow" phenomenon after temporary coronary occlusion in the dog. J Clin Invest 1974;54:1496–1508.

25. Krug A, Du Mesnil de Rochemont W, Korb G. Blood supply to the myocardium after temporary coronary occlusion. Circ Res 1966;19:57–62.

26. Humphrey SM, Gavin JB, Herdson PB. The relationship of ischemic contracture to vascular reperfusion in the isolated rat heart. J Mol Cell Cardiol 1980;12:1397–1406.

27. Forman MB, Puett DW, Virmani R. Endothelial and myocardial injury during ischemia and reperfusion. Pathogenesis and therapeutic implications. J Am Coll Cardiol 1989;13:450–459.

28. Golino P, Ashton JH, Buja M, et al. Local platelet activation causes vasoconstriction of large epicardial arteries in vivo: thromboxane A2 and serotonin are possible mediators. Circulation 1989;79: 154–166.

29. Engler RL, Schmid-Schonbein GW, Pavelec RS. Leucocyte capillary plugging in myocardial ischemia and reperfusion in dog. Am J Pathol 1983;111:98–111.

30. Grech ED, Dodd NJ, Jackson MJ, Morrison WL, Faragher EB, Ramsdole DR. Evidence for free radical generation after primary percutaneous transluminal coronary angioplasty recanalization in acute myocardial infarction. Am J Cardiol 1996;77:122–127.

31. Przyklenk K, Kloner RA. "Reperfusion injury" by oxygen-derived free radicals? Effect of superoxide dismutase plus catalase given at the time of reperfusion on myocardial infarct size, contractile coronary microvasculature, and regional myocardial blood flow. Circ Res 1989;86:86–96.

32. Olafsson B, Forman MB, Puett DW, et al. Reduction of reperfusion injury in the canine preparation by intracoronary adenosine: Importance of the endothelium and the "no reflow" phenomenon. Circulation 1987;76:1135–1145.

33. Campbell CA, Kloner RA, Alker KJ, Braunwald E. Effect of verapamil on infarct size in dogs subjected to coronary artery occlusion with transient reperfusion. J Am Coll Cardiol 1986;8:1169–1174.

34. Taniyama O, Ito H, Iwakura K, et al. Beneficial effect of intracoronary verapamil on microvascular and myocardial salvage in patients with acute myocardial infarction. J Am Coll Cardiol 1997;30:1193–1199.

35. Gibson CM, Murphy SA, Menown I, et al. Determinants of coronary blood flow following thrombolytic administration. J Am Coll Cardiol 1999;34:1403–1412.

36. Dotani I, Dodge TJ, Goel M, et al. Techniques in the angiographic analysis of coronary flow: past, present and future. J Interven Cardiol 1996;9:429–444.

37. Gibson CM, Dodge JT, Rizzo M, et al. Calculating absolute coronary velocity and blood flow by measuring the percutaneous transluminal coronary angioplasty guidewire velocity. Am J Cardiol 1997;80: 1536–1539.

38. Moynihan J, Ryan K, Sparano A, et al. The range of QCA velocities for TIMI grades 2 and 3 flow. J Am Coll Cardiol 1998;31:11A.

39. Kern MJ. A simplified method to measure coronary blood flow velocity in patients: validation and application of a new Judkins-style Doppler tipped angiographic catheter. Am Heart J 1990;120: 1202–1208.

40. Doucette JW, Corl PD, Payne HM, et al. Validation of a Doppler guidewire for intravascular measurement of coronary blood flow velocity. Circulation 1992;85:1899–1906.

41. Kern MJ, Moore JA, Aguirre FV, et al. Determination of angiographic (TIMI Grade) blood flow by intracoronary Doppler flow velocity during acute myocardial infarction. Circulation 1996;94:1545–1552.

42. Goel M, Martin NE, Rizzo MJ, McLean C, Daley WL, Dodge T. Variation in velocity proximal and distal to stenoses following thrombolysis: Implications for angiographic assessment of TIMI flow grades. Circulation 1996;94:I-441.

43. Moynihan JL, Rizzo MJ, Ryan KA, et al. Comparison of angiographically derived velocity to Doppler velocity. Intervention in Acute Coronary Syndromes Course, Allegheny University of the Health Sciences, June 1997.

44. Rentrop KP, Blanke H, Karsch KR, Kreuzer H. Initial experience with transluminal recanalization of the occluded infarct related artery in acute myocardial infarction. Comparison with conventionally treated patients. Clin Cardiol 1979;2:92–102.

45. Khaja F, Walton JA Jr, Brymer JF, et al. Intracoronary fibrinolytic therapy in acute myocardial infarction: report of a prospective randomized trial. N Eng J Med 1983;308:1305–1311.

46. Kennedy JW, Ritchie JL, Davis KB, Fritz JK. Western Washington randomized trial of intracoronary streptokinase in acute myocardial infarction. N Eng J Med 1983;390:1477–1482.
47. The TIMI Study Group. The thrombolysis in myocardial infarction (TIMI) trial. N Engl J Med 1985;31:932-936.
48. Verstraete M, Bernard R, Bory M. Randomized trial of intravenous streptokinase in acute myocardial infarction: report from the European Cooperative Study Group for recombinant tissue type plasminogen activator. Lancet 1985;I:842–847.
49. The GUSTO Investigators. An international randomized trial comparing four thrombolytic strategies for acute myocardial infarction. N Engl J Med 1993;329:673–682.
50. The GUSTO Angiographic Investigators. The effects of tissue plasminogen activator, streptokinase, or both on coronary artery patency, ventricular function, and survival after acute myocardial infarction. N Engl J Med 1993;329:1615–1622.
51. Neuhaus KL, Feuerer W, Jeep-Tebbe S, Niederer W, Vogt A, Tebbe U. Improved thrombolysis with a modified dose regimen of recombinant tissue-type plasminogen activator. J Am Coll Cardiol 1989;14: 1566–1569.
52. Neuhaus KL, von Essen R, Tebbe U, et al. Improved thrombolysis in acute MI with front loaded rt-PA: results of the rt-PA-APSAC patency study (TAPS). J Am Coll Cardiol 1992;19:885–891.
53. Carney RJ, Murphy GA, Brandt TR, et al. Randomized angiographic trial of recombinant tissue-type plasminogen activator (alteplase) in myocardial infarction. J Am Coll Cardiol 1992;20:17–23.
54. Cannon CP, Gibson CM, McCabe CH, et al. TNK tissue plasminogen activator compared with front-loaded alteplase in acute myocardial infarction: results of the TIMI 10B trial. Circulation 1998;98: 2805–2814.
55. Cannon CP, McCabe CH, Diver DJ, et al. Comparison of front-loaded recombinant tissue-type plasminogen activator, anistreplase and combination thrombolytic therapy for acute myocardial infarction: results of the Thrombolysis in Myocardial Infarction (TIMI) 4 trial. J Am Coll Cardiol 1994;24: 1602–1610.
56. Cannon CP, McCabe CH, Henry TD, et al. A pilot trial of recombinant desulfatohirudin compared with heparin in conjunction with tissue-type plasminogen activator and aspirin for acute myocardial infarction: results of the Thrombolysis in Myocardial Infarction (TIMI) 5 trial. J Am Coll Cardiol 1994;24. 1602–1610.
57. Bode C, Smalling RW, Berg G, et al. Randomized comparison of coronary thrombolysis achieved with double-bolus reteplase (recombinant plasminogen activator) and front loaded, accelerated alteplase (recombinant tissue plasminogen activator) in patients with acute myocardial infarction. Circulation 1996;94:891–898.
58. The Global Use Of Strategies To Open Occluded Coronary Arteries (GUSTO III) Investigators. A comparison of reteplase with alteplase for acute MI. N Engl J Med 1997;337:1118–1123.
59. Topol EJ, Califf RM, George BS, et al. A randomized trial of immediate versus delayed elective angioplasty after intravenous tissue plasminogen activator in acute myocardial infarction. N Engl J Med 1987;317:581–588.
60. The TIMI Study Group. Comparison of invasive and conservative strategies after treatment with intravenous tissue plasminogen activator in acute myocardial infarction: results of the Thrombolysis In Myocardial Infarction (TIMI) phase II trial. N Eng J Med 1989;320:618–627.
61. Simoons ML, Col J, Betriu A, et al. Thrombolysis with tissue plasminogen activator in acute myocardial infarction: no additional benefit from immediate percutaneous coronary angioplasty. Lancet 1988;1:197–203.
62. Gibson CM, Schweiger M, Sequiera RF, et al. Outcomes of adjunctive PTCA/stenting for TIMI grade 2 flow following thrombolysis. J Am Coll Cardiol 1998;31:231A.
63. Gibson CM, Dodge JT, Goel M, et al. The PTCA guidewire velocity. A new simple method to measure absolute coronary velocity and blood flow. Am J Cardiol 1997;80:1536–1539.
64. Grines CL, Browne KF, Marco J, et al. A comparison of immediate angioplasty with thrombolytic therapy for acute myocardial infarction. N Engl J Med 1993;328:685–691.
65. DeBoer MJ, Hoorntje JCA, Ottervenger JP, Reiffers S, Suryapranata H, Zijlstra F. Immediate coronary angioplasty versus intravenous streptokinase in acute myocardial infarction: left ventricular ejection fraction, hospital mortality and reinfarction. J Am Coll Cardiol 1994;23:1004–1008.
66. Gibbons RJ, Holmes DR, Reeder GS, Bailey KR, Hopfenspirger MR, Gersh BJ. Immediate angioplasty compared with the administration of a thrombolytic agent followed by conservative treatment for myocardial infarction. N Engl J Med 1993;328:685–691.

67. Ribeiro EE, Silva LA, Carneiro R, et al. Randomized trial of direct coronary angioplasty versus intravenous streptokinase in acute myocardial infarction. J Am Coll Cardiol 1993;22:376–381.
68. The Global Use Of Strategies To Open Occluded Coronary Arteries (GUSTO IIb) Angioplasty Substudy Investigators. A clinical trial comparing primary coronary angioplasty with tissue plasminogen activator for acute myocardial infarction. N Engl J Med 1997;336:1621–1628.
69. Topol EJ, Ellis SG, Califf RM, Betriu A. Primary coronary angioplasty versus thrombolysis. N Engl J Med 1997;336:1168–1170.
70. Weaver WD, Simes RJ, Betriu A, et al. Comparison of primary coronary angioplasty and intravenous thrombolytic therapy for acute myocardial infarction. J Am Med Assoc 1997;278:2093–2098.
71. Ribichini F, Steffino G, Dellavalle A, Meinardi F, Vado A, Feola M, Uslenghi E. Primary angioplasty versus thrombolysis in inferior acute myocardial infarction with anterior ST segment depression: a single center randomized study. J Am Coll Cardiol 1996;27:221A.
72. Garcia E, Elizaga J, Soriano J, et al. Primary angioplasty versus thrombolysis with t-PA in anterior myocardial infarction. J Am Coll Cardiol 1997;29:389A.
73. Gibson CM, Marble SJ, Rizzo MJ, et al. Pooled analysis of primary stenting in acute MI in 1,357 patients. Circulation 1997;96:I-340.
74. Kawai C, Yoshiki Y, Hosoda S, et al. A prospective, randomized, double-blind multicenter trial of a single bolus injection of the novel modified tPA E6010 in the treatment of acute myocardial infarction: comparison with native tPA. J Am Coll Cardiol 1997;29:1447–1453.
75. Vogt A, von Essen R, Tebbe U, Feuerer W, Appel KF, Neuhaus KL. Impact of early perfusion status of the infarct-related artery on short-term mortality after thrombolysis for acute myocardial infarction: retrospective analysis of four German multicenter studies. J Am Coll Cardiol 1993;21:1391–1395.
76. Karagounis L, Sorensen SG, Menlove RL, Moreno F, Anderson JL for the TEAM-2 Investigators. Does Thrombolysis in Myocardial Infarction (TIMI) perfusion grade 2 represent a mostly patent artery or a mostly occluded artery? Enzymatic and electrocardiographic evidence from the TEAM-2 study. J Am Coll Cardiol 1992;19:1–10.
77. Anderson JL, Karagounis LA, Becker LC, Sorensen SG, Menlove RL for the TEAM-3 Investigators. TIMI perfusion grade 3 but not grade 2 results in improved outcome after thrombolysis for myocardial infarction. Ventriculographic, enzymatic, and electrocardiographic evidence from the TEAM-3 study. Circulation 1993;87:1829–1839.
78. Lincoff AM, Ellis SG, Galeana A, et al. Is a coronary artery with TIMI grade 2 flow "patent"? Outcome in the Thrombolysis and Angioplasty in Myocardial Infarction (TAMI) trial. Circulation 1992;86:I-268.
79. Gibson CM, Murphy SA, Rizzo, MJ, et al. The relationship between the TIMI frame count and clinical outcomes following thrombolytic administration. Circulation 1999;99:1945–1950.
80. Gibson CM, Goel M, Cohen DE, et al. Six month angiographic and clinical outcomes following IIb/IIIa blockade with tirofiban. J Am Coll Cardiol 1998;32:28–34.
81. Gibson CM, Rizzo MJ, McLean C, et al. The TIMI frame count and restenosis: faster is better. J Am Coll Cardiol 1997;29:201A.
82. Rizzo MJ, Dotani I, McLean C, et al. Persistent myoglobin elevation is associated with slower flow in patent culprit arteries following successful thrombolysis. J Am Coll Cardiol 1997;29:132A.
83. Gibson CM, Sparano A, Ryan K, et al. A new angiographic method to calculate coronary velocity and its relationship to clinical outcomes after thrombolysis. J Am Coll Cardiol 1998;31:12A.

II   DIAGNOSIS

5

Emergency Department Presentations of Acute Cardiac Ischemia

J. Hector Pope, MD and Harry P. Selker, MD

CONTENTS

INTRODUCTION

In the United States, the leading cause of death is acute myocardial infarction (AMI) with as many as 1.1 million patients having MIs annually *(1)*, about half of whom come to emergency departments (EDs). In addition, nearly twice as many patients come to EDs with unstable angina pectoris (UAP). A confirmed diagnosis of the same will be found in only 25% of patients who present to the ED with symptoms suggestive of acute cardiac ischemia (ACI) *(2)*. Fortunately, the missed diagnosis rate for AMI and UAP in this setting is about 2% each *(3)*. Clinicians have the task of identifying, treating, and hospitalizing (in the appropriate unit) those patients with true ACI, to avoid filling hospital telemetry, stepdown units, and coronary care units (CCUs) with the large majority of patients who do not have ACI.

For many years, the diagnosis of ACI was of more prognostic than therapeutic importance. Over the past three decades, physicians' diagnostic and triage decisions for patients with suspected cardiac ischemia have reflected two tendencies. First, clinicians have tended to admit all patients with even a low suspicion of acute ischemia as the

From: *Contemporary Cardiology: Management of Acute Coronary Syndromes, Second Edition*
Edited by: C. P. Cannon © Humana Press Inc., Totowa, NJ

number of acute interventions for treating dysrhythmias and preventing or limiting the size of AMI has grown. As a result, clinicians have generally admitted nearly all (92–98%) patients presenting with AMI *(4–9)*, as well as nearly 90% of those presenting ACI (i.e., including those with AMI as well as those with UAP) *(6,7,10)*. The conscious strategy of maintaining a high diagnostic sensitivity, i.e., that any error be toward overdiagnosis, has the intended effect: among patients with AMI who seek attention in EDs, the diagnosis is generally missed in 2% *(3)*. High diagnostic sensitivity has been achieved at the cost of admitting many patients who do not have ACI (low diagnostic specificity). Only 18–42% (typically about 30%) of the 1.5 million patients admitted annually to CCUs *(9)* actually experience AMI *(7,12–16)*, and only 50–60% have ACI *(6,7,10,12)*.

Investigating the causes, progression, and treatment of ACI continues to be a national research priority. This research continues to produce substantial progress in the areas of prevention, diagnosis, and treatment of ACI, as well as advances in understanding its molecular and cellular aspects. Over the past decade, there has been a virtual revolution in our understanding of both the pathophysiology and the management of coronary artery disease *(17)*. The conversion of a stable atherosclerotic lesion into a ruptured plaque with thrombosis has provided a unifying hypothesis for the etiology of acute coronary syndromes. Our understanding of ACI has evolved from this thesis. Thus, UAP (i.e., rest angina, new-onset angina, and increasing angina) and AMI are now well appreciated as parts of a "continuum" of myocardial ischemia. The overarching diagnosis of ACI has provided a framework for understanding the pathogenesis, clinical features, treatment, and outcome of patients across the spectrum of myocardial ischemia. For ED triage, the diagnosis of ACI better identifies patients for CCU or telemetry/stepdown unit admission than does the diagnosis of AMI alone. This is partly due to the difficulty in differentiating UA from infarction, and partly by intent, because it helps to reverse ischemia and prevent frank infarction. In fact, for patients with ACI and prolonged chest pain, but without infarction, the medium- and long-term mortality may be as poor or worse than for those who actually have AMI *(3,18)*. In clinical medicine, much research has been focused on the early diagnosis and treatment of ACI. This research has shown that early diagnosis and treatment of UAP is beneficial and may prevent AMI.

For clinical reasons, to promote the optimal use of a limited resource and to reduce unnecessary expenditure, research has focused on improving physician's diagnostic and triage accuracy. However, there remains a need for improved methods of diagnosis that can reduce unnecessary hospitalization for patients incorrectly presumed to have acute ischemia without increasing the number of patients with acute ischemia who are sent home inappropriately *(19,20)*. To this end, and as mandated by Congress, in 1991 the National Heart, Lung, and Blood Institute of the National Institutes of Health instituted the National Heart Attack Alert Program (NHAAP) to focus on issues related to the rapid recognition and response to patients with symptoms and signs of ACI in emergency settings and made reports in 1997 *(19)* and 2000 *(21)* on technologies for identifying ACI in such settings.

This chapter will discuss the state of the art regarding the diagnosis of ACI in the emergency setting by reviewing the role of clinical features, standard electrocardiogram (ECG) analysis, and newer technological adjuncts available to supplement clinical judgment when evaluating patients with suspected ACI, one of emergency medicine's

Table 1
Key Methodologic Issues for Applicability of Study Results

Representative patient sample.
Representative prevalence of ischemic heart disease.
Broad patient inclusion criteria, not just chest pain.
Study setting includes a range of settings.
Diagnostic end point includes unstable angina as well as acute infarction.
Completeness of follow-up.
Follow-up data appropriate and significant.
Validation of findings in generalizable clinical trials.

high-risk presentations. Some methodologic pitfalls inherent in this type of research will be considered first.

METHODOLOGIC ISSUES

Consideration of the specific methods used in studies of patients with ACI is vital when critically reviewing studies of the diagnosis and triage of ED patients with suspected ACI (Table 1). Central to any study is whether the patient sample studied is representative of ED patients seen in actual practice. Also, the positive predictive value (i.e., the proportion of patients that actually have ACI among all those with a positive test or attribute) of a symptom, sign, or test result depends on the prevalence of ischemic heart disease in the study population (22). Thus, the proportion of patients with false-positive results will be higher (and positive predictive value lower) in a population with a low prevalence of ischemia (all ED patients) compared with a population with a high prevalence (CCU patients). Even studies carried out in EDs may not be comparable when ACI prevalence is significantly different. Inclusion criteria can limit studies of ED patients if, for example, only patients with chest pain are studied (23–25) compared with the use of broad entry criteria including multiple symptoms that could be anginal equivalents, such as any chest discomfort, epigastric pain, arm pain, shortness of breath, dizziness, or palpitations (26). Study setting (e.g., urban vs rural or teaching vs community hospital) can also affect the applicability of any findings to various practice settings.

Aside from the study sample, other methodologic issues warrant attention, including the appropriateness of the measured diagnostic end point. Some past ED studies have focused on identifying or predicting only AMI, but identifying UAP is also important for monitoring and early therapy, especially when it is considered that on the order of 9% of patients admitted with new-onset or UAP progress to infarction (27,28). Completeness of follow-up must be considered. Studies with substantial numbers of patients lost to follow-up may have ascertainment bias, especially when the participation rate among eligible patients is not high. Also important is the type of follow-up data collection; for example, the occurrence of AMI will be underestimated if follow-up evaluation does not include biomarker determination results.

Finally, validation of the findings of clinical studies is critical, especially for prediction rules and diagnostic aids: findings may be center- or data-dependent. The ideal validation study is a prospective trial of a finding's or prediction rule's effects on patient care in diverse settings (29).

CLINICAL PRESENTATION

Chest Discomfort

Of all the symptoms for which patients seek emergency medical care, chest pain or chest discomfort is one of the most common and complex. Published reports suggest that up to 7% of visits to the ED involve complaints relating to chest discomfort *(30)*. The complaint of chest discomfort encompasses a wide specturm of conditions that range from insignificant to high risk in terms of threat to the patient's life, including but not limited to ACI (AMI and UAP), thromboembolic disease (pulmonary embolism), aortic dissection, pneumothorax, pneumonia, myocarditis, and pericarditis. Chest discomfort may be perceived as pain or as sensations such as tightness, pressure, or indigestion, or as discomfort most noticeable for its radiation to an adjacent area of the body. Elderly or diabetic patients may have altered ability to specifically localize discomfort. Individuals and cultural groups vary in their expression of pain and ability to communicate with health professionals, so that presentation may range from merely bothersome to cataclysmic for conditions that seem nearly equivalent when objective criteria are matched. The level of discomfort does not necessarily correlate with the severity of illness, making identification of potentially life-threatening conditions very difficult in some patients. Because of the serious nature of many conditions presenting with chest discomfort and the potential for significant reduction in morbidity and mortality with early diagnosis and treatment, clinical policies have been developed to guide clinicians with their initial evaluation of chest discomfort emphasizing prompt triage, assessment, and initiation of therapy *(31)*. Such clinical policies will not be reviewed here other than those that apply to ACI.

It is sometimes difficult to distinguish cardiac from noncardiac chest discomfort, even though chest pain is the hallmark of ACI. Taking the time to elicit the exact character of the sensation (i.e., without prompting the patient if possible) and any pattern of radiation (if present) can be helpful. Typically, the chest discomfort of acute ischemia has a deep visceral character, preventing the patient from localizing the discomfort to a specific region of the chest. It is often described as a pressure-like heavy weight on the chest, a tightness, a constriction about the throat, and/or an aching sensation, not affected by respiration, position, or movement, that comes on gradually, reaches its maximum intensity over a period of 2 to 3 min, and lasts for minutes or longer rather than seconds. In our study of 10,689 ED patients with suspected ACI *(2)* (Tables 2–6, and see Tables 9–11), we found that the 76% of patients presenting with the complaint of chest pain or discomfort (including arm, jaw, or equivalent discomfort) had a 29% incidence of ACI at final diagnosis (10% AMI, 19% UAP); in 69% of patients, chest pain or discomfort was the chief complaint, and this group had a 31% incidence of ACI (10% AMI, 21% UAP); in 21% of patients, it was the only complaint, and this group had a 32% incidence of ACI (9% AMI, 23% UAP). Furthermore, the same study showed that chest pain or discomfort, as chief complaint or presenting symptom, was more frequently associated with a final diagnosis of ACI (88% ACI vs 62% non-ACI; 92% ACI vs 71% non-ACI, respectively; $p = 0.001$). Sharp, stabbing, or positional pain is less likely to represent ischemia *(32)* but does not exclude it: Lee et al. *(33)* found that among ED patients with sharp or stabbing pain, 22% had acute ischemia (5% AMI, 17% UAP). Among those with partially pleuretic pain, 13% had acute ischemia (6% AMI, 7% UAP), and among the group with fully pleuritic pain, none were shown to have acute ischemia.

Table 2
Clinical Presentation Features of ED Patients ($N = 10,689$)

Clinical feature	All (%)
Mean age (yr) (SD)	59 (16)
Gender (% female)	48
Ethnic Group	
White	62
Black	32
Hispanic	5
Other	1
Chief complaint (%)	
Chest pain	69
Presenting symptoms (%)	
Chest pain	76
Shortness of breath	56
Abdominal pain	14
Nausea	28
Vomiting	10
Dizziness	28
Fainting	6
Past medical history (%)	
Diabetes	21
Myocardial infarction	26
Angina pectoris	37
Diagnosis (%)	
Confirmed angina pectoris	15
Confirmed acute infarction	8
Other	77
Mortality (%)	
30-day mortality	2.5

Data from ref 2.

Notably, 7% of the patients whose pain was fully reproduced by palpation nonetheless had acute ischemia (5% AMI, 2% UAP), and 24% of patients with pain partially reproduced with palpation had ischemia (6% AMI, 18% UAP).

Combinations of variables improved discrimination in these patients (24). In patients with sharp or stabbing pain that was also pleuritic, positional, or reproducible by palpation, 3% had UAP and none had AMI. Furthermore, if these same patients had no history of ischemic heart disease, none had acute ischemia. It should be noted that the "partially" and "fully" groups were subjective and small in number.

Exact location of chest pain is not significantly different in patients with or without AMI (34), but chest pain that radiates to the arms or neck does increase the likelihood (35–37). In the study by Sawe (34), which looked at admitted patients with AMI, 71% had pain radiation to arms and/or necks; pain radiated in 39% of patients admitted without AMI. Consistent with the classical description, 33% of patients who proved to have infarction had radiation to both arms, 29% to the left arm only, and 2% to the right arm only (34).

Table 3
Final Diagnosis for Patients by Chief Complaint and Presenting Symtoms[a]

	Final diagnosis ACI (%)			Final diagnosis not ACI				
	No.[b]	AMI	UAP	Total ACI	Non-ACI cardiac	GI	MS	Other	Total Non-ACI
Chief complaints								
Chest pain	7335	10	21	31	33	10	16	11	69
Shortness of breath	1682	6	5	11	53	3	2	31	89
Abdominal pain	47	2	2	4	19	60	2	15	96
Nausea/vomiting	47	11	4	15	23	26	0	36	85
Dizziness/fainting	584	2	2	4	33	5	1	58	96
Presenting symtoms								
Chest pain	8127	10	19	29	34	9	15	13	71
Shortness of breath	5843	8	16	24	41	7	10	18	76
Abdominal pain	1333	6	9	15	29	29	8	18	85
Nausea	2850	10	16	26	32	15	9	18	74
Vomiting	1003	13	10	23	28	19	7	22	77
Dizziness	2599	5	11	16	37	10	10	28	84
Fainting	571	4	2	6	38	3	4	49	94

[a]Abbreviations: ACI, acute cardiac ischemia; AMI, acute myocardial infarction; UAP, unstable angina pectoris; GI, gastrointestinal; MS, musculoskeletal.
[b]Total number of patients with chief complaint or presenting symtom.
Data from ref. 2.

Some investigators feel that a significant number of patients with cardiac ischemia can present with abdominal pain as their chief complaint (23,24). However, in our series of ED patients (2), we found that 14% of study patients had this complaint; this group had a 15% incidence of ACI at final diagnosis (6% AMI, 9% UAP), but <1% complained of abdominal pain as their chief or only complaint and had a 4% incidence of ACI (2% AMI, 2% UAP). In the same study, abdominal pain as a chief complaint or presenting symptom was associated with a higher incidence of a non-ACI final diagnosis (0.6% non-ACI vs 0.1% ACI; 16% non-ACI vs 9% ACI, respectively; $p = 0.001–0.002$). Esophageal reflux and motility disorders are common masqueraders of ACI. In a study of all patients discharged from a CCU with undetermined causes of chest pain, over half had esophageal dysfunction (38). When these patient's presenting complaints were compared with those of patients without ACI, those with esophageal disorders were more likely to complain of a lump in their throat, acid taste, overfullness after eating, a hacking cough, and chest pain that caused awaking at night; they were less likely to report effort-related chest pain, a history of nitroglycerin use, or reliable chest pain relief with its use.

Anginal Pain Equivalents

Dyspnea, present in about one-third of patients with infarction in some series (24,35,39) is the most important angina equivalent. We found in our multicenter ED trial (2) that 16% of patients with suspected ACI presented with a chief complaint of shortness of breath and had an 11% incidence of ACI at final diagnosis (6% AMI, 5% UAP); in 8%,

Table 4

Comparison of Patients With and Without a Final Diagnosis of ACI: Clinical Features, Chief Complaints, Presenting Symptoms, and Past Medical History[a]

| | Total no. | Final diagnosis ACI | | | Final Diagnosis not ACI | | | | | Total vs total non-ACI p value[b] |
		AMI (894)	UAP (1645)	Total ACI (2539)	Non-ACI cardiac (3916)	GI (962)	MS (1268)	Other (2004)	Total non-ACI (8150)	
Clinical features										
Mean age (SD)	(10,689)	65 (13)	65 (13)	65 (13)	58 (17)	56 (15)	49 (14)	58 (16)	57 (16)	0.001[c]
Gender (% Female)	(10,689)	36	47	43	48	52	52	52	50	0.001
Ethnic Group (%)	(10,661)									0.001
White		76	75	75	60	55	45	62	58	
Black		20	21	21	34	38	46	33	36	
Hispanic		3	3	3	5	5	8	5	6	
Other		2	1	1	1	2	1	1	1	
Chief complaints (%)										
Chest pain	(10,689)	82	92	88	62	73	93	40	62	0.001
Shortness of breath	(10,684)	12	5	7	23	5	2	26	18	0.001
Abdominal pain	(10,686)	0.1	0.1	0.1	0.2	2.9	0.1	0.3	0.6	0.002
Nausea/vomiting	(10,685)	0.6	0.1	0.3	0.3	1.2	0	0.8	0.5	0.15
Dizziness/fainting	(10,682)	2	1	1	5	3	0	17	7	0.001
Presenting symptoms (%)										
Chest pain	(10,689)	88	95	92	70	79	96	52	71	0.001
Shortness of breath	(10,493)	56	57	56	62	43	45	55	56	0.5
Abdominal pain	(9,422)	11	8	9	11	43	10	13	16	0.001
Nausea	(10,152)	34	29	30	25	44	22	28	27	0.003
Vomiting	(9,913)	16	7	10	8	21	6	12	10	0.8
Dizziness	(9,222)	17	20	19	29	29	23	40	31	0.001
Fainting	(8,920)	3	1	2	7	2	2	16	8	0.001
Past medical history (%)										
Diabetes	(10,281)	30	32	31	20	18	12	18	18	0.001
History of MI	(10,396)	37	50	45	25	16	12	18	20	0.001
History of angina	(10,328)	43	73	63	33	28	23	24	29	0.001

[a]Abbreviations: see footnote to Table 3.
[b]p values from chi-square test comparing total ACI vs total non-ACI unless noted otherwise.
[c]p value from Student's t-test.
Data from ref. 2.

127

Table 5
Comparison of Patients With and Without a Final Diagnosis of ACI: by Physical Findings[a]

		Final diagnosis ACI			Final Diagnosis not ACI					Total vs total non-ACI p value[b]
	Total no.	AMI (894)	UAP (1645)	Total ACI (2539)	Non-ACI cardiac (3916)	GI (962)	MS (1268)	Other (2004)	Total non-ACI (8150)	
Physical findings										
Pulse										
Median atrial rate	(7,164)	78	75	76	80	75	74	80	78	0.001c
Blood pressure										
Systolic (SBP)										
Median 1st	(10,675)	144	148	147	144	141	138	140	141	0.001c
Median highest	(10,676)	154	154	154	150	148	140	148	149	0.001c
Median lowest	(10,675)	111	125	120	123	128	127	125	124	0.001c
Diastolic										
Median 1st	(10,596)	84	80	82	82	82	80	80	81	0.5c
Median from highest SBP	(10,619)	88	83	84	84	84	82	84	84	0.7c
Median from lowest SBP	(10,557)	69	72	70	73	77	77	74	74	0.001c
Pulse pressures										
Initial	(10,596)	60	64	62	60	59	54	58	58	0.001c
Highest	(10,619)	68	70	70	65	61	58	63	63	0.001c
Lowest	(10,556)	44	51	50	49	50	50	50	50	0.001c
Rales (%)	(10,387)									0.001
None		71	78	76	76	73	93	95	82	
Basilar		19	17	18	18	6	4	14	3	
<Basilar		8	4	6	8	1	1	4	5	
Entire lung		2	0	1	1	0	0	1	1	
S3 gallop (%)	(8,769)	5	2	3	5	1	1	1	3	0.3

[a]Abbreviations: see footnote to Table 3.
[b]p-values from chi-square test comparing total ACI vs total non-ACI unless noted otherwise.
[c]p-value from Wilcoxon rank-sum test.
Data from ref. 2.

128

Table 6
Summary Statistics for Blood Pressure Stratified by Killip Classes (1–3) vs Killip Class 4

| | Final diagnosis AMI | | |
	Killip classes 1–3 (n = 860)	Killip class 4 (n = 34)	p-value[a]
Systolic blood pressure (SBP)			
Median 1st	145	120	0.001
Median highest	155	137	0.001
Median lowest	111.5	90.5	0.001
Diastolic blood pressure			
Median 1st	84	69	0.002
Median from highest SBP	88	80	0.12
Median from lowest SBP	70	60	0.11

[a]p-value from Wilcoxon rank-sum test.
Data from ref. 2.

this was the only complaint, with a 10% incidence of ACI (5% AMI, 5% UAP). However, a final diagnosis of ACI was not more frequent in patients with a presenting symptom of shortness of breath (56% ACI vs 56% non-ACI; $p = 0.5$); as a chief complaint, shortness of breath was more commonly associated with a final diagnosis of non-ACI (18% non-ACI vs 7% ACI; $p = 0.001$), possibly reflecting a high prevalence of patients with lung disease in the study population. Yet, because 4–14% of AMI patients (23,24,26) and 5% of UA patients present only with sudden difficulty breathing (1), ACI should be considered as a cause of unexplained shortness of breath.

Both diaphoresis and vomiting, when associated with chest pain, increase the likelihood of infarction (15,29,35). Diaphoresis occurs in 20–50% of AMI patients (36,40). One study showed that the presence of nausea without vomiting did not discriminate, but vomiting was significantly more frequent in patients who "ruled in" (35). Our study (2) found nausea in 28% of patients with suspected ACI: patients with nausea as a presenting symptom had a 26% incidence of ACI at final diagnosis (10% AMI, 16% UAP); patients with nausea or vomiting as chief complaint (2%) had a 15% incidence of ACI (11% AMI, 4% UAP); and <1% of patients had nausea or vomiting as their only symptom. The same study found vomiting present in 10% of patients: patients with vomiting as a presenting symptom had a 23% incidence of ACI (13% AMI, 10% UAP); patients with vomiting as the chief or only complaint had <1% incidence. Furthermore, we showed that a chief complaint of nausea or vomiting was more frequently associated with a final diagnosis of non-ACI (0.5% non-ACI vs 0.3% ACI; $p = 0.15$), yet a presenting complaint of nausea was more commonly associated with a final diagnosis of ACI (30% ACI vs 27% non-ACI; $p = 0.004$); a presenting complaint of vomiting did not show this association (10% ACI vs 10% non-ACI; $p = 0.7$). In a CCU study, 43% of patients with Q wave infarction but only 4% of patients with non-Q wave infarctions or prolonged angina had vomiting (41).

So-called soft clinical features, such as fatigue, weakness, malaise, dizziness, and "clouding of the mind" are surprisingly frequent, occurring in 11–40% of patients with AMI (29,34,35,39). Prodromal symptoms (those occurring in the preceding days or weeks) are also frequent: 40% report unusual fatigue or weakness, 20–39% dyspnea, 14–20% "emotional changes," 20% change in appearance (i.e., "looked pale"), and 8–10% "dizziness" *(24,39)*. In our series *(2)*, we found that 28% of patients with suspected ACI presented to the ED with dizziness and had a 16% incidence of ACI (5% AMI, 11% UAP); in 5% of study patients dizziness was their primary complaint, with a 4% incidence of ACI (2% AMI, 2% UAP), and in 1% of patients it was their only symptom (2% AMI, 0% UAP). In the same study, dizziness or fainting as a chief complaint were more commonly associated with a final diagnosis of non-ACI (7% non-ACI vs 1% ACI, $p = 0.001$); similarly, dizziness or fainting as presenting symptoms were more frequently associated with final diagnoses of non-ACI (31% non-ACI vs 19% ACI; 8% non-ACI vs 2% ACI; respectively; $p = 0.001$). ECG evaluation is very helpful in low-prevalence patients with these vague complaints.

Atypical Presentations

Few studies address what proportion of ED patients with ACI present with atypical symptoms, a group for whom the diagnostic/triage decision is often most problematic. Among hospitalized patients with AMI, 13–26% had no chest pain or had chief complaints other than chest pain (i.e., dyspnea, extreme fatigue, abdominal discomfort, nausea, or syncope) *(23,24)*. In our ED study of 10,689 patients *(2)* presenting with a wide range of clinical symptoms, we found that 31% of patients with suspected ACI presented without chest pain, with a 26% incidence of ACI at final diagnosis (18% infarction, 8% unstable angina), and had chief complaints other than chest pain (i.e., shortness of breath, abdominal pain, nausea, vomiting, dizziness, or fainting).

Among ED patients, no single atypical symptom is of overwhelming diagnostic importance, although combinations of symptoms can identify high-risk patients who should be admitted regardless of ECG findings. In our series, we ranked atypical presenting symptoms in decreasing order of association with ACI at final diagnosis as follows: nausea (26%), shortness of breath (24%), vomiting (23%), dizziness (16%), abdominal pain (15%), and fainting (65%) *(2)*.

Data from community-based epidemiologic studies *(25,42–44)* suggest that 25–30% of all Q wave infarctions go clinically unrecognized: half were truly silent, and half were associated with atypical symptoms in retrospect *(25,42)*. Because Q waves often resolve (in the Framingham Study), 10% of patients discharged after anterior infarction and 25% of those discharged after inferior infarction lost their Q waves within 2 yr, the true incidence was underestimated *(45)*.

The rate of erroneous discharge from the ED of patients with AMI may be a marker for atypical cases, but such studies are limited by inclusion criteria, small numbers, and lack of complete follow-up. Rates of 2% *(46)*, 4% *(9)*, and as high as 8% *(8)* have been reported. In our ED series *(3)*, patients with suspected ACI reported rates of erroneous discharge of 2% (2.1% AMI, 2.3% UAP). Significantly, the early mortality (30-d) for these "missed " AMIs may be as high as 10–33% *(3,8,9)*.

Finally, in a large ED of patients with unstable angina, Pope et al. *(3)* found that 2.3% were not hospitalized. Over three-fourths of the patients were evaluated by an attending physician, and more than one-fourth by a consulting cardiologist. Although there was disagreement over the interpretation of 16% of the ECGs on subsequent review by an experienced cardiologist, this was not believed to be clinically significant in any of the cases. Given that most of the patients who were not hospitalized had Canadian Cardio-vascular Society class 3 d angina with new symptoms or symptoms that changed within 3 d before presentation, inaccuracies in the clinician assessment of the dynamic nature of anginal symptoms may have contributed to the failure to hospitalize patients with UA.

PAST MEDICAL HISTORY

In addition to the presenting clinical features, the presence of a coronary artery disease risk factor has traditionally been considered diagnostically helpful in the ED setting. Not surprisingly, in our ED series (2), an association was shown between patient having a past history of diabetes mellitus (31% ACI vs 18% non-ACI; $p = 0.001$), MI (45% ACI vs 20% non-ACI; $p = 0.001$), or angina pectoris (63% ACI vs 29% non-ACI; $p = 0.001$), and a final diagnosis of ACI; however, these findings require careful interpretation. From the Framingham Study, it is well known that the risk for developing ischemic heart disease is increased over decades by male gender, advancing age, a smoking habit, hypertension, hypercholesterolemia, glucose intolerance, ECG abnormalities, a type A personality, a sedentary life style, and a family history of early coronary artery disease (24,47,48). Clinicians customarily assess these factors when providing preventive care, because they predict the incidence of future coronary disease. However, coronary risk factors were established to provide an estimate of risk over years. Thus, the Framingham Study showed that hypertension increases the risk of ischemic heart disease 2-fold over 4 yr (25), but only a very small portion of this risk applies to the few hours of the ED patient's acute illness. A patient's report of coronary risk factors is also subject to biases and inaccuracies. This history is presumably less reliable than the methods used to assign risk in longitudinal studies.

Indeed, in a multicenter study, Jayes et al. (49) found that most of the classical coronary risk factors have little predictive value for ACI when used in the ED setting. Except for diabetes and a positive family history in men, no coronary risk factor significantly increased the likelihood that a patient had acute ischemia. Diabetes and family history each confer only about a 2-fold relative risk for acute ischemia in men, whereas chest discomfort, ST-segment abnormalities, and T-wave abnormalities confer relative risks of about 12-, 9-, and 5-fold, respectively. Because these results run counter to the prevailing clinical wisdom, it is possible that physicians who give risk factor history great weight may inappropriately diagnose and/or triage ED patients, an issue that deserves further attention and investigation.

Finally, a past history of medication use for coronary disease increases the likelihood that the current chest pain is ACI. Not surprisingly, in the Boston City Hospital and the multicenter predictive instrument trials, a history of nitroglycerin use was found to be one of the most powerful predictors of ACI (6). Nonetheless, nitrates can cause dramatic relief of chest pain from esophageal spasms (50), and thus, the details of the history must be noted carefully.

PHYSICAL EXAMINATION

The physical examination is generally not very helpful in diagnosing ACI when compared with the value of historical data and ECG findings, except when it points to an alternate process. On the other hand, clinicians must not be lulled into a sense of security by chest pain that is partially or fully reproduced by palpation, because 11% may have infarction or unstable angina *(26)*. Table 5 shows a comparison of patients with and without a final diagnosis of ACI by physical findings from our series *(2)*. We found the pulse rate to be lower in patients with a final diagnosis of ACI vs those with a final diagnosis of non-ACI ($p = 0.02$), but this difference was not considered clinically significant.

Pulse rate observation in isolation appeared to be generally not helpful in ACI identification. First, the patient's pulse rate could be slowed by the presence of β-blockers as part of a prior treatment regime or by coincident vagal stimulation from ACI (i.e., reflex bradycardia and vasodepressor effects associated with inferoposterior wall ACI) or diagnostic/therapeutic procedures in the ED (i.e., phlebotomy, intravenous access). Second, the patient's pulse may be increased by adrenergic excess from just having to come to the ED and everything that accompanies such a visit, in addition to the adrenergic excess (i.e., tachycardia and increased peripheral vascular resistance) associated with possible on-going ACI.

In our series of ED patients *(2)*, median first and highest systolic blood pressures (SBP) were higher in patients with a final diagnosis of ACI. This suggested to us that the adrenergic excess associated with ACI might be greater than that associated with non-ACI diagnoses. However, to use this hypothesis as a predictive factor, clinicians must have some idea of their patient's baseline blood pressure, which is not the case in most ED evaluations. Thus, the usefulness of this observation may be limited.

In the same series *(2)*, in addition to the effect of adrenergic release during acute ischemia, the higher initial and highest pulse pressures found in patients with a final diagnosis of ACI may also reflect the lower compliance of the ischemic left ventricle. Of relevance to those who are candidates for thrombolytic therapy, excess pulse blood pressure (the extent to which a patient's pulse pressure exceeded 40 mmHg for patients with SBP of >120 mmHg) places these patients at increased risk of thrombolysis-related intracranial hemorrhage *(29)*.

We discovered that median first, median highest, and median lowest SBPs of patients with AMI, who subsequently were classified as Killip class 4 (cardiogenic shock), were above the threshold of this classification (SBP ≤ 90 mmHg) for these three blood pressure observations. This suggests that the adrenergic excess associated with ACI may be greater than that associated with non-ACI diagnoses. More importantly, although the number of such patients in this analysis was relatively small, it did suggest that patients with ACI can present with apparently "normal" blood pressures and can go on to develop cardiogenic shock.

Abnormal vital signs and certain combinations of these have been shown to be critically important observations in clinical outcome prediction. The reported probability of infarction decreases with a normal respiratory rate *(35)* and increases with diaphoresis *(13)*, but other signs mainly help identify high-risk patients with infarction *(51)*. In the predictive instrument for AMI mortality proposed by Selker et al. *(52)*, blood pressure, pulse, and their interaction figured prominently in three of the six clinical variables used to develop the prediction instrument.

In our series *(2)*, rales (of any degree), but not S3 gallops, were more frequently seen in patients with a final diagnosis of ACI. This finding is not surprising, as several clinical syndromes of pump failure can complicate ACI. Our failure to find association between an S3 gallop rhythm and ACI at final diagnosis is surprising, but it may have

Table 7
Limitations of Electrocardiography

Single brief sample
Lack of perfect detection
Baseline patterns
Interpretation
Clinical context
Imperfect sensitivity and specificity

to do with a failure to document this finding consistently in the medical record on the part of the ED physicians at study sites.

ELECTROCARDIOGRAM
Standard 12-Lead ECG

A complete summary of evidence related to the diagnostic utility of the standard ECG was recently published *(19,21)*, and this background will not be repeated here. However, the NHAAP's Working Group on Evaluation of Technologies for Identifying ACI *(21)* found that most studies evaluated the accuracy of the technologies and only a few evaluated the clinical impact of routine use. Furthermore, they concluded that although the standard ECG is a safe, readily available, and inexpensive technology with a relatively high sensitivity for AMI, it is not highly sensitive or specific for ACI. However, the ECG remains an integral part of the evaluation of patients with chest pain and the Working Group recommended that it remain the standard of care for evaluating patients with chest pain in the ED.

The ECG provides essential information when the diagnosis is not obvious by symptoms alone *(53)*, despite one study noting that the results of the ECG infrequently changed triage decision based on initial clinical impressions *(54)*. The generally dominant weights given to ECG variables in mathematical models for predicting ACI substantiate this impression *(6,7,10,15,16)*. Moreover, the initial ECG is increasingly important in intra-hospital triage, because of its value in predicting complications of AMI *(55–57)*.

Despite its central role in the evaluation of patients with suspected ACI, there are fundamental limitations in the standard ECG (Table 7). First, it is a single brief sample of the whole picture of the changing supply and demand characteristics of unstable ischemic syndromes. If a patient with UAP is temporarily pain free when the ECG is obtained, the resulting tracing may poorly represent the patient's ischemic myocardium.

Second, 12-lead electrocardiography is limited by its lack of perfect detection *(58)*. Small areas of ischemia or infarction may not be detected; conventional leads do not examine satisfactorily the right ventricle *(59)* or posterior basal or lateral walls well (i.e., AMIs in the distribution of the circumflex artery) *(60,61)*.

Third, some ECG baseline patterns make interpretation difficult or impossible including prior Q waves, early repolarization variant, left ventricular hypertrophy, bundle-branch block, and dysrhythmias *(62)*. Lee et al. *(9)* demonstrated that when the current ECG shows ischemic findings, availability of a prior comparison ECG improved triage.

Fourth, ECG waveforms are frequently difficult to interpret causing disagreement among readers, so-called missed ischemia. In a study of AMI patients sent home, ECGs tended to show ischemia or infarction not known to be old, with 23% of the missed diagnoses owing to misread ECGs *(8)*. Jayes et al. *(63)* compared ED physician readings of ECGs with formal interpretations by expert electrocardiographers and calculated sensitivities of 0.59 and 0.64 and specificities of 0.86 and 0.83 for ST-segment and T-wave abnormalities, respectively. Both McCarthy et al. *(18)* and a review of litigation in missed AMI cases *(64)* emphasized this factor of incorrect ECG interpretation. In the largest study to date of ACI in the ED, Pope et al. *(3)* found that although the rate of missed diagnoses of ACI (2.1% AMI, 2.3% UAP) was low, there was a small but important incidence of failure by the ED clinician to detect ST-segment elevations of 1 to 2 mm in the ECGs of patients with myocardial infarction (11%). Correct ECG interpretation by ED physicians is doubly important today because of the need to use interventions such as thrombolytic agents and percutaneous coronary angioplasty appropriately in ACI.

Fifth, the implications of the ECG findings must be interpreted in their clinical context, a process done intuitively by clinicians and formally stated in Bayesian analysis. When symptoms alone strongly suggest ischemia, a normal or minimally abnormal ECG will not substantially decrease the probability of ischemia. Conversely, when the presentation is inconsistent with acute ischemia, an abnormal ECG, unless diagnostic abnormalities are present, will only modestly increase the likelihood of ischemia. Bayes' rule tells us that the ECG will have the greatest impact when symptoms are equivocal *(65)*. This is illustrated by Table 8, which shows the probability of acute ischemia for combinations of history and ECG findings among 2801 emergency patients *(66)*; this formed the basis for the Acute Ischemic Heart Disease Predictive Instrument *(6)*.

Finally, the ECG suffers from imperfect sensitivity and specificity for ACI. When interpreted according to liberal criteria for MI (i.e., ECGs that show any of the following as positive for AMI: nonspecific ST-segment or T-wave changes abnormal but not diagnostic of ischemia; ischemia, strain, or infarction, but changes known to be old; ischemia or strain not known to be old; and probable AMI), the ECG operates with relatively high (but not perfect) sensitivity (99%) for AMI, at the cost of low specificity (23%; positive predictive value 21%; negative predictive value 99%). Conversely, when interpreted according to stringent criteria for AMI (only ECGs that show probable AMI), sensitivity (61%) drops and specificity equals 95% (positive predictive value 73%; negative predictive value, 92%) *(67)*.

Despite its usefulness, the ECG is insufficiently sensitive to make the diagnosis of ACI consistently. The ECG should not be relied on to make the diagnosis, but rather should be included with history and physical examination characteristics to identify patients who appear to have a high risk for ACI (i.e., a supplement to, rather than a substitute for, physician judgment). In "rule out AMI" patients, a negative ECG carries an improved short-term prognosis *(55,68–71)*. Providing the interpreter with old tracings would intuitively seem to be of value because baseline abnormalities make current evaluation difficult, yet, Rubenstein and Greenfield *(72)*, in a study of 236 patients presenting to EDs with the complaint of chest pain, found that only a small proportion might have benefited from having a previous baseline ECG available (5% might have avoided unnecessary admission). Furthermore, there was no patient for whom a baseline ECG would have aided in avoiding an inappropriate discharge. ECG sampling

Table 8
The Original ACI Predictive Intrument's Probabilities of Acute Ischemia for ED Patients

Question: Chest pain or pressure or left arm pain?	ECG Abnormalities (%)					
	ST0 T0	ST— T0	ST0 ↑↑↓	STT↑↓ T0	ST— ↑↑↓	ST↑↓ T↑↓
Answer: Yes, chief complaint.						
History						
No heart attack *and* no NTG use	19	35	42	54	62	70
Either heart attack *or* NTG use *(not both)*	27	46	53	64	73	85
Both heart attack *and* NTG use	37	58	65	75	80	90
Answer: Yes, but not chief complaint.						
History						
No heart attack *and* no NTG use	10	21	26	36	45	64
Either heart attack *or* NTG use (*not both*)	16	29	36	48	56	74
Both heart attack *and* NTG use	22	40	47	59	67	82
Answer No.						
History						
No heart attack *and no* NTG use	4	9	12	17	23	39
Either heart attack *or* NTG use *(not both)*	6	14	17	25	32	51
Both heart attack *and* NTG use	10	20	25	35	43	62

Key to ECG abnormalities (must be in two loads, excluding aVR); ST—, ST-segment "straightening;" ST↑↓, ST segment elevated at least 1 mm or depressed at least 1 mm; T↑↓, T wave "hyperacute" (>50% of R wave) or inverted at least 1 mm; ST0/T0, above-specified changes absent.

Directions: To determine a given patient's probability of acute ischemia, start by answering the questions at the top of the chart about the presence of chest pain and whether or not it is the chief complaint. This will lead to one of the three large boxes or probability values. Under the History heading are questions regarding history of heart attack or nitroglycerine (NTG) use. Choose the row that corresponds to the patient's report of none, one, or both of these historical features. Then to find the specific probability value, move across the appropriate row to the column corresponding to the ECG ST-segment and T-wave changes for the given patient. For example, for a patient with a chief complaint of chest pain, no history of heart attack or nitroglycerine use, and 1 mm of ST-segment depression and T-wave inversion, the probability of true ACI would be 78%. (Reproduced from McCarthy BD, Wong JB, Selker HP: Detecting acute cardiac ischemia in the emergency department: A review of the literature. *J Gen Intern Med* 5:365–373. Reprinted with permission of Blackwell Science, Incorporated.

Note: Specific definitions of clinical features (questions) for original ACI predictive intrument are modified for use in this chart.

should be periodic, not just static. The pitfalls of not ordering ECGs in younger, atypical patients and of misinterpretation should be anticipated. Finally, clinicians should not be reluctant to obtain a second opinion, by fax transmission if necessary, for difficult tracings (Table 9).

ST-Segment and T-Wave Abnormalities

ST-segment and T-wave abnormalities are the sine quo non of ECG diagnosis of ACI. Numerous studies *(58,71,73)* have found that 65–85% of CCU patients with ST-segment elevation alone will have had an infarction. Other investigators found that if both Q waves and ST-segment elevation were present, 82–94% actually sustained AMI *(58)*. However, it must be remembered that ST-segment elevation can occur in the absence of ischemia (i.e., "early repolarization" variant, pericarditis, left ventricular hypertrophy,

Table 9
Comparison of Patients With and Without Electrocardiographic (ECG) Data

Clinical Feature (no.)	With ECG data (%) (n = 8545)	Without ECG data (%) (n = 2144)	p value
Mean age (yr) (SD) (10,689)	58.6 (16.1)	58.9 (16.0)	0.4
Gender (% female) (10,689)	49	47	0.12
Ethic Group (10,661)			0.001
White	62	61	
Black	33	31	
Hispanic	4	7	
Other	1	1	
Presenting Symptoms			
Chest pain (10,689)	76	77	0.2
Shortness of breath (10,493)	56	55	0.8
Past medical history			
Diabetes (10,281)	21	21	0.7
Myocardial infarction (10,396)	26	26	0.5
Angina pectoris (10,328)	36	39	0.010
Diagnosis (10,689)			0.013
Confirmed angina pectoris	15	15	
Confirmed acute infarction	8	10	
Other			
Mortality (10,116)			
30-d mortality	2.4	2.8	

Data from ref. 2.

and previous infarction even in the absence of a ventricular aneurysm) (74). Conversely, we have shown in our series (2) that a large percentage of patients with ACI (20% AMI, 37% UAP) can present with initial normal ECGs.

In our study of ED patients with suspected ACI (2) (Table 10), we found that ST-segment elevation of either 1 to 2 mm or 2+ mm was more frequently associated with a final diagnosis of ACI (9% ACI vs 7% non-ACI; 5% ACI vs 1% non-ACI, respectively; $p = 0.001$). A full 30% of patients with ST-segment elevation of 1 mm or greater had a final diagnosis of AMI. In addition, in a study of missed diagnosis of ACI in the ED (3), Pope at al. found a small but important incidence of failure by the ED clinician to detect ST-segment elevations of 1 to 2 mm in the electrocardiograms of patients with AMI (11%). This incidence represents an important and potentially preventable contribution to the failure to admit such patients.

Table 10
Comparison of Patients With and Without a Final Diagnosis of ACI by Electrocardiographic Findings[a]

	Total no.	Final diagnosis ACI			Final Diagnosis not ACI					Total vs total non-ACI p value[b]
		AMI (894)	UAP (1645)	Total ACI (2559)	Non-ACI cardiac (3916)	GI (262)	MS (1268)	Other (2004)	Total non-ACI (8150)	
ST-segment	(8,545)									0.001
Normal		42	74	63	78	85	83	83	81	
Elevated 1–2 mm		16	6	9	8	8	8	6	7	
Elevated 2+ mm		14	1	5	1	0	1	1	1	
Depressed 0.5–1 mm		14	12	12	9	5	3	8	7	
Depressed 1–2 mm		10	6	8	2	1	1	2	3	
Depressed 2+ mm		5	1	2	1	0	0	0	0	
T-waves	(8,545)									0.001
Normal		38	48	44	57	66	73	61	61	
Flat		14	20	18	20	21	17	20	20	
Inverted 1–5 mm		37	30	32	21	13	9	17	17	
Inverted 5+ mm		2	1	1	0	0	0	0	0	
Elevated		10	1	4	1	1	1	1	1	
Q waves	(8,545)	29	23	25	13	8	6	11	11	0.001
Normal ST/T, no Q	(8,545)	20	37	31	46	55	63	50	51	0.001

[a]Abbreviation; see footnote to Table 3.
[b]p values from chi-square test comparing total ACI vs total non-ACI, unless noted otherwise.
Data from ref. 2.

137

ST-segment depression usually indicates "subendocardial ischemia." If these abnormalities are new, persistent, and marked, the likelihood of AMI increases. About 50–67% of admitted patients with new or presumed new isolated ST-segment depression have infarctions (59,73); even more patients have probable ischemia. We found that all degrees of ST-segment depression (0.5, 1, 1 to 2, and 2+ mm) were more commonly associated with a final diagnosis of ACI (12% ACI vs 7% non-ACI; 8% ACI vs 3% non-ACI; 2% ACI vs 0% non-ACI, respectively; $p = 0.001$). A full 19% of patients with ST-segment depression of at least 0.5 mm or greater had a final diagnosis of AMI. It should also be remembered that ST-segment depression may occur in non-ischemic settings, including patients who are hyperventilating, those taking digitalis, those with hypokalemia, and those with left ventricular strain (without voltage criteria) (74).

Inverted T-waves may reflect acute ischemia; one study showed that isolated T-wave inversion occurred in 10% of CCU admissions, of whom 22% had AMI (75). T-wave changes may reflect prior myocardial damage or left ventricular strain (74). Our study (2) found that certain T-wave patterns (inverted 1–5 mm, inverted 5+ mm, or elevated) were more frequently associated with a final diagnosis of ACI (32% ACI vs 17% non-ACI; 1% ACI vs 0% non-ACI; 4% ACI vs 1% non-ACI, respectively; $p = 0.001$). Flattened T-waves did not have the same associated with an ACI final diagnosis (18% ACI vs 20% non-ACI; $p = 0.001$). Furthermore, 39% of patients with inverted T-waves of at least 1 mm or greater had a final diagnosis of AMI.

Q Waves

Q waves are diagnostic of myocardial infarction, but what is the age of the Q wave? In the MILIS study of admitted CCU patients, isolated new or presumed new inferior or anterior Q waves were associated with acute infarction in 51 and 77% of patients, respectively (58). Other findings of the MILIS study should be kept in mind: 12% of healthy young men have inferior Q waves (74–76), pathologic Q waves can be from a previously unrecognized infarction and can mask new same-territory ischemia; Q waves alone do not identify ACI and are rarely the sole manifestation of AMI (6% in the MILIS study); and, finally, infarction can occur in the absence of Q waves (77,78). In our ED study (2), we showed that Q waves were more commonly associated with a final diagnosis of ACI (25% ACI vs 11% non-ACI; $p = 0.001$) and that 29% of patients with Q waves present on their ECGs had a final diagnosis of AMI.

Nondiagnostic ECG Patterns

"Nondiagnostic" ST-segment and T-wave abnormalities may be defined as follows: not having ≥1 mm (0.1 mV) ST-segment elevation or depression in two contiguous leads, not having new T-wave inversion in two contiguous leads, absence of significant Q waves (>1 mm deep and 0.3 s duration) in two contiguous leads, not having second- or third-degree heart block, and not having a new conduction abnormality (bundle-branch block, etc.). These are the most difficult to interpret and can result in overdiagnosis (no comparison ECG available) and underdiagnosis (baseline abnormality obscuration of ischemia) (79). Lee et al. (33) found that emergency patients with chest pain and nondiagnostic ECG abnormalities had a low risk of AMI but a significant risk of ACI. Pope et al. (3) found that 53% of ED patients with a missed diagnosis of AMI had normal or nondiagnostic electrocardiograms, as did 62% of patients with a missed diagnosis of unstable angina.

Normal ECG

Among ED patients with normal ECGs (i.e., lacking Q waves, primary ST-segment and T-wave abnormalities, and criteria for nondiagnostic abnormalities), 1 *(33)* to 6% *(79)* have been found to have AMI. Among admitted patients with normal ECGs, 6–21% had AMI *(12,75,78–80)*. Of patients discharged home with a normal ECG, only 1% had acute infarction *(74)*. Patients with a normal ECG and a suggestive clinical presentation still have a significant risk of ACI, especially if the ECG was obtained when the patient was pain free. On the other hand, a truly normal ECG in a patient unlikely to have acute ischemia provides strong evidence against ACI *(33)*.

In our series, patients with normal ST-segment and T-waves and no Q waves more commonly had a final diagnosis of non-ACI, yet 20% of these patients had AMI and 37% had UAP at final diagnosis.

Prehospital 12-Lead ECG

The NHAAP Working Group on Evaluation of Technologies for Identifying ACI *(21)* found that the diagnostic accuracy of prehospital ECG for AMI and ACI, as expected, is similar to that of the standard 12-lead ECG, which is the standard of care in the management of patients suspected of having ACI (Tables 11 and 12). The accumulation of evidence is substantial in both the total sample size and quality, and the data have been gathered from patient populations with few exclusion criteria. The evidence shows that obtaining a prehospital ECG does not prolong time in the field or delay transport to the ED. In addition, prehospital ECG-guided thrombolytic therapy can be administered 45 min to 1 h earlier than hospital-based thrombolytics. Prehospital thrombolysis has a modest but significant impact on early mortality, with approx 60 patients requiring prehospital treatment compared to hospital thrombolysis to save one additional life in the short term. Short-term, beneficial effects of thrombolysis on left ventricular ejection fraction have not been reported in randomized trials. The long-term survival benefits of prehospital thrombolysis remain uncertain. Although it has promise, the Working Group *(17a)* believed that its best use would be in areas with long emergency medical system (EMS) transport times and perhaps in conjunction with prehospital thrombolytic therapy. Its routine use was not recommended.

Continuous ECG/Serial ECG

The Working Group *(17a)* found that only two studies have evaluated the test performance of continuous/serial 12-lead ECG in the ED, but there was no clinical impact study (Tables 11 and 12). One study by Gibler et al. *(84)* included a large retrospective population of 1010 participating in a 9-h protocol. The "serial ECG" consisted of a 20-s interval between readings. The second study *(77)* included patients from a veterans' hospital in which two ECGs were taken 4 h apart. The prevalences of ACI in these studies were very different (4 and 40%, respectively) given the low-risk populations. The sensitivity for ACI was low (21 and 25%, respectively) and the specificity was high (92 and 99%, respectively). With the limitations and the varied source of data, a conclusion about the utility of this technology cannot be drawn at this time.

Nonstandard Leads ECG

The data on the diagnostic performance of nonstandard lead ECG from the four studies reported vary too much to draw any firm conclusion *(21)*. The studies used 15, 18, 22, and 24 leads and were conducted with selected patients for admission (Tables 11 and 12). The prevalence is reflective of this selective population: it ranged between 22 and 65% for AMI. There are no clinical impact studies on nonstandard ECGs.

Exercise Stress ECG

The data on the diagnostic performance of exercise stress testing to detect ACI in the ED are limited to only two studies *(83,84)* (Table 11 and 12).The overall data include a small sample size of a low-risk population. Although the diagnostic performance is encouraging, it would be premature to make conclusions regarding this technology until additional high-quality studies are conducted.

There are also limited data on the clinical impact of exercise testing for ACI. Two studies *(85,86)* had no cardiac events and included very small sample sizes, 28 and 35, respectively. Adding a third study *(83)*, these investigations comprised a total of only 272 subjects and are of low methodological quality; the clinical impact of this technology is unclear.

BIOCHEMICAL MARKERS OF MYOCARDIAL NECROSIS

Creatine Kinase, Single and Serial Measurements

The amount of evidence on creatine kinase (CK) as a single test administered at presentation to patients in the ED is large *(21)* (Tables 11 and 12). The evidence suggests that the sensitivity of a single CK reading for AMI is low (36%), and specificity is modest (88%). Limited evidence suggests that the sensitivity of the test depends on the duration of the patient's symptoms; sensitivity increases with longer symptom duration. Test performance across studies did not appear to vary by type of hospital, inclusion criteria, AMI prevalence, or test threshold.

Only two studies have evaluated serial CK testing *(87, 88)*. Both used broad inclusion criteria, but enrolled populations in which the prevalence of AMI was moderate to high. Test sensitivity was high (95–99%) in serial tests performed over about 15 h after presentation to the ED (or from the onset of symptoms), but was only modest (69%) in the one study that drew serial samples for 4 h. Test specificity was modest in both studies (68 and 84%).

As a single test, CK is insensitive and only modestly specific for AMI. Serial testing appears to have higher sensitivity, although the specificity remains modest. However, the evidence is insufficient to evaluate serial CK measurements over a short time. Because high serum CK levels represent infarcted myocardium, CK has not been evaluated for diagnosing ACI in the ED. There are no clinical impact studies for CK.

Creatine Kinase Subunit, Single and Serial Measurements

As is the case with CK, the total sample size and number of studies on a single creatine kinase subunit (CK-MB) measurement at presentation to the ED are large *(21)* (Tables 11 and 12). The evidence suggests that the sensitivity of single CK-MB for AMI is low (47%), although specificity is high (96%). Studies reported a broad range of sensitivity for diagnosing AMI. Again, as is the case for CK, limited evidence suggests that the sensitivity of CK-MB depends on the duration of the patient's symptoms; sensitivity increases with longer symptom duration. In general, studies reported a narrow range (92–99%) of test specificity. Test performance across studies did not appear to vary by type of hospital, inclusion criteria, AMI prevalence, or test threshold.

The total sample size and number of studies of serial tests for CK-MB in the ED setting are large. Overall, serial testing has a modest sensitivity (87%) and high specificity (96%) for AMI. However, test sensitivity is strongly related to the timing of serial testing. All studies that performed serial testing for at least 4 h after presentation to the ED (or until at least 8 h after symptom onset) found test sensitivity to be greater than 90%. Conversely, all studies that performed serial testing to, at most, 3 h found test sensitivity to be less than 90%. The pooled sensitivity for serial testing to at least 4 h is 96%; pooled sensitivity for serial testing until 3 h is only 81%. In general, test specificity was in a narrow range across studies and was above 90%.

CK-MB as a single test is only modestly sensitive and specific for AMI; however, serial testing performed over 4–9 h is highly sensitive and highly specific. Because serum CK MB levels represent infarcted myocardium, CK-MB has not been tested for diagnosing ACI in the ED. There are no clinical impact studies for CK-MB.

Troponin T and Troponin I

The evidence for the diagnostic performance of troponin T is substantial in diagnosing AMI but rather limited in diagnosing ACI *(21)* (Tables 11 and 12). Data for troponin I are limited, but its performance is similar to that of troponin T. The sensitivity of presentation troponin T for diagnosing AMI in the ED is poor, but improves substantially if serial measurements are obtained for up to 6 h after ED presentation. Most likely, the sensitivity is better for patients who have had symptoms for longer periods of time. The specificity of troponin T for AMI is in the range of 90%.

Myoglobin

The diagnostic performance of myoglobin has been well studied for diagnosing AMI, but not for diagnosing ACI *(21)* (Table 11 and 12). The sensitivity of myoglobin for diagnosing AMI in the ED is poor when a single initial measurement is obtained, but sensitivity improves greatly if a second measurement is obtained 2–4 h after the first one. However, the sensitivity for patients only recently symptomatic is poor, and a second measurement in 2–4 h may still not be sufficiently sensitive to be useful. Specificity is very good, but not excellent, depending on the extent to which other reasons for elevated myoglobin are excluded *a priori*. A doubling of myoglobin levels as soon as 1 to 2 h after the initial measurement is almost perfectly sensitive for AMI.

The evidence suggests that a normal myoglobin value 2 h after presentation may be used safely to rule out AMI. A doubling of myoglobin as early as 1–2 h after the baseline measurement establishes a diagnosis of AMI. A small study *(89)* suggests that normal myoglobin and CK-MB values 2 h after presentation completely rule out AMI. The incremental value of CK-MB compared to myoglobin alone cannot be evaluated given the small sample sizes. In a much larger study, Kontos *(90)* found no advantage for myoglobin over baseline and 3-h CK-MB values.

Table 11
Summary of Test Performance Studies of Diagnostic Technologies for ACS in the ED

Technology	Condition studied	Number of studies (subjects)	Population category of studies[a]	Studies prevalence range %	Sensitivity[b] (95% CI) %	Specificity[b] (95% CI) %	Diagnostic odds ratio[b] (95% CI)	Overall quality of evidence
Prehospital ECG	ACI	5 (4311)	I/II	46–92	76 (54–89)	88 (67–96)	23 (6.3–85)	B
	AMI	10 (4481)	I/II	14–51	68 (59–76)	97 (89–92)	104 (48–224)	B
Continuous/serial ECG	ACI	2 (1271)	III	4–40	21–25[c]	92–99[c]	3.8–45[c]	C
	AMI	1 (261)	III	11	39[c]	88[c]	4.9[c]	B
Nonstandard lead ECG	ACI	1 (52)	IV	48	96[c]	41[c]	17[c]	B
	AMI	4 (897)	IV	22–65	59–83[c]	76–93[c]	10–19[c]	B
Exercise stress ECG	ACI	2 (312)	III	6–10	70–100[c]	82–93[c]	11–320[d]	B
CK (presentation)	AMI	12 (3195)	I/II/III/IV	7–41	37 (31–44)	87 (80–91)	3.9 (2.7–5.7)	B/C
CK (serial)	AMI	2 (786)	I	26–43	69–99[c]	68–84[c]	12–220[c]	C
CK-MB (presentation)	ACI	1 (1042)	III	20	23[c]	96[c]	7.2[c]	C
	AMI	19 (6425)	I/II/III/IV	6–42	42 (36–48)	97 (95–98)	25 (18–36)	B
CK-MB (serial)	ACI	1 (1042)	III	20	31[c]	95[c]	8.5[c]	C
	AMI	14 (11,625)	I/II/III/IV	1–43	79 (71–86)	96 (95–97)	140 (65–310)	B
Myoglobin (presentation)	AMI	18 (4172)	I/II/IV	6–62	49 (43–55)	91 (87–94)	11 (8.0–15)	B/C
Myoglobin (serial)	AMI	10 (1277)	I/II/IV	11–41	89 (80–94)	87 (80–92)	84 (44–160)	B
Troponin I (presentation)	AMI	4 (1149)	II/III/IV	6–39	39 (10–78)	93 (88–97)	11 (3.4–34)	B
Troponin I (serial)	AMI	2 (1393)	III/IV	6–9	90–100[c]	83–96[c]	230–460[c]	A/B
Troponin T (presentation)	AMI	6 (1348)	II/III/IV	6–78	39 (26–53)	93 (90–96)	9.5 (5.7–16)	C
Troponin T (serial)	AMI	3 (904)	I/III/IV	5–78	93 (85–97)	85 (76–91)	83 (33–210)	B
CK-MB and myoglobin combination (presentation)	AMI	3 (2283)	II/IV	9–28	83 (51–96)	82 (68–90)	17 (7.6–40)	B/C
CK-MB and myoglobin combination (serial)	AMI	2 (291)	IV	11–20	100[d]	75–91[d]	4.3–14[d]	A/B

Table 11 (*continued*)

Summary of Test Performance Studies of Diagnostic Technologies for ACS in the ED

Technology	Condition studied	Number of studies (subjects)	Population category of studies[a]	Studies prevalence range %	Sensitivity[b] (95% CI) %	Specificity[b] (95% CI) %	Diagnostic odds ratio[b] (95% CI)	Overall quality of evidence
P-selectin	ACI	1 (263)	II	33	35[d]	79[d]	2.0[d]	B
	AMI	1 (263)	II	8.4	45[d]	76[d]	2.6[d]	B
	AMI	3 (397)	I/III	3–30	93 (81–97)	66 (43–83)	20 (7–62)	B
Rest echocardiography	ACI	2 (228)	III	3–30	70 (43–88)	87 (72–94)	20 (9–48)	C
Stress echocardiography	AMI	1 (139)	III	4	90[d]	89[d]	68[d]	C
Sestamibi (rest)	ACI	3 (702)	III	9–17	81 (74–87)	73 (56–85)	18 (11–29)	B
	AMI	3 (702)	III	2–12	92 (78–98)	67 (52–79)	26 (6–113)	B
ACI-TIPI	ACI	4 (5496)	I	17–34	86–95[c,e]	78–92[d,e]	61–69[d,e]	A
Goldman chest pain protocol	AMI	3 (5359)	I	12–20 (ACI 27–30)	88–91[d]	70–74[d]	20–23[d]	A
Algorithm/Protocols			No data from prospective studies					
Computer-based decision aids	AMI	6 (3606)	I/II/III	7–42	52–98[d]	58–96[d]	4.4–904	A

95% CI, 95% confidence interval; ACI, acute cardiac ischemia; ACI-TIPI, acute cardiac ischemia time-insensitive predictive instrument; AMI, acute myocardial infarction; CK, creatine kinase; ECG, electrocardiograph.

[a] See text for definitions of population categories.

[b] Results from meta-analysis of several studies using random-effects calculations unless otherwise indicated.

[c] For purposes of calculation of diagnostic odds ratio, 0.5 was added to cells with 0 subjects.

[d] Point estimate from single study or a range of reported values, meta-analysis not performed.

[e] ACI-TIPI is not designed to provide sensitivity and specificity. Reported values here represent overall physician diagnostic performance.

Table 12
Summary of Clinical Impact Studies of Diagnostic Technologies for ACI in the ER

Technology	Condition studied	Number of studies (subjects)	Population category[a]	Prevalence %	Clinical outcomes studied	Clinical impact[b]	Quality of evidence[c]
Prehospital ECG	ACI	approx 10	I/II	46–100	Time to thrombolysis, ejection fraction, mortality.	11	A
	AMI	(approx 8000)d		15–51			
Continuous or serial ECG		No study				Not known	
Non-standard lead ECG		No study				Not known	
	AMI			0–1			
Exercise stress ECG	ACI	3 (272)	III	0–6	Feasibility and safety.	Not known	C
CK (single/serial)		No study				Not known	
CK-MB (single)		No study	6.4			Not known	
	AMI						
CK-MB (serial)	ACI	1 (1042)	III	20	Additional admissions or discharges of ACI and non-ACI patients.	++	C
Myoglobin (single/serial)		No study				Not known	
Troponin I or T		No study				Not known	
Other Biomarkers		No study				Not known	
Rest echocardiography		No study				Not known	
Stress echocardiography		No study				Not known	
Sestamibi imaging		No study				Not known	
ACI-TIPI	ACI	4 (14,394)	I	17–59	CCU admission rate, inappropriate discharge.	+++	A
Goldman chest pain protocol	AMI	1 (1921)	II	6.6	Hospitalization rate, length of stay, estimated costs.	– / +	A

Table 12 (*continued*)
Summary of Clinical Impact Studies of Diagnostic Technologies for ACI in the ER

Technology	Condition studied	Number of studies (subjects)	Population category[a]	Prevalence %	Clinical outcomes studied	Clinical impact[b]	Quality of evidence[c]
Algorithm/protocols	ACI	2 (602)	III	6–9	Length of stay, hospital charges, 30-d and 150-d mortality.		
Computer-based decision aids	ACI AMI	1 (977)	III 30	48	30-d mortality.	Not known Not known	B A

ACI, acute cardiac ischemia; ACI-TIPI, acute cardiac ischemia time-insensitive predictive instrument; AMI, acute myocardial infarction; CK, creatine kinase; ECG, electrocardiograph.

a See text for definitions of population categories.

b Clinical impact scores range from low (+) to high (+++)

c Quality of evidence scores range from low (C) to high (A)

d Different outcomes analyzed involved different number of studies and patients.

Other Biomarkers

Studies on P-selectin, malondialdhyde-modified low-density lipoprotein, C-reactive protein, B-type natriuretic peptide, and pregnancy-associated plasma protein A (PAPP-A) are just beginning to appear (Tables 11 and 12). There is only one ED study of P-selectin that reported low sensitivity and low specificity for AMI. In the future, tests for neurohormonal activation (B-type natriuretic peptide) and inflammation (C-reactive protein, PAPP-A) may augment our ability to identify patients with acute cardiac ischemia who are at risk for adverse events. The use of these markers could potentially augment our ability to reserve the most expensive and aggressive therapies for patients who have the highest risk.

CARDIAC IMAGING

Echocardiography

The total sample size and the number of studies evaluating echocardiography for the diagnosis of ACI are small *(17a)* (Tables 11 and 12). Limited evidence suggests that resting echocardiography has high sensitivity (93%) although only modest specificity (66%) for AMI. The availability of previous echocardiograms for comparison may improve the specificity *(91)*. But even if this improved specificity were verified with additional studies, the need for previous echocardiography would limit its applicability in the general ED setting. In addition, the data pertain mostly to patients with normal or nondiagnostic ECGs. The data for stress dobutamine echocardiography is even more limited, one study suggests that it may be the next diagnostic step for patients with a negative resting echocardiogram, normal ECG, and normal enzyme levels. There is no clinical impact study for this technology.

Technetium-99m Sestamibi Myocardial Perfusion Imaging

Data on the diagnostic accuracy of resting Tc-99m sestamibi imaging in the ED is limited, and there are still no data on its clinical impact (Tables 11 and 12). The test has been used in selected patient populations that generally have a low-to-moderate risk of ACI, no history of MI, and a presenting ECG nondiagnostic for ACI. Thus, the generalizability of the current evidence is limited, and the test should be reserved for these circumscribed populations. In these patients, the test has excellent sensitivity for AMI, and very good, but not perfect, sensitivity for coronary disease in general. Specificity is modest for AMI, and although it may be a little better for ACI, it is still far from excellent.

COMPUTER-BASED DECISION AIDS

Acute Cardiac Ischemia Time-Insensitive Predictive Instrument

The acute cardiac ischemia time-insensitive predictive instrument (ACI-TIPI) *(26)* computes a 0–100% probability that a given patient has ACI (i.e., either AMI or UAP) (Tables 11 and 12). Applicable to any ED patient presenting with any symptom suggestive of ACI, it is based on a logistic regression equation that uses presenting symptoms and ECG variables. Originally in handheld calculator form, it is now incorporated into conventional ECGs so that the patient's ACI-TIPI probability is printed with the standard ECG header text. In large controlled interventional trials in a wide range of hospitals, its use by ED physicians has been shown to reduce unnecessary admissions of patients without ACI and patients with stable angina, while not reducing appropriate hospitalization for patients with ACI. It has also been shown to help the triage speed and accuracy of less-trained and less-supervised residents. The wider dissemination and use of ACI-TIPI could result in significant positive impact on the triage of ACI patients in the ED.

Goldman Chest Pain Protocol

The Goldman Chest Pain Protocol (7) is based on a computer-derived model using recursive partitioning analysis to predict myocardial infarction in patients with chest pain (Tables 11 and 12). It has good sensitivity (about 90%) for AMI, but it was not developed to detect UAP as well. In a clinical impact study of "low-intensity, nonintrusive intervention" performed at a teaching hospital ED (16), no differences in hospitalization rate, length of stay, or estimated costs was demonstrated between the experimental group, which used the protocol, and the control group.

Other Computer-Based Decision Aids

Several investigators have reported various computer-based decision aids to diagnose AMI (Tables 11 and 12). The artificial neural network by Baxt et al. (92) was found to have high sensitivity and high specificity for AMI in a prospective study, but the clinical impact has not been demonstrated.

Table 11 (21) summarizes the results of all the diagnostic performance studies evaluated, and Table 12 (21) summarizes the clinical impact studies.

IDENTIFYING ACUTE CARDIAC ISCHEMIA IN PATIENT SUBGROUPS: GENDER, MINORITIES

Knowing whether gender influences the likelihood that a given ED patient is having ACI, and whether any specific presenting clinical features are differentially associated with ACI in women compared with men, can aid clinicians in the accurate diagnosis of ACI. The incidence of AMI in the general population has been shown to be higher in men than women (93–96), but until recently, it has not been clear whether this gender difference holds among symptomatic patients who come to the ED.

Several studies have looked at gender differences in the presentation of patients with AMI (97–101). In a retrospective analysis of patients with confirmed AMI, women had higher rates of atypical presentations such as abdominal pain, paroxysmal dyspnea, or congestive heart failure (CHF) (42,93,102–104). In a group of ED patients with typical presentations, such as chest pain, the prevalence of AMI was lower in women (33,105). However, in another study of ED patients with chest pain, when adjustments were made for other presenting clinical features (specifically ECG), the gender difference was no longer significant (100). From these results, it is difficult to assess whether the gender-specific differences in AMI prevalence among symptomatic ED patients were the result of gender-specific biology or limitations in a particular study's patient selection.

Zucker et al. (106), in a study of 10,525 patients ≥30 yr old who presented to the ED with chest pain or other symptoms suggestive of ACI, found that AMI was almost twice as common in men as women (10 vs 6%). Among women with ST-segment elevation or signs of CHF, however, AMI likelihood was similar to that in men with these characteristics. This finding suggests that the presence of CHF should be given substantial weight in assessing the likelihood of AMI in women presenting to the ED with symptoms suggestive of ACI. Pope et al. *(3)* found that among the patients with AMI who present to the ED, women were more likely than men to have been discharged. In addition, among all patients with ACI, women under the age of 55 yr were at highest risk for not being hospitalized.

Blacks have high levels of risk factors for coronary artery disease but how this finding influences diagnosis in patients presenting to the ED with symptoms suggesting ACI is not well understood *(107,108)*. Studies that have included only patients with chest pain and not other symptoms suggestive of ACI, have found no significant differences in presentation, natural history, or final diagnosis of AMI between black and white patients *(109)*. Evaluating chest pain and establishing the diagnosis of coronary heart disease in blacks is often difficult given the presence of excess hypertension and left ventricular hypertrophy and the increased occurrence of out-of-hospital cardiac arrest in blacks *(110–113)*. Furthermore, the paradoxical finding of severe chest pain without significant angiographic coronary artery disease complicates diagnosis and treatment of blacks with symptoms suggestive of ACI *(107,110)*. In another analysis of the ACI-TIPI Trial data, Maynard et al. *(114)* found that black patients were 8–10 yr younger and that a higher percentage were women than was the case among white patients, which may partially explain why physicians might be less inclined to suspect the presence of ACI in black patients. Finally, Pope et al. *(3)* found that among patients with ACI, the adjusted risk of being sent home was more than 2× as high among nonwhites as among whites; among those with AMI, the risk was more than 4× as high among nonwhites as among whites. In this study, 5.8% of the black patients with AMI were not hospitalized, as compared with 1.2% of the white patients with infarction.

CLINICAL OUTCOMES

Each year in the United States, approx 9 million patients with chest pain or other symptoms suggesting ACI (i.e., IMIR Study inclusion symptoms) *(23)* present to EDs *(115)*. These patients can have various clinical outcomes ranging from discharge home to hospital admission after thrombolytic therapy. Table 13 shows the final diagnosis for the ACI-TIPI Trial *(2)* control subjects by ED triage disposition. These data were employed to develop a flowchart (Fig. 1) to represent the diagnoses and triage dispositions of ED patients presenting with chest pain or other symptoms suggestive of ACI.

The flowchart demonstrates that of all such patients, only 23% of patients (hospital range 12–34%) had ACI at final diagnosis, of which 94% were hospitalized and 6% were sent home. Conversely, 77% did not have ACI at final diagnosis, of which 59% were hospitalized and 41% were sent home. In the ACI group of patients, 36% of patients had AMI and 64% had UAP. This represented, respectively, 8% and 15% of the overall group. In the AMI group, 97% were hospitalized and 3% were sent home; in the UAP group, 92% were hospitalized and 8% were sent home. Of those with AMI, 27% received thrombolytic therapy, representing 2% of the overall group.

Our work with Pozen et al. *(6)* from 1979–1981, at the same hospitals as the present report, demonstrated a 7% ED discharge rate for patients with a final diagnosis of ACI; McCarthy et al. *(18)* found that 2% of these subjects had AMI at final diagnosis. In the mid-1980s, Lee at al. *(9)* reported a 4% AMI discharge rate. Our study found a 6% discharge rate for ACI and a 3% AMI discharge rate, demonstrating stability of these figures over the decade. The proportions of AMI and UAP in our present study (36% AMI,

Table 13
Final Diagnosis (%) for ACI-TIPI Trial Control Subjects by
ED Triage Disposition (N = 5951)[a]

Triage disposition	AMI (n = 496) Control	UAP (n = 898) Control	Non-ACI (n = 4557) Control
Home	3	8	41
Ward	1	2	6
Telemetry	31	61	43
CCU	66	29	10

[a]Abbreviations: (ACI-TIPI), acute cardiac ischemia-time-sensitive predictive instrument; ED, emergency department; AMI, acute myocardial infarction; UAP, unstable angina pectoris; CCU, coronary care unit.

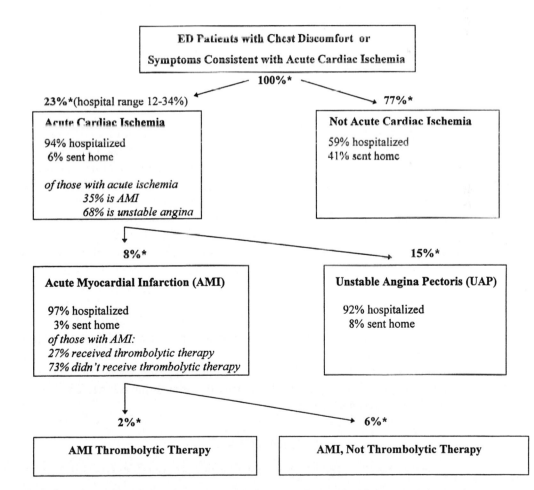

Fig. 1. Flowchart illustrating diagnoses and triage dispositions of patients presenting to the emergency department (ED) with chest pain and other symptoms suggesting acute cardiac ischemia (AMI). *, percent of total ED patients in the control group with chest pain or symptoms consistent with ACI.

64% UAP) were essentially identical to those from our work with Pozen et al. *(6)* in 1979–1984 (35% AMI, 65% UAP). Finally, in an analysis of the ACI-TIPI Trial data for failure to make the diagnosis of ACI, we found that the missed diagnosis rate for ACI was 2.2% (2.1% for AMI, 2.3% for UAP) *(3)*.

CONCLUSIONS

Our better understanding of coronary syndromes allow us to appreciate UAP and AMI as part of a continuum of ACI. ACI is a life-threatening condition whose identification can have major economic and therapeutic importance as far as threatening dysrhythmias and preventing or limiting MI size. The identification of ACI continues to challenge the skill of even experienced clinicians, yet physicians continue (appropriately) to admit the overwhelming majority of patients with ACI; in the process, they admit many patients without acute ischemia *(2)*, still overestimating the likelihood of ischemia in low risk patients because of magnified concern for this diagnosis for both prognostic and therapeutic reasons.

Studies of admitting practices from a decade ago yielded useful clinical information, but showed that neither clinical symptoms nor the ECG could reliably distinguish most patients with ACI from those with other conditions. Most studies have evaluated the accuracy of various technologies for diagnosing ACI, yet only a few have evaluated the clinical impact of routine use. The prehospital 12-lead ECG has moderate sensitivity and specificity for the diagnosis of ACI. It has demonstrated a reduction of the mean time to thrombolysis by 33 min and short-term overall mortality in randomized trials. In the general ED setting, only the ACI-TIPI has demonstrated, in a large multicenter clinical trial, a reduction in unnecessary hospitalizations without decreasing the rate of appropriate admission for patients with ACI. The Goldman chest pain protocol has good sensitivity for AMI, but has not been shown to result in any differences in hospitalization rate, length of stay, or estimated costs in the single clinical impact study performed. Its applicability to patients with UAP has not been evaluated. Single measurement of biomarkers at presentation to the ED has poor sensitivity for AMI, although most biomarkers have high specificity. Serial measurements can greatly increase the sensitivity for AMI while maintaining their excellent specificity. Biomarkers cannot identify most patients with UAP. Finally, diagnostic technologies to evaluate ACI in selected populations, such as echocardiography, sestamibi perfusion imaging, and stress ECG, may have very good to excellent sensitivity; however, they have not been sufficiently studied.

Our clinical outcome data provide a useful point of reference for clinicians regarding the diagnosis and triage dispositions of ED patients presenting with chest pain or other symptoms suggestive of ACI. In general, of all such patients, only 23% will have ACI. Of those with ACI, one-third will have AMI and two-thirds will have UAP. This represents, 8% and 15% of this overall group.

REFERENCES

1. Cardiovascular disease statistics, heart and stroke A to Z guide. American Heart Association, Dallas, 1998;pp. 1–2.
2. Pope J, Ruthazer R, Beshansky J, Griffith J. Clinical features of emergency department patients presenting with symptoms of acute cardiac ischemia: A multicenter study. J Thromb Thrombolysis 1998; 6:63–74.

3. Pope J, Aufderheide T, Ruthazer R, Woolard R. Missed diagnoses of acute cardiac ischemia in the emergency department. N Engl J Med 2000;342:1163–1170.

4. Van de Does E, Lubson J, Pool J, et al. Acute coronary events in a general practice: objectives and design of the Imminent Myocardial Infarction Rotterdam Study. Heart Bull 1976;7:91.

5. McCaig L. National Hospital Ambulatory Care Survey. 1992 Emergency Department Summary. Advanced Data 1994;245:1–12.

6. Pozen M, D'Agostino R, Selker H, Sytkowski P. A predictive instrument to improve coronary care unit admission practices in acute ischemic heart disease: a prospective multicenter clinical trial. N Engl J Med 1984;310:1273–1278.

7. Goldman L, Weinberg M. A computer-derived protocol to aid in the diagnosis of emergency room patients with acute chest pain. N Engl J Med 1982;307:588–596.

8. Schor S, Behar S, Modan B, Drory J. Disposition of presumed coronary patients from an emergency room; a follow-up study. JAMA 1976;236:941–943.

9. Lee T, Rouan G, Weisberg M, et al. Clinical characteristics and natural history of patients with acute myocardial infarction sent home from the emergency room. Am J Cardiol 1987;60:219–224.

10. Pozen M, D'Agostino R, Mitchell J, et al. The usefulness of a predictive instrument to reduce inappropriate admissions to the coronary care unit. Ann Intern Med 1980;92:238–242.

11. Selker H, Pozen M, D'Agostino R. Optimal identification of the patient with acute myocardial ischemia in the emergency room. In: Calif R, Wagner G, eds. Acute Coronary Care: Principles and Practice. Martinus Nijhoff, Boston, 1985, pp. 289–298.

12. Bloom B, Peterson O. End results, costs, and productivity of coronary care units. N Engl J Med 1973; 288:72–78.

13. Eisenberg J, Horowitz L, Busch R, Arvan D. Diagnosis of acute myocardial infarction in the emergency room: a prospective assessment of clinical decision making and usefulness of immediate cardiac enzyme determination. J Community Health 1979;4:190–198.

14. Fuchs R, Scheidt. S. Improved criteria for admission to coronary care units. JAMA 1981;246: 2037–2041.

15. Tierney W, Roth B, Psaty B, et al. Predictors of myocardial infarction in emergency room patients. Crit Care Med 1985;13:526–531.

16. Goldman L, Cook E, Brand D, et al. A computer protocol to predict myocardial infarction in emergency department patients with chest pain. N Engl J Med 1988;318:707-803.

17. Cannon CP. Management of coronary syndromes. In: Cannon CP, ed. Contempory Cardiology. Humana Press, Totowa, 1999.

18. McCarthy B, Beshansky J, D'Agostino R, Selker H. Missed diagnoses of acute myocardial infarction in the emergency department: Results from a multicenter study. Ann Emerg Med 1993;22: 579–582.

19. NIH National Heart Attack Alert Program Working Group on the Diagnosis of Acute cardiac Ischemia Report. Ann Emerg Med 1997;29:1–87.

20. McCarthy B, Wong J, Selker H. Detecting acute cardiac ischemia in the emergency department: a review of the literature. J Gen Intern Med 1990;5:365–373.

21. Evaluation of Technologies for Identifying Acute Cardiac Ischemia in Emergency Departments, Evidence Report,Technology Assessment, Number 26; Agency for healthcare Research and Quality, www.ahrq.gov, May,2001 AHRQ publication No. 01-E006.

22. Rifkin R, Hood WJ. Bayesian analysis of electrocardiographic exercise stress testing. N Engl J Med 1979;297:681–686.

23. Uretsky B, Farquhar D, Berezin A, Hood WJ. Symptomatic myocardial infarction without chest pain: prevalence and clinical course. Am J Cardiol 1977;40:498–503.

24. Kinlen L. Incidence and presentation of myocardial infarction in an English community. Br Heart J 1973;35:616–622.

25. Marglois J, Kannel W, Feinlieb M, Dawber T, McNamara P. Clinical features of unrecognized myocardial infarction-silent and symptomatic. Am J Cardiol 1973;32:1–6.

26. Selker H, Beshansky J, Griffith J, et al. Use of the Acute Cardiac Ischemia Time-Insensitive Predictive Instrument (ACI-TIPI) to assist with triage of patients with chest pain or other symptoms suggestive of acute cardiac ischemia. Ann Intern Med 1998;129:845–855.

27. Russell R. Unstable angina pectoris:National Cooperative Study Group to compare medical and surgical therapy: IV. Results in patients with left anterior descending coronary artery disease. Am J Cardiol 1981;48:517–524.

28. Krause K, Hutter AJ, DeSanctis R. Acute coronary insufficiency. Course and follow-up. Circulation 1972;45 and 46(Suppl. I):166–171.

29. Wasson J, Sox H, Neff R, Goldman L. Clinical prediction rules: applications and methodological standards. N Engl J Med 1985;313:793–799.

30. llaham M. Current Practice of Emergency Medicine. B.C. Decker, Philadelphia, 1991, p. 438.

31. Americian College of Emergency Physicians: Clinical policy for the initial approach to adults presenting with a chief complaint of chest pain with no history of trauma. Ann Emerg Med 1995;25: 274–299.

32. Short D. Diagnosis of slight and subacute coronary attacks in the community. Br Heart J 1981;45: 299–310.

33. Lee T, Cook E, Weisberg M, Sargent R. Acute chest pain in the emergency room: identification and examination of low-risk patients. Arch Intern Med 1985;145:65–69.

34. Sawe U. Pain in acute myocardial infarction. A study of 137 patients in a coronary care unit. Acta Med Scand 1971;190:79–81.

35. Sawe U. Early diagnosis of acute myocardial infarction with special reference to the diagnosis of the intermediate coronary symdrome: a clinical study. Acta Med Scand 1972;520(Suppl.):1–76.

36. Levene D. Chest pain-prophet of doom or nagging necrosis? Acta Med Scand 1981;644(Suppl):11–13.

37. Sievers J. Myocardial infarction. Clinical features and outcome in three thousand thirty-six cases. Acta Med Scand 1964;406(Suppl):1–120.

38. Areskog M, Tibbling L, Wranne B. Oesophageal dysfunction in non-infarction coronary care unit patients. Acta Med Scand 1979;205:279–282.

39. Alonzo A, Simon A, Feilieb M. Prodromata of myocardial infarction and sudden death. Circulation 1975;52:1056–1062.

40. Nattel S, Warnica J, Ogilivie R. Indications for admission to a coronary care unit in patients with unstable angina. Can Med Assoc J 1980;122:180–184.

41. Ingram D, Fulton R, Portal R, P'Aber C. Vomiting as a diagnostic aid in acute ischemic cardiac pain. BMJ 1980;281:636–637.

42. Kannel W, Abbott R. Incidence and prognosis of unrecognized myocardial infarction: an update on the Framingham Study. N Engl J Med 1984;311:1144–1147.

43. Rosenman R, Friedman M, Jenkins C, et al. Clinically unrecognized myocardial infarction in the Western Collaborative Group Study. Am J Cardiol 1967;19:776-782.

44. Grimm R, Tillinghast S, Daniels K, et al. Unrecognized myocardial infarction;experience in the Multiple Risk Factor Intervention Trial (MRFIT). Circulation 1987;75(Suppl. II):116-118.

45. Kannel W. Unrecognized myocardial infarction. Prim Cardiol 1986:93–103.

46. McCarthy B, Beshansky J, D'Agostino R, Selker H. Can missed diagnoses of acute myocardial infarction in the emergency room be reduced? Clin Res 1989;37:779A.

47. Gordon T, Sorlie P, Kannel W. Coronary Heart Disease, Atherothrombotic Brain Infarction, Intermittent Claudication-A Multivariate Analysis of Some factors Related to Their Incidence: Framinghamm Study, 16-Year Follow-up. US Goverment Printing Office,Washington, 1971.

48. Truett J, Cornfield J, Kannel W. A multivariate analysis of the risk of coronary artery diisease in Framingham. J Chron Dis 1967;20:511–524.

49. Jayes RL, Beshansky J, D'Agostino R, et al. Do patient's coronary risk factor reports predict acute cardiac ischemia in the emergency department? A multicenter study. J Clin Epidemiol 1992;45: 621–626.

50. Orlando R, Bozymski E. Clinical and manometric effects of nitroglycerin in diffuse esophageal spasm. N Engl J Med 1973;289:23–25.

51. Killip T, Kimball J. Treatment of myocardial infarction in a coronary care unit. A two year experience with 250 patients. Am J Cardiol 1967;20:457–464.

52. Selker H, Griffith J, D'Agostino R. A time-insensitive predictive instrument for acute myocardial infarction mortality: a multicenter study. Med Care 1991;29:1196–1211.

53. Selker H. Electrocardiograms and decision aids in coronary care triage: the truth but not the whole truth. J Gen Intern Med 1987;2:67–70.

54. Hoffman J, Igarashi E. Influence of electrocardiographic findings on admission decisions in patients with acute chest pain. Am J Med 1985;79:699–707.

55. Brush J, Brand D, Acampora D, et al. Use of the initial electrocardiogram to predict in-hospital complications of acute myocardial infarction. N Engl J Med 1985;312:1137–1141.

56. Slater D, Hlatky M, Mark D, et al. Outcome in suspected acute myocardial infarction with normal or mininally abnormal admission electrocardiographic findings. Am J Cardiol 1987;60:766–770.

57. Stark M, Vacek J. The initial electrocardiogram during admission for myocardial infarction; use as a predictor of clinical course and facility utilization. Arch Intern Med 1987;147:843–846.

58. Rude R, Poole W, Muller J, et al. Electrocardiographic and clinical criteria for recognition of acute myocardial infarction based on analysis of 3,697 patients. Am J Cardiol 1983;52:936–942.

59. Lopez-Sendon J, Coma-Canella I, Alcasena S, et al. Electrocardiographic findings in acute right ventricluar infarction:sensitivity and specificity of electrocardiographic alterations in right precordial leads V4R,V5R,V1,V2,V3. Am Coll Cardiol 1985;19:1273–1279.

60. Wrenn K. Protocols in the emergency room evaluation of chest pain: do they fail to diagnose lateral wall myocardial infarction? J Gen Intern Med 1987;2:66–67.

61. Nestico P, Hakki A, Iskandrian A, et al. Electrocardiographic diagnosis of posterior myocardial infarction revisited. J Electrocardiol 1986;19:33-40.

62. Fisch C. Electrocardiography, exercise stress testing, and ambulatory monitoring. In: Kelly W, ed. Textbook of Internal medicine. Lippincott, Philadelphia, 1989, pp. 305–316.

63. Jayes R, Larsen G, Beshansky J, et al. Physician electrocardiogram reading in the emergency department: accuracy and effect on triage decosions: findings from a multicenter study. J Gen Intern Med 1992;7:387–392.

64. Rusnak R, Stair T, Hansen K, et al. Litigation against the emergency physician: common features in cases of missed myocardial infarction. Ann Emerg Med 1989;18:1029–1034.

65. Griner P, Mayewski R, Mushlin A, et al. Selection and interpretation of diagnostic tests and procedures: principles and applications. Ann Intern Med 1981;94.557–592.

66. Selker H. Sorting out chest pain: identifying acute cardiac ischemia in the emergency room setting, an approach based on the acute ischemia heart disease predicitive instrument. Emerg Decisions 1985;1:8–17.

67. NIH National Heart Attack Alert program Working Group on the Diagnosis of Acute cardiac Ischemia Report. Ann Emerg Med 1997;29:1–87.

68. Bell M, Montarello J, Steele P. Does the emergency room electrocardiogram identify patients with suspected myocardial infarction who are at low risk of acute complications? Aust N Z J Med 1990;20:564–569.

69. Zalenski R, Sloan E, Chen E, et al. The emergency department ECG and immediate life-threatening complications in initially uncomplicated suspected myocardial ischemia. Ann Emerg Med 1988;17:221–226.

70. Cohen M, Hawkins L, Geeenburg S, et al. Usefulness of ST-segment changes in ≥2 leads on the emergency room electrocardiogram in either unstable angina pectoris or non-Q-wave myocardial infarction in predicting outcome. Am J Cardiol 1991;67:1368–1373.

71. Fesmire F, Percy RF, Wears R, et al. Initial ECG in Q wave and non-Q-wave myocardial infarction. Ann Emerg Med 1989;18:741–746.

72. Ruberstein L, Greenfield S. The baseline ECG in the evaluation of acute cardiac complaints. JAMA 1980;244:2536–2539.

73. Miller D, Kligfield P, Schreiber T, et al. Relationship of prior myocardial infarction to false-positive electrocardiographic diagnosis of acute injury in patients with chest pain. Arch Intern Med 1987;147:257–261.

74. Goldberger A. Myocardial Infarction Electrocardiographic Differential Diagnosis. C.V. Mosby, St. Louis, 1979.

75. Granborg J, Grande P, Pederson A. Diagnostic and prognostic significance of transient isolated negative T-waves in suspected acute myocardial infarction. Am J Cardiol 1986;57:203–207.

76. Fisch C. Abnormal ECG in clinically normal individuals. JAMA 1983;250:1321–1323.

77. DeWood M, Stifer W, Simpson C, et al. Coronary arteriographic findings soon after non-Q-wave myocardial infarction. N Engl J Med 1986;315:417–423.

78. Kennedy J. Non-Q-wave myocardial infarction. N Engl J Med 1977;315:451–453.

79. Behar S, Schor S, Kariv I, et al. Evaluation of electrocardiogram in emergency room as a decision-making tool. Chest 1977;71:486–491.

80. McGuinness J, Begg T, Semple T. First electrocardiogram in recent myocardial infarction. BMJ 1976;2:449–451.

81. Gibler W, Runyon J, Levy R, et al. A rapid diagnostic and treatment center for patients with chest pain in the emergency department. Ann Emerg Med 1995;25:1–8.

82. Hedges J, Young G, Henkel G, et al. Serial ECGs are less accurate than serial Ck-MB results for emergency department diagnosis of myocardial infarction. Ann Emerg Med 1992;21:1445–1450.

83. Kirk J, Turnipseed S, Lewis W, et al. Evaluation of chest pain in low-risk patients presenting to the emergency department: the role of immediate exercise testing. Ann Emerg Med 1998;32:1–7.
84. Lewis W, Amsterdam E, Turnipseed S, al e. Immediate exercise testing of low-risk patients with known coronary artery disease presenting to the emergency department with chest pain. J Am Coll Cardiol 1999;33:1843–1847.
85. Tsakonis J, Shesser R, Rosenthal R, et al. Safety of immediate treadmill testing in selected emergency department patients with chest pain: a preliminary report. Am J of Emerg Med 1991;9:557–559.
86. Kerns J, Shaub T, Fontanarosa P. Emergency cardiac stress testing in the evaluation of emergency department patients with atypical chest pain. Ann Emerg Med 1993;22:794–798.
87. Gerhardt W, Waldenstrom J, Horder M, et al. Creatine kinase and creatine kinase B-subunit activity in serum in cases of suspected myocardial infarction. Clin Chem 1982;28:277–283.
88. Roxin L, Cullhed I, Groth T, et al. The value of serum myoglobin determinations in the early diagnosis of acute myocardial infarction. Acta Med Scand 1984;215:417–425.
89. Montague C, Kircher T. Myoglobin in the early evaluation of acute chest pain. Am J Clin Pathol 1995; 104:472–476.
90. Kontos M, Anderson F, Schmidt K, et al. Early diagnosis of acute myocardial infarction in patients without ST-segment elevation. Am J Cardiol 1999;83:155–158.
91. Mohler Er, Ryan T, Segar D, et al. Clinical utility of troponin T levels and echocardiography in the emergency department. Am Heart J 1998;135:253–260.
92. Baxt W, Skora J. Prospective validation of artificial neural network trained to identify acute myocardial infarction. Lancet 1996;347:12–15.
93. Lerner D, Kannel W. Patterns of cornoary heart disease morbidity and mortality in the sexes: a 26-year follow-up of the Framingham pupulation. Am Heart J 1986;111:383–390.
94. Smith W, Kenicer M, et al. Prevalence of coronary heart disease in Scotland: Scottish Heart Health Study. Br Heart J 1990;64:295–298.
95. Elveback L, Connolly D. Coronary heart disease in residents of Rochester, Minnesota, V: prognosis of patients with CAD based on initial manifestation. Mayo Clin Proc 1985;60:305–331.
96. Seeman T, Mendes deLeon C, et al. Risk factors for coronary heart disease among older men and women: a prospective study of community-dwelling elderly. Am J Epidemiol 1993;138: 1037–1049.
97. Maynard C, Weaver W. Treatment of women with acute MI: new findings from the MITI Registry. J Myocard Ischemia 1992;4:27–37.
98. Sharpe P, Clark N, Janz N. Differences in the impact and management of heart disease between older women and men. Women Health 1991;17:25–34.
99. Sullivan A, Holdright D, Wright C, et al. Chest pain in women: clinical, investigative, and prognostic features. BMJ 1994;308:883–886.
100. Cunningham M, Lee T, Cook E, et al. The effect of gender on the probability of myocardial infarction among emergency department patients with acute chest pain. J Gen Intern Med 1989;4:392–398.
101. Liao Y, Lui K, Dyer A, et al. Sex differential in the relationship of electrocardiographic ST-T abnormalities to risk of coronary death: 11.5 year follow-up findings of the Chicago heart association detection project in industry. Circulation 1987;75:347–352.
102. Lusiani L, Perrone A, et al. Prevalence, clinical features, and acute course of atypical myocardial infarction. Angiology 1994;45:49–55.
103. Fiebach N, Viscoli C, Horwitz R. Differences between women and men in survival after myocardial infarction: biology or methology? JAMA 1990;263:1092–1096.
104. Dittrich H, Gilpin E, Nicod P, et al. Acute myocardial infarction in women:influence of gender on mortality and prognostic variables. Am J Cardiol 1988;62:1–7.
105. Murabito JM, Anderson KM, Kannel WB, Evans JC, Levy D. Risk of coronary heart disease in subjects with chest discomfort: the Framingham Heart Study. Am J Med 1990;89:297–302.
106. Zucker D, Griffith J, Beshansky JR, Selker HP. Presentations of acute myocardial infarction in men and women. J Gen Intern Med 1997;12:79–87.
107. Maynard C, Fisher L, Passamani E, et al. Blacks in the Coronary Artery Surgery Study (CASS): risk factors and coronary artery disease. Circulation 1986;74:64–71.
108. Cooper R, Ford E. Comparability of risk factors for coronary artery disease among black and whites in the NHANES-I epidemiologic follow-up study. Ann Epidemiol 1992;2:637–645.
109. Johnson P, Lee T, Cook E, et al. Effect of race on the presentation and management of patients with acute chest pain. Ann Intern Med 1993;118:593–601.

110. Curry C, Lewis J. Cardiac anatomy and function in hypertensive blacks. In: Hall W, Sanders E, Shulman N, eds. Hypertension in Blacks. Year Book Medical Publishers, Chicago, 1985, pp. 61–67.

111. Lenfant C. Report of the NHLBI working group on research in coronary artery disease in blacks. Circulation 1994;90:1613–1623.

112. Becker L, Han B, Meyer P, et al. Racial differences in the incidence of cardiac arrest and subsequent survival. N Engl J Med 1993;329:600–606.

113. Cowie M, Fahrenbruch C, Cobb L, et al. Out-of-hospital cardiac arrest:racial differences in outcome in Seattle. Am J Public Health 1993;83:955–959.

114. Maynard C, Beshansky J, Griffith J, et al. Causes of chest pain and symptoms suggestive of acute cardiac ischemia in African-American paients presenting to the emergency department: a multicenter study. J Natl Med Assoc 1997;89:665–671.

115. Van de Does E, Lubson J, Pool J, et al. Acute coronary events in a general practice: objectives and design of the Imminent Myocardial Infarction Rotterdam Study. Heart Bull 1976;7:91.

6

Early Identification and Treatment of Patients with Acute Coronary Syndromes

Mary M. Hand, MSPH, RN and
Costas T. Lambrew, MD

CONTENTS

INTRODUCTION

Coronary heart disease is the single largest cause of morbidity and mortality in the United States. Each year, approx 1.1 million people in the United States will suffer an acute myocardial infarction (MI)—650,000 of these will be first attacks and 450,000 will be recurrent. Nearly 500,000 will result in death, half dying before reaching a hospital *(1,2)*.

Mortality from acute MI has been dramatically reduced through successful myocardial reperfusion strategies with thrombolytics or primary percutaneous transluminal coronary angioplasty (PTCA). The 6.3% mortality in the Global Use of Strategies to Open Occluded Coronary Arteries (GUSTO) I trial is approximately half the mortality for patients with acute MI reported in the immediate prethrombolytic era *(3)*. Early achievement of reperfusion of the infarct-related artery is directly related to reduced mortality and morbidity—through myocardial salvage and reduction of the degree of left ventricular dysfunction *(4)*.

The issue of time to treatment with these artery-opening therapies has been of great interest, in particular since the advent of thrombolytic therapy. There is clear evidence from both the original animal work and extensive clinical trials with all agents supporting a time-dependent relationship between early reperfusion and outcome *(5)*. The time benefit curve is very steep, with maximum benefit accruing to those patients who are

From: *Contemporary Cardiology: Management of Acute Coronary Syndromes, Second Edition*
Edited by: C. P. Cannon © Humana Press Inc., Totowa, NJ

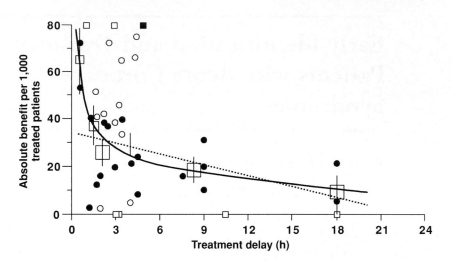

Fig. 1. Absolute 35-d mortality reduction vs treatment delay. Small closed dots, information from trials included in the FTT analysis; open dots, information from additional trials; small squares, data beyond scale of XY cross—the linear (34.7–1.6×) and nonlinear (19.4–0.6 × + 29.3 x − 1) regression lines are fitted within these data and weighted by the inverse of the variance of the absolute benefit for each data point; black squares, average effects in six time to treatment groups (area of squares inversely proportional to the variance of absolute benefits). Reproduced with permission from Boerma et al. The Lancet 1996;348:771–775.

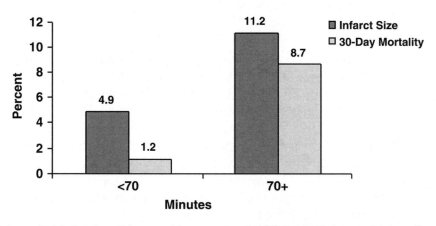

Fig. 2. Myocardial Infarction, Triage, and Intervention (MITI) Trial: 30-d mortality benefits.

reperfused within the first 1 to 2 h after symptomatic occlusion. Analysis of clinical trials provides evidence that equates 1 h of delay in reperfusion to an increase in absolute mortality by approx 1%, or 10 lives per 1000, and this is a linear relationship in the first 4–6 h following symptom onset *(5,6)* (Fig. 1). Also, the classic Myocardial Infarction, Triage, and Intervention (MITI) trial, examining prehospital vs hospital-initiated thrombolysis, found that all patients who received this treatment, within 70 min of symptom onset, experienced a 30-d mortality rate of only 1.2% compared to 8.7% for those treated 70 min or more. Similarly, infarct size was 4.9% for those treated within 70 min vs 11.2% for those treated thereafter *(7)* (Fig. 2). Given the clear cut relationship between delay and mortality, a 30-min delay will result in 5 lives lost per 1000, and a 1-h delay results in 10 lives lost per 1000 *(5,6)*. Therefore, it is imperative that time be considered as much of an adjunct to the treatment of patients with acute MI, as proposed by Cannon et al., as drugs that have been shown to have efficacy in reducing mortality *(8)*.

Unfortunately, the full potential of reperfusion and other therapies is not realized by patients who need these treatments, because many patients do not reach the hospital on time to benefit from them. Approximately one in five patients with acute MI present to the hospital within 1 h of symptom onset, whereas slightly less than one-quarter of patients delay seeking care by 6 or more hours, with no change in these distributions over time *(9)*. The National Registry of Acute Myocardial Infarction-2 analysis of data on 272,651 patients showed that only 31% were eligible for reperfusion therapy. Of these eligible patients, 41% were considered ineligible because symptoms of acute MI were present for more than 6 h prior to diagnosis *(10)*.

National Heart Attack Alert Program

The new treatments and the synergistic effect of time on their effectiveness, coupled with ongoing patient and system delays, gave the impetus for the National Heart, Lung, and Blood Institute's (NHLBI's) consideration, in the late 1980s, of establishing a national education program dedicated to coordinating efforts to improve emergency care for patients with acute MI and their outcomes *(9)*. The NHLBI launched the National Heart Attack Alert Program (NHAAP) in June 1991, with the first meeting of its Coordinating Committee comprised of approx 40 healthcare providers, voluntary, and federal liaison representatives involved in some aspect of care of the acute MI patient in the hospital or in the community. The NHAAP's overarching goal is to promote early identification and treatment of patients with acute MI and to reduce the incidence of (and improve survival from) sudden cardiac death in the community. The scope of program was expanded in 1997 to include all patients with acute coronary syndromes, i.e., unstable angina, as well as acute myocardial infarction. Paramount to the program's goal is the reduction of delays associated with each of three phases ultimately leading to rapid treatment of these patients. At the time the NHAAP was started, patient-associated delays were noted to be the most significant component of total delays ranging from 2.5–6 h in reported studies. Delays related to the emergency medical services (EMS) system response and transportation of the patient to the hospital were also noted, and also very disturbing was delays in the early identification and treatment of patients suitable for reperfusion therapy once the patient arrived in the emergency department. Hospital delays were found to be in the range of 60–90 min in several well-conducted clinical trials. It became evident that the magnitude of delay in the emergency department was not appreciated by most physicians until times from patient arrival to treatment were actually recorded *(11)*.

It was also apparent that patient-mediated delay was an area that was not well understood, yet represented one of the most significant (and challenging) components of delay. Furthermore, early program advisors felt that the existing understanding of the design and implementation of efficient and cost-effective public education campaigns was not sufficient to warrant such a national effort at that time. They were also concerned that EMS and hospital emergency departments would be overrun by patients who responded to an improperly developed public education campaign *(11)*.

On the advice of its early advisors, the NHAAP stimulated the Rapid Early Action for Coronary Treatment (REACT) research program at the NHLBI, to examine the impact of community-wide education regarding symptoms of a heart attack and the importance of accessing EMS. The NHAAP deferred immediate public and patient education efforts pending the results of REACT.

The NHAAP Coordinating Committee and the program's early advisors recommended that, while research was underway that would ultimately inform the NHAAP's public education "arm," it was imperative to first address delays associated with the emergency medical community who would be responding to patients who ultimately present in response to a public education campaign. Thus, during its first nearly 8 yr, the NHAAP focused largely on educating healthcare providers, notably in emergency departments and EMS systems, about the importance of rapid recognition and treatment of individuals with symptoms and signs of a heart attack. The NHAAP published issue papers and reports highlighting: (i) the rapid identification and treatment of acute MI patients in the emergency department setting (12); and (ii) EMS issues that potentially impact on rapid recognition and treatment of these patients (13–15). In addition, the program reviewed the diagnostic performance and clinical impact data for a number of technologies used in diagnosing patients with acute cardiac ischemia in the emergency department (16–19). Subsequently, it issued a position paper on chest pain centers and programs (20) and convened a symposium with the National Library of Medicine and the Agency for Health Care Policy and Research to explore the role of new information technology in expediting the recognition, diagnosis, and treatment of patients with acute MI (21). To address patient delay pending development of a public educational campaign, the NHAAP published a review paper on patient and bystander factors associated with treatment-seeking delay (22), as well as recommendations directed to providers for educational strategies to reduce prehospital delay in their patients at high risk for a heart attack (23,24). In 1998, the NHAAP released a report that described the community as the "ultimate coronary care unit", and encouraged all settings, where patients may present with a cardiac emergency, to plan for a timely and effective response (25).

This chapter reviews the three fundamental areas where timely identification and treatment of patients with an acute MI are critical to their outcomes as identified by NHAAP, and addresses the implications for policies and educational efforts by providers, institutions, and communities.

REDUCING DELAYS IN THE HOSPITAL

The NHAAP concentrated its initial efforts on addressing delays associated with healthcare provider recognition and treatment, notably in the emergency department setting. The program convened a working group, co-chaired by a cardiologist and an emergency medicine physician, to examine emergency department processes related to the care of these patients and identify delays to timely treatment. The working group concluded that patients presenting with symptoms consistent with acute MI, with ST-segment elevation on the initial electrocardiogram (ECG) and who had no contraindications to reperfusion therapy could effectively and safely be identified and treated within 30 min after emergency department arrival (12). The working group also recommended that in order to examine, process, and track improvement through a continuous quality improvement effort, the time from emergency department arrival to initiation of reperfusion therapy would have to be recorded for each patient, since the

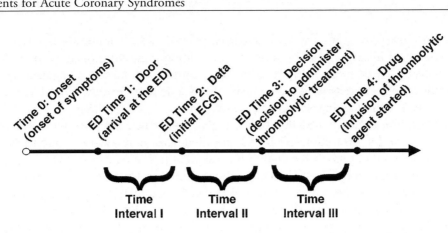

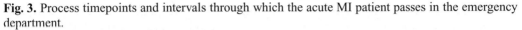

Fig. 3. Process timepoints and intervals through which the acute MI patient passes in the emergency department.

purpose of tracking reductions in delay over time related to changes in the process of identification and treatment.

Analyzing the Process of Care in the Emergency Department: the "Four Ds"

The working group identified four critical time points in the care of these patients and termed them the "four D's." (Fig. 3). "Door" is the time of arrival and registration of the patient in the emergency department. "Data" refers to the time that the first ECG showing ST-segment elevation is recorded, since this electrocardiographic finding is clearly the trigger for consideration of reperfusion therapy. "Decision," the third D, is the time when the decision to proceed with reperfusion therapy is made (the drug is ordered). The fourth D, "Drug," is when the thrombolytic infusion is actually begun. The elapsed time between the patient's emergency department arrival and initiation of thrombolytic drug is then referred to as "door-to-drug time." In the case of patients receiving balloon angioplasty, the interval is referred to as the "door-to-balloon" *(26)* or "door-to-dilation" time *(20)*. The working group analyzed the process of care in the emergency department, based on the four D's, identifying the potential for delays.

DOOR

Once the patient arrives in the emergency department, the initial encounter with the nurse or registration representative should be focused on clinical symptoms and not on the collection of demographic information *(12)*. If a patient complains of chest pain, then triage to a high category with an ECG done within 5 min and physician assessment within 10 min should be expected.

While substernal chest pain remains the cornerstone of patient history for acute MI diagnosis, two recent reports from a large series of patients provide rich additional information as to how patients may present. Goldberg et al. *(27)* reported on the symptom profiles of patients presenting with a complaint of chest pain and a hospital-admission diagnosis of suspected acute myocardial ischemia and a discharge diagnosis of acute MI or unstable angina in 43 hospitals in 20 communities throughout the United States during collection of baseline data for a larger community intervention trial. They noted that four other "cardinal" symptoms of a heart attack or unstable angina—dyspnea (49%), arm pain (46%), sweating (35%), and nausea (33%)—were commonly reported by men *and* women of all ages in addition to the presenting complaint of chest pain. Patients with acute MI were more likely to complain of arm pain, sweating, nausea, vomiting, and indigestion. Patients with a diagnosis of unstable angina were more likely to complain of neck pain, dizziness, and palpitations *(27)*.

Furthermore, in nearly 435,000 patients with confirmed MI from the National Registry of Myocardial Infarction (NRMI) 2 (enrolled from June 1994 to March 1998), 33% (one in three) did not have chest pain on presentation to the hospital. This group of MI patients was on average 7 yr older than those with chest pain (74.2 vs 66.9%); and a higher proportion of them were women (49 vs 38%) and patients with diabetes mellitus (32.6 vs 25.4%) or prior heart failure (26.4 vs 12.3%). Also, MI patients without chest pain had a longer delay before hospital presentation (mean 7.9 vs 5.3 h), were less likely to be diagnosed as having confirmed MI at the time of admission (22.2 vs 50.3%), and were less likely to have received thrombolysis or primary angioplasty (25.3 vs 74.0%), aspirin (60.4 vs 84.5%), β-blockers (28.0 vs 48.0%), or heparin (53.4 vs 83.2%). MI patients without chest pain had a 23.3% in-hospital mortality rate compared with 9.3% among patients with chest pain *(28)*.

DATA

Locating an ECG machine in the emergency department will reduce door-to-data time. Acquisition of the 12-lead ECG should be possible within 5 min, 24 h a day, 7 d a week. If this cannot be accomplished effectively using technical staff, then emergency department personnel, including nurses or physicians, should be trained to acquire a high-quality 12-lead ECG. The nurse should have authority to order the 12-lead ECG, rather than waiting for a physician assessment and order.

DECISION

Once the ECG is available, it should be delivered to the physician for interpretation rather than placed on the chart or at the nurse's desk. In the Time to Thrombolysis Substudy of the NRMI, the median door-to-decision times and door-to-drug times were significantly longer when a consultation by a cardiologist was performed, and these times were substantially longer for those patients who had a bedside consultation compared to those whose consultation occurred by phone *(29)*. Fax consultation for the purpose of interpreting the ECG significantly reduces data-to-decision time and, therefore, median door-to-drug time *(30)*. Contacting the primary care physician before initiating thrombolytic therapy substantially delays door-to-drug time *(29)*. Consultation particularly contributes to delays around the decision to treat women with a thrombolytic agent and in initiation of drug therapy *(29)*. In another study, the median time interval from hospital arrival to initiation of thrombolytic therapy was longer in the consultation group (49 vs 35 min, $p = 0.0001$). A door-to-drug interval of ≤30 min was seen in only 23.8% of the consultation group vs 40.4% of the no consultation group *(31)*.

DRUG

Preparation of the drug in the emergency department as opposed to the pharmacy can result in substantial decrease in door-to-drug time with a difference in one study being 61.5 as opposed to 84.6 mean min *(30)*. Furthermore, waiting to initiate drug infusion in the cardiac intensive care unit results in the greatest delay, 75 min, compared to 50 min when the infusion is begun in the emergency department *(30)*. Extensive written informed consent is not appropriate for a patient with severe chest pain who is suffering an acute MI. The patient may be appropriately informed verbally of benefit and risk within 1 to 2 min by the physician, since reperfusion therapy, like many others in medical emergencies, is now standard of care. There is no evidence that patients who qualify for thrombolytic therapy should be transferred to a tertiary care hospital or center for initiation of drug, since the delay related to transfer will invariably increase mortality. Rural hospitals and community hospitals in urban settings must be capable of treating patients with acute MI with thrombolytic drugs according to the same standards for early diagnosis and treatment as the cardiology centers. Telephone and fax consultation with cardiologists in other hospitals may be appropriate to facilitate care in difficult cases.

Thus, it is imperative that the process of assessing patients with chest pain, acquiring the 12-lead ECG, and making decisions to initiate reperfusion therapy be seamless and consistent. Furthermore, for patients with clear cut clinical symptoms of acute MI and unequivocal evidence of ST elevation on the ECG with no question of contraindications, the responsibility to order and initiate thrombolytic therapy should be delegated by protocol to the emergency medicine physician. Waiting for the cardiologist has been found to result in significant delays *(12)*.

Protocols for assessment of such patients and initiation of thrombolytic therapy have consistently and dramatically reduced door-to-drug times. The experience from several different institutions was that, prior to initiation of a protocol, door-to-drug times were between 69 and 76 median min and were reduced to between 21 and 29 min following protocol development and implementation *(4,29,32)*. Use of critical pathways can facilitate reduction in door-to-drug or door-to-balloon times for patients with acute coronary syndromes *(33,34)*.

Even though the NHAAP emergency department working group recommended that hospitals reduce door-to-needle time to 30 min or less *(12)*, it was only subsequent to this recommendation that the relationship between door-to-needle time and mortality was examined in a registry of 85,589 patients at over 1400 hospitals with ST-segment-elevation MI who were treated with thrombolysis. Door-to-needle times ≤30 min were present in only 33% of patients and were less common in women, elderly, and nonwhites. While the results showed that there was no significant increase in mortality for patients with door-to-needle times of ≤30 min compared with patients whose door-to-needle times were 31–60 min, the adjusted odds ratio of death was significantly increased by 11% for patients with door-to-needle times of 61–90 min ($p = 0.01$) and increased by 23% for patients with door-to-needle times of >90 min. Additional analysis showed a 13–23% increase in the odds for developing an ejection fraction <40% as door-to-needle time increased >30 min ($p = 0.001$ for each time point). These data show that a delay in door-to-needle time >60 min, which is present in about 27% of the patients, was associated with an 11–23% increase in mortality and in the development of left ventricular dysfunction post-MI, the first direct evidence that efforts to reduce door-to-needle time are warranted to improve outcome after thrombolysis *(35)* (Figs. 4 and 5).

The relationship between symptom-onset to balloon time and door-to-balloon time was examined in a cohort of 27,080 patients with ST-segment-elevation MI or left bundle-branch block, who were treated with primary angioplasty and reported to the

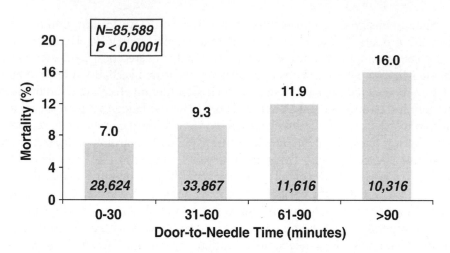

Fig. 4. NRMI-2: Thrombolysis—door-to-needle time vs mortality.

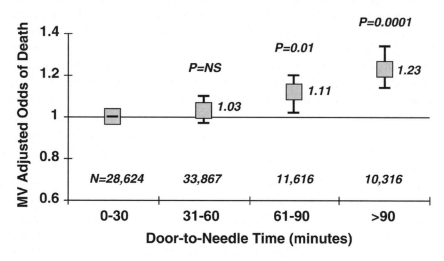

Fig. 5. NRMI-2: Thrombolysis—door-to-needle time vs. mortality.

Second NRMI, from 1994 to 1998 in 661 community and tertiary care hospitals in the United States. The median time from the onset of chest pain to hospital arrival was 1.6 h, and the median time from onset of chest pain to primary angioplasty was 3.9 h. Unadjusted mortality was higher in the patients treated later, but the multivariate-adjusted odds of in-hospital mortality did not increase over the 24-h period (Figs. 6 and 7). The door-to-balloon time, however, showed that the adjusted odds of mortality were significantly increased by 41–62% for patients with door-to-balloon times longer than 2 h (present in nearly 50% of the cohort) *(36)* (Figs. 8 and 9).

Thus, both door-to-needle and door-to balloon times appear to be important quality of care indicators, and efforts to improve processes of care to achieve these optimal treatment times should rigorously continue. Furthermore, door-to-balloon times should be considered when choosing between thrombolysis and primary percutaneous coronary intervention *(36)*.

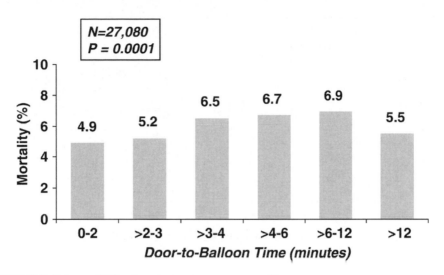

Fig. 6. NRMI-2: Primary PCI—time-to-treatment vs mortality.

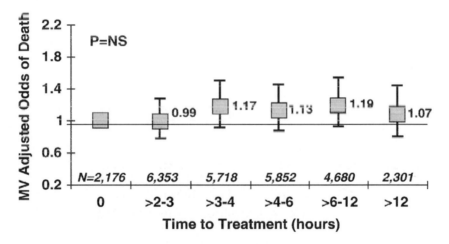

Fig. 7. NRMI-2: Primary PCI—time-to-treatment vs mortality.

It is very clear that reductions in delay can only occur if times are recorded consistently on every patient, and door-to-drug time trends are monitored by quarterly analysis of these data. Significant reductions in door-to-drug times may drift back to unacceptable levels should a multidisciplinary quality improvement team not meet on a regular basis to review times to diagnosis and treatment for the purpose of improving the process. Feedback of these times to participating physicians, nurses, and technologists is critical in improving performance and outcomes. In the NRMI, median door-to-drug time has fallen from 60 min in 1990, when the Registry was initiated, to 34 min in 1999 *(37)* (Fig. 10). The Health Care Financing Administration (now the Centers for Medicare and Medicaid Services) reported that between 1994 and 1995, the median time from emergency department arrival to thrombolytic therapy was 46 min, and by the 1998 to 1999 time period, the median time had decreased to 39 min *(38)*. This is a result of continuing surveillance and feedback of these data to the team involved in caring for these patients.

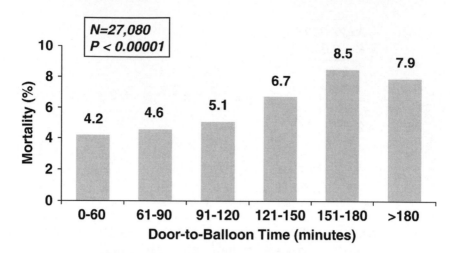

Fig. 8. NRMI-2: Primary PCI—door-to-balloon time vs mortality.

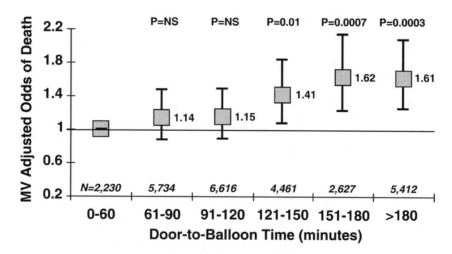

Fig. 9. NRMI-2: Primary PCI—door-to-balloon time vs mortality.

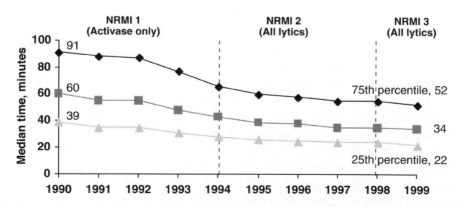

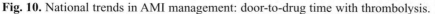

Fig. 10. National trends in AMI management: door-to-drug time with thrombolysis.

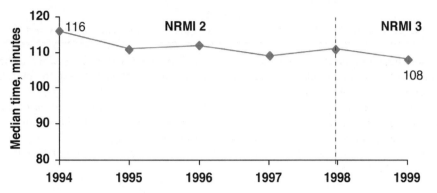

Fig. 11. National trends in AMI management: door-to-balloon time in PPTCA.

The NRMI reported a reduction in median door-to-balloon time for PTCA from 116 min in 1994 to 108 min in 1999 *(37)* (Fig. 11). The Health Care Financing Administration reported that between 1994 and 1995, the median time from hospital arrival to primary angioplasty was 120 min, and by 1998 to 1999, the median time had decreased to 108 min *(38)*. If patients arrive at a hospital without angioplasty capability, there can be no justification on the basis of studies of effectiveness in the community for the delay in reperfusion incurred by the transfer of such patients to angioplasty-capable hospitals. These patients, if they cannot be dilated within 90 min or less (±30 min) as recommended by the most recent American College of Cardiology (ACC) American Heart Association (AHA) Guidelines *(19)*, should be treated with thrombolytics at the receiving hospital.

Currently, there are more than 1200 chest pain centers in the United States *(40)*. The NHAAP, having observed the development and growth of chest pain centers in emergency departments with special interest, created a task force to evaluate such centers and make recommendations to assist emergency physicians in emergency departments (including those with chest pain centers) in providing comprehensive management of patients with acute coronary syndromes *(20)*.

They cited three distinct types of programs in chest pain centers:

1. A heart attack program for the rapid treatment of acute MI in patients with ST-segment elevation on the 12-lead ECG.
2. A diagnostic (observational) program to exclude the diagnosis of acute MI or unstable angina in patients with a low-to-moderate probability of having these conditions.
3. An outreach program to educate patients in the chest pain center and in the broader community about early evaluation for chest pain or related symptoms of a heart attack and the importance of risk factor identification and control.

The task force recommended certain points that should be kept in mind when developing chest pain centers or programs to evaluate patients with symptoms of acute coronary syndromes. These recommendations are shown in Table 1. The authors concluded that in the final analysis the criteria for all approaches and strategies must be the optimal care and clinical outcomes of patients. The organization and designation of a separate chest pain center are worthwhile only to the extent the center demonstrably furthers that goal. It is not the name "chest pain center" that counts, but the program of care in place *(20)*.

Table 1
National Heart Attack Alert Program Recommendations for Chest Pain Centers and Programs

- Address the need to identify accurately and efficiently patients with acute cardiac ischemia (ACI) among the large, and likely increasing, numbers of patients presenting to emergency departments with symptoms suggestive of ACI.
- Make clear to the public, patients, and providers that the goal is to provide prompt evaluation and effective care to all patients with symptoms that may represent ACI: chest pain or discomfort, shortness of breath, nausea, dizziness/fainting, or abdominal pain; a focus only on chest pain is potentially misleading, since as many as 25% of patients presenting with ACI will not have chest pain.
- In outreach efforts, emphasize the general principles of patient response to important symptoms and not direct patients to a particular hospital during an acute episode; instead, encourage them to call 9-1-1 to seek rapid treatment.
- Base care, as much as possible, on the use of approaches and technologies for which evidence supports safety and effectiveness, such as those supported in the NHAAP ACI Diagnostic Technologies Working Group report, its update, or by subsequently published prospective evaluations.
- Use operational processes that facilitate care of all presenting patients, incorporating attention to the "4 Ds" (to reduce door-to-drug time with reperfusion therapies) *(12)* and treatment particularly for those needing reperfusion and anti-ischemic therapy.
- In a continuous quality improvement program, monitor process indicators (measures of appropriateness of emergency department triage, treatment, and outcomes) using forms and systems such as those utilized by continuous improvement cycles.
- Coordinate the care of patients, particularly those discharged without a diagnosis of ACI, to ensure that test results are communicated to the patient's primary care or follow-up physician.

Reprinted from ref. *20.*

PREHOSPITAL ACTIONS AND REDUCING TREATMENT DELAYS

Several prehospital strategies related to transport and care can affect patient outcomes.

Ambulance Transport

How patients with acute MI symptoms get to the hospital has ramifications on how quickly they are evaluated and treated at the hospital. Surprisingly, calling an ambulance for heart attack symptoms is not frequently done. The Atherosclerosis Risk in Communities study reported that the percentage of MI patients arriving at the hospital by ambulance changed little from 1987 to 1998, going from 36 to 40% *(41)*. The REACT research program revealed that the average rate of EMS use was only 33% in both the 10 intervention and 10 control communities at the study's baseline assessment *(42)*. The NRMI-2 compared the baseline characteristics and initial management for 772,586 patients from April 1994 to March 1998 presenting by ambulance vs self-transport (excluding those in cardiogenic shock, over 6 h from symptom onset to hospital arrival, or who were transferred in). Only one of two patients with MI was transported to the hospital by ambulance *(43)*.

Use of the EMS system by calling 9-1-1 or the equivalent local emergency number (which dispatches an ambulance) is associated with significantly faster delivery of acute reperfusion therapies. In the aforementioned NRMI-2 study, the mean door-to-thrombolytic time was 54.7 min in those who were brought to the hospital by ambulance vs 66.9 min in those who self-transported. The mean door-to-balloon time was 141.7 min vs 173 min for those who arrived by ambulance vs those who self-transported, respectively (43).

REACT investigators reported a significant association of early reperfusion therapy with ambulance use. Of 3013 selected study patients who received reperfusion treatment, 1195 (40%) were transported via EMS personnel. The adjusted rate of reperfusion within 6 h of symptom onset was significantly greater for acute MI patients transported via EMS personnel (36 vs 24%) (44).

Prehospital ECGs

Performing an ECG in the field and transmitting it to the emergency department speeds the care of patients with acute MI. Obtaining a prehospital ECG has been shown to be feasible and results in a diagnostic quality ECG. Based on a systematic review and meta-analysis, Lau and his colleagues found that obtaining a 12-lead ECGs did not prolong the time in the field or delay transport to the emergency department (18). Prehospital 12-lead ECGs were shown in both randomized and nonrandomized studies, to clearly result in significant reductions in time to treatment with thrombolysis, ranging between 20 and 60 min (18).

In the largest retrospective study of 70,763 patients from a large registry of acute MI patients, including 3768 patients with prehospital 12-lead ECGs, the median time from symptom onset to hospital arrival was surprisingly prolonged in patients who had a prehospital 12-lead ECG (152 vs 91 min), although the median time from hospital arrival to therapy was shortened both for thrombolysis (30 vs 40 min) and for primary angioplasty (92 vs 115 min) in the prehospital 12-lead ECG group. The prehospital 12-lead ECG group was more likely to have reperfusion therapy by thrombolysis or angioplasty, angiography, and coronary artery bypass grafting than the control group. In-hospital mortality was 8% in the prehospital ECG group vs 12% in the control group ($p <$ 0.001), and the beneficial effect on survival also remained present in multivariate analyses adjusting for various predictors of mortality (45).

Prehospital Thrombolysis

Administering fibrinolytics in the field has also been studied as a way of reducing time-to-treatment for acute MI. A meta-analysis of prehospital fibrinolysis trials summarized by the European Myocardial Infarction Project Group, showed a 17% relative improvement in outcome associated with out-of-hospital fibrinolytic therapy. The greatest improvement was observed when therapy was initiated 60–90 min earlier than in the hospital (46). The US Myocardial Infarction Triage and Intervention trial showed no significant difference in mortality between prehospital and in-hospital fibrinolysis. As noted, a retrospective analysis showed that any patient treated within a median time of 70 min, either before or after hospital arrival, had a significantly improved outcome. It appeared that the window of time from hospital arrival to treatment was shortened for the in-hospital patients due to the protocol of advance notification of staff (7). Pooled results of six randomized trials of over 6000 patients found a significant 58-min reduction in time to fibrinolytic administration ($p = 0.007$) and decreased all-cause hospital mortality with prehospital thrombolysis (OR 0.83; CI 0.70–0.98) (47).

All considered, the AHA Committee on Emergency Cardiovascular Care, the Evidence Evaluation Conference, and the international Guidelines 2000 Conference expert panel members recommend prehospital fibrinolytic therapy only when a physican is present or prehospital transport time is $\geq$ 60 min. They prefer instead that EMS systems focus on early diagnosis and rapid transport, rather than delivery of therapy (48).

REDUCING DELAYS IN PATIENT RECOGNITION AND ACTION

The greatest delay in initiating reperfusion therapy for patients with ST-segment elevation acute MI is patient-mediated delay. The median delay between symptom onset and hospital arrival ranges between 2 and 6.4 h (23). In the Gruppo Italiano per lo Studio della Streptochinasi nell' Infarcto Miocardico (GISSI) I Trial, 10.9% of patients were treated with intravenous streptokinase within the first hour after onset of symptoms (49). In both the Thrombolysis in Myocardial Infarction (TIMI) 2 and GUSTO I trials, only 3% of patients were treated within the first hour (50,51).

Goff et al. (52) reported on prehospital delay times for the largest and most representative sample of US patients admitted to a hospital for evaluation of suspected acute cardiac ischemia and discharged with a coronary heart disease-related diagnosis from the REACT trial. In this study population, the overall median delay time was 2 h (means differed across communities, ranging from 133 to 156 min) with substantially longer delays on the order of 30–45 min for the geometric mean for several important subgroups, including non-Hispanic blacks vs non-Hispanic whites (by 43 min), among older than among younger patients (by 14 min for each 10-yr increment in age), and among Medicaid recipients than among the privately insured (by 41 min). Delay time was longer, but not significantly so among Hispanics vs non-Hispanic whites and among both the disabled and homemakers vs the employed (52).

High-Risk Patients

Prior to embarking on a public education campaign, the NHAAP targeted high risk patients for education by the medical community (23,24). This group continues to be an important patient population for education about early recognition and response to acute MI. Over 12 million patients in the United States have a history of an MI, angina pectoris, or both, divided approximately evenly between males and females. People who survive the acute stage of a heart attack have a chance of illness and death that is 1.5–15 times higher than that of the general population, depending on their sex and clinical outcomes. The risk of another heart attack, sudden death, angina pectoris, heart failure, and stroke, for both men and women in this group, is substantial (1). Within 6 yr after a recognized heart attack, 18% of men and 35% of women will have another heart attack. Furthermore, 7% of men and 6% of women will experience sudden death (1). It is recommended that these high-risk patients receive specific instructions from their caregivers on recognition of symptoms, including an understanding that symptoms of a recurrent MI may not be the same as those of a previous event. They are also to be instructed on what to do in terms of taking nitrates and taking an aspirin, and are urged to call 9-1-1. These recommendations are to be shared not only with the patient, but also with family, and written as a reinforcement to both patient, family members, and others who may be around the patient when symptoms occur (23,24) (Fig. 12).

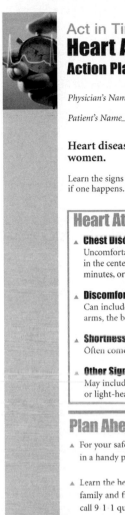

Act in Time to
Heart Attack Signs
Action Plan

Physician's Name _____

Patient's Name _____ *Date* _____

Heart disease is the top killer of men and women.

Learn the signs of a heart attack and the steps to take if one happens. You can save a life–maybe your own.

Treatment can stop a heart attack in its tracks.

Clot-busting drugs and other artery-opening treatments work best to stop a heart attack if given *within 1 hour* of the start of symptoms.

Heart Attack Warning Signs

▲ **Chest Discomfort**
Uncomfortable pressure, squeezing, fullness, or pain in the center of the chest that lasts more than a few minutes, or goes away and comes back.

▲ **Discomfort in Other Areas of the Upper Body**
Can include pain or discomfort in one or both arms, the back, neck, jaw, or stomach.

▲ **Shortness of Breath**
Often comes with or before chest discomfort.

▲ **Other Signs**
May include breaking out in a cold sweat, nausea, or light-headedness.

Minutes Matter

▲ If you or someone else is having heart attack warning signs:

Call 9-1-1

▲ **Don't wait more than a few minutes— 5 minutes at most—to call 9-1-1.**

▲ If symptoms **stop completely** in less than 5 minutes, you should still call your health care provider.

Plan Ahead

▲ For your safety, fill in this action plan and keep it in a handy place.

▲ Learn the heart attack warning signs. Talk with family and friends about them and the need to call 9 1 1 quickly.

▲ Talk with your health care provider about your risk factors for heart attack–and how to reduce them.

Information To Share With Emergency Medical Personnel/Hospital Staff

Medicines you are taking: _____

_____

Medicines you are allergic to: _____

_____

If symptoms *stop completely* in less than 5 minutes, you should still call your health care provider. Phone number during office hours.

_____

Phone number after office hours:

_____

Person You Would Like Contacted If You Go to the Hospital

Name: _____

Home phone number: _____

Work phone number: _____

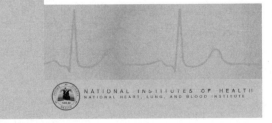

NATIONAL INSTITUTES OF HEALTH
NATIONAL HEART, LUNG, AND BLOOD INSTITUTE

Fig. 12a.

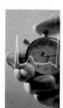

How To Reduce Your Chance of a Heart Attack

To find your risk for a heart attack, check the boxes that apply to you:

☐ A family history of early heart disease
(Father or brother diagnosed before age 55)
(Mother or sister diagnosed before age 65)

☐ Age (Men 45 years or older; Women 55 years or older)

☐ High blood cholesterol

☐ High blood pressure

☐ One or more previous heart attacks, angina, bypass surgery or angioplasty, stroke, or blockages in neck or leg arteries

☐ Overweight

☐ Physical inactivity

☐ Cigarette smoking

☐ Diabetes

The more risk factors you have, the greater your risk for a heart attack.

Reduce Your Risk of a Heart Attack by Taking Steps To Prevent or Control Risk Factors

High blood pressure
▲ Have your doctor check your blood pressure.
▲ Aim for a healthy weight.
▲ Become physically active.
▲ Follow a healthy eating plan, including food lower in salt and sodium.
▲ Limit alcoholic beverages.
▲ Take medication, if prescribed.

High blood cholesterol
▲ Get your blood cholesterol level checked once every 5 years. (Check it more often, if necessary.)
▲ Learn what your numbers mean.
▲ Follow a low-saturated fat and low cholesterol eating plan.
▲ Become physically active.
▲ Aim for a healthy weight.
▲ Take medication, if prescribed.

Cigarette Smoking
▲ Stop smoking now or cut back gradually.
▲ If you can't quit the first time, keep trying.
▲ If you don't smoke, don't start.

Overweight
▲ Maintain a healthy weight. Try not to gain extra weight.
▲ If you are overweight, try to lose weight slowly, 1/2 to 1 pound a week.

Diabetes
▲ Find out if you have diabetes.
▲ Get your blood sugar level checked by your doctor.

Physical inactivity
▲ Become physically active.
▲ Do 30 minutes of moderate-level physical activity, such as brisk walking, on most and preferably all days of the week.
▲ If necessary, break 30 minutes into periods of at least 10 minutes each.

In partnership with: American Heart Association®
Fighting Heart Disease and Stroke

 This material is based on original content developed as part of the Rapid Early Action for Coronary Treatment (REACT) research program, funded by the National Heart, Lung, and Blood Institute, National Institutes of Health, Bethesda, Maryland.

 U.S. DEPARTMENT OF HEALTH AND HUMAN SERVICES
Public Health Service
National Institutes of Health
National Heart, Lung, and Blood Institute

NIH Publication No. 01-3669
September 2001

Fig. 12b.

Patients/Public

Extensive information into the problem of patient delay and implications for potentially reducing this delay became available with the results of the REACT research program, which were reported in 1998 at the AHA's Scientific Sessions. REACT was a 4-yr, multisite community intervention study funded by the NHLBI to learn more about whether patient delays in seeking care for heart attack symptoms could be reduced through a community-wide heart attack awareness campaign to educate providers, patients, and the public about heart attack symptoms and appropriate action steps, and to determine the impact on patient-associated delay time and on EMS systems. The REACT study comprised five academic field centers and a coordinating center at New England Research Institute. Each field center identified two community pairs matched on demographic characteristics totaling 20 communities (10 pairs) of medium-sized population. One community of each pair was randomized to a multifaceted education program or "intervention" for the public, patients, and healthcare providers; the remaining community of each pair served for comparison receiving no organized education program. The main hypothesis was that community-based intervention of 18 mo duration would reduce patient delay in seeking treatment for a suspected acute MI. The time period of concern was from symptom onset to arrival at the hospital emergency department. The community-wide intervention was developed by the investigators during a 1-yr planning phase. The main intervention components were: (*i*) community organization to mobilize the community and enlist support of medical and nonmedical community leaders and agencies; (*ii*) community education to promote awareness, knowledge, beliefs, skills, behavioral intentions, self-efficacy, and behaviors of high-risk individuals, family members, and the general public through mass media, small media, group programs, and magnet events; (*iii*) provider education to increase providers' knowledge, behavioral capacity, and self-efficacy, and their delivery of patient education; and (*iv*) patient education for high-risk patients and their families to promote knowledge, behavioral capacity, self-efficacy, and behaviors for quick action for acute MI *(42)*.

REACT results revealed that delay time reduction, the primary outcome measure, was not observed in the 10 intervention communities, compared with the 10 reference communities. There appeared to be a secular trend in improving patient delay times, although delay times still varied based on region and demographic characteristics of target groups. However, average use of the EMS system by the primary study population, those with an acute cardiac diagnosis, was 33% at the study's baseline in all 20 communities. In those communities receiving the educational intervention, the odds of EMS use increased steadily and significantly in the intervention communities, with a net 20% increase in EMS use in the intervention compared with the reference communities *(42)*.

Despite the lack of statistical significance for the primary outcome measure (patient delay from symptom onset to hospital arrival), REACT investigators reported a number of findings from focus groups that were conducted to inform the study's intervention and from follow-up surveys of patients discharged from the emergency department or from the hospital, after admission for an acute cardiac diagnosis. These findings provide an updated science base for understanding the phenomenon of why patients delay when faced with heart attack symptoms, and have implications for public education in this area.

Expectations about Heart Attack Symptoms

REACT focus groups found that, overwhelmingly, participants expected that heart attack symptoms would correspond to common Hollywood movie portrayals as sharp crushing chest pain or collapse, such as a cardiac arrest. They thought there would be no doubt about the nature of the event that was occurring. This was in sharp contrast to the actual experience of heart attack symptoms described by participants (53).

In addition to expecting a dramatic chest clutching presentation, knowledge of the complex array of heart attack symptoms, even the more common ones, is lacking in the American public. A random-digit-dialed telephone survey conducted among 1294 adult respondents in 20 communities from the REACT research program revealed that knowledge of chest pain as a presenting heart attack symptom was high and relatively uniform (89.7%). However, knowledge of some of the other associated symptoms was suboptimal. Only two-thirds (67.3%) identified arm pain as a symptom; shortness of breath was cited by half (50.8%) of the respondents, sweating was named by one-fifth (21.3%) of those surveyed, and other heart attack symptoms were less common. The median number of correct symptoms reported was 3 (of 11). Significantly higher mean numbers of correct symptoms were reported by non-Hispanic whites than by other racial or ethnic groups, by middle-aged persons than by older and younger persons, by persons with higher socioeconomic status than by those with lower, and by persons with previous experience with heart attack than by those without. Thus knowledge of chest pain (even though there is a misconception that it will be dramatic in nature) as an important heart attack symptom is high and relatively uniform; however, knowledge of the complex constellation of heart attack symptoms is deficient in the US population, especially in low socioeconomic and racial or ethnic minority groups. The authors concluded that at the earliest stages, delay in the recognition of symptoms as being caused by a heart attack, may be due to inadequate knowledge of heart attack symptoms or misattribution of the symptoms to another, noncardiac, and potentially less severe cause. They recommended that efforts to reduce delay in seeking medical care among persons with heart attack symptoms should address these deficiencies in knowledge (54).

Uncertainty about Symptoms

In addition, REACT focus group patients reported feeling uncertain about what the symptoms meant when they experienced them. Heart attack patients described a gradual process of symptom development, self-evaluation and self-treatment, and reevaluation and reappraisal over several hours. While they realized something was wrong, they reported taking a "wait and see" approach to the initial symptoms, hoping they would decline or cease. Elderly patients in particular often attributed the symptoms to other chronic conditions (53).

Perception of Heart Attack Risk

The majority of women in the focus groups believed heart attacks were a male problem. Older women (over age 65) did not link their health conditions to increased risk of a heart attack, especially after menopause. Men at higher risk due to the presence of one or more risk factors, discounted their personal risk if they were receiving regular health care for a chronic condition. Men were more likely than women to say that they were too young to experience a heart attack, perceiving it as a phenomenon of the elderly (53).

Lack of Knowledge of Current Treatments and Timely Care

The REACT focus groups also demonstrated that few were aware of the benefits of early treatment, including reperfusion therapy, and of accessing EMS. Although lacking knowledge, most participants were positive about EMS/9-1-1 with the exception of many African-American participants in the rural South and some Hispanic participants in Texas who perceived EMS services in their area to be inadequate *(53)*.

Calling 9-1-1

REACT investigators reported, based on a random-digit-dial survey conducted in 20 US communities at baseline, that nearly 90% of respondents said they would use EMS during a witnessed cardiac event. However, when they conducted a follow-up survey of chest pain patients presenting to participating emergency department's and either released or admitted to the hospital with a confirmed coronary event, the average proportion of patients who used EMS was 23% with significant geographic differences (range 10–48%). Most victims were driven by someone else (60.4%) or drove themselves to the hospital (15.6%). These findings indicate that, in general, community members recognize the benefit of EMS transport when acting as a bystander to a public cardiac event, but individuals personally experiencing symptoms of an acute MI often choose not to use EMS services. This implies there is a huge discrepancy between what people say they will do and what they actually do in the face of a cardiac event *(55)*.

Embarrassment about False Alarms

People also cited that fear of feeling embarrassed if their symptoms turned out to be a "false alarm", or a perception that they were not sick enough, was a deterrent to calling an ambulance. They also expressed a reluctance to "bother" physicians or EMS unless "really sick." The cost of health care or lack of insurance was not viewed as a barrier to seeking care in emergency situations. Many needed "permission" from others, such as their healthcare provider, spouse, or other family member to take rapid action *(53)*.

Calling a Physician

When patients call a physician for consultation about symptoms, rather than calling EMS, delay time is significantly increased (56–60). Physicians may not be readily available at the time of the call (leading to delays while office or telephone service staff try to reach them) or they may give advice that increases the delay to treatment *(23)*. REACT investigators reported that EMS use was decreased during a cardiac event if patients took an aspirin/antacid or communicated with a doctor before going to the hospital *(55)*.

Provider Discussions with Patients

A survey of patients who presented to hospital emergency departments in REACT communities, who were subsequently released from the emergency department, reported minimal discussion with health professionals or family about what to do in the event of heart attack symptoms prior to their admission. Few felt they knew what to do in case of an MI, even though emergency department staff generally reassured them about the appropriateness of coming in for evaluation of their symptoms (an important finding to convey to patients). About 25% of these released patients reported they were told to call their personal physician if symptoms return. Less than 10% said they were told explicitly to call EMS/9-1-1, although about half reported being told to "go to the emergency department " if symptoms returned.

Surveys of released patients also showed that, although many knew about chest pain as a symptom, few were aware of the other heart attack symptoms. Only about 55–60% were aware of thrombolytic drugs, which is about the same as the general public *(61)*.

A REACT survey of patients admitted to a hospital with an acute cardiac diagnosis found that few talked with healthcare providers about what to do in case of MI symptoms and the need to act quickly, either prior to admission (less than 10%) or after discharge (less than 3%). However while in the hospital, approximately half were talked to about MI symptoms, and half or more were addressed about the need to get to the emergency department quickly. Over 40% were given something to read or watch about MI. Thus, most talking about MI symptoms and the need to react quickly occurred in the hospital *(61)*.

Heart Attack Awareness Campaign

Now that REACT is completed, the NHAAP considered the results in terms how they can best inform the program's public education efforts. The NHAAP has revised the intervention materials created for the REACT research program, for national dissemination, and developed partnerships that could extend the reach of the materials. The program, working with its Coordinating Committee, identified key audiences that should be targeted: women, the elderly, minority groups—patients discharged from the hospital with an acute coronary event or released from the emergency department having been ruled out—and high-risk communities (e.g., those with a high prevalence of coronary heart disease.) The NHAAP intends to market revised REACT materials and to reach these defined audiences through working with strategic partners to get them to use the heart attack message and materials in their community outreach, patient education, and professional education programs.

In addition to revising the intervention materials used in REACT, a significant feature of the NHAAP's planning for its public education activities has been to work with the AHA to fine-tune the symptom message about heart attack warning signs as well as to agree on the action steps while ensuring a science-based approach. The public education materials and Web sites of both organizations reflect this work—they use the identical message about warning signs.

The program's revision of the REACT materials resulted in the "Act in Time To Heart Attack Signs" campaign which was officially launched on September 10 at a press conference, tied to an editorial in the journal *Circulation*. The *Circulation* editorial announced a joint call to action with the AHA to urge physicians to educate their patients about heart attack warning signs and the need to call 9-1-1 immediately. In it, both Dr. Claude Lenfant, Director, NHLBI, and Dr. David Faxon, AHA President, stress that doctor–patient discussions can deliver a powerful message about heart attack warning signs and the steps to take to minimize delay time *(62)*

The Act In Time campaign goal is to reduce delay in seeking emergency care for heart attack symptoms, employing findings from REACT to inform its strategy and messages. It targets patients, the general public (with the aforementioned targets in particular), and physicians with the basic heart attack recognition message and the recommended action steps.

The Act In Time materials include a booklet, a wallet-sized reminder card, a 1-h course with an educational video, a new Web site, and a coordinated set of materials for doctors and other healthcare providers. These include a poster, a laminated quick reference card, and a tear-off prescription pad for patient education.

Based on the findings from REACT, the Act In Time campaign seeks to dispel the misconceptions and fears reported by the REACT investigators and to urge people to learn the warning signs and make an action plan so they can act quickly in case of a heart attack (Fig. 12). It targets patients, the general public, and physicians.

In planning and conducting the campaign, the NHLBI is working in partnership with other organizations. They are the key to conducting a sustained campaign that has a broad reach and high visibility. The NHAAP's work with AHA is also being carried out under a broad partnership with organizations dedicated to helping achieve the objectives of Healthy People 2010, which is the federal government's blueprint for building a healthier nation. Healthy People objectives include raising awareness of heart attack symptoms, increasing the number of patients treated in the first hour of symptoms, and improving the timeliness of defibrillation for sudden cardiac arrest.

CONCLUSIONS

In summary, delays in early identification and treatment of acute MI patients with reperfusion therapy result in significant loss of myocardium and significant, quantifiable increases in mortality. While patient-mediated delays have yet to be resolved, delays in the emergency department have been effectively addressed by a continuous quality improvement (CQI) program that includes gathering of data on door-to-drug time, the frequency with which all patients, as well as subgroups of patients are treated, with reperfusion therapy, the use and kind of adjunctive drugs, and outcomes. A 30-min door-to-drug time as recommended by the NHAAP, can be achieved safely and effectively through a CQI program that continuously scrutinizes the process of care in relationship to time. As recommended in the ACC/AHA guidelines, primary angioplasty for ST-segment elevation left bundle-branch block MI should be performed when dilatation can be effected within 90 min of hospital arrival, and in hospitals with a volume of angioplasty experience at the individual operator and institutional level that exceeds the minimal figures *(39)*. Protocols which designate the process as well as the responsibility for implementation will facilitate early identification and treatment of patients with ST-segment elevation acute MI. Elements of hospital process that are driven by hospital policy and "turf" issues without benefit to the patient significantly delay reperfusion therapy and result in worse outcomes. A seamless patient-oriented protocol will promote a team approach to the care of these patients, which will result in best-expected outcomes.

Transport of patients by EMS leads to earlier treatment in the emergency department, as does identification through prehospital 12-lead ECGs that are transmitted to the hospital. Ideally, the physician–cardiology community should be involved in the EMS planning process for input into key issues that impact on timely treatment, such as diversion practices.

When talking with patients about recognizing and responding to a possible heart attack, providers need to be aware of the common misconceptions and knowledge deficiencies. They should dispel the myth of the "Hollywood" heart attack, acknowledging that while some heart attacks are sudden and intense and involve collapse, most start slowly with mild pain or discomfort. Providers also need to explain that, in addition to chest discomfort, patients may experience a feeling of being short of breath; sweating; pain in the arms, back, neck, jaw, or stomach; a feeling of being "sick to your stomach" or lightheaded. Providers should promote the notion of, "when in doubt, check it out", acknowledging that it is normal to be uncertain about what is wrong or embarrassed or afraid about calling 9-1-1, leading to untoward delays in getting help. In addition, providers can stress that the only way to know for sure is to be evaluated in a hospital emergency department. It is important that they also emphasize that patients will be taken seriously and treated respectfully if they come to the emergency department with possible heart attack signs, even "false alarms." Providers should actively address the benefits of artery-opening treatment and the importance of getting treatment quickly to stop a heart attack in its tracks. Furthermore, the role of early treatment in preventing death or severe heart muscle damage that will affect the quality of life should be directly explained. Patients should be reminded that heart attacks are the number one cause of death among women (as well as men) and that the risk increases greatly with age, especially after menopause. Finally, providers need to discuss individual patient's heart attack risk and what to do if faced with possible heart attack warning signs—including family and friends in the discussions—and develop an action plan with patients in advance.

Early patient recognition and action by calling 9-1-1 can result in early heart attack care by the healthcare system, the best kind short of prevention.

REFERENCES

1. American Heart Association. 2002 Heart and Stroke Statistical Update. American Heart Association, Dallas, 2001.
2. National Heart, Lung, and Blood Institute, Morbidity and Mortality Chart Book. National Heart, Lung, and Blood Institute, National Institutes of Health, Bethesda, 2000.
3. The GUSTO Investigators. An international randomized trial comparing four thrombolytic strategies for acute myocardial infarction. N Engl J Med 1993;329:673–682.
4. Cannon CP. Time to treatment of acute myocardial infarction revisited. Curr Opin Cardiol 1998;13: 254–266.
5. Timm TC, Ross R, McKendall GR, Braunwald E, Williams DO, and the TIMI Investigators. Left ventricular dysfunction and early cardiac events as a function of time to treatment with t-PA: a report from TIMI II [abstract]. Circulation 1991;84:II-230.
6. Newby LK, Rutsch WR, Califf RM, et al. Time from symptom onset to treatment and outcomes after thrombolytic therapy. J Am Coll Cardiol 1996;27:1646–1655.
7. Brouwer MA, Martin JS, Maynard C, et al. Influence of early prehospital thrombolysis on mortality and even-free survival (the Myocardial Infarction Triage and Intervention [MITI} Randomized Trial). Am J Cardiol 1996;78:497–502.
8. Cannon CP, Antman FM, Walls R, Braunwald E. Time as an adjunctive agent to thrombolytic therapy. J Thromb Thrombolysis 1994;1:27–34.
9. Goldberg RJ, Gurwitz JH, Gore JM. Duration of, and temporal trends (1994-1997) in, prehospital delay in patients with acute myocardial infarction: the second National Registry of Myocardial Infarction. Arch Intern Med 1999;159:2141–2147.
10. Barron HV, Bowlby LJ, Breen T, et al. Use of reperfusion therapy for acute myocardial infarction in the United States: data from the National Registry of Myocardial Infarction 2. Circulation 1998;97: 1150–1156.
11. Proceedings of the National Heart, Lung, and Blood Institute Symposium on Rapid Identification and Treatment of Acute Myocardial Infarction. U.S. Department of Health and Human Services. U.S. Government Printing Office 1991;281–846:40018.

12. National Heart Attack Alert Coordinating Committee, 60 Minutes to Treatment Working Group. Emergency department: rapid identification and treatment of patients with acute myocardial infarction. Ann Emerg Med 1994;23;311–329.

13. Ornato JP, Atkins JM, Horan M, et al. Staffing and equipping emergency medical services systems: rapid identification and treatment of acute myocardial infarction. U.S. Department of Health and Human Services, Public Health Service, National Institutes of Health, National Heart, Lung, and Blood Institute. NIH Publication No. 93-3304, September 1993.

14. Atkins J, Glass C, MacLeod B, Madewell W, Shade B, National Heart Attack Alert Program Coordinating Committee Access to Care Subcommittee Writing Group. 9-1-1: rapid identification and treatment of acute myocardial infarction. U.S. Department of Health and Human Services, Public Health Service, National Institutes of Health, National Heart, Lung, and Blood Institute. NIH Publication No. 94-3302, May 1994.

15. Clawson JJ, Atkins JM, Francis CK, et al. Emergency medical dispatching: Rapid identification and treatment of acute myocardial infarction. U.S. Department of Health and Human Services, Public Health Service, National Institutes of Health, National Heart, Lung, and Blood Institute. NIH Publication No. 94-3287, July 1994.

16. Selker HP, Zalenski RJ, Antman EM, et al. An evaluation of technologies for identifying acute cardiac ischemia in the emergency department: a report from a National Heart Attack Alert Program Working Group. Ann Emerg Med 1997;29:13–87.

17. Selker HP, Zalenski RJ, Antman EM, et al. An evaluation of technologies for identifying acute cardiac ischemia in the emergency department: executive summary of a National Heart Attack Alert Program Working Group report. Ann Emerg Med 1997;29:1–12.

18. Evaluation of Technologies for Identifying Acute Cardiac Ischemia in Emergency Departments. Evidence Report/Technology Assessment No. 26. Summary (AHRQ Publication No. 01-E006) and full evidence report (AHRQ 01-E006). [AHRQ Publications Clearinghouse].

19. Ornato JP, Selker HP, Zalenski RJ. Diagnosing acute cardiac ischemia in the emergency department: a report from the National Heart Attack Alert Program. Ann Emerg Med 2001;37:450–452.

20. Zalenski, RJ, Selker HP, Cannon CP, et al. National Heart Attack Alert Program position paper: chest pain centers and programs for the evaluation of acute cardiac ischemia. Ann Emerg Med 2000;35:462–471.

21. Symposium Proceedings. New Information Technology and the National Heart Attack Alert Program: setting a 5-year agenda. Cosponsored by the National Heart, Lung, and Blood Institute; National Library of Medicine; Agency for Health Care Policy and Research. National Institutes of Health, National Heart, Lung, and Blood Institute. NIH Publication No. 99-4089. September 1999.

22. Dracup K, Alonzo AA, Atkins JM, et al. Patient/bystander recognition and action: rapid identification and treatment of acute myocardial infarction. U.S. Department of Health and Human Services, Public Health Service, National Institutes of Health, National Heart, Lung, and Blood Institute. NIH Publication No. 93-3303, September 1993.

23. Dracup K, Alonzo AA, Atkins JM, et al. The physician's role in minimizing prehospital delay in patients at high risk for acute myocardial infarction: recommendations from the National Heart Attack Alert Program. Ann Intern Med 1997:126:645–651.

24. National Heart Attack Alert Program Coordinating Committee Working Group on Educational Strategies to Prevent Prehospital Delay in Patients at High Risk for Acute Myocardial Infarction. Educational Strategies to Prevent Prehospital Delay in Patients at High Risk for Acute Myocardial Infarction. National Institutes of Health, National Heart, Lung, and Blood Institute. NIH Publication No. 97-3787. September 1997.

25. National Heart Attack Alert Program Coordinating Committee, Access to Care Subcommittee. Access to timely and optimal care of patients with acute coronary syndromes—community planning considerations: a report by the National Heart Attack Alert Program. J Thromb Thrombolysis 1998;6:19–46.

26. Cannon CP. Time to treatment: a crucial factor in thrombolysis and primary angioplasty. J Thromb Thrombolysis 1996;3:249–255.

27. Goldberg R, Goff D, Cooper L, et al. Age and sex differences in presentation of symptoms among patients with acute coronary disease. Coron Artery Dis 2000;11:399–407.

28. Canto JG, Shlipak MG, Rogers WG, et al. Prevalence, clinical characteristics, and mortality among patients with myocardial infarction presenting without chest pain. JAMA 2000;283:3223–3229.

29. Lambrew CT, Bowlby LJ, Rogers WJ, et al. Factors influencing the time to thrombolysis in acute myocardial infarction. Arch Intern Med 1997;157:2577–2582.

30. Lambrew CT, Weaver WD, Rogers WJ, et al. Hospital protocols and policies that may delay early identification and thrombolytic therapy of acute myocardial infarction patients. J Thromb Thrombolysis 1996;3:301–306.
31. Al-Mubarak N, Rogers WJ, Lambrew CT, Bowlby LJ, French WJ. Consultation before thrombolytic therapy in acute myocardial infarction. Am J Cardiol 1999;83:89–93,A8.
32. Lambrew CT. Emergency Department triage of patients with non-traumatic chest pain. Acc Curr J Rev 1995;4:61–62.
33. Cannon CP. Critical pathways for management of patients with acute coronary syndromes. An assessment by the National Heart Attack Alert Program. Am Heart J 2002;143:777–789.
34. Cannon CP, Johnson EG, Cermignani M, Scirica BM, Sagarin MJ, Walls RM. Emergency department thrombolysis critical pathway reduces door-to-drug times in acute myocardial infarction. Clin Cardiol 1999;22:17–20.
35. Cannon CP, Gibson CM, Lambrew CT, et al. Longer thrombolysis door-to-needle times are associated with increased mortality in acute myocardial infarction: an analysis of 85,589 patients in the National Registry of Myocardial Infarction 2 & 3. J Am Coll Cardiol 2000;35(Suppl. A):376A.
36. Cannon CP, Gibson CM, Lambrew CT, et al. Relationship of symptom-onset-to-balloon time and door-to-balloon time with mortality in patients undergoing angioplasty for acute myocardial infarction. JAMA 2000;283:2941–2947.
37. Rogers WJ, Canto JG, Lambrew CT, et al. Temporal trends in the treatment of over 1.5 million patients with myocardial infarction in the US from 1990 through 1999: the National Registry of Myocardial Infarction 1, 2 and 3. J Am Coll Cardiol 2000;36:2056–2063.
38. Burwen DR, Galusha DH, Lewis JM, Krumholz HM, Bedinger MR, Radford MJ. National trends in the quality of care for acute myocardial infarction (AMI) between 1994–1995 and 1998-1999, Health Care Financing Administration, Baltimore, MD, and Qualidigm, Middletown, CT. Presented at the American College of Cardiology 50th Annual Scientific Sessions, Orlando, FL, March 20, 2001.
39. Ryan TJ, Anderson JL, Antman EM, et al. 1999 update ACC/AHA guidelines for the management of patients with acute myocardial infarction: a report of the American College of Cardiology/American Heart Association Task Force on Practice Guidelines (Committee on Management of Acute Myocardial Infarction). J Am Coll Cardiol 1999;34:890–911.
40. Bahr RD. Milestones in the development of the first chest pain center and development of the new Society of Chest Pain Centers and Providers. Fourth National Congress of Chest Pain Centers in Emergency Departments. Heart attack: the public health challenge for the new millennium. A supplement to Maryland Medicine. Spring 2001:106–108.
41. Rosamond W. Trends in mortality due to coronary heart disease and trends in incidence of survival after, and medical care for hospitalized acute myocardial infarction: the Atherosclerosis Risk In Communities (ARIC) Study 1987-1998, National Heart, Lung, and Blood Institute, Surveillance Working Group, Bethesda, MD, 2001.
42. Luepker RV, Raczynski JM, Osganian S, et al. Effect of a community intervention on patient delay and emergency medical service use in acute coronary heart disease: the Rapid Early Action for Coronary Treatment (REACT) trial. J Am Med Assoc 2000;284:60–67.
43. Canto JG, Zalenski R, Ornato JP, et al. Utilization of the emergency medical system among patients with myocardial infarction in the reperfusion era: results from the NRMI-2. J Am Coll Cardiol 2001;20A.
44. Hedges JR, Mann NC, Meischke H, Robbins M, Goldberg R, Zapka J. Assessment of chest pain onset and out-of-hospital delay using standardized interview questions: the REACT Pilot Study. Rapid Early Action for Coronary Treatment (REACT) Study Group. Acad Emerg Medi 1998;5:773–780.
45. Canto JG, Rogers WJ, Bowlby LJ, et al. The prehospital electrocardiogram in acute myocardial infarction: is its full potential being realized? National Registry of Myocardial Infarction 2 Investigators. J Am Coll Cardiol 1997;29:498–505.
46. The European Myocardial Infarction Project Group. Prehospital thrombolytic therapy in patients with suspected acute myocardial infarction. N Engl J Med 1993;329:383–389.
47. Morrison LJ, Verbeek Pr, McDonald AC, Sawadsky BV, Cook DJ. Mortality and prehospital thrombolysis for acute myocardial inaction: a meta-analysis. JAMA 2000;283:2686–2692.
48. Guidelines 2000 for Cardiopulmonary Resuscitation and Emergency Cardiovascular Care. International Consensus on Science. Supplement to Circulation 2000;102(8).
49. Gruppo Italiano per lo Studio della Streptochinasi nell' Infarcto Miocardico (GISSI). Effectiveness of Intravenous Thrombolytic Treatment in Acute Myocardial Infarction. Lancet 1986;1:397–401.

50. The TIMI Study Group. Comparison of invasive and conservative strategies after treatment with intravenous tissue plasminogen activator in acute myocardial infarction. Results of the Thrombolysis in Myocardial Infarction (TIMI) Phase II Trial. N Engl J Med 1989;320:618–627.

51. The GUSTO Investigators. An international randomized trial comparing four thrombolytic strategies for acute myocardial infarction. N Engl J Med 1993;329:673:682.

52. Goff DC, Feldman HA, McGovern PG, et al. Prehospital delay in patients hospitalized with heart attack symptoms in the United States: the REACT trial. Am Heart J 1999;138:1046–1057.

53. Finnegan JR, Meischke H, Zapka JG, et al. Patient delay in seeking care for heart attack symptoms: Findings from focus groups conducted in five U.S. regions. Prev Med 2000;31:205–213.

54. Goff DC, Sellers DE, McGovern PG, et al. Knowledge of heart attack symptoms in a population survey in the United States: the REACT Trial. Rapid Early Action for Coronary Treatment. Arch Intern Med 1998;158:2329–2338.

55. Brown AL, Mann NC, Daya M, et al. Demographic, belief and situational factors influencing the decision to utilize emergency medical services among chest pain patients. Circulation 2000;102:173–178.

56. Alonzo AA. The impact of the family and lay others on care-seeking during life-threatening episodes of suspected coronary artery disease. Soc Sci Med 1986;22:1297–311.

57. Simon AB, Feinleib M, Thompson HK Jr. Components of delay in the pre hospital phase of acute myocardial infarction. Am J Cardiol 1972;30:476–482.

58. Schroeder JS, Lamb IH, Hu M. The prehospital course of patients with chest pain: analysis of the prodromal, symptomatic, decision-making, transportation and emergency room periods. Am J Med 1978; 64:742–748.

59. Leitch JW, Birbara T, Freedman B, Wilcox I, Harris PJ. Factors influencing the time from onset of chest pain to arrival at hospital. Med J Aust 1989;150:6–10.

60. Gray D, Keating NA, Murdock, Skene AM, Hampton JR. Impact of hospital thrombolysis policy on out-of-hospital response to suspected myocardial infarction. Lancet 1993;341:654–657.

61. REACT Investigators. NHAAP Coordinating Committee meeting, May 1999.

62. Faxon D, Lenfant C. Timing is everything. Motivating patients to call 9 1 1 at onset of acute myocardial infarction. Circulation 2001;104:1210–1211

7

Serum Markers for Diagnosis and Risk Stratification in Acute Coronary Syndromes

L. Kristin Newby, MD, W. Brian Gibler, MD, Robert H. Christenson, PhD, and E. Magnus Ohman, MD

INTRODUCTION

Increasingly, both economic and clinical pressures necessitate accurate diagnosis and risk stratification of patients presenting to Emergency Departments (EDs) with suspected or actual acute coronary syndromes. Of the more than 6 million patients who present to EDs in the United States each year for evaluation of chest pain or anginal-equivalent symptoms, only about 15% are identified as having an acute myocardial infarction (MI). Conversely, the conventional evaluation, which includes a history, physical examination, and screening electrocardiogram (ECG) and creatine kinase (CK)-MB, may miss up to 25% of acute MIs at presentation. When unstable angina and nonacute coronary artery disease (CAD) presentations are accounted for, 40% of patients with chest pain do not have an underlying coronary etiology for their symptoms. The challenge is to identify both this group and the group at higher risk as early as possible, to pro-

From: *Contemporary Cardiology: Management of Acute Coronary Syndromes, Second Edition*
Edited by: C. P. Cannon © Humana Press Inc., Totowa, NJ

mote rapid treatment of those who may benefit from specific medical or interventional approaches and to avoid costly hospitalization and testing in those at low risk.

This chapter will discuss the evaluation and management of patients with suspected acute coronary syndromes and the use of serum cardiac markers of myocardial necrosis for diagnosis and risk stratification in all chest pain populations. Focus will be placed on the use of cardiac markers in conjunction with the Chest Pain Unit concept for efficient evaluation and triage of patients with chest pain.

INITIAL EVALUATION OF CHEST PAIN IN THE ED

Perhaps the greatest diagnostic and triaging challenge for the ED physician lies in the evaluation of patients presenting with chest pain. The tools immediately available, which are limited in their sensitivity and specificity for acute coronary ischemia, include the initial history, the physical examination, and the 12-lead ECG.

The History and Physical Examination

In the setting of chest pain, the physician's impression of the symptoms as definitely, probably, probably not, or not angina, along with key historical features of prior MI, sex of the patient, age, and number of risk factors (diabetes, smoking, hypercholesterolemia, and hypertension), help establish the likelihood of coronary artery disease *(1)*.

Chest pain or pressure or epigastric burning discomfort, often with radiation to the neck, arms, shoulders, or jaw, is the most common description of ischemic pain *(2–5)*. Dyspnea, diaphoresis, nausea, and vomiting may accompany these symptoms or, in less typical presentations, occur as the sole manifestation of ischemia *(4,6)*. Less often, ischemic pain may be described as sharp or pleuritic *(4,5)*. Older patients and diabetics are more likely to have atypical clinical presentations of ischemia; this warrants increased attention to evaluation of their symptoms *(7)*.

The physical examination is nonspecific for establishing the diagnosis of acute coronary ischemia, but the presence of an S4 or S3 gallop, rales, or hypotension, or the development of transient or worsening mitral regurgitation during symptoms, are important in risk stratification and can support this diagnosis or one of underlying coronary disease *(1,4,8–10)*. If chest pain is reproduced with palpation or movement, it should not lead to a false sense of security about the etiology of symptoms as noncardiac. In one study by Tierney et al., 15% of patients with acute MI complained of tenderness on chest wall palpation *(4)*, and Lee and colleagues found that to be completely certain that chest wall pain was not due to acute coronary ischemia, the pain must be described as sharp or stabbing and be completely reproduced by palpation *(5)*.

The 12-Lead ECG

The 12-lead ECG is usually the earliest available objective test for the presence or absence of cardiac ischemia and can provide important diagnostic and prognostic information in patients with chest pain. In the presence of ST-segment elevation on the 12-lead ECG, the diagnosis of acute MI is confirmed in over 90% of cases by serial CK-MB testing *(11,12)*. Unfortunately, only about 10% of all acute MIs present with ST-segment elevation on the initial ECG; most are confirmed only in retrospect, by serial tracings showing the development of new Q waves or by serial CK-MB testing *(11,13,14)*. The initial 12-lead ECG is further limited in that it provides only a static image of what is usually a dynamic ischemic process and that it has limited ability to evaluate for

Table 1
Likelihood of Significant CAD in Patients with Symptoms Suggesting Unstable Angina

High likelihood (e.g., 0.85–0.99)	Intermediate likelihood (e.g., 0.15–0.84)	Low likelihood (e.g., 0.01–0.14)
Any of the following features:	Absence of high likelihood features and any of the following:	Absence of high or intermediate likelihood features, but may have:
• History of prior MI or sudden death or other known history of CAD.	• Definite angina: males < 60 or females < 70 yr of age.	• Chest pain classifies as probably not angina.
• Definite angina: males ≥ 60 or females ≥ 70 yr of age.	• Probable angina: males ≥ 60 or females ≥ 70 years of age.	• One risk factor other than diabetes.
• Transient hemodynamic or ECG changes during pain.	• Chest pain probably not angina and 2 or 3 risk factors other than diabetes.[a]	• T-wave flattening or inversion < 1mm in leads with dominant R-waves.
• Variant angina (pain with reversible ST-segment elevation)	• Extracardiac vascular disease.	• Normal ECG.
• ST-segment elevation or depression ≥ 1 mm.	• ST-segment depression 0.05–1 mm.	
• Marked symmetrical T-wave inversion ≥ 1 mm in multiple precordial leads.	• T-wave inversion ≥ 1 mm in leads with dominant R-waves.	

[a]Coronary artery disease risk factors include diabetes, smoking, hypertension, and elevated cholesterol.

ischemia in the posterior basal and lateral walls. Despite the lack of diagnostic sensitivity of the initial ECG for acute MI, it can support the overall clinical impression of underlying coronary artery disease (for example, the presence of Q waves) and can provide prognostic information. Dynamic ST-segment elevation or depression and T-wave changes predict a higher short-term risk of death or MI and can be used along with the clinical evaluation to risk-stratify patients presenting with chest pain into high-, moderate-, and low-risk categories for initial triage (1,15–19) (Tables 1 and 2).

Analysis of presenting ECGs from patients in the Global Use of Strategies To Open Occluded Arteries in Acute Coronary Syndromes (GUSTO-IIa) trial showed that the presenting ECG category (ST-segment elevation, ST-segment depression, T-wave inversion/normal, or confounding ECG factors) was an important predictor of short-term mortality in a logistic regression model (20). The highest-risk group included patients with ECG confounders that obscured interpretation of the ST-segment (left bundle-branch block, paced rhythm, or left ventricular hypertrophy), who had a 30-d mortality of 11.6%, followed by ST-segment depression (8.0%), ST-segment elevation (7.4%), and finally, the very-low-risk T-wave inversion/normal group, with a 30-d mortality of only 1.2%. The relationship of the baseline ECG findings with mortality and nonfatal cardiac events in the GUSTO-IIa population is shown in Table 3. A similar gradation

Table 2
Short-Term Risk of Death or Nonfatal MI in Patients with Unstable Angina

High risk	Intermediate risk	Low risk
At least one of the following features must be present:	No high risk feature, but must have any of the following:	No high or intermediate risk feature, but may have any of the following features:
• Prolonged ongoing (>20 min) rest pain.	• Prolonged (>20 min) rest angina, now resolved, with moderate or high likelihood of CAD.	• Increased angina frequency, severity, or duration.
• Pulmonary edema, most likely related to ischemia.	• Rest angina (>20 min or relieved with rest or sublingual nitroglycerin).	• Angina provoked at a lower threshold.
• Angina at rest with dynamic ST-segment changes ≥ 1 mm.	• Nocturnal angina.	• New onset angina with onset 2 wk to 2 mo prior to presentation.
• Angina with new or worsening MR murmur. • Angina with S3 or new and/or worsening rales.	• Angina with dynamic T-wave changes.	• Normal or unchanged ECG.
	• New onset CCSC III or IV angina in the past 2 wk with moderate or high likelihood of CAD.	
• Angina with hypotension.	• Pathologic Q waves or resting ST-segment depression ≤ 1 mm in multiple lead groups (anterior, inferior, lateral).	
	• Age > 65 yr.	

Abbreviations: MR, mitral regurgitation; CAD, coronary artery disease; CCSC, Canadian Cardiovascular Society Class.

of risk by initial ECG characteristics occurred in studies of chest pain patients by Brush and colleagues *(21)* and Villanueva et al. *(8)*. In 12,124 acute coronary syndrome patients enrolled in the GUSTO-IIb trial, Savonitto and colleagues showed that as for 30-d events, the baseline ECG correlated with mortality at 6 mo. In their analysis, patients with T-wave inversion had the lowest mortality (3.4%), followed by ST-segment elevation (6.8%), ST-segment depression (8.9%), and combination ST-segment elevation and depression (9.1%) *(22)*.

In summary, using the conventional tools of the history, the physical examination, and the initial ECG evaluation, the sensitivities of ED physicians for admitting acute MI and unstable angina patients are 92–98% and 90%, respectively *(23–27)*. Specificity is low, however, as only about 30–40% of admitted patients ultimately are found to have an acute coronary syndrome as the etiology for their symptoms *(28,29)*. In the Thrombolysis in Myocardial Infarction (TIMI) IIIb study of conservative vs early interventional care in patients meeting clinical and ECG criteria for unstable angina, 18% of patients were found to have no significant CAD at cardiac catheterization *(30)* (Fig. 1).

Table 3
Characteristics and Outcomes by Admission Electrocardiographic Category[a]

	ST elevation (n = 435)	ST depression (n = 88)	T-Wave depression normal (n = 163)	Electrocardiographic confounders[b] (n = 69)[b]	P
Baseline characteristics					
Duration of chest pain (h)	3.0 (1.7, 4.7)	2.9 (1.5, 5.6)	2.1 (0.8, 4.5)	2.6 (1.0, 4.0)	0.093
CK-MB > 7 ng/mL	143 (32.9)	30 (34.1)	44 (27.0)	28 (40.6)	0.218
TnT > 0.1 ng/mL	138 (31.7)	43 (48.9)	49 (30.1)	39 (56.5)	<0.0001
30-D outcomes[c]					
Death	32 (7.4)	7 (8.0)	2 (1.2)	8 (11.6)	0.010
MI	366 (84.1)	50 (56.8)	83 (50.9)	46 (66.7)	<0.0001
Bypass surgery	63 (14.5)	23 (26.1)	32 (19.6)	7 (10.1)	0.016
Angioplasty	142 (32.6)	20 (22.7)	53 (32.5)	21 (30.4)	0.319
Composite outcome[d]	393 (90.3)	67 (76.1)	114 (69.9)	51 (73.9)	<0.0001

[a]Values are medians (25th, 75th percentiles) or frequencies (percentages).
[b]Bundle-branch block, ventricular hypertrophy, idioventricular, or paced rhythms.
[c]Multiple outcomes are possible.
[d]The occurrence of death, MI, or revascularization by 30 d.
Adapted from ref. 20.

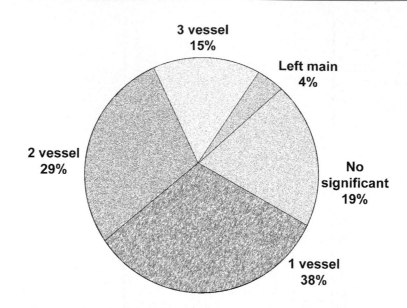

Fig. 1. Extent of coronary artery disease in 720 patients with unstable angina or non-Q wave infarction who underwent angiography in TIMI IIIb. Data from ref. *30*.

Conversely, 2–10% of patients sent home from the ED after initial evaluation of their symptoms will actually have had an unrecognized acute MI *(25,31–33)*; up to 25% of these are due to misinterpretation of the initial 12-lead ECG *(25,32)*. Approximately 25% of patients sent home from the ED with an unrecognized MI may die *(25,31,32)*. This figure, coupled with the recognition that the leading cause of malpractice litigation against ED physicians (about 20% of awards), is related to misdiagnosis of acute MI in this minority of patients *(34)*, creates understandable pressure for ED physicians to admit a large proportion of the chest pain patients they see. This practice pattern leads to significant drains on limited in-hospital resources, including beds and nursing staff, and results in an estimated $600 million in hospital costs annually for patients without a coronary etiology for their symptoms *(35)*.

STRATEGIES TO IMPROVE DIAGNOSTIC ACCURACY OF INITIAL CHEST PAIN EVALUATION

To improve the diagnostic accuracy of the ED physician for acute coronary syndromes, many evaluation strategies and diagnostic adjuncts to the traditional history, physical examination, and baseline ECG have been developed. The use of diagnostic decision aids (algorithms, predictive instruments, and neural networks) that incorporate and synthesize the information gleaned from the presenting history, physical examination, and the initial ECG will be discussed in more detail in Chapter 8. The use of serial ECGs or continuous 12-lead ECG monitoring for ST-segment shifts, as well as both acute echocardiographic and sestamibi nuclear imaging, offer promise in facilitating diagnosis and triage in the ED setting. However, they remain limited by availability of services and technical expertise in many facilities. Research addressing the diagnostic ability and cost of such strategies will be needed before widespread use can be promoted.

Serial ECG Analysis and Continuous ST-Segment Trend Monitoring

Because the process of ischemia is a dynamic one, the initial 12-lead ECG, which captures only a static image of the process at one time point, may miss patients with significant underlying ischemic disease. The use of serial ECG tracings over 3 to 4 h or with a change in symptoms is one method for diagnosing the cause of the symptoms and detecting early ischemia that might prompt intervention, including thrombolytic therapy, in a patient who was initially not a candidate. However, detection of changes in serial ECGs that warrant intervention is infrequent; in addition, an overall strategy of serial ECGs has been shown to have a lower sensitivity and specificity than serial CK-MB testing over the same interval *(36)*.

Some ischemic changes may be silent, technical and logistic limitations may prevent obtaining 12-lead ECGs that are truly diagnostic of the ongoing process, and serial ECGs even at 3- to 4-h intervals may miss diagnostic changes. The use of continuous 12-lead ECG monitoring for ST-segment trends attempts to circumvent these problems. Patients are hooked to an instrument that samples a 12-lead ECG in the usual configuration every 20 s and repeatedly compares it to the previously acquired tracing for changes in the ST-segment (elevation or depression) of ≥0.1 mV. At this point, an alarm sounds and a 12-lead ECG is printed for review. If there are no alarm ECGs, serial 12-lead ECGs are saved approx every 20 min and can be used for later review. This method creates a dynamic record of the patient's course; diagnostic changes are picked up that would otherwise have been missed by static 12-lead ECG evaluation.

In retrospective studies of the use of continuous ST-segment trend monitoring in the ED setting, the sensitivity and positive predictive value were low in overall low prevalence chest pain ED populations *(37,38)*. The use of the technology is limited by patient comfort (patients cannot be ambulatory during the time of monitoring), and baseline artifact related to patient movement can make interpretation inaccurate. In addition, the financial expense of such a monitoring system may be prohibitive. Although the potential for this technology is clear, the National Heart Attack Alert Program Working Group has recommended further prospective studies of its benefit and cost-effectiveness before widespread use in the general ED chest pain population *(39)*. The ongoing Prognostic Accuracy of Cardiac Troponin Studies and Holter ST Monitoring (PACTS) trial was designed to answer these questions. This 1000 patient multicenter study will evaluate the prognostic utility and cost-effectiveness of ST-segment trend monitoring alone and in combination with cardiac troponin I measurement in 1000 patients who present with non-ST-segment elevation acute coronary syndromes.

IMAGING IN THE ED

Acute Echocardiographic Imaging

In the setting of acute coronary ischemia, insufficient blood flow to the myocardium results in abnormalities of wall motion and abnormalities of normal systolic wall thickening. Echocardiographic imaging can detect these abnormalities but cannot distinguish ischemia from acute infarction. However, in patients with chest pain without clear ischemia on ECG and atypical or low risk clinical features, echocardiographic imaging may help clarify the diagnosis. In general, the greatest value has been shown in young male patients without prior cardiac history. Small studies in highly selected populations of patients without known CAD or prior infarction have shown sensitivities from 86–92% and specificities from 53–90% depending on the timing of the ECG with chest pain symptoms and whether acute MI or acute coronary ischemia was the endpoint *(39)*. In a larger study of unselected chest pain patients, Sabia and colleagues reported that 94% of studies were technically adequate with a sensitivity of 93% and a specificity of 57% for acute MI *(40)*.

When considering the use of echocardiographic imaging for diagnosis of MI in ED chest pain patients, keep in mind that obtaining good images of all segments of the myocardium is critical for the accuracy of this means of evaluation. In addition, assessing wall motion abnormalities due to ischemia in patients with prior infarction or left bundle-branch block or after bypass surgery is challenging due to baseline abnormalities of wall motion. Specialized equipment and highly trained individuals capable of performing and interpreting the studies are necessary on-site 24 h a day. The use of telemedicine interpretation of ED ECGs as described by Trippi and colleagues *(41)* could obviate the need to have a cardiologist available on-site for interpretation.

Although early work offers promise, it is not clear that echocardiography adds to the diagnostic accuracy of simpler and more routine ECG and cardiac marker evaluation. At least one small study in the ED setting has shown no advantage from the addition of echocardiographic imaging in the evaluation of chest pain patients *(42)*. Further studies in this group will be needed to assess echocardiography's effect on clinical outcomes, as well as its cost-effectiveness.

Nuclear Imaging

The National Heart Attack Alert Program Working Group has recently published a summary and analysis of the published literature on the use of nuclear perfusion imaging in the ED for the evaluation of chest pain patients *(39)*. In general, the reported sensitivities and specificities of ^{99}Tc sestamibi imaging for predicting acute MI in these studies was >90% and in the 80–90 % range, respectively. Positive and negative predictive values in these studies were also high. In addition, their review of the literature suggests that negative sestamibi imaging in the ED identifies a population at low risk for both short- and long-term cardiac events.

Similar to the case with echocardiographic imaging, the widespread use of nuclear imaging for evaluation of chest pain patients in the ED is limited by the need for 24-h availability of personnel trained in the use of radioisotopes and nuclear imaging techniques, as well as someone to interpret the results in real time. Furthermore, the cost-effectiveness of using nuclear imaging alone or in conjunction with other diagnostic aids such as serial ECGs or ST-segment trend monitoring or cardiac marker analysis has yet to be demonstrated. However, in a study that compared the use of ^{99}Tc sestamibi imaging with troponin I (TnI) analysis for detection of acute MI or the need for revascularization in 424 ED patients with chest pain, Kontos and colleagues concluded that the 2 tests provided complementary information *(43)*. [99]Tc sestamibi imaging identified more patients for revascularization than TnI, but the sensitivity for detecting MI in the low risk population was similar for both strategies. TnI was more specific for the diagnosis of MI than the nuclear imaging strategy, however.

MARKERS OF MYOCARDIAL NECROSIS

The use of cardiac markers in the ED setting is now commonplace and provides additional valuable information to that from the initial ECG, history, and physical examination. For most available markers, the quantitative assay time is 20 min or less, and the overall turnaround time is within 1 to 2 of ordering the test. The development of bedside qualitative assays for various markers or panels of markers promises not only to shorten the overall time to test result, but also to place the testing and result reporting in the hands of the caregivers, a feature that should aid in rapid decision-making in the ED. The use of individual bedside testing assays for cardiac troponin I (cTnI) and troponin T (cTnT) has been studied in several large trials for chest-pain evaluation in the emergency department and for acute ST-segment elevation MI *(44–46)*. In a study of 609 chest pain patients, van Lente and colleagues directly compared bedside qualitative cTnT testing (cut point 0.2 ng/mL) with in-laboratory quantitative testing using the same cut point, finding comparable performance in identifying patients at increased risk for cardiac events *(44)*.

The likelihood of a positive cardiac marker result drawn in the ED in a patient with true myocardial necrosis depends on the release and clearance properties of the marker, the time since symptom onset, and the sensitivity of the marker assay. While a positive marker result identifies a patient at higher risk who should be admitted to a closely monitored setting (if not a cardiac care unit [CCU]) *(47)*, a negative result should not be the sole determinant of whether a patient is released from the ED. This is especially important if other high risk features supporting the diagnosis of unstable angina or possible acute MI have been identified. Almost 50% of patients with an ultimate diagnosis of acute MI will be missed by a single screening CK-MB test obtained on presentation to the ED, and the combination of the initial ECG and CK-MB will miss about 25% of patients with acute MI *(48)*. Research is ongoing to determine the best marker or combination of markers to evaluate chest pain in the emergency setting. The markers of myocardial necrosis that are currently available to the ED physician are discussed in the following section; their properties are summarized in Table 4 and Fig. 2.

The Ideal Marker

An ideal marker of cardiac injury should be both cardiac-specific and have zero blood concentration in the absence of myocardial injury. It should become elevated in the serum soon after the onset of an episode of chest pain to allow the detection of high-risk patients as early as possible and should remain elevated for many hours to allow detection in patients who delay in seeking evaluation. Persistent elevation of a marker for several days could aid in diagnosis and risk stratification of patients with periodic symptoms or those presenting to the ED well after the episode that prompted evaluation. The ideal cardiac marker assay would be inexpensive, have rapid in-laboratory and reporting turnaround times, or be available at the bedside, where ordering, testing, and results feedback would be in the hands of the caregivers.

The most commonly used markers of myocardial necrosis include myoglobin, CK, the cardiac-specific isoenzyme of CK (CK-MB), CK-MB subforms (MB1 and MB2), and cTnI and cTnT. Although none of these individual markers meets all characteristics of the ideal marker, a combination of the individual assays into a panel of tests could

Table 4
Characteristics of Various Biochemical Markers of Myocardial Necrosis

	Myoglobin	Total CK	CK-MB (mass)	MB2/ MB1	cTnT	cTnI
Molecular weight (kDa)	17.8	85	85	NA	33	23.5
Cardiac-specific	No	No	++	++	+++	+++
Affected by renal function	Yes	No	Yes	No	Yes	Yes
Initial detection	1–3 h	4–8 h	3–4 h	3–4 h	4–6 h	4–6 h
Duration of elevation	18–24 h	12–24 h	24–36 h	Unknown	10–14 d	7–10 d
Laboratory assay time, min[a]	8–20	10–20	8–30	25	45[b]	8–25
Bedside assay	Yes	Yes	Yes	No	Yes	Yes

Abbreviations: CK, creatine kinase; cTnT, cardiac troponin T; cTnI, cardiac troponin I; LDH, lactate dehydrogenase; NA, not available; h, hours; d, days; ++, very specific; +++, extremely specific.

[a]The times listed represent on-instrument duration only and do not take into account sample transport or specimen handling. Specimen handling routinely includes accessioning, labeling, centrifugation, and aliquoting, which typically requires about 15 min.

[b]12-Min assay currently in final phase of FDA approval process.

Adapted from Newby LK, Christenson RH, Ohman EM. Role of troponin and other markers of myocardial necrosis in risk stratification. In: Topol EJ, ed. Acute Coronary Syndromes. Marcel Dekker, New York, 1998, pp. 405–435.

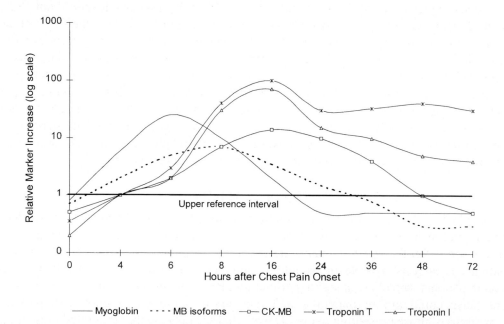

Fig. 2. Relative marker increase over time. Adapted with permission from Newby LK, Christenson RH, Ohman EM. Role of troponin and other markers of myocardial necrosis in risk stratification. In: Topol EJ, ed. Acute Coronary Syndromes. Marcel Dekker, New York, 1998, pp. 405–435.

cover all needs efficiently. Because of the superiority of these markers (alone or in combination), lactate dehydrogenase (LDH) has largely fallen out of use as a marker of myocardial necrosis. The in-laboratory assay times for all of these markers are within 15–20 min, and bedside assays are available for most.

Although the use of cardiac markers (including bedside assays) in chest pain patients has been shown to be of prognostic importance, and Downie and colleagues *(49)* showed that in the CCU setting, bedside assessment of myocardial necrosis was feasible and allowed for more rapid management decisions, the question remains whether point-of-care testing can measurably shorten ED evaluation time. In their study of point-of-care testing of routine chemistries in the ED, Parvin and colleagues *(50)* found no significant difference in ED length of stay through physician use of bedside point-of-care testing, even after adjusting for differences in presenting conditions. Further study of the effect of point-of-care testing of cardiac markers on ED length of stay, rapidity of treatment decisions, and, ultimately, outcome vs standard testing will be needed.

Myoglobin

Myoglobin is a 17.8-kDa heme protein common to all striated muscle; therefore, it is not cardiac-specific. Owing to its small size, it may be detected in the serum within 1–3 h after the onset of ischemic symptoms. Despite a lack of specificity, myoglobin has high diagnostic sensitivity; thus, a negative myoglobin during this time frame has excellent negative predictive value *(51,52)*. Because of rapid renal clearance, myoglobin remains elevated above the reference range for only 12–18 h. This makes it less useful as a diagnostic marker in later presentations of acute coronary syndromes. Because it is eliminated renally, it may be elevated (in the absence of cardiac muscle injury) in patients with chronic renal insufficiency; it also may be falsely elevated in patients with skeletal muscle trauma or even after strenuous exercise. These factors limit the use of myoglobin alone as a diagnostic marker for patients with suspected acute MI.

Creatine Kinase

CK is an 85-kDa enzyme found in all striated muscle cells, where it catalyzes the phosphorylation of creatine to creatine phosphate. There are three isoenzymes of CK, each composed of two subunits (M and B): CK-MM, the predominant form in striated muscle (cardiac and skeletal); CK-MB, most common in the heart; and CK-BB, most common in the brain but also found in the gut and kidney. Sensitivity for acute MI is greater than 90% by 6 h, and total CK may be detectable in the serum as early as 4 h after the onset of symptoms. Because assays for total CK detect all three isoenzymes, however, total CK is not cardiac-specific.

The reference range for total CK assays depends on the patient's age, sex, and race, and levels of total CK may be falsely elevated in many pathological and other conditions *(13,53)*. Therefore, it is a relatively nonspecific marker that alone has limited utility for the diagnosis of myocardial injury.

Creatine Kinase-MB

Although CK-MM is the predominant isoenzyme of CK in both cardiac and skeletal muscle, CK-MB is relatively cardiac-specific, with only small amounts (up to 5%) detected by immunoassay in skeletal muscle. However, CK-MB may be produced in increased amounts in skeletal muscle after trauma or in inflammatory conditions.

Because the CK-MB isoform is found predominantly in cardiac muscle, it is more specific for the diagnosis of myocardial injury and, therefore, provides a distinct advantage over total CK. It becomes elevated within 3 to 4 h after the onset of ischemic myocardial injury and returns to baseline within 24–36 h. Therefore, although it provides a nearly ideal timing profile for a marker of major myocardial necrosis, it remains limited in its ability to detect small amounts of myocardial damage (infarctlets) that may be prognostically important but obscured by background release from normal turnover of skeletal muscle cells.

CK-MB Subforms

In the bloodstream, CK-MB exists predominantly in equilibrium between two forms, the tissue form (MB2) and the circulating seroconverted form (MB1). As cardiac muscle cells die, the MB2 subform is released and converted to MB1 in the serum by carboxypeptidase cleavage of the N-terminal lysine on the M subunit. During an acute MI, large amounts of MB2 are released, increasing the ratio of MB2 to MB1 as well as the absolute amount of circulating MB2. Puleo and colleagues have shown that an absolute level of MB2 > 1 U/L and an MB2/MB1 ratio of ≥1.5 are very sensitive markers of myocardial necrosis (33). Using the CK-MB subform assay, myocardial necrosis can be detected as early as 3 h after the onset of ischemic symptoms. The use of the MB subform assay has the same limitations in specificity as does CK-MB, but it has excellent sensitivity and negative predictive value in patients presenting with chest pain.

The Troponins

The troponins (T, I, and C) are a group of three distinct proteins that are part of the contractile apparatus of all striated muscle. TnT (33 kDa) provides the structural component that links the troponin complex with tropomyosin to the actin filament. TnI (23.5 kDa) is the regulatory subunit involved in the contraction–relaxation process and TnC (18 kDa) is a calcium-binding subunit. TnI and TnT each exist in three isoforms—skeletal (slow- and fast-twitch) and cardiac—that are readily identified as distinct amino acid sequences recognized by immunoassay techniques. This provides the basis for the cardiac specificity of TnI and TnT assays for the diagnosis of myocardial injury. As yet, no tissue-specific isoforms of TnC have been identified.

cTnI is not expressed in skeletal muscle, even during fetal development. However, there is coexpression of the cardiac and skeletal muscle isoforms of TnT in fetal muscle of both types (54). In normal adults, TnT isoforms are not coexpressed, but in stressed human hearts, there may be re-expression of the skeletal isoform (55). Re-expression of the cardiac isoform has occurred in animal models of skeletal muscle injury (56) and has been detected on biopsy of regenerating skeletal muscle in humans (57). It is unknown if these findings represent a clinical or diagnostic disadvantage for cTn.

Unlike myoglobin, total CK, and CK-MB, which exist solely in the soluble state in the cytosol of muscle cells, only about 6% of cTnT and 2 to 3% of cTnI exists in soluble form in the cytosol of the cardiac muscle cell. The remainder is structurally bound in the contractile apparatus. Because of early release of the cytosolic pool, cTnI and cTnT are detectable about 3 to 4 h after the onset of myocardial injury. Somewhat earlier release of cTnT compared with cTnI after myocardial necrosis has been documented (58–60). No studies have directly compared the timing of the rise of cTnT vs cTnI in myocardial injury, but it has been shown that cTnT rises earlier than CK-MB mass in these patients *(61)*. Conversely, studies with one assay show that cTnI rises later than, or at the earliest concurrently with, CK-MB mass in myocardial injury patients *(54,59)*. As suggested by Christenson and colleagues in their comparison of cTnI vs cTnT in acute coronary syndrome patients, these differences may have important implications for use of the Tns for diagnosis in the ED chest pain population and for determining prognosis in acute coronary syndrome patients *(62)*.

After myocardial necrosis, cTnI remains elevated for 7–10 d and cTnT for up to 14 d, likely reflecting sustained release of the structurally bound components. Because of the sustained elevation of the Tns, detection of recurrent events is more difficult. However, the troponin assays do offer the advantage that remote events may be detected in patients who present several hours to days after symptoms occur.

Like CK-MB, and to a variable extent (greater with cTnT than with cTnI), these markers may be "falsely" elevated in patients with end-stage renal disease, particularly those on hemodialysis *(65–74)*. This elevation may be related to the risk of CAD *(75,76)*, but extensive outcomes correlation is not available. Pending further study, the interpretation of the results of Tn testing in chest pain patients with end-stage renal disease must be done with caution.

CARDIAC MARKERS IN PATIENTS WITH HIGH-RISK FEATURES ON INITIAL EVALUATION

ST-Segment Elevation Acute MI

Although the diagnosis of acute MI is later confirmed by serial CK-MB testing in over 90% of patients presenting to the ED with chest pain and ST-segment elevation on the initial ECG *(11,12)*, cardiac marker testing can provide useful information about the size of the myocardial infarction as well as short- and long-term risk stratification.

In both the prethrombolytic and thrombolytic eras, studies have shown a correlation between infarct size and residual left ventricular function and serum CK or CK-MB concentrations *(77–80)*. These findings have also been linked to differences in both death and nonfatal outcomes, as shown by Christenson and colleagues in an analysis of 145 patients who received accelerated alteplase *(81)*. They showed that the area under the CK-MB release curve was inversely correlated with both ejection fraction ($r = 0.21$, $p = 0.04$) and infarct-zone left ventricular function ($r = 0.21$, $p = 0.04$). In addition, there was a trend ($r = 0.12$, $p = 0.16$) toward higher rates of congestive heart failure and death in patients with larger CK-MB areas.

Plasma α-hydroxybutyrate dehydrogenase is not a standard marker of myocardial necrosis, but in a substudy of the Global Utilization of Streptokinase and TPA (alteplase) for Occluded Coronary Arteries (GUSTO-I) trial, Baardman and colleagues showed that infarct size so measured correlated with infarct-artery TIMI flow grade at 90-min angiography. They also showed that smaller infarcts were correlated with accelerated alteplase or combined alteplase streptokinase treatment *(82)*. These findings provide mechanistic support for the correlation between TIMI grade 3 flow at 90-min angiography and improved survival seen in the GUSTO-I angiographic substudy *(83)* and the higher overall survival of alteplase-treated patients in the GUSTO-I trial *(84)*.

The use of cTnT for risk stratification in patients presenting with ST-segment elevation acute MI has been studied by several groups. In the GUSTO-IIa TnT substudy, a single cTnT measure at baseline provided significant information for predicting short-term mortality, even when the baseline ECG showed ST-segment elevation *(20)*. In this group, patients who were cTnT-positive ($\geq$1 ng/mL) at baseline had a 30-d mortality of 13%, compared with 4.7% in those who were cTnT-negative on presentation. Similarly, in a 3-yr follow-up study of patients with acute ST-segment elevation MI, Stubbs and colleagues showed that patients who were cTnT-positive ($\geq$0.2 ng/mL) had a significantly higher mortality rate (32%) than patients who were cTnT-negative (13%) *(85)*.

Most recently, in a substudy of the Global Use of Strategies To Open Occluded Coronary Arteries (GUSTO-III) trial, Ohman and colleagues evaluated the use of a qualitative bedside rapid assay for cTnT at presentation for risk stratification of patients with ST-segment elevation MI *(46)*. Overall, 8.9% of patients were cTnT-positive at baseline. In general, patients who were positive at baseline had longer symptom duration, were slightly older, were more likely to have diabetes, prior angina, and Killip class >II, and more often had anterior MI. Both in-hospital and 30-d mortality (14.4 and 15.6%, respectively) were higher in the cTnT-positive patients than in the cTnT-negative patients (5.5 and 6.3%, respectively). In addition, the rates of nonfatal in-hospital events, including congestive heart failure and cardiogenic shock, were higher in TnT-positive patients. When the results of the baseline cTnT test were added to an established mortality model developed by Lee and colleagues *(86)*, the TnT result contributed significantly ($\chi^2 = 22$, $p = 0.001$) though slightly less than the clinical predictors of Killip class, heart rate, age, and infarct location *(87)*.

These results suggest that cTnT can be used to identify at presentation a subgroup of patients with ST-segment elevation acute MI who are at higher risk for both in-hospital complications as well as short- and long-term mortality. The challenge will be to identify medical or interventional treatments that can be applied early in this subgroup of patients to mitigate their risk.

Myoglobin has also been studied for a possible role in risk stratification, particularly to attempt to identify patients at low-risk of mortality after thrombolysis for ST-segment elevation MI. Srinivas and colleagues have shown that myoglobin levels $\leq$239 ng/mL at 12 h can separate such patients into groups at low risk for 30-d mortality (1.4%) compared with 9.1% 30-d mortality in those with higher levels *(88)*. In a multivariable model, including age, sex, infarct artery location, and 90-min TIMI flow grade of CK-MB, TnI, and myoglobin measured at various time points, only the 12-h myoglobin added significantly in identifying low-risk patients. Similar to the use of markers to identify high-risk patients, identification of low-risk groups after ST-segment elevation MI could aid clinical management and discharge decisions. Prospective validation of the utility of such measures remains to be undertaken, however.

Non-ST-Segment Elevation Acute Coronary Syndromes

The history, physical examination, and baseline ECG all can be used to risk-stratify patients with non-ST-segment elevation acute coronary syndromes. Woodlief and colleagues developed a regression model in 1384 patients in the GUSTO-IIa trial that identified age, Killip class, systolic blood pressure, and previous hypertension as significant predictors of 30-d mortality *(89)*. In 393 patients with unstable angina, Calvin and colleagues found previous infarction, lack of β-blocker or calcium-channel blocker therapy, ST-segment depression on the presenting ECG, and diabetes to be predictors of death or acute MI *(90)*.

As described previously, in the absence of ST-segment elevation on the initial ECG, the diagnosis of acute MI vs unstable angina is largely made, in retrospect, on the basis of serial CK-MB testing. However, because even small infarcts as measured by CK-MB sampling confer worse outcomes, and the best outcomes in these patients are likely to be obtained when specific treatments are started early, it is clearly important to identify these groups as soon as possible. The use of the sensitive specific cardiac markers discussed previously may aid in diagnosis, risk stratification, and management of this diverse group of patients as well. Specifically, TnT and TnI have now been studied extensively as indicators of prognosis in patients with non-ST-segment elevation acute coronary syndromes.

In an enzyme substudy of the Fragmin during Instability in Coronary Artery Disease (FRISC) trial, cTnT was measured at baseline in 976 patients who presented within 12 h of symptom onset *(91)*. At 5 mo there was a correlation between the combined rate of death or MI and the level of TnT measured in the serum at baseline; cTnT < 0.06 ng/mL, 4.3%; 0.06–0.18 ng/mL, 10.5%; >18 ng/mL, 16.1%. The cTnT level, age, hypertension, number of antianginal drugs, and ECG changes were identified in multivariable analysis as the most important independent predictors of risk in this population of unstable angina patients.

The GUSTO-IIa TnT substudy evaluated the use of a single baseline measure of cTnT compared with the baseline ECG and CK-MB as a risk marker in 855 patients across the spectrum of acute coronary syndromes *(20)*. Of the 755 patients who had all three studies at baseline, 36% were cTnT positive and 32% had elevated CK-MB. As in the FRISC analysis, the probability of short-term mortality correlated with the serum concentration of cTnT at baseline; when the result of the cTnT test was considered as a dichotomous variable, 30-d mortality was 11.8% in the cTnT-positive patients compared with 3.9% in cTnT-negative patients. This relationship of TnT status to outcome held across all ECG categories (ST-segment elevation, ST-segment depression, T-wave inversion/normal, and confounding factors), and the incidence of in-hospital complications was also higher in the cTnT-positive patients. When the result of the baseline ECG, cTnT, and CK-MB were evaluated in an unadjusted mortality model, baseline cTnT had the largest χ^2 value, followed by the ECG and the CK-MB. However, when the mortality model was adjusted for the presence of the other two variables (which were forced in first), the ECG was the strongest predictor of 30-d mortality ($\chi^2 = 11.5, p = 0.009$), followed by the baseline cTnT result ($\chi^2 = 9.2, p = 0.027$). In the adjusted model, the baseline CK-MB added no significant information after the ECG and cTnT results were considered.

TnI also has been evaluated as a risk marker in acute coronary syndrome patients. In a retrospective analysis of serum from 1404 acute coronary syndrome patients enrolled in the TIMI-3 trial, cTnI was positive in 41% of patients *(92)*. The risk of mortality increased with increasing levels of cTnI; when troponin I status (positive > 0.04 ng/mL) was analyzed as a dichotomous variable, mortality was significantly higher in positive than in negative patients (3.7 vs 1.0%). In a multivariable mortality model, ST-segment depression ($p < 0.001$), age >65 yr ($p = 0.026$), and the baseline cTnI status ($p = 0.03$) were independent predictors of mortality.

Newby and colleagues have shown that obtaining serial measures of TnT adds significantly to the result of the baseline measure in determining the risk of both in-hospital and 30-d events in the same GUSTO-IIa TnT substudy population *(93)*. Further, the results of both baseline and serial cTnT testing remained predictive of events in the GUSTO-IIa TnT substudy cohort at 1 yr (mortality 14.2% in baseline cTnT-positive patients vs 5.8% in negative patients; 9.6 vs 5.6% for any positive). Similarly, Stubbs and colleagues showed a significant relationship between baseline cTnT measures and death, combined death/MI, and revascularization at a median follow-up of 3 yr *(94)*. However, when the event rates between 30 d and 1 yr were evaluated, there was no significant difference in mortality over this period for either the baseline or any positive result on serial testing. Based on these results, the increased risk identified by cTnT testing in acute coronary syndrome patients appears to be for events that occur early, suggesting that the next step is to identify treatment strategies that can favorably alter this risk when applied early.

Analyses of Tn testing in populations of unstable angina patients enrolled in several large clinical trials suggest that Tn measurement shortly after presentation may be useful to define subgroups of patients who would benefit most from early medical or percutaneous intervention strategies. Such use of Tn testing may improve clinical outcome as well as facilitate cost-effective use of expensive medical and interventional therapies.

The FRISC study of a low molecular weight heparin treatment strategy suggested that Tn-positive subgroups achieved greater benefit from treatment than Tn-negative patients. In the FRISC study, cTnT-positive ($\geq$0.1 ng/mL) patients had greater reduction in the 40-d incidence of death or MI (14.2 vs 7.4%) with long-term administration of dalteparin than did those who were cTnT-negative (<0.1 ng/mL) where there was no difference with or without treatment *(95)*. A similar analysis in 1265 unstable angina patients receiving percutaneous intervention who were randomized to treatment with abciximab or placebo in the Chimeric c7E3 Antiplatelet Therapy in Unstable Angina Refractory to Standard Treatment (CAPTURE) trial suggested that cTnT analysis might be used to identify a subgroup of patients who would realize the most benefit from abciximab treatment *(96)*. This evaluation showed a 60% reduction in death or nonfatal MI at 6 mo among cTnT-positive patients treated with abciximab. However, among patients who were cTnT-negative, there was no benefit of abciximab treatment relative to placebo.

Similar results have been reported by both the Platelet Receptor Inhibition in Ischemic Syndrome Management (PRISM) and the PARAGON-B TnT Substudy investigators with 2 small-molecule glycoprotein IIb/IIIa inhibitors, tirofiban and lamifiban, respectively *(97,98)*. In PRISM, 2222 patients were randomized to treatment with tirofiban plus aspirin vs heparin plus aspirin had Tn levels determined at a mean of 8.4 h after symptom onset. Among patients who were cTnI-positive, the rate of death or MI was 4.3% among tirofiban-treated patients compared with 13.0% among those receiving standard therapy with heparin and aspirin. Among cTnI-negative patients, there was no difference in the occurrence of death or MI by treatment group. Results were similar for TnT, and importantly, this differential treatment effect was observed for both medically treated patients and those treated with percutaneous coronary revascularization. In the PARAGON B TnT substudy, the 30-d rate of death or non-fatal MI was 19.0% in cTnT-positive patients who received placebo compared with 11.0% in those who received lamifiban. The corresponding results among cTnT-negative patients were 10.3% for placebo and 9.6% for lamifiban, suggesting that the majority of the overall reduction of events in lamifiban-treated patients (9.9%) vs placebo (9.9%) occurred among cTnT-positive patients. A systematic overview of these results is displayed in Fig. 3.

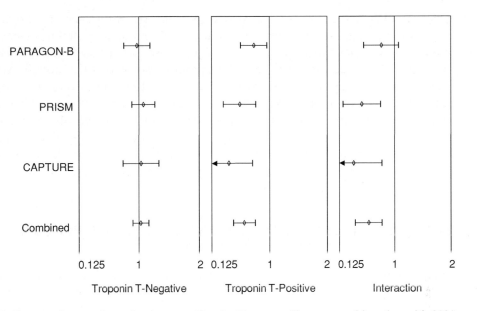

Fig. 3. Systematic overview of treatment effect by Tn status. Shown are odds ratios with 95% confidence intervals for death or MI among Tn-negative and Tn-positive patients and for interaction of Tn status with treatment effect for PRISM, CAPTURE, PARAGON-B, and combined trials. Values to left of 1.0 indicate a benefit of GP IIb/IIIa inhibition. Reprinted with permission from ref. *98*.

Comparisons of TnT with TnI as risk markers have been attempted. However, the lack of standardized assays and use of different cut-off values for the same assay in different studies make the results difficult to interpret. Luscher and colleagues compared cTnT with cTnI by the Sanofi assay in 491 patients with unstable angina and found them to identify similar groups of patients at high risk for 30-d death or MI *(99)*.

Using the Dade Stratus II cTnI assay at a cut point of 1.5 ng/mL in comparison to cTnT in the GUSTO-IIa TnT substudy cohort, both markers when measured at baseline predicted 30-d mortality, but cTnT provided the most prognostic information. In a mortality model with the ECG and the other marker forced in first, only cTnT still provided additional prognostic information *(62)*. Further, the area under the receiver operator characteristics (ROC) curve, which is independent of the cut point used for an assay, was larger for cTnT compared to cTnI (0.68 vs 0.64).

Serial bedside tests for cTnT and cTnI at baseline and 4 h were evaluated by Hamm and colleagues with similar performance (sensitivity and negative predictive value) by both markers. In a logistic regression model, both markers were strong predictors of 30-d death or MI and remained so even after ST-segment depression on the initial ECG was forced into the model first *(45)*. The individual chi-square for cTnI in this model was larger, however.

The results of these studies suggest that the prognostic information demonstrated in individual studies of cTnT or cTnI should not be generalized to other assays or testing conditions. Differences in analytical characteristics and measurement precision for the different cTnI assays may translate into important differences in their ability to risk-stratify the acute coronary syndrome patient. Differences in the characteristics of the marker proteins themselves, including the timing and magnitude of release after both myocardial necrosis and injury, may also translate into the differences in prognostic ability seen in individual studies performed under different testing circumstances and in different patient populations. In an effort to update and standardize the diagnosis of MI and the use of cardiac marker assays, the European Society of Cardiology/American College of Cardiology Joint Committee for the Tn testing, but also on assay precision and standardization *(100)*. They have recommended that each assay should be defined as positive at values above the 99th percentile of normal controls and also that acceptable imprecision should be reflected by a coefficient of variation ≤10%. Further study with standardized assays under well-defined clinical circumstances will be needed to characterize whether there are any important differences between these markers in diagnosis and risk stratification.

THE ROLE OF CHEST PAIN UNITS IN THE EVALUATION OF PATIENTS WITH CHEST PAIN

Because symptoms, the physical examination, and the initial ECG and cardiac marker evaluations are often inconclusive, Chest Pain Units have been devised as one strategy to optimize diagnosis and management in low- to moderate-risk chest pain patients while maintaining reasonable costs of care and avoiding the inherent medicolegal problems of patients who are sent home with undetected MIs.

In general, Chest Pain Units use protocol-driven strategies for observation and "rule-out" of MI in low- to moderate-risk patients—those without clear ischemic changes on the initial ECG, with negative initial cardiac marker assessment, and without high-risk clinical features. These centers provide for more rapid and earlier detection of and therapeutic intervention for acute MI missed by initial evaluation, or the development of an unstable clinical course, than routine admission might allow. Most provide for continuous observation either in or adjacent to the ED with serial sampling of cardiac markers (usually CK-MB, MB subforms, or Tns) every 3–4 h and serial ECG or continuous ST-segment monitoring over a period of 9–12 h. Cardiac evaluation and later risk stratification with exercise stress testing are often included before release in patients who have ruled-out.

In one of the earliest studies of rule-out strategies, Lee and colleagues showed that in the absence of recurrent chest pain and with negative CK-MB enzymes, a 12-h period was sufficient to exclude the diagnosis of acute MI in 99.5% of low-risk patients *(101)*. Similarly, Gibler and colleagues showed that serial sampling of CK-MB over a period of 9 h was sufficient to eliminate the diagnosis of MI in nearly 100% of patients *(28,29)*. In study of a 12-h short-stay observation strategy, Gaspoz et al. showed that if serial CK-MBs were negative in a patient with no recurrent chest pain or ECG changes, the risk of later MI or death was less than 1% *(102)*. In a randomized trial of 9 h of rule-out observation in the Chest Pain Unit vs conventional care, Gomez and colleagues showed no significant difference in outcome between the management strategies *(103)*.

At many sites, the use of Chest Pain Centers or Chest Pain Units has eased the pressure on the ED physician to commit high-cost cardiac care unit resources or release the patient. Several groups have shown the safety of this approach, as well as significant reductions in costs and charges with such short-stay observation strategies (Table 5). In their randomized study, Gomez and colleagues showed a 40% reduction in charges for Chest Pain Unit observation vs conventional care *(103)*. Gaspoz and colleagues showed reductions in hospital costs of care of $7274 and $2785 for the comparison of a proto-

Table 5
Length of Stay and Financial Implications of Chest Pain Unit Rule-Out Protocols

Protocols (reference)	Reduction in length of stay (d)	Cost reduction ($)[a]
Gaspoz (101)		
CCU	4.0	7274 (76%)
Step-down	2.0	2104 (52%)
Wards	3.0	2785 (63%)
Gomez (100)	0.5	981 (47%)
Mikhail (103)	ND	1470 (62%)
DUMC Chest Pain Program (102)	2.3	1765 (47%)

DUMC, Duke University Medical Center; ND, no data recorded.
[a]For hospital stay except Gaspoz, which reflects total costs through 6 mo.
Adapted from Newby LK, Califf RM. Identifying patient risk: the basis for rational discharge planning after acute myocardial infarction. J Thromb Thrombol 1996;3:107–115.

col-driven short-stay strategy vs a CCU- or floor-based strategy, respectively (104). In our own experience at Duke University Medical Center, the use of a Chest Pain Unit compared with conventional admission and rule-out has resulted in a 2.3-d shorter length of stay and a 47% reduction in hospital costs (105). In their chest pain rule-out program, Mikhail and colleagues found hospital costs fell from an average of $2364 before institution of the program to $894 using their protocol (106). They also demonstrated the cost-effectiveness of routine stress testing in patients who had ruled-out for MI. The cost of identifying one patient with CAD after a negative rule-out was $3125; for identifying one patient with disease that warranted bypass surgery or angioplasty, the cost was $10,714. The projected cost/yr of life saved was <$2000.

Cardiac Markers in the Chest Pain Unit

Newer markers, such as the cTns and CK-MB subforms, could further enhance the process of care in the low to moderate risk undifferentiated chest pain population. With markers that are more sensitive, cardiac-specific, and (in some cases) detected earlier than CK-MB, the standard observation time for definitive rule-out of MI could be reduced from 9–12 h to 6–8 h.

The duration of symptoms before presentation varies widely from patient to patient. In the ED or Chest Pain Unit, then, for the earliest and most sensitive and specific diagnosis of myocardial necrosis, the use of a panel of markers that includes myoglobin or MB subforms as a very early marker, CK-MB mass (4–6 h), and TnT or TnI (4–8+ hours) could be ideal (Fig. 4). The Diagnostic Marker Cooperative Study prospectively compared the sensitivity and specificity of myoglobin, CK-MB subforms, CK-MB mass, and cTnI and cTnT at various times from symptom onset across the spectrum of patients presenting to EDs with chest pain. Of 995 patients, 12.5% had MI by CK-MB mass assay. Overall, the sensitivity for detecting MI was highest for the CK-MB subform assay either alone or in combination with a Tn. At 6 h, sensitivity was highest (91%) for CK-MB subforms followed by myoglobin (78%) (107).

In a study of 190 ED patients with chest pain, Levitt and colleagues evaluated the use of CK-MB alone, myoglobin alone, or a combination of myoglobin and CK-MB at base-

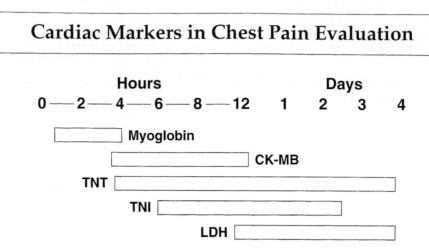

Fig. 4. Overlapping time frames of markers.

Table 6
Predictive capabilities of serum enzymes in the ED

Serum marker value	Sensitivity	Specificity	Positive predictive value	Negative predictive value
Myoglobin	90.59 (69.6–98.8)	88.4 (83.6–93.2)	48.59 (27.9–61.9)	98.79 (95.4–99.8)
CK-MB	81.0 (58.1–94.5)	99.4 (96.8–100)	94.4 (72.7–99.9)	97.7 (94.2–99.4)
Combination	100 (83.2–100.0)	91.2 (85.9–95.0)	58.3 (39.3–73.7)	100 (97.6–100.0)

Presented as % (95% confidence intervals).
A positive serum myoglobin test is defined as a level 88.7 ng/mL or higher, and a positive serum CK-MB as 11.9 ng/mL or higher, at either the time of ED presentation or 3 h later. The combination test is defined as positive if either of the above two tests is positive. Adapted from ref. *42*.

line and 3 h for diagnosis of acute MI in the ED *(42)*. Considering a positive result if the marker was positive at either time point, myoglobin was more sensitive than CK-MB but less specific, and the combination of the results of both markers was most sensitive and specific. The sensitivity, specificity, and positive and negative predictive values of the individual markers and the combination of markers are shown in Table 6. In a similar study of 101 ED patients with chest pain, Kontos et al. showed that when patients with diagnostic ECGs were excluded, the sensitivity and specificity of a combination of myoglobin and CK-MB mass results at baseline were 80 and 84%, respectively, for the diagnosis of acute MI, and were superior to those for either marker alone *(108)*. The combination of the markers' results on serial sampling at 0 and 4 h had both sensitivity and specificity of 100%, suggesting that a combination of markers could identify or exclude the diagnosis of acute MI as early as 4 h after ED presentation.

The Biochemical Markers of Acute Coronary Syndromes (BIOMACS) Study Group evaluated the use of serial testing of CK-MB, myoglobin, and cTnT alone or in combination, and at different discriminatory levels to confirm or exclude the diagnosis of acute MI within 6 h of presentation in 142 patients with chest pain and nondiagnostic ECGs *(52)*. They concluded that no markers alone or in combination could safely

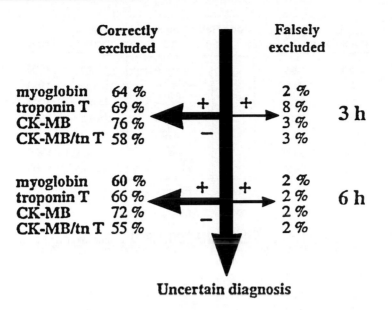

	Correctly excluded			Falsely excluded	
myoglobin	64 %			2 %	
troponin T	69 %	+	+	8 %	3 h
CK-MB	76 %			3 %	
CK-MB/tn T	58 %	−		3 %	
myoglobin	60 %			2 %	
troponin T	66 %	+	+	2 %	6 h
CK-MB	72 %			2 %	
CK-MB/tn T	55 %	−		2 %	

Uncertain diagnosis

Fig. 5. Percentage of correctly and falsely excluded acute MI in all patients (59 with and 83 without infarction) 3 and 6 h after admission. Reproduced with permission from ref. 52.

exclude the diagnosis of acute MI with certainty on admission, but that by monitoring a combination of myoglobin with CK-MB or cTnT, MI could be excluded in up to 72% by 6 h with a low rate of patients falsely excluded (Fig. 5). For the diagnosis of MI, no single marker regardless of the discriminatory level used combined high sensitivity and specificity, but the combination of myoglobin and CK-MB or myoglobin and cTnT on serial testing had sensitivities of 92 and 82%, respectively, at 2 h, and 98% for both combinations at 6 h. Specificities of the combinations were 98 and 94%, respectively, at 2 h, and 93 and 82%, respectively, at 6 h.

Small studies have investigated the potential of some of the newer cardiac markers in diagnosis and risk stratification in the low to moderate risk Chest Pain Unit population. Puleo and colleagues showed that the use of CK-MB subforms in the evaluation of chest pain patients had excellent negative predictive value to rule-out MI *(33)*. Trahey and colleagues reported that serial sampling of CK-MB subforms over a 6-h period followed by diagnostic exercise testing was sufficient to rule-out the diagnosis of MI in their Chest Pain Unit patients and to stratify patients with a negative stress test into a low-risk group with only a 1.3% risk of later MI or recurrent ischemia *(109)*.

TnT testing also shows promise for risk stratification in the low to moderate risk Chest Pain Unit population. In a meta-analysis of published reports of cTnT testing in chest pain patients without documented MI, Wu and colleagues calculated an odds ratio for prediction of the need for coronary revascularization of 4.4 (95% confidence interval 3.0–6.5) in cTnT-positive patients *(110)*. A similar meta-analysis revealed an odds ratio for death or infarction of 4.3 (95% confidence interval 2.8–6.8) in cTnT-positive patients (Fig. 6). In an analysis of 439 consecutive patients assigned to observation in the Duke University Chest Pain Unit, 10% of patients were cTnT-positive on serial testing over 8 h *(63)*. A positive cTnT result identified a group at higher risk for significant (>75% stenosis) underlying CAD (89%) and multivessel disease (67%) than those found in the cTnT-negative

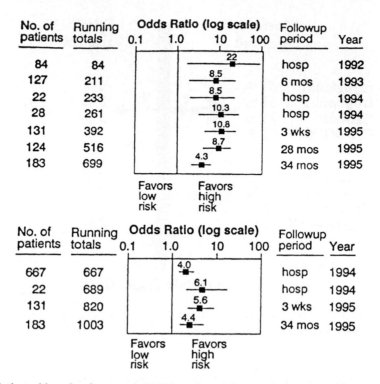

Fig. 6. Cumulative odds ratios for use of cTnT in patients without infarction for an outcome of infarction or cardiac death (top) or for an outcome of coronary artery revascularization (bottom). Squares indicate the actual values; lines indicate the 95% confidence intervals. Reproduced with permission from ref. *107.*

group (49 and 29%, respectively). Furthermore, serial testing of TnT over an 8-h period (compared to CK-MB analysis over 12 h) detected the only patients who were CK-MB-positive. No patient who was cTnT-negative at 8 h later had positive CK-MB. In short-term follow-up (mean 21 d), there were no deaths in either group, but at 2 yr mortality was 27% in the cTnT-positive group compared with 7% in the cTnT-negative patients.

Hamm and colleagues recently reported the use of serial bedside testing for cTnT and cTnI at baseline and at 4 h after presentation in the ED with acute chest pain *(45)*. In their outcome study of 773 consecutive patients presenting within 12 h of onset of symptoms and without ST-segment elevation on initial ECG, the use of qualitative monoclonal antibody-based bedside assays for cTnT and cTnI identified by 4 h after presentation 94 and 100%, respectively, of patients later determined to have MI by follow-up CK and CK-MB testing. Among unstable angina patients, 22% were positive by TnT and 36% by TnI bedside testing. Importantly, the 30-d risks of death or nonfatal MI in patients negative for TnT or TnI were only 1.1 and 0.3%, respectively. These results may be further enhanced by development of a cTnT device having a lower cutoff (0.08 vs 0.2 ng/mL) and greater cardiac specificity.

In a recent study of 1005 patients from six chest pain units in U.S. hospitals, the Chest Pain Evaluation by Creatine Kinase-MB, Myoglobin, and Troponin I (CHECKMATE) Investigators demonstrated the utility of multimarker strategies (MMS) of cardiac marker testing at the point-of-care compared with single marker testing in the local lab-

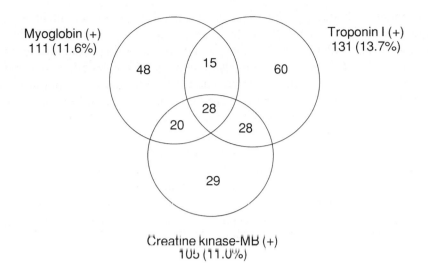

Fig. 7. Overlap of myoglobin, CK-MB, and TnI positivity during sampling. Reprinted with permission from ref. *111*.

oratory *(111)*. In that study, MMS-1, which combined myoglobin, an early marker, with cTnI and CK-MB, later but specific markers, identified more positive patients at baseline (18.9%) or on serial testing (23.9%) than either a two marker strategy (MMS-2), with CK-MB and cTnI (14.3 and 18.8%, respectively), or the single marker local laboratory strategy of CK-MB testing (5.2 and 8.8%, respectively), $p = 0.001$ for all comparisons. As shown in Fig. 7, among chest pain unit patients, no single marker, even with serial testing, was able to detect all patients at risk for subsequent cardiac events. Only 40% of patients were positive by more than one marker, and 21% of patients were positive only by myoglobin. The median time to detection of positive patients by MMS-1 was also shorter (2.5 h) compared with single marker local laboratory testing (3.4 h, $p = 0.0001$). Importantly, MMS-1 was also the best strategy for discriminating patients at risk for mortality and death or MI at 30 d.

As these studies suggest, the use of very specific cardiac markers or panels of markers and new testing strategies can identify early a subset of patients (of those who present without high risk features) who might benefit from earlier intervention. The challenge for future research in this area will be to identify which medical or interventional strategies can modify the future risk these patients face. Further, because these markers also identify a low risk population earlier than conventional testing might allow, the potential exists for further reductions in length of stay and expensive diagnostic testing, thus amplifying the cost savings possible through the use of Chest Pain Units.

CONCLUSION

For evaluation of the thousands of patients with acute nontraumatic chest pain who present to ED each year, serum markers of myocardial injury (alone or in combination) will continue to play an increasingly important role, not only in diagnosis and triage decisions, but also in identifying patients who are at increased risk for adverse outcomes in both the short and long term. In both regards, their utility extends across the spectrum of low, moderate, and high risk patients as defined by the initial clinical assessment. As an adjunct to the basic history, physical examination, and baseline ECG, the use of cardiac markers, particularly the Tns, can provide crucial information for initial and later risk stratification. The use of serial measurements of cardiac markers not only increases their sensitivity and negative predictive value for acute infarction, but also, in the case of the Tns, adds to prognostic ability. With the identification of patients who are negative on serial testing, particularly those with low risk features, length of hospital stay for evaluation can be reduced and in-hospital resources can be better allocated, with substantially decreased costs. However, perhaps the most important feature of the cardiac markers in risk assessment of chest pain patients is that in patients with positive marker studies, the majority of the risk for adverse events is incurred early. Thus, the challenge for the future investigations will be to define the management and treatment strategies (medical and interventional) that, when applied early in marker-positive patients, will reduce their likelihood of adverse events.

REFERENCES

1. Braunwald E, Mark DB, Jones RH, et al. Unstable angina: diagnosis and management. Clinical Practice Guideline No. 10, AHCPR Publication 94-0602. Agency of Health Care Policy and Research and the National Heart, Lung and Blood Institute, Rockville, MD, 1994.
2. McCarthy BD, Wong JB, Selker HP. Detecting acute cardiac ischemia in the Emergency Department: a review of the literature. J Gen Intern Med 1990;5:365–373.
3. Sawe U. Pain in acute myocardial infarction: a study of 137 patients in a coronary care unit. Acta Med Scand 1971;190:79–81.
4. Tierney WM, Fitzgerald J, McHenry R, et al. Physicians' estimates of the probability of myocardial infarction in emergency room patients with chest pain. Med Decis Making 1986;6:12–17.
5. Lee TH, Cook FE, Weisberg M, et al. Acute chest pain in the emergency room: identification and examination of low risk patients. Arch Intern Med 1985;145:65–69.
6. Ingram DA, Fulton RA, Portal RW, P'Aber C. Vomiting as a diagnostic aid in acute ischemic cardiac pain. Br Med J 1980;281:636–637.
7. Uretsky BF, Farquhar DS, Berezin AF, et al. Symptomatic myocardial infarction without chest pain: prevalence and clinical course. Am J Cardiol 1977;40:498–503.
8. Villaneuva FS, Sabia PJ, Afrooktch A, et al. Value and limitations of current methods of evaluating patients presenting to the emergency room with cardiac-related symptoms for determining long-term prognosis. Am J Cardiol 1992;69:746–750.
9. Califf RM, Mark DB, Harrell FE, et al. Importance of clinical measures of ischemia in the prognosis of patients with documented coronary artery disease. J Am Coll Cardiol 1988;11:20–26.
10. Betriu A, Heras M, Cohen M, Fuster V. Unstable angina: outcome according to clinical presentation. J Am Coll Cardiol 1992;19:1659–1663.
11. Rude RE, Poole WK, Muller JE, et al. Electrocardiographic and clinical criteria for the recognition of acute myocardial infarction based on analysis of 3,697 patients. Am J Cardiol 1983;52:936–942.
12. Yusuf S, Pearson M, Sterry H, et al. The entry ECG in the early diagnosis and prognostic stratification of patients with suspected acute myocardial infarction. Eur Heart J 1984;5:690–696.
13. Califf RM, Ohman EM. The diagnosis of acute myocardial infarction. Chest 1992;101:106S–115S.
14. Granger C, Moffie I, for the GUSTO Investigators. Under use of thrombolytic therapy in North America has been exaggerated: results of the GUSTO MI registry [abstract]. Circulation 1994;90(Suppl. I):I-324.
15. Karlson BW, Herlitz J, Petterson P, Hallgren P, Strombom U, Hjalmarson A. One-year prognosis in patients hospitalized with a history of unstable angina pectoris. Clin Cardiol 1993;16:397–402.
16. Califf RM, Mark DB, Harrell FE, et al. Importance of clinical measures of ischemia in the prognosis of patients with documented coronary artery disease. J Am Coll Cardiol 1988;11:20–26.
17. Selker HP, Griffith JL, D'Agostino RB. A tool for judging coronary care unit admission appropriateness, valid for both real-time and retrospective use. A time-insensitive predictive instrument (TIPI) for acute cardiac ischemia: a multicenter study. Med Care 1991;29:610–627.

18. Goldman L, Cook EF, Brand DA, et al. A computer protocol to predict myocardial infarction in emergency department patients with chest pain. N Engl J Med 1988;318:797–803.

19. Rouan GW, Lee TH, Cook EF, Brand DA, Weisberg MC, Goldman L. Clinical characteristics and outcome of acute myocardial infarction in patients with initially normal or nonspecific electrocardiograms. A report form the Multicenter Chest Pain Study. Am J Cardiol 1989;64:1087–1092.

20. Ohman EM, Armstrong PW, Christenson RH, et al. Cardiac troponin T for risk stratification in acute myocardial ischemia. N Engl J Med 1996;335:1333–1341.

21. Brush JE, Brand DA, Acampora D, et al. Use of the initial electrocardiogram to predict in-hospital complications of acute myocardial infarction. N Engl J Med 1985;312:1137–1141.

22. Savonitto S, Ardissino D, Granger CB, et al. Prognostic value of the admission electrocardiogram in acute coronary syndromes. JAMA 1999;281:707–713.

23. Goldman L, Weinberg M, Weisberg M, et al. A computer-derived protocol to aid in the diagnosis of emergency room patients with acute chest pain. N Engl J Med 1982;307:588–596.

24. Schor S, Behar S, Modan B, Barell V, Drory J, Kariv I. Disposition of presumed coronary patients from an emergency room: a follow-up study. JAMA 1976;236:941–943.

25. Lee TH, Rouan GW, Weisberg MC, et al. Clinical characteristics and natural history of patients with acute myocardial infarction sent home from the emergency department. Am J Cardiol 1987;60:219–224.

26. Pozen MW, D'Agostino RB, Mitchell JB, et al. The usefulness of a predictive instrument to reduce inappropriate admissions to the coronary care unit. Ann Intern Med 1980;92:238–242.

27. Pozen MW, D'Agostino RB, Selker HP, et al. A predictive instrument to improve coronary care unit admission practices in acute ischemic heart disease: a prospective multicenter clinical trial. N Engl J Med 1984;310:1273–1278.

28. Gibler WB, Lewis LM, Erb RE, et al. Early detection of acute myocardial infarction in patients presenting with chest pain and non-diagnostic ECGs: serial CK-MB sampling in the emergency department. Ann Emerg Med 1990;9:1359–1366.

29. Gibler WB, Young GP, Hedges JR, et al. Acute myocardial infarction in chest pain patients with non-diagnostic ECGs: serial CK-MB sampling in the emergency department. Ann Emerg Med 1992;21:504–512.

30. The TIMI IIIb Investigators. Effects of tissue plasminogen activator and a comparison of early invasive and conservative strategies in unstable angina and non-Q wave myocardial infarction: results of the TIMI IIIb trial. Circulation 1994;89:1545–1556.

31. Rouan GW, Hedges JR, Toltzis R, Golstein-Wayne B, Brand D, Goldman L. A chest pain clinic to improve follow-up of patients released from an urban university teaching hospital emergency department. Ann Emerg Med 1987;16:1145–1150.

32. McCarthy BD, Behansky JR, D'Agostino RB, Selker HP. Missed diagnoses of acute myocardial infarction in the emergency department: results from a multicenter study. Ann Emerg Med 1993;22:579–582.

33. Puleo PR, Meyer D, Wathen C, et al. Use of a rapid assay of subforms of creatine kinase MB to diagnose or rule out acute myocardial infarction. N Engl J Med 1994;331:562–608.

34. Rusnak RA, Stair TO, Hansen K, Fastow JS. Litigation against the emergency physician: common features in cases of missed myocardial infarction. Ann Emerg Med 1989;18:1029–1034.

35. Cardiology Preeminence Roundtable. Perfecting the Perfect MI Rule-out: Best Practices of Emergency Evaluation of Chest Pain. The Advisory Board Company, Washington, DC, 1994.

36. Hedges JR, Young GP, Henkel GF, et al. Serial ECGs are less accurate than serial CK-MB results for emergency department diagnosis of myocardial infarction. Ann Emerg Med 1992;21:1445–1450.

37. Gibler WB, Runyon JP, Levy RC, et al. A rapid diagnostic and treatment center for patients with chest pain in the emergency department. Ann Emerg Med 1995;25:1–8.

38. Gibler WB, Sayre MR, Levy RC, et al. Serial 12-lead electrocardiographic monitoring in patients presenting to the emergency department with chest pain. J Electrocardiol 1994;26:S238–S243.

39. Selker HP, Zalenski RJ, Antman EM, et al. An evaluation of technologies for identifying acute cardiac ischemia in the Emergency Department: executive summary of a National Heart Attack Alert Program Working Group Report. Ann Emerg Med 1997;29:1–87.

40. Sabia P, Afrookteh A, Touchstone DA, et al. Value of regional wall motion abnormality in the emergency room diagnosis of acute myocardial infarction: a prospective study using two-dimensional echocardiography. Circulation 1991;84:I85–I92.

41. Trippi JA, Lee KS, Kopp G, Nelson D, Kovacs R. Emergency echocardiography telemedicine: an efficient method to provide 24-hour consultative echocardiography. J Am Coll Cardiol 1996;27:1748–1752.

42. Levitt MA, Promes SB, Bullock S, et al. Combined cardiac marker approach with adjunct two-dimensional echocardiography to diagnose acute myocardial infarction in the emergency department. Ann Emerg Med 1996;27:1–7.

43. Kontos MC, Jesse RL, Ornato JP, et al. Comparison between technetium-99m sestamibi imaging and troponin I for identifying patients with acute coronary syndromes [abstract]. Circulation 1997;96 (Suppl. I):I-333.

44. van Lente F, McErlean ES, DeLuca S, et al. Utility of a rapid bedside troponin T compared to quantitative troponin T in patients with suspected coronary syndromes [abstract]. Circulation 1997;96(Suppl. I): I-215.

45. Hamm CW, Goldman BU, Heeschen C, Kreymann G, Berger J, Meinertz T. Emergency room triage of patients with acute chest pain by means of rapid testing of cardiac troponin T or troponin I. N Engl J Med 1997;337:1648–1653.

46. Ohman EM, Armstrong PW, Weaver WD, et al. Prognostic value of whole-blood troponin T testing in patients with acute myocardial infarction in the GUSTO-III trial [abstract]. Circulation 1997;96(Suppl. I):I-216.

47. Hoekstra JW, Hedges JR, Gibler WB, Rubison M, Christensen RA. Emergency Department CK-MB: a predictor of ischemic complications. Acad Emerg Med 1994;1:17–28.

48. Young GP, Green TR. The role of a single ECG, creatine kinase and CKMB in diagnosing patients with acute chest pain. Am J Emerg Med 1993;11:444–449.

49. Downie AC, Frost PG, Fielden P, Joshi D, Dancy CM. Bedside measurement of creatine kinase to guide thrombolysis on the coronary care unit. Lancet 1993;341:452–454.

50. Parvin CA, Lo SF, Deuser SM, Weaver LG, Lewis LM, Scott MG. Impact of point-of-care testing on patients' length of stay in a large emergency department. Clin Chem 1996;42:711–717.

51. Roxin LE, Culled I, Groth T, Hallgren T, Venge P. The value of serum myoglobin determinations in the early diagnosis of acute myocardial infarction. Acta Med Scand 1984;215:417–425.

52. Lindahl B, Venge P, Wallentin L, on behalf of the BIOMACS Study Group. Early diagnosis and exclusion of acute myocardial infarction using biochemical monitoring. Coron Artery Dis 1995;6:321–328.

53. Bais R, Edwards JB. Creatine kinase. Crit Rev Clin Lab Sci. 1982;16:291–335.

54. Adams JE, Abendschein DR, Jaffe AS. Biochemical markers of myocardial injury. Is MB creatine kinase the choice for the 1990s? Circulation 1993;88:750–763.

55. Anderson PAW, Malouf NN, Oakeley AE, Pagani ED, Allen PD. Troponin T isoform expression in humans. Circ Res 1991;69:1226–1233.

56. Saggin L, Gorza L, Ausoni S, Schiaffino S. Cardiac troponin T in developing, regenerating and denervated rat skeletal muscle. Development 1990;110:547–554.

57. Bodor GS, Survant L, Voss EM, Smith S, Porterfield D, Apple FS. Cardiac troponin T composition in normal and regenerating human skeletal muscle. Clin Chem 1997;43:476–484.

58. Mair J, Dienstl F, Puschendorf B. Cardiac troponin T in the diagnosis of myocardial injury. Crit Rev Clin Lab Sci 1992;29:31–57.

59. Adams JE III, Bodor GS, Davita-Roman VG, et al. Cardiac troponin I. A marker with high specificity for cardiac injury. Circulation 1993;88:101–106.

60. Bodor GS, Porter S, Landt Y, Ladenson JH. Development of monoclonal antibodies for an assay of cardiac troponin I and preliminary results in suspected cases of myocardial infarction. Clin Chem 1992;38:2203–2214.

61. Wu AHB, Valdes R Jr, Apple FS, et al. Cardiac troponin T immunoassay for diagnosis of acute myocardial infarction. Clin Chem 1994;40:900–907.

62. Christenson RH, Duh SH, Newby LK, et al. Cardiac troponin T and cardiac troponin I: relative value in short-term risk stratification of patients with acute coronary syndromes. Clin Chem 1998;44: 494–501.

63. Newby LK, Ohman EM, Granger BB, et al. Comparison of cardiac troponin T versus creatine kinase-MB for risk stratification in a Chest Pain Evaluation Unit. Am J Cardiol 2000;85:801–805.

64. Wu AHB, Feng YJ, Contois JH, Pervaiz S. Comparison of myoglobin, creatine kinase-MB, and cardiac troponin I for diagnosis of acute myocardial infarction. J Clin Lab Sci 1996;26:291.

65. Bhayana V, Gougoulias T, Cohoe S, Henderson AR. Discordance between results for serum troponin T and troponin I in renal disease. Clin Chem 1995;14:312–317.

66. Li D, Keffer J, Corry K, et al. Nonspecific elevation of troponin T levels in patients with chronic renal failure. Clin Biochem 1995;28:474–477.

67. Frankel WL, Herold DA, Zeigler TW, Fitzgerald RL. Cardiac troponin T is elevated in asymptomatic patients with chronic renal failure. Am J Clin Pathol 1996;106:118–123.

68. Croitoru M, Taegtmeyer H. Spurious rises in troponin T in end-stage renal disease. Lancet 1995;346: 974.

69. Hossein-Nia M, Nisbet J, Merton GK, Holt DW. Spurious rises of cardiac troponin T. Lancet 1995; 346:1558.

70. Escalon JC, Wong SS. False-positive cardiac troponin T levels in chronic hemodialysis patients. Cardiology 1996;87:268–269.

71. Hafner G, Thome-Kromer B, Schaube J, et al. Cardiac troponins in serum in chronic renal failure. Clin Chem 1994;40:1790–1791.

72. Katus HA, Haller C, Muller-Bardorff M, et al. Cardiac troponin T in end-stage renal disease patients undergoing chronic maintenance hemodialysis. Clin Chem 1995;41:1201–1203.

73. Li D, Jailal I, Keffer J. Greater frequency of increased cardiac troponin T than cardiac troponin I in patients with chronic renal failure. Clin Chem 1996;42:114–115.

74. Braun SL, Baum H, Neumeier D, Vogt W. Troponin T and troponin I after coronary artery bypass grafting: discordant results in patients with renal failure. Clin Chem 1996;42:781–783.

75. Haller C, Zehelein J, Remppis A, et al. Cardiac troponin T in patients with renal failure [abstract]. J Am Coll Cardiol 1997;29:234A.

76. Apple FS, Sharkey SW, Hoeft P, et al. Prognostic value of serum cardiac troponin I and T in chronic dialysis patients: a 1-year outcomes analysis. Am J Kidney Dis 1997;29:399–403.

77. Sobel BE, Bresnehan GF, Shell WE, Yoder RD. Estimation of infarct size in man and its relation to prognosis. Circulation 1972;46:640–648.

78. Sobel BE, Roberts R, Larson KB. Estimation of infarct size from serum MB creatine phosphokinase activity: applications and limitations. Am J Cardiol 1976;37:474–485.

79. Thompson PL, Fletcher EE, Katavatis V. Enzymatic indices of myocardial necrosis, influence on short- and long-term prognosis after myocardial infarction. Circulation 1979;59.113–119.

80. Grande P, Hansen BF, Christianson C, Naestoft J. Estimation of acute myocardial infarct size in man by serum CK-MB measurements. Circulation 1982;65:756–764.

81. Christenson RH, O'Hanesian MA, Newby LK, et al. Relation of area under the CK-MB release curve and clinical outcomes in myocardial infarction patients treated with thrombolytic therapy [abstract]. Eur Heart J 1995;16(Suppl.):75.

82. Baardman T, Hermens WT, Lenderink T, et al. Differential effects of tissue plasminogen activator and streptokinase on infarct size and on rate of enzyme release: influence of early infarct related artery patency. The GUSTO Enzyme Substudy. Eur Heart J 1996;17:237–246.

83. The GUSTO Angiographic Investigators. The effects of tissue plasminogen activator, streptokinase or both on coronary-artery patency, ventricular function, and survival after acute myocardial infarction. N Engl J Med 1993;329:1615–1622.

84. Simes RJ, Topol EJ, Holmes DR, et al. Link between angiographic substudy and mortality outcomes in a large randomized trial of myocardial reperfusion. Importance of early and complete infarct artery reperfusion. Circulation 1995;91:1923–1928.

85. Stubbs P, Collinson P, Moseley D, Greenwood T, Noble M. Prognostic significance of admission troponin T concentrations in patients with myocardial infarction. Circulation 1996;94:1291–1297.

86. Lee KL, Woodlief LH, Topol EJ, et al. Predictors of 30-day mortality in the era of reperfusion for acute myocardial infarction. Results from an international trial of 41,021 patients. Circulation 1995;91: 1659–1668.

87. Ohman EM, Armstrong PW, White HD, et al. Risk stratification with a point-of-care troponin T test in acute myocardial infarction. Am J Cardiol 1999;84:1281–1286.

88. Srinivas VS, Cannon CP, Gibson CM, et al. Myoglobin levels at 12 hours identify patients at low risk for 30-day mortality after thrombolysis in acute myocardial infarction: a Thrombolysis in Myocardial Infarction 10B substudy. Am Heart J 2001;142:29–36.

89. Woodlief LH, Lee KL. Validation of a mortality model in 1384 patients with acute myocardial infarction [abstract]. Circulation 1995;92(Suppl. I):I-776.

90. Calvin JE, Klein LW, Van den Berg BJ, et al. Risk stratification in unstable angina: prospective validation of the Braunwald classification. JAMA 1995;273:136–141.

91. Lindahl B, Venge P, Wallentin L, for the FRISC Study Group. Relation between troponin T and the risk of subsequent cardiac events in unstable coronary artery disease. Circulation 1996;93: 1651–1657.

92. Antman EM, Tanasijevic MJ, Thompson B, et al. Cardiac-specific troponin I levels to predict the risk of mortality in patients with acute coronary syndromes. N Engl J Med 1996;335:1342–1349.

93. Newby LK, Christenson RH, Ohman EM, et al. Value of serial troponin T measures for early and late risk stratification in patients with acute coronary syndromes. Circulation 1998;98:1853–1859.

94. Stubbs P, Collinson P, Moseley D, Greenwood T, Noble M. Prospective study of the role of cardiac troponin T in patients admitted with unstable angina. Br Med J 1996;313:262–264.

95. Lindahl B, Venge P, Wallentin L, for the Fragmin in Unstable Coronary Artery Disease (FRISC) Study Group. Troponin T identifies patients with unstable coronary artery disease who benefit from long-term antithrombotic protection. J Am Coll Cardiol 1997;29:43–48.

96. Hamm CW, Heeschen C, Goldmann B, et al. Benefit of abciximab in patients with refractory unstable angina in relation to serum troponin T levels [published correction appears in N Engl J Med 1999;341:548]. N Engl J Med 1999;340:1623–1629.

97. Heeschen C, Hamm CW, Goldmann B, et al. Troponin concentrations for stratification of patients with acute coronary syndromes in relation to therapeutic efficacy of tirofiban. Lancet 1999;354: 1757–1762.

98. Newby LK, Ohman EM, Christenson RH, et al. Benefit of glycoprotein IIb/IIIa inhibition in patients with acute coronary syndromes and troponin T-positive status: the PARAGON-B Troponin T substudy. Circulation 2001;103:2891–2896.

99. Luscher MS, Thygeson K, Ravkilde J, Heickendorff L. Applicability of cardiac troponin T and I for early risk stratification in unstable coronary artery disease. Circulation 1997;96:2578–2585.

100. The Joint European Society of Cardiology/American College of Cardiology Committee. Myocardial infarction redefined—a consensus document of the Joint European Society of Cardiology/American College of Cardiology Committee for the Redefinition of Myocardial Infarction. J Am Coll Cardiol 2000;36:959–969.

101. Lee TH, Juarez G, Cook EF, et al. Ruling out acute myocardial infarction: a prospective multicenter validation of a 12-hour strategy for patients at low risk. N Engl J Med 1991;324:1239–1246.

102. Gaspoz JM, Lee TH, Cook EF, Weisberg MC, Goldman L. Outcomes of patients who were admitted to a new short stay unit to "rule-out" myocardial infarction. Am J Cardiol 1991;68:145–149.

103. Gomez MA, Anderson JL, Karagounis LA, Muhlestein JB, Moores FB, for the ROMIO Study Group. An emergency department-based protocol for rapidly ruling out myocardial ischemia reduces hospital time and expense: results of a randomized study (ROMIO). J Am Coll Cardiol 1996;28:25–33.

104. Gaspoz JM, Lee TH, Weinstein MC, et al. Cost effectiveness of a new short-stay unit to "rule-out" myocardial infarction in low risk patients. J Am Coll Cardiol 1994;24:1249–1259.

105. Newby LK, Califf RM. Identifying patient risk: the basis for rational discharge planning after acute myocardial infarction. J Thromb Thrombol 1996;3:107–115.

106. Mikhail MG, Smith FA, Gray M, Britton C, Fredericksen SM. Cost-effectiveness of mandatory stress testing in Chest Pain Center patients. Ann Emerg Med 1997;29:88–98.

107. Zimmerman J, Fromm R, Meyer D, et al. Diagnostic marker cooperative study for the diagnosis of myocardial infarction. Circulation 1999;99:1671–1677.

108. Kontos MC, Anderson FP, Hanbury CM, Roberts CS, Miller WG, Jesse RL. Use of the combination of myoglobin and CK-MB mass for the rapid diagnosis of acute myocardial infarction. Am J Emerg Med 1997;15:14–19.

109. Trahey TF, Dunevant SL, Thompson AB, et al. Early hospital discharge of chest pain patients using creatine kinase MB isoforms and stress testing-a community hospital experience [abstrac]. Circulation 1996;94(Suppl. I):I-569.

110. Wu AHB, Lane PL. Metaanalysis in clinical chemistry: validation of cardiac troponin T as a marker for ischemic heart diseases. Clin Chem 1995;41:1228–1233.

111. Newby LK, Storrow AB, Gibler WB, et al. Bedside multimarker testing for risk stratification in Chest Pain Units: The Chest Pain Evaluation by Creatine Kinase-MB, Myoglobin, and Troponin I (CHECK-MATE) Study. Circulation 2001;103:1832–1837.

8 Technologies to Diagnose Acute Ischemia

Robert J. Zalenski, MD, MA, Joseph Lau, MD, and Harry P. Selker, MD, MSPH

CONTENTS

INTRODUCTION

As the most common cause of death in this country, acute myocardial infarction (AMI) has deservedly been the subject of substantial efforts of clinicians, scientists, governmental and other agencies, and the public in efforts to reduce its devastating impact. Although very significant progress continues to be made, The National Heart, Lung, and Blood Institute (NHLBI) of the National Institutes of Health (NIH) recognized the need for a concerted and coordinated effort to reduce mortality and morbidity

From: *Contemporary Cardiology: Management of Acute Coronary Syndromes, Second Edition*
Edited by: C. P. Cannon © Humana Press Inc., Totowa, NJ

in this country from AMI and, in 1991, initiated the National Heart Attack Alert Program (NHAAP).

Detecting AMI and unstable angina pectoris (UAP) in the emergency department (ED) is a most challenging task, and the consequences of a missed diagnosis can be very detrimental to both patients and physicians alike. The high prevalence of disease and resulting common, atypical presentations, and the poor sensitivity or specificity of the clinical exam have led to the use of many technologies to assist in establishing an accurate diagnosis. Recognizing this central and growing role of diagnostic technologies for AMI and for acute cardiac ischemia (ACI) in general (including both UAP and AMI) in emergency settings, which represent patients' entry points into the health care system, the NHAAP Working Group on Evaluation of Technologies for Identifying Acute Cardiac Ischemia in the Emergency Department was formed in 1994 *(1,2)* to assess the utility of diagnostic technologies for ACI/AMI in the ED. A systematic assessment of the literature commenced in 1998 *(3–6)*. This update, termed the Systematic Review, was performed by the New England Medical Center Evidence-based Practice Center under contract to the Agency for Healthcare Research and Quality, Rockville, Maryland. This chapter utilizes the assessments of the Systematic Review on the diagnostic performance and impact on care of those technologies and updates its base of scientific evidence. The technologies reviewed address the diagnosis of ACI (i.e., both AMI and UAP), as this is the condition that must be identified in the treatment of patients with AMI and potential AMI. The review included technologies directed at the diagnosis of ACI in the ED; methods primarily directed at prognostic or risk stratification of such patients are not addressed.

WORKING GROUP METHODS

A systematic review and evaluation of the scientific literature related to these technologies was undertaken based on Medline and related electronic literature searches and supplemented by the scientists' understanding of the literature and ongoing research. Relevant English literature on each technology was reviewed, summarized, and analyzed. For each technology, studies were formally evaluated and then rated. The quality of evidence provided by the relevant studies was rated as A, B, C, or NK as follows: A (least bias), prospective controlled clinical trials of high quality (e.g., large randomized controlled trials); B (susceptible to some bias), substantial clinical studies (e.g., prospective cohort studies); C (likely to have significant bias), limited studies or evidence (e.g., case series, small clinical studies); or NK, not known (e.g., expert opinion or case reports only).

Based on these reviews, each technology, for its primary purpose, was rated in terms of its diagnostic performance for identifying ACI/AMI in actual use and its demonstrated clinical impact. Diagnostic performance indicates the accuracy of the technology and is measured by sensitivity, specificity, or receiver-operating characteristic curve, for ACI or AMI. Clinical impact indicates its demonstrated impact on diagnosis, triage, treatment, or outcome (e.g., mortality) when used by clinicians in actual practice. Performance in each of these two dimensions was rated as: +++ (very accurate diagnosis/large clinical impact), ++ (moderately accurate/medium impact), + (modestly accurate/small impact), NK (not known), or NE (not effective). When there were sufficient numbers of studies available for a specific technology, a meta-analysis was per-formed to quantify diagnostic performance or clinical impact.

In assigning these ratings, each technology was evaluated on the basis of its per-formance of its primary diagnostic purpose of general ED detection (G), early detection (E), and detection in specific subgroup (S). These designations are noted in Table 14, which appears at the end of this summary.

The Systematic Review's conclusions and ratings for each diagnostic technology follow. The ratings of the Systemic Review reflect its estimation of the accuracy or impact of the test in actual practice in the ED. These assessments incorporate the quality of the literature, the magnitude or effect size of the reported findings, and considerations of generalizability and feasibility.

STANDARD ELECTROCARDIOGRAM

The primary purpose of the standard electrocardiogram (ECG) is to detect ACI in broad symptomatic ED populations. However, there are several fundamental limitations in the standard ECG. First, it is a single brief sample from a highly varied domain. Because unstable ischemic syndromes have rapidly changing demand and supply char-acteristics, a single ECG may not adequately represent the entire picture *(7)*. If a patient with unstable angina is (temporarily) pain-free at the time the ECG is obtained, the resulting normal tracing will poorly represent the patient's ischemic myocardium. A tracing taken minutes later may have a very different appearance. Second, 12-lead elec-trocardiography is limited because of its lack of perfect detection in areas of the myocardium it samples. Small areas of ischemia or infarction may not be detected. Addi-tionally, the conventional leads do not directly examine the right ventricle *(8)* or the pos-terior basal or lateral walls very well. AMIs in the distribution of the circumflex artery are likely to have a nondiagnostic ECG *(9,10)*. Third, some ECG baseline patterns make the ECG tracing difficult or impossible to interpret. These findings include early repo-larization, left ventricular hypertrophy, bundle-branch block, and arrhythmias *(11)*. Also, prior Q waves can mask zones of reinfarction, although the presence of any sig-nificant abnormality in a patient with chest pain or other related symptoms should gen-erally be considered positive.

Fourth, the wave forms of ECGs are often difficult to interpret, and thus, there is much disagreement among readers. Such nonagreement frequently includes cases of missed ischemia. This has been studied by Lee and colleagues *(12)* in their review of patients with AMI who were sent home. The ECGs of such discharged patients tended to have ischemia or infarction not known to be old; 23% of missed diagnoses were due to misread ECGs. These patients were younger, were less likely to have prior infarct or angina, and had more atypical symptoms.

In spite of these shortcomings, the standard ECG functions as an integral component of the evaluation of patients with acute chest pain and should continue to be incorpo-rated in strategies that incorporate other clinical characteristics such as historical and physical examination parameters. The ECG is not a perfectly sensitive test, and it should always be considered a supplement to, rather than a substitute for, physician judgment. The Systematic Review recommends the ECG continue to be considered the standard of care in the evaluation of chest pain in the ED patient. The results of the Working

Table 1
Standard ECG[a]

ED diagnostic performance		ED clinical impact	
Quality evidence	Accuracy (max = +++)	Quality of evidence	Impact
A	++	Standard of care	Standard of care

[a]For abbreviations and gradings in Tables 1–13, see footnotes to Table 14.

Group's final ratings of the quality of evidence evaluating this technology and of its ED diagnostic performance and clinical impact are shown in Table 1.

PREHOSPITAL ECG

The primary test purpose for the prehospital ECG is the early detection of AMI with acute ST-segment elevation. Additional important issues are whether the prehospital ECG reduces the time to an appropriate intervention for ST-segment elevation AMI detected in the prehospital setting and whether the intervention yields clinical benefit. A 12-lead prehospital ECG is obtained at the scene or in the ambulance and a preliminary ECG interpretation is printed out in the ambulance. The ECG is then sent to the hospital via cellular telephone through a modem, which takes approx 20 s. Error-free data transmission is ensured by an interactive method of data transfer (13). The following patients are eligible for prehospital ECGs: cooperative adult patients with a complaint of chest pain or other symptoms of heart attack, with systolic blood pressure >90, and without malignant dysrhythmias (ventricular tachycardia or fibrillation, or second/third-degree atrioventricular block) (14).

A prospective evaluation demonstrated that 91.4% of prehospital chest pain patients met these eligibility criteria (15). From 3–5% of prehospital patients with complaints of chest pain may be identified as candidates for thrombolytic therapy, which comprises one-half or more of all patients receiving thrombolytic therapy (14,16,17). Multiple studies have shown the feasibility of performing prehospital 12-lead ECGs (13–25). Diagnostic quality ECGs can be acquired and successfully transmitted in approx 70% of prehospital chest pain patients eligible for 12-lead ECGs (15). ECG acquisition increases the time spent at the scene of an emergency an average of 3.9 min over control (15). Additionally, there is no difference between the information collected in the prehospital setting and that received by cellular transmission at the base station (13). Diagnostic accuracy was evaluated in 11 studies with a total of 7508 patients by meta-analysis (4). Data were available for ACI in 5 studies and for AMI in 8 studies. For ACI, the pooled sensitivity was 76% (95% confidence interval [CI]: 54–89%), the specificity was 88% (95% CI: 67–96%), and the diagnostic odds ratio was 23. For AMI, the sensitivity was 68%, specificity of 97%, and diagnostic odds ratio of 104.

Prehospital ECG's Effect on Hospital-Based Time to Treatment

Several studies have demonstrated significant reductions in hospital-based time to treatment with thrombolytic therapy for AMI patients identified prior to patient arrival with prehospital 12-lead electrocardiography (20,21,23,26). Kereiakes et al. (20)

demonstrated that the median hospital delay to treatment was 64 min for patients transported by automobile, 55 min for patients transported by local ambulance, 50 min for patients transported by the emergency medical services (EMS) system with a prehospital ECG obtained but not transmitted to the receiving hospital, and 30 min for patients transported by the EMS system who had a 12-lead ECG transmitted from the field. Specialized EMS system transport alone did not facilitate in-hospital initiation of thrombolytic therapy; a significant reduction in hospital time delay to treatment was observed only in patients transported by the emergency medical system who had cellular transmission of a prehospital 12-lead ECG from the field. Karagounis et al. *(21)* demonstrated a statistically significant 20-min time reduction to hospital-based treatment with thrombolytic therapy in AMI patients identified by prehospital 12-lead ECG.

Prehospital ECG and Prehospital Thrombolysis

The Myocardial Infarction Triage and Intervention (MITI) trial randomized 360 prehospital AMI patients to receive either prehospital or hospital-based thrombolytic therapy *(27)*. Using prehospital 12-lead ECGs and a paramedic contraindication checklist, the MITI trial demonstrated that 353 (98%) of the 360 patients enrolled had subsequent evidence of AMI. Two percent of patients had nondiagnostic abnormalities on the initial ECG. Prehospital identification of patients eligible for thrombolysis by paramedics reduced the hospital treatment time from 60 min (for patients not in the study) to 20 min (for study patients allocated to begin treatment in the hospital). Since this was not a comparable group by definition, it is only suggestive of the potential benefit of a protocol-driven prehospital thrombolytic program.

The MITI trial also showed that administration of thrombolytics occurred 33 min earlier in the prehospital group than in the hospital group, although the investigators found no significant differences overall in mortality, ejection fraction, or infarct size between the prehospital group and the hospital treatment group. Although there was no improvement in outcome associated with initiating treatment before hospital arrival, treatment within 70 min of symptom onset was associated with a statistically significant lowered mortality rate of 1.2% *(24)*.

A number of other studies outside the United States have demonstrated that it is possible to accurately identify thrombolytic candidates in the prehospital setting *(24,25,28–38)*. The Grampion Region Early Anistreplase Trial *(34)* conducted in northern Scotland demonstrated a median time difference of 130 min between prehospital and hospital-based treatment with thrombolytic therapy. This trial demonstrated a statistically significant 52% relative reduction in 1-yr mortality. Furthermore, significantly fewer Q wave (smaller) MIs were seen in patients treated with prehospital thrombolytic therapy compared with patients treated in the hospital *(34)*. A meta-analysis of seven trials of out-of-hospital thrombolysis showed a 16% (95% CI: 2–27%) reduction in the risk of death *(4)*.

In summary, prehospital identification of thrombolytic candidates through the use of prehospital 12-lead electrocardiography has been shown in almost every study to significantly reduce hospital-based time to treatment. This time savings is perceived as beneficial, but has not, by itself, demonstrated a reduction in mortality. Prehospital treatment with thrombolytic therapy may result in a significant mortality reduction if the time savings is in the area of 1 h or more. Recent meta-analyses of diagnostic tests have

Table 2
Prehospital ECG

| ED diagnostic performance | | ED clinical impact | |
Quality evidence	Accuracy (max = +++)	Quality of evidence	Impact
B	++	A	++

found excellent accuracy and of treatment effects showed that prehospital thrombolysis can reduce hospital mortality in AMI (4). The results of the Systematic Review's final ratings of the quality of evidence evaluating this technology and of its ED diagnostic performance and clinical impact are in Table 2.

CONTINUOUS 12-LEAD ECG

A typical instrument for continuous ST-segment monitoring is microprocessor-controlled and fully programmable (39). It can continuously acquire a new 12-lead ECG every 20 s and analyzes the ST-segments. The initial ECG is defined as the pretrigger ECG. If ST-segment elevation or depression occurs 0.2 mV in a single lead or 0.1 mV in two leads as compared with the pretrigger ECG, the device enters a potential alarm state. If four sequential ECGs have met the threshold criteria, then an alarm sounds and a 12-lead ECG is printed for physician review. This ECG then becomes the new pretrigger ECG for future ST-segment comparisons. Typically, a 12-lead ECG is saved every 20 min as well as any alarm ECGs. One can also print two-dimensional graphs of ST-segment trends (magnitude vs time) for the 12 individual leads or the average ST-segment magnitudes for the four regional groupings: anterior (V_1–V_3), inferior (II, III, AVF), low lateral (V_4–V_6), and high lateral (I, AVL).

The practice of monitoring dysrhythmias in suspected cardiac patients became the standard of care when electrical and chemical defibrillation demonstrated the potential to terminate dysrhythmias. Similarly, with the advent of specific proven modalities to treat both AMI (with thrombolytics or angioplasty) and myocardial ischemia (with anticoagulants, vasodilators, circulation support devices, and angioplasty), there are sound reasons to evaluate and test the continuous 12-lead ECG.

There are two questions that continuous electrocardiography could address: first, it could aid in the early detection of potential candidates for thrombolysis or angioplasty while undergoing monitoring in the ED. This may occur in patients with suspected AMI whose initial ECG is nonspecific, but whose second ECG has at least 0.1 mV of ST-segment elevation in two contiguous leads. Second, in subgroups of ED patients, it could improve the diagnosis of ACI by detecting ST-segment changes that confirm the diagnosis of unstable angina or non-Q wave AMI. Since approx 50% of the patients with chest pain and AMI present to the ED without ST-segment elevation, and nearly 20% of these patients develop in-hospital electrocardiographic evidence of transmural infarction, continuous serial ECGs with ST-segment trend monitoring may identify the patient population most likely to benefit from rapid interventions following detection of electrocardiographic criteria diagnostic for AMI (40).

Table 3
Continuous 12-Lead ECG

ED diagnostic performance		ED clinical impact	
Quality evidence	Accuracy (max = +++)	Quality of evidence	Impact
B	+	NK	NK

In a retrospective study, Gibler et al. *(41)* used ECG/ST-segment trend monitoring to monitor 1010 patients in a chest pain evaluation and treatment program located in the ED. Of 52 patients with cardiac disease, 11 had evidence of ischemia or evolving AMI by ST-segment trend monitoring. As this population had a low prevalence of acute ischemic coronary syndrome, it is hypothesized that such a monitoring device may actually demonstrate a higher utility in a population with greater disease prevalence. In a recent prospective study of serial 12-lead ECGs, automated 12-lead ECGS were monitored every 20 s and printed at least every 20 min during a mean period of 128 min in the ED while awaiting hospital admission *(40)*. The sensitivity of ST-segment elevation was increased by 16.2% from 45.6% to 61.8% ($p < 0.001$) with no decrease in specificity. Serial ECGs made a substantial impact on care as shown by the treatment of 21 of 34 patients (62%) with new ST-segment elevation with reperfusion therapy.

There have been no large randomized controlled prospective ED or coronary care unit (CCU) studies evaluating this technology. Cost-benefit analysis of this technology has not been accomplished. Although ED ST-segment monitoring holds the potential to detect silent myocardial ischemia and MI reduce missed ischemic diagnoses, and provide the earliest evidence for coronary occlusion in patients presenting with preinfarction angina, larger prospective studies are required to make this assessment. The results of the Systematic Review's *(3)* final ratings of the quality of evidence evaluating this technology and of its ED diagnostic performance and clinical impact are shown in Table 3.

NONSTANDARD ECG LEADS

The standard 12-lead ECG is a less-than-perfect predictor of AMI. The sensitivity of ST-segment elevation for AMI is approx 50% *(42)*, and up to 30% of AMI patients have nonspecific or normal ECGs.

One of the explanations offered for these limitations is that the 12-lead ECG poorly detects posterior wall *(43)* and right ventricular infarction (RVI) *(8)*. These areas of the myocardium are not directly interrogated by standard leads but are assessed by posterior leads V_7, V_8, and V_9 and right-sided leads V_{4R}, V_{5R}, and V_{6R} *(44)*.

Posterior AMI is one of the most commonly missed ECG findings, and this may be explained by the lack of direct ECG examination *(45)*. In their study, Seyal and Swiryn *(46)* found that 6% (13 out 250) of infarctions are isolated to the posterior basal surface of the left ventricle.

Posterior and right-sided leads are acquired using the same electrocardiograph as standard leads. For right-sided leads, the lead placement is just the reverse of standard

Table 4
Nonstandard ECG Leads

	ED diagnostic performance		ED clinical impact	
	Quality evidence	Accuracy (max = +++)	Quality of evidence	Impact
Nonstandard ECG leads	B	+	NK	NK

left-sided leads (i.e., midclavicular line, fifth intercostal space for V_{4R}, anterior axillary line for V_{5R}, and midaxillary line for V_{6R}). Posterior leads continue in the same horizontal plane as the precordial leads (i.e., fifth intercostal space, but continue on to the posterior axillary line for V_7, midscapular line for V_8, and paraspinal for V_9) (44).

A plethora of articles assess the diagnostic value of V_{4R} and other right-sided leads to detect RVI (8,47–51). There is a consensus that within this context, right-sided leads detect RVI with a sensitivity of 80–90% and a specificity of 80%. More recently, Zehender and colleagues (47) showed that right ventricular leads are independent predictors of in-hospital and long-term prognosis in inferior wall AMI.

Posterior wall AMI usually occurs in the setting of inferior AMI, but occurs as an isolated phenomenon about 5% of the time. Posterior leads occasionally have been reported to assist in the diagnosis of AMI. However, detecting "true" posterior wall AMI from the numerous noninfarct cases is difficult, partly because it is an uncommon finding.

Although the literature has documented that the standard 12-lead ECG is insensitive for detecting posterior AMI, there have been only occasional reports comparing findings on the standard 12-lead to posterior leads. In a multicenter study of the diagnostic accuracy of an ECG that contained three right ventricular and three posterior leads against the standard 12 lead, 533 patients were enrolled (44). Sensitivity for the diagnosis of AMI was improved with the 18-lead ECG, by 8.5%, but specificity decreased by 6.5%. This was largely due to high false-positive rates for isolated ST-segment elevation in the right ventricular (RV) leads. Posterior leads had better specificity, comparable to the 12-lead ECG. Logistic regression analysis found that RV leads had independently contributed to the diagnosis of AMI; posterior leads just missed standard levels of significance ($p = 0.055$), indicating a small level of impact.

In summary, sampling RV leads is clinically practical, uses the universally available 12-lead ECG, and appears to increase the sensitivity and specificity for detection of right ventricular infarction (a strong, independent predictor of major complications and in-hospital mortality in patients with inferior AMI). Such leads have the potential to improve severity classification of AMIs, help refine the process of risk-benefit assessment for emergency interventions, possibly provide an indication for thrombolytic treatment, and avoid nitrate-induced hypotension in patients with RVI. Sampling posterior leads has improved the sensitivity of the ECG for posterior AMI, but the effect size is small. Right ventricular leads do not contribute to the diagnosis of AMI generally, but only to the diagnosis of RVI. The results of the Systematic Review's (3) final ratings of the quality of evidence evaluating these technologies and of their ED diagnostic performance and clinical impact are shown in Table 4.

ECG EXERCISE STRESS TEST

After ruling out an AMI or an unstable angina, a graded exercise test *(52)* prior to discharge from the ED may assist in the diagnosis of coronary artery disease (CAD) and result in more appropriate referral *(53–61)*. In a study of patients evaluated in a chest pain center located in the ED, 791 of 1010 patients underwent graded ECG exercise stress testing after 9 h of nondiagnostic serial ECG/ST-segment trend monitoring; 0-, 3-, 6-, and 9-h creatine kinase isoenzyme-cardiac muscle subunit (CK-MB) testing; and resting echocardiography *(41)*. None of the patients undergoing ECG exercise stress testing suffered an adverse event while being tested. Of these 791 patients, 782 (98.9%) had a negative or nondiagnostic ECG stress test, and the positive predictive value was 44% (4 out of 9) for CAD. Thirty-day follow-up revealed a 0.1% AMI rate and 0.5% all-cause mortality rate. Two recent prospective studies have shown that this approach has high diagnostic accuracy and is cost-effective. In a study of 317 patients at low probability of AMI by the Goldman computer protocol who met the attending physician's threshold for admission, four serial CK-MBs, three serial ECGs, and clinical re-evaluations were performed *(57)*. A total of 224 patients (71%) were negative for ACI and underwent treadmill exercise testing, and two-thirds of these (148 out of 224) had conclusively negative tests. The overall sensitivity of the protocol with treadmill testing was 90% (CI. 72.3–97.4%), specificity 50.5% (95% CI: 44.6–56.4%), and negative predictive value 98% (95% CI: 94.2–99.6%). Patient satisfaction with the protocol was higher than a randomly selected group of controls *(58)*. A randomized controlled cost subsidy showed that the total cost per patient for the accelerated diagnostic protocol was 27% less than hospital admission ($1528 vs $2095, $p < 0.001$) *(59)*.

A second study of 502 patients evaluated with myoglobin, CK-MB, serial ECGs, and provocative testing (with imaging in appropriate subgroups) showed a 100% sensitivity for AMI at 5-mo follow-up for the 410 (86%) of patients discharged; 8.7% (44 out of 502) of patients had a final diagnosis of ACI, and 58% of these were only detected by stress testing *(60)*. An average cost savings of 62% was reported. Another randomized trial of 100 low-risk patients assigned to either an ED-based rapid rule-out protocol or routine hospital care found significant reductions in length of stay (11.9 vs 22.8 h), and initial ($893 vs $1349) and 30-d costs ($898 vs $1522, all p values < 0.001) *(61)*. Thus, the ED-based protocol was found to be less costly even with the inclusion of mandatory provocative testing. ECG exercise stress testing in the ED can be incorporated into a protocol to evaluate patients with low- to moderate-risk chest pain. The assessment of the Systemic Review's final ratings *(3)* of the quality of evidence evaluating this technology and of its ED diagnostic performance and clinical impact are shown in Table 5.

ACUTE CARDIAC ISCHEMIA TIME-INSENSITIVE PREDICTIVE INSTRUMENT

The ACI time-insensitive predictive instrument (ACI-TIPI) represents the next generation of ACI predictive models developed by Selker and colleagues *(62,63)*. The ACI-TIPI, like the original ACI predictive instrument *(64,65)*, provides the ED physician with the 0–100% probability that a given patient truly has ACI to supplement the ED triage decision. The variables used for the ACI-TIPI are (*i*) age; (*ii*) sex; (*iii*) the presence or absence of chest pain or pressure or left arm pain; (*iv*) whether chest pain or pressure is

Table 5
ECG Exercise Stress Test

ED diagnostic performance		ED clinical impact	
Quality evidence	Accuracy (max = +++)	Quality of evidence	Impact
B	++	C	NK-NE

the patient's most important presenting symptom; (*v*) the presence or absence of ECG Q waves; (*vi*) the presence and degree of ECG ST-segment elevation or depression; and (*vii*) the presence and degree of ECG T-wave elevation or inversion. Its diagnostic performance has been tested in large studies that included ED *(62,66)* and EMS *(67)* patients and has been demonstrated to be diagnostically equivalent to the earlier version *(62)*, except for a slightly higher sensitivity for AMI. Thus, it should be comparable to the original ACI predictive instrument *(62)*, with two advantages for clinical use. First, its incorporation into the conventional computerized electrocardiograph allows direct measurement of details of the ECG waveform without the need for physician interpretation, with automatic printing of the ACI probability on the ECG header (Fig. 1). Second, its "time-insensitivity" makes it valid for retrospective review and assessment of care as well as for real-time ED clinical care.

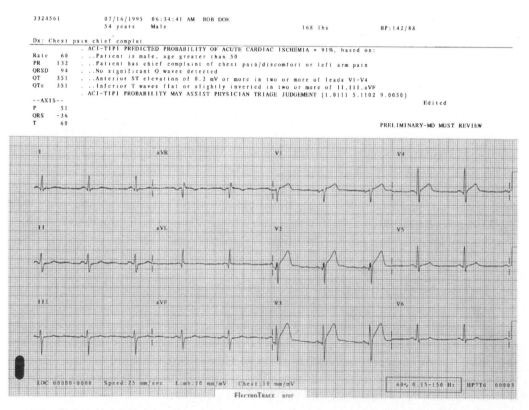

Fig. 1. ACI-TIPI

Table 6
ACI-TIPI

ED diagnostic performance			ED clinical impact	
Quality evidence	Accuracy (max = +++)		Quality of evidence	Impact
A	+++		A	+++

Two published early trials have shown impact on the speed and accuracy of ED triage *(66,68)*. The trial of clinical impact on ED triage decision making of a 10,689-patient multicenter controlled clinical trial showed the diagnostic performance of the ACI-TIPI electrocardiograph by itself and by ACI-TIPI risk groups to be very good and showed that its use improved patient ED triage *(69)*. In terms of its actual impact on ED care, for patients without ACI in hospitals with low telemetry capacities, the use of the ACI-TIPI decreased CCU admissions by 16% and increased ED discharges to home by 7% ($p = 0.09$). Moreover, for patients seen by residents without supervising attending physicians, the ACI-TIPI's use reduced CCU admissions by 31%, reduced telemetry admissions by 19%, and increased discharged to home by 18% ($p = 0.005$).

For patients with stable angina pectoris, in hospitals with low telemetry bed capacities, the ED use of the ACI-TIPI reduced CCU admission by 50%, increased telemetry admissions by 25%, and increased ED discharges to home by 10% ($p = 0.04$). At hospitals with high telemetry capacities, the use of the ACI-TIPI reduced telemetry admissions by 14% and increased ED discharges to home by 101% ($p = 0.03$) (the level of discharge seen in hospitals with lower telemetry unit capacities). Across all hospitals, the ACI-TIPI reduced CCU admission by 26% and increased ED discharges to home by 48% ($p = 0.04$). Finally, for patients with AMI or UAP, at both the low- and high-capacity hospitals, and with both supervised and unsupervised residents, the ACI-TIPI's ED use did not change the appropriate admission of 96% of patients to either CCU or telemetry beds.

The overall results of the Systematic Review's final ratings of the quality of evidence evaluating this technology and of its ED diagnostic performance and clinical impact are shown in Table 6.

GOLDMAN CHEST PAIN PROTOCOL

The Goldman chest pain protocol is a computer-derived decision aid and was developed to assist physicians in using routinely collected clinical and test data in the ED in identifying patients likely to be having an AMI who therefore require triage to the CCU. A statistical technique of recursive partitioning was used to divide the study's subjects into subgroups by ED data elements of the history, physical examination, and ECG into having proportions of AMI higher or lower (Fig. 2) *(70,71)*.

The protocol was developed using prospectively collected data on patients presenting to the ED with acute chest pain *(71)*. AMI was used as the outcome on which to base triage to the CCU, given that the risk of emergent complications early in the admission is 17% compared with 0.5% in patients without AMI. Recursive partitioning was used to develop a decision tree with the probability of ruling in for an AMI as the outcome

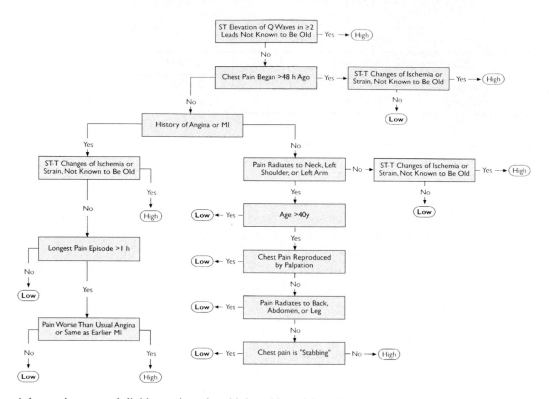

*chest pain protocol divides patients into high and low risks of AMI on the basis of a recursive parti-
tioning model. It uses routinely collected and interpreted history, physical examination, and electrocardiographic data. Reproduced with permission from ref. 57. [Zalenski RJ, McCarren M, Roberts
RR, et al. An evaluation of a chest pain diagnostic protocol to excluded acute cardiac ischemia in the
emergency department. Arch Intern Med 1997;157:1085–1091. ©1997 American Medical
Association.

of each branch. The protocol was prospectively validated in a population of 4770
patients who presented with chest pain *(70)*. Follow-up of the 2232 patients who were
discharged from the ED was performed by either physical examination, follow-up
measurement of CK, or telephone to determine whether an AMI had occurred after discharge from the ED. Diagnostic performance for AMI compared with that of physicians
for the same patients is shown in Table 7.

These data show the sensitivity of the protocol for predicting AMI with triage to the
CCU to be the same as that of physicians, but with higher specificity than physicians.
It was projected that 11.5% of patients without AMI would have been triaged elsewhere
had the protocol been used.

A prospective trial used a time series study design to determine the impact of the protocol on the triage and outcomes of patients presenting to the ED at the Brigham and
Women's Hospital in Boston *(72)*. The time series design used six 14-wk cycles, consisting of a 5-wk control and/or intervention period separated by 2-wk wash-out cycles.
Risk estimates and triage recommendations were provided to physicians in a nonobtru-
sive fashion. Rates of admissions during intervention and control periods were
unchanged in the hospital (52 and 51%, respectively) and in the CCU (10% each). Also,
there were no significant differences in hospital length of stay or average total costs *(72)*.

Table 7
Diagnostic Performance for AMI Compared with that of Physicians for the Same Patients

	Physicians (%)	Protocol (%)	P value
Sensitivity[a]	88	88	NS
Specificity[b]	71	74	<0.00001
Positive predictive value[c]	29	32	0.10
Overall accuracy	73	76	<0.00001

[a]Percentage of patients with AMI admitted to CCU.
[b]Percentage of patients without AMI not admitted to CCU.
[c]Percentage of patients with AMI among the total admitted to CCU.

The Goldman computer-based chest pain protocol was developed using a sound methodology. The fact that it was validated in a large population that included two university and four community hospitals, with at least two of the hospitals having racially diverse populations, supports its potential utility in a diverse patient population. As the protocol currently stands, its greatest potential benefit would likely be in improving physicians' specificity for AMI and avoidance of triage to the CCU with attendant cost savings. However, this impact has not yet been demonstrated in a controlled clinical trial of its use. Also, given that UAP is important with regard to clinical and cost implications, the fact that non-AMI ACI is not addressed by the Goldman protocol is a significant limitation. The protocol cannot be applied to all ED patients with symptoms consistent with ACI. The results of the Systematic Review's final ratings of the quality of evidence evaluating this technology and of its ED diagnostic performance and clinical impact are shown Table 8.

OTHER COMPUTER-BASED DECISION AIDS

These computer-based decision aids, including neural networks, provide examples of a variety of ways to identify patients for CCU admission and to predict MI (73–78), and they are reviewed in the full Systematic Review (3). Models published have some limitations, especially that they often predict AMI rather than ACI, and have not yet been demonstrated to be safe and effective in actual use. Although each has some promise, including very encouraging performance in their preliminary studies, at this point, none can be considered ready for clinical use. The results of the Systematic Review's final ratings of the quality of evidence evaluating these technologies and of their ED diagnostic performance and clinical impact are shown in Table 9.

CREATINE KINASE

CK-MB measurements are traditionally obtained early in the ED course of a patient admitted to the hospital for suspected AMI or ACI (79–82). The utility of the assay in the ED as a one-time test is limited because levels do not significantly increase until 4–6 h after the onset of AMI (79). In a meta-analysis of 10 studies of 2504 ED patients, the presenting CK-MB had a sensitivity of only 44% (95% CI: 35–53%), but a specificity of 96% (95% CI: 94–97%) (6). Serial CK-MB performs significantly better. In a meta-analysis of seven studies of 3229 ED patients, the sensitivity of serial CK-MB meas-

Table 8
Goldman Chest Pain Protocol

ED diagnostic performance		ED clinical impact	
Quality evidence	Accuracy (max = +++)	Quality of evidence	Impact
A	For AMI: +++ For UAP: NE	A	+

Table 9
Other Computer-Based Decision Aids

ED diagnostic performance		ED clinical impact	
Quality evidence	Accuracy (max = +++)	Quality of evidence	Impact
A	++	NK	NK

urements was 80% (95% CI: 61–91%) *(6)*. It is important to be fully aware that CK and CK-MB do not identify patients with ACI, because they do not identify UAP. Patients with UAP comprise about half of patients with ACI. Underscoring this is the study by Hedges et al., which showed that even serial CK-MB measurements had a sensitivity of only 31% for ACI *(83)*.

Despite improvements in the diagnostic performance and practicality of CK and CK-MB assays, there is no randomized controlled clinical impact trial showing that these tests are effective for decisions to send a patient home or to the appropriate level of care of admission for patients with suspected ACI, either as one-time or serial tests. The Systematic Review found only one study that showed a small but important clinical effect of serial CK-MB testing on triage decisions *(83)*. Further prospective trials with follow-up of all (including nonadmitted) patients are needed before a strategy incorporating CK-MB into medical decision making can be fully evaluated. The results of the Systematic Review's final ratings of the quality of evidence evaluating this technology and of its ED diagnostic performance and clinical impact are shown in Table 10.

OTHER BIOCHEMICAL TESTS

Myoglobin, an early marker of AMI *(84–85)*, and the cardiac troponins T and I, which are medium and late markers *(86–88)* specific for myocyte damage, hold promise to improve the identification of patients with AMI and minor myocardial injury. The Systematic Review examined myoglobin in its assessment of biomarkers in ACI *(6)*. The reviewers found that in five studies of 831 ED patients, serial myoglobin had a sensitivity of 90% (95% CI: 78–96%) and a specificity of 92% (95% CI: 82–97%) *(6)*. In 10 studies of 1395 ED patients, a single presentation myoglobin had a sensitivity of only 49% (95% CI: 41–57%) *(6)*. As was found in studies of serial vs single (presentation) values of CK-MB, myoglobin, although an early marker, cannot be used as a one-time

Table 10
CK

	ED diagnostic performance		ED clinical impact	
	Quality evidence	Accuracy (max = +++)	Quality of evidence	Impact
Single test	A	For AMI: + For UAP: NE	NK	NK
Multiple tests over time	A	For AMI: +++ For UAP: NE	C	++

test. Like all other markers, the sensitivity of a single presenting troponin for AMI is low (approx 40%). In serial troponin I or T studies, sensitivities for AMI ranged from 90–100%. Troponin has become the de facto standard for the diagnosis of AMI. Studies suggest that the cardiac troponins can add predictive value to CK-MB measurements (89–91). This is likely due to their ability to detect smaller amounts of myocardial necrosis, amounting to the identification of AMI in some cases of rest angina (92).

Serum protein testing will likely include a panel of multiple markers, which provide utilized marker kinetics to optimize the diagnosis of AMI, regardless of time of presentation to the ED. An early sensitive marker such as myoglobin, when combined with CK-MB and troponin-T or -I, could provide the clinician with critical information necessary to make decisions in the emergency setting. Two studies assessed by the Systematic Review tested a combination strategy. The studies enrolled 291 patients and CK-MB and myoglobin testing were performed at presentation and 3 or 4 h later. This combination had a 100% sensitivity in both studies and specificities of 91 and 75%, respectively (6). Sensitivity of a single presentation testing of combined CK-MB and myoglobin in three studies of 2283 patients had a sensitivity of 83% (95% CI: 51–96%) and specificity of 82% (95% CI: 68–90%). Thus serial testing, over a 3- or 4-h period, provides the best diagnostic outcomes for the detection of AMI. The results of the Systematic Review's final ratings of the quality of evidence evaluating these technologies and of their ED diagnostic performance and clinical impact are shown in Table 11.

ECHOCARDIOGRAM

Resting echocardiography is examined in the Systematic Review's report (5). Its theoretical appeal for the diagnosis of ACI in the ED is based on the relationship between regional myocardial wall motion abnormalities and cardiac ischemia. When the myocardium becomes ischemic, there is a nearly immediate alteration in wall motion, and the wall becomes hypokinetic or dyskinetic (93). However, there are some caveats regarding its use in the ED. When looking for ACI, it still has a high enough false-negative rate to preclude discharging all patients with a negative echo. For the purpose of ruling in or ruling out AMI, echocardiography has not been shown to be able to be either acquired or interpreted by ED personnel. Considerable expertise is needed for data acquisition and interpretation (94–95).

The Systematic Review examined three high-quality (grade B, susceptible to some bias) studies of 397 patients in the ED and found an overall sensitivity for AMI of 93%

Table 11
Other Biochemical Tests

	ED diagnostic performance		ED clinical impact	
	Quality evidence	Accuracy (max = +++)	Quality of evidence	Impact
Troponin-T and troponin-I	B+	For AMI: +++ For UAP: NE	NK	NK
Myoglobin	B	For AMI: +++ For UAP: NE	NK	NK

Table 12
Echocardiogram

ED diagnostic performance		ED clinical impact	
Quality evidence	Accuracy (max = +++)	Quality of evidence	Impact
For ACI: C	+	NK	NK
For AMI: B	++	NK	NK

(range 81–97%), with a specificity of 66% (range 43–83%) *(96–98)*. Resting echocardiography for the diagnosis of ACI was evaluated in two studies of 228 patients, whose overall quality of evidence was rated as C (likely to have significant bias). The sensitivity was 70% (range 43–99%) and specificity was 87% (range 72–94%) *(5)*. Although echocardiography in the ED shows initial promise, there are no data demonstrating that it can effectively triage patients in large clinical settings. The results of the Systematic Review's final ratings of the quality of evidence evaluating this technology and of its ED diagnostic performance and clinical impact are shown in Table 12.

SESTAMIBI AND OTHER TECHNETIUM-99M PERFUSION AGENTS

Technetium-99m-sestamibi (^{99m}Tc sestamibi) is an excellent perfusion tracer *(99–105)*, with advantageous physical characteristics compared with thallium-201 *(100,102)*. Its availability, excellent imaging properties, and stable tracer distribution with time make it a practical agent for ED use *(103–105)*. There is minimal redistribution after its initial coronary flow-related distribution in the myocardium *(99,100)*; thus images made up to 1–4 h after injection will still reflect myocardial blood flow as it was at the time of injection *(103)*. Although large-scale trials are not yet published, the available data indicate that ^{99m}Tc sestamibi is a promising agent for use in the ED evaluation of selected patients with chest pain.

In pooled data of 1571 patients from the ED reveal that sestamibi has a range in sensitivity for AMI of 92–100%, with a range of specificity from 49–84% *(5)*. For ACI, its pooled sensitivity was 89% (95% CI: 73–96%) and pooled specificity was 77%(95%

Table 13
Sestamibi and Other Technetium-99m Perfusion Agents

ED diagnostic performance		ED clinical impact	
Quality evidence	Accuracy (max = +++)	Quality of evidence	Impact
B	++	NK	NK

CI: 63–87%) *(5)*. There are as of now no data on its clinical impact. However, a multi-center randomized trial, known as ERASE, will be published soon.

To date, sestamibi has been used in a small number of centers that have considerable expertise *(105)*. It is not certain that the technique will have good generalized applicability, particularly as a screening test in lower risk ED patients without ongoing chest pain or when used by less experienced interpreters. Until more evidence is available, it cannot yet be recommended for general use. The results of the Systematic Review's final ratings of the quality of evidence evaluating this technology and of its ED diagnostic performance and clinical impact are shown in Table 13.

CONCLUSIONS AND RECOMMENDATIONS
Summary of Clinical Recommendations Based on Demonstrated Diagnostic Performance and Clinical Impact

Recommendations regarding the use of a technology should be based on both ED diagnostic performance and clinical impact data obtained in high-quality or substantial studies. Of the various test technologies evaluated in the sections, however, only four met this highly desirable standard of evaluation. A summary of clinical recommendations based on demonstrated diagnostic performance and clinical impact is provided in Table 14.

The prehospital ECG was found to have good (++) diagnostic performance based on evidence from good-quality prospective studies (B). This technology was judged to have a moderate clinical impact (++) based on high-quality (A) clinical studies. Although this technology has promise in both speeding the diagnosis of ACI and permitting field thrombolyis, the latter will only be realized in areas with long EMS transport times. The general implementation of prehospital ECGs is recommended.

The second technology for which data are available on both its ED diagnostic performance and clinical impact is the Goldman chest pain protocol. An important caveat, however, is that this protocol was designed only for AMI detection and not the more general detection of ACI in the form of UAP. Its diagnostic performance for AMI has been demonstrated to be excellent (+++) in multicenter high-quality studies (A). However, in a high-quality prospective study (A), it has only a very small effect (+) on clinical care. Further studies of clinical impact are desirable.

The third diagnostic technology on which there are studies of both diagnostic performance and clinical impact is the ACI-TIPI. In high-quality (A) studies of both diagnostic performance and clinical impact, the ACI-TIPI achieved a large (+++) effect. The general implementation of the ACI-TIPI is recommended.

Table 14
Summary Ratings of Diagnostic Technologies for ACI for ED Use

Technology	Primary diagnostic use	ED diagnostic performance		Demonstrated ED clinical impact	
		Quality evidence	Accuracy (max = +++)	Quality of evidence	Impact
Standard ECG	G	A	++	Standard of Care	Standard of Care
ACI-TIPI	G	A	+++	A	+++
Prehospital ECG	E	B	++	A	++
Goldman chest pain protocol	G	A	For AMI: +++ For UAP: NE	A	+
CK, multiple tests over time	S	A	For AMI: +++ For UAP: NE	C	++
Sestamibi	S	B	++	NK	NK
CK, single test	S	A	For AMI: + For UAP: NE	NK	NK
ECG exercise stress test	S	B	++	C	NK-NE
Echocardiogram	S	AMI: B ACI: C	For AMI: ++ For ACI: +	NK NK	NK NK
Other computer-based decision aids	G	A	++	A	NK
Troponin-T and troponin-I	S	B+	For AMI: +++ For UAP: NE	NK	NK
Myoglobin	S	B	For AMI: +++ For UAP: NE	NK	NK
Nonstandard ECG leads	S	B	+	NK	NK
Continuous 12-lead ECG	S	B	+	NK	NK

Key:
AMI = acute myocardial infarction
UAP = unstable angina pectoris
G = general detection of ACI
E = early detection
S = detection in subgroup

Diagnostic rating:
A = highest-quality (least bias)
B = high-quality (some bias)
C = significant bias
NK = not known
NE = not effective

Clinical impact rating:
+++ = very accurate/ large clinical impact
++ = moderately accurate/ medium impact
+ = modestly accurate/ small impact
NK = not known
NE = not effective

Note: The technologies are listed in order of the Systematic Review's ratings of diagnostic accuracy and demonstrated clinical impact, and alphabetically among equivalent ratings, with the exception of standard ECG, which is considered to be a standard of care.

The final diagnostic technology, serial CK-MB testing, has been studied in high-quality (A) studies and been found to be highly (+ + +) accurate for the diagnosis of AMI (but not ACI). It has been only evaluated in one study (C), and was found to have a moderate (+ +) effect on triage decisions. Additional studies of high quality are needed to assess its impact are needed.

Summary of Clinical Recommendations Based on Demonstrated Diagnostic Performance but without Data on Clinical Impact

All technologies reviewed had some published evidence of diagnostic performance and nine technologies had no studies of actual impact on clinical care (i.e., all clinical impact grade NK). The Working Group strongly advises that, with the exception of the standard 12-lead ECG (see immediately below), diagnostic performance alone is an insufficient basis for recommendation for general use. This is from the long experience of numerous examples of technologies that have excellent or good diagnostic performance, but negligible or even negative clinical impact when tested under conditions of actual use.

The standard 12-lead ECG has been shown in many studies to have very good, although not perfect, diagnostic performance in the ED. Given that the ECG is part of standard ED evaluation, in the view of the Working Group, a trial to demonstrate its clinical impact would be neither necessary nor ethical. Indeed, the 12-lead ECG should be part of the very initial evaluation of any ED or EMS patient with symptoms suggestive of ACI.

Although they have not yet been demonstrated to actually improve clinical care in high-quality studies, blood biochemical tests of myocardial necrosis have undergone prospective testing of their diagnostic performance for the detection of AMI. Available data suggest that the use of a single biomarker test yields insufficient performance for use in ED triage, but that the use of multiple tests over several or more hours has very good diagnostic performance for AMI. Combinations of differing assays, such as myglobin and CK-MB, performed serially have been found to yield excellent diagnostic performance. Myoglobin may be best suited to complement either CK-MB or a cardiac troponin in combination testing. It is important to bear in mind that none of the biomarkers have good sensitivity for UAP, which raises the possibility of missing this form of ACI if triage is dependent on such tests. Given the paucity of prospective trials of the impact of these tests on ED triage (level of admission or discharge), they cannot yet be recommended for general ED triage use at this time, although they are very useful for the diagnosis of AMI in observation units or in-hospital care.

Echocardiography, well studied in other settings, has undergone several studies in the ED, which have generally shown moderate diagnostic performance for initial ED evaluation. Given this, and that its actual impact on ED care has not been evaluated, this technology cannot be recommended for general ED use at this time.

Sestamibi and other technetium-99m perfusion agents have been studied in the ED setting, and although the overall diagnostic performance of sestamibi has been promising, it has not been sufficiently tested to recommend its general ED use. Whether sestamibi will be found to be more helpful when evaluated for special subgroups, and when tested for its actual impact on care, remains to be seen. At this point, its general ED use cannot be recommended.

As an extension of the standard ECG, nonstandard ECG leads have undergone some limited testing in the ED for detecting AMI, and another prospective trial was just completed. The good-quality (B) studies indicate that there is a small improvement (+) in diagnostic accuracy afforded by these leads. Since their impact on care has not been studied, nonstandard ECG leads cannot yet be recommended for general use. In a similar fashion, good-quality (B) studies of continuous ECGs have also found that they make a modest improvement in the accuracy of the ECG, but their impact on care has not been studied. Therefore, this modality cannot be recommended for general use at this time.

ACKNOWLEDGMENTS

The authors wish to thank the members of the Technologies Working Group, Elliott M. Antman, MD, Tom P. Aufderheide, MD, Sheilah Ann Bernard, MD, Robert O'Bonow, MD, W. Brian Gibber, MD, Michael D. Hagen, MD, Paula Johnson MD, MPH, Robert A. McNutt, MD, Joseph Ornato, MD, J. Sanford Schwartz, MD, Jane D. Scott, ScD, MSN, Paul A. Tunick, MD, W. Douglas Weaver, MD, and the NHLBI staff, Mary M. Hand, MSPH, RN, Michael Horan, MD, ScM, John Clinton Bradley, MS, and Pamela A. Christian, RN, MPA, for their efforts in preparing the report on which this chapter is based. The authors are also indebted to the updated assessment provided by the New England Medical Center Evidence-based Practice Center under contract to the Agency for Healthcare Research and Quality, Rockville, Maryland. Dr. Joseph Lau is the principal investigator.

REFERENCES

1. Selker HP, Zalenski RJ, Antman EM, et al. An evaluation of technologies for identifying acute cardiac ischemia in the emergency department: a report from a National Heart Attack Alert Program Working Group. Ann Emerg Med 1997;29:13–87.
2. Selker HP, Zalenski RJ, Antman EM, et al. An evaluation of technologies for identifying acute cardiac ischemia in the emergency department: executive summary of a National Heart Attack Alert Program Working Group report. Ann Emerg Med 1997;29:1–12.
3. Lau J, Loannidis JPA, Balk EM, et al. Diagnosing acute cardiac ischemia in the Emergency Department: a systematic review of the accuracy and the clinical effect of current technologies. Ann Emerg Med 2001;37:453–460.
4. Loannidis JPA, Salem D, Chew PW, Lau J. Accuracy and clinical effect of out-of-hospital electrocardiography in the diagnosis of acute cardiac ischemia: a meta-analysis. Ann Emerg Med 2001;37:461–470.
5. Loanndis JPA, Salem D, Chew PW, Lau J. Accuracy of imaging technologies in the diagnosis of acute cardiac ischemia in the Emergency Department: a meta-analysis. Ann Emerg Med 2001;37:471–477.
6. Balk EM, Loannidis JPA, Salem D, Chew PW, Lau J. Accuracy of biomakers to diagnose acute cardiac ischemia in the Emergency Department: a meta-analysis. Ann Emerg Med 2001;37:478–494.
7. Bilodeau L, Theroux P, Gregoire J, Gagnon D, Arsenault A. Technetium-99m sestamibi tomography in patients with spontaneous chest pain: correlations with clinical, electrocardiographic and angiographic findings. J Am Coll Cardiol 1991;7:1684–1691.
8. Lopez-Sendon J, Coma-Canella I, Alcasena S, Seoane J, Gamallo C. Electrographic findings in acute right ventricular infarction: sensitivity and specificity of electrographic alteration in right precordial lead V_4R, V_3R, V_1, V_2, and V_3. J Am Coll Cardiol 1985;6:1273–1279.
9. Wrenn KD. Protocols in the emergency room evaluation of chest pain: do they fail to diagnose lateral wall myocardial infarction? J Gen Intern Med 1987;2:66–67.
10. Nestico PF, Hakki AH, Iskandrian AS, Anderson GJ. Electrographic diagnosis of posterior myocardial infarction revisited: a new approach using a multivariate discriminant analysis and thallium-201 myocardial scintigraphy. J Electrocardiol 1986;19:33–40.
11. Fisch C. Electrocardiography, exercise stress testing, and ambulatory monitoring. In: Kelley WN (ed). Textbook of Internal Medicine. J.B. Lippincott Company, Philadelphia, 1989, pp. 305–316.
12. Lee TH, Rouan GW, Weisberg MC, et al. Clinical characteristics and natural history of patients with acute myocardial infarction sent home from the emergency room. Am J Cardiol 1987;60:219-224.

13. Grim P, Feldman T, Martin M, Donovan R, Nevins V, Childers RW. Cellular telephone transmission of 12-lead electrocardiograms from ambulance to hospital. Am J Cardiol 1987;60:715–720.

14. Aufderheide TP, Keelan MH, Hendley GE, et al. Milwaukee Prehospital Chest Pain Project—Phase I: feasibility and accuracy of prehospital thrombolytic candidate selection. Am J Cardiol 1992;69: 991–996.

15. Aufderheide TP, Hendley GE, Woo J, Lawrence S, Valley V, Teichman SL. A prospective evaluation of prehospital 12-lead ECG application in chest pain patients. J Electrocardiol 1992;24S:8–13.

16. Weaver WD, Eisenberg MS, Martin JS, et al. Myocardial Infarction Triage and Intervention Project— Phase I: patient characteristics and feasibility of prehospital initiation of thrombolytic therapy. J Am Coll Cardiol 1990;15:925–931.

17. Aufderheide TP, Kereiakes DJ, Weaver WD, Gibler WB, Simoons ML. Planning, implementation, and process monitoring for prehospital 12-lead ECG diagnostic programs. Prehospital Disaster Med 1996; 11:162–171.

18. Aufderheide TP, Hendley GE, Thakur RK, et al. The diagnostic impact of prehospital 12-lead electro-cardiography. Ann Emerg Med 1990;19:1280–1287.

19. Aufderheide TP, Haselow WC, Hendley GE, et al. Feasibility of prehospital r-TPA therapy in chest pain patients. Ann Emerg Med 1992;21:379–383.

20. Kereiakes DJ, Gibler WB, Martin LH, Pieper KB, Anderson LC. Relative importance of emergency medical system transport and the prehospital electrocardiogram on reducing hospital time delay to therapy for acute myocardial infarction: a preliminary report from the Cincinnati Heart Project. Am Heart J 1992;123:835–840.

21. Karagounis L, Ipsen SK, Jessop MR, et al. Impact of field-transmitted electrocardiography on time to in-hospital thrombolytic therapy in acute myocardial infarction. Am J Cardiol 1990;66:786–791.

22. O'Rourke MF, Cook A, Carroll G, Gallagher D, Hall J. Accuracy of a portable interpretive ECG machine in diagnosis of acute evolving myocardial infarction. Aust N Z J Med 1992;22:9–13.

23. Foster DB, Dufendach JH, Barkdoll CM, Mitchell BK. Prehospital recognition of AMI using inde-pendent nurse/paramedic 12-lead ECG evaluation: impact on in-hospital times to thrombolysis in a rural community hospital. Am J Emerg Med 1994;12:25–31.

24. Koren G, Weiss AT, Hasin Y, et al. Prevention of myocardial damage in acute myocardial ischemia by earlier treatment with intravenous streptokinase. N Engl J Med 1985;313:1384–1389.

25. Fine DG, Weiss AT, Sapoznikov D, et al. Importance of early initiation of intravenous streptokinase therapy for acute myocardial infarction. Am J Cardiol 1986;58:411–417.

26. Aufderheide TP, Lawrence SW, Hall KN, Otto LA. Prehospital 12-lead electrocardiograms reduce hos-pital-based time to treatment in thrombolytic candidates [abstract]. Acad Emerg Med 1994;1: A13–A14.

27. Weaver WD, Cerqueira M, Hallstrom AP, et al. Prehospital-initiated vs hospital-initiated thrombolytic therapy. The Myocardial Infarction and Intervention Trial. JAMA 1993;270:1211–1216.

28. Bippus PH, Storch WH, Andresen D, Schroder R. Thrombolysis started at home in acute myocardial infarction: feasibility and time-gain. Circulation 1987;76(Suppl. IV):IV-122.

29. Holmberg S, Hjalmarson A, Swedberg K, et al. Very early thrombolysis therapy in suspected acute myocardial infarction. Am J Cardiol 1990;65:401–407.

30. Oemrawsingh PV, Bosker HA, Vanderlaarse A, Manger Cats V, Bruschke AV. Early reperfusion by initi-ation of intravenous streptokinase prior to ambulance transport. Circulation 1988;78(Suppl. II):II-110.

31. Castaigne A, Herve C, Duval-Moulin AM, et al. Prehospital use of APSAC: results of placebo-con-trolled study. Am J Cardiol 1989;64:30A–33A.

32. Bossaert LL, Demey HE, Colemont LJ, et al. Prehospital thrombolytic treatment of acute myocardial infarction with anisoylated plasminogen streptokinase activator complex. Crit Care Med 1988;16: 823–830.

33. Roth A, Barbash GI, Hod H, et al. Should thrombolytic therapy be administered in the mobile inten-sive care unit in patients with evolving myocardial infarction? A pilot study. J Am Coll Cardiol 1990; 15:932–936.

34. Rawles J. On behalf of the GREAT group. Halving of mortality at 1 year by domiciliary thrombolysis in the Grampian Region Early Anistreplase Trial (GREAT). J Am Coll Cardiol 1994;23:1–5.

35. The European Myocardial Infarction Project Group. Prehospital thrombolytic therapy in patients with suspected acute myocardial infarction. N Engl J Med 1993;329:383–389.

36. BEPS Collaborative Group. Prehospital thrombolysis in acute myocardial infarction: the Belgian emi-nase prehospital study (BEPS). Eur Heart J 1991;12:965–967.

37. Risenfors M, Gustavsson G, Ekstrom L, et al. Prehospital thrombolysis in suspected acute myocardial infarction: results from the TEAHAT Study. J Intern Med 1991;229(Suppl. 1):3–10.
38. Weiss A, Fine D, Applebaum D, et al. Prehospital coronary thrombolysis. A new strategy in acute myocardial infarction. Chest 1987;92:124–128.
39. Fesmire FM, Smith EE. Continuous 12-lead electrocardiograph monitoring in the emergency department. Am J Emerg Med 1993;11:54–60.
40. Fesmire FM, Percy RF, Bardoner JB,Wharton DR, Calhoun FB. Usefulness of automated serial 12-lead ECG monitoring during the initial emergency department evaluation of patients with chest pain. Ann Emerg Med 1998;31:3–11.
41. Gibler WB, Runyon JP, Levy RC, et al. A rapid diagnostic and treatment center for patients with chest pain in the emergency department. Ann Emerg Med 1995;25:1–8.
42. Rude RE, Poole WK, Muller JE, et al. Electrocardiographic and clinical criteria for recognition of acute myocardial infarction based on analysis of 3697 patients. Am J Cardiol 1983;52:936–942.
43. Rich MW, Imburgia M, King TR, Fischer KC, Kovach KL. Electrocardiographic diagnosis of remote posterior wall myocardial infarction using unipolar posterior lead V_9. Chest 1989;96:489–493.
44. Zalenski RJ, Rydman RJ, Sloan EP, et al. Value of posterior and right ventricular leads in comparison to the standard 12-lead electrocardiogram in evaluation of ST-segment elevation in acute myocardial infarction. Am J Cardiol 1997;79:1579–1585.
45. Perloff JK. The recognition of strictly posterior myocardial infarction by conventional scale electrocardiography. Circulation 1964;30:706–718.
46. Seyal MS, Swiryn S. True posterior myocardial infarction. Arch Intern Med 1983;143:983–985.
47. Zehender M, Kasper W, Kauder E, et al. Right ventricular infarction as an independent predictor of prognosis after acute inferior myocardial infarction. N Engl J Med 1993;328:981–988.
48. Braat SH, Bruguda P, den Dulk K, van Ommen V, Wellens HJ. Value of lead V_{4R} for recognition of the infarct coronary artery in acute myocardial infarction. Am J Cardiol 1984;53:1538–1541.
49. Candell-Riera J, Figueras J, Vaile V, et al. Right ventricular infarction: relationships between ST segment elevation in V_{4R} and hemodynamic, scintigraphic, and echocardiographic findings in patients with acute inferior myocardial infarction. Am Heart J 1981;101:281–287.
50. Klein HO, Tordiman T, Ninio R, et al. The early recognition of right ventricular infarction: diagnostic accuracy of the electrocardiographic V_{4R} lead. Circulation 1983;67:558–565.
51. Ramires JAF, Solimene MC, Savioli RM, et al. Mortality is not increased with inferior infarction associated with right ventricular infarction and atrioventricular block. Cor Heart Dis 1993;4:965–970.
52. Froelicher VF, Marcondes GD. Manual of Exercise Testing. Year Book Medical Publishers, Chicago, 1989, p. 332.
53. Gaspoz JM, Lee TH, Cook EF, Weisberg MC, Goldman L. Outcome of patients who were admitted to a new short-stay unit to "rule-out" myocardial infarction. Am J Cardiol 1991;68:145–149.
54. Lewis WR, Amsterdam EA. Utility and safety of immediate exercise testing of low-risk patients admitted to the hospital for suspected acute myocardial infarction. Am J Cardiol 1994;74:987–990.
55. Kerns JR, Shaub TF, Fontanarosa PB. Emergency cardiac stress testing in the evaluation of emergency department patients with atypical chest pain. Ann Emerg Med 1993;22:794–798.
56. Tsakonis JS, Shesser R, Rosenthal R, Bittar GD, Smith M, Wasserman AG. Safety of immediate treadmill testing in selected emergency department patients with chest pain: a preliminary report. Am J Emerg Med 1991;9:557–559.
57. Zalenski RJ, McCarren M, Roberts RR, et al. An evaluation of a chest pain diagnostic protocol to excluded acute cardiac ischemia in the emergency department. Arch Intern Med 1997;157: 1085–1091.
58. Rydman RJ, Zalenski RJ, Roberts RR, et al. Patient satisfaction with an emergency department Chest pain observation unit. Ann Emerg Med 1997;29:109–115
59. Roberts RR, Zalenski RJ, Mensah EK, et al. Cost of an emergency department-based accelerated diagnostic protocol vs. hospitalization in patients with chest pain: a randomized controlled trial. JAMA 1997:278:1670–1676.
60. Mikhail MG, Smith FA, Gray M, Britton C, Frederiksen SM. Cost-effective of mandatory stress testing testing in chest pain center patients. Ann Emerg Med 1997;29:88–98.
61. Gomez MA, Anderson JL, Karagounis LA, Muhlestein JB, Mooers FB for the ROMIO Study Group. An emergency department-based protocol for rapidly ruling out myocardial ischemia reduces hospital time and expense: results of a randomized study (ROMIO). J Am Coll Cardiol 1996;28: 25–33.

62. Selker HP, Griffith JL, D'Agostino RB. A tool for judging coronary care unit admission appropriateness, valid for both real-time and retrospective use. A time-insensitive predictive instrument (TIPI) for acute cardiac ischemia: a multicenter study. Med Care 1991;29:610–627 [erratum 1992;30:188].

63. Selker HP, D'Agostino RB, Laks MM. A predictive instrument for acute ischemic heart disease to improve coronary care unit admission practices: a potential on-line tool in a computerized electrocardiograph. J Electrocardiol 1988;21:S11–S17.

64. Pozen MW, D'Agostino RB, Mitchell JB, et al. The usefulness of a predictive instrument to reduce inappropriate admissions to the coronary care unit. Ann Intern Med 1980;92:238–242.

65. Pozen MW, D'Agostino RB, Selker HP, Sytkowski PA, Hood WB Jr. A predictive instrument to improve coronary-care-unit admission practices in acute ischemic heart disease. Aprospective multicenter clinical trial. N Engl J Med 1984;310:1273–1278.

66. Cairns CB, Niemann JT, Selker HP, Laks MM. A computerized version of the time-insensitive predictive instrument. Use of the Q wave, ST segment, T wave and patient history in the diagnosis of acute myocardial infarction by the computerized ECG. J Electrocardiol 1992;24:S46–S49.

67. Aufderheide TP, Rowlandson I, Lawrence SW, Kuhn EM, Selker HP. Test of the acute cardiac ischemia time-insensitive predictive instrument (ACI-TIPI) for prehospital use. Ann Emerg Med 1996;27: 193–198.

68. Sarasin FP, Reymond JM, Griffith JL, et al. Impact of the acute cardiac ischemia time-insensitive predictive instrument (ACI-TIPI) on the speed of triage decision making for emergency department patients presenting with chest pain: a controlled clinical trial. J Gen Intern Med 1994;9:187–194.

69. Selker HP, Beshansky JR, Griffith JL, et al. Use of the acute cardiac ischemia time-insensitive predictive instrument (ACI-TIPI) to assist emergency department triage of patients with chest pain or other symptoms suggestive of acute cardiac ischemia: a multicenter controlled clinical trial. Ann Intern Med 1998;129:845–855.

70. Goldman L, Cook EF, Brand DA, et al. A computer protocol to predict myocardial infarction in emergency department patients with chest pain. N Engl J Med 1988;318:797–803.

71. Goldman L, Weinberg M, Weisberg M, et al. A computer-derived protocol to aid in the diagnosis of emergency room patients with acute chest pain. N Engl J Med 1982;307:588–596.

72. Lee TH, Pearson SD, Johnson PA, et al. Failure of information as an intervention to modify clinical management. A time-series trial in patients with acute chest pain. Ann Intern Med 1995;122:434–437.

73. Aase O, Jonsbu J, Liestfl K, Rollag A, Erikssen J. Decision support by computer analysis of selected case history variables in the emergency room among patients with acute chest pain. Eur Heart J 1993; 14:433–440.

74. Jonsbu J, Aase O, Rollag A, Liestol K, Erikssen J. Prospective evaluation of an EDB-based diagnostic program to be used in patients admitted to hospital with acute chest pain. Eur Heart J 1993;14: 441–446.

75. Tierney WM, Roth BJ, Psaty B, et al. Predictors of myocardial infarction in emergency room patients. Crit Care Med 1985;13:526–531.

76. Dilger J, Pietsch-Breitfeld B, Stein W, et al. Simple computer assisted diagnosis of acute myocardial infarction in patients with acute thoracic pain. Methods Inf Med 1992;31:263–267.

77. Baxt WG. Use of an artificial neural network for the diagnosis of myocardial infarction. Ann Intern Med 1991;115:843–888.

78. Baxt WG, Skora J. Prospective validation of artificial neural network trained to identify acute myocardial infarction. Lancet 1996;347:12–15.

79. Lee TH, Weisberg MC, Cook EF, Daley K, Brand DA, Goldman L. Evaluation of creatine kinase and creatine kinase-MB for diagnosing myocardial infarction. Clinical impact in the emergency room. Arch Intern Med 1987;147:115–121.

80. Viskin S, Heller K, Gheva D, et al. The importance of creatine kinase determination in identifying acute myocardial infarction among patients complaining of chest pain in an emergency room. Cardiology 1987;74:100–110.

81. Wu AHB, Gornet TG, Harker CC, Chen HL. Role of rapid immunoassays for urgent ("stat") determinations of creatine kinase isoenzyme MB. Clin Chem 1989;35:1752–1756.

82. Gibler WB, Lewis LM, Erb RE, et al. Early detection of acute myocardial infarction in patients presenting with chest pain and nondiagnostic ECGs: serial CK-MB sampling in the emergency department. Ann Emerg Med 1990;19:1359–1366 [erratum 1991;20:420].

83. Hedges JR, Gibler WB, Young GP, et al. Multicenter study of creatine kinase-MB use: effect on chest pain decision making. Acad Emerg Med 1996;3:7–15.

84. Vaidga HC. Myoglobin. Lab Med 1992;23:306–310.

85. Gibler WB, Gibler CD, Weinshenker E, et al. Myoglobin as an early indicator of acute myocardial infarction. Ann Emerg Med 1987;16:851–856.
86. Katus HA, Scheffold T, Remppis A, Zehlein J. Proteins of the troponin complex. Lab Med 1992;23: 311–317.
87. Adams JE III, Bodor GS, Davila-Roman VG, et al. Cardiac troponin I: a marker with high specificity for cardiac injury. Circulation 1993;88:101–106.
88. Katus HA, Remppis A, Nuemann FJ, et al. Diagnostic efficiency of troponin-T measurements in acute myocardial infarction. Circulation 1991;83:902–912.
89. Ohman EM, Armstrong PW, Christenson RH, et al. Cardiac troponin T levels for risk stratification in acute myocardial ischemia. GUSTO IIA Investigators. N Engl J Med 1996;335:1333–1341.
90. Antman EM, Tanasijevic MJ, Thompson B, et al. Cardiac-specific troponin I levels to predict the risk of mortality in patients with acute coronary syndromes. N Engl J Med 1996;335:1342–1349
91. Hamm CW, Goldmann BU, Heeschen C, Kreymann G, Berger J, Meinertz T. Emergency room triage of patients with acute chest pain by means of rapid testing for cardiac Troponin T or Troponin I. N Engl J Med 1997;337:1648–1653.
92. Hamm CW, Braunwald E. A classification of unstable angina revisited. Circulation 2000;102: 118–122.
93. Hauser G, Gangadharan V, Ramos R, Gordon S, Timmis GC. Sequence of mechanical, electrocardiographic and clinical effects of repeated coronary artery occlusion in human beings: echocardiographic observations during coronary angioplasty. J Am Coll Cardiol 1985;5:193–197.
94. Gardner CJ, Brown S, Hagen-Ansert S, et al. Guidelines for cardiac sonographer education: report of the American Society of Echocardiography Sonographer Education and Training Committee. J Am Soc Echocardiogr 1992;5:635–639.
95. Pearlman AS, Gardin JM, Martin RP, et al. Guidelines for optimal physician training in echocardiography. Recommendations of the American Society of Echocardiography Committee for Physician Training in Echocardiography. Am J Cardiol 1987;60:158–163.
96. Peels CH, Visser CA, Funke-Kupper AJ, Visser FC, Roos JP. Usefulness of two-dimensional echocardiography for immediate detection of myocardial ischemia in the emergency room. Am J Cardiol 1990;65: 687–691.
97. Sabia P, Afrookteh A, Touchstone DA, Keller MW, Esquivel L, Kaul S: Value of regional wall motion abnormality in the emergency room diagnosis of acute myocardial infarction: a prospective study using two-dimensional echocardiography. Circulation 1991;84(Suppl. I):I85–I92.
98. Kontos MC, Arrowood JA, Jesse RL, et al. Comparison between 2-dimensional echocardiography and myocardial perfusion imaging in the emergency department in patients with possible myocardial ischemia. Am Heart J 1998;136:724–733.
99. Ritchie JL, Bateman TM, Bonow RO, et al. Guidelines for clinical use of cardiac radionuclide imaging. A report of the American Heart Association/American College of Cardiology Task Force on Assessment of Diagnostic and Therapeutic Cardiovascular Procedures, Committee on Radionuclide Imaging, developed in collaboration with the American Society of Nuclear Cardiology. Circulation 1995;91: 1278–1303.
100. Zaret BL, Wackers FJ. Nuclear cardiology. N Engl J Med 1993;329:775–783,855–863.
101. Van Train KF, Garcia EV, Maddahi J, et al. Multicenter trial validation for quantitative analysis of same-day rest-stress technetium-99m-sestamibi myocardial tomograms. J Nucl Med 1994;35: 609–618.
102. Berman DS, Kiat HS, Van Train KF, Germano G, Maddahi J, Friedman JD. Myocardial perfusion imaging with technetium-99m-sestamibi: comparative analysis of available imaging protocols. J Nucl Med 1994;35:681–688.
103. Varetto T, Cantalupi D, Altieri A, Orlandi C. Emergency room technetium-99m sestamibi imaging to rule out acute myocardial ischemic events in patients with nondiagnostic electrocardiograms. J Am Coll Cardiol 1993;22:1804–1808.
104. Hilton TC, Thompson RC, Williams HJ, Saylors R, Fulmer H, Stowers SA. Technetium-99m sestamibi myocardial perfusion imaging in the emergency room evaluation of chest pain. J Am Coll Cardiol 1994;23:1016–1022.
105. Tatum JL, Jesse RL, Kontos MC, et al. Comprehensive strategy for the evaluation and triage of the chest pain patient. Ann Emerg Med 1997;29:116–125.

III | ST-Segment Elevation Myocardial Infarction

9 Thrombolytic Therapy

Jeffrey L. Anderson, MD and
James S. Zebrack, MD

CONTENTS

INTRODUCTION

Prevalence and Impact

At the beginning of the 21st century, cardiovascular (CV) disease remains the leading cause of death *(1)*. Over 12,400,000 Americans are living with clinical coronary heart disease (CHD), and this year, an estimated 1,100,000 Americans will have a fatal or nonfatal acute myocardial infarction (AMI). CV disease was responsible for 950,000 deaths in the United States in 1998, accounting for over 40% of all deaths, and CHD was the leading cause of cardiovascular death, claiming 460,000 lives. Half of CHD deaths (a quarter million/yr) are directly related to AMI. Death occurs suddenly, out-of-hospital, in 220,000 annually, and most of these deaths are triggered by coronary ischemia *(2–4)*. Indeed, at least one-half of AMI-related deaths occur within 1 h of onset of symptoms and before reaching a hospital emergency department *(5)*. Although CV mortality rates declined between 1980 and 1992 in men, they increased over the same

From: *Contemporary Cardiology: Management of Acute Coronary Syndromes, Second Edition*
Edited by: C. P. Cannon © Humana Press Inc., Totowa, NJ

period in women, and for the past 10 yr, they have failed to decline or have increased in men as well *(1)*. Thus, the impact of CV disease, and AMI specifically, continues to be great.

Over 5 million people visit U.S. emergency departments each year for evaluation of chest pain and related symptoms, and almost 1.5 million are hospitalized for an acute coronary syndrome (ACS) *(6,7)*. ACS patients on presentation are triaged into ST-elevation AMI and non-ST elevation AMI/unstable angina categories *(8,9)*. In 1990, ST-elevation AMI accounted for 55% of AMIs, whereas in 1999, it had declined to 37% *(10)*. The cause of this redistribution is uncertain, but it likely involves changes in patient demographics and preventive care.

Acute reperfusion (achieved by thrombolysis or coronary angioplasty) has marked a significant conceptual and practical advance for therapy of ST-segment elevation (STE)-AMI *(11)*. With broad application of reperfusion therapy, 30-d mortality rates from STE-AMI have progressively declined (from 20–30% to 5–10%) *(10,12,13)*.

History

It has now been almost a century since Herrick in the United States *(14)* and Obrastzow and Straschesko in the Soviet Union *(15)* described the clinical syndrome of acute coronary occlusion. Coronary thrombosis as a precipitating event was postulated. However, it was not until 1980 that coronary thrombosis, as the mechanism of abrupt coronary occlusion, was demonstrated. In a landmark study, DeWood and colleagues *(16)* performed coronary angiography in the early hours of AMI and found coronary occlusion to be present in 87% of patients studied within 4 h of symptom onset. The nature of the occlusion was shown to be thrombotic at emergency coronary bypass surgery.

A basis for early reperfusion therapy was laid by the late 1970s in classical studies by Reimer, Jennings, and colleagues *(17,18)*. In a canine model of coronary occlusion and reperfusion, myocardial cell death began within 15 min of occlusion and proceeded rapidly in a wave front from endocardium to epicardium. Myocardial salvage could be achieved by releasing the occlusion within a narrow time frame *(<3–6 h)*. The degree of salvage was inversely proportional to the duration of ischemia and occurred in a reverse wave front from epicardium to endocardium. The extent of necrosis could be modified by changing metabolic demands and varying collateral blood supply as well as the duration of occlusion.

Pathophysiologic Considerations

Improved understanding of pathophysiologic events leading to coronary thrombosis has been forthcoming over the past two decades. Pathologic, angiographic, and angioscopic observations have suggested the concept that erosion, fissuring, or rupture of a vulnerable atherosclerotic plaque is the initiating mechanism of coronary occlusion, resulting in coronary spasm, intraplaque hemorrhage, and occlusive luminal thrombosis *(19–23)*. Additional studies have suggested that plaque erosion or rupture most frequently occurs in lipid-laden plaques with the endothelial cap weakened by internal metalloproteinase activity derived primarily from macrophages *(24–26)*.

When the plaque ruptures, elements in the bloodstream are exposed to plaque matrix elements, including collagen and the intensely thrombogenic lipid core with its associated macrophage-derived tissue factor *(24)* (Fig. 1). The result is stimulation of platelet

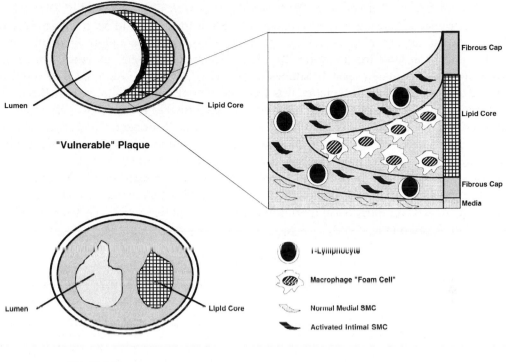

"Vulnerable" Plaque

"Stable" Plaque

Fig. 1. Schematic diagram showing comparison of the characteristics of "vulnerable" and "stable" plaques. Vulnerable plaques often have a well-preserved lumen because plaques grow outward initially. The vulnerable plaque typically has a substantial lipid core and a thin fibrous cap separating the thrombogenic materials such as macrophage-derived tissue factor from the blood. The nonspecific inflammatory process leads to recruitment and activation of macrophages and smooth muscle cells (SMCs), which release collagenases, degrading the protective cap. At sites of plaque rupture or erosions, increased concentration of inflammatory cells may be found, with active uptake of lipids to create foam cells. By contrast, stable plaque has a relatively thick fibrous cap protecting the often-smaller lipid core from contact with the blood. Adapted with permission from ref. *24.*

adhesion, activation, and aggregation; secretion of vasoconstrictive and thrombogenic mediators; thrombin generation; and fibrin formation, causing vasospasm and the formation of a platelet- and fibrin-rich thrombus. The result is reduction (non-STE-ACS) or interruption (STE-AMI) of coronary blood flow with rapid onset of myocardial cell dysfunction and death. These and other observations set the stage conceptually and scientifically for the evaluation of reperfusion therapies in clinical AMI.

DISCOVERY AND EARLY CLINICAL APPLICATION OF THROMBOLYTICS

Early Work

In 1933, Tillet and Garner *(27)* reported the discovery of a streptococcal fibrinolysin. They observed the ability of filtrates of streptococcal cultures to lyse human clots. Streptokinase (SK) was subsequently characterized as reviewed by Sherry *(28)*. SK was first successfully applied clinically for the liquefaction of a pleural clot, reported in 1949

(29). Use of SK in AMI began in 1954, and the first series was reported in 1958 *(30).* This experience suggested that intravenous (IV) SK infusions could be given safely and that treatment begun within 14 h of symptom onset could lead to a more favorable hospital course than later treatment (at 20–72 h), which resulted in outcomes similar to those of no treatment. At least 17 studies of IV SK in AMI were reported over the following two decades, but acceptance was limited by poor understanding of AMI pathophysiology and the role of SK and poor study design with treatment delays *(31–35).* The largest and most promising of these early studies was the European Cooperative Study Group report in 1979 *(31).* Among 315 AMI patients, 6-mo mortality was substantially lower in those receiving a 24-h infusion of SK than placebo (16 vs 31%, $p < 0.01$). Bleeding was observed more frequently with SK, but was mostly minor. An overview of the eight major early-era trials of IV SK of acceptable randomized design suggested a significant (20%) reduction in mortality among 3275 patients *(33).* This set the stage for further development.

Intracoronary Thrombolysis

Despite the promise of these early studies, the primary mechanism of benefit (coronary thrombolysis) was not clearly understood until angiographic demonstrations between 1976 and 1981 *(16,36–38).* These observations led to feasibility studies of clinical thrombolysis with intracoronary (IC) SK under angiographic monitoring *(39–41).* A high rate of coronary occlusion (>80%) was confirmed during the early hours of AMI, and the ability of SK to achieve early reperfusion with a success rate of approx 75% was demonstrated *(41).* Application was generally safe, and clinical outcomes were favorable. Based on these promising results, randomized studies of IC thrombolysis were undertaken.

Anderson et al. *(42)* first demonstrated in 1983 the beneficial potential of IC SK in the setting of AMI based on a randomized study–design. Fifty patients with AMI were enrolled within a mean of 2.7 h of symptom onset and were randomized to receive either standard coronary care or immediate catheterization with IC SK, begun an average of 4 h after symptom onset. In the intervention group, perfusion was achieved in 79% after a mean of 30 min of SK infusion. The intervention strategy was associated with statistically significant relief of ischemic discomfort (quantified by morphine requirement), prevention of heart failure (Killip class), and improvement in functional recovery by hospital discharge (measured by radionuclide left ventricular ejection fraction). Cardiac markers—creatine kinase (CK), CK-MB, lactate dehydrogenase (LDH), LDH-1—peaked earlier, STE resolved more rapidly, and Q wave development was more limited in the SK group. Echocardiographic wall motion score improved in the intervention group, and convalescent thallium perfusion studies showed a smaller defect (infarct) size with the reperfusion strategy. A smaller (n = 40) concurrently published randomized study treated patients later (at >6 h after symptom onset) and demonstrated relief of ischemic pain but found no improvement in global or regional myocardial function *(43).*

Randomized studies of intermediate size followed and suggested the potential for mortality benefit. The Western Washington Trial *(44)* randomized 250 patients with AMI to IC SK or standard therapy (IV nitroglycerin). Early reperfusion was documented in 69% of SK-treated patients vs 12% of controls ($p < 0.01$) at a mean of about 6.5 h after symptom onset. Ischemic pain was relieved in the SK group, but improvement in global and regional cardiac function was not shown. However, 30-d mortality was reduced: 3.7% in SK vs 11.2% in control patients ($p < 0.02$). Mortality after 1 yr also was lower with the reperfusion strategy (8.2 vs 14.7%), although the difference was no longer significant ($p = 0.1$) (45). However, within the SK group, mortality was only 2.5% among those achieving early reperfusion compared to 16.7% in those with partial or no reperfusion ($p < 0.01$). Mortality in the partial and/or no reperfusion SK group was similar to the untreated group. This observation provided the first clinical evidence that the mechanism of thrombolytic benefit is related to the achievement of early reperfusion.

Additional evidence for a survival benefit of IC SK came from a Dutch study of 533 patients (46). Interpretation of the study was complicated by the use of IV SK in the last 117 patients followed by angiography and additional IC SK if needed to achieve reperfusion. This evolving thrombolytic strategy was associated with reduced mortality at both 1 mo (5.9 vs 11.7%, $p < 0.03$) and 1 yr (8.6 vs 15.9%, $p < 0.001$).

IC urokinase (UK) also was tested in AMI and, along with SK, was approved for IC infusion to achieve recanalization in coronary artery thrombosis (41,47,48). Reperfusion rates similar to those reported for SK (range, 62–94%) were achieved by a wide range of infusion rates (2000–24,000 U/min) (41). A randomized comparison of IC UK (total average dose of 500,000 IU) and IC SK found the two drugs to produce comparable rates of recanalization (47). UK was associated with smaller reductions in circulating fibrinogen and a lower incidence of bleeding and allergic complications.

The positive results in these IC thrombolysis trials were counterbalanced by variable results in subsequent studies (49). In a meta-analysis of nine randomized trials of IC SK involving approx 1000 patients, Yusuf et al. (19) found an 18% overall mortality reduction, but the confidence intervals (CI) were wide (44% reduction to 19% increase), and the difference was not significant. The variability in results, the logistic difficulties, and the time delays inherent to IC SK administration (believed to be the cause of suboptimal outcomes) stimulated the reevaluation of IV SK as a more practical, universally applicable approach to thrombolytic therapy.

Intravenous Thrombolysis

Schröder et al. (50) tested a strategy of short-term (1 h), high-dose (0.5–1.5 million units [MU]) infusions of SK given to patients at an early time (within 12 h) of symptom onset. In their initial clinical trial, a baseline angiographic study was followed by a 0.5 MU SK infusion. After 1 h, occluded coronary arteries from 11 of 21 patients (52%) had opened, and total patency rate (adding those with initial subtotal occlusions) was 62%. In a subsequent study, 93 patients were treated with 1.5 MU over 1 h. Early angiography was not performed, but an 84% later patency rate (in the fourth wk) was shown. Serum CK-MB concentrations peaked early (within 10–12 h after therapy), consistent with the pattern seen with angiographically demonstrated recanalization, and myocardial salvage was suggested by improved function in the infarct zone. A successful recanalization pattern was more frequently observed for patients treated within 3 h than later. The safety profile of IV SK in these doses, including bleeding rates, was acceptable.

Several small to intermediate-sized randomized trials of IV vs IC SK followed these feasibility studies (35,51–54). These trials generally supported "equivalence" between the two routes of administration with little difference in coronary patency at 24 h and no significant difference in clinical outcome by route of administration.

The potential utility of IV SK in the modern era of investigation was further supported by a larger randomized trial (Intravenous Streptokinase in Acute Myocardial Infarction, $n = 1741$ patients), which observed an 11% mortality reduction with IV SK, from 7.1% to 6.3% *(55)*. This favorable trend did not achieve statistical significance, however.

In parallel with these, other studies investigated effects on ventricular function. An overview of results suggested functional improvement (myocardial salvage) when therapy was begun early (within 3 to 4 h). Results were inconsistent or negative for later therapy *(41)* as predicted by animal models *(17,18)*. In 12 studies, SK was begun within 4 h of symptom onset. An increase in infarct-zone ventricular function was observed in each study, and an increase in global function (ejection fraction) was noted in 9 of these studies *(41,56)*. By contrast, if therapy was begun more than 4 h after symptom onset (6 studies), regional wall motion rarely improved (in only one study) and global ejection fraction was unchanged *(41,56)*. When functional improvement occurred in patients given later therapy, it appeared to be based on collateral or residual antegrade blood flow and other factors slowing the rate of necrosis *(57,58)*. Consistent improvement in function was observed when reperfusion interventions occurred within 2 h *(58–60)*. Given the variability in functional response and the potential importance of other mechanisms (such as remodeling), the focus shifted to large mortality trials for the assessment of clinical thrombolytic benefit.

OVERVIEW OF THROMBOLYTIC AGENTS

General Mechanisms of Action

All of the so-called thrombolytic (more specifically, fibrinolytic) agents are either direct or indirect activators of plasminogen, a circulating fibrinolytic proenzyme *(61)*. Plasminogen is converted by plasminogen activators or activator complexes to plasmin, the active fibrinolytic enzyme form, by cleavage of the arginine 560–valine 561 bond. Plasmin has relatively broad proteolytic properties, degrading fibrin, fibrinogen, prothrombin, and factors V and VII. Plasminogen activator-induced fibrinolysis may then act to disrupt forming thrombus and lead to reperfusion.

Six thrombolytic agents have been approved and marketed for use in the United States, although UK is approved only for IC delivery. These agents differ in several properties, including structure, fibrin specificity, speed and duration of action, and antigenicity, as summarized in Table 1.

FDA-Approved Thrombolytics

STREPTOKINASE

The first fibrinolytic agent to be discovered and applied clinically, SK is a 415-amino acid protein of bacterial origin that shares homology with several serine proteinases *(62,63)* and is the prototype of an indirect-acting agent. As with other thrombolytics, SK induces fibrinolysis by activating the body's intrinsic fibrinolytic system (plasminogen–plasmin). On administration, SK rapidly combines with circulating plasminogen in an equimolar (1:1) ratio to form a SK-plasminogen activator complex. A catalytic site

Table 1

Characteristics of FDA Approved Intravenous Thrombolytic agents

	SK (streptokinase)	APSAC (anistreplase)	tPA (alteplase)	rPA (reteplase)	TNK-tPA (tenecteplase)
Dose	1.5 MU in 30–60 min	30 U in 5 min	100 mg in 90 min[a]	10 U + 10 U, 30 min apart	30–50 mg[b] over 5 s
Circulating half-life (min)	≅20	≅100	≅4	≅16	≅20
Antigenic	Yes	Yes	No	No	No
Allergic reactions	Yes	Yes	No	No	No
Systemic fibrinogen depletion	Severe	Severe	Mild-Moderate	Moderate	Minimal
ICH	≅0.4%	≅0.6%	≅0.7%	≅0.8%	≅0.7%
Patency (TIMI-2/3) rate, 90 min[c]	51%	≅70%	≅73–84%	≅83%	≅77–88%
Lives saved/100 treated	≅3[c]	≅3[d]	≅4[e]	≅4	≅4
Cost per dose (approx U.S. dollars)	300	1700	1800	2200	2200

[a]Accelerated tPA given as follows: 15 mg bolus, then 0.75 mg/kg over 30 min (maximum, 50 mg), then 0.50 mg/kg over 60 min (maximum 35 mg).
[b]TNK is dosed by weight (supplied in 5 mg/mL vials): <60 kg = 6 mL; 61–70 kg = 7 mL; 71–80 kg = 8 mL; 81–90 kg = 9 mL; >90 kg = 10 mL.
[c]Based on Granger et al. (94) and Bode et al. (74)
[d]Patients with STE or BBB, treated in <6 h.
[e]Based on the finding from the GUSTO trial that tPA saves 1 more additional life/100 treated than does SK.

on plasminogen in the activator complex is activated, leading to conversion of free circulating plasminogen in the region of the activator complex to plasmin. Similarly, the SK-plasminogen complex itself is autocatalytically cleaved to form SK-plasmin, but this form of the complex retains its activator activity. The in vivo half-life of the SK-plasminogen–plasmin activator complex is approx 23 min.

SK is antigenic and has little fibrin specificity, so that substantial systemic lytic effect occurs in clinically applied doses. The generation of circulating fibrinogen degradation products (FDPs) (which exert antiplatelet and antithrombotic effects) and the depletion of circulating fibrinogen and α-1-antiplasmin, along with other clotting factors, provide long-acting (up to 1 to 2 d) antithrombotic actions that far exceed the time-course of fibrinolytic effects. This may explain why the addition of IV heparin to SK and aspirin increases bleeding risk but provides little additional benefit.

UROKINASE

A native protein responsible for part of the proteolytic activity in human urine was first reported in 1861 and was shown to have specificity for fibrin (64,65). It was later established that renal parenchymal cells are responsible for UK production. Contemporary clinical formulations of UK have been obtained from human kidney cells grown in culture and are primarily of the low molecular weight form (33,000 Da), whereas that purified from human urine is of higher molecular weight (55,000 Da). The therapeutic efficacy of the two molecular species in clinical applications is very similar. UK, unlike SK, is a direct-acting proteolytic agent (trypsin-type serine proteinase). UK contains 410 amino acid residues in two polypeptide chains connected by a disulfide bridge.

UK activity is not found in the circulation under normal conditions. When present, UK directly converts plasminogen to plasmin through enzymatic cleavage at the L-arginine 560–valine 561 site (the identical site of attack of SK); no additional cofactors are required. A single bolus of UK is cleared from the circulation with a half-life of 14–16 min by degradation to inert metabolites in the liver. UK is nonantigenic.

For AMI, UK has been approved only for IC use in a dose of 6000 IU a minute for periods up to 2 h or until lysis of the coronary arterial thrombus is observed. Heparin therapy is recommended concurrently with UK. UK also has been tested by the iv route in doses of 2 to 3 MU (generally administered as a bolus plus a short-term infusion regimen). However, iv UK is less well studied than iv SK or tissue-type plasminogen activator (tPA), and its mortality benefits have been less well-established (66). Hence, tPA is generally used when a nonantigenic agent with less systemic-fibrinolytic activity than SK is desired.

Clinically, UK has been most frequently used in catheter-directed infusions to remove thrombus and restore patency in appropriately selected cases of venous, arterial, and graft thromboses, and intravenously for massive pulmonary embolism (64). Recently, however, UK has become unavailable in the U.S. market.

ANISTREPLASE

Anistreplase (anisoylated plasminogen streptokinase activator complex, or APSAC) was the first custom-designed biochemically modified fibrinolytic agent to be developed (67,68). It was designed to allow rapid delivery (a 2- to 5-min injection), rapid onset, more prolonged duration of action, and improved plasma stability and fibrin binding compared with SK. However in doses used clinically, it retains the antigenic and nonspecific systemic thrombolytic effects of SK.

APSAC is synthesized by complexing SK with lys-plasminogen and reversibly acylating the complex by reacting it with the anisoyl group of a special acylating agent, producing a molecule of 131,000-Da molecular weight. Placed in aqueous solution or plasma, APSAC deacylates by a simple ester hydrolysis reaction, a rate-limiting process that follows first-order kinetics. APSAC's fibrinolytic activity has a half-life of approx 105 min in plasma. The commonly used clinical dosage of 30 U of APSAC corresponds to approx 1.1 MU of SK.

TISSUE-TYPE PLASMINOGEN ACTIVATOR

tPA is the primary physiologic (intrinsic) plasminogen activator in the circulation (69). A two-subunit form can be generated by limited proteolytic cleavage. Both single and two-chain forms activate plasminogen with approx similar catalytic efficacy and biologic potency (70). tPA demonstrates partial fibrin selectivity in comparison to SK in that tPA generates greater plasmin and fibrinolytic activity locally, in the neighborhood of thrombus, than systemically. The result is relatively less plasminemia, fibrinogenolysis, and general (systemic) proteolysis than SK. tPA is subject to inhibition by a circulating plasminogen activator inhibitor (PAI-1), and its activity is rapidly cleared from the circulation with a half-life of <5 min (71). tPA is nonantigenic and, unlike SK, may be reutilized without concern about interference with activity by neutralizing antibodies (72). tPA is manufactured for clinical application using recombinant technology as alteplase (rtPA).

RECOMBINANT PLASMINOGEN ACTIVATOR

Reteplase (recombinant plasminogen activator, or rPA) became the first clinically available mutant (modified) form of native plasminogen activator (73–75). rPA is a deletion mutant of alteplase (rtPA) in which the finger, epidermal growth factor, and kringle-1 domains have been deleted. As a result of structural and biosynthetic modifications, rPA, compared to tPA, is nonglycosylated, smaller, and less fibrin-specific (with lower fibrin affinity and more readily reversible binding), but it has an extended half-life (13–18 min). The slower clearance allows rPA to be given in a double-bolus regimen (two boluses separated by 30 min) compared with the 90-min infusion for rtPA. Following the demonstration of a favorable (at least "equivalent") effect on clinical events in AMI compared to SK (73), rPA received market approval in the U.S. in 1997. An apparent advantage in establishment of early patency compared with tPA in a relatively small study (74) was not associated with a superior mortality outcome in a large (15,000 patients), randomized AMI trial, Global Utilization of Streptokinase and tPA for Occluded Coronary Arteries (GUSTO) III (75).

TENECTEPLASE

Tenecteplase (TNK-tPA) is a genetically engineered, triple-site substitution variant of tPA (76). At amino acid 103, threonine is replaced by asparagine, adding a glycosylation site; at site 117, asparagine is replaced by glutamine, removing a glycosylation site; and at a third site (296–299), four amino acids (lysine, histidine, arginine, and arginine) are replaced by four alanines. The first two changes decrease clearance rate (half-life of 20 min), allowing for single bolus dosing (77–79). The third change confers greater fibrin

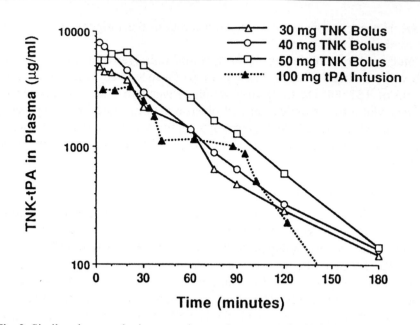

Fig. 2. Similar pharmacologic properties are demonstrated with bolus doses of TNK compared to the standard 90-min infusion of tPA. Adapted with permission from ref. *83.*

specificity *(77)* and resistance to PAI-1 *(77,80,81)*. Given these favorable properties, clinical testing of TNK-tPA was undertaken in the Thrombolysis in Myocardial Infarction (TIMI) 10A trial *(77)*. Doses tested ranged from 5 to 50 mg. TNK-tPA showed a slower plasma clearance rate, approximately one-third or less of that previously observed with tPA. The corresponding plasma half-life of elimination of TNK-tPA ranged from 11 to 20 min, compared to 3.5 min for tPA *(82)*. These results were replicated in the TIMI 10B trial *(78,83)*. After bolus TNK-tPA, plasma levels are maintained over time, so that the curve approximates that of the tPA bolus–infusion regimen (Fig. 2).

Selected Investigational Fibrinolytics

Prourokinase

In the early 1980s, a glycosylated, single chain form of UK-type plasminogen activator (scuPA) was isolated from human urine and cell culture media and characterized biochemically as a proenzyme form of the active two-chain urokinase (tcuPA). Prourokinase (proUK) was of interest in part because it appeared to be more fibrin-specific than UK. This effect is believed to be mediated by the preferential conversion of scuPA to active tcuPA at the fibrin surface *(11)*. The circulating half-life of natural and recombinant scuPA is 4 and 8 min, respectively, with predominant hepatic clearance *(84)*. A phase 2 study of glycosylated proUK produced in mouse hybridoma cells suggested promising coronary patency rates *(85)*, but further development for AMI has not been undertaken.

Saruplase

Saruplase is a recombinant nonglycosylated form of human proUK with less fibrin specificity and stability than glycosylated proUK *(11)*. Elimination is biphasic, with an initial half-life of 6–9 min. Administration has been by bolus (20 mg) plus infusion (60 mg/60 min). Saruplase has undergone comparative clinical studies with SK and tPA *(86–88)*. Saruplase achieves early (60–90 min) coronary patency rates greater than SK and similar to 3-h tPA infusions. Mortality rates were at least equivalent to SK but intracranial hemorrhage rates were greater. An application for clinical use was rejected by the European Medical Evaluation Agency (EMEA).

LANOTEPLASE

Lanoteplase (nPA) is a tPA mutant with deletions of the epidermal growth factor, the fibronectin finger domain, and the amino acid 117 glycosylation site *(11)*. The result is slower clearance (half-life, 37 min), allowing for bolus injection, but decreased fibrin specificity. In comparative studies with tPA, nPA achieved equivalent patency rates *(89)* and similar 30-d mortality rates *(90)*, but an increase in intracranial hemorrhage was observed (1.13 vs 0.62%). It is believed that the dosing strategy of both nPA and heparin may have contributed, but further development of nPA is uncertain.

STAPHYLOKINASE

Staphylokinase (SAK) is a single-chain, 136 amino-acid protein secreted by strains of *Staphylococcus aureus* and manufactured for clinical use by recombinant DNA technology *(91,92)*. The SAK–plasmin complex is fibrin selective, efficiently activating plasminogen while bound to fibrin at the thrombus surface. SAK has shown at least equivalent reperfusion potential and greater fibrin specificity than accelerated dose tPA in phase 2 studies. SAK is antigenic, inducing neutralizing antibodies within 1 wk. A peglyated form has been generated to increase half-life and allow for bolus dosing.

CLINICAL EFFICACY OF THROMBOLYTIC AGENTS
Coronary Recanalization and Patency Profiles

Based on theoretic considerations and clinical observations, it is believed that the establishment and maintenance of coronary perfusion is the major mechanism of thrombolytic benefit in AMI ("open artery hypothesis"). Given the difficulty in performing adequately sized mortality trials, angiographic studies have first been undertaken during development of thrombolytic regimens. These have assessed the recanalization (reperfusion) and patency profiles of the infarct-related coronary artery in response to thrombolytic therapy.

RECANALIZATION (REPERFUSION) VS PATENCY

The earliest series of studies assessed coronary patency at baseline and, for those initially showing total coronary occlusion, the ability of thrombolytic regimens to recanalize ("reperfuse") through the site of obstruction on subsequent angiography (generally at 60–90 min). Larger and more recent studies have omitted the baseline angiogram in favor of rapid administration of iv therapy and have compared coronary patency between regimens at 60–90 min and later. Because spontaneous (re)perfusion (grade 2 or 3 flow) has occurred in approx 15–20% of patients studied angiographically in the early (<4–6) h of AMI, coronary patency rates are generally higher than recanalization rates *(93,94)*. Although recanalization rates may be a better indicator of pharmacologic activity, patency rates may correlate better with patient outcome, are easier to obtain, and form the basis of the present discussion.

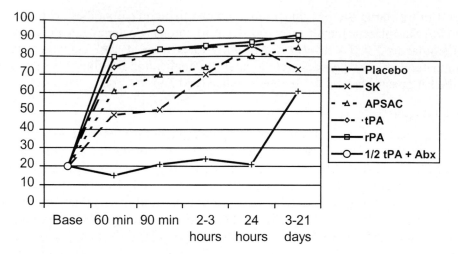

Fig. 3. Pooled angiographic patency rates (TIMI 2 + 3 flow) over time with no thrombolytic agent, SK, APSAC, tPA, rPA, TNK, and combination therapy of half-dose tPA and abciximab.

CORONARY PERFUSION (PATENCY) PROFILES

A pooled analysis of 58 studies ($n = 14,124$ angiographic observations) formed the basis for an overall profile of patency rates of several commonly used reperfusion regimens (Fig. 3) *(94)*. In the absence of thrombolytic therapy, spontaneous perfusion was observed early after STE-AMI in only 15–21% of patients at 60–90 min after study entry. No further increases were observed within the first day, but subsequent follow-up demonstrated gradually increasing patency rates (to about 60% by 3 wk) associated with spontaneous, aspirin, or heparin-facilitated intrinsic thrombolysis.

All thrombolytic regimens improved early patency rates although the speed of thrombolysis varied. SK (generally, 1.5 MU over 1 h) achieved the lowest patency rates at 60 and 90 min (48 and 51%, respectively). Intermediate and roughly similar rates of patency were achieved by APSAC and 3-h tPA infusions (about 60% at 60 min and 70% at 90 min). Accelerated (90 min) tPA bolus–infusion regimens achieved higher patency rates (74 and 84%, respectively). Patency profiles of newer tPA variants given by bolus injection have been similar to tPA. Combination therapy with reduced dose accelerated tPA (or bolus tPA variants) and abciximab (or another platelet glycoprotein IIb/IIIa inhibitor) has improved patency rates further, up to 91 and 94%, respectively *(79)*.

In contrast to the differing early patency profiles observed among various regimens, patency rates at 3–24 h and beyond have been found to be generally similar among standard thrombolytics, averaging 80–85% *(94)*. Reocclusion rates have been generally higher after fibrin-specific therapy (e.g., tPA) than after nonfibrin-specific (systemically active) agents (13 vs 8%, $p = 0.002$), especially in the absence of optimal concurrent IV heparin with fibrin-specific therapies.

The validity of these composite patency rates, generated from many studies of varying design and size, was confirmed by the single large GUSTO angiographic substudy *(95)*. This substudy, embedded within the much larger (41,021 patients) GUSTO mortality trial *(96)*, also enabled clear demonstration of the importance of early (90 min) TIMI grade 3 (complete) perfusion compared with TIMI grade 2 (incomplete) and lower grades (TIMI 0,1) as an accurate predictor of mortality outcomes. Specifically, the GUSTO Angiographic Study ($n = 2431$ patients) demonstrated a 90-min patency rate (TIMI grades 2/3) of 81% for accelerated-dose tPA and heparin, compared with 54% for SK and subcutaneous (sc) heparin ($p < 0.001$ vs tPA) and 60% for SK with iv heparin ($p < 0.001$ vs tPA). At 180 min, patency rates were the same in the four treatment groups and remained constant over 7 d of observation (range, 72–86%). Reocclusion rates in the study were similar among regimens (about 6%).

PATENCY/MORTALITY CORRELATIONS

The achievement of early complete TIMI grade 3 perfusion, recognized recently to be a better predictor of outcome, was specifically evaluated in GUSTO *(96)*. Rates of complete (grade 3) perfusion at 90 min were 54% with accelerated tPA, 29% with SK plus SC heparin, and 32% with SK plus iv heparin ($p < 0.001$ for comparison of SK groups with tPA). Differences in measures of left ventricular function and mortality paralleled differences in rates of patency at 90 min: ventricular function was best in those with normal (grade 3) flow irrespective of treatment. Likewise, mortality at 30 d was lowest among those with normal (TIMI 3) flow at 90 min (4.4%), highest (8.9%) among those with absent flow ($p = 0.009$), and intermediate in those with partial (TIMI 2) flow (7.4%). In a formal predictive model that was based on patency differences, the correlation between predicted and observed mortality rates was 0.97, providing strong evidence for the importance of early and complete infarct artery patency in determining mortality outcomes *(97)*.

Placebo or Nonthrombolytic Controlled Mortality Studies of Intravenous Thrombolytics

During the late 1980s, a few key placebo or nonthrombolytic controlled studies were performed that firmly established the basis for a survival benefit of iv thrombolysis *(49,98–100)*. These studies are summarized in Table 2 *(100)* and discussed below.

GRUPPO ITALIANO PER LO STUDIO DELLA STREPTOCHINASI NELL'INFARTO MYOCARDIO (GISSI)

The Italian GISSI study was the first adequately powered and designed mortality study in the modern era of thrombolysis to establish a survival benefit for iv fibrinolytic therapy *(101)*. GISSI enrolled 11,806 patients with presumed AMI within 12 h of symptom onset who had ST-segment deviation (elevation or depression) on electrocardiogram (ECG) and assigned them to receive 1.5 MU of iv SK over 1 h or standard therapy alone. Treatment was unblinded. The primary end point was 21-d mortality, which could be assessed in 11,712 patients. Aspirin was not routinely given, and heparin use was left to the physician's discretion. Most patients (about 90%) showed STE, and 94% were confirmed to have suffered AMI by discharge. Coronary angiography and coronary interventions were rarely used. Overall, a relative mortality risk reduction of 19% was observed ($p = 0.0002$). Survival benefit was time-dependent: relative risk reduction was not significant for treatment begun after 6 h, but it averaged 26% for therapy begun within 3 h ($p = 0.0005$) and, in an exploratory analysis, 51% ($p < 0.0001$) in a subgroup treated within 1 h of symptom onset. Other subgroup analyses demonstrated benefit specifically in patients with anterior infarction (relative risk [RR] = 0.75), with no

Table 2
Large Mortality Trials Comparing Standard Therapy with tPA or Streptokinase

End points	GISSI (101)[a]		ISIS-2 (103)[b]		ASSET (107)[c]	
Drug (n patients)	SK (5860)	Control (5852)	SK (8592)	Control (8595)	3-h tPA (2512)	Placebo (2493)
Death (%)	10.7	13.0	9.2	12.0	7.2	9.8
Reinfarction (%)	4.1	2.1	2.8	2.4	3.9	4.5
Any stroke (%)	0.2[d]	NR	0.7	0.8	1.1	1.0
Hemorrhagic stroke (%)	NR	NR	0.1	0	0.3	0.08
Major bleeds (%)	0.3[d]	NR	0.5	0.2	1.4	0.5

[a]End points measured at 21 d; included patients without STE.

[b]End points measured at 35 d; death = vascular mortality; included patients without STE. Study also included a factorial randomization to aspirin.

[c]Endpoints measured at 30 d; included patients without STE.

[d]Major bleeds and stroke attributed by investigator to SK. Nonfatal stroke at 6 mo was 0.7% in each group (102).

NR = not reported.

SK = Streptokinase.

previous MI (RR = 0.75), with Killip class I or II (RR = 0.80), and of age <65 yr (RR = 0.72). A trend also favored treatment in more elderly patients. Thus, GISSI, published in 1986, suggested that iv SK was safe and conferred a significant early survival benefit in AMI (at least among patients presenting within 6 h of symptom onset who generally had STE). Moreover, mortality benefits appeared to be maintained in the long term (102).

SECOND INTERNATIONAL STUDY OF INFARCT SURVIVAL (ISIS-2)

ISIS-2, an even more ambitious test of IV thrombolysis, followed in 1988 (103) and confirmed and extended the observations of GISSI. ISIS-2 used a 2-by-2 factorial design to assess the effects of iv SK (1.5 MU over 1 h), aspirin (162 mg/d on admission and daily for 1 mo), both, or neither in 17,187 patients entering 417 hospitals worldwide with suspected AMI within 24 h of symptom onset. The primary end point was vascular death at 5 wk. In the double placebo group, the mortality rate was 13.2%. The odds of dying were reduced by SK alone (by 25%, $p < 0.0001$) and also by aspirin alone (by 23%, $p < 0.0001$). Additive benefit occurred with the combination of SK and aspirin (42% odds reduction, $p < 0.00001$). When SK and aspirin were given early (within 4 h of symptom onset), a 53% odds reduction in mortality was achieved. Benefits were time-dependent, although less so than in GISSI. Subgroup analyses demonstrated lower mortality rates with thrombolytic therapy in the same subgroups shown to benefit in GISSI and, in addition, in those presenting with bundle-branch block (BBB), with inferior infarction, and at all ages (including those > 70 yr old). A notable exception was the group presenting with ST-segment depression. A small excess (0.1%) of confirmed cerebral hemorrhage was observed with SK, as were larger excesses in hypotension, presumed allergic reactions, and minor bleeds. Overall, therapy was regarded as safe, and IV SK was "established" in a broad group of patients with AMI. Importantly, ISIS-2 also established antiplatelet therapy with aspirin, given on admission and daily thereafter, as a routine part of AMI management.

APSAC INTERVENTION MORTALITY STUDY (AIMS)

Contemporary with ISIS-2 (1988), AIMS established a substantial survival benefit of IV APSAC in a multicenter trial from the United Kingdom (104,105). Patients under 70 with STE were entered within 6 h of AMI onset and randomized to APSAC (30 U) or placebo. The primary end points were 30-d and 1-yr mortality. Aspirin was not routinely used, but iv heparin was begun after 6 h. Patients were subsequently given warfarin for at least 3 mo. AIMS was stopped early because of efficacy. In the final analysis of 1258 patients, 30-d mortality was reduced from 12.1% in the placebo group to 6.4% in the APSAC group (odds reduction 51%, 95% CI: 26–67%, $p = 0.0006$) (105). After 1 yr, mortality reductions persisted (17.8% with placebo, 11.1% with APSAC, odds reduction 43%, CI: 21–59%, $p = 0.0007$) (105). All subgroups benefited.

The need for adjunctive IV heparin added to aspirin after APSAC was addressed by the first Duke University Clinical Cardiology Study (DUCCS-1) (106). DUCCS-1, of intermediate size, found no difference in clinical end points other than a higher rate of bleeding in AMI patients assigned to IV heparin compared with no heparin. Hence, current recommendations for heparin with APSAC follow those for its parent drug SK (9), derived from a larger experience including GUSTO-1 (95), which demonstrated no advantage of concomitant iv over sc heparin with SK.

ANGLO-SCANDINAVIAN STUDY OF EARLY THROMBOLYSIS (ASSET)

Shortly after ISIS-2, ASSET provided evidence of a survival benefit with rtPA (107). ASSET enrolled 5013 patients with suspected AMI (ECG confirmation not required) within 5 h of symptom onset and randomized them to double-blind therapy with rtPA, 100 mg over 3 h together with IV heparin, 5000 U, then 1000 U/h for 1 d, or placebo plus heparin. Aspirin was not routinely given. The primary end points were 1- and 6-mo mortality. Thirty-day mortality was significantly lower in the rtPA than the placebo group (7.2 vs 9.8%, relative risk reduction 26%, 95% CI: 11–39%, $p = 0.001$). Bleeding complication rates were higher with rtPA (1.4 vs 0.4% for major hemorrhage), but total stroke rates were similar (1.1 vs 1.0%).

LATE ASSESSMENT OF THROMBOLYTIC EFFICACY (LATE) STUDY

Earlier studies had conclusively demonstrated the benefit of IV thrombolytic therapy begun within 6 h of onset of symptoms. The LATE study aimed to assess the more controversial question of treatment effects of a randomized double-blind comparison of iv rtPA (100 mg over 3 h) with matching placebo in patients with symptoms of 6–24 h duration and ECG criteria consistent with AMI (108). A total of 5711 patients were entered and randomized to rtPA or placebo plus oral aspirin. iv heparin was recommended for 48 h. The primary end point, 35-d mortality, was reduced by 14.1% (95% CI: 0–28%). Mortality reductions occurred primarily in the prespecified patient group given treatment within 12 h of symptom onset (8.9 vs 12.0%, RR reduction 26%, CI: 6–45%, $p = 0.023$). The results of LATE suggested that the time window for thrombolysis (with rtPA) should be extended to at least 12 h from symptom onset for patients with AMI. An overview of "late" studies with SK also supported a survival benefit up to 12 h (109,110).

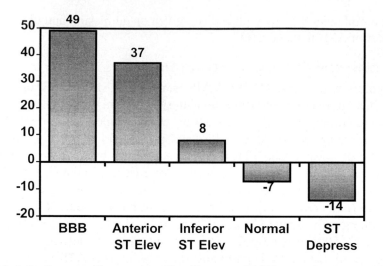

Fig. 4. Thrombolytic therapy effect on mortality (lives saved/1000 treated) as reported in the FTT Collaborative Group (using SK, APSAC, UK, and 3-h tPA), by admission ECG. Patients presenting with BBB and anterior segment elevation derived the most benefit from thrombolytic therapy. Patients with inferior STE derived much less benefit, whereas those with ST-segment depression or with normal or nonspecific ECG showed trends toward harm. Adapted from ref. *110.*

FIBRINOLYTIC THERAPY TRIALISTS' (FTT) COLLABORATIVE GROUP REPORT

By 1990, the benefit of IV thrombolytic therapy in appropriate AMI patients was regarded as established, ending the era of placebo (or nonthrombolytic)-controlled trials *(110,111)*. To maximize information gained from these trials, the FTT collaborative group pooled the nine major trials that had randomized 1000 or more patients *(110)*. The FTT database included 58,600 patients. Overall, an 18% reduction in 5-wk mortality (from 11.5 to 9.6%) was observed with fibrinolytic therapy, a highly significant result ($p < 0.0001$). Most patients (approx 45,000) presented with STE or BBB on ECG, and benefit was concentrated in these groups. Within the group with BBB on admission ECG, 49 lives were saved per 1000 patients treated. Within the STE group, greater benefit was observed in those with anterior (37 saved/1000) than with inferior STE only (8 saved/1000). Combined or other site STE showed intermediate benefit (27 saved/1000). No mortality benefit was observed for patients presenting with normal ECGs or ST depression; indeed, thrombolysis caused a slight adverse trend (7 and 14 more deaths/1000 treatments, respectively) (Fig. 4). The mortality reductions seen in the STE and BBB groups showed time dependence: absolute benefits declined from about 40 lives saved/1000 for treatment within the first h, to 20–30 for h 2–12, to 7 for h 13–24.

When other studies that evaluated very early therapy (i.e., emergency ward or paramedic-based) are included, even greater benefits are observed. Boersma et al. *(112)* reappraised very early therapy based on a database of 50,246 patients derived from all randomized trials of 100 or more patients published between 1983 and 1993. Overall, a nonlinear relation of treatment delay to benefit was observed (Fig. 5). These results clearly demonstrated a time dependency of benefit, particularly when large numbers of patients are treated within the first 1 or 2 "golden hours".

The FTT collaborative group analysis provides important information on therapy for patients over age 75, for whom relatively few data are available in single randomized

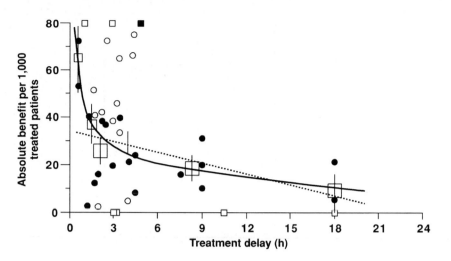

Fig. 5. Absolute reduction in 35-d mortality decreased as time-to-treatment increases. Small closed dots represent data from trials included in the FTT analysis, open dots represent information from additional trials, and small squares represent trials with absolute benefit >80 lives/1000 treated. The linear and nonlinear regression lines are fitted within these data and weighted by the inverse of the variance of the absolute benefit for each data point. The six black squares represent the average effect by time-to-treatment at six different time points (area of the squares are inversely proportional to the variance of the absolute benefit). Reproduced with permission from ref. *112*.

trials. For these patients, proportionate mortality reductions were less (the trend to benefit was not significant) although the absolute mortality reduction was still preserved.

Mortality reductions were little influenced by systolic blood pressure or heart rate except at their extremes. Hypotension (systolic blood pressure < 100 mmHg on presentation) was associated with greater AMI risk overall, but also with greater absolute mortality reductions with therapy (60 lives saved/1000 treated; $p < 0.001$). During persistent hypotension (cardiogenic shock), the effectiveness of thrombolytic therapy is unclear *(113)*. Intra-aortic balloon pumps are associated with lower mortality in the presence of thrombolytic therapy during cardiogenic shock *(114)*; however, emergent revascularization is preferred when available.

Benefits of thrombolytic therapy also were confirmed by FTT for other high-risk groups, including those with prior MI (absolute reduction of 1.6 vs 2.0% for those without prior MI) and diabetes (absolute reduction of 3.7 vs 1.5% for those without diabetes). The absolute benefit of thrombolytics in the currently era may be even greater, as the FTT data are derived primarily from SK, APSAC, and 3-h tPA infusions, which have been shown inferior to accelerated tPA, and these trials have included patients with ECG criteria now known to not benefit from thrombolytic therapy.

Comparative Trials of Thrombolytic Regimens

тPA Vs SK

There are three large mortality trials comparing tPA with SK. These trials are summarized in Table 3 and discussed below (115).

GISSI-2/International Study Group Trial. The GISSI-2/International Study was the first adequately powered mortality study to compare tPA with SK and also to explore the

Table 3
Comparative Mortality Trials of tPA vs SK or APSAC

End points	GISSI-2/ International (116,117)		ISIS-3 (118)[a]			GUSTO-1 (96)[a]		
Drug (n patients)	SK (10,396)	3h tPA (10,372)	SK (13,607)	3h tPA (13,569)	APSAC (13,599)	SK (20,173)	Accel. tPA (10,344)	SK/tPA (10,328)
Death (%)	8.5	8.9	10.6	10.3[a]	10.5	7.3	6.3[a]	7.0
Reinfarction (%)	3.0	2.6	3.5	2.9[a]	3.6	3.7	4.0	4.0
Any stroke (%)	0.9	1.3*	1.0	1.4[a]	1.3	1.3	1.6	1.7
Hemorrhagic stroke (%)	0.3	0.4	0.2	0.7[a]	0.6	0.5	0.7[a]	0.9
Non-CNS bleeds (%)	0.9	0.6[a]	4.5	5.2[a]	5.4	6.0	5.4[a]	6.1

[a]$p < 0.05$; statistical comparisons are only listed for SK vs tPA.

effect of sc heparin *(116,117)*. Patients with suspected AMI of <6 h duration (12,490 from the Italian GISSI-2 centers and 8,401 from the balance of the International Study centers; total 20,891) were randomly allocated to tPA (100 mg given over 3 h) or SK (1.5 MU over 30–60 min), given open-label (unblinded). In a factorial fashion, patients also were randomly allocated to sc heparin (12,500 U twice daily beginning 12 h after the start of thrombolytic therapy) or no heparin. Aspirin (325 mg/d) was given in all treatment groups. Early β-blockade was encouraged. The primary efficacy endpoint, in-hospital mortality, occurred in 8.5% of SK and 8.9% of tPA patients (RR 1.05, 95% CI: 0.96–1.16, $p = NS$) *(116)*. Mortality rates were 8.5% for the sc heparin and 8.9% for the no heparin group (RR 0.95, 95% CI: 0.86–1.04, $p = NS$). Definite hemorrhagic stroke was reported in 0.3% of the SK and 0.4% of the tPA group. A small excess of major bleeds was seen with sc heparin (1.0 vs 0.5%), but heparin did not affect the incidence of stroke or reinfarction. A combined in-hospital endpoint of death or severe left ventricular function, measured in the GISSI-2 cohort *(117)*, also did not differ by thrombolytic (SK 22.5%, tPA 23.1%).

Third International Study of Infarct Survival (ISIS-3). ISIS-3 was the second adequately powered mortality comparison between SK and tPA (given as duteplase) and between sc heparin and no heparin *(118)*. The thrombolytic APSAC also was evaluated. A total of 41,299 patients from 914 hospitals worldwide with a diagnosis of suspected AMI were entered within 24 h of the onset of symptoms (median 4 h) and randomly allocated to SK (1.5 MU infusion over 1 h), tPA (duteplase, 0.6 MU/kg infused over 4 h), or APSAC (30 U over 3 min). Aspirin (162 mg) was given on admission and daily. Patients also were allocated to sc heparin (12,500 IU), starting at 4 h and given twice daily for 7 d, or no heparin, in a second randomization. Study drug was administered in an open-label (unblinded) fashion. The primary end point, mortality at 35 d, occurred in a similar percentage of the three treatment groups (SK 10.6%, APSAC 10.5%, tPA 10.3%). Six-month mortality also showed no differences among thrombolytic regimens (SK 14.0%, APSAC 13.7%, tPA 14.1%).

The addition of sc heparin reduced mortality modestly during the first wk (7.4 vs 7.9%, $p = 0.06$), but the difference diminished by 35 d (10.3 vs 10.6%, $p − NS$), and 6-mo mortality was almost equivalent (0.1% difference) in each heparin group. Combining the heparin results of ISIS-3 and GISSI-2 strengthened the conclusion that a modest benefit occurred during wk 1 (avoidance of 5 deaths/1000 patients, $p < 0.01$) with loss of benefit during follow-up (5 wk, 6 mo). Duteplase was associated with fewer reports of allergy or hypotension but a higher rate of cerebral hemorrhage than the other regimens.

Unresolved Issues after GISSI-2 and ISIS-3. The failure to show a survival advantage of tPA over SK was surprising, given tPA's more rapid reperfusion profile *(93–95,110,120)*. In attempting to explain this paradox, several possibilities were raised *(121,122)*, including the following: heparin dosing was inadequate (sc instead of iv) *(123,124)*; tPA was not front-loaded *(94)*; treatment was begun too late to show differential salvage; and, STE on ECG to insure appropriate patient selection was not required. These concerns led to GUSTO *(96)*.

GUSTO. GUSTO tested the hypothesis that more aggressive thrombolytic strategies would produce earlier reperfusion and result in improved survival. Importantly, tPA was given as an accelerated regimen with iv heparin, and patients were enrolled early (within 6 h, mean 2.7) and were required to show STE on ECG. GUSTO randomized 41,021 patients from 15 countries to: (*i*) IV SK 1.5 MU/1 h with sc heparin; (*ii*) 1.5 MU SK with iv heparin, titrated to achieve an aPTT between 60 and 85 s; (*iii*) accelerated-dose tPA (15-mg bolus, 0.75 mg/kg up to 50 mg over 30 min, then 0.5 mg/kg to 35 mg over 60 min, for a maximum of 100 mg over 90 min) and iv heparin; or (*iv*) a combination of tPA 1 mg/kg and SK 1 MU, given concurrently over 60 min with iv heparin. The primary endpoint, 30-d mortality, was modestly but significantly lowered with accelerated tPA (6.3%), representing a 14% risk reduction ($p = 0.001$) compared with the SK strategies (7.3%). SK outcomes did not differ by heparin regimen. The combined strategy (tPA plus SK) gave an intermediate outcome.

The risk of hemorrhagic stroke was modestly higher with tPA (0.7%) than SK (0.5%). However, even after combining death with nonfatal disabling stroke, tPA continued to be favored (event rates 6.9 vs 7.8%, $p = 0.006$).

In an angiographic substudy embedded within GUSTO ($n = 2431$ patients), the patency rate (TIMI grades 2 + 3) of the infarct-related artery at 90 min was found to vary inversely with mortality rates in the overall study, being highest in the tPA plus heparin regimen (81%), intermediate with combined tPA and SK (73%), and lowest with SK with either iv (60%) or sc heparin (53%) *(95)*. Differences were accounted for by differences in complete (TIMI grade 3) reperfusion rates (54%, 38%, 32%, and 29%, respectively). Later patency rates tended to equalize among therapeutic strategies and were not predictive of mortality outcomes. A formal predictive model was developed for mortality assuming that thrombolytic therapy achieved its survival benefit through increasing coronary artery patency at 90 min *(97)*. The close match between predicted and observed 30-d mortality rates (correlation coefficient = 0.97) further supported the early achievement of complete perfusion as the major mechanism of survival benefit.

T-PA Vs APSAC

tPA-Eminase AMI Study (TEAM-3). The third Thrombolysis trial of Eminase in AMI (TEAM-3) compared APSAC (30 U/2–5 min) and tPA, given in a standard (3 h) infusion, in 325 AMI patients with symptoms of <4 h duration and electrocardiographic STE *(125)*. Coronary patency rates were high after both APSAC (89%) and tPA (86%; $p = 0.4$) (90-min patency rates were not measured), and clinical event rates were generally comparable although bleeding occurred more frequently after APSAC. However, the primary end point, left ventricular ejection fraction, was higher after tPA, both at discharge (54 vs 51%; $p = 0.04$) and at 1 mo (54 vs 50%; $p = 0.002$)

tPA-APSAC Patency Study (TAPS). This German angiographic study compared accelerated tPA with APSAC in 421 AMI patients *(126)*. Early patency rates were higher with tPA (73 vs 60% at 60 min; $p = 0.05$; 84 vs 70% at 90 min; $p = 0.0007$) including rates of complete (TIMI grade 3) perfusion (72 vs 54% at 90 min). By contrast, re-occlusion within 1 to 2 d occurred more frequently after tPA (10 vs 3%), and later patency rates did not differ between the regimens. Bleeding was more frequent after APSAC, given with aggressively dosed iv heparin. Mortality rates were lower with tPA, although the study was not powered for survival comparisons.

TIMI-4 Trial. TIMI-4 compared APSAC, front-loaded tPA, or combination thrombolytic therapy in 382 patients enrolled within 6 h of AMI onset with STE or new left bundle-branch block (LBBB) *(127)*. Double-blind therapy was with front-loaded tPA (up to 100 mg/90 min), APSAC (30 U/2–5 min), or a combination of tPA (up to 50 mg) and APSAC (20 U) with aspirin and iv heparin. Coronary patency rates were higher in tPA- than APSAC-treated patients, both at 60 (78 vs 60%; $p = 0.02$) and 90 min (84 vs

Table 4
Comparative Mortality Trials of tPA with Bolus Thrombolytics

End points	ASSENT-II (133)		GUSTO-III (75)		In-TIME-II (90)	
Drug (n patients)	tPA (8488)	TNK (8461)	tPA (4921)	rPA (10,138)	tPA (5022)	nPA[a] (10,038)
Death (%) at 30 d	6.15	6.18	7.24	7.47	6.61	6.75
Reinfarction (%)	3.8	4.1	4.2	4.2	5.5	5.0
Any stroke (%)	1.66	1.78	1.79	1.64	1.53	1.87
Hemorrhagic stroke (%)	0.94	0.93	0.87	0.91	0.64[b]	1.12[b]
Major bleed (%)	5.94[b]	4.66[b]	1.2	0.95	0.6	0.5

[a]TNK, tenecteplase; rPA, reteplase; nPA, lanoteplase.
[b]$p < 0.05$ for comparison.

73%, $p = 0.02$), including complete (grade 3) perfusion (60 vs 45% at 90 min, $p <$ 0.01). An "unsatisfactory outcome," the primary end point, occurred in 41% of tPA, 49% of APSAC ($p = 0.2$ vs tPA), and 54% of combination patients ($p = 0.06$). Mortality rates were lowest after tPA. Bleeding was more frequent in APSAC-containing regimens. TIMI-4 added to the GUSTO angiographic study (95) in supporting the early open-artery hypothesis of benefit and in favoring tPA over SK or APSAC.

COMPARATIVE TRIALS WITH NEWER BOLUS THROMBOLYTICS

Three bolus-administered mutants of tPA have been compared to wild-type tPA (rtPA) and (for rPA) to SK. Results of the three largest trials are summarized in Table 4.

RPA VS SK OR TPA

International Joint Efficacy Comparison of Thrombolytics Trial (INJECT). INJECT randomized 6010 AMI patients in double-blind fashion to reteplase (two 10-MU boluses given 30 min apart) or SK (1.5 MU over 1 h) (73). The 35-d primary mortality end point was reached by 9.0% of rPA and 9.5% of SK patients—a nonsignificant absolute reduction of 0.5% (95% CI: −1.98% to + 0.96%). Based on the premise that a new thrombolytic agent should achieve a mortality rate no worse than 1% more than a standard regimen (i.e., SK) with 95% confidence ("equivalence"), rPA was approved by the Food and Drug Administration (FDA) in 1996.

Reteplase Vs Alteplase Patency Investigation During AMI (RAPID-2). RAPID-2 compared rPA and its parent drug, tPA, in an angiographic patency study in 324 AMI patients (74). At the primary, 90-min end point, infarct-related artery patency was 83% with rPA vs 73% with tPA ($p = 0.03$), and respective TIMI grade 3 rates were 60 vs 45% ($p = 0.01$). However, very early patency rates (at 30 min) tended to favor tPA. On the basis of this favorable patency comparison, a mortality trial, GUSTO-III, was undertaken.

GUSTO-III. GUSTO-III, an international multicenter trial, tested whether rPA could reduce mortality compared with accelerated rtPA in 15,059 AMI patients presenting within 6 h of symptom onset with STE (75). Both therapies were given with aspirin (160 mg, then 160–325 mg daily) and IV heparin (5000 U, then 800–1000 U/h, adjusted to a target activated partial thromboplastin time (aPTT) of 50–70 s). The study had over 85% power to detect the expected >20% relative mortality reduction with rPA, based on patency differences observed in RAPID-2 *(74)*. However, mortality rates at 30 d did not differ: 7.50% for rPA compared with 7.28% for rtPA ($p = 0.64$, ratio 1.03, 95% CI: 0.91–1.18). The incidence of hemorrhagic stroke was similar for rPA and rtPA (0.93 vs 0.85%). Other outcomes also were similar. Thus, rPA is not superior in its survival benefits to tPA.

GUSTO-III emphasized the hazard of using a surrogate outcome (patency rates) to project small mortality differences. Earlier, a double-bolus regimen of tPA (50 mg + 50 mg administered 30 min apart) also was reported to yield an improved patency outcome compared with the accelerated tPA infusion regimen *(128)*, but a later study failed to show superiority and, in fact, was discontinued owing to increased bleeding *(129)*.

TNK-tPA Vs tPA

TNK-tPA, a fibrin-selective, single bolus fibrinolytic, was evaluated in the TIMI 10A dose finding and TIMI 10B and ASSENT-1 dose confirmation trials *(77,83,130)*. In these phase 1 and 2 studies, a clear dose-response was observed, both for coronary patency and hemorrhage (including intracerebral hemorrhage [ICH] for the 50-mg dose). With limitation and weight-adjustment of TNK-tPA dose and reduction and earlier down-titration of heparin dosing, satisfactory bleeding rates, and comparable TIMI 3 patency rates were demonstrated at 90 min compared with accelerated rtPA.

TIMI-10A. In this first clinical trial of TNK-tPA, ascending doses of 5–50 mg were tested *(77)*. Greater TIMI grade 3 flow rates at 90 min (57–64%) *(77)* and improved better myocardial perfusion *(131,132)* were achieved with 30–50 mg TNK-tPA than with lower doses. A longer half-life of TNK-tPA was confirmed.

Two phase II trials were conducted in the U.S. and Europe to evaluate efficacy (i.e., the rate of grade 3 flow at 90 min, TIMI-10B) *(83)* and safety (i.e., the rate of intracranial hemorrhage, ASSENT-I) *(130)*:

TIMI-10B. TIMI-10B randomized 886 AMI patients to receive either front-loaded tPA or a single 5–10 s TNK-tPA bolus of 30 or 50 mg *(77)*. The 50-mg dose was discontinued due to increased bleeding and replaced with a 40-mg dose. The 40-mg dose produced a similar rate of TIMI grade 3 flow at 90 min as tPA (63 vs 63%, $p = $ NS). TIMI grade 3 flow at 60 min (and 2 or 3 flow) and TIMI frame counts at 90 min also were similar for TNK-tPA and tPA. However, corrected TIMI frame count score improved (more rapid coronary flow) among patients who received higher "weight-corrected" doses (0.5 mg/kg and higher) of TNK-tPA *(132)*. Rates of ICH, initially a concern, decreased later in TIMI-10B and ASSENT-I after institution of a reduced dose heparin protocol *(83)*. This lower dose heparin regimen was selected for the phase-3 study (ASSENT-II). Rates of other serious bleeding (requiring transfusion) were lower with the more fibrin-selective TNK-tPA than tPA.

ASSENT-1. ASSENT-I randomized 3235 patients with AMI to 30, 40, or 50 mg TNK-tPA with the primary goal of determining the rates of intracranial hemorrhage to assist in choosing the most appropriate dose for phase 3 testing *(130)*. Given concerns in TIMI-10B, the 50-mg dose was discontinued early on and replaced by 40 mg, and heparin doses were reduced. ICH occurred in 0.77% of patients overall: 0.94% in the 30 mg arm and 0.62% in the 40 mg arm. Death, death or nonfatal stroke, and severe bleeding complications occurred in a low proportion of patients in all groups. Given the acceptable safety for ICH of TNK-tPA 30–40 mg, given with lower-dose heparin, phase 3 testing was undertaken.

ASSENT-II. The double-blind phase-3 Assessment of the Safety and Efficacy of a New Thrombolytic-2 (ASSENT-II) study was a randomized mortality equivalence trial that compared weight adjusted TNK-tPA (as a bolus over 5–10 s) with accelerated rtPA *(133)*. All patients received aspirin and lower dose heparin. ASSENT-II enrolled 16,950 patients worldwide who presented within 6 h of AMI onset. TNK-tPA dose (range, 30–50 mg) was based on weight adjustment and approximated (in 5-mg increments) 0.53 mg/kg.

The 30-d mortality end point was essentially identical for TNK-tPA (6.17%) and tPA (6.15%) and fulfilled the definition of "equivalence", with a relative risk of 1.00 (90% CI: 0.91–1.10, p for equivalence = 0.028). Only one subgroup stood out: for those treated >4 h after the onset of pain, an apparent survival advantage for TNK-tPA was observed (7.0 vs 9.2% mortality). This result was postulated to relate to TNK-tPA's greater fibrin specificity, in keeping with trends observed in earlier trials *(75,96)*. (It is known that clots become more resistant to fibrinolysis the longer they mature; greater fibrin specificity may enhance a thrombolytic's ability to lyse these older, fibrin-rich clots.)

Relative safety also was favorable in ASSENT-II *(133)*. ICH rates were virtually identical for TNK-tPA and tPA (0.93 vs 0.94%). Total stroke rates also were similar (1.78 vs 1.66%). Reassuringly, ICH rates were lower (not higher) for TNK-tPA vs tPA in the high risk group of low-weight, elderly women. Further, overall major noncerebral bleeding rates were significantly lower with TNK-tPA (4.7 vs 5.9%, p = 0.0002) as were transfusion rates (4.3 vs 5.5%, p = 0.0002) and total bleeding rates. These results may be a consequence of greater fibrin specificity for TNK-tPA and weight adjustment.

Thus, convenience and safety but not mortality advantages were shown to argue for TNK-tPA's utility as an alternative to tPA.

LANOTEPLASE VS TPA

Lanoteplase (nPA), a longer-acting tPA variant, was studied in doses of 15–120 kU/kg in the phase 2 angiographic trial Intravenous nPA for Treating Infarcting Myocardium Early (InTIME) *(89)*. A dose response for 60-min TIMI-3 patency was observed over the three lowest doses but not between 60 and 120 kU/kg, and neither of these doses was superior to rtPA. A subsequent double-blind mortality equivalence trial, InTIME-2, selected the 120 kU/kg dose and randomized 15,078 STE-AMI patients presenting within 6 h to nPA or tPA (2:1 ratio) *(90)*. Although 30-d mortality rates were similar (nPA = 6.77%, tPA = 6.60%), a significantly higher ICH rate occurred in the nPA group (1.13 vs 0.62%). As concerns developed about excessive ICH rates during InTIME-2, heparin down-titration was undertaken earlier (at 3 h) if PTT exceeded 70 s. Reductions in ICH after both nPA and tPA ensued. In an extension study (InTIME-2B, n = 1491), the heparin bolus was omitted, and heparin was initiated with an infusion of 15 U/kg/h (1000 U/h maximum). ICH rates declined further for nPA to 0.87%. These observations have impacted heparin recommendations generally when heparin is given with thrombolytics.

Thus, none of the newer fibrinolytic regimens has surpassed accelerated tPA for survival outcomes. However, the ease of administration of TNK-tPA, together with its reduced transfusion requirements, is likely to lead to its rapid acceptance into clinical use. Lower rates of dosing errors with bolus fibrinolytics such as TNK also may contribute to superior clinical outcomes *(134)*.

Combinations of Thrombolytics with Platelet Glycoprotein IIB/IIIA Inhibitors and New Antithrombins

With the failure of new thrombolytic monotherapies to improve early coronary patency and clinical outcomes compared with tPA, interest has shifted toward combination pharmacotherapies *(135)*. Theoretical arguments have been made for combining fibrinolytics with augmented antiplatelet therapies *(136)*. The platelet membrane glycoprotein (GP) IIb/IIIa, a specific fibrinogen receptor, is the final common pathway in platelet activation and an attractive therapeutic target. Antibodies, peptides, and small molecules have been developed that block the platelet GP IIb/IIIa receptor. These have potent platelet anti-aggregatory effects and have demonstrated efficacy in the setting of non-STE ACS and coronary angioplasty *(137–140)*. In STE-AMI, their utility as adjunctive therapy for patients undergoing direct percutaneous transluminal coronary angioplasty (PTCA) with stenting recently has been shown *(141)*. Given the critical role of platelets in coronary arterial thrombosis, the combination of a fibrinolytic with a GP IIb/IIIa inhibitor has substantial appeal as an approach to improving pharmacologic reperfusion. Results of the two large mortality trials of combination therapy are summarized in Table 5.

TIMI-14

Abciximab, a monoclonal chimeric antibody against GP IIb/IIIa, was tested as conjunctive therapy with lower doses of tPA in the TIMI-14 dose-ranging angiographic trial *(79)*. The combination of half-dose tPA and full-dose abciximab (with reduced doses of heparin) compared with tPA monotherapy produced impressive increments in TIMI-3 flow rates at 60 min (72 vs 43%, $p = 0.0009$) and 90 min (77 vs 62%, $p = 0.01$) with similar bleeding rates. TIMI 2/3 was achieved in an even higher percentage (up to 91–94%).

SPEED

Another angiographic study, Strategies for Patency Enhancement in the Emergency Department (SPEED) tested rPA with abciximab (vs rPA alone) in 2 phases *(140)*. The best combination in phase A (half-dose rPA—5U + 5U 30 min apart—with full dose abciximab) was re-evaluated in phase B with two heparin bolus doses (40 or 60 U/kg). Improved TIMI-3 flow rates were observed with combination therapy, 54 vs 47%, although differences were not significant. Higher rates of bleeding (9.8 vs 3.7%) were observed with combination therapy. SPEED piloted the GUSTO-V AMI outcomes trial.

HART-II

An argument also has been made for substituting an antithrombin more effective than heparin in combination with a fibrinolytic. Low molecular weight heparins (LMWHs) have theoretical advantages over unfractionated heparin *(142)*. Unlike unfractionated heparin, LMWHs interact less with elements in the circulation (plasma proteins, platelets, leukocytes, endothelial cells), have more predictable kinetics, are effective inhibitors of thrombin generation (antifactor Xa activity) as well as thrombin generation (anti-IIa activity), are given in fixed doses without the requirement for monitoring, and have compared well with heparin in clinical trials *(143)*.

The HART II trial was an angiographic trial of 400 patients with AMI given aspirin and accelerated tPA randomized to weight adjusted heparin or enoxaparin 30 mg IV then 1 mg/kg sc at 15 min and every 12 h *(144)*. Coronary patency was greater with enoxaparin than heparin (80 vs 75%), and reocclusion rates were lower (6 vs 10%) without excessive bleeding.

Table 5
Mortality Trials with Combined Thrombolytic and GP IIb/IIIa Inhibitor Therapy

Endpoints	GUSTO-V AMI (145)		ASSENT-3 (146)		
Drug (n patients)	rPA (8260)	1/2 rPA + abciximab (8328)	TNK/heparin (2038)	TNK/enoxaparin (2040)	1/2 TNK + abciximab (2017)
Death at 30 d (%)	6.2	5.9	6.0	5.4	6.6
Reinfarction (%)	3.5	2.3	4.2[d]	2.7[d]	2.2[d]
Any stroke (%)	0.9	1.0	1.5	1.6	1.5
Hemorrhagic stroke (%)	0.6[a]	0.6[b]	0.93	0.88	0.94
Major bleed (%)	2.3[c]	4.6[c]	2.2	3.0	4.3

[a]ICH rate for patients >75 = 1.1%.
[b]ICH rate for patients >75 = 2.1%.
[c]Severe and moderate bleeding combined.
[d]In-hospital events.

Similarly, hirudin, a direct acting antithrombin, and its analogues (e.g., bivalirudin) have been advocated for adjunctive therapy in place of heparin (see below).

GUSTO-V AMI

GUSTO-V AMI was an unblinded mortality study in 16,588 patients with STE-AMI enrolled within 6 h and randomized to standard rPA (10 U + 10 U) or half-dose rPA (5 U + 5 U) plus full-dose abciximab *(145)*. The primary hypothesis, that 30-d mortality rate with combination therapy would be less than with standard thrombolytic therapy, was not confirmed (5.6 vs 5.9%, respectively, $p = 0.43$) although the criterion for non-inferiority was reached. However, of 16 prespecified in-hospital adverse AMI-related outcomes, 14 occurred less frequently with combination therapy. Combined death or nonfatal reinfarction rates (RR, 0.83, $p = 0.001$), nonfatal MI alone ($p < 0.0001$), recurrent ischemia ($p = 0.004$), urgent coronary intervention (RR, 0.64, $p < 0.0001$), ventricular tachycardia or fibrillation, high-grade AV block, and total complications (28.5 vs 31.7%, $p < 0.0001$) were each significantly reduced.

On the other hand, spontaneous bleeding rates and transfusion requirements were increased up to 2-fold with combination therapy ($p < 0.0001$). Moreover, there was a significant ($p = 0.03$) adverse treatment interaction by age for ICH. ICH occurred in 2.1 vs 1.1% for combined vs standard therapy for age >75, whereas the rates were 0.4 vs 0.5%, respectively, for age ≤75 (Fig. 6). *GUSTO-V AMI* was interpreted as validating an alternative reperfusion strategy for patients ≤75 yr old. However, the lack of incremental mortality benefit and the increased bleeding risks were disappointing. Younger patients at higher AMI risk (anterior AMI) arguably might be considered for the GUSTO-V AMI combination regimen although ASSENT-3 suggests another alternative (below).

ASSENT-3

ASSENT-3 was a randomized but unblinded trial of 6095 patients with STE-AMI who were enrolled within 6 h of AMI onset and assigned to one of three regimens: (*i*) TNK-tPA and unfractionated heparin (both weight adjusted); (*ii*) TNK-tPA with the LMWH enoxaparin; or (*iii*) half-dose TNK-tPA with heparin and full-dose abciximab *(146)*. Enoxaparin was given as a 30 mg iv bolus and 1 mg/kg sc repeated every 12 h until hospital discharge or for 7 d. The first two SC doses could not exceed 100 mg. Unfractionated heparin was dosed according to American College of Cardiology/American Heart Association (ACC/AHA) guidelines *(9)*: 60 U/kg bolus (maximum, 4000 U) and 12 U/kg/h initial infusion (maximum, 1000 U/h), adjusted after 3 h to an aPTT of 50–70 s. With abciximab co-therapy, the heparin dose was further reduced to a 40 mg/kg bolus (maximum 3000 U) followed by a 7 U/kg per h initial infusion (maximum, 800 U/h).

The primary efficacy endpoint of ASSENT-3 was the composite of 30-d mortality and in-hospital reinfarction or refractory ischemia. The primary efficacy plus safety endpoint was the efficacy endpoint plus in-hospital ICH or other major bleeding. The efficacy endpoint was significantly lower in both the enoxaparin (11.4%, $p = 0.0002$) and the abciximab co-therapy groups (11.1%, $p < 0.0001$) than the TNK-tPA/heparin group (15.4%) *(146)*. The efficacy plus safety endpoint also was significantly lower with adjunctive enoxaparin (13.7%, $p < 0.004$) and conjunctive abciximab (14.2%, $p = 0.014$) than with unfractionated heparin (17.0%) (Fig. 7), although the advantage of combination therapy was not seen in the elderly. A lesser need for urgent coronary interventions was observed with the two experimental therapies.

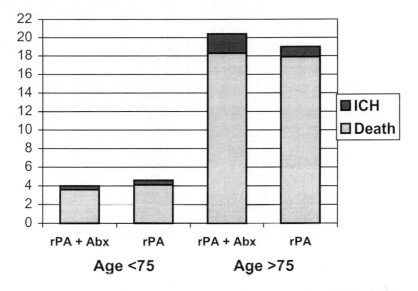

Fig. 6. Percent risk of death or ICH for full dose rPA or half-dose rPA plus abciximab (rPA + Abx) in the GUSTO-V trial. Data from ref. *145*.

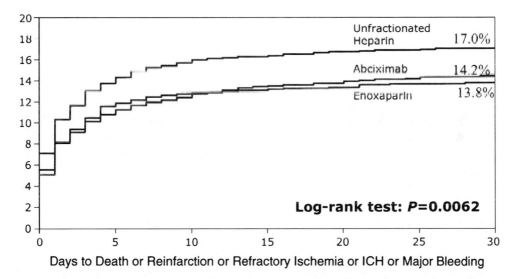

Fig. 7. Kaplan-Meier 30-d survival curves for the end point of death, in-hospital reinfarction, refractory ischemia, or major bleeding from the ASSENT-3 trial. Reproduced with permission from ref *146*.

Despite the positive composite efficacy result with combination abciximab, there was no mortality benefit (6.6 vs 6.0% for TNK-tPA/heparin control). Moreover, significant adverse interactions of treatment with age (RR = 1.30 for >75 yr vs 0.74 for ≤75, p = 0.001) and diabetes (RR = 1.35 with vs 0.74 without diabetes, p = 0.0007) were observed for the efficacy plus safety end point (Fig. 8). More major bleeding complications, transfusions, and thrombocytopenia occurred in the abciximab group (all $p <$ 0.001), and the rates were three times higher in those older than 75 yr.

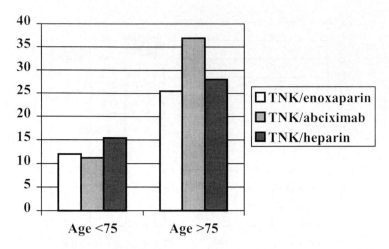

Fig. 8. Thirty-day end point of death, in-hospital reinfarction, refractory ischemia, or major bleeding by age for combination vs control thrombolytic (TNK-tPA) regimens in ASSENT-3. Data from ref. *146.*

In contrast, enoxaparin increased bleeding rates only slightly, and no treatment interactions were seen. Taking into account efficacy and safety, TNK-tPA with adjunctive enoxaparin emerged as the best overall therapy. Ease of administration and lack of need for monitoring advantaged enoxaparin over heparin, and greater safety in the elderly and diabetics distinguished it from the abciximab combination.

ENTIRE: A TEST OF THREE-WAY COMBINATIONS

A combination of half-dose thrombolytic, GP IIb/IIIa inhibition and enoxaparin was studied in ENTIRE-TIMI 23 (Enoxaparin and TNK-tPA with or without GP IIb/IIIa Inhibitor as Reperfusion strategy in STE MI). Preliminary results were presented at the 2001 European Society of Cardiology meetings. A total of 461 patients were enrolled. Patients tended to have higher rates of ST-segment resolution with enoxaparin vs heparin and with combination therapy vs TNK-tPA alone. Rates of major hemorrhage were higher with TNK-tPA combinations. However, bleeding rates trended lower if enoxaparin was used instead of heparin (5.6 vs 7.8%). Although the study was not powered to detect efficacy, the 30-d rates of MI or death were reduced in the enoxaparin groups (14.9% with TNK-tPA/heparin vs 4.4% with TNK-tPA/enoxaparin and 6.2% with half-dose TNK-tPA/abciximab/heparin vs 4.8% with half-dose TNK-tPA/abciximab/enoxaparin).

HERO-2

GUSTO-2B and TIMI-9B trials showed that the direct-acting thrombin inhibitor hirudin was slightly, but not significantly, superior to the less expensive heparin *(147,148).* Hirudin was not developed further for this indication. Recently, a comparison was reported of the less expensive direct thrombin inhibitor bivalirudin (previously, hirulog) to iv heparin as an adjunct to SK in the randomized study, HERO-2, performed in 17,073 AMI patients in 46 countries *(149).* Mortality, the primary end point, was not reduced by bivalirudin compared to heparin (10.8 vs 10.9%) despite reduction in non-fatal reinfarction (2.8 vs 3.6%, $p = 0.004$). Bleeding rates were similar or slightly higher

Table 6
Absolute and Relative Contraindications to Thrombolytic Therapy

Contraindications, absolute:
   Active bleeding or bleeding diathesis.
   Prior hemorrhagic stroke.
   Intracranial or spinal cord tumor.
   Suspected or known aortic dissection.
Contraindications, relative:
   Severe, uncontrolled hypertension (>180/110 mm Hg).
   Anticoagulation with elevated INR.
   Prior ischemic stroke.
   Recent major trauma/surgery.
   Pregnancy.
   Recent noncompressible vascular punctures.
   Recent retinal laser therapy.
   Cardiogenic shock when revascularization is available.

with bivalirudin. Thus, the value of hirudin analogues as adjuncts to fibrinolytics, instead of heparin, continues to be uncertain.

COMBINATION REGIMENS: A SUMMARY

Based on these recent trials of combination therapies, combined enoxaparin and TNK-tPA appears to be the most attractive alternative pharmacological reperfusion strategy at this writing and deserves further study. The role of combined GP IIb/IIIa and thrombolytic therapy, in contrast, is less certain after GUSTO-V and ASSENT-3. Combining GP IIb/IIIa inhibitors with SK has been abandoned because of excessive bleeding rates. Further studies should be limited to younger patients at lower risk of bleeding and high risk of AMI-related complications, and these might include those likely to undergo early percutaneous coronary intervention (PCI). Whether shorter-acting GP IIb/IIIa inhibitors (such as eptifibatide or tirofiban) and further reductions in adjunctive heparin doses can improve the benefit–risk ratio of combination regimens with thrombolytics must await ongoing and future studies.

BLEEDING AND OTHER ADVERSE RISKS OF THROMBOLYTIC THERAPY

Bleeding

Bleeding is the major risk associated with thrombolytic therapy. Absolute and relative bleeding contraindications to thrombolytic therapy are given in Table 6. Fortunately, bleeding is usually manageable with conservative measures, only occasionally requires transfusion, and most frequently (70% of cases) occurs at sites of vascular puncture. In ISIS-3 *(118)*, which did not require angiography, noncerebral bleeding was reported in 4.5% of patients after SK, 5.4% after APSAC, and 5.2% after tPA; hemorrhage required transfusion or was otherwise defined as "major" in only 0.9, 1.0, and 0.8% of patients, respectively. In the FTT overview experience of about 60,000 patients *(110)*, a major bleeding event occurred in 1.1% after thrombolytic therapy compared with 0.4% after control, a small but significant difference ($p < 0.00001$).

Life-threatening internal hemorrhage may occur after thrombolytic therapy, of which ICH is the most important. The fatality rate with ICH is approx 60% (range 44–75%) *(110,150–153)*, and disability is common among survivors. The risk of ICH in clinical trials has averaged about 0.5–1.0% but varies with patient characteristics, particularly advancing age, as well as the specific dose and type of the thrombolytic agent and adjunctive antithrombotic therapies *(150–156)*. Downward adjustment of heparin doses in recent trials has helped to avoid excessive ICH risk with tPA variants *(90,133)*. Increases in ICH associated with thrombolysis are in part offset by decreases in ischemic stroke.

The FTT meta-analysis suggested that for every 1000 patients treated with fibrinolytic agents, therapy causes 7 major noncerebral hemorrhages and 2 nonfatal, noncerebral hemorrhages while preventing 18 deaths by 35 d *(110)*. ISIS-3 compared various older thrombolytic regimens and reported ICH rates of 0.2% for SK, 0.55% for APSAC, and 0.66% for tPA (duteplase) *(118)*. Respective total stroke rates were 1.04, 1.26, and 1.39% (slightly but significantly greater with tPA than SK). In the subsequent GUSTO study *(96)*, rates of ICH were 0.54% with SK and 0.72% with accelerated tPA (alteplase), each with IV heparin. Respective total stroke rates were 1.40 and 1.55%. In a comparison of rPA and tPA, ICH rates were 0.93 and 0.87%, respectively, and total stroke rates 1.68 and 1.81% (p = NS) *(75)*. Similar ICH rates also were found in the phase-3 comparison of TNK-tPA and tPA (0.93 vs 0.94%) *(133)*.

Unacceptable increases in ICH and other bleeding risks have been observed with aggressive adjuvant antithrombotic regimens given together with thrombolytics. Indeed, the GUSTO-IIA, TIMI-9A, and r-Hirudin for Improvement of Thrombolysis (HIT)-III trials *(157–159)* were stopped prematurely and reconfigured because of excessive rates of hemorrhage, including ICH. In the subsequent trials (GUSTO-IIB, TIMI-9B), hemorrhage rates decreased to an expected and acceptable range *(147,148)*. Downward adjustments of heparin dosing were made prior to ASSENT-II (with TNK-tPA) and InTIME-2 (with lanoteplase), as noted above *(90,133,148)*.

In an effort to build a predictive model for ICH, Simoons et al. *(155)* collected information from five clinical study sources providing information on 150 patients with documented ICH after thrombolytic therapy. These were compared with 294 matched controls. A multivariate analysis identified four independent predictors for ICH: age >65 yr (OR: 2.2, CI: 1.4–3.5), weight <70 kg (OR: 2.1, CI: 1.3–3.2), hypertension on admission (OR: 2.0, CI: 1.2–3.2), and use of tPA (alteplase) compared with SK (OR: 1.6, CI: 1.0–2.5). Assuming an overall incidence of ICH of 0.75%, the model predicted incidences of ICH of 0.26, 0.96, 1.32, and 2.17% for those with no, one, two, or three risk factors, respectively. For patients over 75 yr, the risk was predicted to be 1.5% with no other risk factors, climbing to 3.3% with the other two risk factors. Comparing the expected benefits of thrombolytic therapy with these predicted risks may allow the physician to individualize the selection of therapy, which might include a less aggressive thrombolytic or antithrombotic regimen or a primary PCI in those at high risk for ICH.

Allergy, Hypotension, Fever

SK and APSAC are antigenic and potentially allergenic although serious anaphylaxis and bronchoconstriction are rare (incidence <0.2–0.5%) *(96,103,104,110,118,160)*. In ISIS-2, any allergic reaction was observed in 4.4% receiving SK compared to 0.9%

receiving placebo, an absolute excess of 3.5% *(103)*. In the comparative study ISIS-3 *(118)*, any allergic-type reaction was reported after SK in 3.6%, APSAC in 5.1%, and tPA (duteplase) in 0.8% ($p < 0.00001$, SK vs tPA). Most of these reactions were minor; only 0.3% (SK), 0.5% (APSAC), and 0.1% (tPA) required treatment. In GUSTO, severe or "anaphylactic" reactions recurred in 0.6 and 0.2% of SK and tPA patients, respectively *(96)*.

Angioneurotic and periorbital edema have been reported rarely after SK or APSAC. Other rare reactions have included hypersensitivity vasculitis, purpuric rashes, serum sickness, or renal failure due to interstitial nephritis *(63,104,152,161,162)*. These rare reactions appear to be more frequent after repeated administration.

Fever, with or without other associated manifestations of allergic or immune response, has been reported in 5–30% of patients given SK and 5–10% given APSAC. Fever has been reported to respond to acetaminophen.

Hypotension, usually readily managed, occasionally occurs after SK and APSAC. These drugs generate bradykinin, a potent vasodilator. In ISIS-2, "significant" hypotension and/or bradycardia was reported in 10.0% after SK and 2.0% after placebo infusion, an excess of about 8% with SK *(103)*. In the ISIS-3 comparative study, hypotension was reported in 11.8% receiving SK and, similarly, 12.5% receiving APSAC, but a lower percentage (7.1%) receiving tPA *(118)*. Only half of hypotensive episodes required treatment. In GUSTO, rates of reported hypotension were more comparable between SK (13%) and tPA (10%) *(96)*.

Other Associated Adverse Effects

The effect of thrombolytic reperfusion on the incidence of arrhythmias was an early concern. It is now realized that, although transient changes in rhythm may occur at the time of reperfusion, overall, during hospitalization, the incidence of serious ventricular arrhythmias does not increase, and late ventricular fibrillation is reduced.

Reperfusion therapy has been associated with a small increase in re-infarction (absolute excess over control patients of about 1 to 2%). This is primarily accounted for by recurrent occlusive events in the infarct-related artery with infarction of previously salvaged myocardium. Differences in re-infarction rates among thrombolytic agents may be accounted for either by differences in initial salvage rates associated with differences in effective early recanalization and/or by a greater tendency to re-occlusion with one vs another regimen (e.g., after tPA vs SK).

INDICATIONS FOR THROMBOLYTIC THERAPY IN AMI AND CURRENT USE PATTERNS

The 1999 guidelines of the ACC/AHA *(9)* strongly recommend thrombolytic therapy (Class I indication; strong evidence base) for presentations within 12 h of the onset of suggestive clinical features (ischemic chest discomfort or equivalent) with STE (>0.1 mV, 2 or more contiguous ECG leads) or BBB obscuring ST-segment analysis and age ≤75 yr. Thrombolytic therapy also is generally recommended (Class IIa indication; evidence basis suggestive but less firm) for these same features and age >75 yr (in the absence of contraindications). Therapy is considered possibly effective (Class IIb indication; scientific basis weak, opinion divided), i.e., selected use might be considered, for

Table 7
ACC/AHA Guidelines for Management of AMI (9)

	Prerequisites for considering fibrinolytic therapy	Choice/time of fibrinolytic agent	Adjuvant therapy
ACC/AHA 1999	Class I (Available evidence for efficacy and benefit): 1. STE, time to therapy less than 12 h and age ≤75 yr. 2. BBB with history suggestive of MI. Class IIa (Weight of evidence favors use/efficacy and benefit): 1. Age >75 yr with STE or BBB, suggestive history, time <12 h. Class IIb (Usefulness/efficacy is less well established): 1. STE, time to therapy 12–24 h. 2. SBP >180 mmHg, or DBP >110 mmHg with high risk MI. Class III (Evidence for harm): 1. STE, time to therapy >24 h, pain resolved. 2. ST-segment depression.	No specific recommendations: In patients with large area of infarction, early after symptom onset, and at low risk for ICH, may consider the use of tPA. In smaller infarcts with smaller potential of survival benefit and if a greater risk of ICH exists, SK may be the choice. Door to needle time less than 30 min.	Aspirin 160–325 mg/d. β-blockers unless contraindicated or CHF. ACE inhibitors for anterior MI, CHF or EF <40% (alternatively; all patients, reassess need for continued therapy at 6 wk). IV heparin with tPA, rPA, (TNK-tPA) and non-STE-AMI. SC heparin with SK or APSAC unless at high risk for thromboembolism, when IV heparin is preferred.

CHF, congestive heart failure; DBP, diastolic blood pressure; EF, ejection fraction; ICH, intracerebral hemorrhage; SBP, systolic blood pressure; ACE, angiotensin-converting enzyme.

these ECG findings but time 12–24 h or blood pressure on presentation >180 mmHg systolic and/or >110 mmHg diastolic and a high risk AMI. Thrombolysis is not indicated (Class 3 indication; no evidence of benefit or possibility of harm) for those with STE (or BBB) but time to therapy >24 h and ischemic pain resolved and for those with ST-depression (at any time). These recent ACC/AHA guidelines are summarized in Table 7.

Current Use of Fibrinolytics

The National Registry of Myocardial Infarction (NRMI) tracks the use of reperfusion therapies in the U.S., which is accomplished through surveys of over 1400 hospitals. During three phases from 1990–1999, data from 1,514,292 patients with AMI have been assembled *(10–13)*. During the decade, those eligible for thrombolytic therapy (STE or LBBB within 12 h of presentation) fell from 36 to 27%, but eligible patients who actually received reperfusion therapy remained the same (69 vs 70%). Of the patients receiving reperfusion therapy, the use of thrombolytics fell, from 59 to 48%, whereas primary PCI increased, from 12 to 24%. Of those receiving thrombolytic therapy, the mean time from hospital arrival to drug delivery decreased, from 62 min to 38 min.

Under and Over Utilization of Thrombolytic Therapy

A recent Danish study analyzed 3195 AMI patients with indications and 3397 AMI patients without indications for thrombolysis for the appropriate use of thrombolytic therapy *(163)*. Thrombolytic therapy was reportedly overutilized in 13% of subjects, with the most common reason given as presentation after 12 h of onset of symptoms (this analysis was unable to determine individual characteristics in which late use of thrombolytics may have been appropriate). Nevertheless, logistic regression models showed lower 30-d and 4-yr mortality rates among these patients receiving thrombolytics compared to similar patients not treated with thrombolytics. This study also reported thrombolytics to be underutilized in 14% of patients; these patients were older (mean age 72 vs 64 yr) and more likely to have a BBB (17 vs 4.5%) than patients who received thrombolytics. As expected, nonuse of thrombolytics in this group was associated with increased mortality. One-fifth of patients had at least one contraindication to thrombolytic therapy, the most common being prior stroke (52%). Yet 18% of patients with prior stroke received thrombolytics nevertheless. In these subjects with an indication for thrombolytics and a history of stroke, the use of thrombolytic therapy was associated with a 71% reduction in 30-d adjusted mortality (12 vs 32%). Recurrent stroke was more common in patients not treated with thrombolytics (4 vs 2%, p = NS). Thus, physicians appear to be able to select AMI patients without classic inclusion criteria or with exclusion criteria who may benefit from thrombolytic therapy. Many contraindications are relative, and individual assessment is necessary. This study would suggest prior stroke should not be an absolute contraindication; however, definitive data are lacking. Of greater concern is the 20–70% of patients reported in many studies who are eligible for thrombolytic therapy but never receive it.

Thrombolysis in the Elderly

The appropriate use of thrombolytic therapy in the elderly continues to be debated. In a recent analysis of over 37,000 Medicare patients (age >65) with thrombolytic-eligible AMI *(164)*, only 38% received thrombolytic therapy and 4.2% received primary angioplasty. After multivariate adjustments, thrombolytic therapy was not associated with improved 30-d survival (OR: 1.01, CI: 0.94–1.09), whereas primary angioplasty was (OR: 0.79, CI: 0.66–0.94). However, at 1 yr, both thrombolytic therapy (OR: 0.84, CI: 0.79–0.89) and primary angioplasty (OR: 0.71, CI: 0.61–0.83) were associated with lower mortality rates. Another retrospective Medicare analysis *(165)* suggested that thrombolytic therapy may even be harmful in those over 75 yr.

In contrast, a large Swedish registry found a 12% risk reduction in the composite end point of cerebral bleeding and 1-yr mortality *(166)*. Similarly, the FTT overview of randomized trials data for patients over 75 yr reported a trend toward reduced 35-d mortality from 29.4 to 26.0% with thrombolytic therapy *(110)*. Analyses restricted to elderly patients with clear indications for thrombolytic therapy, suggested a greater absolute benefit from thrombolytic therapy than observed in younger patients.

Thrombolytic regimens should be chosen to minimize the risk of ICH, which increases in the elderly *(155)*. Weight adjusting treatment regimens and avoidance of excessive heparin and other adjunctive antithrombotics (e.g., GP IIb/IIIa inhibitors) is important. When safety concerns predominate, primary angioplasty should be considered as a preferred reperfusion strategy.

LBBB AND THROMBOLYSIS

For patients with LBBB not known to be new, the diagnosis of AMI may be obscured, and thrombolytic therapy may be inappropriately withheld. In order to define a prediction rule for evaluating LBBB, the GUSTO-1 investigators evaluated ECG changes in patients with LBBB and AMI and compared them to control LBBB patients without AMI *(167)*. Three ECG criteria proved to have independent value in the diagnosis of AMI: (*i*) STE of 1 mm or more in leads with a positive QRS complex; (*ii*) ST-depression of 1 mm or more in leads V1, V2, or V3; and (*iii*) STE of 5 mm or more with a negative QRS complex. Using an index score, these criteria were shown to have a sensitivity of 36% and a specificity of 96% for AMI in the validation group.

CARDIOPULMONARY RESUSCITATION

Previously, prolonged cardiopulmonary resuscitation (CPR) has been considered a contraindication to thrombolytic therapy. Recently, a small trial evaluated 90 patients who had out-of-hospital cardiac arrest for AMI and did not have return of spontaneous circulation within 15 min *(168)*. During the first study year, patients treated with CPR had return of spontaneous circulation 44% of the time, and 30% were admitted to the intensive care unit (ICU). During the next yr, patients with the above criteria were treated with heparin and tPA, which resulted in improved return of spontaneous circulation (68%, $p = 0.03$) and admission to the ICU (58%, $p = 0.01$) without bleeding complications. Discharge rates from the hospital trended higher in the thrombolytic therapy group (15 vs 8%).

SELECTION OF A REPERFUSION REGIMEN AND ADJUNCTIVE THERAPY

Selection of a Reperfusion Regimen

The selection of a reperfusion regimen is based on the risk of the AMI, a benefit vs risk analysis of therapy, and a consideration of economic constraints. Using these factors, tPA-related thrombolytics have become predominant in the U.S., whereas in Europe and elsewhere, less costly SK is still widely used. These same factors will undoubtedly influence the rate of incorporation of new adjunctive therapies (such as LWMH and platelet GPI) into common practice. A number of algorithms for selecting the reperfusion regimen (i.e., a specific thrombolytic or primary PCI) have been proposed *(9,169,170)*, but none has been prospectively validated and universally accepted.

In the author's view, primary PCI may be viewed as the preferred strategy when readily available (time to PCI, 60–120 min) in experienced centers *(9)*. This is based on an overview of comparative trials, which suggests reduced rates of death, reinfarction, and hemorrhagic stroke with primary PCI as compared to thrombolytics when PCI is performed in a timely fashion by experienced teams with surgical back-up *(171–173)*. Primary PCI is discussed more fully in a subsequent chapter.

In contrast, a differential benefit of PCI has been more difficult to demonstrate in community applications of the two reperfusion strategies, where experience, patient selection, and timing may be suboptimal *(174–176)*. Even in experienced centers, logistic problems for timely PCI often arise (e.g., after hours or laboratories occupied). Thus, in many circumstances, thrombolytic therapy remains the reperfusion strategy of choice.

TNK-tPA, accelerated dose tPA, or rPA may be recommended as a first choice regimen for high risk AMI patients who also have the potential for a large therapeutic benefit, i.e., anterior AMI, BBB-related AMI, or poor-prognosis inferior AMI (i.e., with right ventricular involvement or with anterior reciprocal ST-depression, or with lateral and posterior extension), time <6 h, and age <75 yr (older patients have greater mortality risk, but also have greater bleeding risk and derive less proportionate and absolute benefit from therapy). TNK-tPA offers the advantage of single bolus dosing, a lower transfusion requirement, and may reduce dosing errors *(134)*, yet maintains equivalent survival efficacy compared to tPA. For lower-risk patients, efficacy advantages are less clear, and physician preference, patient safety, cost issues, and availability will guide choice. SK is preferred when cost is an important consideration, although a nonimmunogenic thrombolytic is preferred for patients with a history of prior SK use *(72)*. SK also has a lower risk of ICH if excessive heparin is avoided.

Despite two large trial outcomes *(145,146)*, the role of combination therapies with GP IIb/IIIa inhibitors remains unclear, and recommendations on use cannot be given yet. Combinations tested in GUSTO-V and ASSENT-3 should be avoided in the elderly (>75 yr old) *(145,146)*.

Adjunctive therapy with the LMWH enoxaparin presents another co-therapy option. Based on ASSENT-3 *(146)*, enoxaparin appears to be an attractive alternative to unfractionated heparin as an adjunctive antithrombin with standard dose TNK-tPA. Further testing and assimilation of enoxaparin into official guidelines is anticipated in the near future.

Adjunctive Antiplatelet and Antithrombotic Therapy

Current guidelines strongly recommend (Class I indication) aspirin on admission in a dose of 162–325 mg, preferably chewed *(9)*. Aspirin in then continued in the same dose once daily indefinitely (enteric coated forms are popular). For aspirin allergy, clopidogrel may be used *(9)*.

iv heparin is recommended (Class IIa) with tPA-related fibrinolytics *(9)*, beginning concurrently and given for 48 h, with a target aPTT within12 h of 50–70 s (1.5 to 2 times control) *(120)*. Currently recommended dosing includes a 60 U/kg bolus (maximum 4000 U) followed initially with a 12 U/kg/h infusion (maximum 1000 U/h) with adjustment after 3 h based on aPTT.

iv heparin is not routinely recommended with systemically active (nonfibrin-selective) agents such as SK and APSAC, especially within 6 h of fibrinolysis *(9)*. Rather, sc heparin (7500–12,500 U SC 2× daily until ambulatory) or a LMWH may be given. iv heparin is "probably effective" after 6 h for patients at high risk for further thrombosis or thromboembolism (e.g., those with large or anterior AMI, atrial fibrillation, previous embolus, or known left ventricular thrombus) *(9)*.

An important adjunctive role for the newer antithrombotic agents, including direct antithrombins such as hirudin and hirulog *(145,146,177)*, as replacements for unfractionated heparin, has not yet been established.

INCORPORATING THROMBOLYTIC THERAPY INTO A RAPID TRIAGE AND TREATMENT ALGORITHM

Effective use of thrombolytic therapy (and other reperfusion strategies such as PCI) requires incorporation into an efficiently managed emergency ward-based system *(8,9,178)* that is tailored to each specific hospital's capabilities and strategic preferences (i.e., toward primary PCI or thrombolytic therapy). The importance of developing and implementing such a strategy consistently and efficiently cannot be overemphasized. Outcomes appear to be determined more importantly by the care with which a strategy is developed and implemented than whether thrombolytic therapy or primary PCI forms the preferred approach to reperfusion.

Of the more than 5 million patients presenting with chest pain annually to paramedics or emergency departments, only a small percentage will be candidates for thrombolytic therapy (approx 5–10%) *(179,180)*. However, the importance of rapidly identifying, triaging, and treating these patients cannot be overemphasized. Patients with chest pain are rapidly screened with a targeted history, physical examination, and ECG, within 10 min of arrival. They are then assigned to one of four or five chest pain pathways (definite STE/BBB AMI, unstable angina/non-STE MI, probable unstable angina, possible unstable angina, or noncardiac chest pain) *(8,9)*. In the STE/BBB AMI group, further screening for thrombolytic contraindications is rapidly performed and treatment begun.

REFERENCES

1. American Heart Association. 2001 Heart and Stroke Statistical Update. American Heart Association, Dallas, 2000.
2. Myerburg RJ, Kessler KM, Castellanos A. Sudden cardiac death. Structure, function, and time-dependence of risk. Circulation 1992;85(Suppl. 1):I2–I10.
3. Farb A, Tang AL, Burke AP, Sessums L, Liang Y, Virmani R. Sudden coronary death. Frequency of active coronary lesions, inactive coronary lesions, and myocardial infarction. Circulation 1995;92: 1701–1709.
4. Priori SG, Aliot E, Blomstrom-Lundqvist C, et al. Task Force on Sudden Cardiac Death of the European Society of Cardiology. Eur Heart J 2001;22:1374–1450.
5. Herlitz J, Blohm M, Hartford M, Hjalmarsson A, Holmberg S, Karlson BW. Delay time in suspected acute myocardial infarction and the importance of its modification. Clin Cardiol 1989;12:370–374.
6. National Hospital Discharge Survey, 1996. Detailed diagnoses and procedures. National Center for Health Statistics, Hyattsville, MD, 1998, p. 13.

7. Nourjah P. National Hospital Ambulatory Medical Care Survey: 1997 emergency department summary. National Center for Health Statistics; advance data from Vital and Health Statistics. National Institutes of Health, Hyattsville, MD, 1999, p. 304.

8. Braunwald E, Antman EM, Beasley JW, et al. ACC/AHA guidelines for the management of patients with unstable angina and non-ST-segment elevation myocardial infarction. A report of the American College of Cardiology/American Heart Association Task Force on Practice Guidelines (Committee on the Management of Patients With Unstable Angina). J Am Coll Cardiol 2000;36:970–1062.

9. Ryan TJ, Antman EM, Brooks NH, et al. 1999 update: ACC/AHA guidelines for the management of patients with acute myocardial infarction. A report of the American College of Cardiology/American Heart Association Task Force on Practice Guidelines (Committee on Management of Acute Myocardial Infarction). J Am Coll Cardiol 1999;34:890–911.

10. Rogers WJ, Canto JG, Lambrew CT, et al. Temporal trends in the treatment of over 1.5 million patients with myocardial infarction in the US from 1990 through 1999: the National Registry of Myocardial Infarction 1, 2 and 3. J Am Coll Cardiol 2000;36:2056–2063.

11. Armstrong PW, Collen D. Fibrinolysis for acute myocardial infarction: current status and new horizons for pharmacological reperfusion, part 1. Circulation 2001;103:2862–2866.

12. Hunink MG, Goldman L, Tosteson AN, et al. The recent decline in mortality from coronary heart disease, 1980–1990. The effect of secular trends in risk factors and treatment. JAMA 1997;277: 535–542.

13. Rogers WJ, Canto JG, Barron HV, Boscarino JA, Shoultz DA, Every NR. Treatment and outcome of myocardial infarction in hospitals with and without invasive capability. Investigators in the National Registry of Myocardial Infarction. J Am Coll Cardiol 2000;35:371–379.

14. Herrick JB. Clinical features of sudden obstruction of the coronary arteries. Jama 1912;59:220–228.

15. Obraztsov VP, Strazhesko ND. On the symptomatology and diagnosis of coronary thrombosis. In: Vorobeva VA, Konchalovski MP, eds. Works of the First Congress of Russian Therapists. Comradeship typography of A E Mamontov, 1910, pp. 26–43.

16. DeWood MA, Spores J, Notske R, et al. Prevalence of total coronary occlusion during the early hours of transmural myocardial infarction. N Engl J Med 1980;303:897–902.

17. Reimer KA, Lowe JE, Rasmussen MM, Jennings RB. The wavefront phenomenon of ischemic cell death. 1. Myocardial infarct size vs duration of coronary occlusion in dogs. Circulation 1977;56: 786–794.

18. Reimer KA, Jennings RB. The "wavefront phenomenon" of myocardial ischemic cell death. II. Transmural progression of necrosis within the framework of ischemic bed size (myocardium at risk) and collateral flow. Lab Invest 1979;40:633–644.

19. Falk E. Plaque rupture with severe pre-existing stenosis precipitating coronary thrombosis. Characteristics of coronary atherosclerotic plaques underlying fatal occlusive thrombi. Br Heart J 1983;50: 127–134.

20. Davies MJ, Thomas AC. Plaque fissuring—the cause of acute myocardial infarction, sudden ischaemic death, and crescendo angina. Br Heart J 1985;53:363–373.

21. Mizuno K, Satomura K, Miyamoto A, et al. Angioscopic evaluation of coronary-artery thrombi in acute coronary syndromes. N Engl J Med 1992;326:287–291.

22. Farb A, Burke AP, Tang AL, et al. Coronary plaque erosion without rupture into a lipid core. A frequent cause of coronary thrombosis in sudden coronary death. Circulation 1996;93:1354–1363.

23. Fuster V, Badimon L, Badimon JJ, Chesebro JH. The pathogenesis of coronary artery disease and the acute coronary syndromes (2). N Engl J Med 1992;326:310–318.

24. Libby P. Molecular bases of the acute coronary syndromes. Circulation 1995;91:2844–2850.

25. Shah PK. Inflammation, metalloproteinases, and increased proteolysis: an emerging pathophysiological paradigm in aortic aneurysm. Circulation 1997;96:2115–2117.

26. Shah PK, Galis ZS. Matrix metalloproteinase hypothesis of plaque rupture: players keep piling up but questions remain. Circulation 2001;104:1878–1880.

27. Tillet WS, Garner RL. The fibrinolytic activity of hemoytic streptococci. J Exp Med 1933;58:485–502.

28. Sherry S. The origin of thrombolytic therapy. J Am Coll Cardiol 1989;14:1085–1092.

29. Tillet WS, Sherry S. The effect in patients of streptococcal fibrinolysis (streptokinase) and streptococcal desoxyribonuclease on fibrinous, purulent, and sanguinous pleural exudations. J Clin Invest 1949;28:173–190.

30. Fletcher AP, Alkjaersig N, Smyrniotis FE, et al. Treatment of patients suffering from early acute myocardial infarction with massive and prolonged streptokinase therapy. Trans Assoc Am Phys 1958; 71:287–297.

31. Streptokinase in acute myocardial infarction. European Cooperative Study Group for Streptokinase Treatment in Acute Myocardial Infarction. N Engl J Med 1979;301:797–802.
32. Sharma GV, Cella G, Parisi AF, Sasahara AA. Thrombolytic therapy. N Engl J Med 1982;306: 1268–1276.
33. Stampfer MJ, Goldhaber SZ, Yusuf S, Peto R, Hennekens CH. Effect of intravenous streptokinase on acute myocardial infarction: pooled results from randomized trials. N Engl J Med 1982;307: 1180–1182.
34. Anderson JL. Intravenous thrombolysis and other antithrombotic therapy. In: Anderson JL, ed. Acute Myocardial Infarction: New Management Strategies. Aspen Publishers, Rockville, MD, 1987, pp. 185–217.
35. Anderson JL, Smith BR. Streptokinase in acute myocardial infarction. In: Anderson JL, ed. Modern Management of Acute Myocardial Infarction in the Community Hospital. Marcel Dekker, New York, 1991, pp. 187–215.
36. Chazov EI, Matveeva LS, Mazaev AV, et al. Intracoronary administration of fibrinolysin in acute myocardial infarction (in Russian). Ter Arkh 1976;48:8–19.
37. Rentrop KP, Blanke H, Karsch KR, et al. Acute myocardial infarction: intracoronary application of nitroglycerin and streptokinase. Clin Cardiol 1979;2:354–363.
38. Rentrop KP, Blanke H, Karsch KR, Kreuzer H. Initial experience with transluminal recanalization of the recently occluded infarct-related coronary artery in acute myocardial infarction–comparison with conventionally treated patients. Clin Cardiol 1979;2:92–105.
39. Rentrop P, Blanke H, Karsch KR, Kaiser H, Kostering H, Leitz K. Selective intracoronary thrombolysis in acute myocardial infarction and unstable angina pectoris. Circulation 1981;63:307–317.
40. Ganz W, Ninomiya K, Hashida J, et al. Intracoronary thrombolysis in acute myocardial infarction: experimental background and clinical experience. Am Heart J 1981;102:1145–1149.
41. Anderson JL. Principles of thrombolytic therapy: intracoronary administration. In: Anderson JL, ed. Acute Myocardial Infarction: New Management Strategies. Aspen Publishers, Rockville, MD, 1987, pp. 157–184.
42. Anderson JL, Marshall HW, Bray BE, et al. A randomized trial of intracoronary streptokinase in the treatment of acute myocardial infarction. N Engl J Med 1983;308:1312–1318.
43. Khaja F, Walton JA Jr, Brymer JF, et al. Intracoronary fibrinolytic therapy in acute myocardial infarction. Report of a prospective randomized trial. N Engl J Med 1983;308:1305–1311.
44. Kennedy JW, Ritchie JL, Davis KB, Fritz JK. Western Washington randomized trial of intracoronary streptokinase in acute myocardial infarction. N Engl J Med 1983;309:1477–1482.
45. Kennedy JW, Ritchie JL, Davis KB, Stadius ML, Maynard C, Fritz JK. The Western Washington randomized trial of intracoronary streptokinase in acute myocardial infarction. A 12-mo follow-up report. N Engl J Med 1985;312:1073–1078.
46. Simoons ML, Serruys PW, vd Brand M, et al. Improved survival after early thrombolysis in acute myocardial infarction. A randomised trial by the Interuniversity Cardiology Institute in The Netherlands. Lancet 1985;2:578–582.
47. Tennant SN, Dixon J, Venable TC, et al. Intracoronary thrombolysis in patients with acute myocardial infarction: comparison of the efficacy of urokinase with streptokinase. Circulation 1984;69: 756–760.
48. Yasuno M, Saito Y, Ishida M, Suzuki K, Endo S, Takahashi M. Effects of percutaneous transluminal coronary angioplasty: intracoronary thrombolysis with urokinase in acute myocardial infarction. Am J Cardiol 1984;53:1217–1220.
49. Yusuf S, Wittes J, Friedman L. Overview of results of randomized clinical trials in heart disease. I. Treatments following myocardial infarction. JAMA 1988;260:2088–2093.
50. Schröder R, Biamino G, von Leitner ER, et al. Intravenous short-term infusion of streptokinase in acute myocardial infarction. Circulation 1983;67:536–548.
51. Rogers WJ, Mantle JA, Hood WP Jr, et al. Prospective randomized trial of intravenous and intracoronary streptokinase in acute myocardial infarction. Circulation 1983;68:1051–1061.
52. Anderson JL, Marshall HW, Askins JC, et al. A randomized trial of intravenous and intracoronary streptokinase in patients with acute myocardial infarction. Circulation 1984;70:606–618.
53. Alderman EL, Jutzy KR, Berte LE, et al. Randomized comparison of intravenous versus intracoronary streptokinase for myocardial infarction. Am J Cardiol 1984;54:14–19.
54. Valentine RP, Pitts DE, Brooks-Brunn JA, Williams JG, Van Hove E, Schmidt PE. Intravenous versus intracoronary streptokinase in acute myocardial infarction. Am J Cardiol 1985;55:309–312.

55. A prospective trial of intravenous streptokinase in acute myocardial infarction (I.S.A.M.). Mortality, morbidity, and infarct size at 21 d. ISAM Study Group. N Engl J Med 1986;314:1465–1471.

56. Spann JF, Sherry S. Coronary thrombolysis for evolving myocardial infarction. Drugs 1984;28:465.

57. Smalling RW, Fuentes F, Freund GC, et al. Beneficial effects of intracoronary thrombolysis up to 18 h after onset of pain in evolving myocardial infarction. Am Heart J 1982;104:912–920.

58. Sheehan FH, Mathey DG, Schofer J, et al. Factors that determine recovery of left ventricular function after thrombolysis in patients with acute myocardial infarction. Circulation 1985;71:1121–1128.

59. Mathey DG, Sheehan FH, Schofer J, Dodge HT. Time from onset of symptoms to thrombolytic therapy: a major determinant of mycardial salvage in patients with acute transmural infarction. J Am Coll Cardiol 1985;6:518–525.

60. Sheehan FH, Mathey DG, Schofer J, Krebber HJ, Dodge HT. Effect of interventions in salvaging left ventricular function in acute myocardial infarction: a study of intracoronary streptokinase. Am J Cardiol 1983;52:431–438.

61. Sherry S. Fibrinolysis, Thrombosis and Hemostasis. Lea & Febiger, Philadelphia, 1992, pp. 3–30.

62. Jackson KW, Tang J. Complete amino acid sequence of streptokinase and its homology with serine proteases. Biochemistry 1982;21:6220–6225.

63. Sherry S, Marder MJ. Streptokinase. In: Messerli FH, ed. Cardiovascular Drug Therapy, 2nd ed. W. B. Saunders, Philadelphia, 1996, pp. 1521–1552.

64. Rutherford RB, Comerota AJ. Urokinase. In: Messerli FH, ed. Cardiovascular Drug Therapy. 2nd ed. W B Saunders, Philadelphia, 1990, pp. 1542–1552.

65. W R Bell J. Clinical applications of urokinase, the first tissue plasminogen activating thrombolytic agent. In: Anderson JL, ed. Modern Management of Acute Myocardial Infarction in the Community Hospital. Marcel Dekker, New York, 1991, pp. 251–287.

66. Rossi P, Bolognese L. Comparison of intravenous urokinase plus heparin versus heparin alone in acute myocardial infarction. Am J Cardiol 1991;68:585–592.

67. Ferres H. Preclinical evaluation of anisoylated plasminogen streptokinase activator complex. Drugs 1987;33(Suppl. 3):33 50.

68. Anderson JL, Califf RM. Anisoylated plasminogen-streptokinase activator complex (APSAC). In: Messerli FH, ed. Cardiovascular Drug Therapy. W B Saunders, Philadelphia, 1996, pp. 1553–1567.

69. Tiefenbrunn AJ. Tissue-type plasminogen activator. In: Messerli FH, ed. Cardiovascular Drug Therapy. W. B. Saunders, Philadelphia, 1996:1567–1577.

70. Rijken DC, Hoylaerts M, Collen D. Fibrinolytic properties of one-chain and two-chain human extrinsic (tissue-type) plasminogen activator. J Biol Chem 1982;257:2920–2925.

71. Lucore CL, Sobel BE. Interactions of tissue-type plasminogen activator with plasma inhibitors and their pharmacologic implications. Circulation 1988;77:660–669.

72. Anderson JL. Retreatment with thrombolytic therapy for threatened coronary reocclusion. UpToDate 2001.

73. Randomised, double-blind comparison of reteplase double-bolus administration with streptokinase in acute myocardial infarction (INJECT): trial to investigate equivalence. International Joint Efficacy Comparison of Thrombolytics. Lancet 1995;346:329–336.

74. Bode C, Smalling RW, Berg G, et al. Randomized comparison of coronary thrombolysis achieved with double- bolus reteplase (recombinant plasminogen activator) and front-loaded, accelerated alteplase (recombinant tissue plasminogen activator) in patients with acute myocardial infarction. The RAPID II Investigators. Circulation 1996;94:891–898.

75. A comparison of reteplase with alteplase for acute myocardial infarction. The Global Use of Strategies to Open Occluded Coronary Arteries (GUSTO III) Investigators. N Engl J Med 1997;337: 1118–1123.

76. Keyt BA, Paoni NF, Refino CJ, et al. A faster-acting and more potent form of tissue plasminogen activator. Proc Natl Acad Sci USA 1994;91:3670–3674.

77. Cannon CP, McCabe CH, Gibson CM, et al. TNK-tissue plasminogen activator in acute myocardial infarction. Results of the Thrombolysis in Myocardial Infarction (TIMI) 10A dose-ranging trial. Circulation 1997;95:351–356.

78. Modi NB, Eppler S, Breed J, Cannon CP, Braunwald E, Love T. Pharmacokinetics of a slower clearing tissue plasminogen activator variant, TNK-tPA, in patients with acute myocardial infarction. Thromb Haemost 1998;79:134–139.

79. Antman EM, Giugliano RP, Gibson CM, et al. Abciximab facilitates the rate and extent of thrombolysis: results of the thrombolysis in myocardial infarction (TIMI) 14 trial. The TIMI 14 Investigators. Circulation 1999;99:2720–2732.

80. Benedict CR, Refino CJ, Keyt BA, et al. New variant of human tissue plaminogen activator (TPA) with enhanced efficacy and lower incidence of bleeding compared with recombinant human TPA. Circulation 1995;92:3032–3040.

81. Collen D, Stassen J-M, Yasuda T, et al. Comparative thrombolytic properties of tissue-type plasminogen activator and of a plasminogen activator inhibitor-1-resistant glycosylation variant, in a combined arterial and venous thrombosis model in the dog. Thrombosis and Haemost 1994;72:98–104.

82. Tanswell P, Tebbe U, Neuhaus K-L, Glasle-Schwarz L, Wojcik J, Seifried E. Pharmacokinetics and fibrin specificity of alteplase during accelerated infusions in acute myocardial infarction. J Am Coll Cardiol 1992;19:1071–1075.

83. Cannon CP, Gibson CM, McCabe CH, et al. TNK-tissue plasminogen activator compared with front-loaded alteplase in acute myocardial infarction: results of the TIMI 10B trial. Thrombolysis in Myocardial Infarction (TIMI) 10B Investigators. Circulation 1998;98:2805–2814.

84. Van de Werf F, Vanhaecke J, de Geest H, Verstraete M, Collen D. Coronary thrombolysis with recombinant single-chain urokinase-type plasminogen activator in patients with acute myocardial infarction. Circulation 1986;74:1066–1070.

85. Weaver WD, Hartmann JR, Anderson JL, Reddy PS, Sobolski JC, Sasahara AA. New recombinant glycosylated prourokinase for treatment of patients with acute myocardial infarction. Prourokinase Study Group. J Am Coll Cardiol 1994;24:1242–1248.

86. Randomised double-blind trial of recombinant pro-urokinase against streptokinase in acute myocardial infarction. PRIMI Trial Study Group. Lancet 1989;1:863–868.

87. Bar FW, Meyer J, Vermeer F, et al. Comparison of saruplase and alteplase in acute myocardial infarction. SESAM Study Group. The Study in Europe with Saruplase and Alteplase in Myocardial Infarction. Am J Cardiol 1997;79:727–732.

88. Tebbe U, Michels R, Adgey J, et al. Randomized, double-blind study comparing saruplase with streptokinase therapy in acute myocardial infarction: the COMPASS Equivalence Trial. Comparison Trial of Saruplase and Streptokinase (COMASS) Investigators. J Am Coll Cardiol 1998;31:487–493.

89. den Heijer P, Vermeer F, Ambrosioni E, et al. Evaluation of a weight-adjusted single-bolus plasminogen activator in patients with myocardial infarction: a double-blind, randomized angiographic trial of lanoteplase versus alteplase. Circulation 1998;98:2117–2125.

90. Intravenous NPA for the treatment of infarcting myocardium early; InTIME-II, a double-blind comparison of single-bolus lanoteplase vs accelerated alteplase for the treatment of patients with acute myocardial infarction. Eur Heart J 2000;21:2005–2013.

91. Collen D, Lijnen HR. Staphylokinase, a fibrin-specific plasminogen activator with therapeutic potential? Blood 1994;84:680–686.

92. Vanderschueren S, Barrios L, Kerdsinchai P, et al. A randomized trial of recombinant staphylokinase versus alteplase for coronary artery patency in acute myocardial infarction. The STAR Trial Group. Circulation 1995;92:2044–2049.

93. Chesebro JH, Knatterud G, Roberts R, et al. Thrombolysis in Myocardial Infarction (TIMI) Trial, Phase I: a comparison between intravenous tissue plasminogen activator and intravenous streptokinase. Clinical findings through hospital discharge. Circulation 1987;76:142–154.

94. Granger CB, White HD, Bates ER, Ohman EM, Califf RM. A pooled analysis of coronary arterial patency and left ventricular function after intravenous thrombolysis for acute myocardial infarction. Am J Cardiol 1994;74:1220–1228.

95. The effects of tissue plasminogen activator, streptokinase, or both on coronary-artery patency, ventricular function, and survival after acute myocardial infarction. The GUSTO Angiographic Investigators. N Engl J Med 1993;329:1615–1622.

96. An international randomized trial comparing four thrombolytic strategies for acute myocardial infarction. The GUSTO investigators. N Engl J Med 1993;329:673–682.

97. Simes RJ, Topol EJ, Holmes DR Jr, et al. Link between the angiographic substudy and mortality outcomes in a large randomized trial of myocardial reperfusion. Importance of early and complete infarct artery reperfusion. GUSTO-I Investigators. Circulation 1995;91:1923–1928.

98. Yusuf S, Collins R, Peto R, et al. Intravenous and intracoronary fibrinolytic therapy in acute myocardial infarction: overview of results on mortality, reinfarction and side-effects from 33 randomized controlled trials. Eur Heart J 1985;6:556–585.

99. Yusuf S, Sleight P, Held P, McMahon S. Routine medical management of acute myocardial infarction. Lessons from overviews of recent randomized controlled trials. Circulation 1990;82(Suppl. 3): II117–II134.

100. Granger CB, Califf RM, Topol EJ. Thrombolytic therapy for acute myocardial infarction. A review. Drugs 1992;44:293–325.

101. Effectiveness of intravenous thrombolytic treatment in acute myocardial infarction. Gruppo Italiano per lo Studio della Streptochinasi nell'Infarto Miocardico (GISSI). Lancet 1986;1:397–402.

102. Long-term effects of intravenous thrombolysis in acute myocardial infarction: final report of the GISSI study. Gruppo Italiano per lo Studio della Streptochi-nasi nell'Infarto Miocardico (GISSI). Lancet 1987;2:871–874.

103. Randomised trial of intravenous streptokinase, oral aspirin, both, or neither among 17,187 cases of suspected acute myocardial infarction: ISIS-2. ISIS-2 (Second International Study of Infarct Survival) Collaborative Group. Lancet 1988;2:349–360.

104. Effect of intravenous APSAC on mortality after acute myocardial infarction: preliminary report of a placebo-controlled clinical trial. AIMS Trial Study Group. Lancet 1988;1:545–549.

105. Long-term effects of intravenous anistreplase in acute myocardial infarction: final report of the AIMS study. AIMS Trial Study Group. Lancet 1990;335:427–431.

106. O'Connor CM, Meese R, Carney R, et al. A randomized trial of intravenous heparin in conjunction with anistreplase (anisoylated plasminogen streptokinase activator complex) in acute myocardial infarction: the Duke University Clinical Cardiology Study (DUCCS) 1. J Am Coll Cardiol 1994;23. 11 18.

107. Wilcox RG, von der Lippe G, Olsson CG, Jensen G, Skene AM, Hampton JR. Trial of tissue plasminogen activator for mortality reduction in acute myocardial infarction. Anglo-Scandinavian Study of Early Thrombolysis (ASSET). Lancet 1988;2:525–530.

108. Late Assessment of Thrombolytic Efficacy (LATE) study with alteplase 6- 24 h after onset of acute myocardial infarction. Lancet 1993;342:759–766.

109. Randomised trial of late thrombolysis in patients with suspected acute myocardial infarction. EMERAS (Estudio Multicentrico Estreptoquinasa Republicas de America del Sur) Collaborative Group. Lancet 1993;342:767–772.

110. Indications for fibrinolytic therapy in suspected acute myocardial infarction: collaborative overview of early mortality and major morbidity results from all randomised trials of more than 1000 patients. Fibrinolytic Therapy Trialists' (FTT) Collaborative Group. Lancet 1994;343:311–322.

111. Gersh BJ, Anderson JL. Thrombolysis and myocardial salvage. Results of clinical trials and the animal paradigm—paradoxic or predictable? Circulation 1993;88:296–306.

112. Boersma E, Maas AC, Deckers JW, Simoons ML. Early thrombolytic treatment in acute myocardial infarction: reappraisal of the golden hour. Lancet 1996;348:771–775.

113. Col NF, Gurwitz JH, Alpert JS, Goldberg RJ. Frequency of inclusion of patients with cardiogenic shock in trials of thrombolytic therapy. Am J Cardiol 1994;73:149–157.

114. Sanborn TA, Sleeper LA, Bates ER, et al. Impact of thrombolysis, intra-aortic balloon pump counterpulsation, and their combination in cardiogenic shock complicating acute myocardial infarction: a report from the SHOCK Trial Registry. SHould we emergently revascularize Occluded Coronaries for cardiogenic shocK? J Am Coll Cardiol 2000;36(3 Suppl. A):1123–1129.

115. Zebrack JS, Anderson JL. Fibrinolytic therapy. In: S Yusuf BG, ed. Evidence Based Medicine. British Medical Journal, London, 2002, in press.

116. In-hospital mortality and clinical course of 20,891 patients with suspected acute myocardial infarction randomised between alteplase and streptokinase with or without heparin. The International Study Group. Lancet 1990;336:71–75.

117. GISSI-2: a factorial randomised trial of alteplase versus streptokinase and heparin versus no heparin among 12,490 patients with acute myocardial infarction. Gruppo Italiano per lo Studio della Sopravvivenza nell'Infarto Miocardico. Lancet 1990;336:65–71.

118. ISIS-3: a randomised comparison of streptokinase vs tissue plasminogen activator vs anistreplase and of aspirin plus heparin vs aspirin alone among 41,299 cases of suspected acute myocardial infarction. ISIS-3 (Third International Study of Infarct Survival) Collaborative Group. Lancet 1992;339:753–770.

119. Turpie AG, Robinson JG, Doyle DJ, et al. Comparison of high-dose with low-dose subcutaneous heparin to prevent left ventricular mural thrombosis in patients with acute transmural anterior myocardial infarction. N Engl J Med 1989;320:352–357.

120. Granger CB, Hirsch J, Califf RM, et al. Activated partial thromboplastin time and outcome after thrombolytic therapy for acute myocardial infarction: results from the GUSTO-I trial. Circulation 1996;93: 870–878.

121. Anderson JL, Karagounis LA. Does intravenous heparin or time-to-treatment/reperfusion explain differences between GUSTO and ISIS-3 results? Am J Cardiol 1994;74:1057–1060.

122. de Bono DP, Simoons ML, Tijssen J, et al. Effect of early intravenous heparin on coronary patency, infarct size, and bleeding complications after alteplase thrombolysis: results of a randomised double blind European Cooperative Study Group trial. Br Heart J 1992;67:122–128.

123. Hsia J, Hamilton WP, Kleiman N, Roberts R, Chaitman BR, Ross AM. A comparison between heparin and low-dose aspirin as adjunctive therapy with tissue plasminogen activator for acute myocardial infarction. Heparin-Aspirin Reperfusion Trial (HART) Investigators. N Engl J Med 1990;323: 1433–1437.

124. Verstraete M, Bernard R, Bory M, et al. Randomised trial of intravenous recombinant tissue-type plasminogen activator versus intravenous streptokinase in acute myocardial infarction. Report from the European Cooperative Study Group for Recombinant Tissue-type Plasminogen Activator. Lancet 1985;1:842–847.

125. Anderson JL, Becker LC, Sorensen SG, et al. Anistreplase versus alteplase in acute myocardial infarction: comparative effects on left ventricular function, morbidity and 1-d coronary artery patency. The TEAM-3 Investigators. J Am Coll Cardiol 1992;20:753–766.

126. Neuhaus KL, von Essen R, Tebbe U, et al. Improved thrombolysis in acute myocardial infarction with front-loaded administration of alteplase: results of the rt-PA-APSAC patency study (TAPS). J Am Coll Cardiol 1992;19:885–891.

127. Cannon CP, McCabe CH, Diver DJ, et al. Comparison of front-loaded recombinant tissue-type plasminogen activator, anistreplase and combination thrombolytic therapy for acute myocardial infarction: results of the Thrombolysis in Myocardial Infarction (TIMI) 4 trial. J Am Coll Cardiol 1994;24: 1602–1610.

128. Purvis JA, McNeill AJ, Siddiqui RA, et al. Efficacy of 100 mg of double-bolus alteplase in achieving complete perfusion in the treatment of acute myocardial infarction. J Am Coll Cardiol 1994;23:6–10.

129. A comparison of continuous infusion of alteplase with double-bolus administration for acute myocardial infarction. The Continuous Infusion versus Double-Bolus Administration of Alteplase (COBALT) Investigators. N Engl J Med 1997;337:1124–1130.

130. Van de Werf F, Cannon CP, Luyten A, et al. Safety assessment of single-bolus administration of TNK tissue-plasminogen activator in acute myocardial infarction: the ASSENT-1 trial. The ASSENT-1 Investigators. Am Heart J 1999;137:786–791.

131. Gibson CM, Murphy SA, Rizzo MJ, et al. Relationship between TIMI frame count and clinical outcomes after thrombolytic administration. Thrombolysis In Myocardial Infarction (TIMI) Study Group. Circulation 1999;99:1945–1950.

132. Gibson CM, Cannon CP, Murphy SA, et al. Weight-adjusted dosing of TNK-tissue plasminogen activator and its relation to angiographic outcomes in the thrombolysis in myocardial infarction 10B trial. TIMI 10B Investigators. Am J Cardiol 1999;84:976–980.

133. Single-bolus tenecteplase compared with front-loaded alteplase in acute myocardial infarction: the ASSENT-2 double-blind randomised trial. Assessment of the Safety and Efficacy of a New Thrombolytic Investigators. Lancet 1999;354:716–722.

134. Cannon CP. Thrombolysis medication errors: benefits of bolus thrombolytic agents. Am J Cardiol 2000;85:17C–22C.

135. Anderson JL. Why does thrombolysis fail? Breaking through the reperfusion ceiling. Am J Cardiol 1997;80:1588–1590.

136. Topol EJ. Toward a new frontier in myocardial reperfusion therapy: emerging platelet preeminence. Circulation 1998;97:211–218.

137. Randomised placebo-controlled trial of abciximab before and during coronary intervention in refractory unstable angina: the CAPTURE Study. Lancet 1997;349:1429–1435.

138. Inhibition of platelet glycoprotein IIb/IIIa with eptifibatide in patients with acute coronary syndromes. The PURSUIT Trial Investigators. Platelet Glycoprotein IIb/IIIa in Unstable Angina: Receptor Suppression Using Integrilin Therapy. N Engl J Med 1998;339:436–443.

139. Inhibition of the platelet glycoprotein IIb/IIIa receptor with tirofiban in unstable angina and non-Q-wave myocardial infarction. Platelet Receptor Inhibition in Ischemic Syndrome Management in Patients Limited by Unstable Signs and Symptoms (PRISM-PLUS) Study Investigators. N Engl J Med 1998;338:1488–1497.

140. Trial of abciximab with and without low-dose reteplase for acute myocardial infarction. Strategies for Patency Enhancement in the Emergency Department (SPEED) Group. Circulation 2000;101: 2788–2794.

141. Montalescot G, Barragan P, Wittenberg O, et al. Platelet glycoprotein IIb/IIIa inhibition with coronary stenting for acute myocardial infarction. N Engl J Med 2001;344:1895–1903.

142. Hirsh J, Weitz JI. New antithrombotic agents. Lancet 1999;353:1431–1436.

143. Antman EM, Cohen M, Radley D, et al. Assessment of the treatment effect of enoxaparin for unstable angina/non-Q-wave myocardial infarction. TIMI 11B-ESSENCE meta-analysis. Circulation 1999;100: 1602–1608.

144. Ross AM, Molhoek P, Lundergan C, et al. Randomized comparison of enoxaparin, a low-molecular-weight heparin, with unfractionated heparin adjunctive to recombinant tissue plasminogen activator thrombolysis and aspirin: second trial of Heparin and Aspirin Reperfusion Therapy (HART II). Circulation 2001;104:648–652.

145. Topol EJ. Reperfusion therapy for acute myocardial infarction with fibrinolytic therapy or combination reduced fibrinolytic therapy and platelet glycoprotein IIb/IIIa inhibition: the GUSTO V randomised trial. Lancet 2001;357:1905–1914.

146. Efficacy and safety of tenecteplase in combination with enoxaparin, abciximab, or unfractionated heparin: the ASSENT-3 randomised trial in acute myocardial infarction. Lancet 2001;358: 605–613.

147. Antman EM. Hirudin in acute myocardial infarction. Thrombolysis and Thrombin Inhibition in Myocardial Infarction (TIMI) 9B trial. Circulation 1996;94:911–921.

148. A comparison of recombinant hirudin with heparin for the treatment of acute coronary syndromes. The Global Use of Strategies to Open Occluded Coronary Arteries (GUSTO) IIb investigators. N Engl J Med 1996;335:775–782.

149. White H. Thrombin-specific anticoagulation with bivalirudin versus heparin in patients receiving fibrinolytic therapy for acute myocardial infarction: the HERO-2 randomised trial. Lancet 2001;358: 1855–1863.

150. Carlson SE, Aldrich MS, Greenberg HS, Topol EJ. Intracerebral hemorrhage complicating intravenous tissue plasminogen activator treatment. Arch Neurol 1988;45:1070–1073.

151. Anderson JL, Karagounis L, Allen A, Bradford MJ, Menlove RL, Pryor TA. Older age and elevated blood pressure are risk factors for intracerebral hemorrhage after thrombolysis. Am J Cardiol 1991;68: 166–170.

152. Kase CS, Pessin MS, Zivin JA, et al. Intracranial hemorrhage after coronary thrombolysis with tissue plasminogen activator. Am J Med 1992;92:384–390.

153. De Jaegere PP, Arnold AA, Balk AH, Simoons ML. Intracranial hemorrhage in association with thrombolytic therapy: incidence and clinical predictive factors. J Am Coll Cardiol 1992;19:289–294.

154. Maggioni AP, Franzosi MG, Santoro E, White H, Van de Werf F, Tognoni G. The risk of stroke in patients with acute myocardial infarction after thrombolytic and antithrombotic treatment. Gruppo Italiano per lo Studio della Sopravvivenza nell'Infarto Miocardico II (GISSI-2), and The International Study Group. N Engl J Med 1992;327:1–6.

155. Simoons ML, Maggioni AP, Knatterud G, et al. Individual risk assessment for intracranial haemorrhage during thrombolytic therapy. Lancet 1993;342:1523–1528.

156. Gore JM, Granger CB, Simoons ML, et al. Stroke after thrombolysis. Mortality and functional outcomes in the GUSTO-I trial. Global Use of Strategies to Open Occluded Coronary Arteries. Circulation 1995;92:2811–2818.

157. Randomized trial of intravenous heparin versus recombinant hirudin for acute coronary syndromes. The Global Use of Strategies to Open Occluded Coronary Arteries (GUSTO) IIa Investigators. Circulation 1994;90:1631–1637.

158. Antman EM. Hirudin in acute myocardial infarction. Safety report from the Thrombolysis and Thrombin Inhibition in Myocardial Infarction (TIMI) 9A Trial. Circulation 1994;90:1624–1630.

159. Neuhaus KL, von Essen R, Tebbe U, et al. Safety observations from the pilot phase of the randomized r-Hirudin for Improvement of Thrombolysis (HIT-III) study. A study of the Arbeitsgemeinschaft Leitender Kardiologischer Krankenhausarzte (ALKK). Circulation 1994;90:1638–1642.

160. Johnson ES, Cregeen RJ. An interim report of the efficacy and safety of anisoylated plasminogen streptokinase activator complex (APSAC). Drugs 1987;33(Suppl. 3):298–311.

161. Totty WG, Romano T, Benian GM, Gilula LA, Sherman LA. Serum sickness following streptokinase therapy. AJR Am J Roentgenol 1982;138:143–144.

162. Manoharan A, Ramsay D, Davis S, Lvoff R. Hypersensitivity vasculitis associated with streptokinase. Aust N Z J Med 1986;16:815–816.

163. Ottesen MM, Kober L, Jorgensen S, Torp-Pedersen C. Consequences of overutilization and underutilization of thrombolytic therapy in clinical practice. TRACE Study Group. TRAndolapril Cardiac Evaluation. J Am Coll Cardiol 2001;37:1581–1587.

164. Berger AK, Radford MJ, Wang Y, Krumholz HM. Thrombolytic therapy in older patients. J Am Coll Cardiol 2000;36:366–374.

165. Thiemann DR, Coresh J, Schulman SP, Gerstenblith G, Oetgen WJ, Powe NR. Lack of benefit for intravenous thrombolysis in patients with myocardial infarction who are older than 75 yr. Circulation 2000; 101:2239–2246.

166. Stenestrand U, Wallentin L. Thrombolysis is beneficial in elderly acute myocardial infarctin patients. J Am Coll Cardiol 2001:in press.

167. Sgarbossa EB, Pinski SL, Barbagelata A, et al. Electrocardiographic diagnosis of evolving acute myocardial infarction in the presence of left bundle-branch block. GUSTO-1 (Global Utilization of Streptokinase and Tissue Plasminogen Activator for Occluded Coronary Arteries) Investigators. N Engl J Med 1996;334:481–487.

168. Bottiger BW, Bode C, Kern S, et al. Efficacy and safety of thrombolytic therapy after initially unsuccessful cardiopulmonary resuscitation: a prospective clinical trial. Lancet 2001;357:1583–1585.

169. Simoons ML, Arnold AE. Tailored thrombolytic therapy. A perspective. Circulation 1993;88: 2556–2564.

170. Cairns JA, Fuster V, Gore J, Kennedy JW. Coronary thrombolysis. Chest 1995;108(Suppl. 4): 401S–423S.

171. Michels KB, Yusuf S. Does PTCA in acute myocardial infarction affect mortality and reinfarction rates? A quantitative overview (meta-analysis) of the randomized clinical trials. Circulation 1995;91: 476–485.

172. A clinical trial comparing primary coronary angioplasty with tissue plasminogen activator for acute myocardial infarction. The Global Use of Strategies to Open Occluded Coronary Arteries in Acute Coronary Syndromes (GUSTO IIb) Angioplasty Substudy Investigators. N Engl J Med 1997;336: 1621–1628.

173. Weaver WD, Simes RJ, Betriu A, et al. Comparison of primary coronary angioplasty and intravenous thrombolytic therapy for acute myocardial infarction: a quantitative review. Jama 1997;278: 2093–2098.

174. Weaver WD, Litwin PE, Martin JS. Use of direct angioplasty for treatment of patients with acute myocardial infarction in hospitals with and without on-site cardiac surgery. The Myocardial Infarction, Triage, and Intervention Project Investigators. Circulation 1993;88:2067–2075.

175. Every NR, Parsons LS, Hlatky M, Martin JS, Weaver WD. A comparison of thrombolytic therapy with primary coronary angioplasty for acute myocardial infarction. Myocardial Infarction Triage and Intervention Investigators. N Engl J Med 1996;335:1253–1260.

176. Anderson JL, Karagounis LA, Muhlestein JB. Explaining discrepant mortality results between primary percutaneous transluminal coronary angioplasty and thrombolysis for acute myocardial infarction. Am J Cardiol 1996;78:934–939.

177. Remmen JJ, Verheugt FW. The hotline sessions of the 23rd European congress of cardiology. Eur Heart J 2001;22:2033–2037.

178. Gomez MA, Anderson JL, Karagounis LA, Muhlestein JB, Mooers FB. An emergency department-based protocol for rapidly ruling out myocardial ischemia reduces hospital time and expense: results of a randomized study (ROMIO). J Am Coll Cardiol 1996;28:25–33.

179. Karagounis L, Ipsen SK, Jessop MR, et al. Impact of field-transmitted electrocardiography on time to in-hospital thrombolytic therapy in acute myocardial infarction. Am J Cardiol 1990;66:786–791.

180. Weaver WD, Cerqueira M, Hallstrom AP, et al. Prehospital-initiated vs hospital-initiated thrombolytic therapy. The Myocardial Infarction Triage and Intervention Trial. JAMA 1993;270:1211–1216.

10 Primary Angioplasty

Sorin J. Brener, MD and Eric J. Topol, MD

INTRODUCTION

In the past few years important progress has been made in the field of catheter-based reperfusion for acute ST elevation myocardial infarction (MI). In addition to the emergence of stent implantation as the treatment of choice, important emphasis has been placed on the critical role of preserving an intact microcirculation and pharmacological regimens have evolved to bridge to and facilitate mechanical reperfusion. These innovations will be discussed after a brief review of the key differences between reperfusion strategies, history of catheter-based reperfusion, and its comparison with fibrinolysis.

FIBRINOLYTIC THERAPY VS MECHANICAL REPERFUSION: KEY CONCEPTS AND DIFFERENCES

The use of fibrinolytic therapy, the most widely applied reperfusion therapy, has been extensively investigated in almost 200,000 patients enrolled in randomized clinical trials *(1–4)*. It is logistically ideal for widespread use at almost any medical facility. A few

From: *Contemporary Cardiology: Management of Acute Coronary Syndromes, Second Edition*
Edited by: C. P. Cannon © Humana Press Inc., Totowa, NJ

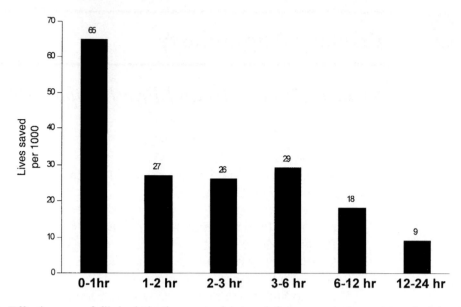

Fig. 1. Effectiveness of fibrinolytic therapy and interval from symptom onset to administration. Adapted from ref. *6*.

key concepts, corroborated by angiographic evaluation and substantial clinical follow-up, have emerged from this vast experience.

Time to Reperfusion

Acute thrombotic coronary occlusion results in a front of ischemia, leading eventually to tissue necrosis *(5)*. The resulting injury depends on the duration of the insult, the rapidity and completeness of reperfusion, presence and extent of collateral circulation, and destruction of microvasculature. Boersma et al. have shown in a systematic evaluation of fibrinolytic therapy that when applied within the first hour of symptom onset, 65 lives/1000 patients treated are saved, as compared to only 29 lives saved, when given 3 h or more from infarct onset *(6)* (Fig. 1). Similar data from the Gruppo Italiano per lo studio della sopravvivenza nell'Infarto Micardico (GISSI)-I trial *(7)* and studies of pre-hospital thrombolytic administration *(8,9)* have focused our attention on the need for very early therapy for acute MI. Regrettably, the same studies showed that only a small fraction (3–5%) of patients present within this "golden hour". In contrast, mechanical reperfusion restores flow almost simultaneously with its successful application. Although earlier mechanical reperfusion is also very desirable, a number of observations suggest that the rather direct relationship between survival and time to reperfusion existent for fibrinolysis applies less stringently in the case of angioplasty. Consistently, there is a 30–60 min additional delay to onset of therapy when comparing angioplasty with fibrinolysis. Cannon et al. *(10)* examined this complex interaction in the National Registry of Myocardial Infarction (NRMI) II. While there was no significant correlation between time from symptom onset to balloon inflation (total ischemia time) and mortality, there was a direct and steep dependency between hospital delay to angioplasty and mortality, particularly beyond 2 h of delay (Fig. 2). The first statement may not accurately account for intermittent arterial patency, while the latter is confounded by sick

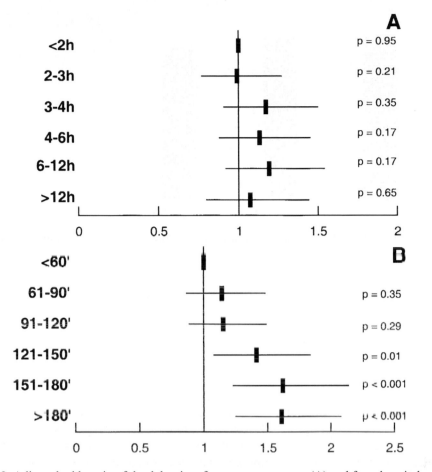

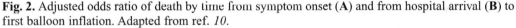

Fig. 2. Adjusted odds ratio of death by time from symptom onset (**A**) and from hospital arrival (**B**) to first balloon inflation. Adapted from ref. *10*.

patients in cardiogenic shock requiring stabilization. Nevertheless, they point to the fact that more reliable reperfusion may atone for a slightly longer delay. Indeed, similar results were obtained from other clinical trials *(11,12)*. Recently, investigators in the Stent versus Thrombolysis for Occluded Coronary Arteries in Patients with Acute Myocardial Infarction (STOP AMI) trial demonstrated that myocardial salvage index was significantly higher for angioplasty than for lysis at any interval from symptom onset and, particularly so, after the initial 3 h *(13)* (Fig. 3).

Quality of Reperfusion

Besides early administration of therapy, complete reperfusion, or Thrombolysis in MI (TIMI) 3 flow in the infarct artery at 90 min is also an extremely potent predictor of improved outcome. The primacy of rapid and sustained infarct artery patency was highlighted in the angiographic substudy of the Global Use of Strategies to Open Occluded Arteries in Acute Coronary Syndromes (GUSTO) I trial *(14)*. As compared with lesser degrees of reperfusion, TIMI 3 flow was associated with a markedly improved survival at 30 d (Fig. 4). Simes et al. *(15)* showed that the differences in the rate of TIMI 3 flow at 90 min among the four fibrinolytic regimens tested in GUSTO I explained almost

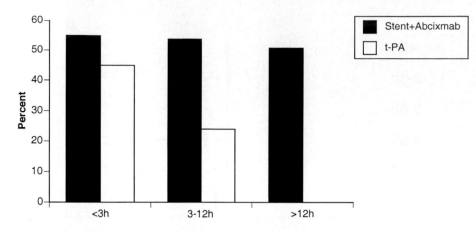

Fig. 3. Reperfusion strategy and myocardial salvage index according to time to treatment. Adapted from ref. *13.*

entirely the differences in mortality among the four groups. Retrospective analyses of other fibrinolytic trials have confirmed this observation *(16,17).* Furthermore, even when brisk antegrade flow is initially achieved with lytic therapy, substantial attrition of the benefit occurs because of intermittent patency (25%), reocclusion (13%), and impaired microvasculature, or "no-reflow" (23%) *(18).* The concept of the "illusion of reperfusion" *(19)* reflects our overestimation of the actual rate of complete reperfusion induced by lytic therapy, which probably occurs in only a quarter of those treated.

Because, as compared with optimal fibrinolytic therapy, primary angioplasty is capable of achieving TIMI 3 flow in 15–35% more patients *(14,20,21),* it is reasonable to expect that this difference in patency rates will translate into clinical benefit. As a mechanistic confirmation of the improved outcome with better patency, the relation between completeness of flow restoration with percutaneous transluminal coronary angioplasty (PTCA) and myocardial salvage was examined by Laster et al. in 180 patients enrolled in the Mayo Clinic Registry of Primary Angioplasty *(22).* TIMI 3 flow was achieved in 163 (91%) patients, TIMI 2 in 13 (7%) patients, and TIMI 0/1 in 4 (2%) patients of the group. Postangioplasty TIMI flow grade was significantly associated with infarct size and degree of myocardial salvage. In a pooled analysis of the four Primary Angioplasty in Myocardial Infarction (PAMI) trials, Stone et al. showed in nearly 2300 patients that TIMI 3 flow after angioplasty is associated with a 6-mo mortality of only 2.6%, while patients with lesser reperfusion had substantially higher mortality (6.1% for TIMI 2 and 22.2% for TIMI 0/1 flow, $p < 0.0001$) *(23).* Furthermore, preangioplasty flow had a significant impact on the ability to achieve TIMI 3 flow after angioplasty (91.5% if TIMI < 3 flow before intervention vs 98.1% if TIMI 3 flow was present), as well as on 6-mo mortality (Fig. 5). As described later in the chapter, this observation becomes important as strategies to facilitate primary angioplasty are developed.

"Temporary Vs Definitive" Reperfusion

The seminal contribution by DeWood et al. *(24)* highlighted the importance of arterial thrombus in the initiation and propagation of the events leading to myocardial necrosis. In the majority of cases, thrombus dissolution induced by lytic agents leaves behind a significant coronary stenosis, which serves as a substrate for recurrent ischemic

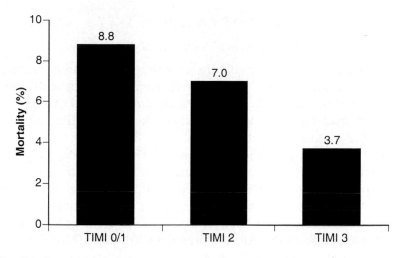

Fig. 4. Mortality (30-d) and 90-min infarct-artery TIMI flow. Adapted from ref. *17*.

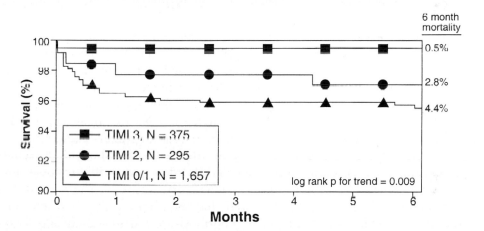

Fig. 5. Impact of pre-angioplasty TIMI flow grade on 6-mo mortality in patients undergoing mechanical reperfusion. Reproduced with permission from ref. *23*.

events. Thus, a large proportion of patients have revascularization procedures before hospital discharge, or within the first few months after an acute MI. This varies with physician preference, availability, and prevailing clinical practice. For example, among the 21,772 patients enrolled in the United States in the GUSTO I trial, 71 and 58% underwent coronary angiography and revascularization, respectively, prior to hospital discharge *(25)*. Successful primary angioplasty virtually eliminates residual high-grade stenoses in the infarct artery, at least until restenosis occurs.

Safety

The hazard of intracranial hemorrhage, especially in elderly patients with uncontrolled hypertension, constitutes another important challenge in the treatment of acute MI with fibrinolytic therapy *(26–28)*. The incidence of hemorrhagic stroke has been substantially reduced when mechanical reperfusion is applied.

PRIMARY ANGIOPLASTY

Observational Series and Registries

Many series reported the results of primary angioplasty in various settings of clinical practice. Most are small in size (<100 patients) and include patients selected for this procedure because of contraindications to lytics or institutional preference *(29–32)*. In these series, comparison with outcome of patients treated with fibrinolytic agents is not possible because of critical selection biases.

O'Keefe et al. reported from the Mid-America Heart Institute, which pioneered the procedure in the United States, on the outcome of 1000 consecutive patients treated with primary angioplasty *(33)*. The mean time from symptom onset to reperfusion was 5.4 ± 4.0 h, and 7.9% of the patients were in cardiogenic shock. Infarct artery patency (not specifically categorized as TIMI 2 or 3 flow) was 94% overall, with lower rates observed for venous bypass grafts (86%). The in-hospital mortality was 7.8% overall, and 44% in those presenting with cardiogenic shock. The global ejection fraction increased from 50% before angioplasty to 57% before discharge. Major bleeding and strokes occurred in 2.8 and 0.5%, respectively. Reocclusion was documented in 13% by angiography in selected patients before hospital discharge.

Rothbaum et al. *(29)* reported on 151 patients who underwent primary angioplasty with a success rate of 87%. In-hospital mortality was 5 and 37% for successful and failed PTCA, respectively. Most of the deaths occurred in patients with cardiogenic shock. Angiographic follow-up, performed in 70% of eligible patients at 6 mo, demonstrated restenosis in 31%. The mortality at an average follow-up of 1.7 yr was 2.2%.

The Primary Angioplasty Registry (PAR) included 271 patients treated within 12 h of symptom onset at six centers with considerable expertise in primary angioplasty *(34)*. Patients with contraindications to lytic therapy, or with cardiogenic shock were excluded from the registry. The procedural success rate (TIMI 3 flow with <50% residual stenosis), assessed by an independent angiographic laboratory, was 92%. The rates of death (4%), reinfarction (3%), and stroke (1%) were very favorable. Only 2% of those discharged from the hospital died during the 6-mo follow-up, and an additional 3% experienced a nonfatal MI *(35)*. Repeat angioplasty was performed in 16% and bypass surgery was necessary in 4%. Systematic protocol-driven repeat angiography was performed in 76% of the patients eligible for it. Almost half the patients (45%) demonstrated angiographic restenosis, including 13% with total occlusion.

The Myocardial Infarction Triage and Intervention (MITI) program in the Seattle area collated a large cohort of consecutive patients with acute MI treated with primary angioplasty (1050) or fibrinolytic therapy (2095) at 19 hospitals, between 1988 and 1994 *(36)*. Despite nonrandomized treatment allocation, the two groups were well matched with respect to age, gender, incidence of anterior infarction, and presence of high-risk characteristics *(21)* (Table 1). As expected, the time to treatment in the PTCA group exceeded that in the lytic group by almost one full hour. The in-hospital mortality was similar in the two groups, 5.5 and 5.6%, respectively. Before hospital discharge, 74 and 32% of lytic-treated patients underwent angiography and angioplasty, respectively. The initial hospitalization was significantly longer and less costly in the lysis group. The mortality at 1 and 3 yr was similar in the two groups (Fig. 6), while the use of repeat angiography and angioplasty remained higher in the angioplasty group at both intervals. The initial choice between lysis and angioplasty was not independently associated with

Table 1
The MITI Registry[a]

Characteristic	Lytic therapy n = 2095	Primary angioplasty n = 1050
Age (yr)	60 ± 12	60 ± 12
Female gender (%)	24	23
Prior infarct (%)	13	15
Prior bypass surgery (%)	6	8
Prior stroke (%)	4	7
Prior GI bleeding (%)[b]	1	3
HR > 100 bpm (%)	10	12
SBP < 100 mmHg (%)	10	12
Current anterior MI (%)	37	34
High risk (%)[c]	55	57
Time to therapy (hr)[b]	1.0 ± 1.0	1.7 ± 1.2

GI, gastrointestinal tract; MI, myocardial infarction; HR, heart rate; SBP, systolic blood pressure.
[a]Adapted from ref. 36.
[b]$p < 0.01$, all others p = NS.
[c]Based on Grines et al. (21).

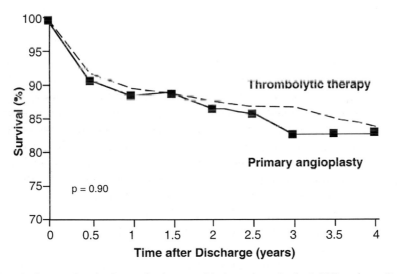

Fig. 6. Survival up to 4 yr in the angioplasty and lytic patients in the MITI registry. Reproduced with permission from ref. 36.

improved survival at 3 yr. Similar results were observed in the NRMI II cohort, in whom the in-hospital mortality (5.2 vs 5.4%), or reinfarction (2.5 vs 2.9%) were comparable for mechanical and pharmacological reperfusion, respectively (37).

Rogers et al. (38) gathered data from the Alabama Registry of Myocardial Ischemia on 1170 acute MI patients, of whom 10 and 19% were treated with primary angioplasty, and lytics, respectively, within 6 h of symptom onset. The average time to treatment was 252 and 184 min, respectively. In the lysis group, 90 and 49% had angiography and angioplasty, respectively, before hospital discharge. The in-hospital mortality was similar in the two groups. At 1 yr, 85 and 88%, respectively, were free from death and reinfarction.

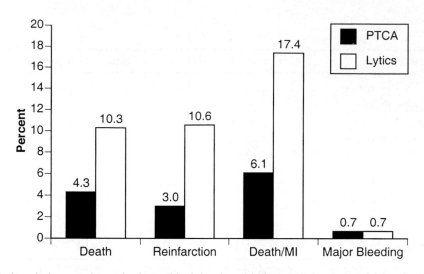

Fig. 7. In-hospital events in angioplasty (black bars) and lytic (white bars)-matched patients from the German Registry of Acute Mycardial Infarction. Adapted from ref. *40*.

The German Multicenter Registry (ALKK) accumulated data on 758 patients treated with primary angioplasty in 1994–95 *(39)*. Time to treatment was almost 6 h from symptom onset, and 17% were in cardiogenic shock. Complete reperfusion (TIMI 3 flow) was achieved in 90%. The overall in-hospital mortality was 11.5%; 3.5 and 50% in those without and with cardiogenic shock, respectively. From the same registry, Zahn et al. reported a comparative analysis of 156 and 437 patients treated with primary angioplasty and lytics, respectively *(40)*, matched by age, gender, infarct location, systolic blood pressure, and delay to treatment. Contraindication to thrombolysis were significantly more common in the angioplasty group. In-hospital death, and death and reinfarction were significantly less common in the angioplasty group, as compared with lytic-treated patients (Fig. 7). The improvement in outcome was apparent by the end of the first 48 h after treatment. The clinical benefit observed in the angioplasty group was strengthened by a low incidence of major bleeding (0.7%) and cerebral hemorrhage (0%).

Ottervanger et al. showed in 600 consecutive patients with 6-mo follow-up angiography after primary angioplasty that over half of the patients had an improvement in ejection fraction, particularly those with anterior infarction, and that the average ejection fraction improved from $44 \pm 11\%$ at discharge to $46 \pm 12\%$ at 6 mo ($p < 0.01$) *(41)*.

As equipment and adjunctive pharmacology improved, the long-term effects of primary angioplasty became more evident. Zahn et al. *(42)* analyzed two large cohorts of patients with acute MI in Germany in two registries, Maximal Individual TheRapy in Acute MI (MITRA) and the Myocardial Infarction Registry (MIR), of nearly 23,000 patients, 9906 of whom were deemed eligible for reperfusion therapy. Fibrinolysis was used in the vast majority ($n = 8759$) and was administered approx 30 min after arrival to the emergency department. The rest ($n = 1370$) underwent primary angioplasty at approx 70 min from arrival. Over the 4-yr period of patient accrual, there was a statistically significant decline in in-hospital mortality among the angioplasty patients ($p = 0.003$ for trend), while lytic-treated patients had no significant change in this outcome (Fig. 8). Furthermore, as compared with fibrinolysis, catheter-based reperfusion was

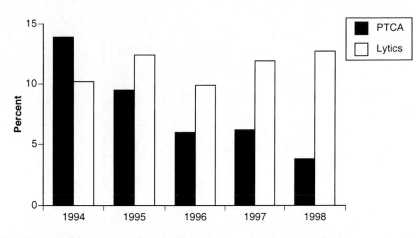

Fig. 8. Mortality in patients treated with fibrinolysis and primary angioplasty over a 4-yr period. Adapted from ref. *42*.

associated with a 46% reduction in the adjusted odds ratio of in-hospital death (95% confidence interval: 0.43–0.67).

Randomized Studies of Primary Angioplasty

Table 2 details the important characteristics of the 10 randomized studies (approx 2700 patients) *(20,21,43–50)* comparing primary angioplasty with various regimens of intravenous fibrinolytic therapy, according to time of publication. All patients were candidates for both interventions and received at least 100 mg of aspirin and an antithrombin agent for at least 2 d after the intervention. Consistently, the first balloon inflation occurred later (17–59 min) than the initiation of lytic therapy. The principal end points were assessed at hospital discharge or 30 d. Some of the studies provided additional follow-up up to 2 yr. According to the overview by Weaver et al. *(51)*, as compared to fibrinolytic therapy, primary angioplasty reduces the relative risk of death by 34%, death plus nonfatal reinfarction by 42%, and nonfatal reinfarction by 47%, by hospital discharge or 30 d. Among the various small trials, there were no differences in outcome among the lytic agents and regimens used. The absolute reduction for the above-mentioned end points was 2.1, 4.6, and 2.4%, respectively (Fig. 9). Except for GUSTO IIb, the studies were insufficiently powered to show a statistically significant difference in mortality or death and reinfarction, respectively, as demonstrated in Fig. 10.

Importantly, as compared to lytic therapy, the rate of stroke was reduced by 65% with primary angioplasty, while the incidence of hemorrhagic stroke was even more drastically affected (93% relative reduction). The difference in stroke was particularly striking in the trials using tissue-type plasminogen activator (tPA) (0.6% for PTCA vs 2.1% for tPA) and less impressive in those using streptokinase (1.0% for PTCA vs 1.6% for streptokinase). Major bleeding episodes (other than intracranial) associated with blood product transfusions were as common in the angioplasty patients (8.8%) as in the lytic group (8.4%).

The Primary Coronary Angioplasty Trials (PCAT) collaborator group followed the patients in the 10 studies mentioned above for at least 6 mo. As shown in Fig. 11, there was a substantial reduction in death and death or reinfarction among angioplasty patients, compared with those receiving pharmacological reperfusion. This advantage

Table 2
Randomized Studies of Primary Angioplasty Vs Fibrinolytic Therapy[a]

Author (reference)	Lytic agent	Duration of sx.	1° End point time	No. patients PTCA	Time to PTCA (min)	No. patients lytics	Time to lytics (min)
Dewood (42)	tPA 4 h	N/A	30 days	46	126	44	84
Grines (21)	tPA 3 h	<12 hr	discharge	195	60	200	32
Zijlstra (44)	SK 1 h	<6 hr	discharge	152	62	142	30
Gibbons (46)	tPA 4 h	<12 hr	discharge	47	45	56	20
Ribeiro (45)	SK 1 h	<6 hr	discharge	50	238	50	179
Zijlstra (50)	SK 1 h	<6 hr	30 days	45	68	50	30
Ribichini (49)	tPA 1.5 h	<6 hr	discharge	41	40	42	33
Grinfeld (48)	SK 1 h	<12 hr	30 days	54	63	58	18
GUSTO IIb (20)	tPA 1.5 h	<12 hr	30 days	565	114	573	72
Garcia (47)	tPA 1.5 h	5 hr	30 d	95	84	94	69

Sk, streptokinase.
[a]Adapted from ref. 51.

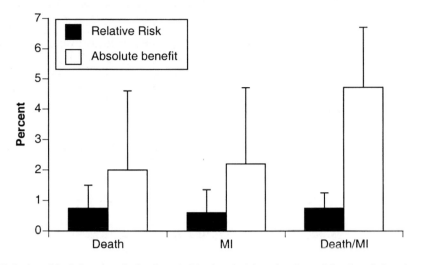

Fig. 9. Relative (black bars) and absolute (white bars) risk reduction of death, reinfarction, and death or reinfarction in 10 randomized trials of primary angioplasty vs lytic therapy. Adapted from ref. *51*.

was evident in all important subgroups, as shown in Fig. 12. The Zwolle Investigators also provided 5-yr follow-up for their cohort and showed an impressive reduction in mortality (13 vs 24% for lysis, *p* < 0.001, 46% relative risk reduction) and in reinfarction (6 vs 22%, *p* < 0.001, 73% relative risk reduction), as well as lower cost and incidence of repeat revascularization *(52)*.

All the trials mentioned above compared balloon angioplasty alone with fibrinolysis. Incorporating the latest advances in mechanical reperfusion (discussed in detail below), the STOP AMI compared the outcome of 71 patients treated with coronary stenting and adjunctive platelet inhibition with abciximab with 69 patients receiving accelerated tPA *(13)*. Beyond clinical outcome, in an attempt to identify the mechanism responsible for the advantage of angioplasty, the investigators measured infarct size and salvage index using serial sestamibi scintigraphy. As shown in Fig. 13, there was a substantial reduction in the incidence of the composite end point of ischemic and hemorrhagic complications in the mechanically reperfused patients. Furthermore, this benefit was linked to a significant reduction in final infarct size (14.3 vs 19.4%, *p* = 0.02). While the salvage index remained rather constant for angioplasty patients (50–55%, regardless of time from symptom onset), patients treated with tPA had a sharp drop-off in efficacy with later reperfusion (45% for therapy within 3 h of onset vs 24% only for patients treated between 3 and 12 h from onset) (Fig. 3).

Even though primary angioplasty appears superior to in-hospital fibrinolysis, data comparing it to prehospital administration are only now emerging. In the Comparison of Angioplasty and Pre-hospital Thrombolysis in MI (CAPTIM) trial, 840 patients with acute MI of less than 6 h were randomized to primary angioplasty (*n* = 421) or early lysis (*n* = 419). The primary end point of death, or re-MI or stroke at 30 d was attained in 6.2 and 8.2% of the two groups, respectively, *p* = 0.29. There were fewer strokes and reinfarctions in the angioplasty group, but nearly twice as many of these patients developed cardiogenic shock, compared with the lytic arm (4.9 vs 2.5%), resulting in an incidence of death of 4.8 and 3.8%, respectively. Both groups completed their assigned reperfusion strategy at nearly identical intervals from symptom onset, 215

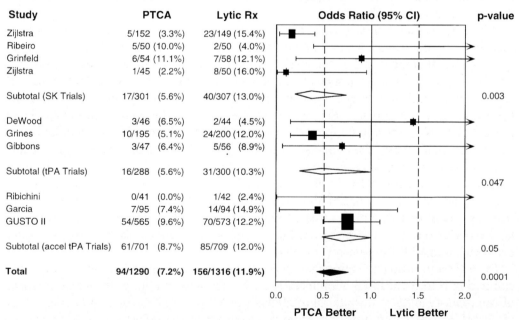

Fig. 10. Relative risk reduction in death (**A**) and death or reinfarction (**B**) in individual randomized trials of primary angioplasty vs lytic therapy. Reproduced with permission from ref. *51.*

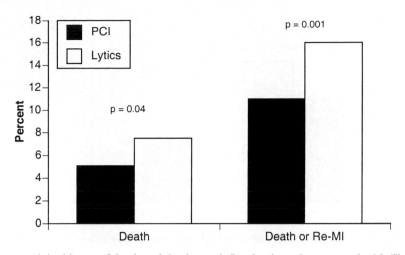

Fig. 11. Six-month incidence of death and death or reinfarction in patients treated with fibrinolysis or mechanical reperfusion. From the PCAT Investigators.

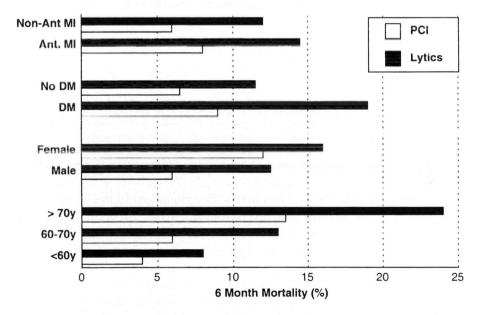

Fig. 12. Benefit of mechanical reperfusion over fibrinolysis in predefined subgroups ($p \leq 0.05$ for all). From the PCAT Investigators.

and 220 min, respectively. A third of the lytic patients required emergency rescue angioplasty *(53)*.

Two other aspects of mechanical reperfusion for acute MI were examined by the PAMI II Investigators in a trial in which all suitable patients received mechanical reperfusion *(54)*. They tested the hypotheses that early angiography identifies patients at high risk of in-hospital death based on coronary anatomy and ventricular function and that intra-aortic counterpulsation (IABP) may improve the patency of the infarct-related artery after primary angioplasty in patients at high risk for recurrent ischemia. One thousand and ninety nine patients were identified within 12 h of symptom onset of acute ST elevation

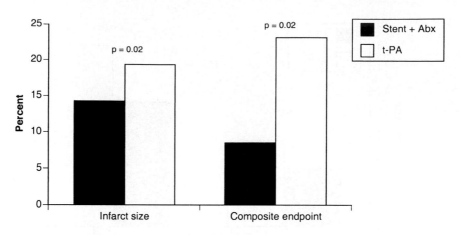

Fig. 13. Six-month outcome in the STOP AMI trial. Data from ref. *13*.

Table 3
Criteria for Low Risk Classification in the PAMI II Study[a]

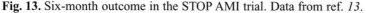

Age < 70 yr
EF > 45%
1 or 2 vessel disease
Native culprit artery
Successful PTCA
No (recurrence of) ventricular arrhythmia

[a]Adapted from ref. *54*.

MI, including fibrinolytic-therapy-ineligible patients. Of the 908 patients entered in the study, emergency angiography identified 437 and 471 patients at high and low risk, respectively, for in-hospital death. The criteria for assignment to the low-risk status are shown in Table 3. The in-hospital event rates are shown in Fig. 14. Importantly, there were no death or reinfarction in the week following discharge in low-risk patients randomized to early discharge without functional testing. Early angiography and angioplasty indeed identified a low-risk group of patients with mortality comparable to that of elective angioplasty patients. IABP did not confer a significant advantage in death, reinfarction, or reocclusion in the high-risk patients. Nevertheless, IABP was associated with a significantly lower need for repeat angiography and repeat PTCA of the infarct-artery in these patients.

ADVANCES IN PRIMARY ANGIOPLASTY: DEVICES AND PHARMACOLOGY

Although the immediate results of primary angioplasty are quite satisfactory, the rate of restenosis and recurrent clinical events remained disappointing. Nakagawa et al. studied survivors of acute MI treated with primary balloon angioplasty from the angiographic standpoint *(55)*. The cumulative rates of restenosis and reocclusion at 3 wk, 4 mo, and 1 yr were 8.8 and 12%, 29 and 14%, 33 and 14%, respectively. Thus, restenosis was very prevalent in this cohort, while reocclusion was less frequent and tended to occur early in the follow-up period (Fig. 15).

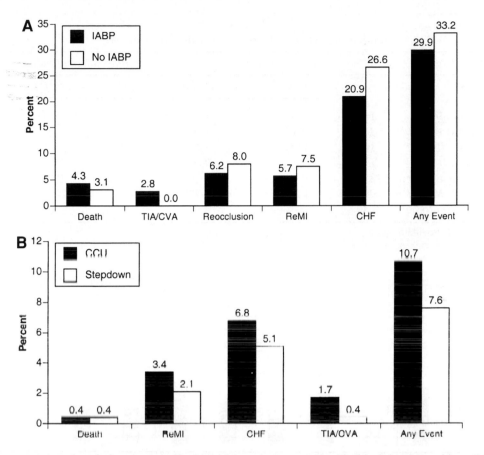

Fig. 14. (A) In-hospital event rates for high risk patients treated with (black bars) or without IABP (white bars) in the PAMI II study. **(B)** In-hospital event rates for low risk patients randomized to intensive care (black bars) or stepdown (white bars) care in the PAMI II study.(Adapted from ref. *54.*)

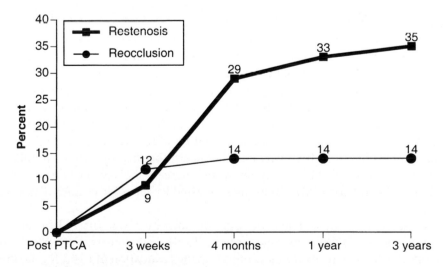

Fig. 15. Incidence of angiographic restenosis and reocclusion in primary angioplasty patients. Reproduced with permission from ref. *55.*

Table 4
Randomized Trials of Coronary Stenting in Acute MI

Study (reference)	N	Death		Composite end point	
		Stent	PTCA	Stent	PTCA
FRESCO (56)	150	0%	1%	9%	28%[a]
STENTIM II (57)	211	3%	1.9%	19%	27%
GRAMI (58)	104	3.8%	7.6%	17%	35%[a]
PASTA (59)	136	5%	7%	21%	46%[a]
Suryapranata (60)	227	2%	3%	5%	20%[a]
STENT PAMI (61)	900	4.2%	2.7%	13%	20%
CADILLAC (63)	2082	3.3%	4.0%	10.9%	15.7%

[a]Author: provide footnote

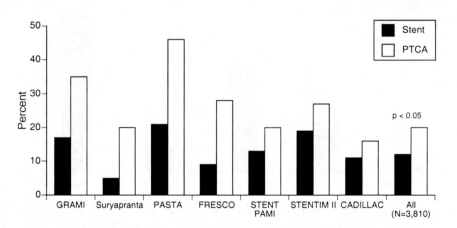

Fig. 16. Six-month incidence of ischemic complications following randomization to stent or balloon angioplasty in acute MI. Adapted from refs. *58–63.*

As coronary stent implantation became the preferred modality of revascularization after the deployment technique and adjunctive dual antiplatelet were perfected, seven randomized trials of stent implantation (and one consecutive series) in acute MI were completed *(56–63)* (Table 4). Important differences existed among the studies with respect to methodology, follow-up, and rate of cross-over. Nevertheless, in aggregate, the results indicate that, at least in low-risk patients, the mortality is very low in both arms and stenting is more effective in preventing reinfarction and repeat infarct artery revascularization (Fig. 16). There was initial concern that deployment of a bulky stent in a thrombus-laden vessel at high pressure would increase the extent of distal embolization and reduce the rate of TIMI 3 flow, as suggested by the STENT PAMI and STENTIM-2 trials.

A partial solution to the problem of distal embolization was offered by the use of aggressive platelet inhibition with glycoprotein IIb/IIIa antagonists. First observed in a small cohort of patients with evolving acute MI in the Evaluation of c7E3 for the Prevention of Ischemic Complications (EPIC) study *(64)*, the benefit of abciximab therapy during primary angioplasty was confirmed in four randomized clinical trials: The Neumann

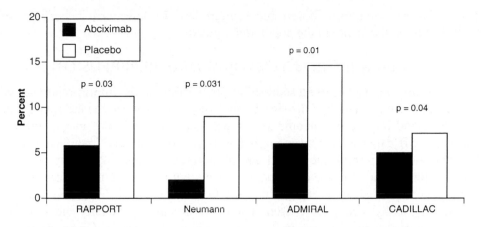

Fig. 17. Thirty-day ischemic events in trials of primary angioplasty with or without abciximab. Adapted from refs. *63* and *65–67*.

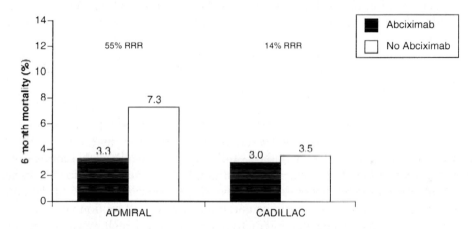

Fig. 18. Incidence of death at 6 mo in the CADILLAC and ADMIRAL trials. Adapted from refs. *63* and *67*.

(Munich) trial, ReoPro and Primary PTCA Organization and Randomized Trial (RAP-PORT), Abciximab before Direct Angioplasty and Stenting in Myocardial Infarction Regarding Long-Term Follow-up (ADMIRAL), and Controlled Abciximab and Device Investigation to Lower Late Angioplasty Complications (CADILLAC) *(63,65–67)*. The incidence of major ischemic events at 30 d was reduced in all trials by abciximab, as shown in Fig. 17. Nevertheless, there was substantial heterogeneity in 6-mo outcome, particularly between the ADMIRAL and CADILLAC studies. Fig. 18 illustrates these differences and highlights the difficulty of comparisons across trials. In ADMIRAL, patients with cardiogenic shock (8%, mortality nearly 80%) were enrolled, while the presence of cardiogenic shock was an exclusion criterion in CADILLAC. Furthermore, nearly a quarter of patients in ADMIRAL received abciximab before angiography, a practice not permitted in CADILLAC. Indeed, the benefit of abciximab was particularly evident in the early treatment group suggesting facilitation of the coronary intervention. Altogether, it appears that abciximab adjunctive therapy reduces early ischemic complications such as abrupt closure, stent thrombosis, and reinfarction. Its long-term benefit is directly dependent upon the acuity of the population treated.

EPICARDIAL AND MYOCARDIAL REPERFUSION

Beyond the importance of reestablishing TIMI 3 flow in the infarct-related artery, we became increasingly aware of the significance of the integrity of the microcirculation in immediate and long-term outcome after reperfusion therapy (68). In general, patients with acute MI experience a systemic hyperactivity of platelets, manifested by slower flow than normal in both the infarct and noninfarct arteries (69). Many retrospective analyses demonstrated worse outcome in patients with impaired microcirculation, even in the presence of adequate epicardial reperfusion (18,70–72). The "no-reflow" phenomenon typically results either from distal embolization of platelet and fibrin thrombus or from destruction of the capillaries by prolonged ischemia. Furthermore, there is spasm and endothelial dysfunction from secretion of vasoactive substances from embolized platelets, as well as reperfusion injury resulting from neutrophil and complement accumulation in the infarcted territory. Distal embolization can be attenuated by adjunctive therapy with platelet IIb/IIIa inhibition. As demonstrated by Neumann et al. (65), patients undergoing angioplasty with abciximab had more improvement in regional and global ejection fraction than those treated with heparin alone. Similar results were obtained in the ADMIRAL study (67). Capillary destruction can be prevented by more rapid reperfusion. Indeed, Sheiban et al. (73) showed that left ventricular systolic function improved gradually only in patients in whom TIMI 3 flow is restored within 4 h of symptom onset. In those with more delayed reperfusion, there was no unfavorable remodeling, with preservation of end-diastolic and end-systolic volumes. Clinical outcome was remarkably similar in all patients with reperfusion. In another analysis of 199 patients with primary angioplasty for acute anterior MI, Iwakura et al. (74) identified the predictors of no-reflow, which occurred in 39% of the cohort. TIMI 0 flow, Q waves, pre-infarct angina and more severe wall motion abnormality on admission were the sole independent predictors of no-reflow, which was associated with a higher peak creatine kinase isoenzyme-cardiac muscle subunit (CK-MB) (3883 ± 2173 vs 1869 ± 1303 IU/L, $p < 0.001$).

Gibson et al. used the myocardial blush apparent after coronary opacification to grade the degree of microvasculature dysfunction after reperfusion. Combining epicardial TIMI flow grade with the Tissue Myocardial Perfusion (TMP) grade, one can better stratify risk of death after reperfusion (75,76) (Fig. 19). Even more importantly, TMP grade can further risk stratify patients with TIMI 3 flow (76) (Fig. 20).

RESCUE AND FACILITATED ANGIOPLASTY

Rescue angioplasty typically refers to catheter-based reperfusion following failed therapy with fibrinolysis. Ellis et al. (77) performed a meta-analysis of 11 series of rescue angioplasty, mostly observational, and found that in patients with moderate and large MIs, there was an advantage in survival (92 vs 87%, $p = 0.01$), reinfarction (3.8 vs 11.7%, $p < 0.05$), and occurrence of heart failure (4.3 vs 11.3%, $p < 0.05$), compared with conservative therapy. The largest randomized trial of rescue angioplasty in patients with TIMI 0 to 1 flow after lytic therapy for acute anterior MI also showed a reduction in the 30-d composite of death, reinfarction, or heart failure (16.6 vs 6.4%, $p < 0.05$)

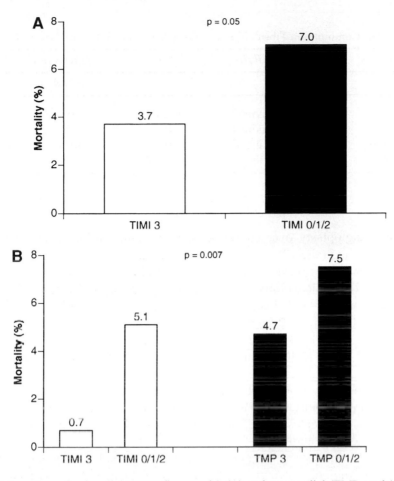

Fig. 19. Integration of epicardial (TIMI flow grade) (**A**) and myocardial (TMP grade) (**B**) perfusion in patients receiving pharmacological reperfusion therapy for acute MI. Adapted from ref. 75.

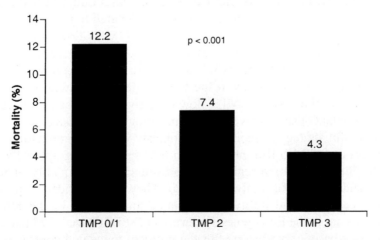

Fig. 20. Impact of TMP grade in patients with TIMI 3 flow after mechanical reperfusion therapy. Adapted from ref. 76.

Table 5
Trials of Combination Fibrinolysis and GP IIb/IIIa Inhibitors in Acute MI

Study (reference)	N	GP IIb/IIIa	Lytic	TIMI 3 flow at 60'	
				Combination	Control
TIMI 14 *(83)*	888	Abciximab	tPA, rPA	63%	45%[a]
SPEED *(84)*	465	Abciximab	rPA	54%	47%
INTRO-AMI *(85)*	649	Eptifibatide	tPA	56%	40%[a]
INTEGRITI *(86)*	189	Eptifibatide	TNK-tPA	67%	N/A

Tnk, tenecteplase.
[a]$p < 0.05$.

favoring rescue angioplasty over conservative management *(78)*. These data reflect mostly the work done in the 1980s and early 1990s, when the success of rescue angioplasty was only 80–90% (TIMI 3 flow without reinfarction). More recently, in the GUSTO III trial *(79)*, patients undergoing rescue angioplasty had a lower mortality at 30 d when abciximab was added compared with standard anticoagulation with heparin (3.6 vs 9.7%, $p = 0.04$). Data from the TIMI 14 study confirm that rescue angioplasty is safe in patients with failed lysis, resulting in a mortality of 5.5% and an incidence of ischemic events of 10.7% at 30 d, considerably better than in historical series of rescue angioplasty *(80)*.

As primary angioplasty is available around the clock in a minority of centers in the United States and the importance of arterial patency before angioplasty has been well established *(23,81)*, strategies geared to achieve arterial patency and thus facilitate angioplasty are intensely studied.

Reduced-dose fibrinolysis as a prelude to angioplasty has been studied in the Plasminogen-activator Angioplasty Compatibility Trial (PACT) *(82)*. It compared the administration of single-bolus tPA (50 mg) or placebo followed by immediate angiography and rescue angioplasty (if TIMI < 3 flow exists) or completion of the pharmacological regimen if normal flow was present. While patients receiving 50 mg tPA had a higher rate of TIMI 2 + 3 flow on initial angiogram than those allocated to placebo (61 vs 34%, $p < 0.001$), there was no difference in the final rate of TIMI 3 flow after rescue angioplasty for TIMI < 3 flow (77 and 79%, respectively). At 30 d, there was no difference in mortality (3.6 vs 3.3%), reinfarction (3.0 vs 2.6%), or major bleeding (12.6 vs 13.5%) between the tPA and placebo groups, respectively. The patients with best recovery of systolic function were those with TIMI 3 flow on arrival to angiography, regardless of whether it was spontaneously achieved or pharmacologically induced.

A more successful strategy to facilitate angioplasty was the combination of reduced dose fibrinolytics and GP IIb/IIIa inhibitors. In four small angiographically controlled trials (Table 5), the combination regimens improved speed and quality of reperfusion compared to standard-dose fibrinolysis *(83–86)*. They also provided important information on the feasibility and utility of facilitated angioplasty. In the Strategies for Patency Enhancement in the Emergency Department (SPEED) trial, 323 patients underwent early catheter-based reperfusion after the protocol-mandated control angiography at 60 min, and 123 did not *(87)*. Compared to patients treated conservatively, those undergoing facilitated angioplasty had significantly less reinfarction, (1.2 vs 4.9%, $p =$

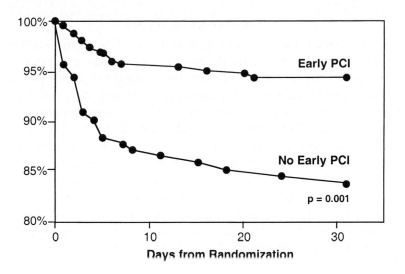

Fig. 21. Clinical outcome of patients undergoing facilitated angioplasty or treated conservatively after combination platelet and fibrin lysis. Reproduced with permission from ref. *87.*

0.003) and a significantly lower incidence of death, reinfarction, or urgent revascularization (Fig. 21). Patients receiving the combination of abciximab and low-dose reteplase (rPA) had a significantly higher incidence of TIMI 3 flow before angioplasty than those receiving abciximab alone or full dose rPA (47 vs 24 vs 39%, $p = 0.05$, respectively) as well as a higher incidence of major bleeding (8.8 vs 2.7 vs 3.6%, respectively, $p = 0.24$).

TARGETED SUBGROUPS FOR PRIMARY ANGIOPLASTY

While primary angioplasty is an alternative to lytic therapy in most reperfusion candidates, certain subgroups of patients are particularly suited for immediate angiography and primary angioplasty, in view of the poor outcome or hazard associated with lytic therapy.

Absolute and Relative Contraindications for Lytic Therapy

In a pooled analysis of eight trials of fibrinolytic therapy, enrolling more than 50,000 patients, only a third of those screened (range 9–51%) were eventually enrolled. Few patients have absolute contraindications to lytic therapy, such as recent bleeding episodes, major surgery, or previous stroke with residual neurological deficits. The common reasons for exclusion were relative contraindications, such as presentation later than 6 h from symptom onset (13–37%), advanced age with its inherent increased risk of intracranial hemorrhage (2–31%), and lack of "classical" electrocardiographic findings (11–62%) *(88,89).* Although the Worcester Heart Attack Study Group reported a 175% increase in the use of lytics in acute MI between 1986 and 1993, still only 25.5% of those screened received the therapy *(90).* Subjects younger than 55 yr were 4.5× more likely to receive it than patients older than 75 yr. Since it is well established that ineligibility for thrombolytic therapy is associated with a 4- to 8-fold increase in 30-d mortality *(91),* such patients should be considered for mechanical reperfusion *(92).*

Cardiogenic Shock

Cardiogenic shock is the result of substantial loss of myocardial function (>40% of left ventricular mass) in 80%, or the development of mechanical complications in 20% of those in whom it occurs *(93,94)*. Historically, cardiogenic shock was associated with an exceedingly poor prognosis, with mortality averaging 70% *(94–96)*. Temporizing measures, such as intra-aortic counterpulsation and inotropic support do not affect survival in the absence of reperfusion. Overall, fibrinolytic agents have not favorably affected the survival in these patients, probably because of poor delivery of the drug to the infarct site. Patients with cardiogenic shock were infrequently enrolled in fibrinolytic trials. In GISSI I *(7)*, 146 and 134 patients with cardiogenic shock (Killip class 4) were randomized to streptokinase and placebo, respectively. The mortality at 21 d was 70% in both groups. In contrast, two other placebo-controlled studies documented a modest mortality reduction in patients assigned to fibrinolysis, as compared to placebo *(97,98)*. In the GISSI II International Study *(99)* the in-hospital mortality of patients with cardiogenic shock assigned to tPA (80 patients, 100 mg over 3 h) or streptokinase (93 patients) was 78 and 65% ($p = 0.04$), respectively. In GUSTO I, 315 patients presented in cardiogenic shock and were evenly distributed among the four lytic regimens *(100)*. Patients assigned to streptokinase-based regimens tended to have a lower mortality than those assigned to tPA (51 vs 57%, respectively). In selected patients who underwent rescue angioplasty, the survival was improved (43%) compared to those who did not undergo revascularization (77%). Obviously, patients who did not undergo emergency angiography and revascularization were more likely to be critically ill, than those referred for intervention.

Mechanical reperfusion for patients with cardiogenic shock has been studied extensively in observational series. Among 539 patients in 16 studies (7–81 patients each) *(93)*, the average mortality was 50%. When reperfusion was successful, the fatality rate was only 35%, while failure to restore flow was associated with a mortality of 84%. None of these studies had an adequate control or alternative therapy arm. An international registry *(94)* prospectively followed 251 patients with cardiogenic shock (8% due to mechanical complications). Among those selected on clinical grounds for emergency angiography and revascularization, the mortality was 51% as compared to 85% in those treated conservatively.

The Should We Emergently Revascularize Occluded Coronaries for Cardiogenc Shock (SHOCK) trial was a randomized trial dedicated to examine the role of immediate revascularization in patients with cardiogenic shock *(101)*. Among 302 patients enrolled, those allocated to early revascularization (angioplasty performed within 1 h of diagnosis in 50%) had a significantly higher survival at 6 mo than those stabilized medically (65 vs 54%, $p = 0.04$), which was maintained at 1 yr (Fig. 22). Particular benefit was observed among those younger than 75 yr.

Thus, because of the generally unsatisfactory results of fibrinolytic therapy and the potential for improved outcome with mechanical reperfusion, this subset of patients represents an important target for primary angioplasty.

Prior Bypass Surgery

These patients tend to have a less favorable result with lytic therapy, especially when saphenous vein grafts are the culprit conduits. In the GUSTO I trial, there was a higher mortality rate in patients with, than without, prior bypass surgery treated with lytics at 30

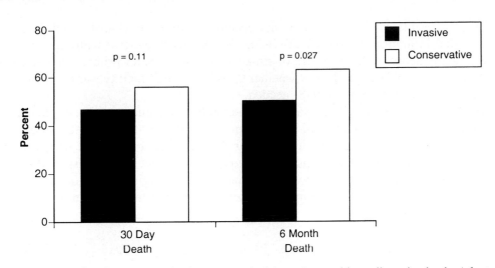

Fig. 22. Impact of early revascularization on survival in patients with cardiogenic shock. Adapted from ref. *101*.

d (10.7 vs 6.7%, respectively). Although not proven in clinical randomized trials, mechanical revascularization when available promptly, may improve outcome in this subgroup.

Diagnostic Uncertainty: Early Triage Angiography

Some patients present with atypical symptoms, or signs, which preclude immediate administration of fibrinolytic therapy, because of the uncertainty that an MI is evolving. Emergency angiography, with subsequent primary angioplasty upon identification of a culprit artery, may afford an immediate diagnosis and therapy and eliminate the risk of exposing the patient to an unneeded and potentially dangerous therapy. McCullough et al. reported on a randomized study of early triage angiography vs conservative therapy in 197 patients ineligible for lytic therapy *(102)*. Revascularization was performed in 52 and 35% of the two groups, respectively. The early angiography group had a significantly lower rate of recurrent ischemia (14 vs 33%) and markedly reduced hospital stay.

Availability of On-Site Facilities

Approximately 20% of the hospitals in the United States are equipped with the facilities and personnel necessary to provide primary angioplasty 24 h/d. Patients having the onset of acute MI in such an institution, or being able to reach it rapidly, are obvious candidates for mechanical revascularization. More controversial is the transfer of candidates for either pharmacological or mechanical therapy from institutions not geared for primary angioplasty to one able to offer this service. For patients who present with cardiogenic shock, or with absolute contraindications to fibrinolytic therapy, consideration for such a transfer is particularly vital.

The Primary Angioplasty in Patients Transferred from General Community Hospitals to Specialized Units with or without Emergency Thrombolysis (PRAGUE) trial randomized 300 patients to streptokinase, streptokinase and transfer for angioplasty, or transfer for primary angioplasty without fibrinolysis, after administration of aspirin and heparin. At 30 d the composite of death, reinfarction, or stroke occurred in 23, 15 and 8%, respectively, $p < 0.001$, demonstrating that transfer is safe and effective *(103)*.

Similar results were obtained in the recently completed Danish Trial in Acute Myocardial Infarction (DANAMI-2) *(103a)*. Among 1,129 patients with high-risk features, the incidence of death, re-MI, or stroke at 30 d was 8% for primary PCI and 14% for lyrics ($p = 0.003$). regardless of whether transfer to a PCI facility was (9 vs 14%, $p = 0.002$) or not (7 vs 12%, $p = 0.048$) needed.

Traditionally, primary PTCA was performed only in institutions with surgical backup. Such an approach is supported by the frequent incidence of multivessel disease discovered during acute angiography, as well as the need to salvage patients with unsuccessful PTCA. Recent advances in the equipment and techniques, especially coronary stents, have minimized the incidence of unsuccessful angioplasty and led to a more aggressive approach, favoring immediate intervention upon the risk of transferring an unstable patient *(103b)*.

TECHNICAL ASPECTS OF PRIMARY ANGIOPLASTY

The patient with an evolving MI should be brought to the catheterization suite as soon as the decision to perform emergency angiography was reached. Aspirin (at least 325 mg) and up to 4000 U (50 U/kg) of heparin should be administered, while obtaining at least two intravenous access lines. Larger doses of heparin may be detrimental if platelet glycoprotein IIb/IIIa inhibitors are to be administered later during the procedure. These agents can even be infused as preparations for angiography are made or in the Emergency Department, in an attempt to enhance patency of the infarct-related artery and facilitate intervention *(67)*. Intravenous nitroglycerin and morphine are helpful in controlling symptoms, if hemodynamic status allows it. Both groins should be prepared for access, in case intra-aortic counterpulsation or percutaneous bypass are needed. Six French arterial sheaths are typically sufficient for most coronary interventions. Regular contrast agents can be used, unless severe left ventricular dysfunction or pulmonary edema exist. Nonionic preparations have been associated with enhanced platelet aggregability *(104)*. A left ventriculogram, preceded by measurement of left ventricular end-diastolic pressure, is very helpful in assessing degree of dysfunction before reperfusion and unsuspected mechanical complications. It is contraindicated in the presence of cardiogenic shock or severe respiratory distress. The noninfarct artery should be visualized first to assess extent of coronary disease and presence of collateral flow. Finally, the suspected infarct-related artery should be engaged with a guiding catheter, in anticipation of primary angioplasty. The size of the occluded artery can be estimated from its proximal portion. Usually, a soft tip wire is sufficient to cross the thrombus-laden lesion. Rarely, a stiffer wire or additional support with a balloon are needed for crossing. Intubation of branches is helpful in ensuring intraluminal guidewire advancement. If doubt persists, the balloon can be advanced distally and a small amount of contrast can be injected via the wire port to assess the distal vessel. Direct stenting should be considered when anatomy permits, particularly if the artery is patent on initial angiogram. Not infrequently, stent implantation results in transient diminution in flow, which usually responds to adenosine (18–48 μg intracoronary) or verapamil (100–200 micrograms intracoronary) or nitroprusside (100–400μg intracoronary). If distal embolization of plaque and thrombus is very profound, support with intra-aortic counterpulsation and intracoronary tPA (10–40 mg) may be helpful in restoring normal flow. Balloon deflation may result in "reperfusion arrhythmia," especially with inferior infarcts. Defibrillation may be necessary and the equipment should be readily available. Rarely, the only way to interrupt the electrical storm is to reinflate the balloon and administer anti-arrhythmic therapy. A pulmonary artery catheter may be placed to facilitate hemodynamic management in patients with complicated procedures. Transvenous temporary pacemakers are rarely needed for treatment of persistent bradycardia or high degree atrioventricular block. Intravenous heparin after the intervention is rarely needed, particularly if the angiographic results is satisfactory and platelet IIb/IIIa inhibition is administered. Standard adjunctive pharmacology, coronary risk factor modification, and rehabilitative care for post-MI patients is subsequently provided.

If the culprit vessel is a venous bypass graft, local infusion of a small dose of tPA may be beneficial, although the risk of distal embolization is high. Platelet activation caused by the lytic agent can further exacerbate the thrombotic tendency and can be attenuated by concomitant platelet IIb/IIIa inhibition. The transluminal extraction catheter (TEC) has been utilized (105) to facilitate thrombus extraction. One hundred patients were prospectively studied, after experiencing lytic failure (40%), postinfarction angina (28%), or cardiogenic shock (11%). A large thrombus was observed in 66% of the patients. The culprit vessel was an occluded saphenous vein bypass in 29%. Recanalization of the infarct artery was achieved in 94%. In-hospital death occurred in 5%. At 6 mo, target vessel revascularization was necessary in 38%, and a disappointing angiographic restenosis rate of 68% was noted. These results tempered the use of this device in the setting of acute MI. Its use may be rejuvenated by the combination of platelet receptor blockade and stenting, following thrombus extraction. More recently, a new suction device (Angiojet™) has been introduced and has shown promising results. In the Vein Graft AngioJet study (VEGAS) II trial, 77% of acute MI patients treated with Angiojet aspiration and stenting achieved TIMI 3 flow, and 75% of them were free of ischemic recurrence at 30 d.

In 5–10% of patients (21), emergency angiography reveals either a patent infarct artery without severe stenosis or severe and diffuse coronary disease (including left main coronary stenosis), which is better suited for surgical revascularization. For the latter case, primary angioplasty may still be indicated, if feasible, to prevent myocardial damage and enable the performance of semielective coronary bypass surgery and use of arterial conduits.

ECONOMIC ASPECTS OF PRIMARY ANGIOPLASTY

The expense incurred in treating patients with primary angioplasty is comprised of the cost of maintaining a 24-h availability for this procedure and the cost of the equipment and resources consumed during the actual procedure. Lieu et al. (106) determined that the additional cost of the procedure is only $1597 if the hospital already has 24-h coverage for acute coronary interventions. In contrast, if night call for the support personnel were a new expense, the cost would increase to at least $3206 for each procedure (assuming 200 patients/yr). A hospital envisioning building a new catheterization suite to provide primary angioplasty services would spend $3866–14,339 for the same volume, per case.

From the PAMI I study, Stone et al. (107) reported the cost analysis of 90% of the patients enrolled in the study. Total hospital charges (including professional fees) were similar in the PTCA and tPA groups. At a mean follow-up of 2.1 yr, there were no significant differences in late events, such as death, reinfarction, revascularization, or recurrence of unstable angina, suggesting similar late resource consumption. Similar results were obtained from the Dutch primary angioplasty study *(108)*. In the Mayo Clinic randomized trial of primary angioplasty and lytic therapy, the in-hospital costs were similar in the two groups, but the late costs were increased in the lytic group, because of increased need for angiography and revascularization *(46)*.

In the PAMI II study, analysis of cost in a small subset of low-risk patients revealed marked savings in those allocated to early discharge, as compared to standard care following primary angioplasty.

The GUSTO IIb Investigators reported the cost analysis in a subset of patients enrolled in the primary angioplasty study (374 out of 1138) *(109)*. The costs were remarkably similar for angioplasty and tPA patients both in-hospital and at 6 mo.

In contrast, the large observational series from the MITI registry *(36)* suggested that both the in-hospital cost and subsequent resource utilization over 3 yr were higher in the angioplasty, as compared to the lytic group.

LIMITATIONS OF PRIMARY ANGIOPLASTY

In order to make percutaneous mechanical revascularization strategy preferable to fibrinolytic therapy in most patients with an evolving MI, the following limitations and obstacles have to be overcome: (*i*) the need for dedicated expert personnel 24 h/d. Hospitals and operators with higher volume of primary angioplasty tend to have the lowest rate of mortality and morbidity *(110,111)*; (*ii*) a longer delay to reperfusion in most instances, especially during off-hours; and (*iii*) intensive resource utilization, especially with the widespread use of coronary stents and potent platelet inhibitors.

These limitations have to be weighed against the potential for more complete reperfusion, avoidance of recurrent ischemic events, faster hospital discharge, and better rehabilitation afforded by primary PTCA. These constraints obviously do not apply to patients who are not candidates for lytic therapy.

CURRENT GUIDELINES FOR PRIMARY ANGIOPLASTY

The American College of Cardiology and American Heart Association Task Force has recently updated the comprehensive recommendations for the management of acute MI *(112)*. Under these guidelines, primary angioplasty is strongly advised (Class I, Level of evidence A) as an alternative to fibrinolytic therapy, "only if performed in a timely (90 ± 30 min from hospital arrival) fashion by individuals skilled in the procedure (>75 PTCA cases/yr) and supported by personnel in high-vol centers (>200 PTCA cases/yr)". It is also recommended for patients younger than 75 yr in cardiogenic shock within 36 h of infarct onset (Class I, Level of evidence A). Less enthusiastic support is offered for its use in patients at risk for bleeding (Class IIa, Level of evidence C). The authors further stress the need for skilled operators who have consistent high rates of success (i.e., TIMI 3 flow in at least 90% of patients, emergency coronary artery bypass graft [CABG] in less than 5%, and overall mortality below 12%).

SUMMARY AND RECOMMENDATIONS

Restoration of brisk antegrade flow in the infarct-related artery is the principal goal in the initial phase of management of acute MI. Consequently, the choice of therapy needs to be tailored to the patient's presenting signs and symptoms, institutional capabilities, timing of presentation, existing comorbid conditions, and patient and physician preference.

The following statements and recommendations are, inherently, assuming "ideal" circumstances and need to be adjusted to the local conditions. There are insufficient data to weigh the benefit of surgical back up in all institutions performing primary angioplasty, against the delay created by trying to secure it.

Primary angioplasty is the preferred reperfusion strategy in patients who present to an experienced facility, where the procedure can be performed (i.e., TIMI 3 flow achieved), within 60–120 min of presentation.

Primary angioplasty is the preferred strategy in patients (<75 yr old) with cardiogenic shock presenting to an institution with the appropriate facilities. Elsewhere, a trial of lytic therapy may be warranted, while transfer to a catheterization laboratory for possible rescue angioplasty is arranged.

Primary angioplasty should be strongly considered in patients with previous bypass surgery, or large infarctions (anterolateral, or extensive inferoposterior involvement), especially with hemodynamic compromise. This is predicated on the ability to perform emergency angiography and angioplasty within 60–120 min of presentation.

Primary angioplasty should be strongly considered in all patients with ST elevation acute MI and absolute contraindications to lytic therapy (bleeding hazard), even if its performance may mandate rapid hospital transfer with appropriate medical supervision.

Emergency angiography and angioplasty (when appropriate) should be undertaken in patients with long presentation delay (>12 h) or in cases of atypical presentations and diagnostic uncertainty.

When anatomy permits, stent implantation should be preferred to balloon angioplasty alone.

Aggressive adjunctive therapy with platelet GP IIb/IIIa inhibitors should be considered in all patients undergoing primary angioplasty, particularly in those at high risk for recurrent ischemia or cardiogenic shock.

REFERENCES

1. Fibrinolytic Therapy Trialists' (FTT) Collaborative Group. Indications for fibrinolytic therapy in suspected acute myocardial infarction: collaborative overview of early mortality and major morbidity results from all randomised trials of more than 1000 patients. Lancet 1994;343:311–322.
2. The GUSTO Investigators. An international randomized trial comparing four thrombolytic strategies for acute myocardial infarction. N Engl J Med 1993;329:673–682.
3. ISIS 3 (Third International Study of Infarct Survival) Collaborative Group. A randomized trial of streptokinase vs tissue plasminogen activator vs. anistreplase and of aspirin plus heparin vs. aspirin alone among 41,299 cases of suspected acute myocardial infarction. Lancet 1992;339:753.
4. Gruppo Italiano per lo Studia della Sopravvivenza nell'Infarto Miocardico. GISSI 2: a factorial randomized trial of alteplase vs streptokinase and heparin vs no heparin among 12,490 patients with acute myocardial infarction. Lancet 1990;336:65.
5. Reimer KA, Vander Heide RS, Richard VJ. Reperfusion in acute myocardial infarction: effect of timing and modulating factors in experimental models. Am J Cardiol 1993;72:13G–21G.
6. Boersma E, Maas CP, Deckers JW, Simoons ML. Early thrombolytic treatment in acute myocardial infarction: reappraisal of the golden hour. Lancet 1996;348:771–775.
7. Gruppo Italiano per lo Studia della Sopravvivenza nell'Infarto Miocardico. Effectiveness of intravenous thrombolytic treatment in acute myocardial infarction. Lancet 1986;1:397–401.
8. Boissel JP. The European Myocardial Infarction Project: an assessment of pre-hospital thrombolysis. Int J Cardiol 1995;49:S29–S37.

9. GREAT Group Invstigators. Feasibility, safety, and efficacy of domiciliary thrombolysis by general practitioners: Grampian Region Early Anistreplase Trial. Br Med J 1992;305:548–553.

10. Cannon CP, Gibson CM, Lambrew CT, et al. Relationship of symptom-onset-to-balloon time and door-to-balloon time with mortality in patients undergoing angioplasty for acute myocardial infarction. JAMA 2000;283:2941–2947.

11. Brener SJ, Ellis SG, Sapp SK, et al. Predictors of death and reinfarction at 30 d after primary angioplasty: the GUSTO IIb and RAPPORT trials. Am Heart J 2000;139:476–481.

12. Berger PB, Ellis SG, Holmes DR Jr, et al. Relationship between delay in performing direct coronary angioplasty and early clinical outcome in patients with acute myocardial infarction: results from the global use of strategies to open occluded arteries in Acute Coronary Syndromes (GUSTO-IIb) trial. Circulation 1999;100:14–20.

13. Schomig A, Kastrati A, Dirschinger J, et al. Coronary stenting plus platelet glycoprotein IIb/IIIa blockade compared with tissue plasminogen activator in acute myocardial infarction. Stent versus Thrombolysis for Occluded Coronary Arteries in Patients with Acute Myocardial Infarction Study Investigators. N Engl J Med 2000;343:385–391.

14. GUSTO Angiographic Investigators. The effects of tissue plasminogen activator, streptokinase, or both on coronary-artery patency, ventricular function, and survival after acute myocardial infarction. N Engl J Med 1993;329:1615–1621.

15. Simes RJ, Topol EJ, Holmes DR Jr, et al. Link between the angiographic substudy and mortality outcomes in a large randomized trial of myocardial reperfusion. Importance of early and complete infarct artery reperfusion. GUSTO-I Investigators. Circulation 1995;91:1923–1928.

16. Lincoff AM, Topol EJ, Califf RM, et al. Significance of a coronary artery with thrombolysis in myocardial infarction grade 2 flow "patency" (outcome in the thrombolysis and angioplasty in myocardial infarction trials). Thrombolysis and Angioplasty in Myocardial Infarction Study Group. Am J Cardiol 1995;75:871–876.

17. Anderson JL, Karagounis LA, Califf RM. Metaanalysis of five reported studies on the relation of early coronary patency grades with mortality and outcomes after acute myocardial infarction. Am J Cardiol 1996;78:1–8.

18. Ito H, Tomooka T, Sakai N, et al. Lack of myocardial perfusion immediately after successful thrombolysis. A predictor of poor recovery of left ventricular function in anterior myocardial infarction. Circulation 1992;85:1699–1705.

19. Lincoff AM, Topol EJ. Illusion of reperfusion. Does anyone achieve optimal reperfusion during acute myocardial infarction? [corrected and republished article originally printed in Circulation 1993 Jun;87(6):1792–1805]. Circulation 1993;88:1361–1374.

20. GUSTO IIb Angioplasty Substudy Investigators. A clinical trial comparing primary coronary angioplasty with tissue plasminogen activator for acute myocardial infarction. N Engl J Med 1997;336:1621–1628.

21. Grines CL, Browne KF, Marco J, et al. A comparison of immediate angioplasty with thrombolytic therapy for acute myocardial infarction. The Primary Angioplasty in Myocardial Infarction Study Group. N Engl J Med 1993;328:673–679.

22. Laster SB, O. Keefe JH J, Gibbons RJ. Incidence and importance of thrombolysis in myocardial infarction grade 3 flow after primary percutaneous transluminal coronary angioplasty for acute myocardial infarction. Am J Cardiol 1996;78:623–626.

23. Stone GW, Cox D, Garcia E, et al. Normal flow (TIMI-3) before mechanical reperfusion therapy is an independent determinant of survival in acute myocardial infarction. Analysis from the Primary Angioplasty in Myocardial Infarction Trials. Circulation 2001;104:636–641.

24. DeWood M, Spores J, Notske R, et al. Prevalence of total coronary occlusion during the early hours of transmural myocardial infarction. N Engl J Med 1980;303:897–902.

25. Pilote L, Miller DP, Califf RM, Rao JS, Weaver WD, Topol EJ. Determinants of the use of coronary angiography and revascularization after thrombolysis for acute myocardial infarction. N Engl J Med 1996;335:1198–1205.

26. De Jaegere PP, Arnold AA, Balk AH, Simoons ML. Intracranial hemorrhage in association with thrombolytic therapy: incidence and clinical predictive factors. J Am Coll Cardiol 1992;19:289–294.

27. Maggioni AP, Franzosi MG, Santoro E, White H, Van de Werf F, Tognoni G. The risk of stroke in patients with acute myocardial infarction after thrombolytic and antithrombotic treatment. Gruppo Italiano per lo Studio della Sopravvivenza nell'Infarto Miocardico II (GISSI-2) and The International Study Group. N Engl J Med 1992;327:1–6.

28. Gore JM, Granger CB, Simoons ML, et al. Stroke after thrombolysis. Mortality and functional outcomes in the GUSTO-I trial. Global Use of Strategies to Open Occluded Coronary Arteries. Circulation 1995;92:2811–2818.

29. Rothbaum D, Linnemeier T, Landin R, et al. Emergency percutaneous transluminal coronary angioplasty in acute myocardial infarction: a 3 year experience. J Am Coll Cardiol 1987;10: 264–272.

30. Ellis S, O'Neill W, Bates E, et al. Implications for patient triage from survival and left ventricular functional recovery analyses in 500 patients treated with coronary angioplasty for acute myocardial infarction. J Am Coll Cardiol 1989;13:1251–1259.

31. Kahn J, Rutherford B, McConahay D, et al. Results of primary angioplasty for acute myocardial infarction in patients with multivessel coronary artery disease. J Am Coll Cardiol 1990;16:1089-1096.

32. Beauchamp G, Vacek J, Robuck W. Management comparison for acute myocardial infarction: direct angioplasty versus sequential thrombolysis-angioplasty. Am Heart J 1990;120:237–242.

33. O'Keefe JH, Bailey WL, Rutherford BD, Hartzler GO. Primary angioplasty for acute myocardial infarction in 1,000 consecutive patients. Results in an unselected population and high-risk subgroups. Am J Cardiol 1993;72:107G–115G.

34. O'Neill W, Brodie B, Ivanhoe R, et al. Primary coronary angioplasty for acute myocardial infarction (the Primary Angioplasty Registry). Am J Cardiol 1994;73:627–634.

35. Brodie BR, Grines CL, Ivanhoe R, et al. Six-month clinical and angiographic follow-up after direct angioplasty for acute myocardial infarction. Final results from the Primary Angioplasty Registry. Circulation 1994;90:156–162.

36. Every NR, Parsons LS, Hlatky M, Martin JS, Weaver DW, for the MITI Investigators. A comparison of thrombolytic therapy with primary coronary angioplasty for acute myocardial infarction. N Eng J Med 1996;335:1253–1260.

37. Tiefenbrunn AJ, Chandra NC, French WJ, Gore JM, Rogers WJ. Clinical experience with primary percutaneous transluminal coronary angioplasty compared with alteplase (recombinant tissue-type plasminogen activator) in patients with acute myocardial infarction. a report from the Second National Registry of Myocardial Infarction (NRMI-2). J Am Coll Cardiol 1998;31:1240–1245.

38. Rogers WJ, Dean LS, Moore PB, Wool KJ, Burgard SL, Bradley EL. Comparison of primary angioplasty versus thrombolytic therapy for acute myocardial infarction. Alabama Registry of Myocardial Ischemia Investigators. Am J Cardiol 1994;74:111–118.

39. Vogt A, Bonzel T, Harmajanz D, et al. PTCA registry of German community hospitals. Arbeitsgemeinschaft Leitender Kardiologischer Krankenhausarzte (ALKK) Study Group. Eur Heart J 1997;18:1110–1114.

40. Zahn R, Koch A, Rustige J, et al. Primary angioplasty versus thrombolysis in the treatment of acute myocardial infarction. Am J Cardiol 1997;79:264–269.

41. Ottervanger JP, Van't Hof AW, Reiffers S, et al. Long-term recovery of left ventricular function after primary angioplasty for acute myocardial infarction. Eur Heart J 2001;22:785–790.

42. Zahn R, Schiele R, Schneider S, et al. Decreasing hospital mortality between 1994 and 1998 in patients with acute myocardial infarction treated with primary angioplasty but not in patients treated with intravenous thrombolysis. Results from the pooled data of the Maximal Individual Therapy in Acute Myocardial Infarction (MITRA) Registry and the Myocardial Infarction Registry (MIR). J Am Coll Cardiol 2000;36:2064–2071.

43. DeWood MA. Direct PTCA vs. intravenous t-PA in acute myocardial infarction: results from a prospective randomized trial. In: Thrombolysis and Interventional Therapy in Acute Myocardial Infarction Symposium. George Washington University, 1990, pp. 28–29.

44. Zijlstra F, de Boer MJ, Hoorntje JC, Reiffers S, Reiber JH, Suryapranata H. A comparison of immediate coronary angioplasty with intravenous streptokinase in acute myocardial infarction. N Engl J Med 1993;328:680–684.

45. Ribeiro EE, Silva LA, Carneiro R, et al. Randomized trial of direct coronary angioplasty versus intravenous streptokinase in acute myocardial infarction. J Am Coll Cardiol 1993;22:376–380.

46. Gibbons RJ, Holmes DR, Reeder GS, Bailey KR, Hopfenspirger MR, Gersh BJ. Immediate angioplasty compared with the administration of a thrombolytic agent followed by conservative treatment for myocardial infarction. The Mayo Coronary Care Unit and Catheterization Laboratory Groups. N Engl J Med 1993;328:685–691.

47. Garcia EJ, Delcan JL, Elizaga J, et al. Primary coronary angioplasty in acute anterior myocardial infarction: immediate results. Revista Espanola de Cardiologia 1994;47:40–46.

48. Grinfeld L, Berrocal D, Belardi J, et al. Fibrinolytics vs primary angioplasty in acute myocardial infarction (FAP): a randomized trial in a community hospital in Argentina [abstract]. J Am Coll Cardiol 1996;27:222A.

49. Ribichini F, Steffenino G, Dellavalle A, et al. Primary angioplasty versus thrombolysis in inferior acute myocardial infarction with anterior ST-segment depression, a single-center randomized study [abstract]. J Am Coll Cardiol 1996;27:221A.

50. Zijlstra F, Beukema WP, van't Hof AW, et al. Randommized comparison of primary coronary angioplasty with thrombolytic therapy in low risk patients with acute myocardial infarction. J Am Coll Cardiol 1997;27:908–912.

51. Weaver WD, Simes RJ, Betriu A, et al. Comparison of primary coronary angioplasty and intravenous thrombolytic therapy for acute myocardial infarction: a quantitative review. JAMA 1997;278:2093–2098.

52. Zijlstra F. Long-term benefit of primary angioplasty compared to thrombolytic therapy for acute myocardial infarction. Eur Heart J 2000;21:1487–1489.

53. Touboul P, Bonnefoy E. Comparison of primary angioplasty and prehospital thrombolysis in the acute phase of myocardial infarction. CAPTIM Study Group. Arch Mal Coeur Vaiss 1998;91 Spec No 2:33–38.

54. Stone GW, Marsalese D, Brodie BR, et al. A prospective, randomized evaluation of prophylactic intra-aortic balloon counterpulsation in high risk patients with acute myocardial infarction treated with primary angioplasty. J Am Coll Cardiol 1997;29:1459–1467.

55. Nakagawa Y, Iwasaki Y, Kimura T, et al. Serial angiographic follow-up after successful direct angioplasty for acute myocardial infarction. Am J Cardiol 1996;78:980–984.

56. Antoniucci D, Santoro GM, Bolognese L, Valenti R, Trapani M, Fazzini PF. A clinical trial comparing primary stenting of the infarct-related artery with optimal primary angioplasty for acute myocardial infarction: results from the Florence Randomized Elective Stenting in Acute Coronary Occlusions (FRESCO) trial. J Am Coll Cardiol 1998;31:1234–1239.

57. Maillard L, Hamon M, Khalife K, et al. A comparison of systematic stenting and conventional balloon angioplasty during primary percutaneous transluminal coronary angioplasty for acute myocardial infarction. STENTIM-2 Investigators. J Am Coll Cardiol 2000;35:1729–1736.

58. Rodriguez A, Bernardi V, Fernandez M, et al. In-hospital and late results of coronary stents versus conventional balloon angioplasty in acute myocardial infarction (GRAMI trial). Gianturco-Roubin in Acute Myocardial Infarction. Am J Cardiol 1998;81:1286–1291.

59. Saito S, Hosokawa G, Tanaka S, Nakamura S. Primary stent implantation is superior to balloon angioplasty in acute myocardial infarction: final results of the primary angioplasty versus stent implantation in acute myocardial infarction (PASTA) trial. PASTA Trial Investigators. Cathet Cardiovasc Intervent 1999;48:262–268.

60. Suryapranata H, van't Hof AW, Hoorntje JC, de Boer MJ, Zijlstra F. Randomized comparison of coronary stenting with balloon angioplasty in selected patients with acute myocardial infarction. Circulation 1998;97:2502–2505.

61. Antoniucci D, Valenti R, Mochi G, et al. Primary stenting in nonselected patients with acute myocardial infarction: the Multilink Duet in Acute Myocardial Infarction (MIAMI) trial. Cathet Cardiovasc Intervent 2000;51:273–279.

62. Grines CL, Cox DA, Stone GW, et al. Coronary angioplasty with or without stent implantation for acute myocardial infarction. Stent Primary Angioplasty in Myocardial Infarction Study Group. N Engl J Med 1999;341:1949–1956.

63. Stone GW, Grines CL, Cox DA, et al. Comparison of angioplasty with stenting, with or without abciximab, in acute myocardial infarction. N Engl J Med 2002;346:957–966.

64. Lefkovits J, Ivanhoe RJ, Califf RM, et al. Effects of platelet glycoprotein IIb/IIIa receptor blockade by a chimeric monoclonal antibody (abciximab) on acute and six-month outcomes after percutaneous transluminal coronary angioplasty for acute myocardial infarction. EPIC investigators. Am J Cardiol 1996;77:1045–1051.

65. Neumann FJ, Blasini R, Schmitt C, et al. Effect of glycoprotein IIb/IIIa receptor blockade on recovery of coronary flow and left ventricular function after the placement of coronary-artery stents in acute myocardial infarction. Circulation 1998;98:2695–2701.

66. Brener SJ, Barr LA, Burchenal JE, et al. Randomized, placebo-controlled trial of platelet glycoprotein IIb/IIIa blockade with primary angioplasty for acute myocardial infarction. ReoPro and Primary PTCA Organization and Randomized Trial (RAPPORT) Investigators. Circulation 1998;98:734–741.

67. Montalescot G, Barragan P, Wittenberg O, et al. Platelet glycoprotein IIb/IIIa inhibition with coronary stenting for acute myocardial infarction. N Engl J Med 2001;344:1895–1903.

68. Topol EJ, Yadav JS. Recognition of the importance of embolization in atherosclerotic vascular disease. Circulation 2000;101:570–580.

69. Gibson CM, Ryan KA, Murphy SA, et al. Impaired coronary blood flow in nonculprit arteries in the setting of acute myocardial infarction. The TIMI Study Group. Thrombolysis in Myocardial Infarction. J Am Coll Cardiol 1999;34:974–982.

70. Ito II, Maruyama A, Iwakura K, et al. Clinical implications of the 'no reflow' phenomenon. A predictor of complications and left ventricular remodeling in reperfused anterior wall myocardial infarction. Circulation 1996;93:223–228.

71. Iliceto S, Galiuto L, Marchese A, et al. Analysis of microvascular integrity, contractile reserve, and myocardial viability after acute myocardial infarction by dobutamine echocardiography and myocardial contrast echocardiography. Am J Cardiol 1996;77:441–445.

72. Wu KC, Zerhouni EA, Judd RM, et al. Prognostic significance of microvascular obstruction by magnetic resonance imaging in patients with acute myocardial infarction. Circulation 1998;97:765–772.

73. Sheiban I, Fragasso G, Rosano GMC, et al. Time course and determinants of left ventricular function recovery after primary angioplasty in patients with acute myocardial infarction. J Am Coll Cardiol 2001;38:464–471.

74. Iwakura K, Ito H, Kawano S, et al. Predictive factors for development of the no reflow phenomenon in patients with reperfused anterior wall acute myocardial infarction. J Am Coll Cardiol 2001;38:472–477.

75. Gibson CM, Cannon CP, Murphy SA, et al. Relationship of TIMI myocardial perfusion grade to mortality after administration of thrombolytic drugs. Circulation 2000;101:125–130.

76. Stone GW, Lansky AJ, Mehran R, et al. Beyond TIMI 3 flow: the importance of restored myocardial perfusion for survival in high risk patients undergoing primary or rescue PTCA [abstract]. J Am Coll Cardiol 2000;35:403A.

77. Ellis SG, Da Silva ER, Spaulding CM, Nobuyoshi M, Weiner B, Talley JD. Review of immediate angioplasty after fibrinolytic therapy for acute myocardial infarction: insights from the RESCUE I, RESCUE II, and other contemporary clinical experiences. Am Heart J 2000;139:1046–1053.

78. Ellis S, da Silva E, Heyndrickx G, et al. Randomized comparison of rescue angioplasty with conservative management of patients with early failure of thrombolysis for acute anterior myocardial infarction. Circulation 1994;90:2280–2284.

79. Miller JM, Smalling R, Ohman EM, et al. Effectiveness of early coronary angioplasty and abciximab for failed thrombolysis (reteplase or alteplase) during acute myocardial infarction (results from the GUSTO-III trial). Global Use of Strategies To Open occluded coronary arteries. Am J Cardiol 1999; 84:779–784.

80. Schweiger MJ, Antman EM, Piana RN, et al. Effect of Abciximab (ReoPro) on early rescue angioplasty in TIMI 14 [abstract]. Circulation 1998;98:I-17.

81. Brodie BR, Stuckey TD, Hansen C, Muncy D. Benefit of coronary reperfusion before intervention on outcomes after primary angioplasty for acute myocardial infarction. Am J Cardiol 2000;85:13–18.

82. Ross AM, Coyne KS, Reiner JS, et al. A randomized trial comparing primary angioplasty with a strategy of short-acting thrombolysis and immediate planned rescue angioplasty in acute myocardial infarction: the PACT trial. Plasminogen-activator Angioplasty Compatibility Trial. J Am Coll Cardiol 1999;34:1954–1962.

83. Antman EM, Giugliano RP, Gibson CM, et al. Abciximab facilitates the rate and extent of thrombolysis: results of the thrombolysis in myocardial infarction (TIMI) 14 trial. The TIMI 14 Investigators. Circulation 1999;99:2720–2732.

84. Strategies for Patency Enhancement in the Emergency Department (SPEED) Group. Trial of abciximab with and without low-dose reteplase for acute myocardial infarction. Circulation 2000;101: 2788–2794.

85. Brener SJ, Adgey AAJ, Vrobel TR, et al. Eptifibatide and low-dose tissue plasminogen plasminogen activator in acute myocardial infarction: The INtegrilin and low-dose Thrombolysis in Acute Myocardial Infarction—INTRO AMI. J Am Coll Cardiol 2002; 39: 377–386.

86. Giugliano RP, Roe MT, Zeymer U, et al. Restoration of epicardial and myocardial perfusion in acute ST-elevation myocardial infarction with combination eptifibatide+reduced-dose tenecteplase: dose-finding results from the INTEGRITI trial [abstract]. Circulation 2001;104.

87. Herrmann HC, Moliterno DJ, Ohman EM, et al. Facilitation of early percutaneous coronary intervention after reteplase with or without abciximab in acute myocardial infarction: results from the SPEED (GUSTO-4 Pilot) Trial. J Am Coll Cardiol 2000;36:1489–1496.

88. Mueller DWM, Topol EJ. Selection of patients with acute myocardial infarction for thrombolytic therapy. Ann Intern Med 1990;113:949–960.

89. Lieu TA, Gurley RJ, Lundstrom RJ, Parmley WW. Primary angioplasty and thrombolysis for acute myocardial infarction: an evidence summary [see comments]. J Am Coll Cardiol 1996;27:737–750.

90. Chandra H, Yarzebski J, Goldberg RJ, et al. Age-related trends (1986-1993) in the use of thrombolytic agents in patients with acute myocardial infarction. The Worcester Heart Attack Study. Arch Intern Med 1997;157:741–746.

91. Cragg D, Friedman H, Bonema J, et al. Outcome of patients with acute myocardial infarction who are ineligible for thrombolytic therapy. Ann Inter Med 1991;115:173–177.

92. Holmes DR Jr, White HD, Pieper KS, Ellis SG, Califf RM, Topol EJ. Effect of age on outcome with primary angioplasty versus thrombolysis. J Am Coll Cardiol 1999;33:412–419.

93. O'Gara PT. Primary pump failure. In: Fuster V, Ross R, Topol EJ, eds. Atherosclerosis and Coronary Artery Disease. 1st ed. Lippicott-Raven, Philadelphia, 1996, pp. 1051–1064.

94. Hochman JS, Boland J, Sleeper LA, et al. Current spectrum of cardiogenic shock and effect of early revascularization on mortality. Results of an International Registry. SHOCK Registry Investigators. Circulation 1995;91:873–881.

95. Califf RM, Bengston JR. Cardiogenic shock. N Eng J Med 1994;330:1724.

96. Goldberg RJ, Gore JM, Alpert JS, et al. Cardiogenic shock after acute myocardial infarction. Incidence and mortality from a community-wide perspective, 1975 to 1988. N Engl J Med 1991;325:1117–1122.

97. AIMS Trial Study Group. Effect of intravenous APSAC on mortality after acute myocardial infarction: preliminary report of a placebo-controlled clinical trial. Lancet 1988;1:545–549.

98. Wilcox RG, van der Lippe G, Olssen CG, et al. Trial of tissue-plasminogen activator for mortality reduction in acute myocardial infarction: Anglo-Scandinavian Study of Early Thrombolysis. ASSET. Lancet 1988;1:525–530.

99. The International Study Group. In-hospital mortality and clinical course of 20,891 patients with suspected acute myocardial infarction randomised between alteplase and streptokinase with or without heparin. Lancet 1990;336:71–75.

100. Holmes DR Jr, Bates ER, Kleiman NS, et al. Contemporary reperfusion therapy for cardiogenic shock: the GUSTO-I trial experience. The GUSTO-I Investigators. Global Utilization of Streptokinase and Tissue Plasminogen Activator for Occluded Coronary Arteries. J Am Coll Cardiol 1995;26:668–674.

101. Hochman JS, Sleeper LA, Webb JG, et al. Early revascularization in acute myocardial infarction complicated by cardiogenic shock. SHOCK Investigators. Should We Emergently Revascularize Occluded Coronaries for Cardiogenic Shock. N Engl J Med 1999;341:625–634.

102. McCullough PA, O'Neill WW, Graham M, et al. A prospective randomized trial of triage angiography in suspected acute myocardial infarction patients who are ineligible for reperfusion therapy [abstract]. Circulation 1996;94:I-570.

103. Widimsky P, Groch L, Zelizko M, Aschermann M, Bednar F, Suryapranata H. Multicentre randomized trial comparing transport to primary angioplasty vs immediate thrombolysis vs combined strategy for patients with acute myocardial infarction presenting to a community hospital without a catheterization laboratory. The PRAGUE study. Eur Heart J 2000;21:823–831.

103a. Coletta A, Thackray S, Nikitin N, Cleland JG. Clinical trials update: highlights of the scientific sessions of The American College of Cardiology 2002: LIFE, DANAMI 2, MADIT-2, MIRACLE-ICD, OVERTURE, OCTAVE, ENABLE 1 & 2, CHRISTMAS, AFFIRM, RACE, WIZARD, AZACS, REMATCH, BNP trial and HARDBALL. Eur J Heart Fail 2002;4:381–388.

103b. Aversano T, Aversano LT, Passamani E, et al. Thrombolytic therapy vs primary percutaneous coronary intervention for myocardial infarction in patients presenting to hospitals without on-site cardiac surgery: a randomized controlled trial. JAMA 2002;287:1943–1951.

104. Grines CL, Schreiber TL, Savas V, et al. A randomized trial of low osmolar ionic versus nonionic contrast media in patients with myocardial infarction or unstable angina undergoing percutaneous transluminal coronary angioplasty. J Am Coll Cardiol 1996;27:1381–1386.

105. Kaplan BM, Larkin T, Safian RD, et al. Prospective study of extraction atherectomy in patients with acute myocardial infarction. Am J Cardiol 1996;78:383–388.

106. Lieu TA, Lundstrom RJ, Ray T, Fireman BH, Gurley RJ, Parmley WW. Initial cost of primary angioplasty for acute myocardial infarction. J Am Coll Cardiol 1996;28:882–889.

107. Stone GW, Grines CL, Rothbaum D, et al. Analysis of the relative cost and effectiveness of primary angioplasty versus tissue-type plasminogen activator: the Primary Angioplasty in Myocardial Infarction (PAMI) Trial. J Am Coll Cardiol 1997;29:901–907.

108. de Boer MJ, van Hout BA, Liem AL, Suryapranata H, Hoorntje JC, Zijlstra F. A cost-effective analysis of primary coronary angioplasty versus thrombolysis for acute myocardial infarction. Am J Cardiol 1995;76:830–833.

109. Mark DB, Granger CB, Ellis SE, et al. Costs of direct angioplasty versus thrombolysis for acute myocardial infarction: results from the GUSTO II randomized trial [abstract]. Circulation 1996;94:I-168.

110. Canto JG, Every NR, Magid DJ, et al. The volume of primary angioplasty procedures and survival after acute myocardial infarction. National Registry of Myocardial Infarction 2 Investigators. N Engl J Med 2000;342:1573–1580.

111. Magid DJ, Calonge BN, Rumsfeld JS, et al. Relation between hospital primary angioplasty volume and mortality for patients with acute myocardial infarction treated with primary angioplasty vs. thrombolytic therapy. JAMA 2000;284:3131–3138.

112. ACC/AHA Task Force. ACC/AHA guidelines for percutaneous coronary intervention. J Am Coll Cardiol 2001;37:2215–2238.

11

Expanding the Access to Percutaneous Coronary Intervention for Patients Admitted to Community Hospitals

Thomas P. Wharton, Jr. and
Nancy Sinclair McNamara

CONTENTS

INTRODUCTION

Interventional therapy is now central to the treatment of patients with acute coronary artery syndromes (ACS): acute ST-segment elevation myocardial infarction (STEMI), non-ST-segment elevation myocardial infarction (NSTEMI), and unstable angina (UA). Most patients with acute myocardial infarction (AMI), however, present to community hospitals that do not have cardiac surgical programs, and thus usually lack the capability to provide percutaneous coronary intervention (PCI) *(1)*. The requirement that PCI be provided only at tertiary cardiac surgery centers has thus limited the widespread application of this optimal therapy for ACS. Extending the benefits of early PCI to this large population of patients with ACS that are admitted to community hospitals requires either transfer to a tertiary surgery center, often emergently, or the performance of PCI on site. A third solution is the ambulance triage of patients with AMI to emergency inter-

From: *Contemporary Cardiology: Management of Acute Coronary Syndromes, Second Edition*
Edited by: C. P. Cannon © Humana Press Inc., Totowa, NJ

vention centers if within a reasonable distance; this is not yet an acceptable practice in most regions of the United States.

PRIMARY PCI IS THE TREATMENT OF CHOICE FOR PATIENTS WITH AMI AT QUALIFIED CENTERS

In a well-known meta-analysis of 10 randomized trials of acute STEMI, primary PCI lowered the rates of death, stroke, and the combined end point of death or reinfarction compared to fibrinolytic therapy (2). The trials in this meta-analysis were performed before the advent of newer fibrinolytic agents and glycoprotein (GP) IIb/IIIa platelet inhibitors and before the widespread use of coronary stenting. More recent randomized studies utilizing these newer modalities continue to demonstrate an even greater clinical superiority of primary PCI in fibrinolytic-eligible patients (3,4). Such randomized studies are usually conducted at experienced, dedicated centers; the applicability of such studies to the "real world" has been questioned.

The most recently reported observational registries confirm that the clinical outcomes of PCI which are reported in randomized trials from research centers, can indeed be broadly reproduced. For example, a current registry of over 2000 PCI procedures in New York State demonstrated outstanding outcomes for primary PCI that did in fact reproduce the results of randomized trials (5). The authors concluded that the mortality rates for PCI in this registry "are, for the most part, similar to those reported by other studies in the literature. Furthermore, the mortality rates reported in this study for primary PCI are lower than the rates reported for fibrinolytic therapy in recent studies." Other recent registry data from the Second and Third National Registries of Myocardial Infarction (NRMI-2 and -3) found that primary PCI at hospitals that performed >16 procedures per year had lower mortality than fibrinolytic therapy. Very interestingly, hospitals that performed fewer procedures than this still had mortality rates with primary PCI that were equal to those with fibrinolytic therapy (6). Another report of pooled registry data for nearly 10,000 patients in two recent registries of AMI in Germany noted a nearly 50% reduction in mortality for patients treated with primary PCI compared to patients treated with fibrinolytic therapy (7). In this report, primary PCI was associated with a lower mortality in all subgroups analyzed; as the mortality of the subgroup increased, the absolute benefit of primary PCI also increased. In addition, over the study period from 1994 to 1998, there was continuous improvement in the rates of death and reinfarction for patients with AMI treated with primary PCI, but no such improvement for patients treated with fibrinolytic therapy (8).

Even if the outcomes of primary PCI and fibrinolytic therapy were equal in lytic-eligible patients, fibrinolytic therapy is not appropriate in around two-thirds of patients with AMI. Patients ineligible for lytic therapy include patients without NSTEMI, even if they have unrelieved/ongoing ischemic symptoms (a higher-risk group), patients who present late, patients with cardiogenic shock, those with prior bypass surgery (9), the elderly, and, of course, patients with bleeding contraindications. Patients that are ineligible for fibrinolytic therapy are at higher risk of death than those eligible (10–12). Such patients may have a considerably improved survival rate when afforded the reperfusion alternative of primary PCI.

For example, data from the NRMI-2 registry suggest that patients with AMI and bleeding contraindications to fibrinolysis may be very appropriate for primary PCI *(13)*. A large registry in Germany has demonstrated that, for patients with AMI that were ineligible for fibrinolytics due to bleeding risk, there was an 11-fold reduction in mortality with primary PCI compared to conservative therapy *(14)*. This same registry also demonstrated a three-fold reduction in mortality for primary PCI compared to fibrinolytic therapy in patients that are normally excluded from randomized trials: those with nondiagnostic ECG, left bundle-branch block, late presentation >12 h, or unknown prehospital delay *(15)*. There was a similar reduction in the combined end points of death, reinfarction, stroke, advanced heart failure, and postinfarction angina for primary PCI in this population.

The elderly represent another group that has suboptimal outcomes with fibrinolytic therapy. A recent analysis of Medicare patients with AMI reported that in patients over 75 yr old, fibrinolytic therapy resulted in worse outcomes than no reperfusion therapy, especially in women *(16,17)*. This elderly population represents almost one-third of patients with acute MI *(17)*. Another analysis has reported that primary PCI improves mortality dramatically compared to fibrinolytic therapy in elderly patients *(18)*.

The most feared complication of fibrinolytic therapy is cerebral hemorrhage. The risk of hemorrhagic stroke is generally less than 1% in patients treated with fibrinolytics. However, a study of Medicare patients identified multiple readily identifiable risk factors for cerebral hemorrhage with fibrinolytic therapy, which included age ≥75 yr, female sex, black race, prior stroke, blood pressure ≥160 mmHg, use of tissue plasminogen activator (tPA) instead of streptokinase, elevated prothrombin time, and low body weight *(19)*. The overall risk was 1.4% in this population. A risk stratification scale developed on the basis of these factors demonstrated a progressively increasing risk of hemorrhagic stroke with increasing numbers of risk factors. For example, a black woman over age 75 weighing under 143 pounds treated with tPA (five risk factors) would have a 4.1% chance of suffering a cerebral hemorrhage! Clearly, for this reason alone, PCI can be regarded as the treatment of choice for ST-elevation AMI in the elderly population with risk factors for intracerebral hemorrhage.

In patients with cardiogenic shock, early intra-aortic balloon counterpulsation and early mechanical revascularization is imperative. Immediate intervention with hemodynamic support at initial presentation can salvage viable myocardium and preserve other hypoperfused organ systems. In the recent Should We Emergently Revascularize Occluded Coronaries for Cardiogenic Shock? (SHOCK) trial, revascularization in under 6 h conferred the best survival advantage compared to fibrinolytic therapy of all descriptors examined *(20)*. Another large series recently reported a dramatically increased survival in patients receiving PCI within the first 2 h *(21)*, confirming the imperative of rapid revascularization for survival in shock. Patients presenting with acute MI and cardiogenic shock should be treated with immediate balloon counterpulsation followed by emergent mechanical revascularization, at the point of first contact wherever possible *(22–28)*. The on-site availability of coronary bypass surgery for such patients in shock is largely moot, since these patients are so critically ill *(29,30)*.

In view of the superiority of primary PCI for treatment of AMI, it is not surprising that the use of primary PCI has increased three-fold in the past decade (from 2.4% to 7.3% of all patients with AMI), while the use of fibrinolytic therapy has declined 40% (from 34.3% to 20.8%), according to data from the first three NRMI registries *(31)*.

EARLY PCI IS THE TREATMENT OF CHOICE FOR
PATIENTS WITH HIGH-RISK ACS

In recent registry data from Washington State, patients with NSTEMI who were admitted to hospitals that favored an early invasive treatment strategy had 30-d and 4-yr mortality rates that were almost 50% lower than those admitted to hospitals that favored a conservative treatment strategy *(32)*. It should be noted that fibrinolytic therapy is not indicated in patients with NSTEMI and may be harmful *(12,33)*.

Previous randomized trials of early aggressive vs conservative approaches in UA and NSTEMI have had conflicting results. These were conducted before the common usage of stents and GP IIb/IIIa antagonists *(34–37)*. The Veterans Affairs Non-Q-Wave Infarction Strategies in Hospital (VANQWISH) trial randomized patients with non-Q wave AMI to an early invasive strategy vs noninvasive risk stratification *(34)*. In VANQWISH, there was an excess risk of the invasive approach, which was entirely a direct result of a high surgical mortality of 11.6% in the invasive group. This operative mortality rate does not reflect current experience, and thus, the conclusions of the VANQWISH study thus cannot be applied to patients at centers with lower operative mortalities. Conversely, the Thrombolysis in Myocardial Infarction (TIMI) 3B trial showed less recurrent ischemia and fewer and shorter hospitalizations at 1 yr in patients randomized to routine early (18–48 h) cardiac catheterization and revascularization, compared to conservative management *(37)*.

The use of early PCI in patients with ACS has been re-examined in two other recent trials and a recently reported registry. The Second Fragmin and Fast Revascularization during Instability in Coronary Artery Disease (FRISC II) trial demonstrated an improvement in the combined rate of death or AMI at 6 mo in patients with high-risk ACS using an early invasive approach compared to a stepwise selective invasive approach *(36)*. This trial also showed that patients with ST-segment depression on admission electrocardiogram (ECG) had more severe coronary disease; in these patients, an early invasive strategy substantially decreased the combined rate of death and AMI. Now, 2-yr follow-up results of FRISC II have demonstrated a 4.2% reduction in death and AMI with the early invasive approach *(38)*. The event curves continued to separate over the 2 yr, even though half of the patients in the conservative arm ultimately underwent revascularization. Patients with ST-segment depression and elevated troponin, at the highest risk, benefited the most: the 1-yr risk of death or AMI was reduced by nearly 50% with the early invasive approach compared to the conservative approach (14 vs 25%, respectively).

The Treat Angina with Aggrastat and Determine Cost of Therapy with an Invasive or Conservative Strategy—Thrombolysis in Myocardial Infarction (TACTICS-TIMI) -18 trial randomized 2220 patients with ACS to early coronary angiography within 4–48 h of presentation vs a more conservative ischemia-guided approach, both groups being treated with tirofiban *(39)*. Enrollment criteria included accelerating angina and either ischemic ECG changes, elevated serum cardiac markers (troponin or creatine kinase isoenzyme-cardiac muscle subunit [CK-MB]), or previous AMI or coronary revascularization. The composite end point of death, acute MI, or rehospitalization for recurrent UA at 6 mo was significantly reduced in patients treated with an early invasive approach (Table 1), with the greatest benefit conferred to patients with ischemic ECG changes or elevated troponin levels.

Table 1

Six-Month Outcomes of TACTICS-TIMI-18: Prospective Randomized Trial Comparing Early Coronary Angiography Vs Ischemia-Guided Therapy in Patients with ACS Treated with Tirofiban *(39)*

	Early invasive strategy (n = 1114)	Conservative strategy (n = 1106)
Combined endpoint[a]	15.9%	19.4%
Death or reinfarction	7.3%	9.5%
Reinfarction	4.8%	6.9%

TIMI, Thrombolysis in Myocardial Infarction; %, percent of patients.
[a]Death, reinfarction, or hospitalization for unstable angina
$p < 0.05$, $p = 0.029$, $p < 0.025$ vs early invasive approach.

These new studies together indicate that patients with NSTEMI or other ACS associated with ischemic ECG changes and/or elevated troponin should be treated with an early invasive strategy within the first 48 h of hospital admission. The findings of these trials are corroborated by a recent report from the Mayo clinic, which found in a retrospective population-based study that early coronary angiography in patients with ACS was independently associated with a reduction in all-cause mortality, particularly in intermediate- and high-risk patients *(40)*.

An economic analysis of the TACTICS study was recently presented. TACTICS demonstrated that, while the initial in-hospital costs were higher with the invasive strategy, the costs incurred in the conservative arm were higher during the 6 mo of followup, largely because of increased rehospitalizations *(41)*. The total 6-mo cost for patients in the aggressive arm was essentially the same as for those in the conservative arm.

THE DELIVERY OF INTERVENTIONAL THERAPY TO PATIENTS WITH ACS MUST BE IMPROVED

While great advances continue to be made in the technology and pharmacology of coronary intervention, much more work needs to be done to improve the delivery of PCI to a greater proportion of patients with ACS, now that the superiority of the interventional approach is being clearly established. According to Medicare data in Michigan, 60% of patients with AMI present to hospitals that do not have cardiac surgical programs *(1)*. Nearly all of these hospitals do not have the capability to provide PCI.

The solution to this problem of improving the access to early PCI for patients with AMI and other high risk ACS requires three interdependent approaches: (*i*) the development of new PCI programs at those nonsurgical hospitals that can meet rigorous requirements, such as those that we have advocated (Tables 2 and 3) *(30)*; (*ii*) the development of systems and transfer agreements at the local hospital level to encourage more frequent and earlier transfer of more patients to emergency intervention centers; and (*iii*) the establishment of guidelines, policies, and protocols to enable and encourage the prehospital ambulance triage of patients with suspected AMI to emergency intervention centers that have 24-h, 365-d PCI capability (analogous to trauma centers).

Because the transfer of ever-increasing numbers of patients with high-risk ACS to tertiary centers, which currently provide PCI, could quickly overload their capacity, even

Table 2

Operator, Institutional, and Angiographic Criteria for Primary PCI Programs at Hospitals without On-Site Cardiac Surgery (30)

1. The operators must be experienced high-vol interventionalists who regularly perform elective intervention.
2. The nursing and technical CCL staff must be experienced in handling acutely ill patients and comfortable with interventional equipment. They must have acquired experience in dedicated interventional laboratories. They participate in a 24-h, 7-d/wk call schedule.
3. The CCL itself must be well equipped, with optimal imaging systems, resuscitative equipment, IABP support, and must be well stocked with a broad array of interventional equipment.
4. The CCU nurses must be adept in the management of acutely ill cardiac patients, including invasive hemodynamic monitoring and IABP management.
5. The hospital administration must fully support the program and enable the fulfillment of the above institutional requirements.
6. Formalized written protocols must be in place for immediate and efficient transfer of patients to the nearest cardiac surgical facility.
7. Primary PCI must be performed routinely as the treatment of choice around the clock for a large proportion of patients with AMI, to ensure streamlined care paths and increased case vol. The institution should expect to perform 3 to 4 primary PCI procedures/mo.
8. Clinical and angiographic selection criteria for the performance of primary PCI and for transfer for emergency CABG must be rigorous (Table 4).
9. There must be an ongoing program of outcomes analysis and formalized periodic case review.

AMI, acute myocardial infarction; CABG, coronary artery bypass graft; CCL, cardiac catheterization laboratory; CCU, cardiac care unit; IABP, intra-aortic balloon pump; PCI, percutaneous coronary intervention.
Adapted from ref. *30*.

Table 3

Selection for Primary PCI and Emergency Aortocoronary Bypass Surgery at Hospitals without On-Site Cardiac Surgery (30)

Avoid intervention in hemodynamically stable patients with:
- Significant ($\geq$60%) stenosis of an unprotected left main coronary artery upstream from an acute occlusion in the left coronary system that might be disrupted by the angioplasty catheter.
- Extremely long or angulated infarct-related lesions with TIMI grade 3 flow.
- Infarct-related lesions with TIMI grade 3 flow in stable patients with three-vessel disease *(56,57)*.
- Infarct-related lesions of small or secondary vessels.
- Lesions in other than the infarct artery.

Transfer for emergent aortocoronary bypass surgery patients with:
- High-grade residual left main or multivessel coronary disease and clinical or hemodynamic instability:
  —After angioplasty of occluded vessels.
  —Preferably with intra-aortic balloon pump support.

PCI, percutaneous coronary intervention; TIMI, Thrombolysis in Myocardial Infarction.
Adapted from ref. *30*.

if all of them did provide primary PCI as first-line therapy for AMI, the second and third approaches above will ultimately depend on the development of more interventional programs at more community hospitals. The need for more interventional facilities can be projected to increase even further in the near future, with the aging of the baby boomers *(42)* and with the increased application of PCI to more patients. This increasing need for coronary intervention may well outstrip the need for more cardiac surgery facilities. Thus, solutions 2 and 3 above will ultimately depend, in part, on solution 1, the uncoupling of PCI programs from cardiac surgery programs.

Though there is an emerging practice in some hospitals in the US to provide primary, urgent, and even elective PCI with off-site surgical backup, there are important regulatory barriers that discourage this practice in many states. It is to be hoped that the new American College of Cardiology/American Heart Association (ACC/AHA) guidelines for PCI will help to discourage these regulatory barriers. The new guidelines state that the superiority and greater applicability of primary PCI for the treatment of AMI has raised the question of whether primary PCI should be performed at institutions . . . [without] on-site cardiac surgery *(43)*. The guidelines recommend primary PCI at hospitals with off-site cardiac surgical backup with a Class IIb indication (usefulness/efficacy less well-established by evidence/opinion), provided that >36 procedures per year are performed at such hospitals by higher-volume interventionalists within 30–90 min of admission and that a proven plan for rapid access to a cardiac surgical center is in place. These guidelines also include tables listing further operator, institutional, and patient selection criteria for the performance of PCI and emergency coronary bypass surgery at such hospitals, based on those that we originally proposed (Tables 2 and 3). Thus they affirm that, when appropriate standards are met, the provision of primary PCI at hospitals with off-site cardiac surgical backup is a reasonable treatment alternative. These guidelines, while still discouraging the performance of nonemergent PCI at nonsurgical hospitals, do add in a discussion of this issue that, "As with many dynamic areas in interventional cardiology, these recommendations may be subject to revision as clinical data and experience increase."

Development of New PCI Programs at Qualified Hospitals with Off-Site Surgical Backup

The need for emergency surgery because of mishap in the catheterization laboratory is very rare today in light of the major technological and pharmacological advances related to PCI. The advent of newer-generation stents and glycoprotein IIb/IIIa platelet inhibitors has lowered the risk of abrupt vessel (re)closure from 2–5%, as reported in the 1980s, to approx 0.4% *(44–48)*. In an analysis of Primary Angioplasty in Myocardial Infarction (PAMI) trials, emergency surgery for failed primary angioplasty was required in only 0.4% of patients *(47)*. The authors of this study concluded: "In concert with the declining incidence of emergent coronary artery bypass graft (CABG) with the use of stents, these data suggest that skilled physicians and personnel may safely perform primary angioplasty at select hospitals without operative facilities (allowing patients to benefit from enhanced survival free from reinfarction and stroke with primary angioplasty compared to fibrinolytic therapy), as long as steps are in place to facilitate surgical revascularization expeditiously by transfer to a nearby tertiary center when necessary."

Table 4

Pooled Results from 6 Published Reports from Primary PCI Programs with Off-Site Cardiac
Surgical Backup (30,53,56–61) compared to the PAR, which Included 6 High-Vol Tertiary
Hospitals (62)

	Programs with off-site backup (n)	PAR hospitals (n) (n = 245)
Median time to reperfusion	86 min (1357)	124 min
Successful PCI	92% (1186)	88%
Reinfarction	2.2% (1419)	3.0%
Stroke	0.5% (1419)	1.0%
Mortality[a]	3.7% (1102)	4.0%
Emergency surgery for procedural complication	0.2% (1419)	1.2%

ED, emergency department; %, percent of patients.
[a]Patients without cardiogenic shock.

Over 850 community hospitals in the United States have cardiac catheterization laboratories but no cardiac surgical programs (49). Often these laboratories are staffed by
experienced interventionalists who perform PCI at surgical centers. At least 75 hospitals in 30 states now perform primary PCI with off-site backup, of which at least 25, in
17 states, also provide nonemergent PCI. Overseas, the British Cardiac Society and
British Cardiovascular Intervention Society together recently issued new guidelines for
PCI (50). These guidelines now allow both emergency and elective PCI to be performed
at hospitals with off-site surgical backup, provided that they have systems in place to
enable patients to be on cardiopulmonary bypass within 90 min of calling the cardiac
surgeon. Regulations in the Netherlands and in Australia are being modified to allow
PCI programs at hospitals without on-site cardiac surgery. Recently, the Cardiac Care
Network of Ontario, Canada, recommended to the Ontario Ministry of Health that pilot
programs be set up to perform PCI at hospitals with off-site surgical backup (51), for
the same reasons that have been cited above.

That primary PCI can be performed safely and effectively at hospitals with off-site
cardiac surgery backup has been demonstrated in many reports (30,52–61). Table 4
shows pooled outcomes from six reported registries of primary PCI at community hospitals with off-site cardiac surgical backup (30,53–61). In the combined experience of
these six community hospital registries, which included a total of 1679 primary PCI procedures, the pooled rates of procedural success, coronary artery bypass surgery for procedural complication, reinfarction, stroke, and mortality in patients without shock were
very similar to the outcomes of patients without shock in the contemporaneous Primary
Angioplasty Registry (PAR) of five high-volume cardiac surgery centers (62). In addition, the time from arrival to emergency department to reperfusion was lower in the hospitals without on-site surgery than those with on-site surgery (86 vs 124 min). The
overall mortality in these registries was 6.4%. Data that discriminate patients with and
without shock are available for 1209 patients in these series. The mortality in 1102
patients without shock was 3.7%. Only two patients (0.16%) out of the 1209 in which
data were available required emergency bypass surgery because of new myocardial jeopardy caused by the interventional procedure.

The excellent results in these six series were, for the most part, achieved before stents and IIb/IIIa platelet inhibitors were in common use. These modalities should further improve the safety of the procedure *(3,63–68)*. In fact, newer-generation stents and platelet GP IIb/IIIa inhibitors have lowered the risk of abrupt vessel (re)closure from 2–5% to around 0.4% *(44–48)*.

It should be added that smaller hospitals with dedicated primary PCI programs may be able to perform primary PCI faster than larger centers *(69)*. Possible reasons for potentially greater efficiency of smaller hospitals may include more direct communication between the emergency physician and the cardiologist with less bureaucracy, decreased travel times if the catheterization team lives nearby, and greater flexibility in a catheterization laboratory schedule that may not be as congested.

The efficacy and safety of primary PCI with off-site cardiac surgical backup has now been demonstrated in the first randomized study of PCI vs fibrinolysis at hospitals with off-site surgical backup. The 453-patient Cardiovascular Patient Outcomes Research Team (C-PORT) trial, the second largest of all prospective randomized trials to date of primary PCI vs fibrinolytic therapy in AMI *(70,70a)*, demonstrated the superiority of primary PCI at those hospitals without cardiac surgery that performed more than 12 procedures per year. Primary PCI at these centers resulted in a reduction of the combined incidence of death, recurrent AMI, and stroke at 6 mo by 42% ($p = 0.04$). There was no significant difference between the two treatment modalities in hospitals that performed fewer procedures. Patient groups that particularly benefited in this trial were women, diabetics, and the elderly. No patient in this trial required emergency surgery for PCI mishap. The investigators concluded that the need for in-house cardiac surgery backup was not supported by the results of the C-PORT study.

Community hospitals that consider offering primary PCI should have experienced high-volume interventionalists on staff who routinely perform elective PCI at intervention centers, an experienced catheterization laboratory staff, a well-equipped laboratory, and established protocols for emergent transfer to surgical centers *(30)*. They should expect to perform at least two to four procedures/mo in order to maintain competence *(5,70,71,72,73)*. Thus, they should offer primary PCI as the first-line treatment of choice for patients that present with AMI with full-time availability of the on-call team on a 24-h, 7-d/wk basis (Table 2). Recent reports indicate that hospitals that perform at least two to four primary PCI procedures/mo have better mortality rates than those that perform fewer, and better than mortality rates for fibrinolytic therapy alone *(5,71–73)*. For example, the NRMI-2 and -3 registries found that patients who received primary PCI at hospitals that performed >16 procedures per year had lower mortality than those receiving fibrinolytic therapy *(5)*. Hospitals that performed <16 procedures per year, nevertheless, had mortality rates with PCI that were still similar to those with fibrinolytic therapy. Patients in this study that were randomized to primary PCI also had fewer strokes and less need for subsequent revascularization.

Development of Systems and Transfer Agreements to Encourage More Frequent and Earlier Transfer of More Patients to Emergency Intervention Centers

As discussed above, current studies support an early invasive approach in patients with high-risk ACS. When such patients present to hospitals without PCI capability, the risk and delay associated with transfer to interventional centers may be more than off-

Table 5
One-Month Outcomes of the PRAGUE Prospective Randomized Trial, Comparing Emergency
Transfer for Primary Angioplasty Vs Fibrinolytic Therapy Vs a Combined Strategy (76)

	Fibrinolysis without transfer (n = 99)	Transfer with fibrinolysis (n = 100)	Transfer without fibrinolysis (n = 101)
Mortality	14%	12%	7%
Reinfarction	10%	7%	1%
Stroke	1%	3%	0%
Combined endpoint[a]	23%	15%	8%

PTCA, percutaneous transluminal coronary angioplasty.
[a]Death, reinfarction, or stroke; %, percent of patients
$p < 0.03, p < 0.002$.

set by the added benefit of coronary intervention, especially in the case of patients with AMI. Because the benefit of primary PCI does not seem to be nearly so time-dependent as the benefit of fibrinolytic therapy (74), a policy of emergent transfer of at least the high-risk and fibrinolytic-ineligible patients with AMI may be a reasonable approach.

There are not many randomized trials that test this approach. The Air-Primary Angioplasty in Myocardial Infarction (AIR-PAMI) trial was a prospective multicenter randomized study of 138 fibrinolytic-eligible patients with high-risk AMI without shock that presented to hospitals which lacked interventional capability (75). Patients were randomized to fibrinolytic therapy versus transfer for PCI without fibrinolytic therapy. The group transferred for PCI had a 38% reduction of the combined end point of death, reinfarction, and stroke compared to patients receiving fibrinolytic therapy on-site (not statistically significant due to lack of recruitment).

Another such trial was the Primary Angioplasty in Patients Transferred from General Community Hospitals to Specialized PTCA Units (PRAGUE) study, which provides more support for immediate transfer for PCI of high-risk AMI patients that present to noninterventional hospitals (76). PRAGUE was a prospective randomized study involving 300 patients with AMI. In PRAGUE, patients with AMI were randomized into three groups: (i) transfer for primary PCI without antecedent fibrinolytic therapy; (ii) transfer for PCI after starting fibrinolytic therapy; and (iii) fibrinolytic therapy without transfer. Patients in the first group that were transferred for PCI without fibrinolytic therapy had significantly lower 30-d incidence of major adverse cardiac events (MACE), which included death, reinfarction, and stroke, than those randomized to the second and third groups (Table 5). There were two episodes of ventricular fibrillation during transfer in the 100 patients that received fibrinolytic agents before transfer; no complications occurred during transfer in the 101 patients not treated with fibrinolytic therapy.

The Second Danish Trial of Acute Myocardial Infarction (DANAMI 2) has randomized two different groups of patients with AMI to fibrinolytic therapy vs primary PCI. Patients presenting to tertiary centers will be randomized to fibrinolytic therapy vs immediate PCI, and patients presenting to community hospitals will be randomized to fibrinolytic therapy vs immediate transfer for PCI. This trial has been halted prematurely, following recommendations from the trial's Safety and Ethical Committee. Results of DANAMI 2 are expected to be announced at the ACC Scientific Sessions in March, 2002.

When primary PCI is delayed in patients with AMI, owing to need for transfer or catheterization laboratory unavailability, lower doses of fibrinolytic agents, especially with platelet GP IIb/IIIa inhibitors, may enhance early patency without jeopardizing PCI outcomes. The Plasminogen Activator Angioplasty Compatibility Trial (PACT) found that treatment with alteplace, compared to placebo before primary PCI in 606 patients, improved early patency rates without increased complications of the procedure *(77)*. This strategy of 'facilitated' coronary intervention is now being studied on a broader scale in several new trials, including the Controlled Abciximab and Device Investigation to Lower Late Angioplasty Complications (CADILLAC) II trial, which will also incorporate the use of GP IIb/IIIa platelet inhibitors *(78)*. In CADILLAC II, 3000 patients with AMI will be randomized to a combination of a fibrinolytic agent and a GP IIb/IIIa platelet inhibitor vs double placebo and then taken to the catheterization laboratory (after transfer, if necessary).

Thus, it is reasonable to recommend that patients with high-risk AMI that present to hospitals without coronary intervention should be transferred emergently to an interventional center for immediate coronary angiography and primary PCI. Patients with ACS that have ischemic ECG changes or elevated cardiac markers should be treated immediately with platelet GP IIb/IIIa inhibitors and transferred for intervention within the first 4–48 h of admission, and more emergently if symptoms or signs of ongoing ischemia do not stabilize quickly.

Although the need is clear for hospitals without interventional capability to establish rapid transfer protocols to interventional centers for their higher-risk AMI patients, the emergent transfer of such patients presents many difficulties. Many community hospitals may be reluctant to transfer patients early in the throes of AMI unless they deteriorate clinically, at which time the risk is much greater. Another problem is that many tertiary centers still do not offer primary PCI as routine first-line care, even for their own patients with AMI, and thus, may not have established protocols to perform immediate PCI on critically ill patients that they accept in transfer. These considerations support the need to expand the availability of centers that are capable of offering primary PCI. Uncoupling PCI from the requirement for on-site coronary bypass surgery will reduce the pressure to open more low-volume surgical programs to support needed new PCI programs.

Establishment of Policies and Protocols to Enable the Prehospital Ambulance Triage of Patients with Suspected AMI to Emergency Intervention Centers

Current registry data in the United States indicate that patients with AMI that present to interventional centers may have improved outcomes compared to patients with AMI that are transferred for primary PCI. The NRMI-2 registry analyzed the outcomes of 10,618 fibrinolytic-eligible patients with AMI that receiving PCI within 6 h of arrival to a center capable of coronary intervention. This registry demonstrated that patients that were transferred for PCI underwent the procedure a mean of 2.3 h later than patients receiving intervention at the point of first presentation and had a significantly higher mortality rate (7.7 vs 5.0%, $p = 0.0001$) *(79)*.

Recently, the AIR-PAMI trial outcomes (cited above) were compared to the PAMI-No Surgery On Site (No S.O.S.) Registry *(80)*. In the No S.O.S. registry, 500 patients, with the same enrollment criteria for high-risk AMI as the AIR-PAMI Trial, received primary PCI at 19 community hospitals with off-site surgical backup. In this comparison, transfer for primary PCI was safe, but the performance of coronary intervention on-site at hospitals without cardiac surgery was associated with shorter delay, higher rates of PCI success, and significantly lower 1-yr mortality than patients transferred for coronary intervention.

These data support the contention that patients with high-risk AMI who are treated with PCI might have better outcomes if triaged by ambulance directly to nearby qualified emergency interventional centers, rather than to the closest acute-care hospital. Emergency intervention centers need not be limited to those with on-site cardiac surgery, as discussed above. Patients with cardiogenic shock should be especially likely to benefit from this approach, since emergency revascularization within the first few hours of presentation improves survival dramatically in this group *(20,21)*.

Establishing a system of routine prehospital ambulance triage of patients with AMI to emergency intervention centers will also present many difficulties. Unlike for major trauma cases, there are no policies or protocols in the United States for ambulance providers to bypass a conventional acute-care hospital to travel further to an emergency intervention center. In many areas of the United States, tertiary centers are widely spaced geographically, some over 3 h from acute-care community hospitals. Many tertiary centers do not offer primary PCI as routine first-line care, even for their own patients. These considerations thus support the need to increase the availability of centers that can offer primary PCI for AMI in broader geographical locations. Uncoupling the requirement for on-site cardiac surgery would enable the establishment of more qualified PCI programs, while at the same time, reducing the pressure to build more low-volume cardiac surgery centers to support coronary intervention.

The practice of prehospital ambulance triage of higher-risk AMI patients to specialized emergency intervention centers for immediate PCI will require a major change in paradigm in the United States. Prehospital ambulance triage of AMI patients is already practiced in Paris, France, and is being studied in another European trial, the Prehospital Infarction Angioplasty Triage (PHIAT) trial. In PHIAT, 213 patients with large AMI as identified by ambulance ECG underwent prehospital triage directly to emergency intervention centers *(81)*. Catheterization laboratory staff were alerted prior to patient arrival. In this trial, investigators achieved a median time of 128 min from symptom onset to admission, and a median time from admission to first balloon inflation of only 38 min. The rapid time from symptom onset to reperfusion was reflected in a very favorable 6-mo mortality of 6%, in a population that included only patients with 'large' AMI; 89% of patients had anterior infarctions. The authors of PHIAT concluded that prehospital ambulance triage is a feasible, effective, and safe way to provide early intervention to patients with large AMI.

CONCLUSIONS

There is a clear need to increase the delivery of coronary intervention for patients with AMI and other high-risk ACS that present to community hospitals, which represent the majority of such patients. In order to expand the access to PCI for such patients, there are three main approaches that are both appropriate and necessary:

1. Programs to provide both primary and nonemergent PCI at qualified hospitals without on-site cardiac surgery should be encouraged, if they can meet rigorous standards such as those outlined in Tables 2 and 3 *(30)*.
2. Protocols for rapid and routine transfer of high risk and fibrinolytic-ineligible patients with AMI and other ACS to centers capable of emergency intervention on a 24-h, 7-d/wk basis. The goal from initial presentation to catheterization laboratory arrival after transfer should and can be less than 1 h *(82,83)*. Appropriate patients for transfer would include those with shock, those at increased risk to develop shock (those with congestive heart failure, hypotension, tachycardia, anterior AMI, or age over 70 yr) *(84)*, and those with contraindications to fibrinolytic therapy, as well as patients treated with fibrinolytic agents who would be appropriate for rescue angioplasty in the event of treatment failure. Such patients should be considered for pro-active transfer to an interventional center after starting fibrinolytic therapy, in order to avoid the delay of waiting for failure of reperfusion prior to initiating the transfer process.

High-risk patients with UA and NSTEMI, which includes those with ischemic ECG changes or elevated cardiac markers, should be treated with platelet GP IIb/IIIa inhibitors and transferred on an urgent basis for intervention within the first 48 h. Those that fail to stabilize quickly should be transferred more emergently.

3. The practice of routine prehospital ambulance triage to centers capable of around-the-clock emergency intervention should be encouraged by new national and local guidelines and policies. In order to provide wider geographic distribution, hospitals without on-site cardiac surgical programs in underserved areas should be encouraged to establish PCI programs, if they can meet the rigorous qualifications in Table 3.

Acute coronary intervention is now the treatment of choice for patients with AMI and high-risk acute coronary syndromes. This best treatment for acute coronary disease must be made more available at the hospitals in the community, which are the hospitals to which most patients with ACS present *(1)*. Improving the delivery of interventional therapy by methods such as those described here can provide a substantial healthcare benefit to society.

REFERENCES

1. Mehta RH, Stalhandske EJ, McCargar PA, et al. Elderly patients at highest risk with acute myocardial infarction are more frequently transferred from community hospitals to tertiary centers: reality or myth? Am Heart J 1999;138:688–695.
2. Weaver WD, Simes J, Betriu A, et al. Comparison of primary coronary angioplasty and intravenous thrombolytic therapy for acute myocardial infarction. JAMA 1997;278:2093–2098.
3. Schömig A, Kastrati A, Dirschinger J, et al. Coronary stenting plus platelet glycoprotein IIb/IIIa blockade compared with tissue plasminogen activator in acute myocardial infarction. N Engl J Med 2000; 343:385–391.
4. Garcia E, Elizaga J, Perez-Castellano N, et al. Primary angioplasty versus systemic thrombolysis in anterior myocardial infarction. J Am Coll Cardiol 1999;33:605–611.
5. Hannan EL, Racz MJ, Arani DT, et al. Short- and long-term mortality for patients undergoing primary angioplasty for acute myocardial infarction. J Am Coll Cardiol 2000;36:1194–1201.
6. Magid DJ, Calonge BN, Rumsfeld JS, et al. Relation between hospital primary angioplasty volume and mortality for patients with acute MI treated with primary angioplasty vs thrombolytic therapy. JAMA 2000;284:3131–3138.

7. Zahn R, Schiele R, Schnieder S, et al. Primary angioplasty versus intravenous thrombolysis in acute myocardial infarction: can we define subgroups of patients benefiting most from primary angioplasty? Results from the pooled data of the maximal individual therapy in acute myocardial infarction registry and the myocardial infarction registry. J Am Coll Cardiol 2001;37:1827–1835.

8. Zahn R, Schiele R, Schnieder S, et al. Decreasing hospital mortality between 1994 and 1998 in patients with acute myocardial infarction treated with primary angioplasty but not in patients treated with intravenous thrombolysis. J Am Coll Cardiol 2000;36:2064–2071.

9. Grines CL, Booth DC, Nissen SE, et al. Mechanism of acute myocardial infarction in patients with prior coronary artery bypass grafting and therapeutic implications. Am J Cardiol 1990;65: 1292–1296.

10. Rogers WJ. Contemporary management of acute myocardial infarction. Am J Med 1995;99:195–206.

11. The TIMI Study Group. Effects of tissue plasminogen activator and a comparison of early invasive and conservative strategies in unstable angina and non-Q-wave myocardial infarction: results of the TIMI IIIB Trial. Thrombolysis in Myocardial Ischemia. Circulation 1994;89:1545–1556.

12. Fibrinolytic Therapy Trialists' (FTT) Collaborative Group. Indications for fibrinolytic therapy in suspected acute myocardial infarction: collaborative overview of early mortality and major morbidity results from all randomised trials of more than 1000 patients. Lancet 1994;343:311–322.

13. Barron HV, Rundle A, Gurwitz J, Tiefenbrunn A. Reperfusion therapy for acute myocardial infarction: observations from the National Registry of Myocardial Infarction 2. Cardiol Rev 1999;7:156–160.

14. Zahn R, Schuster S, Schielel R, et al. Comparison of primary angioplasty with conservative therapy in patients with acute myocardial infarction and contraindications for thrombolytic therapy. Maximal Individual Therapy in Acute Myocardial Infarction (MITRA) Study Group. Cathet Cardiovasc Intervent 1999;46:127–133.

15. Zahn R, Schiele R, Schneider S, et al. Primary dilatation versus thrombolysis in patients with acute myocardial infarct, not included in randomized studies. Results of the MITRA Study: Maximal Individual Optimized Therapy for Acute Myocardial Infarct. Z Kardiol 1999;88:418–425.

16. Thiemann DR, Coresh J, Schulman SP, et al. Lack of benefit for intravenous thrombolysis in patients with myocardial infarction who are older than 75 years. Circulation 2000;101:2239–2246.

17. Berger AK, Schulman KA, Gersh BJ, et al. Primary coronary angioplasty vs thrombolysis for the management of acute myocardial infarction in elderly patients. JAMA 1999;282:341–348.

18. Berger AK, Schulman KA, Gersh BJ, et al. Primary coronary angioplasty vs thrombolysis for the management of acute myocardial infarction in elderly patients. JAMA 1999;282:341–348.

19. Brass LM, Lichtman JH, Wang Y, et al. Intracranial hemorrhage associated with thrombolytic therapy for elderly patients with acute myocardial infarction: results from the Cooperative Cardiovascular Project. Stroke 2000;31:1802–1811.

20. Hochman JS, Sleeper LA, Webb JG, et al. Early revascularization in acute myocardial infarction complicated by cardiogenic shock. N Engl J Med 1999;341:625–634.

21. Brodie BR, Stuckey TD, Muncy DB, et al. Importance of time to reperfusion in patients with acute myocardial infarction with and without cardiogenic shock treated with primary angioplasty (abstract). Circulation 2000;102:II-386.

22. Holmes DR Jr, Topol EJ, Berger PB, et al. Contemporary reperfusion therapy for cardiogenic shock: the GUSTO-I trial experience. The GUSTO-I Investigators. Global Utilization of Streptokinase and Tissue Plasminogen Activator for Occluded Coronary Arteries. J Am Coll Cardiol 1995;26:668–674.

23. Antoniucci D, Valenti R, Santoro GM, et al. Systematic direct angioplasty and stent-supported direct angioplasty therapy for cardiogenic shock complicating acute myocardial infarction: in-hospital and long-term survival. J Am Coll Cardiol 1998;31:294–300.

24. Bengtson J, Kaplan J, Pieper K, et. al. Prognosis in cardiogenic shock after myocardial infarction in the interventional era. J Am Coll Cardiol 1992;20:1482–1488.

25. Stomel RJ, Basak M, Bates ER. Treatment strategies for acute myocardial infarction complicated by cardiogenic shock in a community hospital. Chest 1994;105:997–1002.

26. Kovack PJ, Stomel RJ, Ohman EM, et al. Thrombolysis plus aortic counterpulsation: improved survival in patients who present to community hospitals with cardiogenic shock. J Am Coll Cardiol 1997; 29:1454–1458.

27. Berger PB, Topol EJ, Califf RM, et al. Impact of an aggressive invasive catheterization and revascularization strategy on mortality in patients with cardiogenic shock in the Global Utilization of Streptokinase and Tissue Plasminogen Activator for Occluded Coronary Arteries (GUSTO-I) trial. An observational study. Circulation 1997;96:122–127.

28. Hernandez F, Hernandez P, Tascon JC, et al. Emergency revascularization and hybrid approaches in cardiogenic shock [abstract]. Eur Heart J 1999;20(Suppl.):169.

29. Wharton TP Jr, McNamara NS, Lew D, et al. Cardiogenic shock at community hospitals with no surgery on site: outcomes after primary angioplasty in 101 patients in a multicenter registry [abstract]. Circulation 1998;98:I-307–I-308.

30. Wharton TP Jr, McNamara NS, Fedele FA, et al. Primary angioplasty for the treatment of acute myocardial infarction: experience at two community hospitals without cardiac surgery. J Am Coll Cardiol 1999;33:1257–1265.

31. Rogers WJ, Canto JG, Lambrew CT, Tiefenbrunn AJ. Temporal trends in the treatment of over 1.5 million patients with myocardial infarction in the U.S. from 1990 through 1999. The National Registry of Myocardial Infarction 1, 2 and 3. J Am Coll Cardiol 2000;36:2056–2063.

32. Scull GS, Martin JS, Weaver WD, Every, NR, for the MITI Investigators. Early angiography versus conservative treatment in patients with non-ST elevation acute myocardial infarction. J Am Coll Cardiol 2000;35:895–902.

33. Rogers WJ, Bowlby LJ, Chandra NC, et al. Treatment of myocardial infarction in the United States (1990 to 1993): observations from the National Registry of Myocardial Infarction. Circulation. 1994; 90:2103–2114.

34. Boden WE, O'Rourke RA, Crawford MH, et al. Outcomes in patients with acute non-Q-wave myocardial infarction randomly assigned to an invasive as compared with a conservative management strategy. Veterans Affairs Non-Q-Wave Infarction Strategies in Hospital (VANQWISH) Trial Investigators. N Engl J Med 1998;338:1785–1792.

35. The TIMI Study Group. Effects of tissue plasminogen activator and a comparison of early invasive and conservative strategies in unstable angina and non-Q-wave myocardial infarction: results of the TIMI IIIB Trial. Thrombolysis in Myocardial Ischemia. Circulation 1994;89:1545–1556.

36. Fragmin and Fast Revascularisation during Instability in Coronary Artery Disease Investigators. Invasive compared with non-invasive treatment in unstable coronary-artery disease: FRISC II prospective randomised multicentre study. Lancet 1999;354:708–715.

37. Anderson HV, Cannon CP, Stone PH, et al. One-year results of the Thrombolysis in Myocardial Infarction (TIMI) IIIB clinical trial. A randomized comparison of tissue-type plasminogen activator versus placebo and early invasive versus early conservative strategies in unstable angina and non-Q wave myocardial infarction. J Am Coll Cardiol 1995;26:1643–1650.

38. Wallentin LC. Patients without ST-segment elevation, revascularization. When? For whom? Presented at the European Society of Cardiology XXIII Congress, 2001 September 1–5; Stockholm, Sweden.

39. Cannon CP, Weintraub WS, Demopoulous LA, et al. Comparison of early invasive and conservative strategies in patients with unstable coronary syndromes treated with the glycoprotein IIb/IIIa inhibitor tirofiban. New Engl J Med 2001;344:1879–1887.

40. Mathew V, Farkouh ME, Gersh BJ, et al. Early coronary angiography improves long-term survival in unstable angina. Am Heart J 2001;142:768–774.

41. Weintraub WS. Treat angina with aggrastat and determine cost of therapy with an invasive or conservative strategy (TACTICS)-TIMI 18. Oral presentation during the 50th Annual Scientific Sessions of the American Heart Association, 2001 March 18-21; Orlando, FL.

42. Foot DK, Lewis RP, Pearson TA, Beller GA. Demographics and cardiology, 1950-2050. J Am Coll Cardiol 2000;35:66B–80B.

43. Smith SC Jr, Dove JT, Jacobs AK, et al. ACC/AHA guidelines for percutaneous coronary intervention: executive summary and recommendations: a report of the American College of Cardiology/American Heart Association Task Force on Practice Guidelines (Committee to Revise the 1993 Guidelines for Percutaneous Transluminal Coronary Angioplasty). J Am Coll Cardiol 2001;37:2215–2238.

44. Stone GW, Brodie BR, Griffin JJ, et al. Prospective, multicenter study of the safety and feasibility of primary stenting in acute myocardial infarction: in-hospital and 30-day results of the PAMI stent pilot trial. Primary Angioplasty in Myocardial Infarction Stent Pilot Trial Investigators. J Am Coll Cardiol 1998;31:23–30.

45. Antoniucci D, Santoro GM, Bolognese L, et al. A clinical trial comparing primary stenting of the infarct-related artery with optimal primary angioplasty for acute myocardial infarction. Results of the Florence Randomized Elective Stenting in Acute Coronary Occlusions (FRESCO) trial. J Am Coll Cardiol 1998;31:1234–1239.

46. Loubeyre C, Morice MC, Berzin B, et al. Emergency coronary artery bypass surgery following coronary angioplasty and stenting: results of a French multicenter registry. Cathet Cardiovasc Intervent 1999;48:441–448.

47. Stone GW, Brodie B, Griffin J, et al. "Role of cardiac surgery in the hospital phase management of patients treated with primary angioplasty for acute myocardial infarction." Am J Cardiol 2000;85: 1292–1296.

48. Shubrooks SJ Jr, Nesto RW, Leeman D, et al. Urgent coronary bypass surgery for failed percutaneous coronary intervention in the stent era: is backup still necessary? Am Heart J 2001;142:190–196.

49. The Society for Cardiac Angiography and Interventions. Directory of cardiac catheterization laboratories in the United States. 4th ed. The Laboratory Performance Standards Committee of The Society for Cardiac Angiography and Interventions, Raleigh, NC, 1996.

50. Joint Working Group on Coronary Angioplasty of the British Cardiac Society and British Cardiovascular Intervention Society. Coronary angioplasty: guidelines for good practice and training. Heart 2000;83:224–235.

51. Expert Panel on Invasive Cardiology in Ontario. Cardiac Care Network of Ontario: final report and recommendations. Submitted to the Ontario Ministry of Healty and Long-Term Care, June 2001. Available from URL: (http://www.ccn.on.ca).

52. Vogel J. Angioplasty in the patient with an evolving myocardial infarction: with and without surgical backup. Clin Cardiol 1992;15:880–882.

53. Weaver WD, Litwin PE, Martin JS. Use of direct angioplasty for treatment of patients with acute myocardial infarction in hospitals with and without on-site cardiac surgery. Circulation 1993;88: 2067–2075.

54. Iannone LA, Anderson SM, Phillips SJ. Coronary angioplasty for acute myocardial infarction in a hospital without cardiac surgery. Tex Heart Inst J 1993;20:99–104.

55. Ayres M. Coronary angioplasty for acute myocardial infarction in hospitals without cardiac surgery. J Invasive Cardiol 1995;7(Suppl. F):40F–48F.

56. Weaver WD, Parsons L, Every N. Primary coronary angioplasty in hospitals with and without surgery backup. J Invasive Cardiol 1995;7(Suppl. F):34F–39F.

57. Brush JE, Thompson S, Ciuffo AA, et al. Retrospective comparison of a strategy of primary coronary angioplasty versus intravenous thrombolytic therapy for acute myocardial infarction in a community hospital without cardiac surgery. J Invasive Cardiol 1996;8:91–98.

58. Weaver WD for the MITI Project Investigators. PTCA in centers without surgical backup-outcome, logistics, and technical aspects. J Invasive Cardiol 1997;9(Suppl. B): 20B–23B.

59. Smyth DW, Richards AM, Elliot JM. Direct angioplasty for myocardial infarction: one-year experience in a center with surgical backup 220 miles away. J Invasive Cardiol 1997;9:324–332.

60. Wharton TP Jr, Johnston JD, Turco MA, et al. Primary angioplasty for acute myocardial infarction with no surgery on site: outcomes, core angiographic analysis, and six-month follow-up in the 500-patient prospective PAMI—No S.O.S. Registry [abstract]. J Am Coll Cardiol 1999;33:352A–353A.

61. Ribichini F, Steffenino G, Dellavalle A, et al. Primary angioplasty without surgical back-up at all. Results of a five years experience in a community hospital in Europe [abstract]. J Am Coll Cardiology 2000;35:364A.

62. O'Neill WW, Brodie BR, Ivanhoe R, et al. Primary coronary angioplasty for acute myocardial infarction (the Primary Angioplasty Registry). Am J Cardiol 1994;73:627–634.

63. Stone GW, Brodie BR, Griffin JJ, et al. Prospective, multicenter study of the safety and feasibility of primary stenting in acute myocardial infarction: in-hospital and 30-day results of the PAMI stent pilot trial. Primary Angioplasty in Myocardial Infarction Stent Pilot Trial Investigators. J Am Coll Cardiol 1998;31:23–30.

64. Antoniucci D, Santoro GM, Bolognese L, et al. A clinical trial comparing primary stenting of the infarct-related artery with optimal primary angioplasty for acute myocardial infarction. Results of the Florence Randomized Elective Stenting in Acute Coronary Occlusions (FRESCO) trial. J Am Coll Cardiol 1998;31:1234–1239.

65. Suryapranata H, van't Hof AW, Hoorntje JCA, et al. Randomized comparison of coronary stenting with balloon angioplasty in selected patients with acute myocardial infarction. Circulation 1998;97: 2502–2505.

66. The EPISTENT Investigators. Randomised placebo-controlled and balloon-angioplasty-controlled trial to assess safety of coronary stenting with use of platelet glycoprotein-IIb/IIIa blockade. Lancet 1998;352:87–92.

67. The EPISTENT Investigators. Randomised placebo-controlled and balloon-angioplasty-controlled trial to assess safety of coronary stenting with use of platelet glycoprotein-IIb/IIIa blockade. Lancet 1998;352:87–92.

68. Blankenship JC, Sigmon KN, Pieper KS, et al. Effect of eptifibatide on angiographic complications during percutaneous coronary intervention in the IMPACT (Integrilin to Minimize Platelet Aggregation and Coronary Thrombosis) II Trial. Am J Cardiol 2001;88:969–973.

69. Simpson DE, Boura JA, Grines LL, Grines CL. Predictors of delay from ER to cath with primary PTCA for acute MI [abstract]. J Am Coll Cardiol 2000;3520A.

70. Aversano T, et al. Atlantic cardiovascular patient outcomes research team trial of primary percutaneous coronary intervention vs thrombolysis in acute MI (C-PORT PCI). Oral presented during the 73rd Annual Scientific Sessions of the American Heart Association, 2000 November 12–15, New Orleans, LA.

70a. Aversano T, Aversano LT, Passamani E. Thrombolytic therapy vs primary percutaneous coronary intervention for myocardial infarction in patients presenting to hospitals without on-site cardiac surgery. JAMA 2002;287:1943–1951.

71. Every NR, Maynard C, Schulman K, Ritchie JL. The association between institutional primary angioplasty procedure volume and outcome in elderly Americans. J Invasive Cardiol 2000;12:303–308.

72. Cannon CP, Gibson CM, Lambrew CT, et al. Relationship of symptom-onset-to-balloon time and door-to balloon time with mortality in patient undergoing angioplasty for acute myocardial infarction. JAMA 2000;283:2941–2947.

73. Canto JG, Every NR, Magid DJ, et al. The volume of primary angioplasty procedures and survival after acute myocardial infarction. N Engl J Med 2000;342:1573–1580.

74. Brodie BR, Stuckey TD, Wall TC, et al. Importance of time to reperfusion for 30-day and late survival and recovery of left ventricular function after primary angioplasty for acute myocardial infarction. J Am Coll Cardiol 1998;32:1312–1319.

75. Grines L, Westerhausen DR, et al. A randomized trial of transfer for primary angioplasty versus on-site thrombolysis in patients with high risk myocardial infarction: the Air Primary Angioplasty in Myocardial Infarction study. J Am Coll Cardiology 2002;39:1713–1719.

76. Widimsky P, Groch L, Zelizko M, et al. Multicentre randomized trial comparing transport to primary angioplasty vs immediate thrombolysis vs combined strategy for patients with acute myocardial infarction presenting to a community hospital without a catheterization laboratory. The PRAGUE study. Eur Heart J 2000;2:823–831.

77. Ross AM, Coyne KS, Reiner JS, et al. A randomized trial comparing primary angioplasty with a strategy of short-acting thrombolysis and immediate planned rescue angioplasty in acute myocardial infarction: the PACT trial. PACT investigators. J Am Coll Cardiol 1999;34:1954–1962.

78. Stone GW. Providing facilitated primary PTCA—the CADILLAC II trial. Oral presentation during the Transcatheter Cardiovascular Therapeutics XII 2000 Oct 18-20; Washington, DC.

79. Tiefenbrunn AJ, Chandra NC, Every NR, et al. High mortality in patients with myocardial infarction transferred for primary angioplasty: a report from the National Registry of Myocardial Infarction-2 [abstract]. Circulation 1997;96:I-531.

80. Grines LL, Wharton TP Jr, Balestrini C, et al. Should high-risk acute myocardial infarction patients admitted to non-surgical hospitals be transferred for primary PTCA or receive it on-site? [abstract] Circulation 2000;102:II-386.

81. Ernst N, de Boer MJ, van't Hof AW, et al. Prehospital infarction angioplasty triage (PHIAT): results from the Zwolle myocardial infarction study group [abstract]. J Am Coll Cardiol 2001;37:339A.

82. Timmis SB, Timmis GC, Pica MC, et al. Facilitated primary percutaneous intervention in acute myocardial infarction using glycoprotein IIb/IIIa inhibitors with or without thrombolytic therapy. Circulation 2001;104:II-504.

83. Brodie B, Stuckey T, Hansen C, et al. The effect of time delay on outcomes in patients with acute myocardial infarction transferred from community hospitals for primary angioplasty. Circulation 2001;104:II-630.

84. Hasdai D, Califf RM, Thompson TD, et al. Predictors of cardiogenic shock after thrombolytic therapy for acute myocardial infarction. J Am Coll Cardiol 2000;35:136–143.

12 Antiplatelet and Anticoagulant Therapy

Marc S. Sabatine, MD, MPH and Ik-Kyung Jang, MD

CONTENTS

INTRODUCTION
PLATELET INHIBITION
ANTICOAGULATION
CONCLUSION
REFERENCES

INTRODUCTION

Fifteen years ago the Gruppo Italialono per lo Studio della Streptochianasi nell'Infarto Miocardico (GISSI) trial firmly established the benefit of fibrinolytic therapy in acute myocardial infarction *(1)*. Several years later, the importance of adjunctive antiplatelet therapy with aspirin was demonstrated in the Second International Study of Infarct Survival (ISIS-2) *(2)*. The need for concomitant anticoagulant therapy with heparin remains less clear, but indirect evidence in the setting of fibrin-specific lytics has led to widespread adoption *(3,4)*.

However, pharmacologic reperfusion for acute ST-elevation myocardial infarction is limited by the fact that infarct-related artery patency is achieved in only 60–80% of patients at 90 min, and Thrombolysis in Myocardial Infarction (TIMI) flow grade 3 is achieved in only 30–55% of patients *(5)*. Moreover, even after successful thrombolysis, reocclusion occurs in 5–10% of patients and is associated with increased morbidity and mortality *(5,6)*. Third-generation bolus fibrinolytics such as reteplase and tenecteplase appeared to be more effective than alteplase in angiographic studies *(7–10)*, but these patency data have not translated into lower mortality rates in large phase III clinical trials *(11,12)*.

Thus, attention has shifted to optimizing adjunctive antithrombotic therapy. It is well recognized that there are several important limitations to our current antiplatelet and anticoagulant agents, namely aspirin and unfractionated heparin. Aspirin is only a weak inhibitor of platelet activation, allowing platelet activation to occur by cyclooxygenase-independent pathways *(13)*. Persistent platelet activation leads to platelet aggregation,

From: *Contemporary Cardiology: Management of Acute Coronary Syndromes, Second Edition*
Edited by: C. P. Cannon © Humana Press Inc., Totowa, NJ

creating platelet-rich coronary thrombi which are relatively resistant to thrombolysis *(14)* and to further stimulation of the clotting cascade by providing a catalytic surface for coagulation factor interactions *(15)*. Heparin has several major limitations to being an ideal anticoagulant. First, although heparin is able to inactivate fluid-phase thrombin, it is unable to inactivate fibrin monomer-bound *(16)* or clot-bound *(17)* thrombin. Second, heparin is inactivated by platelet factor 4 and heparinases, both of which are released by activated platelets *(18)*. Third, heparin is a heterogeneous mixture with highly variable pharmacokinetics *(19)*. Fourth, treatment with heparin can be complicated by heparin-induced thrombocytopenia *(20)*.

Along with these pharmacodynamic and pharmacokinetic limitations to our current adjunctive therapy, there is evidence that a hypercoagulable state exists during acute coronary syndromes that may persist as far as 6 mo out *(21)*. Furthermore, thrombolysis may even potentiate this hypercoagulable state. Thrombolytic therapy has been shown to cause platelet activation *(22,23)*, increased thrombin generation *(24–26)*, and increased thrombin activity *(27,28)*, that heparin may not be able to adequately suppress *(25,29–31)*. The mechanisms underlying this hypercoagulable state and its potentiation by thrombolysis are incompletely understood, but may involve clot digestion leading to thrombin liberation *(32)*, reexposure of prothrombotic lesions, or direct effects on the coagulation cascade *(33)*.

Thus, research efforts have focused on developing new antiplatelet and anticoagulant agents that are capable of overcoming the above limitations and achieving higher rates of infarct-related artery patency and lower rates of reocclusion and, thereby, enable us to reduce the morbidity and mortality still associated with acute myocardial infarction.

PLATELET INHIBITION

Platelet Activation and Aggregation

Platelets play a key role in initiating coronary artery thrombosis *(13,34,35)*. Damage to the vessel wall exposes the subendothelial matrix and allows platelet adhesion through glycoprotein (GP) Ib binding to von Willebrand factor (vWF), GP Ia binding to collagen, and other adhesion molecule interactions *(36)*. Platelets can then be activated by a variety of agonists including thrombin, adenosine diphosphate (ADP), collagen, and thromboxane A_2 (TXA_2) (Fig. 1). There are three main signal transduction path-

Fig. 1. A greatly simplified schematic depicting platelet adhesion, activation, and aggregation and the sites of action of antiplatelet agents. Platelet adhesion is mediated primarily by collagen binding to GP Ia and vWF binding to GP Ib. Platelet activation is extremely complex and only incompletely understood. Three major pathways have been identified. One pathway involves stimulation of PLC by agonists such as TXA_2, thrombin, serotonin (5-HT), platelet-activating factor (PAF), and collagen. PLC converts phosphatidylinositol 4,5-bisphosphate (PIP_2) to inositol 1,3,5-triphosphate (IP_3) and diacyl glycerol (DAG). Increased levels of IP_3 causes translocation of calcium from intracellular storage sites to the cytosol, which, with the help of calmodulin, leads to the activation of a variety of enzymes including myosin light chain kinase (MLCK). The other product of PLC activity is DAG, which activates protein kinase C (PKC). These two kinases, MLCK and PKC, phosphorylate, respectively, myosin light chain (MLC) and a 47-kDa protein (p47), ultimately leading to platelet activation. Another pathway involves stimulation of PLA by agonists such as ADP and epinephrine (epi). PLA liberates arachidonic acid (AA) from membrane phospholipids. AA is then converted by cyclooxygenase (CO) to PGH_2, which can then be converted either into TXA_2 by thromboxane synthase (TxS)

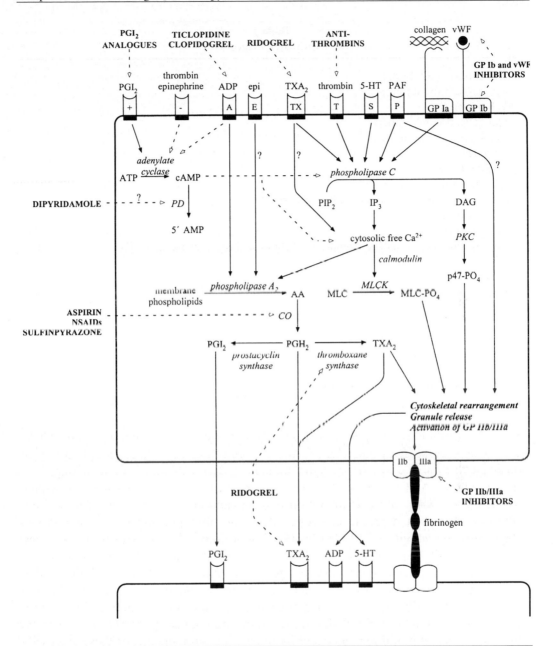

or into PGI_2 by prostacyclin synthase. TXA_2 is a platelet activator and a vasoconstrictor. A third pathway involves adenylate cyclase which, when inhibited by thrombin, ADP, or epi, leads to decreased levels of cyclic adenosine monophosphate (cAMP) and consequent depression of the PLC pathway described above. The end result of activation of any of these three pathways is to induce platelet activation specifically by bringing about cytoskeletal rearrangement, granule release, and the activation of GPIIb/IIIa. Platelet aggregation then occurs through fibrinogen binding to GP IIb/IIIa receptors on different platelets. The sites of action of platelet inhibitors is shown using open arrowheads and dashed lines. Addional abbreviations: (+), receptors which lead to activation of adenylate cyclase; (−), receptors which lead to inhibition of adenylate cyclase; A, ADP receptor; E, epinephrine receptor; TX, TXA_2 receptor; T, thrombin receptor; S, 5-HT receptor; P, PAF receptor; ATP, adenosine triphosphate; 5' AMP, 5' adenosine monophosphate; PD, phosphodiesterase.

Table 1
Antiplatelet Agents

Platelet adhesion inhibitors:
  Glycoprotein Ib inhibitors
  vWF inhibitors
Platelet activation inhibitors:
  Cyclooxygenase inhibitors
    Aspirin
    NSAIDs
    Sulfinpyrazone
  ADP antagonists (i.e., thienopyridine derivatives)
    Ticlopidine
    Clopidogrel
  Thromboxane inhibitors (i.e., synthase inhibitor and receptor antagonist)
    Ridogrel
  Dipyridamole
  Prostacyclin and analogues
  Thrombin inhibitors
Platelet aggregation inhibitors:
  Glycoprotein IIb/IIIa inhibitors
    Monoclonal antibodies (e.g., abciximab)
    Synthetic peptide compounds (e.g., eptifibatide)
    Nonpeptide mimetics (e.g., tirofiban)

ways: (*i*) activation of phospholipase C (PLC) (e.g., by thrombin, collagen, and TXA_2) leads to an increase in intraplatelet calcium concentration and subsequent phosphorylation and activation of downstream signal transducers; (*ii*) activation of phospholipase A_2 (PLA_2) (e.g., by ADP) leads to an increase in arachidonic acid levels with subsequent conversion to TXA_2; and (*iii*) inhibition of adenylate cyclase (e.g., by ADP and epinephrine) leads to a decrease in cyclic adenosine monophosphate (which normally antagonizes the activity of PLC) *(36–39)*. Importantly, platelet activation can occur through both TXA_2-dependent and TXA_2-independent pathways. Regardless of the pathway, platelet activation results in changes in morphology *(36)*, degranulation, induction of procoagulant activity *(15)*, and activation of the glycoprotein IIb/IIIa (GP IIb/IIIa) receptor *(37)*. The final step, platelet aggregation, occurs when fibrinogen molecules bind to the activated GP IIb/IIIa receptor and connect platelets to one another *(40)*. Thus, platelet inhibition can occur by interfering with any one of these steps (Fig. 1 and Table 1) *(41–43)*.

Cyclooxygenase Inhibitors: Aspirin

Pharmacology

Aspirin irreversibly inhibits cyclooxygenase (COX) by acetylating a serine residue at position 529 of the COX polypeptide *(44,45)*. COX converts arachidonic acid into the eicosanoid prostaglandin G_2 (PGG_2), which is the precursor of PGH_2. PGH_2 is either converted into prostacyclin (PGI_2) by prostacyclin synthase or converted into TXA_2 by thromboxane synthase. Which of the two eicosanoids is synthesized depends on whether prostacyclin synthase or thromboxane synthase predominates; the former predominates in endothelial cells and the latter predominates in platelets *(46)*. Because platelets lack the biosynthetic machinery to synthesize new proteins, aspirin inhibits thromboxane synthesis for the lifespan of the platelet (approx 10 d). Conversely, vascular endothelial cells can generate new COX, and therefore, the duration of aspirin's inhibitory effect on prostacyclin synthesis may be shorter *(47)*. Clinically, this translates into aspirin acting as an antiplatelet and anticoagulant agent. However, as thromboxane acts only on one of the platelet activation pathways, aspirin is unable to inhibit platelet activation by mediators such as thrombin that can utilize TXA_2-independent pathways. Interestingly, there is some preliminary evidence that aspirin may have an antithrombotic effect unrelated to inhibition of COX *(48,49)*.

Plasma levels of aspirin are detectable 20–30 min after administration of a single crushed or chewed dose, and platelet inhibition is achieved after approx 60 min *(50)*. Although the current recommendations call for 162–325 mg of aspirin orally daily in acute myocardial infarction *(4)*, it appears that 100 mg of aspirin is probably sufficient to almost completely inhibit the synthesis of thromboxane in individuals both with and without atherosclerotic disease *(51,52)*.

CLINICAL DATA

A meta-analysis of all clinical trials involving aspirin in the treatment of acute myocardial infarction demonstrated that antiplatelet therapy confers statistically significant reductions in nonfatal reinfarction, nonfatal stroke, vascular death, and overall mortality *(53)*. The definitive study in this area is ISIS-2, in which 17,187 patients, who presented within 24 h of the onset of symptoms consistent with acute myocardial infarction, were randomized in a 2-by-2 factorial design to receive streptokinase 1.5 million units (MU) intravenously (iv) over 60 min, aspirin 162.5 mg orally once daily, both, or neither *(2)*. At 5 wk, treatment with aspirin reduced vascular mortality by 20% (from 11.8 to 9.4%, $p < 0.00001$) (Fig. 2) and nonfatal reinfarction by 49% (from 2.0 to 1.0%, $p < 0.00001$). Treatment with aspirin was not associated with any significant increase in major bleeding. Follow-up of the patients in ISIS-2 has shown that these benefits from short-term antiplatelet therapy with aspirin have persisted for several years *(54)*.

Of note, the reductions in vascular mortality seen with streptokinase and aspirin were additive (vascular mortality 13.2% with neither, 10.7% with aspirin alone, 10.4% with streptokinase alone, and 8.0% with both). Moreover, aspirin produced an even greater reduction in the in-hospital reinfarction rate in the group that received fibrinolytic therapy (from 3.8 to 1.8%) than in the group that did not (from 2.9 to 1.9%). It has been shown that fibrinolytic therapy can activate platelets *(22,23)*, and antiplatelet therapy with aspirin may abolish this effect and prevent potential thrombolysis-induced platelet aggregation, coronary artery reocclusion, and reinfarction.

ADP Antagonists: Ticlopidine and Clopidogrel

PHARMACOLOGY

Ticlopidine and clopidogrel are thienopyridine derivatives that inhibit the binding of ADP to its receptor (Fig. 1) *(55)*. There are, in fact, multiple ADP receptors, all of which are part of the membrane-bound nucleotide P2 receptor family. It is believed that ticlopidine and clopidogrel inhibit the $P2T_{AC}$ receptor, which is linked to adenylate cyclase inhibition *(56)*. The thienopyridines can also indirectly inhibit the activity of several other platelet agonists such as arachidonic acid, collagen, thrombin, epinephrine, and

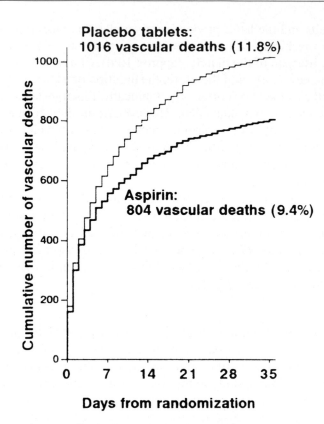

Fig. 2. Cumulative vascular mortality in d 0–35 in the ISIS-2 trial for all patients allocated aspirin vs all patients allocated placebo tablets. Reproduced with permission from ref. *2*.

serotonin. This is thought to occur because the aggregation response to these agonists is augmented by the initial release of ADP from activated platelets. At high concentrations of these agonists, platelet aggregation is ADP-independent, and therefore, ticlopidine and clopidogrel have no significant effect. Unlike aspirin, the ADP antagonists can inhibit platelet aggregation in response to vascular shear stress *(57)*. Observations that ticlopidine can block GP IIb/IIIa-mediated platelet aggregation *(58)* probably reflect a downstream effect of ADP inhibition rather than a direct effect. After starting a standard daily oral maintenance dose of either ticlopidine or clopidogrel, the full antiplatelet effect is not seen for 3–5 d and then persists for 4–8 d after drug discontinuation, consistent with an in vivo metabolite causing irreversible platelet inhibition *(58–60)*. However, administration of an oral loading dose results in antiplatelet effect being apparent after 60–90 min *(61)*.

Gastrointestinal (GI) upset, nausea, vomiting, diarrhea, and rashes occur in approx 10–20% of patients taking ticlopidine; many of the GI side effects can be eliminated by having the patient take ticlopidine with food. The most serious adverse effects are idiosyncratic neutropenia, which has been reported to occur in 1% of patients, and thrombotic thrombocytopenic purpura (TTP), which occurs in <0.1% of patients *(62,63)*. Clopidogrel enjoys a better side effect profile with lower rates of GI and dermatologic adverse reactions and rates of neutropenia and TTP that are roughly comparable to what is seen in the overall population. For these reasons, it has largely supplanted ticlopidine.

CLINICAL DATA

To date, there are few data regarding the efficacy of the ADP antagonists in ST-elevation myocardial infarction. However, two ongoing trials, CLARITY-TIMI 28 and COMMIT, will address this issue. The former is an angiographic study that will examine the effect of clopidogrel on late infarct-related artery patency in patients undergoing fibrinolysis. The latter is a phase III trial that will examine the effect of clopidogrel on mortality in patients undergoing fibrinolysis with a nonfibrin-selective lytic. However, while we await the results of these studies, there are several lines of evidence that support the utility of ADP antagonists as adjunctive antiplatelet therapy in acute coronary syndromes.

The ADP antagonists have become standard of care after intracoronary stent deployment to reduce thrombotic complications. The Intracoronary Stenting and Antithrombotic Regimen (ISAR) trial demonstrated that, compared to anticoagulant therapy, combination antiplatelet therapy with aspirin and ticlopidine resulted in an 86% reduction in stent occlusion, an 82% reduction in reinfarction, a 78% reduction in reintervention, and elimination of severe hemorrhagic complications *(64)*. In a subgroup analysis of 123 patients with stent placement for acute myocardial infarction, antiplatelet therapy resulted in a significant 84% reduction (from 21 to 3.3%, $p = 0.005$) in clinical events defined as cardiac events (cardiac death, reinfarction, reintervention) plus noncardiac events (noncardiac death, stroke, severe hemorrhage) *(65)*. The Stent Anticoagulation Regimen Study (STARS) demonstrated that the incidence of adverse events (death, emergent coronary artery bypass graft [CABG], myocardial infarction, or subacute closure) was significantly lower with aspirin plus ticlopidine (0.6%) as compared to aspirin alone (3.6%, $p < 0.001$) or aspirin plus warfarin (2.4%, $p - 0.01$) *(66)*. Several recent randomized trials suggest that, compared with ticlopidine, clopidogrel offers equivalent efficacy and better safety and tolerability *(67–69)*.

In the Clopidogrel versus Aspirin in Patients at Risk of Ischemic Events (CAPRIE) trial, 19,185 patients who had either a recent ischemic stroke, a myocardial infarction in the past 35 d, or symptoms of peripheral arterial disease were randomized to clopidogrel 75 mg orally once daily or aspirin 325 mg orally once daily *(70)*. Treatment with clopidogrel resulted in a statistically significant 8.7% reduction in the combined primary endpoints of ischemic stroke, myocardial infarction, or vascular death (from 5.83 to 5.32%, $p = 0.043$). More recently, the Clopidogrel in Unstable Angina to Prevent Recurrent Events (CURE) trial demonstrated that in 12,562 patients presenting with unstable angina, the addition of clopidogrel to a standard regimen of aspirin and unfractionated heparin resulted in a 20% reduction in the rate of the composite endpoint of death, myocardial infarction, and stroke (from 11.4 to 9.3%, $p < 0.001$) *(71)*. There was a 38% increase in major bleeding, but no statistically significant increase in life-threatening bleeding.

Glycoprotein IIb/IIIa Inhibitors

PHARMACOLOGY

The glycoprotein IIb/IIIa receptor (GP IIb/IIIa) is a member of the integrin superfamily of heterodimeric adhesion molecules that is found on platelets *(40)*. It is the primary receptor for platelet aggregation through binding to fibrinogen. GP IIb/IIIa contains two domains responsible for the binding of adhesive proteins (Fig. 3) *(72)*.

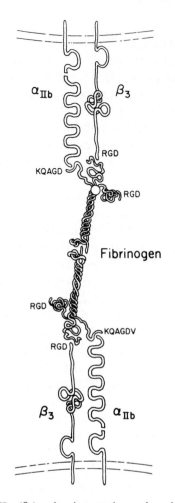

Fig. 3. GP IIb/IIIa structure. The IIIa (β_3) subunit contains a domain whose ligand is the peptide sequence RGD, which is found in each α-chain of fibrinogen. The IIb (α_{IIb}) subunit contains a domain whose ligand is the dodecapeptide HHLGGAKQAGDV, which is found in the γ chain of fibrinogen. Reproduced with permission from ref. *72*.

One domain is on the GP IIIa subunit and its ligand is the peptide sequence RGD. The other domain is on the GP IIb subunit and its ligand is the dodecapeptide HHLGGAKQAGDV. The dodecapeptide is found only in fibrinogen and is located on the γ chain. Conversely, the RGD sequence is found in many peptides including fibrinogen (where it is located on the α chain), fibronectin, vitronectin, vWF, and thrombospondin. GP IIb/IIIa is unable to bind fibrinogen unless the platelet is first activated by an agonist, which then induces a conformational change in GP IIb/IIIa, revealing the binding domain and rendering the molecule a competent fibrinogen binder. Platelet aggregation occurs when two activated platelets bind to the same fibrinogen molecule (each to one end), thereby forming a fibrinogen bridge between the two platelets.

GP IIb/IIIa inhibitors are particularly attractive as antiplatelet agents, because they can block the final step in platelet aggregation triggered by all endogenous platelet activators. There are several types of GP IIb/IIIa inhibitors *(40,73)*. In 1985, a mouse monoclonal antibody against GP IIb/IIIa (known as 7E3) was generated *(74)*; subsequent clinical trials have used abciximab (ReoPro), which is a Fab fragment of a chimeric human–mouse genetic reconstruction of 7E3 (abbreviated c7E3 Fab). Based on the disintegrins, which are natural peptides derived from snake venom that contain either an RGD-based or KGD-based sequence, researchers developed small-molecule GP IIb/IIIa inhibitors including synthetic peptide compounds, such as the cyclic KGD peptide analog eptifibatide (Integrilin) *(75,76)*, and nonpeptide mimetics, such as tirofiban (Aggrastat) *(77,78)*.

There are several important differences in the pharmacokinetics and pharmacodynamics of the currently available GP IIb/IIIa inhibitors. Abciximab has a very high affinity for GP IIb/IIIa and a long half-life (8–12 h), and after discontinuation of the infusion, platelet function returns gradually. In contrast, the small-molecule inhibitors eptifibatide and tirofiban have short half-lives, and platelet function returns quickly after discontinuation of the infusion. Although it has high affinity, abciximab has low specificity and binds to other integrins, including the vitronectin receptor (GP $\alpha_V\beta_3$), which is found on endothelial cells. Whether this is of clinical relevance remains unknown. In contrast, eptifibatide and tirofiban are extremely specific for the GP IIb/IIIa receptor. In addition to the expected side effect of excess bleeding, abciximab has also been associated with profound thrombocytopenia in 0.5–1.0% of cases *(79)* and the development of antimouse antibodies in 5–6% of cases *(80)*. However, in the ReoPro Readministration Registry, retreatment with abciximab was not associated with diminished efficacy or serious side effects, although the cases of thrombocytopenia tended to be more profound *(81)*.

CLINICAL DATA

Primary Angioplasty. All three GP IIb/IIIa inhibitors have been tested extensively in patients undergoing percutaneous coronary interventions (PCIs) and pooled analyses have demonstrated a 33% reduction in the composite of death, myocardial infarction, or the need for urgent revascularization through 30 d *(73)*. The early trials, however, generally excluded patients undergoing intervention in the setting of an acute myocardial infarction.

More recently, though, four trials have examined the efficacy of GP IIb/IIIa inhibitors in patients undergoing primary angioplasty for acute ST-elevation myocardial infarction. In the ReoPro in Acute Myocardial Infarction and Primary PTCA Organization and Randomized Trial (RAPPORT), 483 patients were treated with abciximab or placebo before primary balloon angioplasty. Treatment with abciximab was associated with a 48% reduction in death, reinfarction, or the need for urgent revascularization by 30 d (*p* = 0.03) *(82)*. However, the majority of this benefit derived from a reduction in the need for urgent revascularization. Major bleeding was twice as common in the abciximab group.

As with elective PCI, stenting has now become common in primary angioplasty for ST-elevation myocardial infarction. In the ISAR 2 trial, 401 patients undergoing intracoronary stenting for ST-elevation myocardial infarction were randomized to abciximab or placebo *(83)*. Treatment with abciximab was associated with a 52% reduction in the rate of death, reinfarction, or target lesion revascularization at 30 d (*p* = 0.038). Importantly, the magnitude of the risk reductions for each of the individual components of the composite end point were similar. Moreover, the 5% absolute reduction in the composite end point seen at 30 d persisted through 1 yr of follow-up.

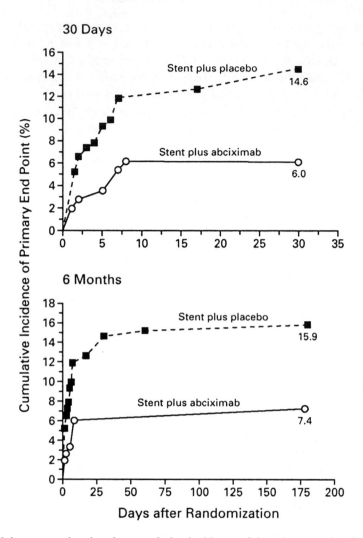

Fig. 4. Kaplan-Meier curves showing the cumulative incidence of the primary end point (death, reinfarction, or urgent target-vessel revascularization) at 30 d and 6 mo in the ADMIRAL trial for patients randomized to stent plus placebo (solid squares) vs stent plus abciximab (open circles). Reproduced with permission from ref. *84.*

Similar results were seen in the 300 patients in the Abciximab Before Direct Angioplasty and Stenting in Myocardial Infraction Regarding Acute and Long-Term Follow-up (ADMIRAL) study, in which treatment with abciximab in patients undergoing primary stenting for ST-elevation myocardial infarction had a 59% reduction in the rate of death, reinfarction, or the need for urgent target vessel revascularization by 30 d (*p* = 0.01) (Fig. 4) *(84)*. Angiographic data demonstrated improved rates of TIMI flow grade 3 in the culprit artery both before and after stenting. The magnitude of the clinical benefits seen with abciximab persisted without attenuation through 6 mo (Fig. 4). Moreover, there was a lower rate of elective target vessel revascularization by 6 mo, raising the possibility that abciximab reduced the rate of restenosis.

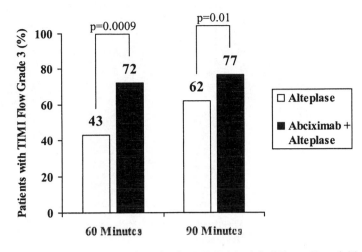

Fig. 5. Proportion achieving TIMI flow grade 3 in the TIMI 14 trial *(87)* at 60 and 90 min for al patients (dose-finding and dose confirmation) randomized to accelerated full-dose alteplase (open bars) vs reduced-dose alteplase (15 mg bolus followed by 35 mg infusion over 60 min) plus abciximab (solid bars).

The results from the CADILLAC study have been published *(85)*. This was a large study in 2082 patients with acute myocardial infarction who were randomized in a 2 × 2 factorial design to balloon angioplasty vs stent and to abciximab vs placebo. Treatment with abciximab resulted in approx 15% reductions in recurrent ischemic events in both the balloon angioplasty and primary stenting arms.

Fibrinolysis. The Thrombolysis and Angioplasty in Myocardial Infarction (TAMI) 8 pilot study first examined the safety and utility of abciximab given after thrombolysis for acute myocardial infarction *(86)*. Patients were treated with accelerated alteplase and aspirin, and were randomized to receive a bolus of abciximab at 15 h, 6 h, or 3 h after the beginning of the alteplase infusion at doses ranging from 0.1 to 0.25 mg/kg. There was no significant difference in the bleeding or thrombocytopenia rates. Although not designed to detect differences in clinical cardiac events (e.g., angina, myocardial infarction, urgent revascularization, or death), this combined end point was seen in 13% of the pooled abciximab group vs 20% of the control group.

TIMI 14 was a large angiographic trial that evaluated the efficacy of full-dose abciximab in conjunction with reduced-dose lytic *(87)*. Ninety-minute angiography revealed that the rates of TIMI flow grade 3 were 32% in patients treated with abciximab alone, 62% in patients treated with alteplase alone, and 77% in patients receiving full-dose abciximab plus reduced-dose alteplase (15-mg bolus, followed by a 35-mg infusion over 60 min) ($p = 0.01$). Moreover, at 60 min, rates of TIMI flow grade 3 were 43% in the alteplase group compared to 72% in the abciximab plus reduced-dose alteplase group ($p = 0.0009$) (Fig. 5).

Major bleeding rates were similar in the alteplase-alone and the abciximab plus reduced-dose alteplase groups. Interestingly, in a very-low-dose heparin arm (bolus of 30 U/kg followed by an infusion at 4 U/kg/h), the rate of 60-min TIMI flow grade 3 was 68% and the major bleeding rate was only 1%. These findings suggest that future optimization of the heparin dose may minimize bleeding complications without significantly compromising efficacy.

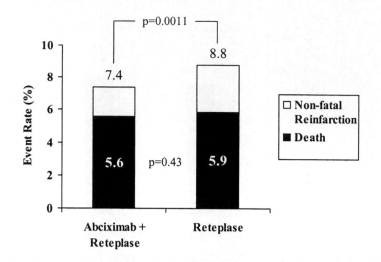

Fig. 6. Proportion of patients with the primary end point of death (solid bars) or the composite end point of death and nonfatal reinfarction (solid and open bars) in the GUSTO V trial *(91)* for patients randomized to abciximab plus reduced-dose reteplase vs reteplase alone.

Abciximab was tested in conjunction with reduced doses of other fibrinolytics. In the Strategies for Patency Enhancement in the Emergency Department (SPEED) *(88)* and the reteplase phase of TIMI 14 *(89)*, combination therapy consisting of full-dose abciximab and reduced-dose reteplase (5 + 5 U) resulted in marginally higher rates of TIMI flow grade 3 at 60–90 min compared to full-dose reteplase alone (54 vs 47% in SPEED and 73 vs 70% in TIMI 14, p = NS for both). In the Enoxaparin and tenecteplase (TNK-tPA) with or without GP IIb/IIIa Inhibitor as Reperfusion Strategy in ST-elevation myocardial infarction (ENTIRE) study, abciximab plus reduced dose TNK-tPA was compared to full-dose TNK-tPA (patients also were randomized to unfractionated heparin vs the low-molecular-weight heparin enoxaparin, discussed below) *(90)*. Combination therapy resulted in similar rates of TIMI flow grade 3, but trends towards higher rates of complete ST-segment resolution by 180 min and lower rates of death or myocardial infarction among patients receiving unfractionated heparin (6.5 vs 15.9%).

The overall promising results with combination reperfusion therapy in pilot studies, coupled with prior observations from the Global Utilization of Streptokinase and tPA for Occluded Coronary Arteries (GUSTO) I angiographic substudy that a 23% improvement in the proportion of patients achieving TIMI flow grade 3 was associated with a 1% absolute decrease in mortality *(5)*, led to GUSTO V, a phase III clinical trial in 16,588 patients comparing abciximab plus reduced-dose reteplase to reteplase alone *(91)*. The 30-d mortality rates were not statistically different between the abciximab plus reduced-dose reteplase (5.6%) and the reteplase alone (5.9%) arms. However, patients receiving combination therapy did have a 16% lower rate of the combined end point of death or nonfatal reinfarction (p = 0.0011; Fig. 6) as well as a 12% lower rate of recurrent ischemia (p = 0.004) and trends toward lower rates of a variety of other end points including malignant arrhythmias and mechanical complications. Although rescue angioplasty was used infrequently, it did occur more often in the reteplase group (8.6 vs 5.6%, p < 0.0001), and this may have minimized potential mortality differences between the two arms. Moderate and severe bleeding was twice as frequent in the combination therapy arm (Fig. 6). Rates of intracranial hemorrhage (ICH) were similar in patients ≤75 yr of age, but twice as high in patients >75 yr of age.

In the Assessment of the Safety and Efficacy of a New Thrombolytic Regimen (ASSENT) III trial, patients were randomized to one of three regimens: full-dose TNK-tPA plus unfractionated heparin, full-dose TNK-tPA plus the low-molecular-weight heparin enoxaparin, or reduced-dose TNK-tPA plus abciximab and unfractionated heparin *(92)*. The 30-d mortality rates were not statistically significantly different between the abciximab and unfractionated heparin treatment groups (6.6 vs 6.0%, $p = 0.4$). However, the rate of the composite end point of death, in-hospital reinfarction, or in-hospital refractory ischemia was lower in the abciximab arm compared with the unfractionated heparin arm (11.1 vs 15.4%, $p < 0.001$). Major bleeding, however, was twice as high in the abciximab arm (4.4%) compared to the unfractionated heparin arm (2.2%).

Analogous to the approach with abciximab, initial studies examining the utility of eptifibatide in pharmacologic reperfusion for ST elevation MI combined different doses of eptifibatide with a full-dose of a fibrinolytic. In IMPACT-AMI, combination therapy with the highest dose of eptifibatide and full-dose alteplase resulted in very high rates of patency (93%) and TIMI flow grade 3 (71%), but this degree of success was not replicated in the dose-confirmation phase, in which combination therapy was not superior to lytic alone *(93)*.

In another trial, patients with acute myocardial infarction were given full-dose streptokinase and different doses of eptifibatide or placebo *(94)*. Treatment with eptifibatide was associated with a higher likelihood of achieving TIMI flow grade 3 in the infarct-related artery at 90 min (50 vs 32%), but at the expense of increased bleeding complications.

In the Integrilin and Reduced Dose Thrombolytic in Acute Myocardial Infarction (INTRO-AMI) study, testing of multiple different combinations of eptifibatide and alteplase in a dose-finding phase led to two regimens being tested in a dose-confirmation phase: a "180/1.33/90" regimen (initial 180 μg/kg bolus, infusion at 1.33 μg/kg/h, and then a second 90 μg/kg bolus 30 min later) and a "180/2.0/90" regimen (with the second bolus 10 min later) *(95)*. Combination therapy using the 180/2.0/90 regimen yielded superior rates of TIMI flow grade 3 compared to alteplase alone (56 vs 40%, $p = 0.04$).

The Integrilin + TNK in AMI (INTEGRITI) angiographic trial examined combinations of eptifibatide and reduced-dose TNK-tPA. A 180/2.0/180 regimen appeared most promising in the dose-finding phase. In the dose-confirmation phase, compared with patients receiving full-dose TNK-tPA alone, there were trends toward higher rates of TIMI flow grade 3 (59 vs 49%, $p = 0.15$) and complete ST resolution (71 vs 61%, $p = 0.08$) in patients receiving combination therapy *(96)*.

In summary, combination therapy with a reduced-dose fibrinolytic and a GP IIb/IIIa inhibitor does offer improvements in infarct-related artery patency, but these have not translated into mortality benefits. It may be that, between rescue angioplasty and improved overall medical therapy (e.g., angiotensin converting enzyme [ACE] inhibitors and statins), small differences in patency do not have a large impact on survival. Nonetheless, the reductions in nonfatal ischemic events seen with combination therapy are clinically important. Moreover, combination therapy offers a more attractive transition to the cardiac catheterization laboratory than does full-dose fibrinolytic therapy without a GP IIb/IIIa inhibitor on board. Studies helping to define the optimal facilitated angioplasty regimen are ongoing.

Other Antiplatelet Agents

NONSTEROID ANTI-INFLAMMATORY DRUGS

Unlike aspirin, nonsteroid anti-inflammatory drugs (NSAIDs) are reversible COX inhibitors. Although studied in the setting of acute myocardial infarction, they have not been shown to be superior to aspirin (97). However, their antiplatelet effects have been highlighted by reports from some (98,99), but not all (100), studies in which patients not on aspirin who were assigned new selective COX-2 inhibitors had higher cardiovascular thrombotic events than did patients assigned to NSAIDs. It should be noted, though, that not all NSAIDs exert the same antiplatelet effect, and there is even some evidence that certain NSAIDs may block aspirin's antiplatelet effect (101).

SULFINPYRAZONE

Sulfinpyrazone is a uricosuric agent structurally related to phenylbutazone. It is a competitive inhibitor of COX but it may inhibit platelets through other mechanisms as well. Although in one study it reduced the rate of reinfarction in patients after myocardial infarction (102), there are no consistent data supporting the utility of sulfinpyrazone in acute coronary syndromes.

DIPYRIDAMOLE

Dipyridamole inhibits platelets through an unknown mechanism: it may act as a phosphodiesterase inhibitor, thereby increasing concentrations of cAMP and maintaining the platelet in its resting state, it may stimulate prostacyclin synthesis, or it may inhibit cellular uptake and metabolism of adenosine (103). Clinically, dipyridamole is a weak antiplatelet agent with no established role in acute coronary syndromes (104).

RIDOGREL

Ridogrel is a thromboxane synthase inhibitor as well as a competitive TXA_2/prostaglandin endoperoxide (PGEND) receptor blocker (105,106). This dual activity allows ridogrel to inhibit platelet activation several ways (Fig. 1). There has been one randomized controlled trial of ridogrel in acute myocardial infraction. In the Ridogrel vs Aspirin Patency Trial (RAPT), 907 patients presenting within 6 h of an acute myocardial infarction were treated with streptokinase 1.5 MU and randomized to re-ceive either ridogrel 300 mg IV bolus, followed by 300 mg orally 2× daily, or aspirin 250 mg IV bolus, followed by 160 mg orally once daily (107). There were no differences in the rates of infarct-related artery patency at predischarge angiography or mortality.

PROSTACYCLIN AND ANALOGUES

Prostacyclin acts both as an antiplatelet agent and as a vasodilator. Its antiplatelet effects are mediated through stimulation of adenylate cyclase. This causes an increase in levels of cAMP, thereby stimulating cAMP-dependent protein kinases, decreasing cytoplasmic calcium levels, and maintaining the platelet in its resting state (108). Receptor down-regulation and unacceptable vasodilatation leading to hypotension have limited the clinical efficacy of current prostacyclin preparations as antiplatelet agents (109).

THROMBIN INHIBITORS

As thrombin is the most potent endogenous platelet activator *(110–112)*, antithrombins should exert an antiplatelet effect. This has been established in experimental models *(113,114)*, and these agents are discussed in detail below.

GLYCOPROTEIN IB AND vWF INHIBITORS

Analogous to the development of GP IIb/IIIa inhibitors to block platelet aggregation, GP Ib and vWF inhibitors are being developed to block platelet adhesion *(42,115,116)*. No clinical data are available at this time. However, there is concern that these inhibitors would significantly interfere with normal hemostasis and produce unacceptable bleeding complications, as seen clinically in GP Ib deficiency (Bernard–Soulier syndrome) and von Willebrand's disease homozygotes.

Summary

- Platelets play a pivotal role in acute coronary syndromes and platelet activation is a complex process with multiple pathways leading to the final common pathway of platelet aggregation.
- Aspirin, a COX inhibitor and a relatively weak platelet antagonist, is the standard of care for antiplatelet therapy in acute coronary syndromes and has been shown to significantly reduce the rates of death and nonfatal reinfarction.
- Ticlopidine and, more recently, clopidogrel, are ADP antagonists that are beneficial when combined with aspirin for intracoronary stent deployment and unstable angina. Studies in the setting of ST-elevation myocardial infarction are ongoing.
- GP IIb/IIIa inhibitors are clearly efficacious in the setting of primary angioplasty or primary stenting, where they reduce the rates of death, cardiac ischemic events, and the need for repeat revascularization. The picture is less clear for pharmacologic reperfusion therapy, where a reduced dose fibrinolytic plus a GP IIb/IIIa inhibitor improves infarct-related artery patency, but not overall mortality. The rate of recurrent ischemic events is decreased, but unfortunately bleeding, especially ICH in the elderly, is increased. Additional data are needed before recommendations can be made.

ANTICOAGULATION

Coagulation Cascade

Thrombin is a glycosylated serine protease that plays a fundamental role in thrombosis *(117)*. Thrombin is generated from prothrombin by the prothrombinase complex, which includes factors Xa, Va, calcium, and phospholipids (Fig. 7). Its main action is to transform fibrinogen into fibrin. Thrombin is one of the most potent endogenous platelet activator *(110–112)*. The active catalytic site lies within a relatively narrow canyon on the molecule's surface (Fig. 8) *(118)*. Adjacent to this site is the substrate recognition site, also known as the anion-binding exosite, to which fibrinogen binds *(118)*. In addition, there is a separate fibrin-binding site *(17)*. Finally, there are several other well-characterized binding sites including an apolar binding site *(119)*, which is involved in both substrate binding as well as platelet attachment via GP Ib, a heparin-binding site, and the primary platelet attachment site, which is an anion-binding exosite similar to the

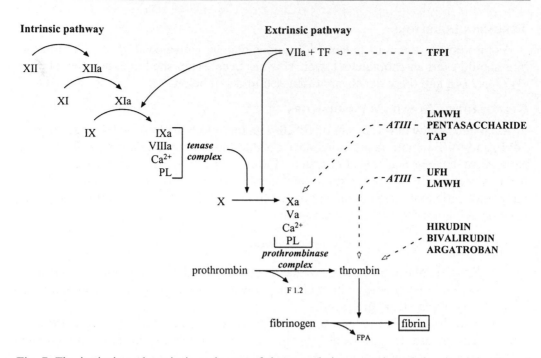

Fig. 7. The intrinsic and extrinsic pathways of the coagulation cascade and the sites of action of antithrombin agents (open arrowheads and dashed lines). Abbreviations: TF, tissue factor; TFPI, tissue factor pathway inhibitor; ATIII, antithrombin III; LMWH, low-molecular weight heparin; TAP, tick anticoagulant peptide; UFH, unfractionated heparin; F1.2, prothrombin fragment 1.2; FPA, fibrinopeptide A.

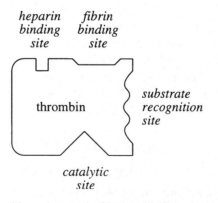

Fig. 8. Simplified depiction of thrombin and several of its key binding sites.

Table 2
Antithrombotic Agents

Indirect thrombin inhibitors:
  Heparin
  LMWHs
Direct thrombin inhibitors:
  Hirudin
  Bivalirudin
  Argatroban
Thrombin generation inhibitors:
  Factor Xa inhibitors
    LMWHs
    Pentasaccharide
    TAP
  TFPI

substrate recognition site, which binds to platelets using a tethered-ligand motif *(111)*. Thrombin inhibition can be achieved either by binding to one of these critical sites or by inhibiting thrombin generation, which is achieved primarily by inhibiting Factor Xa (Fig. 7 and Table 2) *(42,117,120,121)*.

Heparin

PHARMACOLOGY

Heparin is a glycosaminoglycan that contains a unique pentasaccharide sequence with high binding affinity for antithrombin III (ATIII) *(19,122)*. When bound to heparin, ATIII undergoes a conformational change that results in an acceleration of its ability to inactivate both thrombin and factor Xa by acting as a "suicide substrate" (Fig. 9). Heparin also increases the rate of the thrombin-ATIII reaction by greater than 1000-fold by acting as a catalytic template to which both the inhibitor and the protease bind, thereby forming a ternary complex. *(Note:* ternary complex formation is not required for factor Xa inactivation.) Once thrombin binds to ATIII, heparin is released from the complex. There is also some evidence that part of heparin's anticoagulant effect is due to its ability to both stimulate the release and enhance the activity of tissue factor pathway inhibitor *(123–125)*. Heparin molecules that contain fewer than 18 saccharide units (i.e., low-molecular-weight heparins [LMWHs]) are unable to bind thrombin and ATIII simultaneously and are, therefore, unable to form ternary complexes to accelerate thrombin inhibition (see below). Heparin is largely ineffective against fibrin monomer-bound *(16)* or clot-bound *(17)* thrombin (Figs. 9 and 10) and against factor Xa bound in the prothrombinase complex.

Heparin is a heterogeneous mixture of glycosaminoglycans of varying molecular sizes *(126)*. This translates into heterogeneous anticoagulant activity for three reasons. First, only approx 30% of heparin molecules actually contain the specific pentasaccharide sequence mentioned above that is required for ATIII binding *(122)*. Second, the anticoagulant profile of heparin in terms of the ratio of thrombin to factor Xa inhibition is influenced by the chain length *(127)*. Third, the clearance of heparin is proportional to its molecular size *(128)*.

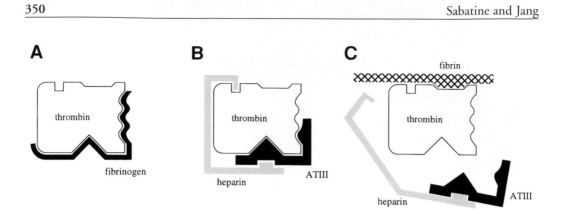

Fig. 9. Interaction between thrombin and heparin. (**A**) Thrombin binding to its natural substrate fibrinogen. (**B**) Inactivation of thrombin by ATIII and heparin. (**C**) Fibrin-bound thrombin is enzymatically active but resistant to inactivation by ATIII and heparin.

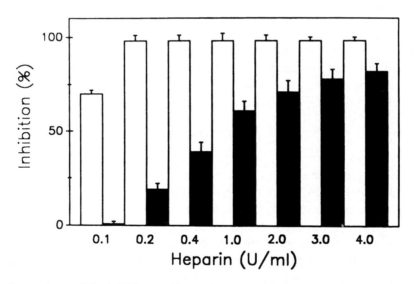

Fig. 10. Comparison of the inhibitory effects of heparin against fluid phase (open bars) and clot-bound (solid bars) thrombin activity. Thrombin or fibrin clots were incubated with citrated plasma in the presence or absence of heparin. FPA levels were then measured by radioimmunoassay, and the percent inhibition of FPA generation was calculated for each inhibitor concentration. Heparin concentrations of 0.2–0.4 U/mL span the therapeutic range for this agent. Reproduced with permission from ref. *17*.

Heparin can be administered either by continuous iv infusion or by intermittent subcutaneous injections with comparable efficacy, although there is a 1–2 h delay in achieving an anticoagulant effect via the subcutaneous route. The half-life of heparin varies depending on the dose given, but is approx 60–90 min.

Heparin-induced thrombocytopenia (HIT) is a well-documented complication of heparin administration *(20)*. HIT type I occurs in approx 10% of patients receiving heparin and is manifested by mild thrombocytopenia occurring within 48 h of the initiation of therapy. The platelet count rarely falls below 100,000/mm³ and returns to normal within 5 d even if heparin therapy is continued. The mechanism is thought to be direct heparin-mediated platelet aggregation. Patients with HIT type I do not go on to have thrombotic complications. In contrast, HIT type II is marked by more severe thrombocytopenia and a greatly increased risk of thrombosis. This syndrome occurs in 1–5% of patients receiving heparin, approximately one-third of whom will go on to develop thrombosis. The platelet count usually starts to decrease after 5–12 d of therapy (and potentially earlier if the patient has been exposed to heparin before) and usually falls by more than 50% or drops to less than 100,000/mm^3. If heparin is discontinued, the platelet count usually returns to normal in 4–10 d. The pathogenesis of this syndrome is believed to be due to antibodies forming against heparin–platelet factor 4 complexes (Fig. 11) (129,130). These immune complexes can then bind to Fc receptors on platelets and trigger platelet activation, thereby releasing more platelet factor 4. Platelet factor 4 can bind to heparin-like molecules on the surface of endothelial cells, providing a target for the above-mentioned antibodies and leading to endothelial cell injury and thrombosis.

Several investigators have reported a "rebound effect" after the cessation of heparin therapy in patients with acute coronary syndromes. In one trial that randomized patients with unstable angina to heparin, aspirin, both, or neither, there was a nearly threefold higher incidence of disease reactivation (i.e., recurrent unstable angina or myocardial infarction) in patients who had received heparin than in the other groups (13 vs 5%) (131). The majority of these recurrences were severe enough to require urgent intervention. Other investigators have noted that after the cessation of heparin in patients with acute coronary syndromes there is a transient increase in prothrombin fragment 1.2 and fibrinopeptide A levels, suggesting that both thrombin generation and activity were increased (132). Similar observations have been made after the discontinuation of heparin in patients undergoing coronary angioplasty (133). The mechanism underlying this rebound phenomenon is unclear but may be due to an accumulation of prothrombotic factors during heparin therapy that then create a hypercoagulable state after the cessation of heparin.

Clinical Data

Trials with No Routine Aspirin. There have been 21 trials enrolling a total of approx 5000 patients that have examined the effects of heparin in acute myocardial infarction in the pre-aspirin era (i.e., pre-ISIS-2). Most of these trials were also in the prethrombolysis era as only 14% of the patients in these trials received thrombolytic therapy. A meta-analysis revealed that treatment with heparin resulted in a statistically significant 25% reduction in mortality (from 14.9 to 11.4%, $p = 0.002$) and a statistically non-significant 18% reduction in reinfarction (from 8.2 to 6.7%, $p = 0.08$) (Fig. 12) (134). Conversely, treatment with heparin was also associated with a near doubling of the major bleeding rate (1.9 vs 0.9%). Two trials (135,136) have examined the role of heparin in patients receiving a thrombolytic but not aspirin (Table 3). Treatment with heparin was associated with a higher infarct-related artery patency rate (136) and a lower mortality rate (135). However, the applicability of these data is limited now that treatment with aspirin has become standard of care.

Trials with Routine Aspirin. There have been six trials (137–143) enrolling approx 68,000 patients that have examined the effects of heparin in acute myocardial infarction in patients who did routinely received aspirin as part of the treatment protocol (Table 3). Ninety-three percent of the patients in these trials received thrombolytic therapy. A meta-analysis (134) revealed that treatment with heparin resulted in marginally statisti-

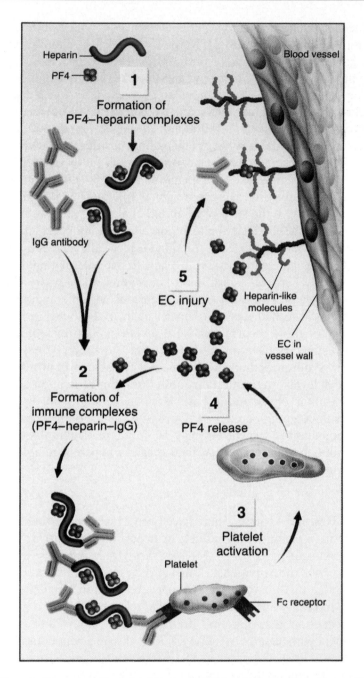

Fig. 11. HIT. Heparin interacts with platelet factor 4 (PF4), which is released in small quantities from circulating platelets to form PF4–heparin complexes (**1**). Specific IgG antibodies react with these conjugates to form immune complexes (**2**) that bind to Fc receptors on circulating platelets. Fc-mediated platelet activation (**3**) releases PF4 from α-granules in platelets (**4**). Newly released PF4 binds to additional heparin, and the antibody forms more immune complexes, establishing a cycle of platelet activation. PF4 can also bind to heparin-like molecules on the surface of endothelial cells (EC) to provide targets for antibody binding, potentially leading to immune-mediated EC injury (**5**) and thrombosis. Reproduced with permission from ref. *130*.

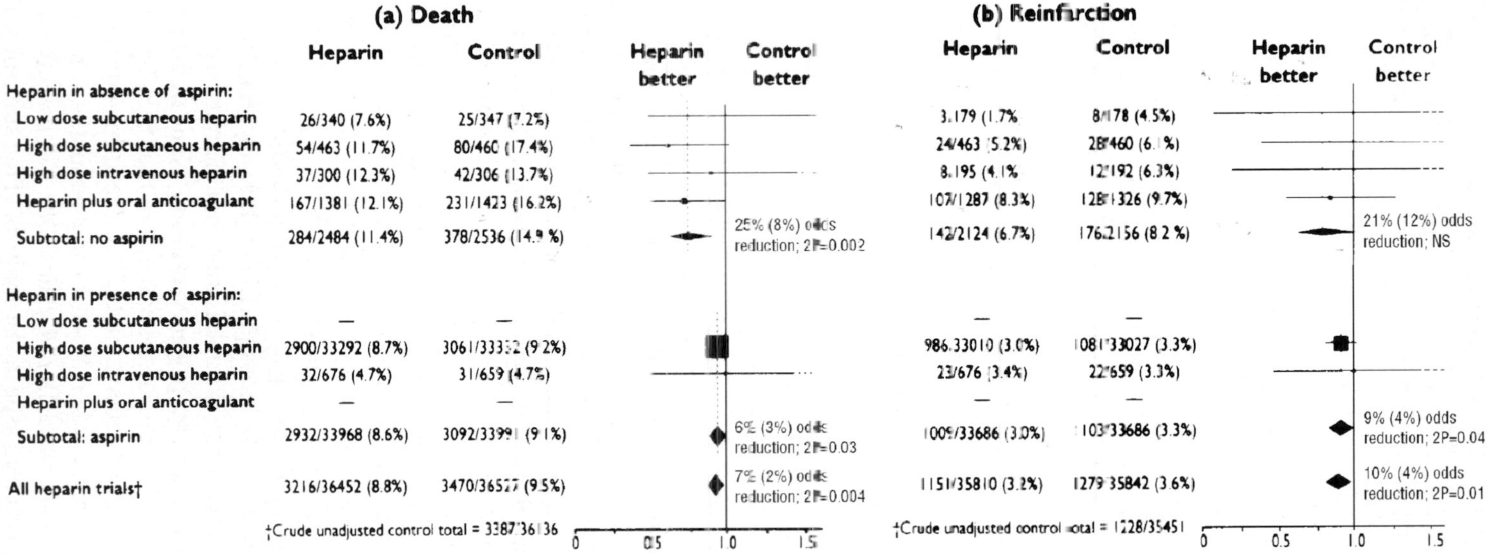

Fig. 12. Meta-analysis of the effects of heparin in the absence and presence of aspirin in patients with suspected acute myocardial infarction. Reproduced with permission from ref. *134*.

Table 3

Randomized Trials of Heparin in Patients Receiving Thrombolysis for
Acute Myocardial Infarction

Trial (reference)	Year	Aspirin	Heparin	Thrombolytic	Patients
SCATI1 (35)	1989	–	SC	± SK	711
Bleich et al. (136)	1990	–	IV	TPA	95
ISIS-2 pilot (137)	1987	±	IV	± SK	619
HART1 (44)	1990	±	IV	TPA	205
GISSI-2 (138,139)	1990	+	SC	SK	20,891
ISIS-3 (140)	1992	+	SC	SK	45,856
DUCCS-1 (143)	1994	+	IV	APSAC	250
OSIRIS (142)	1992	+	IV	SK	128
ECSG-6 (141)	1992	+	IV	TPA	652

Abbreviations: SK, streptokinase; tPA, tissue-type plasminogen activator (alteplase); APSAC, anisoylated plasminogen streptokinase activator complex.

cally significant in-hospital 6% reduction in mortality (from 9.1 to 8.6%, $p = 0.03$) and 9% reduction in reinfarction (from 3.3 to 3.0%, $p = 0.04$) (Fig. 12). Again, treatment with heparin was also associated with an increased major bleeding rate (1.0 vs 0.7%).

Most of the data come from the GISSI-2 trial (138,139) and the ISIS-3 trial (140). During the actual period of heparin treatment in these trials there was a 7% relative reduction in mortality (from 7.3 to 6.8%), but at 35 d, the difference in mortality was no longer statistically significant (2% relative reduction, from 10.2 to 10.0%). There is, however, concern that these two megatrials may have underestimated the beneficial effects of heparin because of the way in which the heparin was administered. In GISSI-2, the heparin was started 12 h after the initiation of fibrinolytic therapy, and in ISIS-3, it was started 4 h after the initiation of fibrinolytic therapy. Moreover, in both trials, the heparin was administered subcutaneously, which further delayed the achievement of an anticoagulated state.

Trials with IV Heparin. Given the fact that patients enrolled in GISSI-2 and ISIS-3 accounted for greater than 95% of the patients included in the above meta-analysis and that there are concerns regarding the efficacy of the heparin regimens in those two megatrials, it is reasonable to undertake a separate inspection of trials that have used intravenous heparin. There have been six randomized controlled trials (136,137,141–144) that have directly examined the effect of iv heparin in patients receiving thrombolytic therapy for acute myocardial infarction (Table 3). A meta-analysis of these trials (145) revealed a statistically nonsignificant 9% reduction in mortality (from 5.6 to 5.1%) (Fig. 13). There was no significant difference in the rates of reinfarction or recurrent ischemia. There was, however, a statistically nonsignificant 42% increase in the rate of severe bleeding with double the rates of stroke and intracranial hemorrhage.

The above trials, however, are a heterogeneous group. None of the patients in the study by Bleich and colleagues (136), half of the patients in the ISIS-2 pilot study (137), and only those patients who did not receive heparin in Heparin-Aspirin Reperfusion Trial (HART) (144) received aspirin, whereas all of the patients in European Cooperative Study Group (ECSG)-6 (141), OSIRIS (142), and Duke University Clinical Cardiology Study (DUCCS)-1 (143) received aspirin. An analysis of the subgroup of patients in these six trials who were given aspirin revealed that heparin had no effect on mortality. In con-

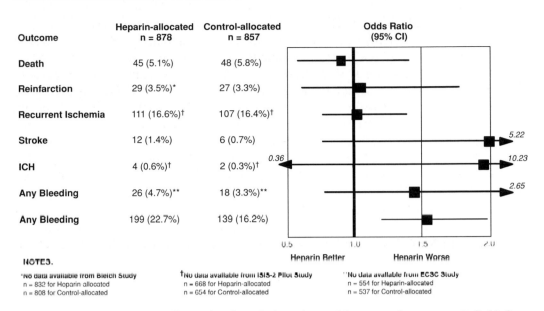

Fig. 13. Meta-analysis of the effects of IV heparin in patients with suspected acute myocardial infarction. Reproduced with permission from ref. *145*.

Table 4
Angiographic Studies Randomizing IV Heparin in Patients Receiving Thrombolysis for Acute Myocardial Infarction

Trial (reference)	Year	Aspirin	Patients	TIMI grade 2 or 3(%)		TIMI grade 3 (%)	
				– Hep	+ Hep	– Hep	+ Hep
Bleich et al. *(136)*	1990	–	95	43	71	38	52
HART *(144)*	1990	±	205	52	82	31	56
ECSG-6 *(141)*	1992	+	652	75	83	66	76

trast, in patients who were not given aspirin, treatment with heparin was associated with a statistically nonsignificant 28% reduction in mortality, similar to the effect seen in the meta-analysis of trials in the pre-aspirin and prethrombolytic era.

When streptokinase is used as the thrombolytic agent, the data from the GUSTO trial demonstrated that treatment with iv heparin conferred no mortality benefit over high-dose subcutaneous heparin *(146)*. Since iv heparin is not superior to subcutaneous heparin (from GUSTO), and subcutaneous heparin is not superior to placebo (from GISSI-2 and ISIS-3), there is indirect data that iv heparin offers no advantage in patients receiving thrombolysis with streptokinase for acute myocardial infarction.

In contrast, when alteplase is used as the thrombolytic agent, iv heparin is a standard part of adjunctive therapy *(4)*. There are two indirect lines of evidence that support this practice. First, several small trials *(136,141,144)* have shown improved infarct-related artery patency (defined as TIMI flow grade 2 or 3) when iv heparin is added to thrombolysis with alteplase (Table 4). More importantly, these trials have also demonstrated a higher percentage of patients achieve TIMI flow grade 3 with the addition of iv heparin to thrombolysis with alteplase. These trials were themselves too small to show a significant difference in mortality or reinfarction. However, extrapolating from the GUSTO-I data showing that TIMI flow grade 3 at 90 min is associated with lower mortality and better left ventricular function at 30 d *(5)*, one can argue that the addition of iv heparin to thrombolysis with alteplase may improve patient outcome. Second, if one analyzes the patients receiving alteplase in GISSI-2, ISIS-3, and GUSTO-I, the mortality rates are 9.8% for alteplase alone, 9.6% for alteplase plus subcutaneous heparin, and 6.3% for alteplase plus iv heparin. Such comparisons are hazardous for several reasons. The mortality rates in general were lower in GUSTO-I than in GISSI-2 or ISIS-3 for comparable groups. More importantly, in GISSI-2 and ISIS-3, the "standard" alteplase infusion was used (100 mg over 3 h), whereas in GUSTO-I, an "accelerated" alteplase infusion *(147)* was used (100 mg over 90 min). Nonetheless, the lowest mortality rate with alteplase was achieved by giving it with iv heparin, and thus, this has become the standard of care.

Trials with More Intensive Intravenous Heparin Regimens. In GUSTO-I, 50% of patients failed to achieve therapeutic anticoagulation. Therefore, a more intensive iv heparin regimen (increasing the upper limit of the target activated partial thromboplastin time [aPTT] to 90 s and increasing the initial infusion of heparin to 1300 U/h for patients weighing 80 kg or more) was initially used in TIMI-9A *(148)*, GUSTO-IIa *(149)*, and HIT-III *(150)*. This resulted in 20% more heparin being administered in GUSTO-IIa than in GUSTO-I. All three trials were stopped prematurely because of an increased rate of ICH and other major bleeding events. Whereas the rate of ICH was 0.7% in GUSTO-I, it was 1.9% in the heparin arm of TIMI-9A and 1.5% in the heparin arm of GUSTO-IIa (for the subset of patients receiving thrombolytic therapy for acute myocardial infarction); there were no ICHs in the heparin arm of HIT-III, but there was a 3.4% rate in the hirudin arm, prompting the termination of that trial. The mean aPTT of patients with ICH was 100 s in TIMI-9A and 110 s in GUSTO-IIa as compared to a mean aPTT of 85 s (both trials) for patients without ICH. An analysis of the aPTTs from patients enrolled in the GUSTO-I trial revealed a lower mortality was associated with aPTT at 12 h between 50 and 70 s; aPTTs higher than this were associated with an increased rate of moderate to severe bleeding, ICH, and, interestingly, reinfarction *(151)*.

In summary, in patients ineligible for thrombolytic therapy, heparin is of proven benefit in patients unable to take aspirin and is of no proven benefit in those taking aspirin. For patients receiving thrombolytic therapy with streptokinase, there is no data that heparin, either subcutaneous or iv, offers any benefit. For patients receiving alteplase, heparin continues to be used based on angiographic data showing higher infarct-related artery patency, but clinical trials demonstrating decreased mortality or reinfarction are lacking. By extension from its use with alteplase, heparin is also routinely used with the new third-generation fibrinolytics reteplase and TNK-tPA. If heparin is to be used, it should be adjusted to achieve an aPTT between 50 and 70 s.

Direct Thrombin Inhibitors

HIRUDIN

Pharmacology. Hirudin is a naturally occurring anticoagulant derived from the saliva of the medicinal leech (Hirudo medicinalis) that has subsequently been produced via recombinant DNA technology *(152)*. It is a 65-amino-acid protein with a molecular weight of 7000 Da that contains two domains: the N-terminal domain binds to and inhibits the active catalytic site of thrombin *(153)* and the C-terminal tail binds to the sub-

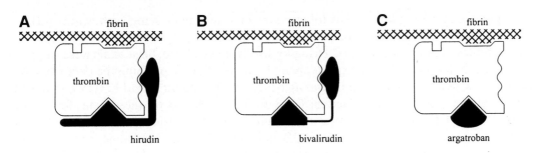

Fig. 14. Interaction between thrombin and direct thrombin inhibitors. Hirudin (**A**) and bivalirudin (**B**) bind to both the catalytic and substrate recognition sites. Argatroban (**C**) binds only to the catalytic site. All of the direct thrombin inhibitors can inactivate clot-bound thrombin and none of them requires the presence of ATIII.

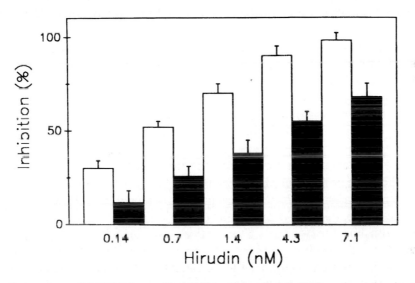

Fig. 15. Comparison of the inhibitory effects of hirudin against fluid phase (open bars) and clot-bound (solid bars) thrombin activity. Thrombin or fibrin clots were incubated with citrated plasma in the presence or absence of hirudin. FPA levels were then measured by radioimmunoassay, and the percent inhibition of FPA generation was calculated for each inhibitor concentration. Reproduced with permission from ref. *17*.

strate recognition site of thrombin *(154)* (Fig. 14). The apolar binding site of thrombin may also be involved in the interaction *(119)*. Unlike heparin, hirudin is a direct thrombin inhibitor and, therefore, does not require the presence of ATIII to neutralize thrombin. Hirudin is uniquely specific for thrombin *(155)*, does not cross-react with the antibodies responsible for HIT, and is not inactivated by platelet factor 4 or heparinases. Hirudin is an extremely potent antithrombin and can inactivate both fluid-phase and clot-bound thrombin, although it is less effective against the latter, requiring approx 10-fold higher doses to achieve comparable degrees of thrombin inhibition (Fig. 15) *(17,156)*.

Clinical Data. After demonstrating promising results in two pilot studies when given as adjunctive antithrombin therapy with alteplase (TIMI-5) *(157)* and streptokinase (TIMI-6) *(158)*, hirudin was compared to heparin in three phase III trials (TIMI-9A *[148]*, GUSTO-IIa *[149]*, and HIT-III *[150]*). In both TIMI-9A and GUSTO-IIa, hirudin was given as a 0.6 mg/kg iv bolus followed by an infusion at 0.2 mg/kg/h, while in HIT-III, a different recombinant hirudin was used and at a slightly lower dose (0.4 mg/kg iv bolus followed by an infusion at 0.15 mg/kg/h). As stated above, these trials were stopped prematurely because of an unexpectedly high rate of ICH. Combining the data from the three trials, treatment with hirudin was associated with a higher rate of ICH (1.6 vs 0.9%) and a higher rate of major bleeding (10.8 vs 7.7%). Based on these data, the TIMI, GUSTO, and HIT investigators altered their anticoagulation protocols with a reduction in the hirudin and heparin doses in TIMI-9B and GUSTO-IIb and a change from alteplase to streptokinase and a change from iv to subcutaneous hirudin and heparin in HIT-4.

In TIMI-9B *(159)*, 3002 patients with acute myocardial infarction were treated with aspirin and either alteplase or streptokinase (at the discretion of the treating physician) and were randomized within 12 h of symptoms to receive anticoagulation for 96 h with either hirudin 0.1 mg/kg iv bolus, followed by an infusion at 0.1 mg/kg/h, or heparin 5000 U iv bolus, followed by an infusion at 1000 U/h. Both anticoagulants were adjusted to achieve an aPTT of 55–85 s. At 24 h, there was a slightly higher rate of death or non-fatal myocardial infarction with hirudin (2.8 vs 2.3%). At 30 d, treatment with hirudin was associated with a 21% higher incidence of death (6.1 vs 5.1%), a 19% reduction in the rate of myocardial infarction (3.6 vs 4.4%), and a 9% higher incidence of the combined end point of death, recurrent myocardial infarction, congestive heart failure, or shock (12.9 vs 11.9%). None of these differences achieved statistical significance. There was also no significant difference in the rates of ICH or other major bleeding events.

In GUSTO-IIb *(160)*, 12,142 patients with acute coronary syndromes were randomized to receive anticoagulation for 72 h with either hirudin or heparin, each dosed according to the same protocol used in TIMI-9B. Of the 12,142 patients, 4131 presented with ST-segment elevation and 74% of those patients received thrombolytic therapy with either alteplase or streptokinase (again, at the discretion of the treating physician). At 24 h, treatment with hirudin (for both ST-elevation and non-ST-elevation patients) was associated with a statistically significant 39% reduction in the combined end point of death or myocardial infarction (from 2.1 to 1.3%). At 30 d, for the patients with ST-segment elevation, there was only a 6% reduction in mortality (from 6.2 to 5.9%), an 18% reduction in myocardial infarction (from 6.0 to 5.0%), and a 14% reduction in the primary combined end point of death or myocardial infarction (from 11.3 to 9.9%). None of these differences achieved statistical significance. For patients with ST-segment elevation, there was no significant difference in the rates of ICH or of severe or moderate bleeding (although for all patients, treatment with hirudin was associated with a 14% higher rate of major bleeding).

In HIT-4, 1208 patients with acute myocardial infarction were treated with streptokinase and were randomized to hirudin 0.2 mg/kg iv bolus, followed by 0.5 mg/kg subcutaneously 2× daily for 5 to 7 d, or a bolus of placebo, followed by heparin 12,500 U subcutaneously 2× daily *(161)*. Thirty-day mortality and reinfarction rates were similar with a 6.8% mortality and a 4.6% reinfarction rate in the hirudin group compared to a 6.4% mortality and a 5.1% reinfarction rate in the heparin group. Data from the angiographic substudy revealed a trend towards higher rates of TIMI flow grade 3 at 90 min with hirudin than with heparin (41 vs 34%, $p = 0.16$) and data from the electrocardiogram (ECG) substudy demonstrated a higher rate of complete ST-segment resolution by 90 min with hirudin than with heparin (28 vs 22%, $p = 0.05$).

Thus, despite promising angiographic data, three large randomized controlled trials have failed to show any statistically significant benefit of hirudin over heparin in terms of mortality or reinfarction (although in the largest trial, GUSTO-IIb, there was a trend showing an approx 18% reduction in reinfarction). There are several possible reasons for the lack of a significant demonstrable benefit with hirudin in these trials *(162)*. First, the trials may have been underpowered, given the relatively low event rates. Calculations by the TIMI-9B investigators, however, showed that the likelihood that a 25% relative superiority of hirudin over heparin failed to be detected in TIMI-9B is less than 1 in 1000 and that the likelihood that even a 10% relative superiority failed to be detected is 1 in 20. Second, hirudin may have been dosed inadequately. However, in GUSTO-IIa, despite a higher dose of hirudin, which was associated with an unacceptably high rate of ICH, the rate of death or myocardial infarction was 11.7% in the hirudin group. Third, the duration of antithrombin therapy may have been inadequate. There is, however, no indication that treatment for 96 h (in TIMI-9B) was clearly superior to treatment for 72 h (in GUSTO-IIb). Fourth, the effects of direct thrombin inhibitors, such as hirudin, may not be durable. In GUSTO-IIb, all of hirudin's beneficial effect on reducing the rate of death or reinfarction was evident at 24 h; subsequent to this, the event-rate curves neither converged nor diverged (this pattern, however, was not seen in TIMI-9B, in which hirudin was associated with mixed results in terms of the rate of death or reinfarction at 24 h). This potential lack of a durable effect has also been noted in other trials using thrombin inhibitors *(163–165)* and stands in contradistinction to the beneficial effects seen with the GP IIb/IIIa inhibitors, which persist even out to 3 yr *(166)*. The mechanistic implication of this observation is that thrombin inhibitors may not be able to "passivate" the arterial surface in order to prevent the generation of platelet thrombi after the treatment is discontinued. Fifth, like heparin, hirudin is not able to inhibit clot-bound thrombin. Sixth, although hirudin may be a more potent inhibitor of thrombin activity, it may be a less potent inhibitor of thrombin generation. Prothrombin fragment 1.2 (F1.2) levels are used as a marker of thrombin generation, and fibrinopeptide A (FPA) levels are used as a marker of thrombin activity. Data show that heparin causes a greater reduction in F1.2 levels than hirudin does, whereas hirudin causes a greater reduction in FPA levels than heparin does *(167,168)*, implying that heparin may possess a greater ability to decrease thrombin generation (potentially through its enhancement of ATIII's inhibition of factor Xa) and hirudin may possess a greater ability to decrease thrombin activity.

BIVALIRUDIN

Pharmacology. Bivalirudin (Angiomax, formerly Hirulog) is a 20-amino acid synthetic peptide with a molecular weight of 873 Da that contains the [D] Phe-Pro-Arg-Pro sequence of the amino terminus of hirudin connected by a polyglycyl link to a 12-amino acid sequence from the carboxy terminus of hirudin *(117,169)*. The former sequence binds to and blocks the catalytic site, while the latter sequence binds to and blocks the substrate recognition site (Fig. 14). Bivalirudin has been shown to be equally active against both fluid-phase and clot-bound thrombin *(17)*, and it is not inhibited by platelet factor 4.

Clinical Data. After promising data was seen in a pilot angiographic study *(170)*, Théroux and colleagues at the Montreal Heart Institute randomized 68 patients presenting with acute myocardial infarction and treated with aspirin and streptokinase to iv heparin, low-dose bivalirudin (0.5 mg/kg/h for 12 h, followed by 0.1 mg/kg/h for 4–6 days), and high-dose bivalirudin (1.0 mg/kg/h for 12 h, followed by a placebo infusion)

(171). The primary end point of TIMI flow grade 3 at 90 min was achieved in 31% of patients who received heparin, 85% of patients who received low-dose bivalirudin, and 61% of patients who received high-dose bivalirudin ($p = 0.008$).

The Hirulog Early Reperfusion/Occlusion (HERO) trial randomized 412 patients presenting with acute myocardial infarction and treated with aspirin and streptokinase to iv heparin, low-dose bivalirudin (0.125 mg/kg IV bolus, followed by an infusion at 0.25 mg/kg/h for 12 h, followed by an infusion at 0.125 mg/kg/h for <60 h), and high-dose bivalirudin (0.25 mg/kg IV bolus, followed by an infusion at 0.5 mg/kg/h for 12 h, followed by an infusion at 0.25 mg/kg/h for <60 h) *(172)*. Again, the primary end point was achievement of TIMI flow grade 3 at 90–120 min. There was a statistically significantly higher percentage of patients achieving TIMI flow grade 3 with high-dose bivalirudin (48%) and low-dose bivalirudin (46%) than with heparin (35%) ($p = 0.03$). Major bleeding was significantly less in the low-dose bivalirudin group (14%) than in the high-dose bivalirudin (19%) or heparin (28%) groups ($p < 0.01$).

Based on the results of HERO-1, the HERO-2 trial was conducted in which patients undergoing fibrinolysis with streptokinase were randomized to bivalirudin (the same high-dose regimen used in HERO-1) or iv unfractionated heparin *(173)*. Thirty-day mortality rates were similar in the bivalirudin (10.8%) and heparin (10.9%) arms and higher than the rates seen in other contemporary lytic trials (approx 6%). However, similar to the results seen with the direct thrombin inhibitor hirudin, treatment with bivalirudin was associated with a 30% reduction in the rate of reinfarction (1.6 vs 2.3%, $p = 0.001$).

ARGATROBAN

Pharmacology. Argatroban is an arginine derivative tripeptide synthetic compound with a molecular weight of 527 Da that is structurally similar to fibrinopeptide A *(117,174–176)*. Argatroban contains a sequence corresponding to the cleavage sequence in fibrinogen and inhibits thrombin by acting as a competitive antagonist, binding to the apolar binding site, and blocking the catalytic site (Fig. 14). Like hirudin, argatroban does not require the presence of ATIII to neutralize thrombin, and it is not inhibited by platelet factor 4 or heparinases. Argatroban is equally effective against fluid phase and clot-bound thrombin (Fig. 16) *(156)*. This is in contrast both to heparin, which is largely ineffective against clot-bound thrombin, and to hirudin, which demonstrates reduced activity against clot-bound thrombin *(17,156,177)*. This may be related to argatroban's relatively small size (Table 5), which may allow it to better penetrate into the interstices of a fibrin clot and, thus, more effectively inhibit fibrin-bound thrombin.

Clinical Data. In the Myocardial Infarction with Novastan and TPA (MINT) trial, 120 patients with acute myocardial infarction presenting within 6 h of symptom onset received alteplase and aspirin and were randomized to receive IV heparin (70 U/kg IV bolus, followed by an infusion at 15 U/kg/h), low-dose argatroban (100 µg/kg IV bolus, followed by an infusion at 1.0 µg/kg/min), or high-dose argatroban (100 µg/kg IV bolus, followed by an infusion at 3.0 µg/kg/min) *(178)*. Treatment with argatroban was associated with a trend towards higher rates of TIMI flow grade 3 at 90 min (58.7% in the high-dose argatroban group and 56.8% in the low-dose argatroban group compared to 42.1% in the heparin group; $p = 0.13$ and 0.20, respectively). In patients who received treatment between 3 and 6 h after the onset of symptoms, the superiority of argatroban was even more striking with TIMI flow grade 3 achieved in 57.1% of the high-dose argatroban patients vs in 20.0% of the heparin patients ($p = 0.03$). There were trends towards

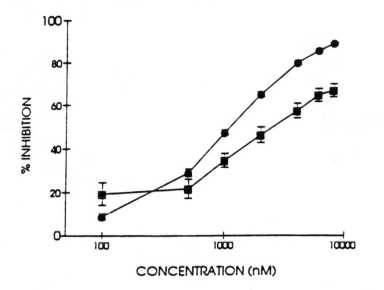

CONCENTRATION (nM)

Fig. 16. Comparison of the inhibitory effects of argatroban against fluid phase (circles) and clot-bound (squares) thrombin activity. Thrombin or fibrin clots were incubated with the chromogenic synthetic substrate S2238 in the presence or absence of argatroban. p-nitro-aniline (p-NA) release was then assayed and the percent inhibition of p-NA release was calculated for each inhibitor concentration. Reproduced with permission from ref. 156.

Table 5
Molecular Weights of Antithrombins

Antithrombin	Molecular weight (Da)
Heparin	average 15,000
Hirudin	7000
LMWHs	4000–6000
Hirulog	873
Argatroban	527

Abbreviations: LMWHs, low-molecular-weight heparins.

less major bleeding in the low-dose argatroban (2.6%) and high-dose argatroban (4.3%) groups than in the heparin group (10.0%).

Low-Molecular-Weight Heparin

PHARMACOLOGY

LMWHs are fragments of standard unfractionated heparin (UFH) produced by controlled depolymerization to yield chains with mean molecular weights of 4000–6000 (179,180). As with UFH, the anticoagulant activity of LMWH is due to the unique pentasaccharide sequence that binds to ATIII, thereby inducing a conformational change that makes the reactive site more accessible to both factor Xa and thrombin. However, unlike UFH, only a small percentage of LMWH contains the sufficient number of polysaccharide residues to be able to act as a catalytic template by binding ATIII and thrombin simultaneously. Thus, LMWH exerts its anticoagulant effect

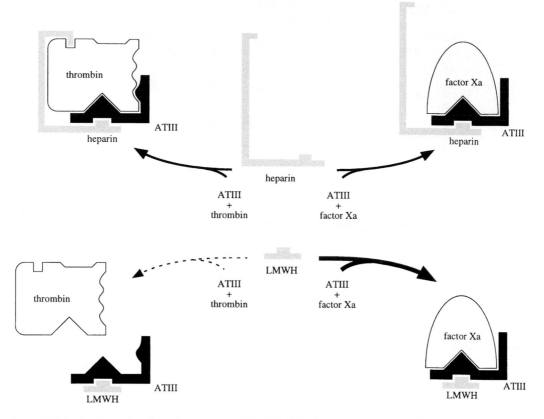

Fig. 17. Mechanism of action of heparin vs LMWH. UFH induces a conformational chane in ATIII, allowing the latter to more readily inhibit thrombin and factor Xa. In the case of thrombin inhibition, UFH also acts as a catalytic template, forming a ternary complex with thrombin and ATIII and accelerating their interaction by greater than 1000-fold. In contrast, LMWH does not contain a sufficient number of polysaccharide residues to act as a catalytic template for ATIII and thrombin, but still can induce the conformational change in ATIII and therefore is primarily a factor Xa inhibitor.

primarily by inhibition of thrombin generation that is achieved by inactivating factor Xa (Fig. 17) *(181)*. Like UFH, LMWH cannot inactivate clot-bound thrombin *(182)*, nor can it inactivate factor Xa once it is part of the prothrombinase complex. LMWHs are resistant to inactivation by platelet factor 4 *(183)*, are less bound by acute phase reactants and vascular endothelial cells, thereby resulting in a more predictable anticoagulation effect *(128,179)*, and are far less likely to trigger HIT *(184)* (although in a patient with HIT and antiplatelet antibodies LMWH may cross-react). The LMWHs have different chemical characteristics, different degrees of anti-Xa:anti-IIa activity, and different effects on tissue factor pathway inhibitor, and thus, should not be considered as a single class of agents *(185)*. The two most-studied LMWHs are enoxaparin (Lovenox) and dalteparin (Fragmin), which have anti-Xa:anti-IIa activity ratios of 3.8 and 2.7, respectively.

CLINICAL DATA

Several studies have shown improved angiographic results in patients receiving LMWH compared with UFH. In the Biochemical Markers in Acute Coronary Syndromes II (BIOMACS II) study, 101 patients with ST-elevation myocardial infarction were treated with streptokinase and aspirin and were randomized to subcutaneous dalteparin or placebo. There was a trend toward higher rates of TIMI flow grade 3 in patients treated dalteparin (68 vs 51%, $p = 0.10$) and a lower rate of recurrent ischemic episodes (16 vs 38%, $p = 0.04$).

Dalteparin (30 U/kg IV bolus and 90 U/kg subcutaneously, followed by 120 U/kg subcutaneously 2× daily for 4–7 d) was compared to IV UFH (for 48 h) in 439 patients undergoing fibrinolysis with alteplase in the ASSENT Plus trial *(186)*. Late angiography after 4–7 d revealed higher rates of patency (87 vs 76%, $p = 0.006$) and a trend towards modestly higher rates of TIMI flow grade 3 (69 vs 63%, $p = 0.16$).

The LMWH enoxaparin was studied in three angiographic trials. In the Acute Myocardial Infarction-Streptokinase (AMI-SK) trial, 496 patients receiving streptokinase for ST-elevation myocardial infarction were randomized to enoxaparin (30 mg IV bolus, followed by 1 mg/kg subcutaneously 2× daily) or placebo *(187)*. Late angiography (d 5–10) revealed higher rates of patency (87.6 vs 71.7%, $p < 0.001$) and TIMI flow grade 3 (70.3 vs 57.8%, $p < 0.01$). Complete ST segment resolution was also higher at both 90 min (15.7 vs 11.1%, $p = 0.012$) and at 180 min (36.3 vs 25.4%, $p = 0.004$).

In the 400 patients undergoing fibrinolysis with alteplase in HART-II, enoxaparin (30 mg IV bolus, followed by 1 mg/kg subcutaneously every 12 h) was compared to iv UFH *(188)*. After 90 min, treatment with enoxaparin resulted in modest trends towards higher rates of patency (80.1 vs 75.1%) and TIMI flow grade 3 (52.9 vs 47.6%) at 90 min. Patients with a patent infarct-related artery at 90 min underwent follow-up angiography at 5–7 d. In this subgroup, treatment with enoxaparin was associated with a trend towards lower rates of reocclusion (5.9 vs 9.8%).

In the ENTIRE study, several enoxaparin regimens (with and without a bolus; different subcutaneous maintenance doses) were compared to iv UFH. There were no significant differences between the enoxaparin regimens. Compared to UFH, enoxaparin resulted in similar rates of TIMI flow grade 3, but a trend towards higher rates of complete ST segment resolution by 180 min. Among patients receiving full dose TNK-tPA, ischemic events (death, nonfatal myocardial infarction) were less frequent in patients receiving enoxaparin (4.4 vs 15.9%, $p = 0.005$).

As detailed above, ASSENT-3 was a phase III trial comparing three pharmacologic reperfusion regimens: full-dose TNK-tPA plus UFH, full-dose TNK-tPA plus the LMWH enoxaparin, or reduced-dose TNK-tPA plus abciximab *(92)*. The 30-d mortality rates did not statistically significantly differ between the groups (5.4% for enoxaparin, 6.6% for abciximab, and 6.0% for UFH, $p = 0.25$) (Fig. 18). However, the rate of the composite end point of death, in-hospital reinfarction, or in-hospital refractory ischemia was lower in the enoxaparin and abciximab arms compared with the unfractionated heparin arm (11.4 and 11.1 vs 15.4%, $p < 0.001$). Major bleeding rates were 3.0% in the enoxaparin arm, 4.3% in the abciximab arm, and 2.2% in the unfractionated heparin arm ($p = 0.0005$).

Thus, compared with using UFH, adjunctive anticoagulation in fibrinolysis using LMWH appears to offer a reduction in ischemic events with only a minimal excess in bleeding. This is in contrast to combining a GP IIb/IIIa inhibitor with a reduced-dose fibrinolytic, which was also associated with a reduction in ischemic events, but with a significant excess in bleeding. However, as discussed above, the latter option does offer an easier transition to the cardiac catheterization laboratory. Despite several studies sug-

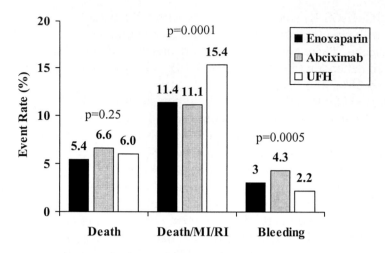

Fig. 18. Proportion of patients with the primary end point of death (left group of bars), the composite end point of death, nonfatal reinfarction, or refractory ischemia (middle group of bars), and the safety end point of major bleeding (right group of bars) in the ASSENT 3 trial *(92)* for patients randomized to full-dose TNK-tPA plus enoxaparin (solid bars) vs reduced-dose TNK-tPA plus abciximab (shaded bars) vs full-dose TNK-tPA plus UFH (open bars).

gesting that patients on LMWH can safely undergo cardiac catheterization *(189)*, uncertainly with regard to this point has, to date, slowed widespread adoption of LMWHs in acute coronary syndromes.

Other Anticoagulants

PENTASACCHARIDE

The unique pentasaccharide sequence found in heparin that is required for binding to and activation of ATIII has been synthesized *(190)*. Several recent studies have shown that pentasaccharide is more efficacious than LMWHs in the treatment of deep vein thrombosis *(191–193)*. In the PENTALYSE study, 333 patients with ST-elevation myocardial infarction undergoing fibrinolysis with alteplase were randomized to UFH or one of several different doses of pentasaccharide *(194)*. Rates of TIMI flow grade 3 in the infarct-related artery at 90 min were comparable across all the groups, but there was a trend towards improved late patency (d 5–7) in the pooled pentasaccharide group vs the UFH group (86 vs 75%, $p = 0.1$).

TICK ANTICOAGULANT PEPTIDE

Tick anticoagulant peptide (TAP) was originally derived from the soft tick (*Ornithodorus moubata*) and is now produced via recombinant DNA technology *(195–197)*. TAP can inhibit factor Xa both in its free form and as part of the prothrombinase complex. In animal models, TAP proved superior to heparin *(198)* and hirudin *(199,200)* in accelerating thrombolysis and preventing acute reocclusion.

TISSUE FACTOR PATHWAY INHIBITOR

Tissue factor pathway inhibitor (TFPI), also known as lipoprotein-associated coagulation inhibitor (LACI), has been examined as a means to block one of the pathways leading to factor Xa generation. TFPI is a 276-amino acid protein containing three

Kunitz-type inhibitor domains *(201–203)*. TFPI can bind and inhibit factor Xa, and the Xa-TFPI complex can inhibit the VIIa-tissue factor complex, which generates factor Xa *(204,205)*. In animal studies, TFPI prevented reocclusion after thrombolysis *(206–208)*, although not effectively as TAP *(209)*.

Thrombin Generation Vs Thrombin Activity

The pattern of reocclusion seen in experiments with thrombin generation inhibitors confirms previous observations that both active thrombin generation and preformed thrombin play a role in reocclusion. Inhibition of prothrombinase prevents further thrombin generation, but leaves preformed clot-bound thrombin to trigger reocclusion once it is exposed during ongoing thrombolysis. Conversely, thrombin inhibition may effectively prevent preformed thrombin from triggered thrombosis, but such therapy must continue until prothrombinase activity has been neutralized by endogenous anticoagulant systems or new thrombin generation will lead to thrombosis. Therefore, inhibition of both thrombin and prothrombinase may allow one to rapidly achieve thrombolysis and prevent reocclusion using the shortest duration of therapy with the lowest systemic effects.

Summary

- Thrombin is a complex molecule that plays a key role in both the coagulation cascade and platelet activation. Multiple agents have been developed in an attempt to block its role in coronary thrombosis.
- In patients not receiving aspirin, heparin has been shown to reduce mortality and nonfatal reinfarctions. In patients receiving aspirin and undergoing thrombolysis, neither subcutaneous nor iv heparin is of proven benefit when streptokinase is used, but iv heparin remains the standard of care when fibrin-specific lytics are used, based primarily on extrapolations from angiographic data. Attempts to use more intensive iv heparin regimens have resulted in unacceptably high rates of bleeding.
- Despite several theoretical advantages and promising angiographic data, direct thrombin inhibitors such as hirudin, bivalirudin, and argatroban have yet to be shown to be superior to heparin. In several large, phase III clinical trials, hirudin and bivalirudin were associated with lower rates of reinfarction, but similar rates of mortality when compared with heparin.
- LMWHs preferentially inhibit factor Xa and, hence, thrombin generation. In a recently completed phase III trial, adjunctive anticoagulation with enoxaparin proved superior to UFH in reducing the composite of death and ischemic events. As more clinical data accumulate on LMWHs and as clinicians become more comfortable with patients on LMWH undergoing coronary interventions, LMWH may supplant UFH as the preferred anticoagulant in fibrinolysis.

CONCLUSION

The current standard for adjunctive therapy with thrombolysis remains aspirin and heparin. Both of these medications came into use more than 50 yr ago when our understanding of the molecular biology underlying acute coronary syndromes was nonexistent. As we have deciphered the mechanisms underlying platelet activation and aggregation and thrombin generation and activity, we now stand at the threshold of a new era in which exquisitely tailored pharmacotherapy can be used to inhibit the pathways leading to coronary artery thrombosis.

Platelet physiology has now been sufficiently dissected to allow us to specifically target and inhibit platelet adhesion, activation, and aggregation. While aspirin remains a vital component of acute myocardial infarction therapy, both ADP antagonists and GP IIb/IIIa inhibitors have emerged as powerful new adjunctive agents. Similarly, we now have at our disposal inhibitors both of thrombin generation and of thrombin activity and we are able to attack both fluid-phase and clot-bound thrombin.

Regardless of whether a patient with ST elevation myocardial infarction undergoes pharmacologic-based or catheter-based reperfusion, intensive antiplatelet therapy and proximal inhibition of the coagulation cascade are likely to be the mainstays of adjuvant therapy. As we continue to refine our knowledge, the next steps will be to design appropriate combinations of agents for each setting.

REFERENCES

1. Gruppo Italiano per lo Studio della Streptochianasi nell'Infarto Miocardico (GISSI). Effectiveness of intravenous thrombolytic treatment in acute myocardial infarction. Lancet 1986;1:65–71.
2. ISIS-2 (Second International Study of Infarct Survival) Collaborative Group. Randomised trial of intravenous streptokinase, oral aspirin, both or neither among 17,187 cases of suspected acute myocardial infarction: ISIS-2. Lancet 1988;2:349–360.
3. Ryan TJ, Anderson JL, Antman EM, et al. ACC/AHA guidelines for the management of patients with acute myocardial infarction. A report of the American College of Cardiology/American Heart Association Task Force on Practice Guidelines (Committee on Management of Acute Myocardial Infarction). J Am Coll Cardiol 1996;28:1328–1348.
4. Ryan TJ, Antman EM, Brooks NH, et al. 1999 update: ACC/AHA Guidelines for the Management of Patients With Acute Myocardial Infarction: Executive Summary and Recommendations: A report of the American College of Cardiology/American Heart Association Task Force on Practice Guidelines (Committee on Management of Acute Myocardial Infarction). Circulation 1999;100:1016–1030.
5. The GUSTO Angiographic Investigators. The effects of tissue plasminogen activator, streptokinase, or both on coronary-artery patency, ventricular function, and survival after acute myocardial infarction. N Engl J Med 1993;329:1615–1622.
6. Ohman EM, Califf RM, Topol EJ, et al. Consequences of reocclusion after successful reperfusion therapy in acute myocardial infarction. Circulation 1990;82:781–791.
7. Smalling RW, Bode C, Kalbfleisch J, et al. More rapid, complete, and stable coronary thrombolysis with bolus administration of reteplase compared with alteplase infusion in acute myocardial infarction. RAPID Investigators. Circulation 1995;91:2725–2732.
8. Bode C, Smalling RW, Berg G, et al. Randomized comparison of coronary thrombolysis achieved with double-bolus reteplase (recombinant plasminogen activator) and front-loaded, accelerated alteplase (recombinant tissue plasminogen activator) in patients with acute myocardial infarction. The RAPID II Investigators. Circulation 1996;94:891–898.
9. Cannon CP, McCabe CH, Gibson CM, et al. TNK-tissue plasminogen activator in acute myocardial infarction. Results of the Thrombolysis in Myocardial Infarction (TIMI) 10A dose-ranging trial. Circulation 1997;95:351–356.
10. Cannon CP, Gibson CM, McCabe CH, et al. TNK-tissue plasminogen activator compared with front-loaded alteplase in acute myocardial infarction: results of the TIMI 10B trial. Thrombolysis in Myocardial Infarction (TIMI) 10B Investigators. Circulation 1998;98:2805–2814.
11. The Global Use of Strategies to Open Occluded Coronary Arteries (GUSTO III) Investigators. A comparison of reteplase with alteplase for acute myocardial infarction. N Engl J Med 1997;337:1118–1123.
12. Assessment of the Safety and Efficacy of a New Thrombolytic (ASSENT-2) Investigators. Single-bolus tenecteplase compared with front-loaded alteplase in acute myocardial infarction: the ASSENT-2 double-blind randomised trial. Lancet 1999;354:716–722.

13. Coller BS. The role of platelets in arterial thrombosis and the rationale for blockade of platelet GPIIb/IIIa receptors as antithrombotic therapy. Eur Heart J 1995;16(Suppl. L):11–15.
14. Jang I-K, Gold HK, Ziskind AA, et al. Differential sensitivity of erythrocyte-rich and platelet-rich arterial thrombi to lysis with recombinant tissue-type plasminogen activator: a possible explanation for resistance to coronary thrombolysis. Circulation 1989;79:920–928.
15. Walsh PN, Schmaier AH. Platelet-coagulant protein interactions. In: Colman RW, Hirsh J, Marder VJ, Salzman EW, eds. Hemostasis and Thrombosis: Basic Principles and Clinical Practice. J.B. Lippincott Company, Philadelphia, 1994, pp. 629–651.
16. Hogg PJ, Jackson CM. Fibrin monomer protects thrombin from inactivation by heparin-antithrombin III: implications for heparin efficacy. Proc Natl Acad Sci USA 1989;86:3619–3623.
17. Weitz JI, Huboda M, Massel D, Maraganore J, Hirsh J. Clot-bound thrombin is protected from inhibition by heparin-antithrombin but is susceptible to inactivation by antithrombin III-independent inhibitors. J Clin Invest 1990;86:385–391.
18. Loscalzo J, Melnick B, Handin R. The interaction of platelet factor 4 and glycosaminoglycans. Arch Biochem Biophys 1985;240:446 455.
19. Hirsh J, Dalen JE, Deykin D, Poller L. Heparin: mechanism of action, pharmacokinetics, dosing considerations, monitoring, efficacy, and safety. Chest 1992;102:337S–351S.
20. Miller ML. Heparin-induced thrombocytopenia. Cleve Clin J Med 1989;56:483–490.
21. Merlini PA, Bauer KA, Oltrona L, et al. Persistent activation of coagulation mechanism in unstable angina and myocardial infarction. Circulation 1994;90:61 68.
22. Fitzgerald DJ, Catella F, Roy L, FitzGerald GA. Marked platelet activation in vivo after intravenous streptokinase in patients with acute myocardial infarction. Circulation 1988;77:142–150.
23. Kerins DM, Roy L, FitzGerald GA, Fitzgerald DJ. Platelet and vascular function during coronary thrombolysis with tissue-type plasminogen activator. Circulation 1989;80:1718–1725.
24. Eisenberg PR, Sobel BE, Jaffe AS. Activation of prothrombin accompanying thrombolysis with recombinant tissue-type plasminogen activator. J Am Coll Cardiol 1992;19:1065–1069.
25. Merlini PA, Bauer KA, Oltrona L, et al. Thrombin generation and activity during thrombolysis and concomitant heparin therapy in patients with acute myocardial infarction. J Am Coll Cardiol 1995;25: 203–209.
26. Genser N, Mair J, Maier J, Dienstl F, Puschendorf B, Lechleitner P. Thrombin generation during infusion of tissue-type plasminogen activator. Lancet 1993;341:1038.
27. Eisenberg PR, Sherman LA, Jaffe AS. Paradoxic elevation of fibrinopeptide A after streptokinase: evidence for continued thrombosis despite intense fibrinolysis. J Am Coll Cardiol 1987;10:527–529.
28. Owen J, Friedman KD, Grossman BA, Wilkins C, Berke AD, Powers ER. Thrombolytic therapy with tissue plasminogen activator or streptokinase induces transient thrombin activity. Blood 1988;72: 616–620.
29. Rapold HJ, de Bono D, Arnold AE, et al. Plasma fibrinopeptide A levels in patients with acute myocardial infarction treated with alteplase. Correlation with concomitant heparin, coronary artery patency, and recurrent ischemia. The European Cooperative Study Group. Circulation 1992;85:928–934.
30. Galvani M, Abendschein DR, Ferrini D, Ottani F, Rusticali F, Eisenberg PR. Failure of fixed dose intravenous heparin to suppress increases in thrombin activity after coronary thrombolysis with streptokinase. J Am Coll Cardiol 1994;24:1445–1452.
31. Seitz R, Blanke H, Prätorius G, Strauer BE, Egbring R. Increased thrombin activity during thrombolysis. Thromb Haemost 1988;59:541–542.
32. Bloom AL. The release of thrombin from fibrin by fibrinolysis. Br J Haematol 1962;82:129–133.
33. Lee CD, Mann KG. Activation/inactivation of human factor V by plasmin. Blood 1989;73:185–190.
34. Fuster V, Badimon L, Badimon JJ, Chesebro JH. The pathogenesis of coronary artery disease and the acute coronary syndromes (Part 1). N Engl J Med 1992;326:242–250.
35. Fuster V, Badimon L, Badimon JJ, Chesebro JH. The pathogenesis of coronary artery disease and the acute coronary syndromes (Part 2). N Engl J Med 1992;326:310–318.
36. Schafer AI. The platelet life cycle: normal function and qualitative disorders. In: Handin RI, Lux SE, Stossel TP, eds. Blood: Principles and Practice of Hematology. J.B. Lippincott Company, Philadelphia, 1995, pp. 1095–1126.
37. Colman RW, Cook JJ, Niewiarowski S. Mechanisms of platelet aggregation. In: Colman RW, Hirsh J, Marder VJ, Salzman EW, eds. Hemostasis and Thrombosis: Basic Principles and Clinical Practice. J.B. Lippincott Company, Philadelphia, 1994, pp. 508–523.

38. Hawinger J, Brass LF, Salzman EW. Signal transduction and intracellular regulatory processes in platelets. In: Colman RW, Hirsh J, Marder VJ, Salzman EW, eds. Hemostasis and Thrombosis: Basic Principles and Clinical Practice. J.B. Lippincott Company, Philadelphia, 1994, pp. 603–628.
39. Handin RI. Platelet membrane proteins and their disorders. In: Handin RI, Lux SE, Stossel TP, eds. Blood: Principles and Practice of Hematology. J.B. Lippincott Company, Philadelphia, 1995, pp. 1049–1067.
40. Lefkovits J, Plow EF, Topol EJ. Platelet glycoprotein IIb/IIIa receptors in cardiovascular medicine. N Engl J Med 1995;332:1553–1559.
41. Schafer AI. Antiplatelet therapy. Am J Med 1995;101:199–209.
42. Verstraete M. New developments in antiplatelet and antithrombotic therapy. Eur Heart J 1995;16: 16–23.
43. Frishman WH, Burns B, Atac B, Alturk N, Altajar B, Lerrick K. Novel antiplatelet therapies for treatment of patients with ischemic heart disease: inhibitors of the platelet glycoprotein IIb/IIIa integrin receptor. Am Heart J 1995;130:877–892.
44. Patrono C. Aspirin as an antiplatelet drug. N Engl J Med 1994;330:1287–1294.
45. Willard JE, Lange RA, Hillis LD. The use of aspirin in ischemic heart disease. N Engl J Med 1992; 327:175–181.
46. Campbell WB. Lipid-derived autacoids: eicosanoids and platelet-activating factor. In: Gilman AG, Rall TW, Nies AS, Taylor P, eds. Goodman and Gilman's The Pharmacologic Basis of Therapeutics. Pergamon Press, New York, 1990, pp. 600–617.
47. Jaffe EA, Weksler BB. Recovery of endothelial cell prostacyclin production after inhibition by low doses of aspirin. J Clin Invest 1979;63:532–535.
48. Hanson SR, Harker LA, Bjornsson TD. Effects of platelet-modifying drugs on arterial thromboembolism in baboons: Aspirin potentiates the antithrombotic actions of dipyridamole and sulfinpyrazone by mechanism(s) independent of platelet cyclooxygenase inhibition. J Clin Invest 1985;75:1591–1599.
49. Gaspari F, Vigano G, Orisio S, Bonati M, Livio M, Remuzzi G. Aspirin prolongs bleeding time in uremia by a mechanism distinct from platelet cyclooxygenase inhibition. J Clin Invest 1987;79: 1788–1797.
50. Hirsh J, Dalen JE, Fuster V, Harker LB, Salzman EW. Aspirin and other platelet-active drugs: the relationship between dose, effectiveness, and side effects. Chest 1992;102 (Suppl. 4):327S–336S.
51. Patrignani P, Filabozzi P, Patrono C. Selective cumulative inhibition of platelet thromboxane production by low-dose aspirin in healthy subjects. J Clin Invest 1982;69:1366–1372.
52. Weksler BB, Pett SB, Alonso D, et al. Differential inhibition by aspirin of vascular and platelet prostaglandin synthesis in atherosclerotic patients. N Engl J Med 1983;308:800–805.
53. Antiplatelet Trialists' Collaboration. Collaborative overview of randomised trials of antiplatelet therapy—I: prevention of death, myocardial infarction, and stroke by prolonged antiplatelet therapy in various categories of patients. BMJ 1994;308:81–106.
54. Baigent C, Collins R. ISIS-2: 4-year mortality follow-up of 17,187 patients after fibrinolytic and antiplatelet therapy in suspected acute myocardial infarction [abstract]. Circulation 1993;88(Suppl. I): I-291.
55. Quinn MJ, Fitzgerald DJ. Ticlopidine and clopidogrel. Circulation 1999;100:1667–1672.
56. Defreyn G, Gachet C, Savi P, Driot F, Cazenave JP, Maffrand JP. Ticlopidine and clopidogrel (SR 25990C) selectively neutralize ADP inhibition of PGE1-activated platelet adenylate cyclase in rats and rabbits. Thromb Haemost 1991;65:186–190.
57. Cattaneo M, Lombardi R, Bettega D, Lecchi A, Mannucci PM. Shear-induced platelet aggregation is potentiated by desmopressin and inhibited by ticlopidine. Arterioscler Thromb 1993;13:393–397.
58. Di Minno G, Cerbone AM, Mattioli PL, Turco S, Iovine C, Mancini M. Functionally thrombosthenic state in normal platelets following the administration of ticlopidine. J Clin Invest 1985;75:328–338.
59. Defreyn G, Bernat A, Delebassee D, Maffrand JP. Pharmacology of ticlopidine: a review. Semin Thromb Hemost 1989;15:159–166.
60. Savi P, Combalbert J, Gaich C, et al. The antiaggregating activity of clopidogrel is due to a metabolic activation by the hepatic cytochrome P450-1A. Thromb Haemost 1994;72:313–317.
61. Seyfarth HJ, Koksch M, Roethig G, et al. Effect of 300- and 450-mg clopidogrel loading doses on membrane and soluble P-selectin in patients undergoing coronary stent implantation. Am Heart J 2002;143:118–123.
62. Gent M, Blakely JA, Easton JD, et al. The Canadian American Ticlopidine Study (CATS) in thromboembolic stroke. Lancet 1989;2:1215–1220.

63. Hass WK, Easton JD, Adams HP, et al. A randomized trial comparing ticlopidine hydrochloride with aspirin for the prevention of stroke in high-risk patients. N Engl J Med 1989;321:501–507.

64. Schömig A, Neumann F-J, Kastrati A, et al. A randomized comparison of antiplatelet and anticoagulant therapy after the placement of coronary-artery stents. N Engl J Med 1996;334:1084–1089.

65. Schömig A, Neumann F-J, Walter H, et al. Coronary stent placement in patients with acute myocardial infarction: Comparison of clinical and angiographic outcome after randomization to antiplatelet or anticoagulant therapy. J Am Coll Cardiol 1997;29:28–34.

66. Leon MB, Baim DS, Popma JJ, et al. A clinical trial comparing three antithrombotic-drug regimens after coronary-artery stenting. N Engl J Med 1998;339:1665–1671.

67. Muller C, Buttner HJ, Petersen J, Roskamm H. A randomized comparison of clopidogrel and aspirin versus ticlopidine and aspirin after the placement of coronary-artery stents. Circulation 2000;101: 590–593.

68. Bertrand ME, Rupprecht HJ, Urban P, Gershlick AH, for the CLASSICS Investigators. Double-blind study of the safety of clopidogrel with and without a loading dose in combination with aspirin compared with ticlopidine in combination with aspirin after coronary stenting : the clopidogrel aspirin stent international cooperative study (CLASSICS). Circulation 2000;102:624–629.

69. Taniuchi M, Kurz HI, Lasala JM. Randomized comparison of ticlopidine and clopidogrel after intra coronary stent implantation in a broad patient population. Circulation 2001;104:539–543.

70. CAPRIE Steering Committee. A randomised, blinded, trial of clopidogrel versus aspirin in patients at risk of ischemic events (CAPRIE). Lancet 1996;348:1329–1339.

71. The Clopidogrel in Unstable Angina to Prevent Recurrent Ischemic Events Trial Investigators. Effects of clopidogrel in addition to aspirin in patients with acute coronary syndromes without ST-segment elevation. N Engl J Med 2001;345:494–502.

72. Hacker LA, Mann KG. Thrombosis and fibrinolysis. In: Fuster V, Verstraete M, eds. Thrombosis in Cardiovascular Disorders. WB Saunders, Philadelphia, 1992, pp. 1–16.

73. Sabatine MS, Jang I-K. The use of glycoprotein IIb/IIIa inhibitors in patients with coronary artery disease. Am J Med 2000;109:224–237.

74. Coller BS. A new murine monoclonal antibody reports an activation dependent change in the conformation and/or microenvironment of the glycoprotein IIb/IIIa complex. J Clin Invest 1985;76: 101–108.

75. Scarborough RM, Naughton MA, Teng W, et al. Design of potent and specific integrin antagonists. Peptide antagonists with high specificity for glycoprotein IIb-IIIa. J Biol Chem 1993;268:1066–1073.

76. Goa KL, Noble S. Eptifibatide. Drugs 1999;57:439–462.

77. Hartman GD, Egbertson MS, Halczenko W, et al. Non-peptide fibrinogen receptor antagonists. 1. Discovery and design of exosite inhibitors. J Med Chem 1992;35:4640–4642.

78. McClellan KJ, Goa KL. Tirofiban. Drugs 1998;56:1067–1080.

79. Berkowitz SD, Harrington RA, Rund MM, Tcheng JE. Acute profound thrombocytopenia after c7E3 Fab (abciximab) therapy. Circulation 1997;95:809–813.

80. Berkowitz SD, Sane DC, Sigmon KN, et al. Occurrence and clinical significance of thrombocytopenia in a population undergoing high-risk percutaneous coronary revascularization. J Am Coll Cardiol 1998;32:311–319.

81. Tcheng JE, Kereiakes DJ, Lincoff AM, et al. Abciximab readministration: results of the ReoPro Readministration Registry. Circulation 2001;104:870–875.

82. Brener SJ, Barr LA, Burchenal JEB, et al. Randomized, placebo-controlled trial of platelet glycoprotein IIb/IIIa blockade with primary angioplasty for acute myocardial infarction. Circulation 1998;98: 731–741.

83. Neumann F-J, Kastrati A, Schmitt C, et al. Effect of glycoprotein IIb/IIIa receptor blockade with abciximab on clinical and angiographic restenosis rate after the placement of coronary stents following acute myocardial infarction. J Am Coll Cardiol 2000;35:915–921.

84. Montalescot G, Barragan P, Wittenberg O, et al. Platelet glycoprotein IIb/IIIa inhibition with coronary stenting for acute myocardial infarction. N Engl J Med 2001;344:1895–1903.

85. Stone GW, Grines CL, Cox DA, et al. Comparison of angioplasty with stenting, with or without abciximab, in acute myocardial infarction. N Engl J Med 2002;346:957–966.

86. Kleiman NS, Ohman EM, Califf RM, et al. Profound inhibition of platelet aggregation with monoclonal antibody 7E3 Fab after thrombolytic therapy: results of the Thrombolysis after Angioplasty in Myocardial Infarction (TAMI) 8 pilot study. J Am Coll Cardiol 1993;22:381–389.

87. Antman EM, Giugliano RP, Gibson CM, et al. Abciximab facilitates the rate and extent of thrombolysis. Results of the Thrombolysis in Myocardial Infarction (TIMI) 14 trial. Circulation 1999;99: 2720–2732.
88. Strategies for Patency Enhancement in the Emergency Department (SPEED) Group. Trial of abciximab with and without low-dose reteplase for acute myocardial infarction. Circulation 2000;101: 2788–2794.
89. Antman EM, Gibson CM, de Lemos JA, et al. Combination reperfusion therapy with abciximab and reduced dose reteplase: results from TIMI 14. The Thrombolysis in Myocardial Infarction (TIMI) 14 Investigators. Eur Heart J 2000;21:1944–1953.
90. Antman EM, Louwerenburg HW, Baars HF, et al. Enoxaparin as adjunctive antithrombin therapy for ST-elevation myocardial infarction: results of the ENTIRE-Thrombolysis in Mycardial Infarction (TIMI) 23 Trial. Circulation 2002;105:1642–1649.
91. The GUSTO V Investigators. Reperfusion therapy for acute myocardial infarction with fibrinolytic therapy or combination reduced fibrinolytic therapy and platelet glycoprotein IIb/IIIa inhibition: the GUSTO V randomised trial. Lancet 2001;357:1905–1914.
92. The Assessment of the Safety and Efficacy of a New Thrombolytic Regimen (ASSENT)-3 Investigators. Efficacy and safety of tenecteplase in combination with enoxaparin, abciximab, or unfractionated heparin: the ASSENT-3 randomised trial in acute myocardial infarction. Lancet 2001;358:605–613.
93. Ohman EM, Kleiman NS, Gacioch G, et al. Combined accelerated tissue-plasminogen activator and platelet glycoprotein IIb/IIIa integrin receptor blockade with integrilin in acute myocardial infarction: results of a randomized, placebo-controlled, dose-ranging trial. Circulation 1997;95:846–854.
94. Simoons ML. Streptokinase with platelet glycoprotein IIb/IIIa blockade (eptifibatide): an angiographic study, Thrombolysis and Interventional Therapy in Acute Myocardial Infarction, Orlando, November 8, 1997.
95. Brener SJ, Vrobel TR, Lopez JF, et al. INTRO AMI: marked enhancement of arterial patency with eptifibatide and low-dose t-PA in acute myocardial infarction. Circulation 1999;100(Suppl.):I-649.
96. Giugliano RP, Roe MT, Zeymer U, et al. Restoration of epicardial and myocardial perfusion in acute ST-elevation myocardial infarction with combination eptifibatide + reduced-dose tenecteplase: dose-finding results from the INTEGRITI trial. Circulation 2001;104(Suppl. II):II-538.
97. Brochier ML, for the Flurbiprofen French Trial. Evaluation of flurbiprofen for prevention of reinfarction and reocclusion after successful thrombolysis or angioplasty in acute myocardial infarction. Eur Heart J 1993;14:951–957.
98. Bombardier C, Laine L, Reicin A, et al. Comparison of upper gastrointestinal toxicity of rofecoxib and naproxen in patients with rheumatoid arthritis. N Engl J Med 2000;343:1520–1528.
99. Mukherjee D, Nissen SE, Topol EJ. Risk of cardiovascular events associated with selective COX-2 inhibitors. JAMA 2001;286:954–959.
100. Konstam MA, Weir MR, Reicin A, et al. Cardiovascular thrombotic events in controlled, clinical trials of rofecoxib. Circulation 2001;104:2280–2288.
101. Catella-Lawson F, Reilly MP, Kapoor SC, et al. Cyclooxygenase inhibitors and the antiplatelet effects of aspirin. N Engl J Med 2001;345:1809–1817.
102. Anturane Reinfarction Italian Study. Sulfinpyrazone in post-myocardial infarction. Lancet 1982;1: 237–42.
103. FitzGerald GA. Dipyridamole. N Engl J Med 1987;316:1247–1257.
104. Gent AE, Brook CGD, Foley TH, Miller TN. Dipyridamole: a controlled trial of its effect in acute myocardial infarction. BMJ 1968;4:366–368.
105. De Clerck F, Bettens J, de Chaffoy de Courcelles D, Freyne E, Janssen PAJ. R 68070: thromboxane synthetase inhibition and thromboxane A_2/prostaglandin endoperoxide receptor blockade combined in one molecule—I. Biochemical profile in vitro. Thromb Haemost 1989;61:35–42.
106. De Clerck F, Bettens J, Van de Water A, Vercammen E, Janssen PAJ. R 68070: thromboxane synthetase inhibition and thromboxane A_2/prostaglandin endoperoxide receptor blockade combined in one molecule—II. Pharmacologic effects in vivo and ex vivo. Thromb Haemost 1989;61:43–49.
107. The RAPT Investigators. Randomized trial of ridogrel, a combined thromboxane A_2 synthase inhibitor and thromboxane A_2/prostaglandin endoperoxide receptor antagonist, versus aspirin as adjunct to thrombolysis in patients with acute myocardial infarction: the Ridogrel versus Aspirin Patency Trial (RAPT). Circulation 1994;89:588–595.
108. Schrör K. Antiplatelet drugs: a comparative review. Drugs 1995;50:7–28.

109. Topol EJ, Ellis SG, Califf RM, et al. Combined tissue-type plasminogen activator and prostacyclin therapy for acute myocardial infarction. J Am Coll Cardiol 1989;14:877–884.

110. Takamatsu J, Horne MD, Gralnick HR. Identification of the thrombin receptor on human platelets by chemical crosslinking. J Clin Invest 1986;77:362–369.

111. Coughlin SR, Vu TKH, Wheaton TI. Characterization of a functional thrombin receptor: issues and opportunities. J Clin Invest 1992;89:351–355.

112. Van Willigen G, Akkerman JW. Regulation of glycoprotein IIb/IIIa exposure on platelets stimulated with alpha-thrombin. Blood 1992;79:82–90.

113. Lumsden AB, Kelly AB, Schneider PA, et al. Lasting safe interruption of endarterectomy thrombosis by transiently infused antithrombin peptide D-Phe-Pro-ArgCH$_2$Cl in baboons. Blood 1993;81:1762–1770.

114. Harker LA, Hanson SR, Runge MS. Thrombin hypothesis of thrombus generation and vascular lesion formation. Am J Cardiol 1995;75:12B–17B.

115. Miller JL, Thiam-Cisse M, Drouet LO. Reduction in thrombus formation by PG-1 (Fab'), an anti-guinea pig platelet glycoprotein Ib monoclonal antibody. Arteriosclerosis Thromb 1991;11:1231–1236.

116. Bellinger DA, Nichols TC, Read MS, et al. Prevention of occlusive coronary thrombosis by a murine monoclonal antibody to porcine von Willebrand factor. Proc Natl Acad Sci USA 1987;84:8100–8104.

117. Lefkovits J, Topol EJ. Direct thrombin inhibitors in cardiovascular medicine. Circulation 1994;90: 1522–1536.

118. Stubbs MT, Bode W. A player of many parts: the spotlight falls on thrombin's structure. Thromb Res 1993;69:1–58.

119. Sonder SA, Fenton JW. Proflavin binding within the fibrinopeptide groove adjacent to the catalytic site of human alpha-thrombin. Biochemistry 1984;23:1818–1823.

120. Rihal CS, Flather M, Hirsh J, Yusuf S. Advances in antithrombotic drug therapy for coronary artery disease. Eur Heart J 1995;16:10–21.

121. Ali MN, Villarreal-Levy G, Schafer AI. The role of thrombin and thrombin inhibitors in coronary angioplasty. Chest 1995;108:1409–1419.

122. Hirsh J. Heparin. N Engl J Med 1991;324:1565–1574.

123. Sandset PM, Abildgaard U, Larsen ML. Heparin induces release of extrinsic coagulation pathway inhibitor (EPI). Thromb Res 1988;50:803–813.

124. Broze GJJ. Tissue factor pathway inhibitor. Thromb Haemost 1995;74.90–93.

125. Huang ZF, Wun T-C, Broze GJJ. Kinetics of factor Xa inhibition by tissue factor pathway inhibitor. J Biol Chem 1993;268:26950 26955.

126. Johnson EA, Mulloy B. The molecular weight range of commercial heparin preparations. Carbohydr Res 1976;51:119–127.

127. Anderson L, Barrowcliffe TW, Holmer E, Johnson EA, Soderstrom G. Molecular weight dependency of the heparin potentiated inhibition of thrombin and activated factor X: effect of heparin neutralization in plasma. Thromb Res 1979;15:531–541.

128. Andersson LO, Barrowcliffe TW, Holmer E. Molecular weight dependency of the heparin potentiated inhibition of thrombin and activated factor X. Effect of heparin neutralization in plasma. Thromb Res 1979;115:531.

129. Visentin GP, Ford SE, Scott JP, Aster RH. Antibodies from patients with heparin-induced thrombocytopenia/thrombosis are specific for platelet factor 4 complexed with heparin or bound to endothelial cells. J Clin Invest 1994;93:81–88.

130. Aster R. Heparin-induced thrombocytopenia and thrombosis. N Engl J Med 1995;335:1374–1376.

131. Théroux P, Waters D, Lam J, Juneau M, McCans J. Reactivation of unstable angina after the discontinuation of heparin. N Engl J Med 1992;327:141–145.

132. Granger CB, Miller JM, Bovill EG, et al. Rebound increase in thrombin generation and activity after cessation of intravenous heparin in patients with acute coronary syndromes. Circulation 1995;91: 1929–1935.

133. Smith AJC, Holt RE, Fitzpatrick K, et al. Transient thrombotic state after abrupt discontinuation of heparin in percutaneous coronary angioplasty. Am Heart J 1996;131:434–439.

134. Collins R, MacMahon S, Flather M, et al. Clinical effects of anticoagulant therapy in suspected acute myocardial infarction: systematic overview of randomised trials. BMJ 1996;313:652–659.

135. The SCATI (Studio sulla Calciparina nell'Angina e nella Trombosi Ventricolare nee'Infarto) Group. Randomised controlled trial of subcutaneous calcium-heparin in acute myocardial infarction. Lancet 1989;2:182–186.

136. Bleich SD, Nichols TC, Schumacher RR, Cooke DH, Tate DA, Teichman SL. Effect of heparin on coronary arterial patency after thrombolysis with tissue plasminogen activator in acute myocardial infarction. Am J Cardiol 1990;66:1412–1417.

137. ISIS (International Studies of Infarct Survival) Pilot Study Investigators. Randomized factorial trial of high-dose intravenous streptokinase, or oral aspirin and of intravenous heparin in acute myocardial infarction. Eur Heart J 1987;8:634–642.

138. Gruppo Italiano per lo Studio della Sopravvivenza nell'Infarto Miocardico. GISSI-2: a factorial randomised trial of alteplase versus streptokinase and heparin versus no heparin among 12,490 patients with acute myocardial infarction. Lancet 1990;336:65–71.

139. The International Study Group. In-hospital mortality and clinical course of 20,891 patients with suspected acute myocardial infarction randomised between alteplase and streptokinase with or without heparin. Lancet 1990;336:71–75.

140. ISIS-3 (Third International Study of Infarct Survival) Collaborative Group. ISIS-3: a randomised comparison of streptokinase vs tissue plasminogen activator vs anistreplase and of aspirin plus heparin vs aspirin alone among 41,299 cases of suspected acute myocardial infarction. Lancet 1992;339: 753–770.

141. de Bono DP, Simoons ML, Tijssen J, et al. Effect of early intravenous heparin on coronary patency, infarct size, and bleeding complications after alteplase thrombolysis: results of a randomised double blind European Cooperative Study Group trial. Br Heart J 1992;67:122–128.

142. Col J, Decoster O, Hanique G, et al. Infusion of heparin conjunct to streptokinase accelerates reperfusion of acute myocardial infarction. Results of a double blind randomized study (OSIRIS). Circulation 1992;86(Suppl. I):I-259.

143. O'Connor CM, Meese R, Carney R, et al. A randomized trial of intravenous heparin in conjunction with anistreplase (anisoylated plasminogen streptokinase activator complex) in acute myocardial infarction: The Duke University Clinical Cardiology Study (DUCCS) 1. J Am Coll Cardiol 1994;23: 11–18.

144. Hsia J, Hamilton WP, Kleiman N, et al. A comparison between heparin and low-dose aspirin as adjunctive therapy with tissue-plasminogen activator for acute myocardial infarction. N Engl J Med 1990;323: 1433–1437.

145. Mahaffey KW, Granger CB, Collins R, et al. Overview of randomized trials of intravenous heparin in patients with acute myocardial infarction treated with thrombolytic therapy. Am J Cardiol 1996;77: 551–556.

146. The GUSTO Investigators. An international randomized trial comparing four thrombolytic strategies for acute myocardial infarction. N Engl J Med 1993;329:673–682.

147. Neuhaus K-L, Feuerer W, Jeep-Tebbe S, Niederer W, Vogt A, Tebbe U. Improved thrombolysis with a modified dose regimen of recombinant tissue-type plasminogen activator. J Am Coll Cardiol 1989;14: 1566–1569.

148. Antman EM, for the TIMI 9A Investigators. Hirudin in acute myocardial infarction: safety report from the Thrombolysis and Thrombin Inhibition in Myocardial Infarction (TIMI) 9A trial. Circulation 1994; 90:1624–1630.

149. The Global Use of Strategies to Open Occluded Coronary Arteries (GUSTO) IIa Investigators. Randomized trial of intravenous heparin versus recombinant hirudin for acute coronary syndromes. Circulation 1994;90:1631–1637.

150. Neuhaus K-L, von Essen R, Tebbe U, et al. Safety observation from the pilot phase of the randomized r-Hirudin for Improvement of Thrombolysis (HIT-III) study. Circulation 1994;90: 1638–1642.

151. Granger CB, Hirsh J, Califf RM, et al. Activated partial thromboplastin time and outcome after thrombolytic therapy for acute myocardial infarction: results from the GUSTO-I trial. Circulation 1996;93: 870–878.

152. Cannon CP, Braunwald E. Hirudin: initial results in acute myocardial infarction, unstable angina and angioplasty. J Am Coll Cardiol 1995;25(Suppl.):30S–37S.

153. Markwardt F. Development of hirudin as an antithrombotic agent. Semin Thromb Hemost 1989;15: 269–282.

154. Krstenansky JL, Mao SJT. Antithrombin properties of the C-terminus of hirudin using synthetic unsulfated N-a-acetyl-hirudin. FEBS Lett 1987;211:10–16.

155. Stone SR, Maraganore JM. Hirudin interactions with thrombin. In: Berliner LJ, ed. Thrombin: Structure and Function. Plenum Press, New York, 1992, pp. 219–256.

156. Berry CN, Girardot C, Lecoffre C, Lunven C. Effects of the synthetic thrombin inhibitor argatroban on fibrin- or clot-incorporated thrombin: comparison with heparin and recombinant hirudin. Thromb Haemost 1994;72:381–386.

157. Cannon CP, McCabe CH, Henry TD, et al. A pilot trial of recombinant desulfatohirudin compared with heparin in conjunction with tissue-type plasminogen activator and aspirin for acute myocardial infarction: results of the Thrombolysis in Myocardial Infarction (TIMI) 5 trial. J Am Coll Cardiol 1994;23: 993–1003.

158. Lee LV. Initial experience with hirudin and streptokinase in acute myocardial infarction: results of the Thrombolysis in Myocardial Infarction (TIMI) 6 trial. Am J Cardiol 1995;75:7–13.

159. Antman EM, for the TIMI 9B Investigators. Hirudin in acute myocardial infarction. Thrombolysis and Thrombin Inhibitors in Myocardial Infarction (TIMI) 9B trial. Circulation 1996;94:911–922.

160. The Global Use of Strategies to Open Occluded Coronary Arteries (GUSTO) IIb Investigators. A comparison of recombinant hirudin with heparin for the treatment of acute coronary syndromes. N Engl J Med 1996;335:775–782.

161. Neuhaus K-L, Molhock GP, Zeymer U, et al. Recombinant hirudin (lepirudin) for the improvement of thrombolysis with streptokinase in patients with acute myocardial infarction: results of the HIT-4 trial. J Am Coll Cardiol 1999;34:966–973.

162. Chesebro JH. Direct thrombin inhibition superior to heparin during and after thrombolysis: dose, duration, and drug. Circulation 1997;96:2118–2120.

163. Serruys PW, Herrman J-P, Simon R, et al. A comparison of hirudin with heparin in the prevention of restenosis after coronary angioplasty. Helvetica Investigators. N Engl J Med 1995;333:757–763.

164. Bittl JA, Strony J, Brinker JA, et al. Treatment with bivalirudin (Hirulog) as compared with heparin during coronary angioplasty for unstable or postinfarction angina. Hirulog Angioplasty Study Investigators. N Engl J Med 1995;333:764–769.

165. Fragmin during Instability in Coronary Artery Disease (FRISC) study group. Low-molecular-weight heparin during instability in coronary artery disease. Lancet 1996;347:561–568.

166. Topol EJ, Ferguson JJ, Weisman III, et al. Long-term protection from myocardial ischemic events in a randomized trial of brief integrin β3 blockade with percutaneous intervention. JAMA 1997;278: 479–484.

167. Zoldhelyi P, Jassens S, Lefevre G, Collen D, Van de Werf F, for the GUSTO-2A Investigators. Effects of heparin and hirudin (CGP 39393) on thrombin generation during thrombolysis for acute myocardial infarction. Circulation 1995;92(Suppl. I):I-740.

168. Rao AK, Sun L, Chesebro JH, et al. Distinct effects of recombinant desulfatohirudin CGP 39,393 and heparin on plasma levels of fibrinopeptide A and prothrombin fragment F1.2 in unstable angina: a multicenter trial. Thromb Haemost 1995;73:1306.

169. Maraganore JM, Bourdon P, Jablonski J, Ramachandran KL. Design and characterization of hirulogs: a novel class of bivalent peptide inhibitors of thrombin. Biochemistry 1990;29:7095–7101.

170. Lidón R-M, Théroux P, Lespérance J, et al. A pilot, early angiographic patency study using a direct thrombin inhibitor as adjunctive therapy to streptokinase in acute myocardial infarction. Circulation 1994;89:1567–1572.

171. Théroux P, Pérez-Villa F, Waters D, Lespérance J, Shabani F, Bonan R. Randomized double-blind comparison of two doses of hirulog with heparin as adjunctive therapy to streptokinase to promote early patency of the infarct-related artery in acute myocardial infarction. Circulation 1995;91: 2132–2139.

172. White HD, Aylward PE, Frey MJ, et al. Randomized, double-blind comparison of hirulog versus heparin in patients receiving streptokinase and aspirin for acute myocardial infarction (HERO). Circulation 1997;96:2155–2161.

173. The Hirulog and Early Reperfusion or Occlusion (HERO)-2 Trial Investigators. Thrombin-specific anticoagulation with bivalirudin versus heparin in patients receiving fibrinolytic therapy for acute myocardial infarction: the HERO-2 randomised trial. Lancet 2001;358:1855–1863.

174. Okamoto S, Hijikata A, Kikumoto R, et al. Potent inhibition of thrombin by the newly synthesized arginine derivative No. 805. The importance of stereo-structure of its hydrophobic carboxamide portion. Biochem Biophys Res Commun 1981;101:440–446.

175. Kikumoto R, Tamao Y, Tezuka T, et al. Selective inhibition of thrombin by (2R,4R)-4-methyl-1-[N2-[(3-methyl-1,2,3,4-tetrahydro-8-quinolinyl)sulfonyl]-arginyl]-2-piperidinecarboxylic acid. Biochemistry 1984;23:85–90.

176. Fitzgerald D, Murphy N. Argatroban: a synthetic thrombin inhibitor of low relative molecular mass. Coron Artery Dis 1996;7:455–458.

177. Lunven C, Gauffeny C, Lecoffre C, O'Brien DP, Roome NO, Berry CN. Inhibition by argatroban, a specific thrombin inhibitor, of platelet activation by fibrin clot-associated thrombin. Thromb Haemost 1996;75:154–160.

178. Jang IK, Brown DFM, Giugliano RP, et al. A multicenter, randomized study of argatroban versus heparin as adjunct to tissue plasminogen activator (TPA) in acute myocardial infarction: Myocardial Infarction with Novastan and TPA (MINT) study. J Am Coll Cardiol 1999;33:1879–1885.

179. Hirsh J, Levine MN. Low molecular weight heparin. Blood 1992;79:1–17.

180. Weitz JI. Low-molecular-weight heparins. N Engl J Med 1997;337:688–698.

181. Samama MM, Bara L, Gerotziafas GT. Mechanisms for the antithrombotic activity in man of low molecular weight heparins (LMWHs). Haemostasis 1994;24:105–117.

182. Weitz J. New anticoagulant strategies. Current status and future potential. Drugs 1994;48:485–497.

183. Melandri G, Semprini F, Cervi V, et al. Comparison of efficacy of low molecular weight heparin (parnaparin) with that of unfractionated heparin in the presence of activated platelets in healthy subjects. Am J Cardiol 1993;72:450–454.

184. Warkentin TE, Levine MN, Hirsh J, et al. Heparin-induced thrombocytopenia in patients treated with low-molecular-weight heparin or unfractionated heparin. N Engl J Med 1995;332:1330–1335.

185. Antman EM. The search for replacements for unfractionated heparin. Circulation 2001;103:2310–2314.

186. Wallentin L. ASSENT Plus, 73th Scientific Sessions of the American Heart Association, New Orleans, LA, November 12–15, 2000.

187. Alonso A. AMI-SK, 50th Annual Scientific Sessions of the American College of Cardiology, Orlando, FL, March 2001, 2001.

188. Ross AM, Molhoek P, Lundergan C, et al. Randomized comparison of enoxaparin, a low-molecular-weight heparin, with unfractionated heparin adjunctive to recombinant tissue plasminogen activator thrombolysis and aspirin: second trial of Heparin and Aspirin Reperfusion Therapy (HART II). Circulation 2001;104:648–652.

189. Young JJ, Kereiakes DJ, Grines CL, for the National Investigators Collaborating on Enoxaparin. Low-molecular-weight heparin therapy in percutaneous coronary intervention: the NICE 1 and NICE 4 trials. J Invasive Cardiol 2000;12 (Suppl. E):E14–E18.

190. Herbert JM, Hérault JP, Bernat A, et al. Biochemical and pharmacological properties of SANORG 32701. Comparison with the "synthetic pentasaccharide" (SR 90107/ORG 31540) and standard heparin. Circ Res 1996;79:590–600.

191. Turpie AGG, Gallus AS, Hoek JA, for the Pentasaccharide Investigators. A synthetic pentasaccharide for the prevention of deep-vein thrombosis after total hip replacement. N Engl J Med 2001;344:619–625.

192. Eriksson BI, Bauer KA, Lassen MR, Turpie AG; Steering Committee of the Pentasaccharide in Hip-Fracture Surgery Study. Fondaparinux compared with enoxaparin for the prevention of venous thromboembolism after hip-fracture surgery. N Engl J Med 2001;345:1298–1304.

193. Bauer KA, Eriksson BI, Lassen MR, Turpie AGG, the Steering Committee of the Pentasaccharide in Major Knee Surgery Study. Fondaparinux compared with enoxaparin for the prevention of venous thromboembolism after elective major knee surgery. N Engl J Med 2001;345:1305–1310.

194. Coussement PK, Bassand JP, Convens C, et al. A synthetic factor-Xa inhibitor (ORG31540/SR9017A) as an adjunct to fibrinolysis in acute myocardial infarction. The PENTALYSE study. Eur Heart J 2001;22:1716–1724.

195. Waxman L, Smith DE, Arcuri KE, Vlasuk GP. Tick anticoagulant peptide is a novel inhibitor of blood coagulation factor Xa. Science 1990;248:593–596.

196. Neeper MP, Waxman L, Smith DE, et al. Characterization of recombinant tick anticoagulant peptide: a highly selective inhibitor of blood coagulation factor Xa. J Biol Chem 1990;265:17746–17752.

197. Vlasuk GP. Structural and functional characterization of tick anticoagulant peptide (TAP): a potent and selective inhibitor of blood coagulation factor Xa. Thromb Haemost 1993;70:212–216.

198. Sitko GR, Ramjit DR, Stabilito II, Lehman D, Lynch JJ, Vlasuk GP. Conjunctive enhancement of enzymatic thrombolysis and prevention of thrombotic reocclusion with the selective factor Xa inhibitor, tick anticoagulant peptide: comparison to hirudin and heparin in a canine model of acute coronary artery thrombosis. Circulation 1992;85:805–815.

199. Lynch JJ Jr, Sitko GR, Mellott MJ, et al. Maintenance of canine coronary artery patency following thrombolysis with front loaded plus low dose maintenance conjunctive therapy. A comparison of factor Xa versus thrombin inhibition. Cardiovasc Res 1994;28:78–85.

200. Nicolini FA, Lee P, Malycky JL, et al. Selective inhibition of factor Xa during thrombolytic therapy markedly improves coronary artery patency in a canine model of coronary thrombosis. Blood Coagul Fibrinolysis 1996;7:39–48.
201. Broze GJJ, Warren LA, Novotny WF, Higuchi DA, Girard JJ, Miletich JP. The lipoprotein-associated coagulation inhibitor that inhibits the factor VII-tissue factor complex also inhibits factor Xa: insight into its possible mechanism of action. Blood 1988;71:335–343.
202. Girard TJ, Warren LA, Novotny WF, et al. Functional significance of the Kunitz-type inhibitor domains of lipoprotein-associated coagulation inhibitor. Nature 1989;338:518–520.
203. Lindahl AK. Tissue factor pathway inhibitor: from unknown coagulation inhibitor to major antithrombotic principle. Cardiovasc Res 1997;33:286–291.
204. Broze GJ, Girard TJ, Novotny WF. Regulation of coagulation by a multivalent Kunitz-type inhibitor. Biochemistry 1990;29:7539–7546.
205. Rapaport SI. The extrinsic pathway inhibitor: a regulator of tissue-factor dependent blood coagulation. Thromb Haemost 1991;66:6–15.
206. Haskel EJ, Torr SR, Day KC, et al. Prevention of arterial reocclusion after thrombolysis with recombinant lipoprotein-associated coagulation inhibitor. Circulation 1991;84:821–827.
207. Abendschein DR, Meng YY, Torr-Brown S, Sobel BE. Maintenance of coronary patency after fibrinolysis with tissue factor pathway inhibitor. Circulation 1995;92:944–949.
208. Kaiser B, Fareed J. Recombinant full-length tissue factor pathway inhibitor (TFPI) prevents thrombus formation and rethrombosis after lysis in a rabbit model of jugular vein thrombosis. Thromb Haemost 1996;76.615–620.
209. Lefkovits J, Nicolini FA, Malycky JL, Rao S, Hart C, Topol EJ. Selective inhibition of factor Xa is more effective than tissue factor-factor VIIa complex blockade at facilitating TPA-induced thrombolysis in the canine model. Circulation 1995;92(Suppl. I):I-740.

13

β-Adrenergic Blockers, Calcium Channel Blockers, and Nitrates

Yerem Yeghiazarians, MD and
Peter H. Stone, MD

CONTENTS

INTRODUCTION
β-ADRENERGIC BLOCKING AGENTS
CALCIUM CHANNEL BLOCKING AGENTS
NITRATES
CONCLUSIONS
ACKNOWLEDGMENT
REFERENCES

INTRODUCTION

During the past two decades the pathophysiologic mechanisms considered responsible for the acute coronary syndromes (ST-segment elevation myocardial infarction [MI], ST-segment depression MI, and unstable angina) have been evolving dramatically. In the mid-to-late 1970s, episodic coronary vasospasm was thought to be responsible for the development of unstable angina and acute MI (AMI) *(1,2)*. In the mid-to-late 1980s and mid-1990s, plaque rupture and subsequent thrombus formation were considered paramount *(3,4)*, and coronary vasoconstriction was considered quite inconsequential. The different acute coronary syndromes were perceived simply to represent different points on a single continuum of plaque rupture and thrombus formation: the continuum ranged from a ruptured plaque with little or no thrombus (often asymptomatic), to a ruptured plaque with moderate thrombus leading to only partial coronary occlusion (unstable angina and MI associated with ST-segment depression), to a ruptured plaque with extensive thrombus and complete occlusion of the artery (MI associated with ST-segment elevation). In the mid-to-late 1990s, however, it has been appreciated that this two-component pathophysiologic model of the acute coronary syndromes may be simplistic and inadequate for some patients. Recent evidence from atherectomy samples, for example, indicate that a substantial number of patients with unstable angina, and perhaps a subset of patients with ST-segment deviation MI as well, may be manifesting disease due to a rapid cellular proliferation of the atherosclerotic plaque itself, with little contri-

From: *Contemporary Cardiology: Management of Acute Coronary Syndromes, Second Edition*
Edited by: C. P. Cannon © Humana Press Inc., Totowa, NJ

bution from either major thrombus formation or vasoconstriction *(5,6)*. These three mechanisms (ruptured plaque, thrombus formation, and rapid cellular proliferation) may also be closely interrelated in a given patient, with a substantial contribution from each.

As the understanding of culprit mechanisms has evolved, the targets of therapeutic intervention have likewise evolved. Because the predominant pathophysiology of the acute coronary syndromes relates to an abrupt cessation of coronary blood flow and myocardial oxygen supply, therapeutic strategies have focused on restoration of coronary blood flow: therapies to limit thrombus formation and enhance thrombus dissolution (thrombolytic therapy, thrombin inhibitors, and platelet inhibitors) and therapies to "debulk" the luminal obstruction mechanically (percutaneous transluminal coronary angioplasty, stent, atherectomy, laser, and so on). A critical foundation in the therapeutic approach to patients with the acute coronary syndromes remains, however, the reduction in myocardial oxygen demand since this approach may limit the amount of infarction for a given amount of ischemia, and it may also widen the window of time within which other therapeutic interventions may be effective. The purpose of this chapter is to focus on the role of the conventional antiischemic therapies, i.e., β-adrenergic blockers, calcium channel blockers, and nitrates, in the management of the acute coronary syndromes. Although an effort is made to review the experience with these agents separately for patients who present with ST-segment elevation compared with those who present with ST-segment depression or unstable angina, this distinction often cannot be made from many of the clinical trials conducted before the thrombolytic era. Entry criteria for most of the older studies included persistent ST-segment elevation or depression ±1.0 mm, whereas many of the newer studies include only those with persistent ST-segment elevation if thrombolytic therapy was administered.

β-ADRENERGIC BLOCKING AGENTS

Mechanisms of Action

β-Blockers function as competitive antagonists to the β-adrenergic receptors on cell membranes. Selective β-1 antagonists act at receptor sites found primarily in the myocardium, inhibiting catecholamine-mediated increases in cardiac contractility and nodal conduction rates. β-2 receptors are found mainly in vascular and bronchial smooth muscle; inhibition at these receptor sites can lead to vasoconstriction and bronchospasm. These β-blockers exert their beneficial effect in the acute coronary syndromes by preventing catecholamine-mediated β-1 activation, leading to decreased contractility and heart rate, thereby improving the oxygen supply/demand balance. These drugs also exert an antiarrhythmic effect, as evidenced by an increase in the threshold for ventricular fibrillation in animals and a reduction in complex ventricular arrhythmias in humans *(7–9)*. Finally, β-blockers may prevent plaque rupture by reducing the mechanical stresses imposed on the plaque *(10)*.

Use in ST-Segment Elevation MI

The β-blockers were among the first therapeutic interventions designed to limit the size of an AMI. In most of these studies, all patients with AMI were included together regardless of the direction of the ST-segment deviation on admission. Norris and colleagues in New Zealand *(11,12)* demonstrated in 1978 that early administration of β-blockers decreased the size of AMI measured enzymatically (as a function of creatine-kinase

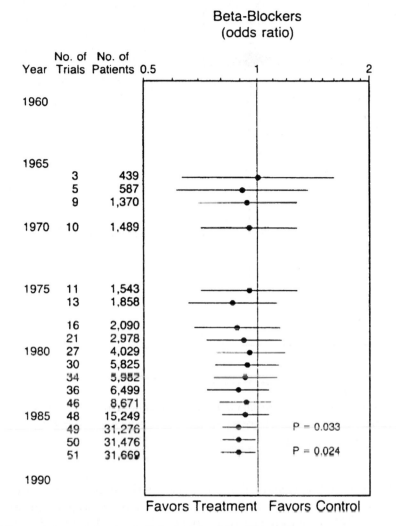

Fig. 1. Results of 51 randomized clinical trials of the effects of oral or iv followed by oral β-blockers for the treatment of AMI (odds ratios and 95% CI for effect of treatment on mortality). Reproduced with permission from ref. *60*.

enzyme release) or by reduction of ST-segment elevation. Some of the early studies of β-blockers to reduce infarct size *(13)* were limited by the lack of appreciation that the window of time within which myocardium may be salvaged was in the range of 6–12 h. In the Multicenter Investigation of the Limitation of Infarct Size (MILIS) study, for example, β-blockers were administered up to 24 h after onset of chest pain *(13)*.

More recent studies using a more appropriate design to administer the β-blocker within an appropriate time window have definitively demonstrated a benefit associated with β-blocker therapy (Fig. 1) *(14,15)*. In the largest trial, the First International Study of Infarct Survival (ISIS-1) *(16)*, over 16,000 patients with suspected MI were treated with immediate intravenous (iv) atenolol, 5–10 mg, within 12 h of the onset of symptoms, followed by 100 mg daily. The mortality difference between those receiving atenolol and the controls was evident by the end of d 1; the 7-d mortality was reduced

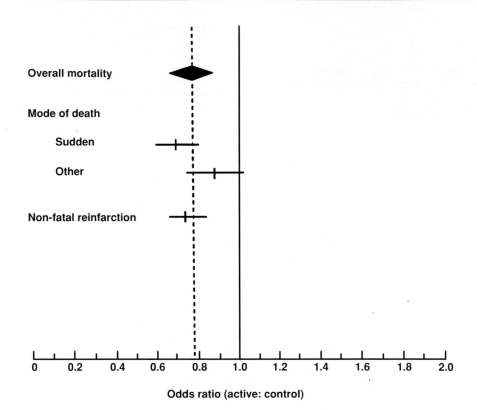

Fig. 2. Sudden death, other death, and nonfatal reinfarction in long-term β-blocker trials that reported these end points separately (odds ratios [active/control], together with approximate 95% confidence ranges). See original article for citation of specific trials. Reproduced with permission from ref. *14*.

from 4.3 to 3.7% ($p < 0.02$). Meta-analyses from 27 randomized trials, totaling about 27,000 patients, indicate that early iv (followed by oral) β-blockers reduced mortality by 13% in the first week (95% confidence interval [CI]:-2–25; $p < 0.02$) *(14,17)*. The mortality reduction was greatest in the first 2 d (about 25%), supporting the value of early initiation of β-blockade *(17)*. Early treatment also reduced nonfatal reinfarction by about 19% (95% CI -5 to -33; $p < 0.01$) and nonfatal cardiac arrest by about 16% (95% CI:-2–30; $p < 0.02$). Composite end points of death, nonfatal reinfarction, and nonfatal arrest were reduced by 16% ($p < 0.001$) *(17)*. Data from the ISIS-1 trial suggest that the reduction in mortality is largely due to prevention of cardiac rupture and ventricular fibrillation *(16)*. Detailed analyses of the results based on various subgroups (initial heart rate, risk category, presence or absence of ventricular arrhythmia, and so on) indicated a benefit in all groups.

When β-blockers are used in conjunction with thrombolytic therapy, they provide incremental benefit, particularly if they can be administered early after the onset of infarct symptoms. In the Thrombolysis in Myocardial Infarction (TIMI)-II trial *(18)*, patients with persisting ST-segment elevation, who were randomized to receive early metoprolol (15 mg iv, followed by oral metoprolol 50 mg twice daily (bid) for 1 d and then 100 mg bid thereafter) in addition to iv alteplase, experienced a 49% lower incidence of subsequent nonfatal reinfarction ($p = 0.02$) and a 27% lower incidence of

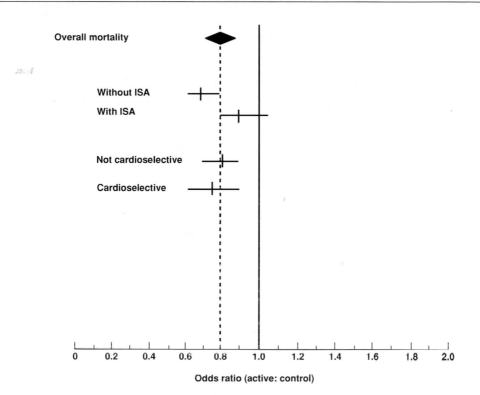

Fig. 3. Mortality in long-term β-blocker trials, by ancillary properties of agent tested (odds ratios [active/control], together with approximate 95% CI. See original article for citation of specific trials. Reproduced with permission from ref. *14*.

recurrent ischemia ($p - 0.005$) compared to those patients randomized to receive metoprolol only orally, beginning 6 d after the acute event. Those patients who were treated within 2 h of symptom onset had the greatest reduction of the composite end point of death or reinfarction compared to those treated to only late oral metoprolol.

A number of studies have classified the mechanism of death as sudden or nonsudden, based on the duration of time from the onset of symptoms to actual death. Sudden death is variably defined as "instantaneous" to "within 2 h of symptoms" and is presumably due to arrhythmias or cardiac rupture; nonsudden deaths are those occurring later after the onset of symptoms, presumably owing to nonarrhythmic causes, such as reinfarction, and may include a few noncardiac deaths. Tabulation of the results from the available studies indicates a highly significant reduction of approx 30% in the incidence of sudden death and a nonsignificant reduction of only about 12% in the incidence of nonsudden death (Fig. 2) *(14)*. The fact that β-blockers were particularly effective in reducing both sudden death and mortality among patients with complex ventricular ectopy at baseline *(19)* suggests that β-blockers exert their beneficial effect primarily by reducing the frequency and severity of arrhythmias *(20)*.

It is striking that the long-term mortality benefits of the β-blockers following an index MI (i.e., secondary prevention) extend to most members of this class of agents *(14)*. There does not seem to be a significant difference agents with or without cardioselectivity (Fig. 3). However, the presence of intrinsic sympathomimetic activity reduced the benefit to

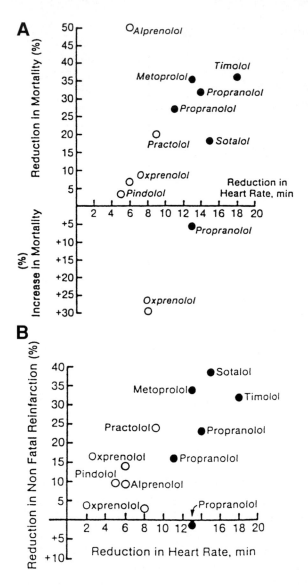

Fig. 4. (A) Relation between reduction in heart rate (difference between treatment groups) and percentage of reduction in mortality in large, prospective, double-blind trials with β-blockers. Open circles, β-blockers with intrinsic sympathomimetic activity: $r = 0.6$; $p < 0.05$. See original article for citation of specific trials. Reproduced with permission from ref. *21*. **(B)** Relation between reduction in heart rate and percentage of reduction in recurrent nonfatal infarctions in large, prospective, double-blind trials with β-blockers. Open circles, β-blockers with intrinsic sympathomimetic activity; $r = 0.59$; $p < 0.05$. See original article for citation of specific trials. Reproduced with permission from ref. *21*.

nonsignificance (odds ratio 0.90; 95% CI: 0.77–1.05) (Fig. 3) *(14)*. Reduction in heart rate appears to be a critical feature associated with the protective effect of β-blockers. Indeed, there is a significant relationship between the magnitude of heart rate reduction observed on the active agent and the magnitude of reduction in mortality (Fig. 4A) *(21)*.

Many of the large-scale clinical trials have also reported the effects of long-term β-blocker use on nonfatal reinfarction. Results from pooled analyses indicate that β-blocker use is associated with an odds ratio of 0.74 (95% CI: 0.66–0.83; $p < 0.001$). As observed for mortality, there is also a significant relationship between the magnitude of reduction in heart rate and the reduction in nonfatal recurrent MI ($r = 0.54$; $p < 0.05$) (Fig. 4B) (21). This observed benefit of reducing nonfatal reinfarction is in addition to the benefit on mortality.

The magnitude of benefit from long-term use of a β-blocker is also dependent on the patient's risk of mortality associated with their index MI (Table 1). Post hoc analyses of data from the Beta Blocker Heart Attack Trial (BHAT) (22) indicate that those MI patients without electrical or mechanical complications experienced only a 6% relative benefit from the use of propranolol. MI patients with electrical complications experienced a 52% relative benefit, those with mechanical complications experienced a 38% relative benefit, and those with both mechanical and electrical complications experienced a 25% relative benefit. Considering the low cost of routine β-blocker use and its substantial benefit, such therapy has a relatively favorable cost-effectiveness ratio: an estimated cost of therapy per year of life saved would be $13,000 in low-risk patients, $3600 in medium-risk patients, and $2400 in high-risk patients (23).

The benefits from routine β-blocker use seem to persist as long as the active agent is continued (24–26). It is, therefore, most appropriate after MI to maintain β-blocker therapy indefinitely in patients who can tolerate it (27). The benefits of a β-blocker in long-term secondary prevention appear to extend to most patient subgroups. The Beta-Blocker Pooling Project (28) combined the results of nine large trials and found that although high-risk patients were most likely to benefit from β-blocker therapy, lower-risk patients also benefited, even though the absolute and relative benefits were small. The experience using β-blockers in the elderly is limited, but available data indicate that the benefit may even be greater in patients older than 50–60 yr than in younger patients. Benefit appeared to be similar in both men and women.

The recently published CAPRICORN trial (29) was a multicenter double-blind randomized controlled trial of 1959 patients with a definite MI 3–21 d prior to enrollment with a left ventricular (LV) ejection fraction of 40% or less, who were receiving concurrent treatment with an angiotensin-converting enzyme (ACE)-inhibitor. Patients were randomly assigned to receive carvedilol or placebo with an upward titration of the dose to a maximum of 25 mg bid. The primary end point was all-cause mortality and hospital admission. After a mean follow-up of 1.3 yr, all-cause mortality was lower in the carvedilol than in the placebo group (12 vs 15%, $p = 0.03$), but there was no significant difference in the co-primary end points of death and hospitalization. In addition, the patients treated with the β-blocker had lower rates of cardiovascular mortality (11 vs 14%, $p = 0.024$) and nonfatal myocardial infarctions (3 vs 6%, $p = 0.014$). The benefits of long-term therapy with carvedilol in post-MI patients complicated by LV dysfunction were in addition to the effects of ACE-inhibitors, which were prescribed in up to 98% of the enrolled patients.

Given the beneficial results of other β-blocker trials in the post-MI setting, the CAPRICORN trial might be generalized to other β-blockers in providing yet another strong evidence that, unless contraindicated, all post-MI patients should be maintained on long-term β-blocker therapy in addition to other proven therapies, such as ACE inhibitors. The side effects from prolonged β-blocker use have generally been minor and are similar to those seen with placebo (30). In studies that report it, the incidence of heart failure is slightly but significantly higher in patients receiving β-blocker (5.9%) than in

Table 1
All-Cause Mortality by Risk and Treatment Groups: β-Blocker Heart Attack Trial[a]

Risk group	Placebo group		Propranolol group				
	No. of patients	Mortality rate (%)	No. of patients	Mortality rate (%)	Absolute efficacy (100)	Relative efficacy (%)	Adjusted relative efficacy (%)
No electrical or mechanical complications	1079	6.6	1047	6.2	0.4	6	-4
Electrical complications only	423	10.9	443	5.2	5.7	-52	-57
Mechanical complications only	202	16.8	201	10.4	6.4	-38	-43
Both electrical and mechanical complications	217	17.1	225	12.9	4.2	-25	-30

[a]Average length of follow-up was 25 mo. Data adjusted for 13 variables predictive of mortality. Reproduced with permission from ref. 20.

patients receiving placebo (5.4%) (pooled odds ratio 1.16; 95% CI: 1.01–1.34) *(14)*. However, even patients with a history of mild or moderate congestive heart failure (CHF) actually experienced greater benefit from β-blockade than did patients without that condition *(20)*.

Use in Patients with Unstable Angina and ST-Segment Depression MI

Many of the studies evaluating the efficacy of β-blockers for AMI were conducted before the era of thrombolytic therapy, and patients were included with either ST-segment elevation or depression on their presenting electrocardiogram (ECG). Since treatment was administered as early as possible after the onset of symptoms, criteria were not available to identify who would evolve a Q wave MI, a non-Q wave MI, or even unstable angina. Most of the experience previously discussed, therefore, concerning patients with "ST-segment elevation MI" actually represents a heterogeneous mixture of "acute coronary syndromes" and is applicable to patients with non-Q wave MI and those with unstable angina as well.

Only one placebo-controlled trial *(31)* specifically examined the effectiveness of β-blockers in unstable angina. In this study, patients not on prior β-blocking therapy were randomized to receive metoprolol, nifedipine, or both. Patients already on β-blockers were randomized to either nifedipine or placebo. The use of β-blockers alone was associated with a 25% reduction in recurrent ischemia or MI at 48 h. This reduction was not statistically significant. However, the addition of nifedipine to existing β-blockade was associated with a 20% reduction in short-term cardiac end points.

Other trials of β-blocker use in unstable angina have been small and uncontrolled *(32–34)*. A meta-analysis of these trials *(35)* showed a 13% reduction in progression from unstable angina to MI, but no significant reduction in mortality. However, a number of randomized trials have shown a clear mortality benefit from β-blockers in other coronary syndromes, including acute MI, stable angina, and postinfarction angina, as discussed above.

Thus, β-blockers remain a cornerstone of the acute treatment of MI. Treatment is generally initiated intravenously, especially if it can be administered within 12 h of symptom onset, followed by continuation using oral formulations. The recent American College of Cardiology/American Heart Association (ACC/AHA) guidelines for the management of patients with AMI are noted in Tables 2 and 3 *(15)*. β-Blockers are consistently useful for secondary prevention following MI *(27)* and should be maintained indefinitely.

CALCIUM CHANNEL BLOCKING AGENTS

Mechanisms of Action

Calcium channel blocking agents inhibit the entry of calcium into vascular smooth muscle cells and myocardial cells during the action potential, which triggers the contractile process. This calcium entry blockade leads to direct effects of vasodilation, negative inotropy, negative chronotropy (decreased heart rate), and negative dromotropy (decreased arteriovenous [AV]-nodal conduction) *(36)*. The systemic vasodilation leads to reflex sympathetic activation, which, in turn, promotes an increase in AV-nodal conductions.

Table 2
Recommendations for the Use of β-Blocker Therapy Administered Early During Acute Myocardial Infarction

Conditions for which there is evidence that treatment is beneficial, useful, and effective.
  Patients without a contraindication to β-adrenoceptor blocker therapy who can be treated within 12 h of onset of infarction, irrespective of administration of concomitant thrombolytic therapy.
  Patients with continuing or recurrent ischemic pain.
  Patients with tachyarrhythmias, such as atrial fibrillation with a rapid ventricular response.
Conditions for which evidence is less well established.
  Non-Q wave MI.
Conditions for which evidence suggests treatment is not useful and may be harmful.
  Patients with moderate or severe left ventricular failure or other contraindications to β-adrenoceptor blocker therapy.

Data from ref. *15*.

Table 3
Recommendations for Long-Term Adminstration of β-Blockers (i.e., Secondary Prevention)

Conditions for which therapy is beneficial, useful, and effective.
  All but low-risk patients without a clear contraindication to β-adrenoceptor blocker therapy; treatment should begin within a few days of the event (if not initiated acutely) and continue indefinitely.
Conditions for which beneficial effects are less well established but weight of evidence favors their use.
  Low risk patients without a clear contraindication to β-adrenoceptor blocker therapy.
Conditions for which evidence suggests treatment is not useful and may be harmful.
  Patients with a contraindication to β-adrenoceptor blocker therapy.

Data from ref. *15*.

The net clinical effects of the calcium channel blockers will be a composite of their direct effects and their reflex-mediated indirect effects. The two major categories of calcium channel blockers, the dihydropyridines (including nifedipine, amlodipine, and nicardipine) and the nondihydropyridines (including diltiazem and verapamil) differ fundamentally: the dihydropyridines have greater vascular selectivity, leading to more peripheral vasodilation, and the potential for increased reflex sympathetic activation, whereas the nondihydropyridines have greater myocardial selectivity with a greater negative inotropic, chronotropic, and dromotropic effect. Both types of calcium channel blockers prevent coronary vasoconstriction and lower blood pressure. Thus, the principal anti-ischemic effects of the calcium blockers are to reduce myocardial oxygen demand by lowering blood pressure (dihydropyridines and nondihydropyridines) and lowering contractility and heart rate (nondihydropyridines only), as well as preventing coronary vasoconstriction if it is present. It should be noted that if reflex sympathetic activation predominates, as may be observed with use of immediate-release dihydropyridines, then the increase in contractility and heart rate may lead to an exacerbation of oxygen supply/demand imbalance. The calcium channel blockers may also exert a fun-

Myocardial infarction

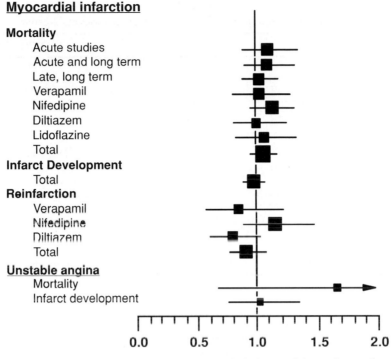

Mortality
    Acute studies
    Acute and long term
    Late, long term
    Verapamil
    Nifedipine
    Diltiazem
    Lidoflazine
    Total
Infarct Development
    Total
Reinfarction
    Verapamil
    Nifedipine
    Diltiazem
    Total
Unstable angina
    Mortality
    Infarct development

0.0   0.5   1.0   1.5   2.0

Typical odds ratio (95% confidence Interval)

Fig. 5. Typical odds of death, infarct development, and reinfarction by disease, type of trials, and drug. Areas of squares are proportional to numbers of patients. *Bars,* 95% confidence intervals. *Portions to left of vertical line (corresponding to odds ratio <1) indicate risk with treatment, portions to right of* vertical line indicate increased risk with treatment. Upper 95% confidence limit for effect on mortality in unstable angina = 6.2. Note that treatment does not seem to reduce risk of any event. See original article for citation of specific trials. Reproduced with permission from ref. *37.*

damental cardioprotective effect of limiting calcium influx during ischemia, thereby limiting the amount of necrosis that ensues from a given ischemic result *(36).*

Use of Calcium Channel Blockers in Patients with MI

Dihydropyridine Calcium Blockers (Nifedipine and Nicardipine)

Early studies investigated the use of calcium channel blockers, particularly the dihydropyridines, for the early treatment of MI, but they were not found to be useful (Fig. 5) *(37).* Patients were generally included regardless of the direction of ST-segment deviation on presentation. The dihydropyridines were studied in particular because they could be safely combined with β-adrenergic blockers without the concern for excessive reduction in myocardial contractility or bradycardia. The available formulation of dihydropyridines in this early era consisted of short-acting nifedipine, and this agent was found to be actually detrimental when used without a β-blocker to blunt the reflex sympathetic activity *(38–42).* When combined with a β-blocker, nifedipine was significantly beneficial in reducing symptomatic manifestations of AMI *(38).* Many of the studies *(17,26,37,43)* may not be methodologically comparable because the doses tested varied,

Table 4
Secondary Prevention Trials of Calcium Channel Blocking Agents[a]

Event and agent	Active	Control	Odds ratio (CI)
Mortality			
Dihydropyridine	379/5137	335/5135	1.16 (0.99–1.35)
Verapamil	244/2644	266/2649	0.91 (0.76–1.10)
Diltiazem	180/1574	181/1577	0.99 (0.80–1.24)
Reinfarction			
Dihydropyridine	138/3838	119/3871	1.19 (0.92–1.53)
Verapamil	138/2606	171/2624	0.80 (0.63–1.01)
Diltiazem	113/1557	142/1560	0.79 (0.61–1.02)

[a]Data are number of events/number of subjects.

and both the underlying disease manifestation and the timing from onset of the acute ischemic manifestation to initiation of the study drug may have been different.

Nevertheless, nifedipine has been uniformly unsuccessful in reducing either mortality or the rate of reinfarction (Fig. 5). A recent update of a pooled analysis (43) of stable coronary patients in a coronary regression trial with either nifedipine (44) or nicardipine (45) showed a trend toward an increase in mortality (7.4 vs 6.5%; odds ratio 1.16; 95% CI: 0.99–1.35; $p = 0.07$) and a nonsignificant increase in reinfarction (3.5 vs 3.1%; odds ratio 1.19; 95% CI: 0.92–1.53) (Table 4).

Nondihydropyridine Calcium Blockers (Verapamil and Diltiazem)

The calcium channel blockers verapamil and diltiazem can be considered together because their net pharmacologic effect is that of slowing the heart rate and, in some instances, reducing myocardial contractility (36), thereby reducing myocardial oxygen demand. These studies are closer to more conventional secondary prevention design, since patients in these studies were treated with the active agent after their index MI was stabilized. A recent pooled analysis by Yusuf and colleagues (43) indicated that verapamil and diltiazem had no effect on mortality following AMI, but that they exerted a significant effect on reducing the rate of reinfarction (6.0 vs 7.5%; odds ratio 0.79; 95% CI: 0.67–0.94; $p < 0.01$) (Table 4). The effect seems similar for both agents.

Although the overall results of trials with verapamil showed no mortality benefits, subgroup analysis showed that immediate-release verapamil initiated several d after AMI in patients who were not candidates for a β-blocking agent may be useful in reducing the incidence of the composite end point of reinfarction and death, provided LV function is well preserved with no clinical evidence of heart failure. In a placebo-controlled trial of almost 1800 patients, verapamil 360 mg/d started in the second wk after AMI and continued for a mean of 16 mo had no effect on mortality compared to the control group, but reduced major event rates (death or reinfarction) from 21.6% in the control group to 18.0% in the active treatment group ($p = 0.03$) (46). In patients without heart failure in the coronary care unit, however, verapamil significantly reduced both mortality (from 11.8% in the control group to 7.7% in the active treatment group; $p = 0.02$) and major events (from 19.7% in the control group to 14.6% in the active treatment group; $p = 0.01$), but there was no effect on either end point among patients who experienced CHF in the coronary care unit *(46)*. Verapamil is detrimental to patients with heart failure or bradyarrhythmias during the first 24–48 h after AMI *(15,47,48)*.

Data from the Multicenter Diltiazem Postinfarction Trial (MDPIT) and the Diltiazem Reinfarction Study (DRS) *(49,50)* suggest that patients with non-Q wave MI or those with Q wave infarction, preserved LV function, and no evidence of heart failure may also benefit from treatment with immediate-release diltiazem. In the DRS, 576 patients with non-Q wave MI were treated with either diltiazem (90 mg every 6 h) or placebo initiated 24–72 h after the onset of MI and continued for 14 d *(50)*. There was no difference in mortality, but diltiazem reduced the rate of reinfarction from 9.3% in the control group to 5.2% ($p < 0.03$) and the rate of refractory postinfarction angina from 6.9% in the control group to 3.5% ($p = 0.03$). In the MDPIT, 2466 patients with a Q wave or non-Q wave MI were treated with either diltiazem (240 mg/d) or placebo 3–15 d after the MI onset and followed for a mean of 25 mo. There was no difference in mortality in the two treatment groups *(49)*. A significant bidirectional interaction was observed, however, between diltiazem and the presence of pulmonary congestion during the index MI (Fig. 6). In the 1909 patients without pulmonary congestion, diltiazem was associated with a significant reduction in cardiac events at 1 yr from 11% in the control group to 8%, whereas in the 490 patients with pulmonary congestion, diltiazem increased the cardiac event rate from 18% in the control group to 26%. A similar pattern was observed with respect to the ejection fraction, which was dichotomized at 40% *(49)*. The results of MDPIT may be confounded by the fact that 53 and 55% of placebo- and diltiazem-treated patients, respectively, received concomitant β-blocker therapy. Also, both the MDPIT and DRS projects were conducted in an era when the use of aspirin was not as prevalent as it is today, raising further uncertainty about the relevance of their findings for contemporary management of AMI *(15)*. Of particular clinical importance is the detrimental mortality effect of diltiazem in patients with LV dysfunction.

It should be emphasized that there have not been studies comparing the efficacy of verapamil or diltiazem with that of a β-blocker. β-Blockers more consistently reduce both mortality and reinfarction and should be recommended for those patients who can tolerate such medication. Verapamil or diltiazem may be a reasonable alternative for those patients who cannot tolerate a β-blocker, but who can tolerate one of the calcium blockers, for example, patients with severe chronic obstructive pulmonary disease or asthma. It should be noted, however, that many patients who cannot tolerate a β-blocker, because of concern of excessive bradycardia or CHF, may experience similar complications from diltiazem or verapamil.

Use of Calcium Blockers in Patients with Unstable Angina

Several small randomized trials have examined the use of nifedipine and diltiazem in unstable angina. A meta-analysis of these trials *(37)* showed no reduction in MI or death rates in patients given calcium antagonists (110 of 561 patients [20%] treated with calcium antagonists developed MI, compared to 104 of 548 [19%] in the control group; death rates were 2.4 and 1.6% for the calcium antagonist and control groups, respectively) (Fig. 5). The largest trial, the Holland University Nifedipine/Metoprolol Trial (HINT) *(31)* described above, was discontinued prematurely because of a trend toward more nonfatal MIs in patients receiving nifedipine alone. When combined with a β-blocking agent, however, patients receiving nifedipine had a decreased rate of MI and death compared with placebo.

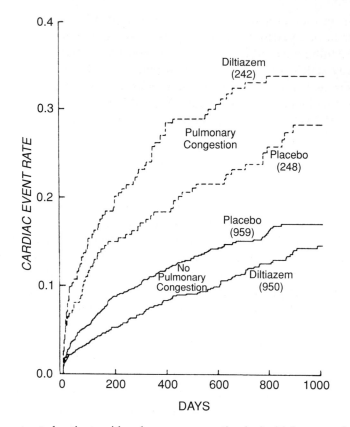

Fig. 6. Diltiazem-treated patients with pulmonary congestion had a higher rate of cardiac events than patients receiving placebo; diltiazem-treated patients without pulmonary congestion had a lower rate of cardiac events than patients receiving placebo. The values in parentheses are numbers of patients.

Several studies, however, have shown symptomatic benefit from calcium antagonists *(50–52)*. Thus, evidence for calcium channel blockers in unstable angina does not suggest any beneficial effect on mortality or progression of MI, but does support their use for relief of refractory symptoms. Because of randomized trials showing an increased risk of death in patients treated with calcium channel blockers in the setting of AMI, particularly in patients with LV dysfunction *(49)*, calcium antagonists should be used only in patients with refractory symptoms despite the use of nitrates and β-blockers.

Calcium blocking agents have also been used successfully to reduce symptoms and possibly decrease morbidity in patients with vasospastic (also known as Prinzmetal's or variant) angina *(53–56)*. Although patients with either Prinzmetal's variant angina or unstable angina may present with rest angina, patients with Prinzmetal's angina are characterized by preservation of exercise capacity without angina. By contrast, patients with unstable angina, who usually have severe epicardial coronary plaques that reduce blood flow, typically have very limiting exertional angina, as well as rest angina. In several small controlled and uncontrolled trials, a significant reduction in angina frequency was reported with the use of calcium antagonists *(53–55)*. There are no data to suggest superior efficacy of any one agent in particular. In one very small trial of patients with refrac-

Table 5

Recommendations for the Use of Calcium Blocker Therapy for the Acute Coronary Syndromes[a]

Conditions for which there is evidence that treatment is beneficial, useful, and effective.

Verapamil or diltiazem may be given to patients in whom β-adrenoceptor blockers are ineffective or contraindicated (i.e., bronchospastic disease) for relief of ongoing ischemia or control of a rapid ventricular response with atrial fibrillation after AMI in the absence of CHF, LV dysfunction, or AV block.

Conditions for which beneficial effects are less well established.

In non-ST-elevation infarction, diltiazem may be given to patients without LV dysfunction, pulmonary congestion, or CHF; it may be added to standard therapy after the first 24 h and continues for 1 yr.

Conditions for which evidence suggests treatment is not useful and may be harmful.

Nefedipine (short-acting) is generally contraindicated in routine treatment of AMI because of its negative inotropic effects and the reflex sympathetic activation, tachycardia, and hypotension associated with its use.

Diltiazem and verapamil are contraindicated in patients with AMI and associated LV dysfunction or CHF.

[a]Abbreviations: AMI, acute myocardial infarction; CHF, congestive heart failure; LV, left ventricular. Data from ref. *15*.

tory angina, the combination of diltiazem and nifedipine was more effective than either agent alone *(55)*, although intolerable side effects precluded the use of both drugs in several of these patients. Because vasospastic angina is due to transient coronary arterial spasm rather than plaque rupture and thrombus, there is no role for antithrombotic or antiplatelet agents. Medical therapy, with an emphasis on nitrates and calcium antagonists titrated to symptom relief, is the mainstay of treatment. However, because most patients with vasospastic angina have some degree of underlying epicardial coronary artery disease, they may occasionally present with AMI due to plaque rupture. These patients should be managed according to standard practice.

The most recent ACC/AHA guidelines concerning use of the calcium channel blockers are shown in Table 5 *(15)*.

NITRATES

Mechanisms of Action

Nitroglycerin remains central to the treatment of coronary artery disease. The clinical effects of nitrates are mediated through several distinct mechanisms, including the following:

1. Dilation of large coronary arteries and arterioles with redistribution to blood flow from epicardial to endocardial regions. Nitroglycerin provides an exogenous source of nitric oxide in vascular endothelium, facilitating coronary vasodilation even when damaged endothelium is unable to generate endogenous nitric oxide production due to coronary artery disease. It is important to emphasize that these coronary vasomotor effects may either increase or decrease collateral flow.

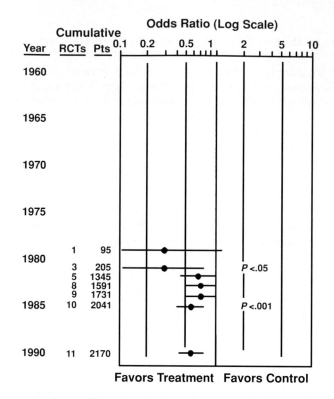

Fig. 7. Cumulative meta-analyses of the use of iv nitroglycerin for AMI. Reproduced with permission from ref. *60.*

2. Peripheral venodilation leads to an increase in venous capacitance and a substantial decrease in preload, thus reducing myocardial oxygen consumption (MVO_2). Nitrates are consequently of particular value in treating patients with LV dysfunction and CHF.
3. Peripheral arterial dilation, typically of a modest degree, may decrease afterload.

In addition, nitrates have been shown to relieve dynamic coronary constriction, including that induced by exercise. Nitrates may also have an inhibitory effect on platelet aggregation in patients with unstable angina *(57)*, although the clinical significance of this finding is unclear.

Use of Nitrates in Patients with ST-Segment Elevation MI

Early studies demonstrated that nitrates may be of value to reduce infarct size and improve regional myocardial function when administered early in the course of AMI (Fig. 7) *(58–60)*. Judgutt et al. *(59)*, for example, found that IV nitroglycerin administered to patients with AMI preserved LV function, particularly in patients with an anterior MI, and led to improved survival. A meta-analysis of these earlier studies prior to the acute reperfusion era indicated that nitrates reduced the odds of death after AMI by 35% (95% CI: 28–49; $p < 0.001$) *(61)*. However, it should also be noted that use of nitroprusside was actually found in early studies to exacerbate MI by causing a coronary steal phenomenon. Routine use of nitroprusside to limit infarct size has led to conflicting results (62–64), and its use cannot be recommended.

The use of nitrate therapy was investigated in the context of routine use of thrombolytic therapy and aspirin with short-term mortality as the primary end point in two recently completed large trials (15). The Gruppo Italiano per lo Studio della Sopravvivenza nell'Infarto Miocardico (GISSI)-3 trial (65) randomly assigned 19,394 patients to a 24-h infusion of nitroglycerin (beginning within 24 h of onset of pain), followed by topical nitroglycerin (10 mg daily) for 6 wk (with patch removed at bedtime, allowing a 10-h nitrate-free interval to avoid tolerance), or control. Approximately 50% of patients in the control group received nitrates on the first d or two at the discretion of their physician. There was an insignificant reduction in mortality at 6 wk in the group randomly assigned to nitrate therapy alone, compared with the control group (6.52 vs 6.92%, respectively). GISSI-3 evaluated lisinopril in a similar fashion; 6-wk mortality was reduced slightly. At both 6-wk and 6-mo follow-up, the combined use of lisinopril and nitrates led to a greater reduction in mortality when compared with the group that received no nitrate therapy or lisinopril alone. The other large trial (66), compared 28-d treatment of controlled-release oral isosorbide mononitrate with placebo control (as well as iv magnesium sulfate vs control and the angiotensin-converting enzyme inhibitor captopril vs placebo control) in a 2-by-2-by-2 factorial design of 58,050 patients with suspected MI. Nitrate therapy in ISIS-4 was associated with a small nonsignificant reduction in 35-d mortality compared with the control group (7.34 vs 7.54%) in the overall comparison. All subgroups examined, including those not receiving short-term nonstudy IV or oral nitrates at entry, failed to demonstrate a significant mortality benefit with nitrate use. In both GISSI-3 and ISIS-4, the power to detect potential beneficial effects of routine nitrate therapy was reduced by the extensive early use (>50%) of nontrial nitrate in the control subjects.

A review of evidence from all pertinent randomized clinical trials does not support routine use of long-term nitrate therapy in patients with uncomplicated AMI (15). However, it is reasonable to use IV nitroglycerin for the first 24–48 h in patients with AMI and recurrent ischemia, CHF, or management of hypertension. It should be continued orally or topically in patients with CHF and large transmural MIs as well. IV administration is recommended in the early stage of AMI, because of its onset of action, ease of titration, and opportunity for prompt termination in the event of side effects (Table 6).

These agents remain of major value in the treatment of recurrent angina or hypertension associated with AMI.

Use of Nitrates in Patients with Unstable Angina

Despite a clear benefit when applied in patients with chronic coronary artery disease or ischemic left heart failure, there are no data from randomized placebo-controlled trials that demonstrate an effect of nitrates with respect to symptom relief or reduction in morbid events in patients with unstable angina. In patients receiving continuous nitrates, tachyphylaxis may be seen as early as 24–48 h after initiation. This problem can be managed by increasing the dose as needed until symptom relief is achieved. Once a patient has been pain-free for 24 h, it is advisable to switch to a topical or oral form of nitrate therapy, with a nitrate-free interval of 6–8 h/d.

Table 6
Recommendations for the Use of Nitrate Preparations for Acute Coronary Syndromes[a]

Intravenous nitroglycerin may be useful for the first 24–48 h in patients with AMI and recurrent ischemia, CHF or management of hypertension.

It should be continued orally or topically in patients with CHF and large transmural MI.

Routine use of long-term nitrate therapy is not recommended in patients with uncomplicated AMI.

[a]Abbreviations: MI, myocardial infarction; CHF, congestive heart failure. Data from ref. *15*.

CONCLUSIONS

- β-Adrenergic blockers are effective in reducing cardiac events in the acute coronary syndromes by lowering heart rate and contractility (i.e., myocardial oxygen demand).
- The benefit of β-blockers in secondary prevention supports indefinite use of these agents following AMI.
- β-Blockers are most effective in improving outcome in patients whose AMI is complicated by electrical or hemodynamic disturbances.
- Calcium channel blockers reduce myocardial oxygen demand by lowering blood pressure dihydropyridines and nondihydropyridines) and lowering contractility and heart rate (nondihydropyridines), as well as preventing coronary vasoconstriction, if it is present.
- Dihydropyridines should not be used without concomitant treatment with a β-blocker, because reflex-mediated increases in sympathetic activation may exacerbate the myocardial supply/demand balance.
- Nondihydropyridines (verapamil or diltiazem) may be given to patients in whom β-blockers are ineffective or contraindicated in the absence of CHF, LV dysfunction, or AV block. IV nitroglycerin may be useful for the first 24–48 h in patients with AMI and recurrent ischemia, CHF, or management of hypertension.
- Routine use of long-term nitrates is not recommended in patients with uncomplicated AMI. These agents can be used in patients with AMI and recurrent ischemia, CHF or for the management of acute hypertension.

REFERENCES

1. Maseri A, Severi S, DeNes M, et al. "Variant" angina: one aspect of a continuous spectrum of vasospastic myocardial ischemia. Pathogenic mechanisms, estimate incidence, clinical and coronarographic findings in 138 patients. Am J Cardiol 1978;42:1019–1035.
2. Oliva PB, Potts DE, Pluss RC. Coronary arterial spasm in Prinzmetal angina. Documentation by coronary arteriography. N Engl J Med 1973;232:745–751.
3. Davies MJ, Thomas AC. Plaque fissuring: the cause of acute myocardial infarction, sudden death, and crescendo angina. Br Heart J 1985;53:363–373.
4. Davies MJ. A macro and micro view of coronary vascular insult in ischemic heart disease. Circulation 1990;82:(Suppl. II):II-38–46.

5. Flugelman MY, Virmani R, Correa R, et al. Smooth muscle cell abundance and fibroblast growth factors in coronary lesions of patients with nonfatal unstable angina. Circulation 1993;88:2493–2500.

6. Arbustini E, DeServi S, Bramucci E, et al. Comparison of coronary lesions obtained by directional coronary atherectomy in unstable angina, stable angina, and restenosis after either atherectomy or angioplasty. Am J Cardiol 1995;75:675–682.

7. Rossi PRF, Yusuf S, Ramsdale D, et al. Reduction of ventricular arrhythmias by early intravenous atenolol in suspected AMI. BMJ 1983;286:506–510.

8. Yusuf S, Sleight P, Rossi PRF, et al. Reduction in infarct size, arrhtyhmias, chest pain and morbidity by early intravenous β-blockade in suspected acute myocardial infarction. Circulation 1983;67(Pt 2): 32–41.

9. Morganroth J, Lichstein E, Byington R, et al. Beta-blocker heart attack trial: impact of propranol therapy on ventricular arrhythmias. Prev Med 1985;14:346.

10. Lee RT, Grodzinsky AJ, Frank EH, et al. Structure-dependent dynamic mechanical behavior of fibrous caps from human atherosclerotic plaques. Circulation 1991;83:1764–1770.

11. Norris R, Clarke ED, Sammel NL, Smith WM, Williams B. Protective effect of propranolol in threatened myocardial infarction. Lancet 1978;2:907 209.

12. Peter I, Norris RM, Clarke ED, et al. Reduction of enzyme levels by propranolol after AMI. Circulation 1978;57:1091 1095.

13. Roberts R, Croft C, Gold HK, et al. Effect of propranolol on myocardial infarct size in a randomized, blinded, multi-center trial. N Engl J Med 1984;311:218–225.

14. Yusuf S, Peto R, Lewis J, et al. Beta-blockade during and after myocardial infarction: an overview of the randomized trials. Prog Cardiovasc Dis 1985;27:335–371.

15. Ryan TJ, Antman EM, Brooks NH, et al. 1999 update: ACC/AHA guidelines for the management of patients with acute myocardial infarction: a report of the American College of Cardiology/American Heart Association Task Force on Practice Guidelines (Committee on Management of Acute Myocardial Infarction) [ACC Practice Guidelines]. J Am Coll Cardiol 1999;34:890-911.

16. First International Study of Infarct Survival Collaborative Group. Randomised trial of intravenous atenolol among 16027 cases of suspected acute myocardial infarction: ISIS-1. Lancet 1986;2:57–66.

17. Yusuf S, Wittes J, Friedman L. Overview of results of randomized clinical trials in heart disease. I. Treatments following myocardial infarction. JAMA 1988;260:2088–2093.

18. The TIMI Study Group. Comparison of invasive and conservative strategies after treatment with intravenous tissue plasminogen activator in acute myocardial infarction results of the thrombolysis in myocardial infarction (TIMI) phase II trial. N Engl J Med 1989;320:618 627.

19. Friedman LM, Byington RP, Capone RJ, et al. Effect of propranolol in postinfarction patients with mechanical or electrical complications. Circulation 1984;69:761.

20. Byington RP, Furberg CD. Beta-blockers during and after acute myocardial. In: Francis A. eds. Modern Coronary Care. Little Brown, Boston,1990, pp. 511 539.

21. Kjekshus JK. Importance of heart rate in determining β-blocker efficacy in acute and long-term AMI intervention trials. Am J Cardiol 1986;57:43F–9F.

22. Furberg CD, Hawkins CM, Lichstein E, for the Beta-Blocker Heart Attack Trial Study Group. Effect of propranolol in postinfarction patients with mechanical or electrical complications. Circulation 1984;69:761–765.

23. Goldman L, Sia BST, Cook EF, et al. Cost and effectiveness of routine therapy with long-term β-adrenergic antagonists after AMI. N Engl J Med 1988;319:152–157.

24. Olsson G, Oden A, Johansson L, Sjogren A, Rehnqvist N. Prognosis after withdrawal of chronic postinfarction metoprolol treatment: a 2–7 year follow-up. Eur Heart J 1988;9:365–372.

25. Olsson G. How long should post MI β-blocker therapy be continued? Primary Cardiol 1991;17: 44–49.

26. Yusuf S, Lessem J, Jha P, Lonn E. Primary and secondary prevention of myocardial infarction and strokes: an update of randomly allocated, controlled trials. J Hypertens 1993;11(Suppl. 4):S61–S73.

27. Stone PH, Sacks FM. Strategies for secondary prevention. In: Manson JE, Ridker PM, Gaziano JM, Hennekens CH, eds. Prevention of Myocardial Infarction. Oxford University Press, New York, 1996, pp. 463–510.

28. Beta-Blocker Pooling Project Research Group. The Beta-Blocker Pooling Project (BBPP): sub-group findings from randomized trials in post-infarction patients. Eur Heart J 1988;9:8.

29. Otterstad J, Ford I. The effect of carvedilol in patients with impaired left ventricular systolic function following an acute myocardial infarction. How do the treatment effects on total mortality and recurrent myocardial infarction in CAPRICORN compare with beta-blocker trials? Eur J Heart Fail 2002;4:501.

30. Beta-Blocker Heart Attack Trial Reseach Group. A randomized trial of propranolol in patients with AMI. I. Mortality results. JAMA 1982;247:1707–1714.

31. Early treatment of unstable angina in the coronary care unit: a randomised, double blind, placebo controlled comparison of recurrent ischaeimia in patients treated with nifedipine or metroprolol or both. Report of the Holland Interuniversity Nifedipine/Metoprolol Trial (HINT) Research Group. Br Heart J 1986;56:400–413.

32. Gottlieb SO, Weisfeld ML, Ouyang P, et al. Effect of the addition of propranolol to therapy with nifedipine for unstable angina pectoris: a randomized, double-blind, placebo-controlled trial. Circulation 1986;73:331–337.

33. Telford AM, Wilson C. Trial of heparin versus atenolol in prevention of myocardial infarction in intermediate coronary syndrome. Lancet 1981;1:1225–1228.

34. Lubsen J, Tijssen JG. Efficacy of nifedipine and metoprolol in the early treatment of unstable angina in the coronary care unit; findings from the Holland Interuniversity Nifedipine/Metoprolol Trial (HINT). Am J Cardiol 1987;60:18A–25A.

35. Yusuf S, Wittes J, Friedman L. Overview of results of randomized clinical trials in heart disease. II. Unstable angina, heart failure, primary prevention with aspirin, and risk factor modification. JAMA 1988;260:2259–2263.

36. Stone PH, Antman EM, Muller JE, Braunwald E. Calcium channel blocking agents in the treatment of cardiovascular disorders. Part II. Hemodynamic effectsand clinical applications. Ann Intern Med 1980;93:886–904.

37. Held PH, Yusuf S, Furberg CD. Calcium channel blockers in acute myocardial infarction and unstable angina: an overview. BMJ 1989;229:1187–1192.

38. Muller JE, Morrison J, Stone PH, et al. Nifedipine therapy in patients with threatened and acute myocardial infarction. A randomized double-blind, placebo-controlled comparison. Circulation 1984; 69:740–747.

39. Sirnes PA, Overskeid K, Pedersen TR, et al. Evolution of infarct size during the early use of nifedipine in patients with AMI: the Norwegian Nifedipine Multicenter Trial. Circulation 1984;70:638–644.

40. Wilcox RG, Hampton JR, Banks DC, et al. Trial of early nifedipine in acute myocardial infarction: the TRENT study. BMJ 1986;293:1204–1208.

41. The Israeli SPRINT Study Group. Secondary Prevention Reinfarction Israeli Nifedipine Trial (SPRINT): a randomized intervention trial of nifedipine in patients with AMI. Eur Heart J 1988;9: 354–364.

42. Goldbourt U, Behar S, Reicher-Reiss H, Zion M, Mandelsweig L, Kaplinsky E. Early administration of nifedipine in suspected AMI: the Secondary Prevention Reinfarction Israel Nifedipine Trial 2 Study. Arch Intern Med 1993;153:345–353.

43. Yusuf S, Held P, Furberg C. Update of effects of calcium antagonists in myocardial infarction or angina in light of the second Danish Verapamil Infarction Trial (DAVIT-II) and other recent studies. Am J Cardiol 1991;67:1295–1297.

44. Lichtlen PR, Hugenholtz PG, Rafflenbenl W, et al. Retardation of angiographic progression of coronary artery disease by nifedipine: results of the International Nifedipine Trial on Antiatherosclerotic Therapy (INTACT). Lancet 1990;335:1109–1113.

45. Waters D, Lesperance J, Francetich M, et al. A controlled clinical trial to assess the effect of a calcium channel blocker upon the progression of coronary atherosclerosis. Circulation 1990;82:1940–1953.

46. Effect of verapamil on mortality and major events after AMI (the Danish Verapamil Infarction Trial II-DAVIT II). Am J Cardiol 1990;66:779–785.

47. Verapamil in AMI. The Danish Study Group on Verapamil in Myocardial Infarction. Eur Heart J 1984; 5:516–528.

48. Held PH, Yusuf S. Effects of β-blockers and calcium channel blockers in acute myocardial infarction. Eur Heart J 1993;14:(Suppl F):18–25.

49. Multicenter Diltiazem Postinfarction Trial Research Group. The effect of diltiazem on mortality and reinfarction after myocardial infarction. N Engl J Med 1988;319:385–392.

50. Gibson RD, Boden WE, Theroux P, et al. Diltiazem and reinfarction in patients with non-Q-wave myocardial infarction. N Engl J Med 1986;315:423–429.

51. Gerstenblith G, Ouyang P, Achuff SC, et al. Nifedipine in unstable angina: a double-blind randomized trial. N Engl J Med 1982;306:885–889.

52. Muller JE, Turi ZG, Pearle DL et al. Nifedipine and conventional therapy for unstable angina pectoris: a randomized double-blind comparison. Circulation 1984;69:728–739.

53. Antman E, Muller J, Goldberg S, et al. Nifedipine therapy for coronary-artery spasm. N Engl J Med 1980;302:1269–1273.

54. Chahine RA, Feldman RL, Giles TD, et al. Randomized placebo-controlled trial of amlodipine in vasospastic angina. J Am Coll Cardiol 1993;21:1365–1370.

55. Prida XE, Gelman JS, Feldman RL, Hill JA, Scott E. Comparison of diltiazem and nifedipine alone and in combination in patients with coronary artery spasm. J Am Coll Cardiol 1987;9:412–419.

56. Schroeder JS, Lamb IH, Briston MR, Ginsburg R, Hung J, McAuley BJ. Prevention of cardiovascular events in the variant angina by long-term diltiazem therapy. J Am Coll Cardiol 1983;1:1507–1511.

57. Diodati J, Theroux P, Latour J-G, et al. Effects of nitroglycerin in therapeutic doses on platelet aggregation in unstable angina pectoris and acute myocardial infarction. Am J Cardiol 1990;66:683–688.

58. Bussmann WD, Passek D, Seidel W, Kaltenbach M. Reduction of CK and CK-MB indexes of infarct size by intravenous nitroglycerin. Circulation 1981;63:615–622.

59. Jugdutt BI, Warnic JW. Intravenous nitroglycerin therapy to limit myocardial infarct size, expansion, and complications: effect of timing, dosage, and infarct location. Circulation 1988;78:1088–1092

60. Antman EM, Lau J, Kupelnick B, Mosteller F, Chalmers TC. A comparison of results of meta-analyses of randomized control trials and recommendations of clinical experts. Treatments for myocardial infarction. JAMA 1992;268:240–248.

61. Yusuf S, Collins R, MacMahon S, Peto R. Effect of intravenous nitrates on mortality in AMI: an overview of the randomized trials. Lancet 1988;1:1088–1092.

62. Durrer JD, Lie KI, Van Capell JFL, Durrer D. Effect of sodium nitroprusside on mortality in AMI. N Engl J Med 1982;306:1121–1128.

63. Cohn J, Franciosa JA, Francis GS, et al. Effect of short-term infusion of sodium nitroprusside on mortality rate in AMI complicated by left ventricular failure. N Engl J Med 1982;306:1129–1135.

64. Passamani ER. Editorial: nitroprusside in myocardial infarction. N Engl J Med 1982;306:1168–1169.

65. GISSI-3. Effects of lisinopril and transdermal glyceryl trinitrate singly and together on 6-week mortality and ventricular function after AMI: Gruppo Italiano per lo Studio della Sopravvivenza nell'infarto Miocardico. Lancet 1994;343:1115–1122.

66. ISIS-4. A randomized factorial trial assessing early oral captopril, oral mononitrate, and intravenous magnesium sulphate in 58,050 patients with suspected AMI. Lancet 1995;345:669–685.

67. Lau J, Antman EM, Jimenez-Silva J, et al. Cumulative meta-analysis of the therapeutic trials for myocardial infarction. N Engl J Med 1992;327:248–254.

14

Angiotensin Converting Enzyme Inhibitors After and During Acute Coronary Syndromes, and, in Particular, Myocardial Infarction

Rodolfo Carrillo-Jimenez, MD,
Charles H. Hennekens, MD, DrPH, *and*
Gervasio A. Lamas MD

CONTENTS

INTRODUCTION

A century ago, Tigerstedt and Bergman *(1)* infused extracts of rabbit kidney into experimental animals and noted a hypertensive response. The chemical effector in the extracts would later be named renin. Years later in another landmark study, Goldblatt et al. *(2)* produced systemic hypertension in dogs by clipping their renal artery, further supporting the hypothesis that the kidneys play a central role in blood pressure regulation. It was not, however, until the 1950s that the blood-borne complement of enzymes and

From: *Contemporary Cardiology: Management of Acute Coronary Syndromes, Second Edition*
Edited by: C. P. Cannon © Humana Press Inc., Totowa, NJ

substrates comprising the renin–angiotensin system would be elucidated. It is clear that renal juxtaglomerular cells secrete renin in response to intravascular volume depletion, decreased serum sodium concentration, and adrenergic stimulation. In the blood stream, renin proteolytically cleaves the prohormone angiotensinogen, produced and secreted by the liver, into the decapeptide angiotensin I. Angiotensin I, in turn, is cleaved into the octapeptide angiotensin II by angiotensin-converting enzyme (ACE), a ubiquitous enzyme present on the surface of endothelial cells. Many of the clinically important effects of the renin–angiotensin system discussed in this chapter are likely to be attributable to the action of angiotensin II on its receptors in multiple organs.

Extensive investigation of the renin–angiotensin system over the last 25 yr has expanded a previously restrictive view of its role as a blood pressure and volume regulator. It appears that an activated renin–angiotensin system is a maladaptive response in many disease states. These include an increased risk of initial and subsequent myocardial infarction (MI), myocardial hypertrophy, development and progression of congestive heart failure, ventricular remodeling following infarction, and ventricular arrhythmias. These observations formed the basis for the evaluation of possible beneficial effects of blockade of the renin–angiotensin system. This chapter will focus on the mechanisms and clinical benefits of ACE inhibition after and during acute coronary syndromes, in particular MI.

MECHANISMS AND EFFECTS OF ACE INHIBITORS AFTER ACUTE CORONARY SYNDROMES, IN PARTICULAR MI

Myocardial Hypertrophy and Its Prognostic Implications

Left ventricular (LV) remodeling following MI, the process by which the infarcted ventricle changes in size and shape, provides a plausible link between neurohormonal activation and postinfarct prognosis. There is ample experimental evidence that angiotensin II plays a role in both mechanical stress-induced, as well as stress-independent, myocyte hypertrophy. For example, Yamazaki et al. *(3)* stretched cardiac myocytes on deformable silicone dishes. This mechanical stress rapidly increased the activity of mitogen-activated protein kinases (MAPKs) and activators. Saralasin, an angiotensin II antagonist peptide, and CV-11974, a specific antagonist to type 1 angiotensin II receptors, both partially inhibited the stretch-induced activities of these enzymes.

However, the application of these concepts to clinical practice is neither simple nor straightforward. Patients do not present with degrees of hypertrophy or remodeling in exact proportion to the calculated hemodynamic stress *(4,5)*. Nonhemodynamic mechanisms may, therefore, help determine the extent of LV hypertrophy. Schunkert et al. *(6)* assessed the effects infusion of angiotensin II had on new protein synthesis in isolated rat hearts. Angiotensin II infusion stimulated protein synthesis, and the signal transduction pathway appeared to involve the type 1 angiotensin II receptor and protein kinase C. It appears that there are significant similarities in the signal transduction pathways induced by both mechanical stimulation of myocytes and that of angiotensin II. Both stimuli employ activation of protein kinase C that in turn leads to phosphorylation and activation of MAPKs. These translocate into the cell nucleus and activate nuclear transcription factors modulating the hypertrophic response. Further evidence in support of the role of angiotensin II as a cardiac growth factor has been developed by showing that angiotensin II causes an increase in protein synthesis without changing the rate of DNA synthesis in cultured myocytes (hypertrophy). Similarly, in cultured cardiac fibroblasts, angiotensin II induces an increase in protein synthesis, DNA synthesis, and cell number (mitoses), independent of hemodynamic or neurohormonal effects *(7)*. These effects are modulated by the angiotensin II type I receptor subtype and can be inhibited by subtype I angiotensin II receptor antagonists *(7)*. Indeed, blockade of the renin–angiotensin system with ACE inhibitors has been shown to regress LV hypertrophy *(8)*. However, the clinical significance in terms of any mortality benefits to be gained from regression of hypertrophy is presently unknown. Thus, the process of postinfarct LV remodeling has been tied to angiotensin II, as well as hypertrophy by morphologic evidence *(9,10)* and experimental studies. The net clinical benefits of the use of ACE inhibitors to prevent remodeling are a logical clinical correlate of these experimental findings.

Evidence from Genetic Studies

Preliminary evidence for the involvement of the renin–angiotensin system in ischemic events also has come from retrospective but not prospective epidemiological studies of the ACE gene in humans. A retrospective case-controlled study of small sample size by Cambien et al. *(11)* suggested a link between polymorphism of the ACE gene with increased risk of MI. This finding, however, was not supported by data of a larger sample size from the Physicians' Health Study studied by Lindpaintner et al. *(12)*, who found no association between the presence of the ACE gene D allele and an increased risk of ischemic heart disease or MI *(12,13)*. This ACE gene polymorphism consists of an insertion (I) or deletion (D) of a 287-bp sequence of DNA. Individuals containing the D/D genotype exhibit plasma ACE levels twice that of individuals containing the I/I genotype *(11)*. The D/D genotype also is more prevalent in middle-aged men with a prior history of MI when compared to age-matched controls *(11)*. An increased incidence of the ACE D/D genotype has been identified in children of patients with a history of MI compared with controls *(14)*. Additional disease states, which have been associated with the D/D genotype include LV hypertrophy *(15)*, hypertrophic cardiomyopathy *(16)*, restenosis after coronary angioplasty *(17)*, and progressive ventricular dilatation following anterior MI *(18)*. Subjects enrolled in the Captopril and Thrombolysis Study (CATS) *(19)* underwent quantitative echocardiography immediately following therapy with streptokinase. After a 1-yr follow-up, both end-systolic and end-diastolic volumes, as well as plasma norepinephrine levels, were greater in the D/D genotype group. Furthermore, these effects were attenuated in patients with the D/D genotype group by therapy with captopril. Also, in a study by Kohno et al. *(20)* ACE inhibitor therapy was administered for >2 yr to 54 patients with hypertension and moderate to severe LV hypertrophy. In 17 patients with the D/D genotype, mean regression in posterior wall thickness and LV mass index was significantly less than in the other patients with I/D or I/I genotypes.

Lindpaintner et al. *(12)* found no association between the presence of the ACE gene D-allele and an increased risk of ischemic heart disease or MI. Explanations advanced in attempt to reconcile the conflicting and variable experimental results hinge on the influences that multiple environmental factors may have on the expression of a particular disease process and variations of genetic backgrounds among differing populations being studied *(12,13)*.

Vascular Endothelial Function and ACE Inhibition

Endothelial cells line the entire inner surface of the vasculature providing a smooth interface between circulating blood and the vessel wall, as well as mediating crucial metabolic functions. As a rich source of vasoactive substances, the endothelium plays a role as an organ system with autocrine, paracrine, and even endocrine functions regulating vascular tone, regional blood flow, and intimal proliferation. Important endothelium-derived vasodilators are prostacyclin, bradykinin, nitric oxide (NO), and endothelium-derived hyperpolarizing factor. These substances have a major role in the evolving concept of early atherosclerosis, as well as that of stable and unstable ischemic syndromes (21).

The predominant tone of a vascular bed is the sum of simultaneously acting vasodilator and vasoconstrictor influences. In normally functioning endothelial cells, a basal rate of production of NO is maintained by the action of the constitutive enzyme NO synthase (22). This basal production, which requires a normal endothelium, maintains a net vascular relaxation. However, various vasoactive substances (i.e., bradykinin, serotonin, adenosine diphosphate, and substance P), as well as the effect of blood's shearing force on the endothelium, can up-regulate NO synthase activity, increasing production and secretion of NO (23–25). NO inhibits cellular growth and migration. In concert with prostacyclin, NO exerts potent anti-atherogenic and antithrombotic properties by preventing platelet aggregation and cell adhesion (21).

The renin–angiotensin system influences endothelial function, and there is evidence that ACE inhibition may improve endothelial function through multiple possible mechanisms. Mancini and co-workers (26) reported on 129 patients with documented coronary atherosclerosis randomized to quinapril or placebo for 6 mo. Coronary endothelial function was assessed with intracoronary infusions of acetylcholine. Quinapril-treated patients had an improvement in endothelial function, when compared to placebo-treated patients. The authors postulated that among other causes, decreased degeneration of NO, and bradykinin-mediated NO release may also play a part.

More recently, Takashi et al. (27) have investigated the potential role of the interactions of ACE inhibitors containing a sulfhydryl (SH) group. Using in vitro techniques that included preparation of human coronary vessels with either nitroglycerin or nicorandil, the investigators studied the effects on the vessels after the addition of either captopril (a SH-group-containing ACE inhibitor) or enalaprilat. Both nitroglycerin and nicorandil exhibited an increase in vasodilatation in the presence of captopril and not in response to enalaprilat. The response may involve the opening of an ATP-sensitive potassium channel and subsequent guanylate cyclase activation. Buikema et al. (28) studied the effects of SH-containing zofenopril vs lisinopril (no-SH group). They found that ACE inhibition with a SH group has a potential advantage in the improvement of endothelial dysfunction through increased activity of NO after release from endothelium. Thus, improvement in endothelial function is an additional possible mechanism to explain the net benefits of ACE inhibitors after and during acute coronary syndromes, in particular MI.

LV Remodeling Following Acute Myocardial Infarction (AMI)

The clinical association of cardiomegaly, congestive heart failure, and decreased survival has been documented extensively (29). Over half a century ago, Waris et al. (30) studied 125 patients who had sustained their first MI. Patients exhibiting cardiac enlargement on chest radiography demonstrated a significantly increased 5-yr mortality. A high proportion of the survivors with an enlarged heart developed New York Heart Association

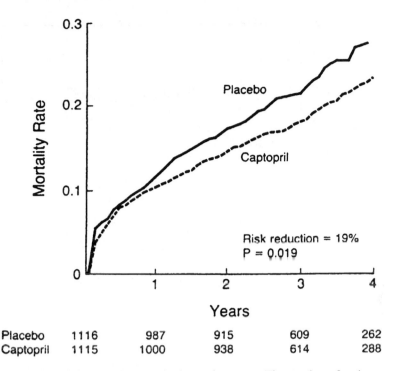

Fig. 1. Cumulative mortality from all causes in the study groups. The number of patients at risk at the beginning of each year is shown at the bottom. Therapy with captopril (within 3–16 d after MI) significantly reduced mortality from all causes compared with the placebo group. The reduction in risk was 19% (95% CI: 3–32%; $p = 0.019$). Data from ref. *34*.

class III angina or congestive heart failure during follow-up. White et al. and St. John Sutton et al. *(31,32)* have demonstrated that after MI, LV volumes predict clinical outcome. This has been further evidenced from higher brain natriuretic peptide (BNP) concentrations early after first MI, which is associated with adverse LV remodeling characteristics. This partially explains why BNP is a strong predictor of outcome after MI *(33)*. Thus, the early clinical impression regarding the importance of cardiac enlargement following MI was correct and provided an impetus for defining mechanisms responsible for the observed topographic alterations, as well as and therapeutic modalities to limit them.

RANDOMIZED TRIALS OF ACE INHIBITORS AFTER ACUTE CORONARY SYNDROMES, IN PARTICULAR MI

SAVE

The Survival and Ventricular Enlargement Study (SAVE) *(34)* was the first large randomized double-blind placebo-controlled trial to evaluate the effects of an ACE inhibitor (captopril) on clinical outcome in survivors of AMI. Patients with ejection fractions (EF) of <40% (average 31%) and no overt congestive heart failure or severe ongoing ischemia were randomized to captopril 3–16 d after infarction (initial oral dose, 6.25–12.5 mg, slowly titrated to 50 mg 3× daily if tolerated) or placebo and were followed for 2–5 yr. Eligibility was confirmed by radionuclide ventriculogram. The SAVE study demonstrated a 19% reduction in all-cause mortality (Fig. 1), 21% for cardiovas-

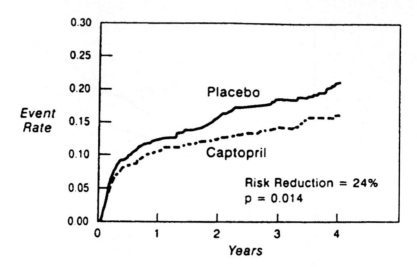

Fig. 2. Life table of cumulative need for revascularization (by either percutaneous coronary angioplasty or coronary artery bypass surgery) after randomization. For this combined analysis, the time to first event was used. Data from ref. *35.*

cular mortality, 37% for development of severe congestive heart failure, and 22% for heart failure requiring hospitalization. Thus, SAVE established the role of ACE inhibition in the treatment of patients after MI with low EFs.

Although the primary end point of SAVE focused on the assessment of survival and prevention of deterioration of LV function, recurrent MI was a prospectively defined and carefully sought end point. The captopril-treated group demonstrated a 25% relative reduction in the risk of recurrent MI. A more detailed analysis for predictors of MI by Rutherford et al. *(35)* demonstrated that LV EF was not a predictor of recurrent MI. Captopril therapy was associated with similarly decreased risk of reinfarction for SAVE patients with EFs above and below the median. Furthermore, captopril therapy also decreased the incidence of angioplasty or bypass surgery (relative reduction in risk 24%, $p = 0.014$) when compared to placebo (Fig. 2). Lamas et al. *(36)* demonstrated that the principal predictor of recurrent infarction was the number of vessels diseased and not revascularized. Captopril therapy reduced the incidence of recurrent infarction in patients with single, as well as multivessel, disease.

SOLVD

Studies of Left Ventricular Dysfunction (SOLVD) randomized 6797 patients in two separate placebo-controlled trials of enalapril in LV dysfunction—a treatment arm *(37)* and a prevention arm *(38)*. All patients had an EF of <35%. Patients in the prevention arm had asymptomatic LV dysfunction, and patients in the treatment arm had clinically established heart failure. Although SOLVD was a trial of patients with chronic LV dysfunction of any etiology, 79% were thought to have an ischemic cardiomyopathy. However, no patient in either trial had unstable angina at the time of enrollment nor had suffered an AMI in the month before enrollment. There was a reduction in risk of MI of 23% and unstable angina of 20% in the enalapril-treated group.

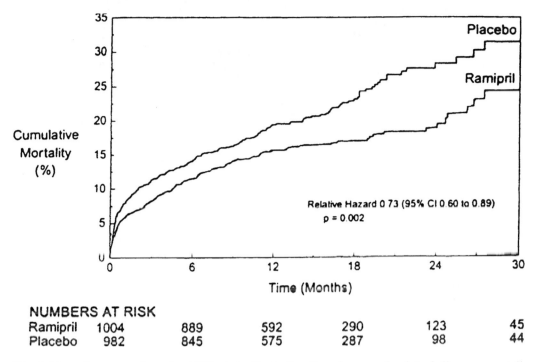

Fig. 3. Mortality curves from the AIRE study illustrating the primary end point of all-cause mortality analyzed by intention to treat. Separation of the curves occurred early, and they continued to diverge throughout the study. There was a 27% overall reduction in risk of death (95% CI: 11–40%; $p = 0.002$) in the ramipril group. Data from ref. *39*.

AIRE

The Acute Infarction Ramipril Efficacy (AIRE) trial *(39)* randomized patients with early pulmonary congestion after infarction (Killip Class >1) to ramipril or placebo. Ramipril was given as 1.25–2.5 mg 2× daily, titrated up to 5 mg 2× daily for an average of 15 mo. There was a 27% reduction in risk of death from all causes (from 23% in placebo patients to 17% in treated patients) (Fig. 3). Furthermore, there was a reduction of 19% in the first occurrence of a prespecified combined end point of death, severe heart failure, MI, or stroke. AIRE required clinical evidence of pulmonary congestion.

TRACE

Echocardiography was used to select patients participating in the Trandolapril Cardiac Evaluation (TRACE) trial *(40)*. Patients were screened within 2-6 d and wall motion index was calculated based on the nine-segment wall motion assessment described by Heger et al. *(41)*, and calculated to select patients with EFs of <35%. In TRACE, approx 39% of all MI patients had an early EF of <35%. There was a significant 22% reduction in mortality after 24–50 mo in patients with LV dysfunction assigned at random to trandolapril 1 mg orally once daily, slowly titrated to 4 mg once daily. As in the other trials, those patients treated with the ACE inhibitor had improved survival (Fig. 4A) and a lower incidence of heart failure (Fig. 4B).

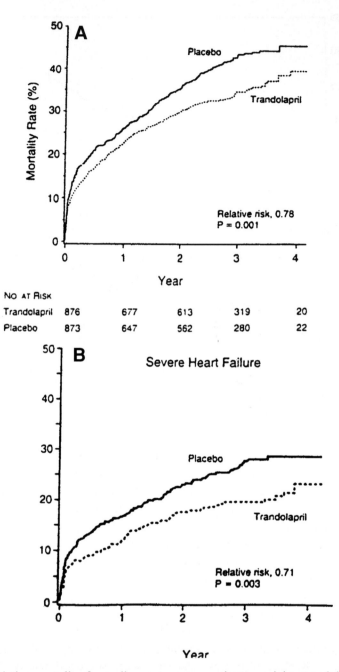

Fig. 4. (A) Cumulative mortality from all causes among patients receiving trandolapril or placebo. Mortality curves diverged early, with estimated mortality at 1 mo of 8.8% in the trandolapril group and 11.2% in the placebo group. The relative risk of death from any cause in the trandolapril group, compared with the placebo group, was 0.78 (95% CI: 0.67–0.91; $p = 0.001$). **(B)** Progression to severe heart failure occurred more often and developed earlier in the placebo group compared with the trandolapril group (relative risk, 0.71; 95% CI: 0.56–0.89; $p = 0.001$). Data from ref. *40*.

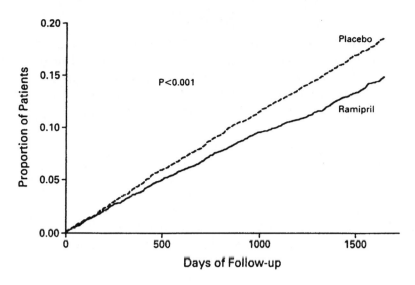

Fig. 5. Estimates of the composite outcome of MI, stroke, or death from cardiovascular causes in the ramipril group and the placebo group. The relative risk of the composite outcome in the ramipril group as compared with the placebo group was 0.78 (95% CI:, 0.70–0.86). Data from ref. *43.*

SMILE

The Survival of Myocardial Infarction Long-Term Evaluation (SMILE) trial *(42)* randomized patients with anterior wall infarctions who had not received thrombolytic therapy. Patients assigned to the ACE inhibitor zofenopril had an improved outcome.

HOPE

The Heart Outcomes Prevention Evaluation Study (HOPE)(43) trial provides the first evidence of clinical benefit in unselected high-risk patients with or without a prior cardiovascular event. This trial evaluated the effect of oral ramipril (10 mg daily) vs placebo in 9297 patients, who either established atherosclerotic disease or diabetes with another cardiovascular risk factor (e.g., hypertension, dyslipoproteinemia, and history of smoking or microalbuminuria). Patient characteristics included diabetes in 39%, coronary artery disease in 80%, peripheral vascular disease in 43%, and a previous cerebrovascular event in 11%. Interestingly, in contrast to previous ACE inhibitor trials, patients were excluded if they had a known history of congestive heart failure or an EF <40%. A significant reduction of 22% (p < 0.001) in the primary end point (a composite end point of MI, stroke, or death from cardiovascular disease (Fig. 5). Also, ramipril treatment showed a significant risk reduction in all-cause mortality, MI, stroke, cardiac arrest, and revascularization procedures in all subgroups. Of note, ACE inhibition appeared to be beneficial independently of the effect on blood pressure.

These findings demonstrate that an important part of the early and late benefit of ACE inhibition relates not only to hemodynamic and cardiac architectural benefits, but also to the prevention of ischemic events. Indeed, perhaps the early benefit may relate more to prevention of early recurrent myocardial ischemia than with other mechanisms.

PEACE

The Prevention of Events with Angiotensin Converting Enzyme Inhibitor (PEACE) (44) trial will randomize 8290 patients to trandolapril or placebo. This trial will further provide important information as to whether ACE inhibition will reduce the incidence of cardiovascular mortality or nonfatal MI in patients with documented coronary artery disease (CAD), including previous MI and a preserved LV function.

RECOMMENDED USE OF ACE INHIBITORS AFTER ACUTE CORONARY SYNDROMES, IN PARTICULAR MI

In the aforementioned randomized trials, maintaining therapy for 2–4 yr will lead to reductions in mortality of 30–70 lives per 1000 patients treated. As suggested by the American College of Cardiology (ACC)/American Heart Association (AHA) guidelines (45,46), ACE inhibitors should be given to all post-MI patients with signs of LV dysfunction with or without symptoms (47). The HOPE trial suggests that all high-risk patients (regardless of whether they experienced MI or LV dysfunction) should receive ACE inhibitors, but these conclusions must be viewed in light of the emerging data from the PEACE trial of patients with prior MI and preserved LV function. Given the totality of current evidence, we recommend the use ACE inhibitors in all patients with prior MI indefinitely, unless results from ongoing trials indicate otherwise. This recommendation includes all post-MI patients regardless of LV function, except in those where there are known contraindications for use.

ACE Inhibition and Aspirin

Both ACE inhibitors and aspirin are recommended for secondary prevention after AMI. Curiously, it had been suggested based on a data-derived hypothesis from SOLVD that there was an adverse interaction and, indeed, several plausible biological mechanisms were postulated (48). However, in subgroup analysis of other trials of ACE inhibitor use after acute coronary syndromes, a deleterious interaction was not consistently found. Furthermore, in observational studies, consistent beneficial additive effects have been observed (49,50). Thus, we currently recommend concomitant use of ACE inhibitors and aspirin in all post-MI patients.

MECHANISMS AND EFFECTS OF ACE INHIBITORS DURING ACUTE CORONARY SYNDROMES, IN PARTICULAR MI

The Renin–Angiotensin System During Coronary Ischemia

A considerable body of evidence exists supporting the link between activation of the renin–angiotensin system and increased risk of MI. The time-course of neurohormonal rise and subsequent decline and the degree of activation are related to the clinical condition and hemodynamic compensation of the patients. In patients whose MI is complicated by congestive heart failure, cardiogenic shock, or arrhythmias, activation of the renin–angiotensin system can be detected within 6 h of symptom onset. In others, elevation of renin and angiotensin II does not occur until after d 1, with peak levels on d 3. The highest levels of renin and angiotensin II are seen in patients who develop heart failure or cardiogenic shock (51) and in those treated with diuretics (52). By d 10, renin and angiotensin II levels return to normal except in patients treated with diuretics, in which renin levels may remain elevated for a longer time period *(51)*. However, even in patients who are hemodynamically compensated, but who have sustained an extensive infarction, higher levels of renin and angiotensin II are generally detected. For example, Vaughan et al. *(52)* studied patients who were 11–30 d after a first anterior wall AMI, who were not taking diuretics, and who did not have overt congestive heart failure. These investigators found mild but significant increases in angiotensin II and renin in patients with the most severe LV dysfunction, as well as in those with a history of pulmonary congestion early after infarction.

Intuitively, it is tempting to speculate that activation of the neuroendocrine system with its attendant vasoconstriction and tachycardia, has some value in supporting hemodynamic stability during the peri-infarct phase. However, except for extreme conditions such as cardiogenic shock or circulatory collapse, neurohormonal activation has detrimental clinical effects on cardiovascular function during the acute and convalescent phases of MI.

Cohn et al. *(53–55)* and Packer et al. *(56)* have clearly shown that higher levels of catecholamines and renin are associated with increased mortality in heart failure patients. The prognostic importance of neurohormonal activation in patients following MI is less apparent but real. Rouleau et al. *(57)* measured neurohormones in 534 patients an average of 12 d after infarction. Multivariate analyses, which included clinical characteristics as well as EF, showed that plasma renin activity and atrial natriuretic peptide independently predicted postinfarct cardiovascular mortality. Plasma renin activity, aldosterone, atrial natriuretic peptide, and arginine vasopressin predicted a broader endpoint of cardiovascular mortality, congestive heart failure, or recurrent infarction. These analyses suggest that an activated neurohormonal system is not merely an epiphenomenon of LV dysfunction, but is directly maladaptive and detrimental to cardiovascular survival. The clinical implications of these analyses are supported by the results of randomized trials of ACE inhibitors. Similarly, the improvement in survival seen in patients treated with β-blockers during and following MI favors at least some direct detrimental effects of unopposed elevations of neurohormones. Thus, despite some data to the contrary, at present neurohormonal activation is considered a cause of poor postinfarct prognosis, and an important therapeutic target.

Interaction of the Renin–Angiotensin System with the Fibrinolytic System and Platelets

Another important proposed mechanism of the renin–angiotensin system in acute coronary syndromes concerns the ability to modulate the plasma fibrinolytic system, which is based on the balance between plasminogen activator inhibitor-1 (PAI-1) and tissue-type plasminogen activator (tPA). tPA is released from endothelial cells and is present in small amounts in plasma where it catalyzes the conversion of plasminogen to plasmin. Plasmin proteolytically degrades fibrin, hence its antithrombotic activity. PAI-1, also secreted mainly from endothelial cells is a major inhibitor of tPA, thereby slowing degradation of the fibrin clot and promoting hemostasis. Both have short plasma half-lives, on the order of 5 min, and their relative concentrations play an integral role in modulation of both thrombosis and fibrinolysis. PAI-1 is elevated in a variety of prothrombotic or ischemic states, including young survivors of MI *(58)*. Angiotensin II stimulates endothelial cells in culture to release PAI *(59,60)*, an observation confirmed in vivo in normal volunteers *(61)*. Furthermore, bradykinin, a vasoactive peptide that is

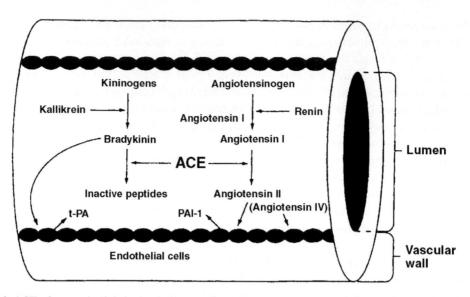

Fig. 6. ACE plays a crucial dual role in the fibrinolytic balance between PAI-1 and tPA. Conversion of angiotensin I to angiotensin II leads to increased expression of PAI-1; degradation of bradykinin inhibits the production of tPA. Inhibition of ACE enhances bradykinin-mediated release of tPA from the endothelium while decreasing angiotensin-II-mediated release of PAI-1. The net effect is a shift in the fibrinolytic balance toward lysis, which is an advantageous condition during acute ischemic syndromes *(59)*.

degraded by ACE, induces dose-dependent increases in circulating plasminogen activator levels *(62)*.

Vaughan et al. studied plasma fibrinolytic balance in patients following anterior MI randomized to ramipril or placebo in the Healing and Early Afterload Reducing Therapy (HEART) study. At d 14 after the infarct, PAI levels were 44% lower in the ramipril-treated group ($p = 0.004$) than in placebo patients. Furthermore, the ratio of circulating PAI to tPA was higher than at baseline in those patients not treated with ACE inhibition *(63)*. Also, Miani et al. *(64)* demonstrated that intracoronary infusion of bradykinin stimulates tPA release without causing any change in PAI-1 levels in the human coronary circulation. An ACE inhibitor augmented this effect. Furthermore, Soejima et al. *(65)* demonstrated that administration of enalapril reduces the increased procoagulant activity in patients with MI associated with inhibition of the activation and accumulation of macrophages and monocytes by reduction of plasma tissue factor (TF), tissue factor pathway inhibitor (TFPI) and monocyte chemoattractant protein-1 (MCP-1) levels. These observations form the basis of a new paradigm for the treatment of acute coronary syndromes.

Protection against intravascular thrombosis depends on the balance between pro-thrombotic influences, such as PAI, and fibrinolytic influences, such as tPA *(66)*. ACE inhibition, through nonhemodynamic humoral mechanisms, may favorably shift this balance towards fibrinolysis and prevention of thrombotic events (Fig. 6). The proposed beneficial effects of ACE inhibition on vascular reactivity and the coagulation system are supported by a recent study *(67)*. In a prospective cohort of 301 patients with non-ST-segment elevation acute coronary syndrome, 53 patients had been pretreated with ACE inhibitors. This intervention significantly reduced the likelihood of troponin I release and was associated with lower maximum troponin I concentrations. These findings were independent of aspirin treatment and not associated with ACE genotype.

Evidence of Antiplatelet Effects

Antiplatelet effects have been found during ACE inhibition in AMI. In a study involving the blood samples of 25 patients with AMI, ACE inhibition was shown to reduce the formation of large platelet aggregates in an experimental perfusion system when compared to the blood samples of the placebo group *(68)*. The authors speculate that this effect might be related to a down-regulation of glycoprotein IIb/IIIa complex on the platelet surface.

Arrythmogenesis

Since activation of the renin–angiotensin system, along with other neurohormones, occurs during the acute and convalescent phases of MI, this system may play an important role in arrhythmogenesis, which is mediated by direct and in direct effects of angiotensin II *(69–71)*. At least five mechanisms are postulated through which angiotensin II may promote cardiac arrhythmias during MI: (*i*) angiotensin II mediates increases in cardiac filling pressures, thereby abnormally increasing wall stress *(72)*; (*ii*) angiotensin II directly produces coronary vasoconstriction and decreases coronary blood flow; (*iii*) angiotensin II enhances sympathetic tone and the effects of circulating catecholamines *(73)*; (*iv*) angiotensin II has direct electrophysiologic effects on cardiac myocytes *(74)*; and (*v*) angiotensin II stimulates the adrenal glands to produce aldosterone, promoting renal salt and water retention and potassium excretion leading to potential electrolyte disturbances, such as hypokalemia *(75)*.

There is ample experimental and some clinical evidence of an antiarrhythmic effect of ACE inhibition. For example, captopril administered before the start of or at the end of experimentally induced ischemia in isolated rat myocardium reduces reperfusion-induced ventricular fibrillation and decreases purine outflow and peak creatine phosphokinase levels during reperfusion *(76)*. Similarly, in the closed chest pig model, captopril (continued beyond the acute phase of experimentally produced ischemia) decreases the inducibility of ventricular arrhythmia by programmed electrical stimulation performed 2 wk after MI *(77)*.

Early captopril treatment after an AMI has been shown to reduce the incidence of late potentials on signal-averaged electrocardiography. This was shown on d 6–30, favorably affecting the antiarrythmogenic profile of this ACE inhibitor *(78)*. Spargias et al. *(79)* analyzed 67 patients from the AIRE trial and found that ramipril therapy was associated with a significant reduction in QT dispersion over a 2-mo period after AMI. This reduction of ventricular repolarization inhomogeneity may be a potential antiarrythmic effect. Furthermore, in 1577 patients from the TRACE study *(80)*, patients with reduced LV function secondary to AMI randomized to trandolapril had a decreased incidence of atrial fibrillation.

While ACE inhibitors clearly reduce sudden cardiac death and all-cause mortality, whether ACE inhibition reduces the incidence of sudden presumably arrhythmic death is less clear. The Multicenter Unsustained Tachycardia Trial (MUSTT) *(81)* randomized 2087 patients with prior MI, nonsustained ventricular tachycardia, and depressed ventricular function. There were no significant differences in total mortality ($p = 0.47$) or arrhythmic death or cardiac arrest ($p = 0.51$) with ACE inhibitor use at discharge over a median 43 mo of follow-up. In 56 patients randomized to ACE inhibitor or placebo for 3 mo after MI, programmed electrical stimulation revealed no significant differences in inducibility of monomorphic sustained ventricular tachycardia *(82)*. However, the incidence of ventricular fibrillation tended to be lower in the ACE inhibitor group. In summary, randomized trials are necessary to better define the possible beneficial role of ACE inhibition in arrhythmogenesis.

Infarct Expansion: Mechanism of Early Remodeling

Immediately after MI, rapidly occurring and complex alterations in the histology of the infarcted segment lead to the morphologic and geometric change termed infarct expansion. Morphologically, infarct expansion is thinning and lengthening of the infarcted segment. Histologic analyses show that infarct expansion may begin within hours to days following acute infarction, prior to the period when phagocytic cells begin debriding the area of necrotic tissue *(83,84)*. Therefore, wall thinning, an essential part of infarct expansion, is not due to removal of necrotic tissues by phagocytic cells, but rather due to slippage and rearrangement of necrotic myocytes, leading to a decrease in the number of cells across the LV wall.

Multiple factors are known to determine the degree to which infarct expansion occurs. Large infarcts involving the anteroapical walls *(85)*, elevated intracardiac pressures *(86)*, and impaired infarct healing *(87)* all increase expansion. Infarct expansion is an important, but transient mechanism for LV dilatation and distortion. As scar tissue forms in infarcted areas, increased tensile strength leads to greater resistance to deforming forces. By 3 wk after infarction, infarct expansion has largely halted.

Infarct expansion and the resulting alterations in LV size and geometry are important physiologic triggers for the late phase of LV remodeling. The law of Laplace relates wall tension to the pressure and shape of the fluid-filled chamber being examined. Wall tension is directly proportional to pressure and inversely proportional to curvature. Thus, at any intracavitary pressure examined, wall tension is lowest for a normally shaped, highly curved LV apex. This principle explains why the LV wall is thinnest at the apex. Furthermore, as apical curvature becomes even greater in systole, wall tension in the normal apex tends to fall, offsetting the systolic rise in wall tension caused by the increase in systolic pressure *(88)*.

These favorable physiologic conditions may be adversely affected by infarct expansion. In an expanded apex, the normal, sharp curvature of the apex is blunted, leading to higher wall tension. Furthermore, and most importantly, the peri-infarct regions are tethered to the akinetic segments. During systole, these peri-infarct regions develop a concave-outward curvature, or anticlastic curve, which also severely increases wall tension *(85)*.

The degree of systolic dysfunction after MI is a key determinant of early and chronic alterations in ventricular topography. With small insults involving <20% of the LV muscle *(89)*, EF and stroke vol remain normal due to compensatory hyperfunctioning of remaining viable tissues. However, with larger impairments of LV function, the ability of remaining viable muscle to compensate is overcome, EF falls, and LV dilatation occurs to maintain stroke vol.

Thus, the morphologic and physiologic forces that lead to progressive LV remodeling in the chronic phase of the infarct are based on the degree of systolic dysfunction, as well as the extent of geometric ventricular derangement. Increases in ventricular wall stress are a physiologic trigger for hypertrophy in noninfarcted myocardium. Thus, a decreased EF following transmural MI results in elevation of end-systolic vol with an attendant increase in end-systolic wall stress. If the infarct has sufficiently compromised systolic function, alterations in local geometry, particularly in the peri-infarct regions, may lead to the development of small peri-infarct segments with an anticlastic curve. These abnormalities in vol and stress all are markedly exaggerated by infarct expansion, if it occurs. Thus, the chronic phase after infarction may be characterized by regional hypertrophy of the noninfarcted segment, as well as progressive LV dilatation and dysfunction. A vicious cycle is set into action, whereby dilation is the catalyst for increased wall stress. Mass-to-vol ratio cannot be normalized, and further dilation ensues.

Strategies to Limit Remodeling

For a long time, infarct scar had been considered an inert tissue. However, utilizing molecular and cellular biologic technologies, we know that infarct scar is composed of biologically active components such as myofibroblasts with contractile behavior and the capacity of producing type I collagen (90). This activity contributes to the formation of fibrous tissue in noninfarcted myocardium. ACE inhibition or angiotensin 1 receptor antagonism has proven effective in attenuating this metabolic activity In the early phase postinfarction, which encompasses the first several days, there is evidence from randomized trials that improvement in loading conditions, either with intravenous (IV) nitroglycerin (91) or with ACE inhibitors, may reduce infarct expansion. However, the data with iv nitroglycerin remain controversial, and the acute impact of early ACE inhibition on LV vol appears small. By contrast, long-term ACE inhibition has demonstrated remarkable benefits in postinfarct patients, particularly in those with LV dysfunction.

In seminal investigations on rats with experimental infarctions, captopril significantly decreased ventricular dilation and prolonged survival (92). The experimental work was rapidly followed by two small clinical trials in humans that first demonstrated that the process of LV remodeling could be attenuated in man by treatment with ACE inhibition (93,94). In the study published by Pfeffer et al. (93), patients with a first anterior infarction and an EF of 45% or less were randomized to captopril or placebo. While captopril attenuated remodeling, treated patients with the most severe LV dilatation had an occluded infarct artery and a large infarct. In a subanalysis of the HEART study, BNP elevation after MI further proved that neurohormonal activation occurs and persists in patients with AMI, even in the presence of preserved LV function. Despite significant clinical effects and benefits on LV remodeling, ramipril use in patients soon after MI has been show to have only a modest impact on BNP levels (95).

The clinically important question of whether tissue-specific ACE inhibitors have more antiremodeling benefit over nontissue-specific ones has been addressed. Konermann et al. (96) randomized 52 patients with their first AMI to receive captopril (nontissue-specific) or fosinopril (tissue-specific) started 7 d after the event. Cine magnetic resonance was done at the beginning of the trial and at 26 wk to assess remodeling. The investigators found that the use of either ACE inhibitor had no major difference in their influence on LV remodeling. However, equivalence must be viewed in the context of the small sample size. In this regard, a meta-analysis of 845 patients with a 3-mo echocardiographic follow-up, de Kam et al. (97), found the very early use (<9 h) of ACE inhibitors after the onset of AMI, LV dilatation was only significantly reduced in those patients in which thrombolysis failed. Other mechanisms may be responsible for the beneficial effects of ACE inhibitors in successfully reperfused patients. Nevertheless, whether there is clinical significance of small (15 mL) differences in LV vol requires testing in large randomized trials.

CLINICAL TRIALS DURING ACUTE CORONARY SYNDROMES, IN PARTICULAR MI

CONSENSUS II

Several years ago, the Cooperative New Scandinavian Enalapril Survival Study II (CONSENSUS II) *(98)* had planned to randomize 9000 patients to determine whether early administration (within 24 h of the onset of symptoms of AMI) of iv enalapril would reduce mortality during a 6-mo follow-up period. Mortality at 6 mo did not differ significantly between groups (9.4% in the placebo group and 10% in the enalapril group, $p = 0.26$). However, the trial was terminated early, after approx 6000 patients were enrolled due to concerns of adverse effects from early hypotension. This side effect, defined as a systolic blood pressure <90 mmHg or diastolic blood pressure <50 mmHg, was observed more commonly in the treatment group than in the placebo group. Furthermore, patients with hypotension appeared to have a poorer clinical outcome. These findings led to an early and erroneous recommendation against the use of intravenous ACE inhibition in acute infarction, particularly when accompanied by thrombolytic therapy with streptokinase, which may itself lead to hypotension via similar enzymatic pathways.

GISSI III

The third Gruppo Italiano della Sopravvivenza nell'Infarcto Miocardico (GISSI-3) study *(99)* randomized 19,394 patients within 24 h of the onset of symptoms of AMI to the long-acting ACE inhibitor lisinopril (initial dose, 5 mg daily, titrated to 10 mg daily if tolerated) for 6 wk. A small (relative risk reduction of 12%, absolute risk reduction of 0.8%) but significant reduction ($p = 0.03$) in mortality was observed at 42 d after infarction only with lisinopril therapy (Fig. 7). Hypotension was the principal side effect, but it did not lead to adverse outcomes.

ISIS IV

The International Study of Infarct Survival (ISIS-4) randomized 58,050 patients within 1 d of infarction to test the effect of 1 mo of captopril therapy, magnesium, or nitrates in a factorial design *(100)*. Patients were assigned to either captopril (titrated from an initial dose of 6.25 mg to as much as 50 mg 2× daily) or placebo for 28 d. There was a significant ($p = 0.02$) benefit of captopril therapy with a relative reduction in mortality risk for captopril-treated patients of 7% at 5 wk and an absolute reduction in risk of 0.5% (Fig. 8). The benefit of early treatment persisted for at least 1 yr.

CCS

The Chinese Cardiac Study (CCS) *(101)* assessed the efficacy of early captopril use on mortality and mortality after AMI. A total of 14,962 patients in China up to 36 h (mean 16.6 h) after the onset of suspected AMI, without clear contraindications, were randomized to either 4 wk of oral captopril (6.25 mg initial dose, 12.5 mg 2 h later, and then 12.5 mg 3× daily) or placebo. Although no significant reduction in the overall 4-wk mortality was found, the incidence of heart failure was significantly reduced in the

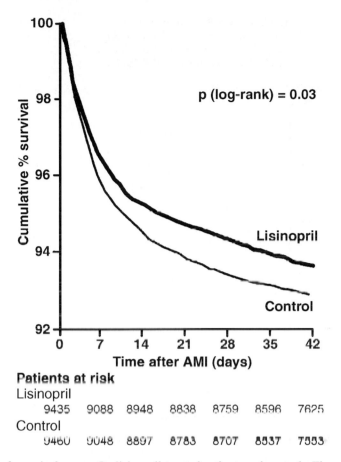

Fig. 7. Six-week survival curves for lisinopril-treated patients and controls. The curves separated early (d 0 to 1) and continued to diverge throughout the next 6 wk, supporting the argument for the early institution of therapy with ACE inhibitors in selected patients. Patients allocated lisinopril had an 11% lower risk of death than the controls (6.3 vs 7.1%). Data from ref. 9.

captopril group (17 vs 18.7%; $p = 0.01$). Also, the anterior wall infarction of captopril treated group was found to have a lower mortality (8.6 vs 10.2%, $p = 0.02$). Thus, early captopril use in AMI was found to prevent about 6 deaths per 1000 patients treated and about 15 deaths due to heart failure per 1000 patients in the first 4 wk with greater benefits. In the subgroup of patients with anterior MI, ACE inhibitor therapy prevented 16 deaths per 1000 patients with no benefit for the inferior infarction group. Furthermore, after analyzing patient subgroups by heart rate at presentation, there were no benefits of ACE inhibition when heart rate is slow or heart block and hypotension are present. This is believed to be due to the parasympathetic effect of ACE inhibition.

These studies have particular clinical relevance because they address the patient during the very acute phase of the infarct, prior to the time when any screening tests or evaluations for LV function could be done. Indeed, their strength is generalizability and ease of application. This strategy led to a significant benefit of 5 lives saved per 1000 patients treated per year, and extended the use of ACE inhibitors to the majority of post-MI patients.

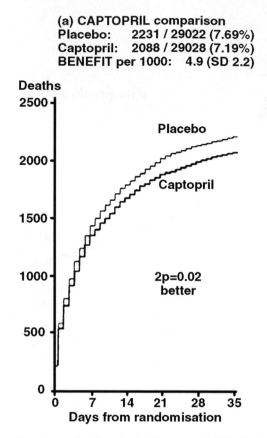

Fig. 8. Effects on mortality during the first 5 wk; there were 7.19% deaths in the captopril group compared with 7.69% deaths in the placebo group. Relative reduction in mortality for captopril-treated patients was 7% absolute risk reduction was 0.5% (95% CI: 0.13–1%; $p = 0.02$) Data from ref. *100*.

The time course of benefit becomes particularly relevant in encouraging the early use of ACE inhibition in patients with MI. In the ISIS-4 and GISSI-3 studies, encompassing 77,444 patients, 219 lives were saved by 4–6 wk of ACE inhibition. Latini and coworkers *(102)* analyzed the time course of the total survival difference between active therapy and control. In both studies, patients were treated within 24 h of presentation. By the end of the first d of therapy, there were already 65 fewer deaths in the treatment arm than in the control group, so that 29.7% of the total difference between groups was already present at the end of d 1. By the end of d 7, the difference between groups had increased to 145 lives, or 66.2% of the total number of lives destined to be saved. The sum total benefit of the remaining weeks of therapy accounted for a minority (33.8%) of lives saved. One must consider whether attenuation of LV remodeling accounts for early survival benefit, or whether any convincing explanation of the early benefit of ACE inhibitor therapy must invoke an anti-ischemic mechanism. Pertinent to the findings of Vaughan and coworkers *(52)* described before, the association of activation of the renin–angiotensin system with greater risk of acute ischemic events has clinical significance. Specifically, if inhibition of the renin–angiotensin system prevents MI and other ischemia through alterations in the fibrinolytic system, then the early benefit of ACE inhibition observed in GISSI-3 and ISIS-4 could be more easily explained.

RECOMMENDED USE OF ACE INHIBITORS DURING ACUTE CORONARY SYNDROMES, IN PARTICULAR MI

As recommended by the ACC/AHA *(45,46)*, ACE inhibition should be started early, when no known contraindications exist, preferably within 24 h in all patients who are suffering an AMI. ACE inhibition should be initiated in the setting of AMI in the absence of hypotension (systolic blood pressure >100 mmHg). Any ACE inhibitor may be used, since the benefits appear to be a class effect *(47)*. However, to avoid hypotension, a small dose of a short-acting agent, such as captopril (6.25 mg), may be used initially, especially in unstable patients or in patients with systolic blood pressure <110 mmHg. An ACE inhibitor should also be given when hypertension persists despite treatment with nitroglycerin and a β-adrenergic antagonist in patients with LV dysfunction or congestive heart failure.

At the present time, treating patients with AMI should include early mechanical or pharmacological reperfusion with thrombolysis, aspirin, β-blockade, and ACE inhibition *(47)*. β-adrenoreceptor blocking agents or thrombolysis with streptokinase may lead to undesirable lowering of blood pressure. Therefore, a cautionary note to be addressed is the potential for hypotension that may occasionally accompany ACE inhibition. Particularly important is the fact that none of the previously mentioned trials were designed to determine optimal dose or frequency of administration of the ACE inhibitor chosen. Targeting dose principles were utilized so clinicians wishing to generate similar results in their own patient population may wish to choose one of the ACE inhibitors studied and administer it in the manner described in hopes of achieving outcomes similar to those in the trials. Also, clinical judgment on the part of the physician plays a key role in determining which patients will benefit from the earliest use of ACE inhibitors.

NEW FRONTIERS

At the present time, most of the beneficial effects of ACE inhibition depend on reduction in angiotensin II levels or activity, although the potential benefit of elevations in bradykinin on venodilation and on the fibrinolytic system should not be discounted. Recently, two new classes of agents have been developed and are being studied in clinical trials, which may prove to have important hemodynamic or anti-ischemic effects possibly equaling or surpassing those of traditional ACE inhibition. Angiotensin II receptor blockers (ARB) such as losartan, valsartan, ibesartan, and candesartan offer selective blockade of the type 1 angiotensin II receptor. This receptor is thought to primarily mediate vasoconstrictive and proliferative effects of angiotensin II. Given the recent appreciation that there are non-ACE pathways for the formation of angiotensin II, direct receptor blockade promises an even more complete reduction of angiotensin II-mediated effects. Preliminary studies suggest some benefits of ARBs in the post-MI setting. However, the reported trials are small, and the positive results do not yet merit widespread clinical application but do support the conduct of several ongoing large-scale trials *(103,104)*.

Spinar et al. *(103)* randomized 201 patients with AMI treated either with direct angioplasty, thrombolysis or heparin alone to captopril or losartan. These patients were followed for 2 wk, and it was found that losartan did not affect diastolic vol but decreased end-systolic vol ($p < 0.001$), resulting in a significant increase in EF and a decrease in

Table 1
Angiotensin-Converting Enzyme Inhibitor

Acute Myocardial Infarction: Selective Clinical Trials[a]					
Study[b]	No.	Duration (d)	Placebo (%)	RR (%)	Lives/1000
SAVE	2231	42	25	19	42
AIRE	2006	15	23	27	57
SMILE	1556	1	8	(22)	18
		12	14	33	41
TRACE	1749	24	42	22	76

[a]Abbreviations: AIRE, Acute Infarction Ramipril Efficacy study; SAVE, Survival and Ventricular Enlargement trial; SMILE, Survival of Myocardial Infarction Long-Term Evaluation trial; TRACE, Trandolapril Cardiac Evaluation trial; RR, risk reduction.

[b]These trials of postinfarct ACE inhibitors studied only high-risk patients: patients with asymptomatic left ventricular dysfunction (SAVE), patients with manifested symptoms of heart failure in the early myocardial infarction period (AIRE), patients with anterior wall myocardial infarction and not receiving thrombolytic therapy (SMILE), and patients with acute myocardial infarction exhibiting wall motion abnormalities (TRACE). Each of these studies have clearly shown a mortality benefit with the use of ACE inhibitors. Data from ref. *102.*

wall-motion index ($p < 0.001$). The authors concluded that ARBs seem to have a more pronounced effect on LV remodeling than ACE inhibitors. Furthermore, in a pilot study by Di Pasquale et al. *(104)*, 99 patients presenting with AMI were randomized to captopril, 75 mg/d plus placebo (50 patients), or to captopril, 75 mg/d plus losartan 12.5 mg as a first dose and 25 mg/d successively. Patients in both groups were similar with regard to age, sex, creatine kinase peak, EF, end-systolic vol, and risk factors. The combination of captopril and losartan had a significantly larger effect in decreasing end-systolic vol at 3 mo than captopril alone during echocardiographic follow-up.

Larger international clinical trials such as Valsartan In Acute Myocardial Infarction trial (VALIANT) *(105)* will further evaluate the role of the addition of ARB to ACE inhibitors or ARB alone in the management of patients with AMI associated with LV dysfunction. The study Optimal Trial in Myocardial Infarction with the Angiotensin II Antagonist Losartan (OPTIMAAL) *(106)* will evaluate the effects of ARB in survival and morbidity when compared to ACE inhibitors in the setting of AMI or reinfarction and heart failure. Of interest, the Evaluation of Losartan in the Elderly (ELITE II) study compared the use of captopril (50 mg 3× daily) to losartan (50 mg daily) in 3152 randomized patients with congestive heart failure, failed to show a mortality benefit of losartan over captopril at 2 yr *(107)*. Thus, while data from large-scale trials are not yet available, ARB might be a useful alternative in the setting of contraindications or patient intolerance to ACE inhibition. Finally, the Candesartan in Heart Failure—Assessment of Reduction in Mortality and Morbidity (CHARM) is a multicenter trial designed to investigate the clinical usefulness of the long-acting angiotensin II type 1 blocker candesartan in a broad spectrum of patients with symptomatic heart failure. CHARM intends to randomize 6500 patients into 3 independent parallel placebo-controlled studies characterized by: (*i*) low LV EF ($>= 40\%$) and ACE inhibitor tolerance, (*ii*) low LV EF and ACE inhibitor intolerance; and (*iii*) normal LV EF and not current use of ACE inhibitor. The primary objective in each trial is to evaluate the effects of candesartan on the combined end point of cardiovascular mortality or congestive heart failure hospitalization *(108)*.

Table 2
Angiotensin-Converting Enzyme Inhibitor Acute

Myocardial Infarction: Broad Inclusion Clinical Trials[a]

Study[b]	No.	Duration (d)	Placebo mortality (%)	RR (%)	Lives/1000
CONSENSUS II	6090	5.0	9.4	Null	—
GISSI-3	19394	1.5	7.1	12.0	8
ISIS-4	58043	1.0	7.6	7.0	5
Chinese	13634	1.0	9.6	9.1	5

[a]Abbreviations: CONSENSUS II, Cooperative New Scandinavian Enalapril Survival study; GISSI-3, Gruppo Italiano per lo Studio della Sopravvivenza nell'Infarto Miocardico; ISIS-4, Fourth International Study of Infarct Survival; RR, risk reduction.

[b]These studies tested the use of ACE inhibitors in a much broader population of patients with acute myocardial infarction not screened for any particular functional or clinical markers of high risk. In all these studies, patients were randomly assigned to receive ACE inhibitors or placebo within 24 h after presentation, except the Chinese study (36 h). Except for the CONSENSUS II, all showed a definite survival benefit with ACE inhibitor therapy. Data from ref. *102*.

Another exciting new pharmacotherapy involves the development of cell surface metalloprotease inhibitors. These agents promise a host of potentially beneficial hemodynamic effects that include inhibition of ACE, inhibition of endopeptidase, and increases in levels of natriuretic peptides. Again, data are inconclusive to suggest whether there is any benefit over standard-of-care ACE inhibition.

At present, based on the totality of evidence, ACE inhibitors represent a mainstay of the therapy of patients during and after acute coronary syndromes, in particular MI.

REFERENCES

1. Tigerstedt R, Bergman PG. The kidneys and the circulation. Scand Arch Physiol 1898;8:223-227-. as translated by Ruskin A., in classics in arterial hypertension. Charles C. Thomas, Springfield, IL, 1956, pp. 273.
2. Goldblatt H, Lynch J, Hanzal RF, Summerville WW. Studies on experimental hypertension. The production of persistent elevation of systolic blood pressure by means of renal ischemia. J Exp Med 1937;59:347–378.
3. Yamazaki T, Komuro I, Kudoh S, et al. Angiotensin II partly mediates mechanical stress-induced cardiac hypertrophy. Circ Res 1995;77:258–265.
4. Drayer JIM, Weber MA, De Young JL. Blood pressure as determinant of cardiac left ventricular muscle mass. Arch Intern Med 1983;143:90–92.
5. Ganau A, Deveraux RB, Pickering TG, et al. Relation of left ventricular hemodynamic load and contractile performance to left ventricular mass in hypertension. Circulation 1990;81:25–36.
6. Schunkert H, Sadoshima JI, Cornelius T, et al. Angiotensin II-induced growth responses in isolated adult rat hearts; evidence for load-independent induction of cardiac protein synthesis by Angiotensin II. Circ Res 1995;76:489–497.
7. Sadoshima JI, Izumo S. Molecular characterization of angiotensin II-induced hypertrophy of cardiac myocytes and hyperplasia of cardiac fibroblasts; critical role of the AT receptor subtype. Circ Res 1993;73:413–423.
8. Linz W, Scholkens BA, Ganten D. Converting enzyme inhibition specifically prevents the development and induces regression of cardiac hypertrophy in rats. Clin Exp Hypertens 1989;11:1325–1350.
9. Mackay RG, Pfeffer MA, Pasternak RC, et al. Left ventricular remodeling following myocardial infarction: a corollary to infarct expansion. Circulation 1986;74:693–702.

10. Mitchell GF, Lamas GA, Vaughan DE, Pfeffer MA. Left ventricular remodeling in the year after first myocardial infarction: a quantitative analysis of contractile segment lengths and ventricular shape. J Am Coll Cardiol 1992;19:1136–1144.

11. Cambien F, Poirier O, Lecerf L, et al. Deletion polymorphism at the angiotensin-converting enzyme gene is a potent risk factor for myocardial infarction. Nature 1992;359:641–644.

12. Lindpaintner K, Pfeffer MA, Kreutz R, et al. A prospective evaluation of an angiotensin-converting enzyme gene polymorphism and the risk of ischemic heart disease. N Engl J Med 1995;332:706–711.

13. Lindpaintner K, Pfeffer MA. Molecular genetics crying wolf? The case of the angiotensin-converting enzyme gene and cardiovascular disease. J Am Coll Cardiol 1995;25:1632–1633.

14. Tiret L, Kee F, Poirier O, et al. Deletion polymorphism in angiotensin-converting enzyme gene associated with parenteral history of myocardial infarction. Lancet 1993;341:991–992.

15. Schunkert H, Hense HW, Holmer SR, et al. Association between a deletion polymorphism of the angiotensin-converting enzyme gene and left ventricular hypertrophy. N Engl J Med 1994;330: 1634–1638.

16. Marian AJ, Yu Q, Workman R, Greve G, Roberts R. Angiotensin-converting enzyme polymorphism in hypertrophic cardiomyopathy and sudden cardiac death. Lancet 1993;342:1085–1086.

17. Ohishi M, Fujii K, Minamino T, et al. A potent genetic risk factor for restenosis. Nat Genet 1994;5: 324–325.

18. Pinto YM, Van Gilst WH, Kingma JH, Schunkert H. Deletion-type allele of the angiotensin-converting enzyme gene is associated with progressive is associated with progressive ventricular dilation after anterior myocardial infarction. J Am Coll Cardiol 1995;25:1622–1626.

19. Kingma JH, Van Gilst WH, Peels CH. Dambrink JHE, Verheught FWA, Wielanga RP. Acute intervention with captopril during thrombolysis in patients with a first anterior myocardial infarction. Eur Heart J 1994;15:898–907.

20. Kohno M, Yokokawa K, Minami M, et al. Association between angiotensin-converting enzyme gene polymorphisms and regression of left ventricular hypertrophy in patients treated with angiotensin-converting enzyme inhibitors. Am J Med 1999;106:544–549.

21. Enseleit F, Hurlimann D, Luscher TF. Vascular protective effects of angiotensin converting enzyme inhibitors and their relation to clinical events. J Cardiovasc Pharm 2001;37(Suppl. 1):S21–S30.

22. Vallance P, Collier J, Moncada S. Effects of endothelium-derived nitric oxide in peripheral arteriolar tone in man. Lancet 1989;2:997.

23. Golino P, Piscione F, Willerson JT, et al. Divergent effects of serotonin on coronary artery dimensions and blood flow in patients with coronary atherosclerosis and control patients. N Engl J Med 1991;324: 641.

24. Nabel EG, Selwyn AP, Ganz P. Large coronary arteries in humans are responsive to changes in blood flow: An endothelium dependent mechanism that fails in patients with atherosclerosis. J Am Coll Cardiol 1990;16:349.

25. Drexler H, Zeiher AM, Wollschläger H, et al. Flow-dependent coronary artery dilatation in humans. Circulation 1989;80:466.

26. Mancini GB, Henry GC, Macaya C, et al. Angiotensin-converting enzyme inhibition with quinapril improves endothelial vasomotor dysfunction in patients with coronary artery disease. The TREND (Trial on reversing endothelial dysfunction) study. Circulation 1996;94:258–265.

27. Takahashi K, Ohyanagi M, Kobayashi S, Iwasaki T, Miyamoto T. Effect of angiotensin-converting enzyme inhibitors and nitroxy groups on human coronary resistance vessels in vitro. J Cardiovasc Pharm 2000;36:417–422.

28. Buikema H, Monnink SH, Tio RA, et al. Comparison of zofenopril and lisinopril to study the role of the sulfhydryl-group in improvement of endothelial dysfunction with ACE-inhibitors in experimental heart failure. Br J Pharm 2000;130:1999–2007.

29. Fuster V, Gersh BJ, Giuliani ER, Tajik AJ, Brandenburg RO, Frye RL. The natural history of idiopathic dilated cardiomyopathy. Am J Cardiol 1981;47:525–531.

30. Waris EK, Siitonen L, Himanka E. Heart size and prognosis in myocardial infarction. Am Heart J 1966;71:187–195.

31. White HD, Norris RM, Brown MA, Brandt PWT, Whitlock RML, Wild CJ. Left ventricular end systolic volume as the major determinant of survival after recovery from myocardial infarction. Circulation 1987;76:44–51.

32. St. John Sutton M, Pfeffer MA, Plappert T, et al. Quantitative two-dimensional echocardiographic measurements are major predictors of adverse cardiovascular events after acute myocardial infarction. The protective effects of captopril. Circulation 1994;89:68–75.

33. Crilley JG, Farrer M. Left ventricular remodeling and brain natriuretic peptide after first myocardial infarction. Heart 2001;86:638–642.
34. Pfeffer MA, Braunwald E, Moye LA, et al. Effects of captopril on mortality and morbidity in patients with left ventricular dysfunction after myocardial infarction: results of the survival and ventricular enlargement trial. N Engl J Med 1992;327:669–677.
35. Rutherford JD, Pfeffer MA, Moyé LA, et al. Effects of Captopril on ischemic effects after myocardial infarction. Circulation 1994;90:1731–1738.
36. Lamas GA, Flaker GC, Mitchell G, et al. The effects of infarct artery patency on prognosis after acute myocardial infarction. The Survival and Ventricular Enlargement Investigators. Circulation 1995;92: 1101–1109.
37. The SOLVD investigators. Effect of enalapril on survival in patients with reduced left ventricular ejection fractions and congestive heart failure. N Engl J Med 1991;325:293–302.
38. The SOLVD investigators. Effects of Enalapril on mortality and development of heart failure in asymptomatic patients with reduced left ventricular ejection fractions. N Engl J Med 1992;327:685–691.
39. The Acute Infarction Ramipril Efficacy (AIRE) study investigators. Effects of ramipril on mortality and morbidity of survivors of acute myocardial infarction with clinical evidence of heart failure. Lancet 1993;542:821–828.
40. Kober L, Torp Pedersen C, Carlsen JE, et al. A clinical trial of the angiotensin-converting enzyme inhibitor trandolapril in patients with left ventricular dysfunction after myocardial infarction. Trandolapril Cardiac Evaluation (TRACE) Study Group. N Engl J Med 1995;333:1670 1676.
41. Heger JJ, Weyman AE, Wann LS, Rogers EW, Dillon JC, Feigenbaum H. Cross-sectional echocardiographic analysis of the extent of left ventricular asynergy in acute myocardial infarction. Circulation 1980;61:1113–1118.
42. Ambrosioni E, Borghi C, Magnani B, for the Survival in Myocardial Infarction long- term evaluation (SMILE) study investigators. The effects of angiotensin-converting enzyme inhibitor Zofenopril on mortality and morbidity after anterior myocardial infarction. N Engl J Med 1995;332:80–85.
43. Yusuf S, Sleight P, Pogue J, Bosch J, Davies R, Dagenais G. Effects of an Angiotensin-converting-enzyme inhibitor, ramipril, on cardiovascular events in high-risk patients. The Heart Outcomes Prevention Evaluation Study Investigators. N Eng J Med 2000;342:145–153.
44. Pfeffer MA, Domanski M, Rosenberg Y, et al. Prevention of events with angiotensin-converting enzyme inhibition (The PEACE study design). Am J Cardiol 1998;82:25H–30H.
45. Ryan TJ, Antman EM, Brooks NH, et al. 1999 Update: ACC/AHA guidelines for the management of patients with acute myocardial infarction. J Am Coll Cardiol 1999;34:890–911.
46. Braunwald E, Antman EM, Beasley JW, et al. ACC/AHA Guidelines for the management of patients with unstable angina and non-ST-segment elevation myocardial infarction. J Am Coll Cardiol 2000;36: 970–1062.
47. Hennekens CH, Albert CM, Godfried SL, Gaziano JM, Buring JE. Adjunctive drug therapy of acute myocardial infarction: evidence from clinical trials. N Eng J Med 1996;335:1660–1667.
48. Peterson JG, Topol EJ, Sapp SK, et al. Evaluation of the effects of aspirin combined with angiotensin-converting enzyme inhibitors in patients with coronary artery disease. Am J Med 2000;109:371–377.
49. Latini R, Tognoni G, Maggioni AP, et al. Clinical effects of early angiotensin-converting enzyme inhibitor treatment for acute myocardial infarction are similar in the presence and absence of aspirin: systematic overview of individual data from 96,712 randomized patients. Angiotensin-converting enzyme inhibitor Myocardial Infarction Collaborative group. J Am Coll Cardiol 2000;3597:1801–1807.
50. Krumholz HM, Chen YT, Wang Y, Radford MJ. Aspirin and angiotensin-converting enzyme inhibitors among elderly survivors of hospitalization for an acute myocardial infarction. Arch Int Med 2001;161:538–544.
51. McAlpine HM, Morton JJ, Leckie B, Rumley A, Gillen G, Dargie HJ. Neuroendocrine activation after acute myocardial infarction. Br Heart J 1988;60:117–124.
52. Vaughan DE, Lamas GA, Pfeffer MA. Role of left ventricular dysfunction in selective neurohumoral activation in the recovery phase of anterior wall acute myocardial infarction. Am J Cardiol 1990;66: 529–533.
53. Cohn JN, Rector TS. Prognosis of congestive heart failure and predictors of mortality. Am J Cardiol 1988;62:25A–30A.
54. Cohn JN, Rector TS, Olivari MT, Levine TB, Francis GS. Plasma norepinephrine, ejection fraction and maximal oxygen consumption as prognostic variables in congestive heart failure. Circulation 1985;72: 285A.

55. Cohn JN, Levine TB, Olivari MT, et al. Plasma norepinephrine as a guide to prognosis in patients with chronic congestive heart failure. N Engl J Med 1984;311:819.
56. Packer M, Lee WH, Kessler PD, Gottlieb SS, Bernstein MS, Kukin ML. Role of neurohumoral mechanisms in determining survival in patients with severe chronic heart failure. Circulation 1987; 75(Suppl. IV):IV-80–IV-92.
57. Rouleau JL, Packer M, Moyè L, et al. Prognostic value of neurohumoral activation in patients with acute myocardial infarction: effect of captopril. J Am Coll Cardiol 1994;24:583–591.
58. Hamsten A, Wiman B, deFaire U, Blombäck M. Increased plasma levels of a rapid inhibitor of tissue plasminogen activator in young survivors of myocardial infarction. N Engl J Med 1985;313:1557–1563.
59. Vaughan DE, Lazos SA, Tong K. Angiotensin II regulates the expression of plasminogen activator inhibitor-1 in cultured endothelial cells. J Clin Invest 1995;95:995–1001.
60. Feener EP, Northrup JM, Aiello LP, King GL. Angiotensin II induces plasminogen activator inhibitor-1 and -2 expression in vascular endothelial and smooth muscle cells. J Clin Invest 1995;95:1353–1362.
61. Ridker PM, Gaboury CL, Conlin PR, Seely EW, Williams GH, Vaughan DE. Stimulation of plasminogen activator in vivo by infusion of angiotensin II. Circulation 1993;87:1969–1973.
62. Brown NJ, Nadeau J, Vaughan DE. Stimulation of tissue-type plasminogen activator in vivo by infusion of bradykinin. Thromb Haemost 1997;77:522–525.
63. Vaughan DE, Rouleau JL, Ridker PM, Arnold JMO, Menapace FJ, Pfeffer MA. On behalf of the HEART study investigators. Effects of Ramipril on plasma fibrinolytic balance in patients with acute anterior myocardial infarction. Circulation 1997;96:442–447.
64. Minai K, Matsumoto T, Horie H, et al. Bradykinin stimulates the release of tissue plasminogen activator in human coronary circulation: effects of angiotensin-converting enzyme inhibitors. J Am Coll Cardiol 2001;37:1565–1570.
65. Soejima H, Ogawa H, Yasue H, et al. Angiotensin-converting enzyme inhibition reduces monocyte chemoattractant protein-1 and tissue factor levels in patients with myocardial infarction. J Am Coll Cardiol 1999;34:983–988.
66. Saksela O, Rifkin DB. Cell-associated plasminogen activation: regulation and physiologic functions. Am Rev Cell Biol 1988;4:93–126.
67. Kennon S, Barakat K, Hitman G, et al. Angiotensin-converting enzyme inhibition is associated with reduced troponin release in non-ST-elevation acute coronary syndromes. J Am Coll Cardiol 2001;38: 724–728.
68. Zurbano MJ, Anguera I, Heras M, et al. Captopril administration reduces thrombus formation and surface expression of platelet glycoprotein IIb/IIa in early postmyocardial infarction stage. Arterioscler Thromb Vasc Biol 1999;19:1791–1795
69. Pitt B. Natural history of patients with congestive heart failure. Potential role of converting enzyme inhibitors in improving survival. Am J Med 1986;81:32–35.
70. Webster MWI, Fitzpatrick MA, Nicholls MG, Ikram H, Wells JE. Effect of enalapril on ventricular arrhythmias in congestive heart failure. A double blind controlled trial. Br Heart J 1984;52:530–535.
71. Linz W, Scholkens BA, Han Y-F. Beneficial effects of the converting enzyme inhibitor ramipril in ischemic rat hearts. J Cardiovasc Pharmacol 1986;8:591–599.
72. Franz MR, Burkhoff D, Yue DT, Sagawa K. Mechanically induced action potential changes and arrhythmia in isolated and in situ canine hearts. Cardiovasc Res 1989;23:213–223.
73. Lown B, Verrier RL. Neural activity and ventricular fibrillation. N Engl J Med 1976;294:1165.
74. Moorman RM, Kirsch GE, Lacerda AE, Brown AM. Angiotensin II modulates cardiac Na+ channels in neonatal rat. Circ Res 1989;65:1804–1809.
75. Reiter MJ, Synhorst DP, Mann DE. Electrophysiological effects of acute ventricular dilatation in the isolated rabbit hearts. Am J Physiol 1993;265:1544–1550.
76. deGraeff PA, de Langen CDJ, Van Gilst WH, et al. Protective effects of captopril against ischemia/reperfusion-induced ventricular arrhythmias in vitro and in vivo. Am J Med 1988;67:67–74.
77. Kingma JH, de Graeff PA, Van Gilst WH, Van Binsbergen E, de Langen CDJ, Wesseling H. Effects of intravenous captopril on inducible sustained ventricular tachycardia one week after experimental infarction in the anesthetized pig. Postgrad Med J 1986;62:159–163.
78. Chiladakis JA, Karapanos G, Agelopoulos G, Alexopoulos D, Manolis AS. Effects of early captopril therapy after myocardial infarction on the incidence of late potentials. Clin Cardiol 2000;23:96–102.
79. Spargias KS, Lindsay SJ, Hall AS, Cowan JC, Ball SG. Ramipril reduces QT dispersion in patients with acute myocardial infarction and heart failure. Am J Cardiol 1999;83:969–971.

80. Pedersen OD, Bagger H, Kober L, Torp-Pedersen C. Trandolapril reduces the incidence of atrial fibrillation after acute myocardial infarction in patients with left ventricular dysfunction. Circulation 1999;100:376–380.

81. Singh SN, Karsik P, Hafley GE, et al. Electrophysiologic and clinical effects of angiotensin-converting enzyme inhibitors in patients with prior myocardial infarction, non-sustained ventricular tachycardia, and depressed left ventricular function. MUSTT investigators. Multicenter Unsustained Tachycardia trial. Am J Cardiol 2001;87:716–720.

82. Tuininga YS, Wiesfeld AC, van Veldhuisen DJ, et al. Electrophysiologic changes of angiotensin-converting enzyme inhibition after myocardial infarction. J Card Failure 2000;6:77–79.

83. Hutchins GM, Bulkley BH. Infarct expansion versus extension: two different complications of acute myocardial infarction. Am J Cardiol 1978;41:1127–1132.

84. Weisman HF, Bush DE, Mannisi JA, Weisfeldt ML, Healy B. Cellular mechanisms of myocardial infarct expansion. Circulation 1988;78:186–201.

85. Mitchell GF, Lamas GA, Vaughan DE, Pfeffer MA. Left ventricular remodeling in the year after first anterior myocardial infarction: a quantitative analysis of contractile segment lengths and ventricular shape. J Am Coll Cardiol 1992;19:1136–1144.

86. McKay RG, Pfeffer MA, Pasternak RC, et al. Left ventricular remodeling following myocardial infarction: a corollary to infarct expansion. Circulation 1986;74:693–702.

87. Brown EJ, Kloner RA, Schoen FJ, Hammerman H, Hale S, Braunwald E. Scar thinning due to ibuprofen administration after experimental myocardial infarction. Am J Cardiol 1983;51:877–883.

88. Burton AC. The importance of the shape and size of the heart. Am Heart J 1957;54:801–810.

89. Herman MV, Gorlin R. Implications of left ventricular asynergy. Am J Cardiol 1969;23:538–547.

90. Sun Y, Weber KT. Infarct scar: a dynamic tissue. Cardiovasc Res 2000;46:250–256.

91. Jugdutt BI, Schwartz-Michorowski BL, Tymchak WJ, Burton JR. Prompt improvement of left ventricular function and preservation of topography with combined reperfusion and intravenous nitroglycerin in acute myocardial infarction. Cardiology 1997;88:170–179.

92. Pfeffer MA, Pfeffer JM. Ventricular enlargement and reduced survival after myocardial infarction. Circulation 1987;75:IV93–97.

93. Pfeffer MA, Lamas GA, Vaughan DE, Parisi AF, Braunwald E. Effects of captopril on progressive ventricular dilatation after anterior myocardial infarction. N Engl J Med 1988;319:80–86.

94. Sharpe N, Murphy J, Smith H, Hannan S. Treatment of patients with symptomless left ventricular dysfunction after myocardial infarction. Lancet 1988;1:255–259.

95. White M, Roleau JL, Hall C, et al. Changes in vasoconstrictive hormones, natriuretic peptides, and left ventricular remodeling soon after anterior myocardial infarction. Am J Cardiol 2001;142:1056–1064.

96. Konermann M, Sanner BM, Altmann C, et al. Is the tissue affinity of ACE inhibitors of relevance for the remodeling of the left ventricular wall following myocardial infarction? Estimations with cine magnetic resonance imaging. Cardiology 2000;94:179–187.

97. de Kam PJ, Voors AA, van den Berg MP, et al. Effect of very early angiotensin-converting enzyme inhibition on left ventricular dilation after myocardial infarction in patients receiving thrombolysis: results of a meta-analysis of 845 patients. J Am Coll Cardiol 2000;36:2047–2053.

98. Swedberg K, Held P, Kjekshus J, Rasmussen K, Ryden L, Wedel H. Effects of early administration of enalapril on mortality in patients with acute myocardial infarction: results of the Cooperative New Scandinavian Enalapril Survival Study II. N Engl J Med 1992;327:678–684.

99. Gruppo Italiano per lo Studio della Sopravvivenza nell'Infarcto miocardico. GISSI-3: effects of lisinopril and transdermal glyceryl trinitrate singly and together on 6-week mortality and ventricular function after acute myocardial infarction. Lancet 1994;343:1115–1122.

100. ISIS-4. Collaborative Group. Fourth international study of infarct survival (ISIS-4): a randomized factorial trial assessing early oral captopril oral mononitrate and intravenous magnesium sulfate in 58,050 patients with suspected acute myocardial infarction. Lancet 1995;345:669–685.

101. Oral captopril versus placebo among 14,962 patients with suspected acute myocardial infarction: a multicenter, randomized, double-blind, placebo-controlled clinical trial. Chinese Cardiac Study (CCS-1) Collaborative Group. Chin Med J 1997;110:834–838.

102. Latini R, Maggioni AP, Flather M, Sleight P, Tognoni G. ACE inhibitor use in patients with myocardial infarction: summary of evidence from clinical trials. Circulation 1995;92:3132–3137.

103. Spinar J, Vitovec J, Spinarova L, et al. A comparison of intervention with losartan or captopril in acute myocardial infarction. Eur J Heart Fail 2000;2:91–100.

104. Di Pasquale P, Bucca V, Scalzo S, Cannizzaro S, Giubilato A, Paterna S. Does the addition of losartan improve the beneficial effects of ACE inhibitors in patients with anterior myocardial infarction? A pilot study. Heart 1999;81:606–611.
105. Pffefer MA, McMurray J, Leizorovicz A, et al. Valsartan in acute myocardial infarction trial (VALIANT): rationale and design. Am Heart J 2000;140;727–750.
106. Dickstein K, Kjekshus J, OPTIMAAL Trial committee and investigators. Optimal Trial in Myocardial Infarction with the Angiotensin II Antagonist Losartan. Comparison of baseline data, initial course, and management: losartan versus captopril following acute myocardial infarction (The OPTIMAAL Trial). OPTIMAAL Trial Steering committee and investigators. Optimal Trial in myocardial infarction with the angiotensin II antagonist losartan. Am J Cardiol 2001;87:766–771.
107. Pitt B, Poole-Wilson PA, Segal R, et al. Effect of losartan compared with captopril on mortality in patients with symptomatic heart failure: randomized trial—the Losartan Heart Failure Survival Study ELITE II. Lancet 2000;355:1582–1587.
108. Swedberg K, Pfeffer M, Granger C, et al. Candesartan in heart failure—assessment of reduction in mortality and morbidity (CHARM): rationale and design. Charm-Programme Investigators. J Card Failure 1999;5:276–282.

15 Risk Stratification

Exercise Testing, Imaging, and
Cardiac Catheterization

Sanjeev Puri, MD, Hani A. Razek, MD, and Bernard R. Chaitman, MD, FACC

CONTENTS

INTRODUCTION

Each year, approx 1.1 million patients in the United States suffer an acute myocardial infarction (AMI) and 440,000 die *(1)*. The number of index vs recurrent MI events is 650,000 and 450,000, respectively. Reperfusion therapy, increased use of adjunctive medication such as aspirin, β-blockers, angiotensin-converting enzyme inhibitors, and lipid lowering therapy coupled with better risk stratification to identify those most likely to benefit from early coronary revascularization has led to significant improved long-term prognosis after MI.

Effective risk stratification after AMI encompasses several phases; emergency triage within the initial hours of symptom onset, the intermediate hospital phase, and the pre-hospital discharge or early (< 3 wk) posthospital discharge phase. The risk estimates for mortality provided in this chapter are based on physiologic information provided by a detailed clinical history, judicious use of certain noninvasive tests, anatomic information provided by coronary angiography in selected patients, and prognostic importance of various treatment options that may favorably impact long-term survival. The focus of this chapter is to review risk stratification procedures in the early postinfarction phase to identify higher risk patients that may benefit from therapeutic treatment strategies that reduce mortality.

From: *Contemporary Cardiology: Management of Acute Coronary Syndromes, Second Edition*
Edited by: C. P. Cannon © Humana Press Inc., Totowa, NJ

Risk Factor	Points
Age 65-74	2
Age >75	3
Killip II-IV	2
Systolic Blood Pressure <100	2
DM, h/o HTN, or h/o angina	1
Anterior STEMI or LBBB	1
Weight < 67 kg	1
Time to treatment >4 hours	1

Risk Score (0 - 14 possible points)

Fig. 1. TIMI risk score for STEMI. Adapted with permission from ref. *2*.

EARLY CLINICAL RISK STRATIFICATION

The use of clinical and electrocardiogram (ECG) variables alone at the time of hospital admission in patients with ST-segment elevation myocardial infarction (STEMI) was examined in the InTIME II database of 14,114 patients treated within 4 h of symptom onset with lanoteplase (nPA) or tissue-type plasminogen activator (tPA), aspirin, and heparin to predict 30-d mortality *(2)*. Ten independent variables accounting for 97% of the overall predictive capacity for increased 30-d mortality risk were included in the Thrombolysis in Myocardial Ischemia (TIMI) risk score for STEMI (Fig. 1). Of the 10 variables, diabetes, history of hypertension, and prior history of angina were grouped as a composite variable for a final variable set of 8 components. The mortality rate was <1% with a score of zero and increased to 35.9% for a score >8 (Fig. 2). The InTIME risk score for patients treated with thrombolytic therapy was tested in the TIMI 9 trial and showed similar prognostic capacity. The authors then tested the score in the National Registries of Myocardial Infarction (NRMI) III registry of 84,029 patients with STEMI. Patients in NRMI III tended to be older, more often female, and have a history of coronary artery disease more often than those in the derivation set; 48% received reperfusion therapy. The risk score showed strong prognostic capacity overall and among patients with acute reperfusion therapy. However, among patients not receiving reperfusion therapy, the risk score underestimated death rates and offered lower discriminatory capacity *(3)*.

Cannon et al. examined the use of a risk score to diagnose patients with acute coronary syndrome and non-STEMI to determine likelihood of developing a non-Q-MI *(4)*. Four of 50 baseline variables independently predicted non-Q-MI. The four risk factors were absence of prior percutaneous transluminal coronary angioplasty (PTCA), chest pain >60 min, ST deviation on presenting ECG, and recent onset angina. The risk of non-Q-MI was 7, 19.6, 24.4, 49.9, and 70.6% for 0, 1, 2, 3, or 4 risk factors, respectively.

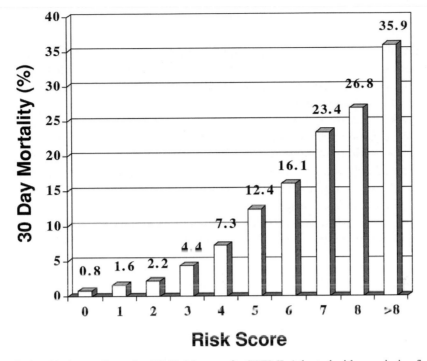

Fig. 2. Predicting 30-d mortality using TIMI risk score for STEMI. Adapted with permission from ref. *2*.

Age

Age is a major risk factor for increased mortality in patients after AMI treated with thrombolytic therapy. In-hospital mortality rates were 28% in patients >85 yr in the community-based NRMI *(5)*, 21% after 30 d in patients >65 yr in the Cooperative Cardiovascular Project, 11.2% in patients ≥ 70 yr in the TIMI II trial after 42 d, and 17.2% in patients >70 yr after 30 d in the Global Use of Strategies To Open Occluded Arteries in Acute Coronary Syndromes (GUSTO)-1 trial *(6–9)*.

By contrast, in-hospital mortality rates were only 3, 3.8, and 1.1% in patients <55 yr, <50 yr, and <45 yr enrolled in the Myocardial Infarction Registry, TIMI II trial, and GUSTO-1 trials, respectively *(5,9–11)*. Older patients are prone to an increased reinfarction rate and readmission for cardiac events *(8)*. Multivessel coronary disease, important comorbid conditions, and aging myocardium with concomitant decreased myocardial reserve explains some of the increased mortality risk compared to younger individuals.

Gender

Women tend to be older than men at the time of first infarction and have a greater prevalence of associated comorbidity *(12,13)*. The 35-d mortality rate for women compared with men was 12.5 vs 8.2% in the Fibrinolytic Therapy Trialists Group *(11)*. In this report, 44% of patients >75 yr were women. Kober et al. *(14)* reported a 1-yr mortality rate of 28% for women and 21% for men in a consecutive series of 6676 patients with AMI; the increased mortality risk in women occurred relatively early (<30 d).

Diabetes Mellitus and Stress Hyperglycemia

Diabetes mellitus increases the relative risk of in-hospital mortality by at least 1.5–2 compared with nondiabetic patients *(15)*. Diabetic women in particular have a relatively poor prognosis, in part related to an increased incidence of congestive heart failure, reinfarction, and recurrent ischemic events *(15–18)*. Late mortality is significantly increased in diabetic compared with nondiabetic patients *(19)*.

Stress hyperglycemia at the time of MI is strongly correlated with mortality rates. In a meta-analysis conducted by Capes et al. *(20)*, data from 15 trials reporting admission glucose concentrations in relation to in-hospital mortality or heart failure rates after AMI were reviewed. In the patients without known diabetes, those with a glucose concentration ≥109–143 mg/dL had a 3.9-fold higher risk of death compared to patients with lower glucose concentrations. At glucose concentrations of ≥143–180 mg/dL, the risk of cardiogenic shock or heart failure was increased 3-fold. In patients with frank diabetes, glucose concentrations ≥180–196 mg/dL were associated with a moderate risk of death (relative risk 1.7).

Race

The 1-yr mortality rate in TIMI II was similar in White, African-American, and Hispanic patients, although the presence of atherosclerotic risk factors was greater in African-American and Hispanics *(21)*. Similar findings were reported in the Charleston Heart Study *(22)* and GUSTO-1 (after 30 d) *(9)*; however, African-American patients had >2-fold increase risk of late death at 1 yr after adjustment for other prognostic factors in the GUSTO-1 *(23)*. Secondary prevention measures are likely to be an area of future research into race related differences in outcome.

Prior MI

The relative mortality risk of patients with a previous MI is approx 1.5× greater than in patients with a first infarction regardless of whether or not the patient is treated with thrombolytic therapy *(9,11)*. The mortality gradient is greatest in patients with major left ventricular (LV) dysfunction prior to the reinfarction event. In TIMI II, a prior vs no prior history of MI was associated with 7.9 vs 4.3% mortality rate after 42 d *(6)*. Multivessel coronary disease was present in 60 vs 28% of patients with prior vs no prior infarction.

Prior Revascularization

In GUSTO-1, the 30-d mortality rate was 10.7% in 41,021 patients who had prior coronary bypass grafting vs 6.7% in those without prior cardiac surgery. The mortality rates were 5.6 vs 7.0% in patients who had prior vs no prior coronary angioplasty *(9)*.

Physical Examination

Hypotension, systolic pressure <100 mmHg, sinus tachycardia (ventricular rate >100 beats/min), a third heart sound, jugular venous distension, and pulmonary rales may indicate significant LV dysfunction and are markers of increased mortality *(2,23–25)*. The physical examination is important in the early recognition of catastrophic mechanical complications such as ventricular septal defect, mitral valve dysfunction, or myocardial rupture.

Pulmonary Edema

Detection of clinical or radiologic evidence of congestive heart failure is a strong indicator of cardiac events. The 1-yr cardiac mortality of patients with acute pulmonary edema approaches 25–30% (26,27). In the acute postinfarct phase, pulmonary edema may represent permanent damage from the infarct and myocardial stunning as a result of the ischemic insult. The finding of clinical evidence of pulmonary congestion as a prognostic indicator is independent of ejection fraction measurements at the time of hospital discharge (28).

Cardiogenic Shock

Cardiogenic shock occurs in approx 7% of patients in the acute infarct setting and is associated with a mortality rate >70% (29,30). Retrospective analyses of thrombolytic trials do not show a significant mortality reduction in patients presenting with cardiogenic shock (11,31,32). In an overview of 386 patients who were treated with coronary angioplasty for cardiogenic shock, Bates and Topol (31) reported an overall reperfusion rate of 73% and inhospital mortality rate of 44%. Emergency coronary bypass grafting in this setting has an associated mortality rate of approx 40% (31). The approximate 60% survival rate after coronary revascularization is better than the expected 70% mortality rate. The SHOCK trial (33) randomized 302 patients with cardiogenic shock <36 h post-MI to conventional medical therapy with thrombolysis or to acute coronary revascularization; 64% of patients received percutaneous coronary intervention (PCI) and 36% received coronary artery bypass graft (CABG). At 6 mo, mortality was significantly lower among patients receiving earlier revascularization compared to conventional therapy (50.3 vs 63.1%) (p < 0.05). Mortality was not significantly different at 30 d. Thus, an early revascularization strategy for patients with cardiogenic shock is associated with improved 6-mo survival rates.

White Cell Count

Elevated white blood cell counts (WBCs) are associated with a higher risk of adverse events after an AMI. In the TIMI 10A and B trials (n = 975), an elevated WBC was associated with resistance to thrombolytic therapy, lower coronary artery patency at 60 and 90 min, worse TIMI myocardial perfusion grades and increased thrombus burden. When the WBC counts were >15,000/μL, the 30-d mortality was 10.4% vs 0–4.9% for WBC counts <15,000/μL. Shock or heart failure was also more common in patients with higher WBC counts (17% vs 0–6%).

C-Reactive Protein

C-reactive protein (CRP) within 6 h of an AMI is predictive of in-hospital adverse coronary events. In a study (34) of 234 patients with AMI who underwent primary angioplasty and stenting, elevated CRP ≥0.3 mg/dL was associated with a 22.4% incidence of coronary reocclusion, reinfarction, target vessel revascularization, and death compared to 4.3% in patients with normal levels. The need for bailout stenting was increased in patients with elevated CRP levels (61 vs 38%).

Cardiac Troponin

Cardiac troponin measurements improve MI detection and allow early risk stratification in acute coronary syndromes. In GUSTO IIA (35), 30-d mortality was 13% among

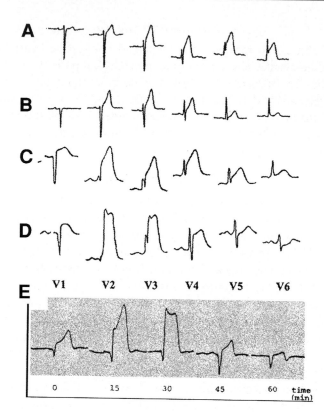

Fig. 3. Prognostic information from ECG patterns. **(A and B)** From patients without distortion of terminal position of the QRS complex. **(C and D)** From patients with terminal QRS distortion (emergence of J point at >50% of R-wave in leads with qR configuration or disappearance of S-wave in leads with Rs configuration). Reproduced with permission from ref. *40*. **(E)** From a patient with anterior infarction with additional STE 15 min after initiation of thrombolysis with final resolution suggestive of favorable clinical outcome. Reproduced with permission from ref. *47*.

patients with STEMI and a positive cardiac troponin T (cTnT) on admission vs 4.7% among those with negative cTnT results. This was confirmed by Giannitsis et al. *(36)*, who reported a 9-mo mortality of 14 vs 3.9% among patients with STEMI and admission cTnT >0.1 ng/mL vs <0.1 mg/mL. Incomplete reperfusion was more common in patients with increased cTnT. In the Fragmin During Instability in Coronary Artery Disease (FRISC) study and other studies of patients with an acute coronary syndrome *(36–38)*, cTnT >0.1 ng/mL predicts a lower likelihood of achieving TIMI III grade flow in the infarct related vessel with thrombolytic therapy or primary PCI.

Increased mortality rates among STEMI patients with elevated admission cTnT may be due to later presentation after symptom onset, microvascular dysfunction, or failure to achieve post procedural TIMI III flow. Higher rates of congestive heart failure and shock are also associated with elevated levels of cardiac troponin *(39)*.

The 12-Lead ECG

ECG findings associated with increased mortality risk include anterior STE, distortion of the terminal portion of the QRS complex (Fig. 3), left bundle-branch block, right bundle-branch block, advanced atrioventricular block, and atrial fibrillation

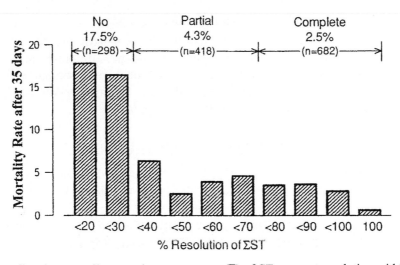

Fig. 4. Thirty-five-day mortality rates by percent sum (Σ) of ST segment resolution within 3 h after start of thrombolysis. Reproduced with permission from ref. *49*.

(9,11,21,40). In GUSTO-1, the 30-d mortality rate was 9.9 vs 5.0% in patients with anterior vs inferior STE. The relative risk of death, reinfarction, or congestive heart failure was 4-fold greater in patients with inferior infarction if ST-segment depression was also noted in the anterior lead group, particularly leads V4–V6 or if evidence of right ventricular involvement was present *(41–45)*. In GUSTO-1, the 30-d mortality rates were 18.7, 17, 14, and 17% for patients with left bundle-branch block, right bundle-branch block, left anterior fascicular block, and left posterior fascicular block, respectively, compared with 6% in patients with a normal conduction pattern *(46)*.

Early resolution of STE (within hours of thrombolysis) is associated with a more favorable prognosis than in patients with persistent STE. Additional STE over and above the initial elevation seen in the first h of thrombolysis with ultimate resolution is also associated with favorable clinical outcome *(47)* (Fig. 3E). The 30- and 180-d mortality rates of patients who had >50% resolution of STE within 4 h of treatment were 3.5 and 5.7% compared to 5.7 and 7.4% in patients without these findings in the Gruppo Italiano per lo Studio della Sopravvienza nell'Infarto Miocardico (GISSI)-2 *(48)*. The International Joint Efficacy Comparison of Thrombolytics (INJECT) study, which compared the effects of reteplase or streptokinase in 6010 patients reported a 35-d mortality rate of 2.5% in patients with complete resolution of STE compared with 17.5% in patients without ST-segment resolution *(49)* (Fig. 4).

LV function can be estimated from the resting ECG at the time of hospital discharge. Silver et al. *(50)* reported a positive predictive value of 98% to estimate LV ejection fraction >40% in patients with new non-anterior Q wave infarction, no previous history of Q wave MI, or congestive heart failure. The findings were validated in 10,756 patients enrolled in GUSTO-1 *(51)*.

New Q waves as compared to absence of new Q waves at the time of presentation to the emergency room are also associated with higher cardiac mortality rates at 30 d (7 vs 2%) and at 5 yr (16 vs 6%) *(52)*.

Early Coronary Angiography

In the acute infarct setting, coronary angiography is usually performed because of hemodynamic instability, persistent chest pain, or evidence of continued infarct artery occlusion and thrombolytic ineligibility (53–57). Clinical trials comparing PTCA with thrombolytic therapy or PTCA in the setting of failed thrombolysis or ineligibility for thrombolytic drugs are discussed in subsequent chapters.

INTERMEDIATE HOSPITAL PHASE

In the intermediate phase of hospitalization (>24 h after admission), low-risk patients who might be candidates for early hospital discharge should be identified (58,59). In TIMI II, absence of significant risk factors at the time of emergency room presentation was associated with a 6-wk mortality rate of only 1.5% (6). In the Thrombolysis and Angioplasty in Acute Myocardial Infarction (TAMI) trials, Mark et al. (60) reported on 708 patients who underwent early coronary angiography and identified 30% of patients at low risk who were discharged on d 4 after the index event. In GISSI-2, 53% of patients were able to perform an exercise test and had an ejection fraction >40%; the 6-mo mortality rate after hospital discharge was <1% (61). In GUSTO, absence of ischemic cardiac complications and need for coronary revascularization or cardioversion was reported in 57.3% of enrolled patients, 30-d mortality rate was 1%, and the 1-yr mortality rate was 3.6% (62). Low-risk patient subsets account for as many as half of all recent postinfarct survivors and may not require extended hospitalization or expensive diagnostic procedures. Active cholesterol lowering therapy as per the National Cholesterol Education Project guidelines, motivation to stop smoking, and identification of social isolation and depression are all part of the postinfarct rehabilitative strategy.

Recurrent ischemic cardiac pain, reinfarction, and congestive heart failure significantly increase mortality risk during the intermediate hospital phase. In TIMI II, reinfarction significantly increased mortality rates after 3 yr of follow-up (63). In the TAMI trials, the in-hospital mortality rate was 21% for reinfarction, 11% for recurrent ischemia, and 4% when neither complication occurred. Congestive heart failure symptoms occurred in 50% of patients who developed reinfarction, 31% of patients who developed recurrent ischemia, and 17% of patients when neither ischemic complication occurred (64). Recurrent in-hospital ischemic cardiac events after infarction are a class I indication for cardiac catheterization according to American College of Cardiology/American Heart Association (ACC/AHA) guidelines (57).

PREDISCHARGE RISK STRATIFICATION

The use of noninvasive testing in the prethrombolytic era for risk stratification after AMI has been extensively reviewed (65–67). The predictive value of noninvasive testing for cardiac events is somewhat less in patients who received thrombolysis or direct coronary angioplasty; the patients tend to be younger, have better preserved left ventricular function, and have less extensive multivessel coronary disease (Fig. 5) (68). A substantial number of patients who undergo early coronary angiography have high-risk anatomy and are subsequently revascularized. This results in a relative low-risk patient population at the time of hospital discharge with a subsequent anticipated lower number of cardiac events to be investigated by noninvasive testing. The 1-yr mortality rates

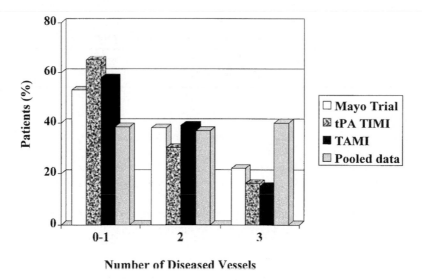

Fig. 5. Comparison of angiographic findings in reperfusion trials with the pooled data from studies done in the prethrombolytic era. Reproduced with permission from ref. *68*.

in patients who survive to hospital discharge range from 2 to 3.3% in the TIMI II and the Should We Intervene Following Thrombolysis? (SWIFT) trials, respectively *(69–71)*. Thus, according to Bayesian theory, noninvasive testing would need to be extremely precise to separate the 98 patients who survive from the 2 to 3 patients that will die in the year following AMI.

Acute coronary syndrome patients with an uncomplicated course that are ambulatory at the time of hospital discharge are generally lower risk individuals, since those with a complicated course have either died or received coronary revascularization procedures. Guidelines for the noninvasive evaluation of low risk patients at or around the time of hospital discharge were reviewed in the 1999 ACC/AHA Update of Acute Myocardial Infarct Guidelines. Three classes of recommendations for the noninvasive evaluation are published. Class I indications are conditions for which there is general evidence or general agreement that a given procedure or treatment is beneficial, useful, and effective. Class II indications are conditions for which there is conflicting evidence or divergent opinion about the usefulness/efficacy of a procedure or treatment. A class IIA guideline indicates the weight of evidence/opinion is in favor of usefulness/efficacy, whereas a class IIB indication is less well established by evidence/opinion. The class III indication are conditions for which there is evidence or general agreement that a procedure/treatment is not useful/effective and in some cases may be harmful. Table 1 illustrates the three different class indications for the use of noninvasive test procedures for lower risk postmyocardial infarct survivors.

Echocardiography

Two-dimensional echocardiogram with Doppler analysis is the preferred noninvasive method for evaluation of overall and regional left and right ventricular systolic and diastolic function, valvular integrity and function, and detecting mechanical complications of AMI. Predischarge LV function assessment is among the most important and accu-

Table 1
Preparation for Discharge from the Hospital

Noninvasive Evaluation of Low Risk Patients
Recommendations

Class I
1. Stress ECG
   a. Before discharge for prognostic assessment or functional capacity (submaximal at 4–6 d or symptom-limited at 10–14 d).
   b. Early after discharge for prognostic assessment and functional capacity (14–21 d).
   c. Late after discharge (3–6 wk) for functional capacity and prognosis if early stress was submaximal.
2. Exercise, vasodilator stress nuclear scintigraphy, or exercise stress echocardiography when baseline abnormalities of the ECG compromise interpretation.[a]

Class IIa
1. Dipyridamole or adenosine stress perfusion nuclear scintigraphy or dobutamine echocardiography before discharge for prognostic assessment in patients judged to be unable to exercise.
2. Exercise 2-dimensional echocardiography or nuclear scintigraphy (before or early after discharge for prognostic assessment).

Class III
1. Stress testing within 2 to 3 d of AMI.
2. Either exercise or pharmacological stress testing at any time to evaluate patients with unstable postinfarction angina pectoris.
3. At any time to evaluate patients with AMI who have uncompensated congestive heart failure, cardiac arrhythmia, or noncardiac conditions that severely limit their ability to exercise.
4. Before discharge to evaluate patients who have already been selected for cardiac catheterization. In this situation, an exercise test may be useful after catheterization to evaluate function or identify ischemia in distribution of a coronary lesion of borderline severity.

[a]Marked abnormalities in the rest ECG as left bundle-branch block (LBBB), LV hypertrophy with strain, ventricular pre-excitation, or a ventricular paced rhythm render a displacement of the ST-segments virtually uninterpretable. For patients taking digoxin or who have <1 mm ST-depression on their resting tracing who undergo standard stress electrocardiographic testing, it must be realized that further ST-depression with exercise may have minimal diagnostic significance.
Adapted with permission from ACC/AHA 1999 MI Guidelines (57).

rate predictors of subsequent cardiac events after AMI. Increased LV vol, extensive LV wall motion abnormalities, and severe depressed LV ejection fraction identify patients at significant increased mortality risk in the 1- to 5-yr follow-up after AMI (Fig. 6 and Table 2) *(28,72–79)*. Assessment of LV diastolic function and LV filling patterns on Doppler echocardiography provide additional information in the setting of AMI. Cerisano et al. report that restrictive filling patterns (short deceleration time and increased early rapid filling wave [E]/filling wave due to atrial contraction [A] ratio) were strong predictors of LV remodeling, and they identified patients at higher risk of progressive LV dilation within 6 mo after MI (Fig. 7) *(80)*. Nijland et al. *(81)* report 1-yr survival rates of 100% for nonrestrictive vs 50% for restrictive mitral valve inflow problems after MI. Patients with a restrictive filling pattern had larger enzymatic infarct

Table 2
Noninvasive Tests, Echocardiography, and Prognostic Value of Resting Wall Motion Abnormalities in Patients with AMI[a]

Study[b] (reference)	Year	No. of patients	Sensitivity (%)	Specificity (%)	PPA (%)	NPV (%)	End points
Gibson et al. (72)	1982	68	79	61	34	92	Cardiogenic shock
Horowitz et al. (73)	1982	43	85	17	69	93	Death, serious arrhythmias, pump failure
Nishimura et al. (74)	1984	61	80	90	89	32	Death, serious arrhythmias, pump failure
Jaarsma et al. (75)	1988	77	88	57	35	95	Severe heart failure
Saabia et al. (76)	1991	30	100	12	46	100	Shock, arrythmias, angina

[a]Abbreviations: PPA, positive predictive accuracy; NPV, negative predictive value.
[b]Thrombolysis was not used in these studies.

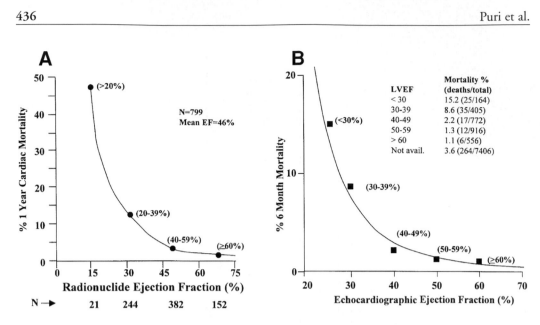

Fig. 6. Effect of LV function on survival following MI; **(A)** Prethrombolytic era; the curvilinear relationship between radionuclide ejection fraction and 1-yr cardiac mortality showing a sharp increase in mortality with ejection fraction <40%. **(B)** Thrombolytic era: although not strictly comparable to panel A, the same curvilinear relationship between echocardiographic ejection fraction and 6-mo mortality rates suggest that the use of thrombolytic therapy shifts the mortality curve to the left. Reproduced with permission from ref. *27*.

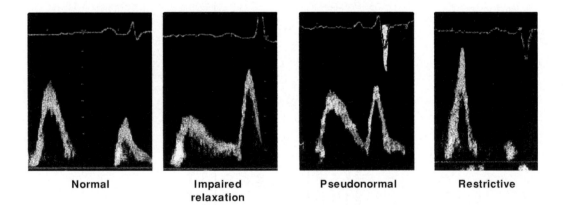

Fig. 7. Pulsed-wave doppler recording of mitral inflow velocities to identify diastolic filling patterns. Normal, DT ≥ 160–240 ms with E/A ratio >1.0; Impaired relaxation, DT ≥240 ms with E/A ratio < 1.0; Pseudonormal, DT 160–200 ms with E/A ratio 1–1.5; Restrictive, DT <160 ms with E/A ratio >1.5. DT, deceleration time; E, early rapid filling wave; A, filling wave due to atrial contraction; ms, milliseconds.

size, larger LV end-diastolic and end-systolic vol indexes, lower ejection fractions, higher wall motion score index, and more frequent symptoms of heart failure than patients without restrictive patterns.

Sakate et al. *(82)* examined 44 patients after MI with cardiopulmonary exercise testing and echo Doppler studies. LV ejection fraction did not correlate to exercise capacity, whereas Doppler echo indices of LV diastolic function correlated with exercise capacity in this cohort of patients with mild cardiac dysfunction. Similar results were reported by Miyashita et al. *(83)*.

Exercise Electrocardiography

The use of exercise electrocardiography provides an estimate of functional capacity after an infarction to prepare patients for cardiac rehabilitation and occupational work evaluation and also provides information regarding adequacy of medical therapy or coronary revascularization therapy and on subsequent cardiac event rates.

Functional capacity and the ability to generate an adequate systolic blood pressure response are major predictors of medium- and long-term mortality after AMI. Patients who are unable to perform an exercise test predischarge because of cardiac causes are high risk subjects with significant increased mortality rates. Inability to complete the exercise protocol because of functional limitations is also associated with a significant increased risk compared to patients able to complete the exercise test *(84–86)*.

In TIMI II, 1-yr mortality was 7.7% in patients unable to perform an exercise test at the time of hospital discharge vs 1.8% in patients who were able to perform the test *(84)*. Similar results were reported by the GISSI-2 investigators *(87)*. Exercise-induced ST-segment depression >1 mm increased the relative mortality risk in patients assigned to the invasive strategy in TIMI II *(84)*.

Approximately 25% of patients who receive thrombolysis AMI have an abnormal exercise test at the time of hospital discharge (Table 3). The frequency of ischemic responses is increased with symptom-limited as opposed to target heart rate or workload-limited tests *(93,94)*. The positive predictive value of exercise-induced ST-segment depression ≥1 mm was 8% in patients who received thrombolysis vs 18% who did not for the end point of recurrent MI or death in a meta-analysis of 54 studies (Fig. 8) *(95)*.

A normal exercise ECG at the time of discharge is associated with a 1-yr mortality rate of <1% with >90% predictive accuracy. Additional noninvasive testing with more expensive modalities in this low-risk patient subset is unlikely to be warranted, since coronary revascularization is unlikely to reduce overall cardiac mortality at 1 yr below 1%. However, no data is available that tests this strategy against 5-yr outcome data. A practical approach to the use of exercise testing in the postinfarct setting adapted from recent ACC/AHA guidelines is illustrated in Fig. 9 *(57,96)*.

Indications for the use of exercise testing after AMI are illustrated in Table 4.

The need to perform exercise electrocardiography in all low risk postinfarct survivors was examined by Bogaty et al. *(97)*. In a study of 121 consecutive patients with acute MI fulfilling low risk criteria, patients were randomized to either: *(i)* a short hospital stay (80 subjects); or *(ii)* conventional stay (40 subjects). Short stay patients with no ischemia on ST-segment monitoring were discharged on d 3, returning for an exercise test 1 wk later. During the patient recruitment phase, 41% of all screened patients with AMI would have been medically eligible for the short stay strategy. Twenty-one percent were not discharged early because of ischemia on ST-segment

Table 3

Selected Exercise Treadmill Studies done in the Thrombolytic Era and Relationship to Prognosis

Studies (reference)	No. of patients	Year	Type of test	Duration of follow-up (mo)	Abnormal test %	Prognostic information	Strongest predictor of cardiac events
Piccalo et al. (88)	157	1992	Symptom Ltd. (12 ± 2 d)	6	33	No variables predictive of mortality.	ST-depression with angina predicted more postinfarct angina.
Chaitman et al. (84)	2502	1993	Submaximal (14 d)	12	13	Mortality for positive test 2.4%; for negative test 1.8%; 7.7% for patients unable to exercise.	Predictor of mortality: inability to exercise.
Stevenson et al. (89)	256	1993	Symptom Ltd. (7–21 d)	6–12	49	Low PPV for new cardiac events (17%) (D, RI, UA, R).	Inability to reach workload of <7 METS.
Arnold et al. (90)	981[b]	1993	Symptom Ltd. (predischarge)	12	24	2.2 RR of mortality for patients unable to exercise.	Systolic BP rise <30 mmHg.
Villela et al. (87) GISSI	6296	1995	Symptom Ltd. (28 d)	6	26	Mortality for positive test 1.7%; for negative test 0.9%; 7.1% for patients unable to exercise.	Predictors for mortality: systolic BP rise <28 mmHg (RR 1.85); symptomatic ischemia (RR 2.54); submaximal positive (RR 2.28); low work capacity (<100 W) (RR 2.05).
Toft et al. (91)	178	1995	Symptom Ltd. (predischarge)	26–50	40	Low PPV for new cardiac events (19%) (D, RI).	ST-segment depression >1 mm and ΔST/ΔHR index.
Khattur et al. (92)	114	1997	Symptom Ltd. (5–8 d)	18	31	Ejection fraction <40%; (PPA 69%) Exercise time <6 METS, PPA 58% for D, RI, UA, CHF, VA.	Exercise time <6 METS.

438

[a]Abbreviations: D, death; RI, reinfarction; UA, unstable angina; CHF, congestive heart failure; VA, ventricular arrhythmia; PPA, positive predictive accuracy; R, revascularization; METS, metabolic equivalents; BP, blood pressure; RR, relative risk; W, Watts; ΔST/ΔHR, change in ST-segment depression vs change in heart rate.
[b]490 out of 981 received thrombolytics.

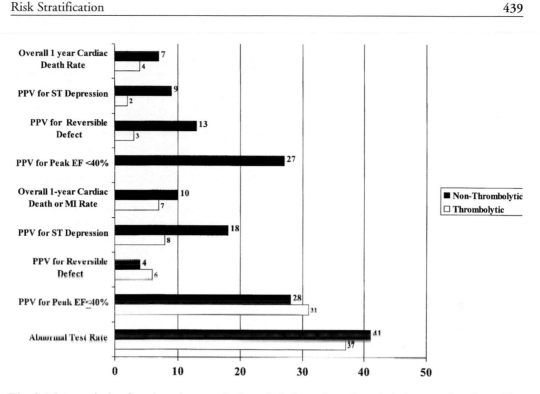

Fig. 8. Meta-analysis of noninvasive tests in thrombolytic- and nonthrombolytic-treated patients. The positive predictive accuracy for cardiac death, reinfarction rate, and rates of abnormal tests are lower in thrombolytic patients. Reproduced with permission from ref. 95.

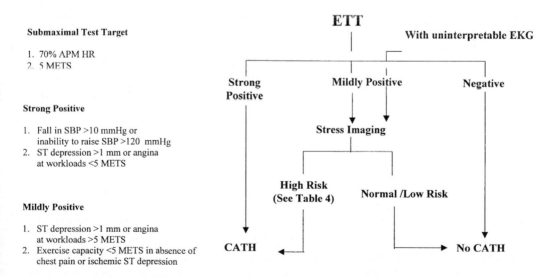

Fig. 9. Use of noninvasive testing with exercise (ETT) to risk-stratify lower risk survivors after MI. Submaximal, rather than symptom-limited, testing should be done if exercise is scheduled early (3–5 d) after the index event. APM HR, age-predicted maximum heart rate; METS, metabolic equivalents. Adapted from ref. 96 with permission.

Table 4
Indications for Exercise Electrocardiography after MI

Recommendations

Class I
1. Before discharge for prognostic assessment, activity prescription, evaluation of medical therapy (submaximal at about 4–7 d).[a]
2. Early after discharge for prognostic assessment, activity prescription, evaluation of medical therapy, and cardiac rehabilitation if the predischarge exercise test was not done (symptom-limited/about 14–21 d).[a]
3. Late after discharge for prognostic assessment, activity prescription, evaluation of medical therapy, and cardiac rehabilitation if the early exercise test was submaximal (symptom-limited/about 3–6 wk).[a]

Class IIa
1. After discharge for activity counseling and/or exercise training as part of the cardiac rehabilitation in patients who have undergone coronary revascularization.

Class IIb
1. Patients with the following ECG abnormalities:
   a. Complete left bundle-branch block.
   b. Pre-excitation syndrome.
   c. LV hypertrophy.
   d. Digoxin therapy.
   e. Greater than 1 mm of resting ST-segment depression.
   f. Electronically paced ventricular rhythm.
2. Periodic monitoring in patients who continue to participate in exercise training or cardiac rehabilitation.

Class III
1. Severe comorbidity likely to limit life expectancy and/or candidacy for revascularization.
2. At any time to evaluate patients with AMI who have uncompensated congestive heart failure, cardiac arrhythmia, or noncardiac conditions that severely limit their ability to exercise.
3. Before discharge to evaluate patients who have already been selected for cardiac catheterization. Although a stress test may be useful after catheterization to evaluate or identify ischemia in the distribution of a coronary lesion of borderline severity, stress imaging tests are recommended.

[a]Exceptions are noted under classes IIb and III.
Adapted with permission from ACC/AHA Exercise Guidelines *(96)*.

monitoring or spontaneous angina. After 6 mo, median total days hospitalized were 7.5 in the standard stay and 3.6 in the short stay group ($p < 0.001$). The findings from this study indicate that the reduced hospital stay strategy for low risk patients after AMI is feasible, resulting in a substantial and sustained reduction in hospitalized days without unfavorable psychosocial consequences or adverse risk of cardiac events. The reduced hospital stay strategy also reduced the number of invasive cardiac procedures performed.

Myocardial Perfusion Imaging

Myocardial perfusion scintigraphy localizes ischemia to a specific myocardial territory and distinguishes peri-infarction ischemia from ischemia at a remote distance from the infarct site. The test is particularly useful in patients who cannot exercise or who have noninterpretable rest ECGs (Fig. 9). The incremental prognostic value using myocardial perfusion scintigraphy to that obtained by exercise ECG alone has not been extensively studied in patients who receive thrombolysis or direct primary coronary angioplasty. In a series of 210 patients who received thrombolytic therapy and were followed for 21 mo, Miller et al. *(98)* reported a 2-yr survival rate free of cardiac events of 86 vs 80% in patients with high- vs low-risk scans. Table 5 illustrates exercise myocardial perfusion studies of patients who received thrombolysis or direct coronary angioplasty and their relationship to prognosis *(98–105)*.

In patients who cannot perform exercise, dipyridamole or adenosine myocardial perfusion imaging can be useful for risk stratification *(106,107)*. Mahmarian et al. *(102)* studied the value of quantitative adenosine thallium-201 myocardial scintigraphy 2–5 d after AMI. Multivariate analysis of the 146 patients, 36% of whom received thrombolytic therapy, revealed that a combination of ejection fraction and extent of myocardial ischemia provided the optimal model for risk stratification. When the extent of myocardial ischemia was < 10% and ejection fraction >40%, 1-yr survival free of rein farction was 94%. In this report, mortality was best predicted by total infarct size. Miller et al. *(108)* showed that infarct size <12% of the left ventricle measured by ^{99m}Tc sestamibi SPECT was associated with no mortality in 274 patients over a 2-yr follow-up (Fig. 10). Characteristics of a high risk nuclear study include: (*i*) reversible defect >10% LV; (*ii*) perfusion defect >20% LV; and (*iii*) increased lung uptake of thallium-201

Exercise or Dobutamine Echocardiography

There are few data reporting the prognostic value of exercise echocardiography after infarction in patients who received thrombolysis or direct PTCA. In three small patient series (<100 patients), exercise echocardiography was associated with a greater sensitivity and specificity for cardiac events than exercise electrocardiography alone *(109–111)*. Smart et al. *(112)* reported sensitivity, specificity, and safety of dobutamine–atropine stress echocardiography 5 ± 2 d after MI in a 232-patient series. Wall motion abnormalities remote from the infarct zone were associated with 97% specificity and 68% sensitivity for multivessel coronary disease. The most sensitive and specific findings for residual infarct-related stenosis were an ischemic response (decrease in wall thickness in more than two contiguous segments at peak dose without improvement at low dose) and a biphasic response (improved wall thickening in more than two contiguous segments from rest to low dose, but decreased wall thickening from low to peak dose). Carlos et al. *(113)* used dobutamine stress echocardiography for risk stratification after acute MI in 214 patients, 121 of whom received thrombolytic therapy. A lower basal wall motion score index (1.55 vs 1.88), higher number of infarcted segments (4.1 vs 1.9), and lower number of dobutamine-responsive segments (1.2 vs 2.9) were associated with an adverse prognosis. Absence of viability was associated with the worst prognosis in multivariate analysis. They also report that dobutamine echocardiography was a better predictor of cardiac events than coronary angiography (Fig. 11). Pierard et al. *(114)* confirmed that wall motion response to dobutamine in a region with rest dysfunction is highly sensitive and specific for predicting the functional recovery of segmental contraction after AMI and recovery of LV function. This was further studied by Picano et al. *(115)*, in 314 medically treated patients from the Echo Dobutamine International Cooperative (EDIC) study who underwent dobutamine stress echocardio-

Table 5

Prognostic Value of Stress Nuclear Imaging Studies in Patients Undergoing Thrombolysis[a]

Studies (reference)	No. of patients	Type of stress	Time after MI (d)	Follow-up (mo)	% ST-depression/ % reversible defects	Cardiac events (%)	Multivariate predictors of cardiac events
Tilkemeier et al. (99)	64/171	Low-level exercise thallium	10 ± 4	12	15/42	D, RI, R (7)	LV enlargement.
Hendel et al. (100)	71	Dipyridamole thallium	10 ± 2	24	NR	D + MI (14)	No clinical or scintigraphic variable.
Bowling et al. (101)	84	Exercise thallium	Predischarge	6	NR	D, MI, UA (13)	Postdischarge angina.
Miller et al. (98)	210	Symptom-limited exercise thallium	9 ± 6	24	15/56	D (3)	Rate pressure product.
Mahmarian et al. (102)	146 (36%) received thrombolytics	Adenosine thallium	5 ± 3	16	NR	D, RI, VA, CHF (33)	Absolute extent of ischemia; EF; total perfusion defect size best predicted death.
Basu et al. (103)	100	Symptom-limited exercise	42	21	39/68	D, RI, UA, CHF (37)	Cardiac events in 89% of patients.
Travin et al. (104)	134/54[b]	Symptom-limited exercise Tc sestamibi	7	15	23/70	D, MI, UA (13)	Event rate 38% in patients with >3 reversible sestamibi defects.
Dakik et al. (105)	71	Symptom-limited exercise thallium	13	24	15/38	D, MI, VA, CHF (37)	EF reversible; perfusion defect size >20%.

[a]Abbreviations: D, death; RI, reinfarction; UA, unstable angina; CHF, congestive heart failure; VA, ventricular arrhythmia; PPA, positive predictive accuracy; R, revascularization; NR, not reported; LV, left ventricle; EF, ejection fraction.
[b]Number of patients with imaging studies/number of patients in study.
[c]All patients received primary PTCA.

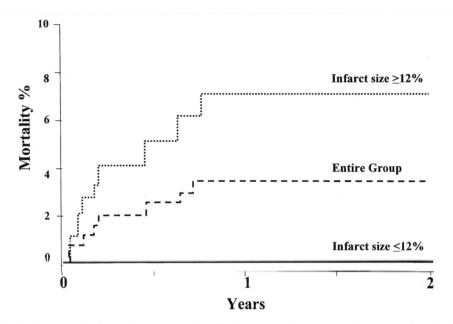

Fig. 10. Influence of infarct size measured by 99mTc sestamibi on mortality during 2-yr follow-up. Two-year mortality was 7% for 137 patients with infarct size >12% and 0% for 137 patients with infarct size <12%. Reproduced with permission from ref. *108.*

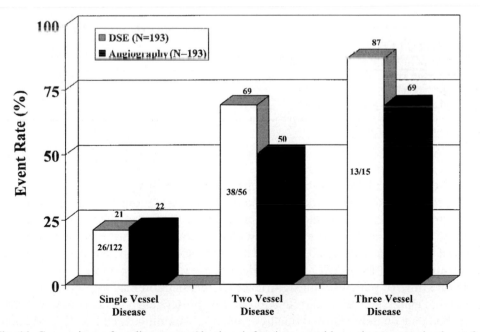

Fig. 11. Comparison of cardiac events (death, reinfarction, unstable angina, congestive heart failure, ventricular arrhythmias) according to extent of coronary artery disease detected by dobutamine echocardiography and coronary angiography. Reproduced with permission from ref. *113.*

Table 6
Prognostic Value of Stress Echocardiography in Patients After MI[a]

Study (reference)	Year	Test	No. of patients	Follow-up (mo)	Cardiac Events		Comments
					Ischemic	Non-ischemic	
Ryan et al. (109)	1987	EX	40	6–10	94	17	D, MI, UA, R
Applegate et al. (110)	1987	EX	67	11	50	13	D, MI, R
Iliceto et al. (116)	1990	Pacing	83	14 ± 12	65	8	D, MI, UA, R
Bolognese et al. (117)	1992	DIP	217	24	16	5	D, MI, UA
Camerici et al. (118)	1993	DIP	190	14 ± 10	52	17	D, MI, UA, R
Picano et al. (119)	1993	DIP	1080	16	5.4	2.8	MI
Quintanta et al. (111)	1995	EX	70	36	27	9	D, MI, R
Carlos et al. (113)	1997	DOB	214	16 ± 6	44	28	D, MI, CHF, UA
Greco et al. (120)	1997	EX	178	17 ± 13	23	14	D, MI, UA
Greco et al. (120)	1997	DOB	178	17 ± 13	24	12	D, MI, UA
Salustri et al. (121)	1999	DOB	245	17 ± 13	23	11	D, MI, UA

[a]Abbreviations: D, death; MI, myocardial infarction; R, revascularization; UA, unstable angina; CHF, congestive heart failure; EX, exercise; DIP, dipyridamole; DOB, dobutamine.

Table 7
Indications for Nuclear/Echocardiogram Stress Testing Based on ACC/AHA Guidelines

1. Uninterpretable ECG.
2. Mild abnormality on exercise treadmill test (ETT).
3. Unable to exercise.
4. MI not treated with acute reperfusion.
5. Myocardial viability assessment.

Data from refs. *57, 96,* and *122.*

graphy. They reported the presence of myocardial viability identified as inotropic reserve after low-dose dobutamine is associated with higher probability of survival. The higher the number of segments showing improvement of function, the better the survival probability. The prognostic information provided by stress echocardiography after AMI is reviewed in Table 6 *(109–111,113,116–121).* Indications for nuclear/echocardiogram stress testing adapted from ACC/AHA guidelines are reviewed in Table 7 *(122).*

Up to one-third of patients with significant LV dysfunction may improve with revascularization. Depressed ventricular function may be present even though coronary blood flow has been adequately restored due to myocardial stunning. Identification of extensive reversible LV dysfunction is of prognostic importance and may help to optimize medical management after MI. Techniques to assess viability include myocardial perfusion imaging, positron emission tomography, contrast magnetic resonance imaging, and dobutamine echocardiography. Evidence of improved contractility at low dose dobutamine in dyssynergic myocardium indicates regions of myocardium that may be improved with coronary revascularization procedures.

Table 8
Indication for Coronary Angiography After MI[a]

Indication	Class[b]
1. Patients with spontaneous episodes of myocardial ischemia or episodes of myocardial ischemia provoked by minimal exertion.	I
2. Before definitive therapy of mechanical complications of MI (acute MR, VSD, pseudoaneurysm).	I
3. Persistent hemodynamic instability.	I
4. MI suspected to have occurred by a mechanism other than thrombotic occlusion at an atherosclerotic plaque.	IIa
5. Survivors of AMI with depressed LV systolic function (LV EF <40%), CHF, prior revascularization, or malignant ventricular arrhythmia.	IIa
6. Survivors of AMI who had clinical heart failure during acute episode but subsequently demonstrated preserved LV function.	IIa

[a]Abbreviations: MI, myocardial infarction; AMI, acute myocardial infarction; MR, mitral regurgitation; VSD, ventricular septal defect; LV, left ventricular; EF, ejection fraction; CHF, congestive heart failure.

[b]Class I, evidence that the given procedure is beneficial, useful, and effective; class IIa, weight of evidence in favor of usefulness.

Adapted with permission from the ACC/AHA 1999 Guidelines (57).

Coronary Angiography

Ellis et al. (123) randomized 87 patients treated with thrombolysis who had a negative noninvasive risk stratification workup to medical therapy or coronary angioplasty (4–14 d). After a 12-mo follow-up, survival free of MI was 97.8% in patients who did not receive PTCA compared to 90.5% in patients ($p = 0.07$). Mark et al. (124) compared the use of angiography, angioplasty, and survival rates of patients enrolled in GUSTO-1 from the U.S. and Canada. The rate of coronary angiography was 72 vs 25%, coronary angioplasty 29 vs 11% and 1-yr survival rate 90.7 vs 90.3% in the U.S. vs Canada, respectively. In the Survival and Ventricular Enlargement (SAVE) trial, 31% compared with 12% of American vs Canadian patients underwent coronary revascularization. The 1-yr mortality rates, however, were virtually identical (11%) (125). Results were similar in 240,989 patients surveyed in 1073 U.S. hospitals from 1990–1993 (126). The indications for cardiac catheterization after MI adapted from ACC/AHA guidelines are illustrated in Table 8.

Evaluation for Electrical Instability

The risk of sudden cardiac death in survivors of MI with normal ejection fraction is low, whereas patients with an ejection fraction <35–40% have a 10% risk of sudden cardiac death over 3.5 yr; 6–8% in the first yr and 2–4%/yr thereafter (127). In GISSI 2, the prevalence of frequent ventricular ectopy (>10 PVC/h) was 20% in 8676 patients, which is not significantly different than the frequencies reported in the prethrombolytic era (128). The predictive accuracy for cardiac events is lower in the postthrombolytic patient (Table 9) (128–132).

In GUSTO, Singh et al. (133) reported lower heart rate variability (HRV) 24 h after AMI in patients with anterior vs nonanterior MI (SDANN 53 ± 21 vs 63 ± 24 ms; $p < 0.005$), increased HRV with TIMI II flow low frequency [LF] 5.3 ± 1.0 vs 4.8 ± 1.2 ms²; $p < 0.01$), and lower HRV in those who died at 1 yr compared to survivors.

Table 9
Prevalence of Frequent PVCs (>10/h), Risk of SCD, Sensitivity, Specificity, and PPA of
Frequent PVCs to Predict SCD and Sustained Ventricular Arrhythmias[a]

Study (reference)	Year	No. of patients	Prevalence (%)	SCD (%)	Sensitivity (%)	Specificity (%)	PPA (%)
Moss et al. (129)	1979	940	23	5.9	42	78	11
Bigger et al. (130)	1984	819	15	6.6	55	72	12
Mukharji et al. (131)	1984	533	15	4.6	67	47	8
Maggioni et al. (128)	1993	8626	20	0.9	42	80	3
McClements et al. (132)	1993	301	26	4.3	38	74	6

Abbreviations: SCD, sudden cardiac death; PPA, positive predictive accuracy; PVCs, premature ventricular couplets.
[a]After thrombolysis.

Low-amplitude (<25 V) late potentials along with increased filtered QRS duration (>120 ms) are suggestive evidence of slowed and fragmented conduction. Absence of these findings in the postinfarct setting is associated with a 96–99% negative predictive value for sustained ventricular tachycardia or sudden death after 1 yr (132,134–137). The combined use of ambulatory ECG variables, signal-averaged ECG, and HRV leads to a greater positive predictive accuracy for cardiac events (134–136).

Programmed electrical stimulation inducing monomorphic ventricular tachycardia with cycle length >230 ms performed 2–4 wk after MI patients with ejection fraction <35% is a good predictor of spontaneous sustained ventricular tachycardia (138,139). Pedretti et al. (140) reported a sensitivity of 81% and specificity of 97% for inducibility of ventricular tachycardia to predict future arrhythmia in patients after MI who had two or more of the following: ejection fraction <40%, late potentials, or high-grade ectopy. Zoni-Barriso et al. (139), using up to two extra stimuli for induction of monomorphic ventricular tachycardia, found inducibility to have a sensitivity, specificity, and positive predictive accuracy of 55, 99, and 67%, respectively, for arrhythmic event. Patients were selected if they had either ejection fraction <40%, late potentials, or complex ventricular arrhythmias. Lack of inducibility in this high-risk population carries a better prognosis. The Multicenter Automatic Defibrillator Implantation Trial (MADIT) showed that in a select group of patients enrolled 4 wk to 2 yr after MI (with ejection fraction <35%, an episode of nonsustained ventricular tachycardia, and nonsuppressible ventricular tachyarrhythmia during electrophysiologic study) randomization to automatic implantable cardioverter-defibrillator was associated with significantly improved survival rates compared to conventional therapy (141). The Multicenter Unsustained Tachycardia Trial (MUSTT) (142) showed that electrophysiologically guided therapy with implantable defibrillators, but not with antiarrhythmic drugs in patients with coronary disease, LV ejection fraction <40%, and asymptomatic, nonsustained ventricular tachycardia reduced the risk of cardiac arrest and sudden death from arrhythmia. The use of noninvasive predictors of sudden cardiac death to select candidates for electrophysiologic studies to identify the highest risk patient for sudden cardiac death after AMI is shown in Fig. 12.

Arrhythmia Evaluation for Risk of SCD After MI

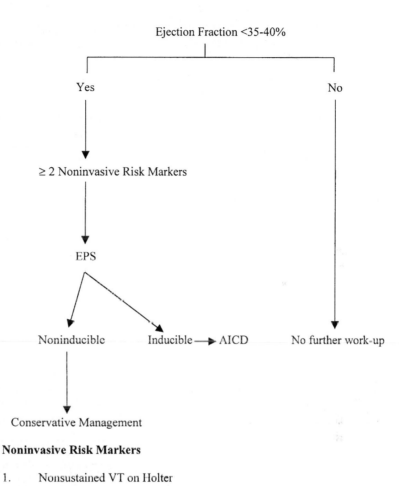

Ejection Fraction <35-40%

Yes   No

≥ 2 Noninvasive Risk Markers

EPS

Noninducible   Inducible ⟶ AICD   No further work-up

Conservative Management

Noninvasive Risk Markers

1.   Nonsustained VT on Holter

2.   Low heart rate variability

3.   Late potentials

Fig. 12. Use of noninvasive electrophysiologic markers to identify high risk patients for electrophysiologic studies and evaluation for risk of sudden cardiac death after MI.

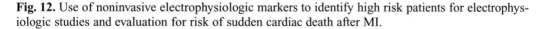

CONCLUSION

Using mostly data from the thrombolytic era, a logical sequence of clinical and noninvasive test procedures has been provided to risk-stratify postinfarct survivors into high and lower risk populations. The highest risk patients should be considered for early coronary angiography and revascularization therapy if clinically indicated, and the lowest risk patients could be managed medically. However, all risk stratification algorithms that are developed based on noninvasive testing will continue to evolve as ongoing clinical outcome studies and consensus statements are tested. Presently, the strategy given in Fig. 13

Clinical Indications of High Risk at Predischarge

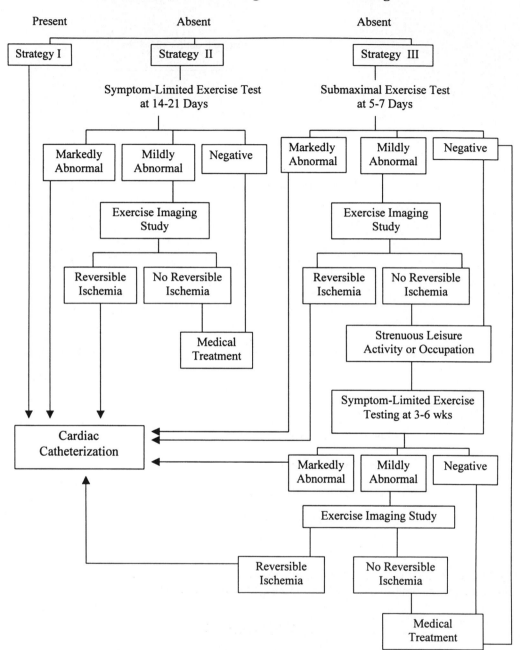

Fig. 13. Overall strategy to risk-stratify postinfarct survivors and identify optimal candidates for cardiac catheterization or continue medical management. Reproduced with permission from ref. *57.*

and Table 1 can be used to assess cardiac risk after AMI in the postthrombolytic/ direct angioplasty era.

REFERENCES

1. American Heart Association. 2001 heart and stroke facts. American Heart Association, 2001.
2. Morrow DA, Antman EM, Charlesworth A, et al. TIMI risk score for ST-elevation myocardial infarction: a convenient, bedside, clinical score for risk assessment at presentation. An Intravenous nPA for Treatment of Infarcting Myocardium Early II Trial Substudy. Circulation 2000;102:2031–2037.
3. Morrow DA, Antman EM, Parsons L, et al. Application of the TIMI risk score for ST-elevation MI in the National Registry of Myocardial Infarction 3. JAMA 2001;286:1356–1359.
4. Cannon CP, Thompson B, McCabe CH, et al. Predictors of non-Q-wave acute myocardial infarction in patients with acute ischemic syndromes: an analysis from the Thrombolysis in Myocardial Ischemia (TIMI) III investigators. Am J Cardiol 1995;75:977–981.
5. Gurwitz JH, Gore JM, Goldberg RJ, Rubison M, Chandra N, Rogers WJ. Recent age-related trends in the use of thrombolytic therapy in patients who have had acute MI. National Registry of Myocardial Infarction. Ann Intern Med 1996;124:283–291.
6. Hillis LD, Forman S, Braunwald E, and the Thrombolysis in Myocardial Infarction (TIMI) Phase II Co-investigators. Risk stratification before thrombolytic therapy in patients with acute myocardial infarction. J Am Coll Cardiol 1990;16:313–315.
7. Normand ST, Glickman ME, Sharma RG, McNeil BJ. Using admission characteristics to predict short-term mortality from myocardial infarction in elderly patients. Results from the Cooperative Cardiovascular Project. JAMA 1996;275:1822–1828.
8. Rouleau JL, Talajic M, Sussex B, et al. Myocardial infarction patients in the 1990s—their risk factors, stratification and survival in Canada: The Canadian Assessment of Myocardial Infarction (CAMI) Study. J Am Coll Cardiol 1996;27:1119–1127.
9. Lee KL, Woodlief LM, Topol EJ, Weaner D, Bertrin J, Califf RM. Predictors of 30 day mortality in the era of reperfusion for acute myocardial infarction. Results from international trial of 41,021 patients. Circulation 1995;91:1659–1663.
10. Aguirre FV, McMahon RP, Mueller H, et al. Impact of age on clinical outcome and postlytic management strategies in patients treated with intravenous thrombolytic therapy. Results from the TIMI II study. Circulation 1994;90:78–86.
11. Fibrinolytic Therapy Trialists' (FTT) Collaborative Group. Indications for fibrinolytic therapy in suspected acute myocardial infarction: collaborative overview of early mortality and major morbidity results from all randomized trials of more than 1000 patients. Lancet 1994;343:311–322.
12. Vaccarino V, Krumholz HM, Berkman LF, Horwitz RI. Sex differences in mortality after myocardial infarction. Is there evidence for an increased risk for women? Circulation 1995;91:1861–1871.
13. Weaver WD, White HD, Wilcox RG, et al. Comparisons of characteristics and outcomes among women and men with acute myocardial infarction treated with thrombolytic therapy. GUSTO-1 Investigators. JAMA 1996;275:777–782.
14. Kober L, Torp-Pedersen C, Ottesen M, et al. Influence of gender on short- and long-term mortality after acute myocardial infarction. Am J Cardiol 1996;77:1052–1056.
15. Stone PH, Muller JE, Hartwell T, et al. The effect of diabetes mellitus on prognosis and serial left ventricular function after acute myocardial infarction: contribution of both coronary disease and left ventricular dysfunction to the adverse prognosis. The MILIS Study Group. J Am Coll Cardiol 1989;14:49–57.
16. Granger CB, Califf RM, Young S, et al. Outcome of patients with diabetes mellitus and acute myocardial infarction treated with thrombolytic agents. The Thrombolysis and Angioplasty in Myocardial Infarction (TAMI) Study Group. J Am Coll Cardiol 1993;21:920–925.
17. Aronson D, Rayfield EJ, Chesebro JH. Mechanisms determining course and outcome of diabetic patients who have had acute myocardial infarction. Ann Intern Med 1997;126:296–306.
18. Abbot RD, Donaue R, Kannel WB. The impact of diabetes on survival following myocardial infarction in men vs. women: the Framingham Study. JAMA 1988;260:3456–3460.
19. Abbud ZA, Shindler DM, Wilson AC, Kostis JB. Effect of diabetes mellitus on short-and long-term mortality rates of patients with acute myocardial infarction: a statewide study. Myocardial Infarction Data Acquisition System Study Group. Am Heart J 1995;130:51–58.

20. Capes SE, Hunt D, Malmberg K, Gerstein HC. Stress hyperglycemia and increased risk of death after myocardial infarction in patients with and without diabetes: a systematic overview. Lancet 2000;355: 773–778.

21. Taylor HA, Chaitman BR, Rogers WJ, et al. TIMI Investigators. Race and prognosis after myocardial infarction. Results of the Thrombolysis in Myocardial Infarction (TIMI) Phase II Trial. Circulation 1993;88: 1484–1494.

22. Keil JE, Sutherland SE, Knapp RG, Lackland DT, Gazes PC, Tyroler HA. Mortality rates and risk factors for coronary disease in black as compared with white men and women. N Engl J Med 1993;329:73–78.

23. Califf RM, Pieper KS, Lee KL, et al. Prediction of 1-year survival after thrombolysis for acute myocardial infarction in the Global Utilization of Streptokinase and TPA for Occluded Coronary Arteries Trial. Circulation 2000;101:2231–2238.

24. Killiip T III, Kimball JT. Treatment of myocardial infarction in a coronary care unit. A two year experience with 250 patients. Am J Cardiol 1967;20:456–464.

25. Forrester JS, Diamond G, Chatterjee K, Swan HJ. Medical therapy of acute myocardial infarction by application of hemodynamic subsets. N Engl J Med 1976;295:1356–1362.

26. Multicentre Postinfarction Research Group. Risk stratification and survival after myocardial infarction. N Engl. J Med 1983;309:331–336.

27. Volpi A, DeVita C, Franzosi MG, et al. Determinants of the 6-month mortality in survivors of myocardial infarction after thrombolysis: results of the GISSI-2 database. Circulation 1993;88: 416–429.

28. Warnowicz MA, Parker H, Chetlin MD. Prognosis of patients with acute pulmonary edema and normal ejection fraction after acute myocardial infarction. Circulation 1983;67:330–334.

29. Califf RM, Bengtson JR. Cardiogenic shock. N Engl J Med 1994;330:1724

30. O'Gara PT. Primary pump failure. In: Fuster V, Ross R, Topol E, eds. Atherosclerosis and Coronary Artery Disease. Raven Press, New York, 1995, p. 1051.

31. Bates ER, Topol EJ. Limitations of thrombolytic therapy for acute myocardial infarction complicated by congestive heart failure and cardiogenic shock. J Am Coll Cardiol 1991;18:1077.

32. Holmes DR, Bates ER, Kleiman NS, et al. Contemporary reperfusion therapy for cardiogenic shock: the GUSTO-1 trial experience. J Am Coll Cardiol 1995;26:668.

33. Hochman JS, Sleeper LA, Webb JG, et al. Early revascularization in acute myocardial infarction complicated by cardiogenic shock. N Eng J Med 1999;341:625–634.

34. Tomoda H, Aoki N. Prognostic value of C-reactive protein levels within six hours after the onset of acute myocardial infarction. Am Heart J 2000;140:324–328.

35. Ohman EM, Armstrong PW, Christenson RH, et al. Cardiac Troponin T levels for risk stratification in acute myocardial ischemia. N Engl J Med 1996;335:1333–1341.

36. Giannitsis E, Muller-Bardorff M, Lehrke S, et al. Admission Troponin T levels predict clinical outcome, TIMI flow, and myocardial tissue perfusion after primary percutaneous intervention for acute ST-segment elevation myocardial infarction. Circulation 2001;104:630–635.

37. Giannitsis E, Lehrke S, Weigand UK, et al. Risk stratification in patients with inferior acute myocardial infarction treated by percutaneous coronary interventions: the role of admission troponin T. Circulation 2000;102:2038–2044.

38. Ramanathan K, Stewart JT, Theroux P, French JK, White HD. Admission troponin T level may predict 90 minute TIMI flow after thrombolysis. Circulation 1997;96(Suppl. I):I-270.

39. Matetzky S, Sharir T, Domingo M, et al. Elevated Troponin I level on admission is associated with adverse outcome of primary angioplasty in acute myocardial infarction. Circulation 2000;102: 1611–1616.

40. Birnbaum Y, Herz I, Sclarovsky S, et al. Prognostic significance of the admission electrocardiogram in acute myocardial infarction. J Am Coll Cardiol 1996;27:1128–1132.

41. Bates ER, Clemmensen PM, Califf RM, et al. Precordial ST segment depression predicts a worse prognosis in inferior infarction despite reperfusion therapy. The Thrombolysis and Angioplasty in Myocardial Infarction (TAMI) Study Group. J Am Coll Cardiol 1990;16:1538–1544.

42. Wong CK, Freedman SB, Bautovich G, Bailey BP, Bernstein L, Kelly DT. Mechanisms and significance of precordial ST-segment depression during inferior wall acute myocardial infarction associated with severe narrowing of the dominant right coronary artery. Am J Cardiol 1993;71:1025.

43. Peterson ED, Hathaway WR, Zabel KM, et al. Prognostic significance of precordial ST segment depression during inferior myocardial infarction in the thrombolytic era: results in 16,521 patients. J Am Coll Cardiol 1996;28:305–312.

44. Birnbaum Y, Herz I, Sclaraovsky S, Ziotikamien B, Chetrit A, Barbash G. Prognostic significance of different patterns of precordial ST segment depression in inferior wall acute myocardial infarction. J Am Coll Cardiol 1995;343A.

45. Zehender M, Kasper M, Kauder E, et al. Right ventricular infaction as an independent predictor of prognosis after acute inferior myocardial infarction. N Engl J Med 1993;218:981–988.

46. Newby KH, Natale A, Krucoff MW, et al. The incidence and clinical relevance of bundle branch block in patients with acute myocardial infarction treated with thrombolytic agents. J Am Coll Cardiol 1995; 343A.

47. Shecter M, Rabinowitz B, Beker B, Motro M, Barbash G, Kaplinski E. Additional ST segment elevation during the first hour of thrombolytic therapy, an electrocardiographic sign predicting a favorable clinical outcome. J Am Coll Cardiol 1992;20:1460–1464.

48. Mauri F, Maggioni AP, Franzosi MG, et al. A simple electrocardiographic predictor of the outcome of patients with acute myocardial infarction treated with a thrombolytic agent. A Gruppo Italiano per lo Studio della Sopravvienza nell'Infarto Miocardico (GISSI-2)-Derived Analysis. J Am Coll Cardiol 1994;24:600–607.

49. Schroder R, Wegscheider K, Schroder K, Dissmann R, Meyer-Sabellek W, for the INJECT Trial Group. Extent of early ST segment elevation resolution: a strong predictor of outcome in patients with acute myocardial infarction and a sensitive measure to compare thrombolytic regimens. A substudy of the International Joint Efficacy Comparison of Thrombolytics (INJECT) Trial. J Am Coll Cardiol 1995; 26:1657–1664.

50. Silver MT, Rose GA, Paul SD, O'Donnell CJ, O'Gara PT, Eagle KA. A clinical rule to predict preserved left ventricular ejection fraction in patients after myocardial infarction. Ann Intern Med 1994; 121:750–756.

51. Shaw LJ, Peiper K, Peterson ED, Eagle KA, Wagner GS, Califf RM. Optimization of resources by efficient use of readily available simple clinical measures in a high-risk post-myocardial infarction population. Presented at the 13th Annual Meeting of the Association for Health Service Research, Atlanta, GA, June 9–11, 1996.

52. Andrews J, French JK, Manda SO, White HD. New Q waves on the presenting electrocardiogram independently predicts increased cardiac mortality following a first ST-elevation myocardial infarction. Eur Heart J 2000;21:647–653.

53. Brodie BR, Weintraub RA, Stuckey TD, et al. Outcomes of direct coronary angioplasty for acute myocardial infarction in candidates and non-candidates for thrombolytic therapy. Am J Cardiol 1991; 67:7–12.

54. Himbert D, Juliard JM, Steg PG, et al. Primary coronary angioplasty for acute myocardial infarction with contraindication to thrombolysis. Am J Cardiol 1993;71:377–381.

55. Michels KB, Yusuf S. Does PTCA in acute myocardial infarction affect mortality and reinfarction rates? A quantitative overview (meta-analysis) of the randomized clinical trials. Circulation 1995;91: 476–485.

56. Ellis SG, Ribeiro da Silva E, Heyndrickx GR, et al. Randomized comparison of rescue angioplasty with conservative management of patients with early failure of thrombolysis for acute anterior myocardial infarction. Circulation 1996;90:2280–2284.

57. Ryan TJ, Antman EM, Brooks NH, et al. 1999 Update: ACC/AHA guidelines for the management of patients with acute myocardial infarction: a report of the American College of Cardiology/American Heart Association Task Force on Practice Guidelines (Committee on Management of Acute Myocardial Infarction). J Am Coll Cardiol 1999;34:890–911.

58. Reeder GS. Identification and management of the low-risk patient after myocardial infarction. ACC Curr J Rev 1997;May/June:27–31.

59. Peterson ED, Shaw LJ, Califf RM. Risk stratification after myocardial infarction. Ann Intern Med 1997;126:561–582.

60. Mark DB, Sigmon K, Topol EJ, et al. Identification of acute myocardial infarction patients suitable for early hospital discharge after aggressive intervention therapy: results from the Thrombolysis and Angioplasty in Acute Myocardial Infarction Registry. Circulation 1991;83:1186–1193.

61. Villela A, Maggioni AP, Villela M, et al. Prognostic significance of maximal exercise testing after myocardial infarction treated with thrombolytic agents: the GISSI-2 database. Lancet 1995;346: 523–529.

62. Newby KL, Califf RM, Guerci A, et al. Early discharge in the thrombolytic era: an analysis of criteria for uncomplicated infarction from the GUSTO trial. J Am Coll Cardiol 1996;27:625–632.

63. Mueller HS, Forman SA, Menegns MA, Cohen LS, Knatterud GL, Braunwald E. Prognostic significance of nonfatal reinfarction during 3 year follow-up: results of the TIMI phase II trial. J Am Coll Cardiol 1995;26:900–907.
64. Barbagelata A, Granger CB, Topol EJ, et al. Frequency, significance and cost of recurrent ischemia after thrombolytic therapy for myocardial infarction. Am J Cardiol 1995;76:1007–1013.
65. Figuerdo V, Cheitlin MD. Risk stratification. In: Julain DG, Braunwald E, eds. Management of Acute Myocardial Infarction. W.B. Saunders, London, 1994, pp. 361–391.
66. Theroux P, Juneau M. Exercise and pharmacologic testing after acute myocardial infarction. In: Francis GS, Alpert JS, eds. Coronary Care. Little, Brown, Boston, 1993, pp. 615–628.
67. DeBusk RF. Specialized testing after recent acute myocardial infarction. Ann Intern Med 1989;110:470.
68. Topol EJ, Bates ER, Walton JA Jr, et al. Coronary angiography after thrombolytic therapy for acute myocardial infarction. Ann Intern Med 1991;114:877–885.
69. The TIMI Study Group. Comparison of invasive and conservative strategies after treatment with intravenous tissue plasminogen activator in acute myocardial infarction: results of the Thrombolysis in Myocardial Infarction (TIMI) Phase II Trial. N Engl J Med 1989;329:618–627.
70. Williams DO, Braunwald E, Knatterud G, TIMI Investigators. One-year results of the Thrombolysis in Myocardial Infarction Investigation (TIMI) Phase II Trial. Circulation 1992;85:533–542.
71. SWIFT (Should We Intervene Following Thrombolysis?) Trial Study Group. SWIFT trial of delayed elective intervention versus conservative treatment after thrombolysis with anistreplase in acute myocardial infarction. BMJ 1991;302:555–560.
72. Gibson RS, Bishop HL, Stamm RB, Crampton RS, Beller GA, Martin RP. Value of early two-dimensional echocardiography in patients with acute myocardial infarction. Am J Cardiol 1982;49:1110–1119.
73. Horowitz RS, Morganroth J, Parrotto C, Chun CC, Soffer J, Pauletto FJ. Immediate diagnosis of acute myocardial infarction by two-dimensional echocardiography. Circulation 1982;65:323–329.
74. Nishimura RA, Tajek AJ, Shub C, Miller FA, Ilstrip DM, Harrison CE. Role of two-dimensional echocardiography in the prediction of inhospital complications after acute myocardial infarction. J Am Coll Cardiol 1984;4:1080–1087.
75. Jaarsma W, Visser CA, Eemgevan MJ, Verhengt FW, Kupper AJ. Predictive value of two-dimensional echocardiography and hemodynamic measurements on admission with acute myocardial infarction. J Am Soc Echocardiogr 1988;1:187–193.
76. Saabia P, Abbott RD, Afrookteh A, Keller MW, Touchstone DA, Karl S. Importance of two dimensional echocardiographic assessment of left ventricular function in patients presenting to emergency room with cardiac related symptoms. Circulation 1991;84:1615–1624.
77. White HD, Norris RM, Brown MA, Brandt PW, Whitlock RM, Wild CJ. Left ventricular end-systolic volume as the major determinant of survival after recovery from myocardial infarction. Circulation 1987;76:44.
78. Reeder GS, Gibbons RJ. Acute myocardial infarction: risk stratification in the thrombolytic era. Mayo Clin Proc 1995;70:87–94.
79. Pilote L, Silberberg J, Lisbona R, Sniderman A. Prognosis in patients with low left ventricular ejection fraction after myocardial infarction. Circulation 1989;80:1636.
80. Cerisano G, Bolognese L, Carrabba N, et al. Doppler-derived mitral deceleration time: an early strong predictor of left ventricular remodeling after reperfused anterior acute myocardial infarction. Circulation 1999;99:230–236.
81. Nijland F, Kamp O, Karreman AJ, Van Eenige MJ, Visser CA. Prognostic implications of restrictive left ventricular filling in acute myocardial infarction: a serial doppler echocardiographic study. J Am Coll Cardiol 1997;30:1618–1624.
82. Sakate Y, Yoshiyama M, Hirata K, et al. Relationship between Doppler-derived left ventricular diastolic function and exercise capacity in patients with myocardial infarction. Jpn Circ J 2001;65:627–631.
83. Miyashita T, Okano Y, Takaki H, Satoh T, Kobayashi Y, Goto Y. Relation between exercise capacity and left ventricular systolic versus diastolic function during exercise in patients after myocardial infarction. Coron Artery Dis 2001;12:217–225.
84. Chaitman BR, McMahon RP, Terrin M, et al. Impact of treatment strategy on predischarge exercise test in the Thrombolysis in Myocardial Infarction (TIMI) II trial. Am J Cardiol 1993;71:131–138.
85. Dominguez H, Torp-Prdersen C, Koeber L, Rask-Madsen C. Prognostic value of exercise testing in a cohort of patients followed for 15 years after acute myocardial infarction. Eur Heart J 2001;22:300–306.

86. Dorn J, Naughton J, Imamura D, Trevisan M. Prognostic value of peak exercise systolic blood pressure on long-term survival after myocardial infarction. Am J Cardiol 2001;87:213.

87. Villella A, Maggioni AP, Villella M, et al. Prognostic significance of maximal exercise testing after myocardial infarction treated with thrombolytic agents: the GISSI-2 database. Lancet 1995;346: 523–529.

88. Piccalo G, Pirelli S, Massa D, Cipriani M, Sarullo FM, De Vita C. Value of negative predischarge exercise testing in identifying patients at low risk after acute myocardial infarction treated by systemic thrombolysis. Am J Cardiol 1992;70:31–33.

89. Stevenson R, Umachandran V, Ranjandayalan K, Wilkinson P, Marchant B, Timms AD. Reassessment of treadmill stress testing for risk stratification in patients with acute myocardial infarction treated with thrombolysis. Br Heart J 1993;70:415–420.

90. Arnold AE, Simoons ML, Detry JM, et al. Prediction of mortality following hospital discharge after thrombolysis for acute myocardial infarction: is there a need for coronary angiography? The European Cooperative Study Group. Eur Heart J 1993;14:306–315.

91. Toft E. Neilson G, Mortenson B, Dalsgaard D, Mansen JB, Rasmussen K. The prognostic value of exercise testing early after myocardial infarction in patients treated with thrombolytics. Eur Heart J 1995;16:1177–1180.

92. Khattar RS, Basu SK, Ranal V. Senior R, Lahiri A. Prognostic value of predischarge exercise testing, ejection fraction and ventricular ectopic activity in acute myocardial infarction treated with streptokinase. Am J Cardiol 1996;78:136–141.

93. Juneau M, Colles P, Theroux P, et al. Symptom-limited versus low level exercise testing before hospital discharge after myocardial infarction. J Am Coll Cardiol 1992;20:927–933.

94. Jain A, Myers GH, Sapin PM, O'Rourke RA. Comparison of symptom-limited and low level exercise tolerance tests early after myocardial infarction. J Am Coll Cardiol 1993;22:1816–1820.

95. Shaw LJ, Peterson ED, Kesler K, Hasselblad V, Califf RM. A metaanalysis of predischarge risk stratification after acute myocardial infarction with stress electrocardiographic, myocardial perfusion and ventricular function imaging. Am J Cardiol 1996;78:1327–1337.

96. Ritchie JL, Gibbons RJ, Cheitlin MD, et al. ACC/AHA guidelines for exercise testing. A report of the American College of Cardiology/American Heart Association Task Force on Practice Guidelines (Committee on Exercise Testing). J Am Coll Cardiol 1997;30:260–315.

97. Bogaty P, Dumont S, O'Hara GE, et al. Randomized trial of noninvasive strategy to reduce hospital stay for patients with low-risk myocardial infarction. J Am Coll Cardiol 2001;37:1289–1296.

98. Miller TD, Gersh BJ, Christian TF, Bailey KR, Gibbons RJ. Limited prognostic value of thallium-201 exercise treadmill testing early after myocardial infarction in patients treated with thrombolysis. Am Heart J 1995;130:259–266.

99. Tilkemeier PL, Guiney TE, LaRaia PJ, Boucher CA. Prognostic value of predischarge low-level exercise thallium testing after thrombolytic treatment of acute myocardial infarction. Am J Cardiol 1990; 66:1203–1207.

100. Hendel RC, Gore JM, Alpert JS, Leppo JA. Prognosis following interventional therapy for acute myocardial infarction utility of dipyridamole thallium scintigraphy. Cardiology 1991;79:73–80.

101. Bowling BA, Aljuni SC, Puchrowicz S, Juni JE, Grines CE. Assessing the utility of exercise nuclear scintigraphy after reperfusion following myocardial infarction. Circulation 1992;86(Suppl. I):I-136.

102. Mahmarian JJ, Mahmarian AC, Marks GF, Pratt CM, Verani MS. Role of adenosine thallium-201 tomography for defining long-term risk in patients after acute myocardial infarction. J Am Coll Cardiol 1995;25:1333–1340.

103. Basu S, Senior R, Dore C, Lahiri A. Value of thallium 201 imaging in detecting adverse cardiac events after myocardial infarction and thrombolysis: a follow up of 100 consecutive patients. BMJ 1996;313: 844–848.

104. Travin MI, Dessouki A, Cameron T, Heller GV. Use of exercise technetium-99m sestamibi SPECT imaging to detect residual ischemia and for risk stratification after acute myocardial infarction. Am J Cardiol 1985;75:665–669.

105. Dakik MA, Mahmarian JK, Kimball KT, Koutelow MG, Medrano R, Verani MS. Prognostic value of exercise Tl-201 tomography in patients treated with thrombolytic therapy during myocardial infarction. Circulation 1996;94:2735–2742.

106. Leppo JA, O'Brien J, Rothendler JA, Getchell JD, Lee VW. Dipyridamole thallium 201 scintigraphy in the prediction of future cardiac events after acute myocardial infarction. N Engl J Med 1984;310: 1014–1018.

107. Brown KA, O'Meara J, Chambers CE, Plante DA. Ability of dipyridamole-thallium-201 imaging one to four days after acute myocardial infarction to predict inhospital and late recurrent ischemic events. Am J Cardiol 1990;65:160–167.

108. Miller TD, Christian TF, Hopfenspirger MR, Hodge DO, Gersh BJ, Gibbons RJ. Infarct size after acute myocardial infarction measured by quantitative tomographic 99mTc sestamibi imaging predicts subsequent mortality. Circulation 1995;92:334–341.

109. Ryan T, Armstrong WF, O'Donnell JA, Feigenbaum H. Risk stratification after acute myocardial infarction by means of exercise two-dimensional echocardiography. Am Heart J 1987;114:1305–1316.

110. Applegate RJ, Dell'Italia LJ, Crawford MH. Usefulness of two-dimensional echocardiography during low-level exercise testing early after uncomplicated acute myocardial infarction. Am J Cardiol 1987; 60:10–14.

111. Quintana M, Lindvall K, Ryden L, Brolund F. Prognostic value of predischarge exercise stress echocardiography after acute myocardial infarction. Am J Cardiol 1995;76:1115–1121.

112. Smart SC, Knickelbine T, Stoiber TR, Carlos M, Wynsen JC, Sagar KB. Safety and accuracy of dobutamine-atropine stress echocardiography for the detection of residual stenosis of the infarct-related artery and multivessel disease during the first week after acute myocardial infarction. Circulation 1997;95:1394–1401.

113. Carlos ME, Smart SC, Wynsen JC, Sagar KB. Dobutamine stress echocardiography for risk stratification after myocardial infarction. Circulation 1997;95:1402–1410.

114. Pierard LA, De Landsheere CM, Berthe C, Rigo P, Kulbertus HE. Identification of viable myocardium by echocardiography during dobutamine infusion in patients with myocardial infarction after thrombolytic therapy: comparison with positron emission tomography. J Am Coll Cardiol 1990;15: 1021–1031.

115. Picano E, Sicari R, Landi P, et al. Prognostic value of myocardial viability in medically treated patients with global left ventricular dysfunction early after an acute uncomplicated myocardial infarction: a dobutamine stress echocardiographic study. Circulation 1998;98:1078–1084.

116. Iliceto S, Caiali C, Ricci A. Prediction of cardiac events after uncomplicated myocardial infarction by cross-sectional echocardiography during transesophageal atrial pacing. Int J Cardiol 1990;28:95–103.

117. Bolognese L, Rossi L, Sarasso G, et al. Silent versus symptomatic dipyridamole-induced ischemia after myocardial infarction: clinical and prognostic significance. J Am Coll Cardiol 1992;19:953–959.

118. Camerici, Picano E, Landi P. Prognostic value of dipyridamole echocardiography early after myocardial infarction in elderly patients. J Am Coll Cardiol 1993;22:1809–1815.

119. Picano E, Pingitore A, Sicari R, et al. Stress echocardiographic results predict risk reinfarction early after uncomplicated acute myocardial infarction: large-scale multicenter study. J Am Coll Cardiol 1995;26:908.

120. Greco CA, Salustri A, Seccareccia F, et al. Prognostic value of dobutamine echocardiography early after uncomplicated acute myocardial infarction: a comparison with exercise electrocardiography. J Am Coll Cardiol 1997;29:261–267.

121. Salustri A, Ciavatti M, Seccareccia F, Palamara A. Prediction of cardiac events after uncomplicated acute myocardial infarction by clinical variables and dobutamine stress test. J Am Coll Cardiol 1999; 34:435–440.

122. Ritchie JL, Bateman TM, Bonow RO, et al. Guidelines for clinical use of cardiac radionuclide imaging: report of the American College of Cardiology/American Heart Association Task Force on Assessment of Diagnostic and Therapeutic Cardiovascular Procedures (Committee on Radionuclide Imaging) developed in collaboration with the American Society of Nuclear Cardiology. J Am Coll Cardiol 1995; 25:521–527.

123. Ellis SG, Mooney MR, George GS, et al. Randomized trial of late elective angioplasty versus conservative management for patients with residual stenoses after thrombolytic treatment of myocardial infarction. Circulation 1992;86:1400–1406.

124. Mark DB, Naylor CD, Hlatky MA, et al. Use of medical resources and quality of life after acute myocardial infarction in Canada and the United States. N Engl J Med 1994;331:1130–1135.

125. Rouleau JL, Moye LA, Pfeffer MA, Arnold JM, for the SAVE investigators. A comparison of management patterns after acute myocardial infarction in Canada and United States—the SAVE investigators. N Engl J Med 1993;328:779–784.

126. Rogers WJ, Bowlby LJ, Chandra NC, et al. Treatment of myocardial infarction in the United States (1990-1993). Observations from National Registry of Myocardial Infarction. Circulation 1994;90: 2103–2114.

127. Pfeffer MA, Braunwald E, Moye LA on behalf of the SAVE investigators. Effect of Captopril on mortality and morbidity in patients with left ventricular dysfunction after myocardial infarction. N Engl J Med 1992;327:669–667.

128. Maggioni AP, Zuanetti G, Franzosi MG, et al. Prevalence and prognostic significance of ventricular arrhythmia after acute myocardial infarction in the fibrinolytic era. GISSI-2 results. Circulation 1993; 87:312–322.

129. Moss AJ, Davis HJ, DeCamilla J, Bayer LW. Ventricular ectopic beats and their relation to sudden and nonsudden cardiac deaths after myocardial infarction. Circulation 1979;60:998–1003.

130. Bigger JT, Fleiss JL, Kleiger R, Miller JP, Rolnitzky LM and the Multicenter Post-Infarction Research Group. The relationships among ventricular arrhythmias, left ventricular dysfunction and mortality in the 2 years after myocardial infarction. Circulation 1984;69:250–258.

131. Mukharji J, Rude RE, Poole WK. The MILIS study group. Risk factors for sudden death after acute myocardial infarction. Two year follow-up. Am J Cardiol 1984;54:31–36.

132. McClements BM, Adgey AAJ. Value of signal-averaged electrocardiography, radionuclide ventriculography, Holter monitoring and clinical variables for prediction of arrhythmic events in survivors of acute myocardial infarction in the thrombolytic era. J Am Coll Cardiol 1993;21:1419–1427.

133. Singh N, Mironov D, Armstrong PW, Ross AM, Langer A, for the GUSTO ECG Substudy Investigators. Heart rate variability assessment early after acute myocardial infarction. Pathophysiological and prognostic correlates. Circulation 1996;93:1388–1395.

134. Farrell TG, Bashir Y, Cripps T, et al. Risk stratification for arrhythmic events in postinfarction patients based on heart rate variability, ambulatory electrocardiographic variables and the signal-averaged electrocardiogram. J Am Coll Cardiol 1991;18:687–697.

135. Reinhardt L, Makijarvi M, Fetsch T, et al. Noninvasive risk modeling after myocardial infarction. Am J Cardiol 1996;78:627–632.

136. Fei L, Copie X, Malik M, Camm AJ. Short-and long-term assessment of heart rate variability for risk stratification after acute myocardial infarction. Am J Cardiol 1996;77:681–684.

137. Denes P, el-Sherif N, Katz R, et al. Prognostic significance of signal-averaged electrocardiogram after thrombolytic therapy and/or angioplasty during acute myocardial infarction (CAST substudy). Cardiac Arrhythmia Suppression Trial (CAST) SAECG Substudy Investigators. Am J Cardiol 1994;74: 216–220.

138. Richards DA, Blyth K, Ross DL, Uther JD. What is the best predictor of spontaneous ventricular tachycardia and sudden death after myocardial infarction? Circulation 1991;83:756–763.

139. Zoni-Berisso M, Molini D, Mela GS, Vecchio C. Value of programmed ventricular stimulation in predicting sudden death and sustained ventricular tachycardia in survivors of acute myocardial infarction. Am J Cardiol 1996;77:673–680.

140. Pedretti R, Etro MD, Laporta A, Braga SS, Caru B. Prediction of late arrhythmic events after acute myocardial infarction from combined use of noninvasive prognostic variables and inducibility of sustained monomorphic ventricular tachycardia. Am J Cardiol 1993;71:1131–1141.

141. Moss AJ, Hall J, Cannom DS, et al. Improved survival with an implanted defibrillator in patients with coronary disease at high risk for ventricular arrhythmia. N Engl J Med 1996;335:1933–1940.

142. Buxton AE, Lee KL, Fisher JD, et al. A randomized study of the prevention of sudden death in patients with coronary artery disease. N Engl J Med 1999;341:1882–1890.

IV NON-ST-SEGMENT ELEVATION MYOCARDIAL INFARCTION

16 Anticoagulant Therapies

Marc Cohen, MD

CONTENTS

INTRODUCTION

The underlying precipitant of unstable angina non-ST-segment elevation myocardial infarction (UA/NSTEMI) is the ruptured or fissured coronary plaque, or endothelial erosion, which elicits a complex interaction between the coagulation cascade and platelets to form a thrombus. The majority of these disruptions and resulting thrombi cause only insignificant obstruction to coronary blood flow. However, a large thrombus can cause a significant impediment to coronary flow resulting in ischemia. This thrombus may resolve spontaneously with restoration of blood flow, or propagate to cause further ischemia. Often, this process can lead to complete occlusion of the vessel precipitating a myocardial infarction (MI) *(1–9)*.

Since 1980, when DeWood et al. *(9)* proved that MI was the result of in vivo thrombus formation, great resources have been expended to understand and curtail coronary thrombosis. A number of antiplatelet and anticoagulant regimens have been investigated that include aspirin, clopidogrel, glycoprotein IIb/IIIa antagonists, indirect thrombin inhibitors (heparin, low-molecular-weight heparin [LMWH] and pentasaccharide), direct thrombin inhibitors, and thrombolytics in acute coronary syndromes (ACS). The core of the problem lies within the ruptured plaque itself. Cellular and lipid elements such as tissue factor, surface-bound von Willebrand factor, and types I and III collagen are exposed, activating the intrinsic and extrinsic coagulation cascades. These pathways lead to the activation of thrombin, which, among a number of activities, cleaves fibrinogen to fibrin, activates factor XIII to stabilize the fibrin clot, and activates factors V and VIII in a positive feedback loop to accelerate thrombin's own generation. Simultaneously, thrombin as well as collagen, adenosine diphosphate (ADP), von Willebrand fac-

From: *Contemporary Cardiology: Management of Acute Coronary Syndromes, Second Edition*
Edited by: C. P. Cannon © Humana Press Inc., Totowa, NJ

tor, thromboxane A_2, and local shear forces activate platelets. There is then an exocytosis of the platelets' α and dense granules, releasing ADP and thromboxane A_2 which, in turn, feeds back to accelerate local platelet activation. Activated platelets then expose glycoprotein IIb/IIIa receptors that allow platelets to bind fibrin to form a thrombus (1–5).

A number of randomized clinical trials have established the beneficial role of antiplatelet agents, such as aspirin, ticlopidine, clopidogrel in UA/NSTEMI (10–14). Several anticoagulation regimens have been investigated as well, and these include the indirect thrombin inhibitor heparin and LWMHs and direct thrombin inhibitors. In patients treated with aspirin plus unfractionated heparin (UFH) or LMWH, a meta-analysis revealed a 33% reduction in the risk of MI or death compared with those treated only with aspirin (15). For patients pretreated with aspirin, the combination of aspirin plus short-term UFH or LMWH appears to halve the risk of MI or death. However, longer term use of LMWH or UFH (beyond the first 7 d) does not seem to provide additional benefit (16). Yet despite antiplatelet and anticoagulant therapy, approx 7–12% of patients with UA go on to suffer MI within 14 d (15). Furthermore, a significant proportion of patients with NSTE ACS, being aggressively treated with aspirin and either UFH or LMWH, experience recurrent angina prompting urgent revascularization, MI or death, within the first 24 h, 48 h, and 8 d of hospital admission, respectively (17). The 1-yr mortality of patients with UA is 5–14%, with half of the deaths occurring within the first 4 wk (15). Thus, there remains great interest in improving the efficacy of the current antiplatelet and anticoagulant therapy. The following is a synopsis of the data generated in the investigation of new anticoagulant therapies.

UNFRACTIONATED HEPARIN

Of the available anticoagulant regimens for ACS, UFH is the oldest, most widely available, and until recently was the standard by which new anticoagulant agents were judged (18). Heparin was first identified in 1916. In 1939, investigators found that its anticoagulant properties required the presence of a cofactor that was later named antithrombin III (ATIII) (19). Heparin binds to the lysine site of ATIII and produces a conformational change at the arginine reactive center, converting ATIII from a slow to a rapid inhibitor of thrombin (factor IIa) (Fig. 1). Heparin then dissociates from the complex to be re-utilized (18,19). Commercial preparations of UFH are heterogeneous with compounds ranging in molecular weight from 3000–30,000 Da. One-third of these molecules with the essential pentasaccharide sequence bind ATIII and are responsible for the majority of heparin's anticoagulant effect. The remaining two-thirds have little anticoagulant effect at therapeutic doses (19).

The heparin–antithrombin III complex inactivates factors IIa (thrombin), Xa, XIIa, XIa, and IXa. Thrombin is $10\times$ more sensitive to the heparin–ATIII complex than is factor Xa (19). However, the inactivation of thrombin requires that both ATIII and long-chain heparin bind to thrombin. The inactivation of factor Xa can be accomplished with short or long chains of heparin. Heparin moieties less than 5400 Da are unable to bind thrombin and ATIII simultaneously, but can bind factor Xa if they contains the correct pentasaccharide. As such, UFH exerts the majority of its anticoagulant properties through thrombin inactivation. Unfortunately, the anticoagulant effect of heparin is modified by platelets, fibrin, vascular surfaces, and plasma proteins. Platelet-bound factor Xa is inaccessible to UFH. Thrombin, when bound to fibrin, is also protected from

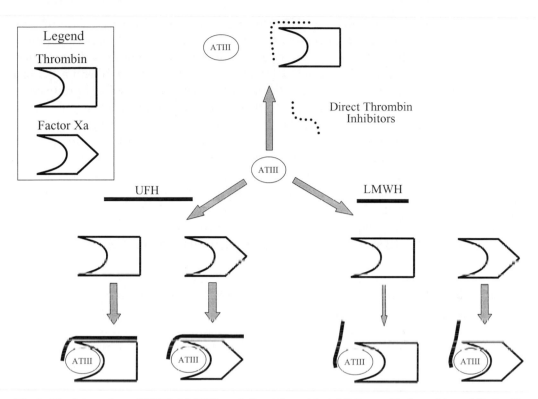

Fig. 1. The interaction of UFH, LMWH, and direct thrombin inhibitors with thrombin and factor Xa to inhibit thrombus formation.

inactivation by the heparin–ATIII complex. Finally, heparin binds to, and is inactivated by, a number of plasma proteins, including vitronectin and other acute phase reactant proteins *(19)*. Therefore, despite its compelling anticoagulant properties, its use in the platelet-rich arterial thrombus may be somewhat limited.

From 1962–1973, six randomized trials encompassing 3800 patients with ACS were conducted involving UFH, as well as warfarin and phenindione, either alone or in combination *(19)*. Pooling of the data from these trials showed a 22% reduction in total mortality ($p < 0.002$). Another overview of 5700 patients treated with heparin alone demonstrated a 16% reduction in mortality as well *(20)*.

The first randomized, placebo-controlled trial of UFH in 1981 by Telford and Wilson *(21)* showed a significant reduction (vs placebo) in the incidence of MI (15 vs 3%) after 7 d of intravenous heparin. Theroux et al. *(22)* performed a placebo-controlled randomized trial evaluating aspirin alone vs heparin alone vs a combination of the two in 479 patients with acute UA. The incidence of refractory angina decreased by 63% in the heparin group and 53% in the combination group, but there was no change in the group receiving aspirin alone. The incidence of MI was reduced in the group receiving aspirin (3%, $p = 0.01$), UFH (0.8%, $p = 0.001$), and combination therapy (1.6%, $p = 0.003$) vs placebo (12%). As compared with aspirin, UFH was associated with a relative risk of 0.47 for refractory angina ($p = 0.006$), 0.25 for MI ($p = 0.52$), and 0.52 for any event ($p = 0.10$). The combination of aspirin and UFH was only slightly superior to aspirin alone and was worse than UFH alone. Thus, there was a trend towards the superiority of

UFH over aspirin in the treatment of UA. However, as a result of the efficacy of both drugs in UA, the study was under-powered to show a benefit of combination therapy.

Theroux et al. then continued their study (23), altering the design to evaluate aspirin alone in comparison with UFH alone, deleting the placebo and combination therapy arms. During the study period, MI occurred in 0.8% of patients in the UFH group compared with 3.7% in the aspirin group ($p = 0.035$). An extended factorial analysis of the 479 patients in the first trial and 245 patients in the second trial was performed. Four of 362 patients receiving UFH therapy experienced a fatal or nonfatal MI compared with 23 of 362 patients who did not (odds ratio 0.16, $p < 0.005$). Eleven of 366 patients who received aspirin suffered an event, compared with 16 of 358 patients who did not receive aspirin (odds ratio 0.66, $p =$ NS). Bleeding complications were seen in 4 aspirin-treated patients compared with 15 heparin-treated patients ($p = 0.008$). The degree of risk reduction with UFH in comparison with aspirin exceeded 75%.

In the interim, the RISC Group (12) had published data showing that aspirin (75 mg daily), and not UFH (delivered in intermittent boluses), decreased the risk for MI in patients with UA. The results of this study should be qualified by the fact that heparin was delivered by intermittent boluses and the average dose of heparin was only 15,000 U/d. There was no adjustment of the dose on the basis of activated partial thromboplastin time (aPTT), making it likely that many patients had subtherapeutic anticoagulation. Additionally, patients were randomized up to 72 h after the last episode of chest pain, with the average time to randomization being 33 h. This resulted in the selection of a less acute cohort with lower-risk unstable coronary syndromes.

In another study of patients with refractory UA (24), where heparin was administered by continuous infusion, Neri Serneri et al. found that there was a significant decrease in the number of anginal attacks (71–77%), silent ischemia (84–94%), and total duration of ischemia (81–86%) compared with baseline ($p < 0.001$). Neither aspirin alone nor alteplase significantly reduced these endpoints.

In a later study (25), Neri Serneri et al. randomized patients with UA to subcutaneous UFH, intravenous heparin, or aspirin. The study design called for all patients to receive aspirin for 3 d prior to taking the study drug. Patients begun on heparin were taken off aspirin on d 4. After 72 h of the study drug, aspirin alone was found to have no effect on the number of anginal attacks, total ischemic episodes, or the duration of ischemia. Heparin, however, significantly lowered all three end points, whether given subcutaneously or intravenously. Analysis would suggest that those receiving heparin actually also benefited from the residual effects of 3 d of aspirin. Similarly, Theroux et al. (26) observed a rebound of clinical symptoms after heparin discontinuation. Of note, this study also showed a trend suggesting that continuation of heparin therapy (12,500 IU subcutaneously daily) for at least 4 wk may be useful in patients with UA. A similar trend was not observed in the aspirin group.

In the Antithrombotic Therapy in Acute Coronary Syndromes (ATACS) Trial (27), 214 nonprior aspirin users with UA were randomized to aspirin (162.5 mg daily) alone, or aspirin plus UFH (aPTT adjusted) for 5 d followed by 12 wk of coumadin. Of the 214 patients, 147 had UA, 46 had a non-Q wave myocardial infarction (NQWMI), and 16 had a Q wave myocardial infarction (QWMI). At 14 d, 27% of patients receiving aspirin alone reached a primary end point of recurrent angina, or MI, or death, compared with 10% in the combination therapy group ($p = 0.004$). In the subset of patients with UA, a primary end point was attained in 29% of the aspirin group compared with 21% of the heparin group. Major bleeding was observed in 2.9% of the combination group, but not in those taking aspirin alone. By the end of 12 wk of therapy, 25% of those solely on aspirin experienced a primary end point compared with 13% assigned to the aspirin and heparin group ($p = 0.06$). Pooling data from the ATACS, RISC, and Theroux studies produced an estimated relative risk of 0.44 for infarction or death among patients treated with combination anticoagulant and antiplatelet therapy in comparison with aspirin alone (27).

Holdright et al. (28), using Holter electrocardiogram (ECG) detection of ischemia, published results discordant with those above in a single-blind study of 285 patients with UA randomized to aspirin (150 mg daily) or aspirin plus intravenous aPTT-adjusted UFH. ST-segment monitoring was performed for the first 48 h of therapy. No significant difference between the two groups was noted for episodes of ischemia, total duration of ischemia, nor for secondary end points of MI or death.

Finally, in a meta-analysis (15) of 6 trials involving 1353 patients with UA and NSTEMI, the incidence of MI or death during combination therapy with heparin and aspirin was shown to be 7.9% compared to 10.4% in those on aspirin alone at 2 wk. This represents a risk reduction of 0.67 ($p - 0.057$). Risk of recurrent ischemic pain was 17.3% compared with 22.6% ($p = 0.08$), respectively. Major bleeding occurred in 0.4% and 1.5% ($p = NS$), respectively. Heparin had no effect on the rate of revascularization.

Thus, although there are some data showing that heparin is superior to aspirin alone in the treatment of patients with UA, the superiority of aspirin plus heparin over aspirin alone is not as strongly supported. Additionally, it is also clear that aspirin, when used in conjunction with heparin, reduces the incidence of rebound ischemic episodes that appear to cluster around 9.5 h after termination of the heparin infusion (27). Because UA represents a heterogeneous collection of ischemic pathology with varying degrees of risk for infarction and death, the potential benefit of heparin across these different groups probably differs. However, even when most would advocate the use of heparin, there is considerable disagreement as to the optimal duration of therapy. Although UFH continues to be viewed as a clinically important anticoagulant, the nomograms its use is based on need to be adjusted for the clinical variables that affect aPPT, the syndrome being treated, and any medications, other than UFH, that might affect hemostasis. Thus a guidance is required in view of the fact that different situations require different approaches regarding the use of UFH. For example, the dosage of UFH for the treatment of venous thromboembolic disease does not appear to be appropriate for subjects with ACS. This becomes important when UFH is used together with thrombolytic agents, because of the increased risk of intracranial hemorrhage. In view of this, recent American College of Cardiology/American Heart Association (ACC/AHA) Guidelines recommend that patients with acute MI receive an initial bolus of heparin at 60 U/kg (maximum, 4000 U), followed by alteplase (12 U/kg/h). Where intravenous heparin is given for the treatment of NSTEMI and UA, an initial bolus of 60–70 U/kg (maximum, 5000 U) followed by a 12–15 U/kg/h infusion is suggested. The aim is to reach an aPTT of 50–70 s (29).

LOW-MOLECULAR-WEIGHT HEPARIN

To date, combination anticoagulant therapy with intravenous heparin and aspirin remains a common standard of care for hospitalized patients with UA and NSTEMI (15,28). Unfortunately, a significant failure rate still exists, with 32% of UA patients requiring coronary revascularization with 4 d of hospital admission (only 12% of which are considered periprocedural) and the peak risk of recurrent angina prompting urgent revasularization, MI, or death occurring in the first 24 h, 48 h, and 8 d, respectively *(17)*. The rate of failure, however, is likely secondary to the unpredictable anticoagulant response to standard UFH, as well as neutralization by serum proteins and activated platelets.

The last decade has seen the introduction and immense benefits of LMWH. Standard UFH is a heterogeneous mixture of sulfated polysaccharides with an average molecular weight of 12,000–15,000 Da and a range from 5000–30,000 Da. LMWH is comprised of molecules averaging 4000–6500 Da, depending on the preparation *(30–33)*. Importantly, heparin molecules less than 5400 Da lack the ability to bind thrombin and ATIII simultaneously. Therefore, its predominant effect is the inactivation of factor Xa rather than factor IIa (Fig. 1). As such, the anti-Xa to antithrombin ratio of LMWH ranges from 1.5–3.9 depending on the preparation *(30,31)*.

LMWH has several clear advantages over UFH. First, its effective half-life is approx 4 h, which allows twice daily dosing. Because it does not bind to plasma proteins, such as platelet factor four and von Willebrand factor, it cannot be neutralized, and its anticoagulant response is much less erratic than that of UFH. Therefore, laboratory monitoring is not required. Furthermore, LMWH remains active in a platelet-rich environment because it can bind platelet-bound factor Xa. Unlike UFH, it does not increase vascular permeability and inhibit platelet function *(30,31)*. Finally, heparin-induced thrombocytopenia occurs much less frequently with LMWH than with UFH *(30,33)*.

LMWH was first reported to have benefits over UFH in the prophylaxis of deep-venous thrombosis in orthopedic patients *(34)*. Since then, several blinded randomized trials have demonstrated that LMWH is as good as UFH in the treatment of deep-venous thrombosis *(35–39)*.

In arterial diseases, Edmonson et al. *(40)* observed better peripheral artery bypass graft patency with LMWH than standard aspirin plus dipyridamole. Kay et al. *(41)* compared LMWH (nadroparin) to placebo in patients with ischemic stroke and found a favorable dose-dependent effect of twice daily LMWH given for 10 d with respect to neurodeficit at 6 mo without a significant increase in rates of hemorrhagic transformation of the infarct ($p = 0.005$).

Given these studies, there was great enthusiasm to utilize LMWH in acute ischemic syndromes such as UA. Gurfinkel et al. *(42)* studied UA patients ($n = 219$) in an open-label study. Patients were randomized to aspirin alone, aspirin plus aPTT-adjusted UFH, and aspirin plus the LMWH nadroparin (214 UIC/kg anti-Xa) 2× daily, subcutaneously for 5–7 d after presentation. The combination of aspirin plus LMWH was superior to aspirin only with respect to recurrent angina ($p = 0.03$), nonfatal MI ($p = 0.01$), and urgent revascularization ($p = 0.01$). This combination was also superior to aspirin and UFH with respect to recurrent angina ($p = 0.002$) and myocardial ischemia ($p = 0.04$). Additionally, patients receiving LMWH were less likely to suffer hemorrhagic complications than those receiving intravenous UFH ($p = 0.01$).

The Fragmin During Instability in Coronary Artery Disease (FRISC) Group *(43)* examined the efficacy of LMWH ($n = 1506$) in patients with UA or NQWMI. It was a double-blinded randomized parallel-group multicenter trial comparing aspirin alone (75 mg daily) with aspirin plus dalteparin (120 IU/kg 2× daily) for 5–7 d, followed by dalteparin (7500 IU subcutaneously daily) for the next 35–45 d. The primary end point of death and new MI was decreased by 48% (an absolute decrease of 3%) in the first 6 d

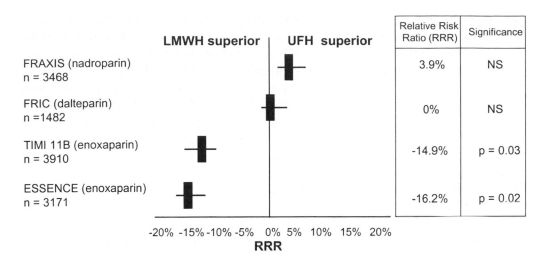

	Relative Risk Ratio (RRR)	Significance
FRAXIS (nadroparin) n = 3468	3.9%	NS
FRIC (dalteparin) n =1482	0%	NS
TIMI 11B (enoxaparin) n = 3910	-14.9%	p = 0.03
ESSENCE (enoxaparin) n = 3171	-16.2%	p = 0.02

Fig. 2. Superior cardiac outcomes of LMWHs vs UFH. Composite end points at 14 d in the FRAX-IS, FRIC, TIMI 11b, and ESSENCE studies. Reproduced with permission from Cohen M. Semin Thromb Hemost 1999;25(Suppl. 3):113–212.

by dalteparin. The rates of urgent revascularization also decreased significantly. At 40 d, the benefit of LMWH persisted, but subgroup analysis showed this only to extend to nonsmokers. There was evidence of a rebound in ischemic events when the dose was changed from twice to once daily.

Thus, the FRISC study showed that aspirin plus LMWH was better than aspirin plus placebo. The Fragmin in Unstable Coronary Artery Disease (FRIC) study *(44)* compared aspirin plus LMWH with aspirin plus aPTT-adjusted intravenous UFH. Patients with UA or NQWMI (*n* = 1482) were randomly assigned, in an open-label fashion, either 2× daily subcutaneous dalteparin (120 IU/kg) or aPTT-adjusted intravenous UFH, in addition to aspirin. In the second phase, patients in both groups were randomized to one daily injection of dalteparin (7500 IU) or placebo in a double-blinded fashion. The composite end point of death, MI, or recurrent angina was 9.3% in the dalteparin group and 7.6% in the UFH group. The combined end points of death and MI for the 2 groups were 3.9 and 3.6%, respectively. In the prolonged treatment phase, there was no difference in the composite end point of death, MI, or recurrent angina (12.3% in both groups) with a relative risk ration (RRR) of 0% (Fig. 2). The authors speculated that although dalteparin did not provide prolonged benefit at this dose, it might with twice-daily treatment. This was examined in the FRISC II study *(45)*, in which patients with unstable coronary artery disease, who had received treatment with open-label dalteparin for at least 5 d, were randomly assigned to continue with double-blind twice-daily subcutaneous dalteparin (120 IU/kg) or placebo in addition to aspirin for 3 mo. At 30 d, there was a significant decrease in the composite end point of death or MI in the dalteparin versus placebo groups (3.1 and 5.9%), while the decrease was not significant at 3 mo (6.7 and 8.0%, respectively). In the total cohort, there was a decrease in death, MI, or revasularization at 3 mo in the dalteparin and placebo groups (29.1 and 33.4%, respectively). The initial benefits were not sustained at the 6-mo follow-up.

In the Enoxaparin vs Unfractionated Heparin for Unstable Angina and Non-Q Wave Myocardial Infarction (ESSENCE) Trial *(46)*, 3171 patients with rest UA and NQWMI were randomly assigned subcutaneous enoxaparin (1 mg/kg) 2× daily or continuous aPTT-adjusted intravenous UFH for 2–8 d in a double-blind placebo-controlled fashion. After 14 d of therapy, the risk of death, MI, or recurrent angina was significantly lower in patients assigned to enoxaparin compared with UFH (16.6 vs 19.8%, $p = 0.019$) with a RRR of 16.2% ($p = 0.02$) in favor of enoxaparin (Fig. 2). This difference remained significant at 30 d (19.8 vs 23.3%, $p = 0.016$). The secondary end point of death or MI was reached at 14 d in 4.9% of the enoxaparin group compared to 6.1% of the UFH group ($p = 0.13$), and at 30 d, by 6.2% of the enoxaparin group compared to 7.7% of the UFH group ($p = 0.08$). Furthermore, at 30 d, the need for coronary revascularization was significantly lower in patients assigned to enoxaparin (27.1 vs 32.2%, $p = 0.001$). There was no difference between the two groups with regard to major hemorrhagic complications.

In a 1-yr follow-up survey of the ESSENCE study (47) the primary composite end point of death, MI, or recurrent angina was significantly lower among patients randomized to receive enoxaparin compared with those receiving UFH (32.0 vs 35.7%, $p = 0.022$). In addition, a trend toward a lower incidence of the secondary composite end point of death or MI was detected (11.5 vs 13.5%, $p = 0.082$). There was also a significant reduction in the enoxaparin treatment group with respect to the need for diagnostic catheterization (55.8 vs 59.4%, $p = 0.036$), and the need for coronary revascularization was significantly lower in the enoxaparin treatment group (35.9 vs 41.2%, $p = 0.002$).

Therefore, the ESSENCE Study is the first to show a significant benefit of LMWH over standard UFH that is sustained over 1 yr. These results are contrary to those of the FRIC Study. This may be a result of a number of factors. One major difference is the choice of LMWH preparation. Enoxaparin has an anti-Xa:anti-IIa activity ratio of 3:1 compared with 2:1 for dalteparin. In addition, the levels of von Willebrand Factor, a marker of both platelet stimulation and clinical adverse outcome (48), have been shown to be reduced significantly more by enoxaparin compared to both dalteparin and UFH (49). These differences are discussed in more detail below, but it should also be noted that the open-label nature of the FRIC Study (in-hospital phase), make it difficult to compare these two studies head-to-head.

The Thrombolysis in Myocardial Infarction (TIMI) 11A investigators (50) showed that enoxaparin 1.0 mg/kg 2× daily is the optimal dose, because the risk of major hemorrhage was almost 3-fold less than with 1.25 mg/kg 2× daily. Importantly, there was no difference in the composite end point of death, MI, or recurrent ischemia.

The TIMI 11B trial (51) was initiated to assess the benefits of an extended course of anticoagulant treatment with enoxaparin compared with UFH for the prevention of death and cardiac ischemic events in individuals with UA/NQWMI and to confirm enoxaparin's superiority over UFH in UA/NSTEMI patients. In this study, 3910 patients were randomly assigned UFH intravenously for a minimum of 3 d and a maximum of 8 d, followed by either subcutaneous placebo injections or uninterrupted treatment with enoxaparin during both an acute and an outpatient phase. The acute phase of the study was designed to assess whether enoxaparin was superior to UFH in preventing events during hospitalization and for a limited period thereafter, whereas the outpatient phase addressed the question of whether there was a potential benefit in continuing the administration of enoxaparin for a further 35 d following discharge from hospital. Treatment in the acute phase consisted of an initial intravenous bolus of 30 mg followed by injections of 1.0 mg/kg every 12 h. The outpatient phase involved 40-mg injections every 12 h for patients weighing less than 65 kg and 60 mg for patients weighing more than or equal to 65 kg. The primary end point of the study was the composite of all-cause mortality, recurrent MI, or the need for urgent revascularization. Of the 3910 patients enrolled, 1957 received UFH and 1953 received enoxaparin. The primary end point was reached by 8 d in 14.5% of patients in the UFH treatment group and 12.4% of the patients in the enoxaparin treatment group, with a RRR of 14.5% ($p = 0.03$) in favor of enoxaparin (Fig. 2). The difference between groups was significant ($p = 0.048$). By 43 d, the primary end point had been reached in 19.5% of the UFH group and 17.3% of the enoxaparin group ($p = 0.048$). The rates of major hemorrhage in the two treatment groups did not differ during the first 72 h or the entire initial hospital stay. However, during the outpatient phase, there was a significantly higher occurrence of major hemorrhage in the enoxaparin treatment group compared with the placebo group (2.9 vs 1.5%, $p = 0.021$). From these findings it was concluded that for the acute treatment of UA/NQMI patients, enoxaparin is superior to UFH in reducing the triple composite end point without causing significant increases in the rate of major hemorrhage.

Although both TIMI 11B and ESSENCE independently indicated the superiority of enoxaparin over UFH in reducing the primary composite end point, neither study was sufficiently powered to detect statistically significant treatment effects on end points other than the composite end points selected. To address this, a prospectively planned meta-analysis was to provide more robust estimates of the treatment effects of enoxaparin on death and serious cardiac ischemic events, either on their own or in various combinations, especially death and nonfatal MI in patients with UA/NQWMI (52). Enoxaparin was found to be associated with a 20% reduction in death and serious ischemic events that appeared within the first few d of treatment: this benefit was maintained up to 43 d. The treatment effect of enoxaparin occurs within 48 h and a quantitatively similar relative treatment effect was observed at d 2 and d 43. The 1-yr follow-up of TIMI 11B-ESSENCE (53), in which event rates for the composite end point of death, nonfatal MI, and urgent revascularization, and its individual components were assessed, revealed a significant treatment benefit of enoxaparin on the event rate at 1 yr ($p = 0.08$). The event rate was 25% in the UFH group and 23.3% in the enoxaparin group, representing an absolute difference of 2.5%.

The objective of the Fraxiparine in Ischaemic Syndrome (FRAXIS) study (54) was to assess the short-term benefit of the LMWH nadroparin in comparison with UFH for patients with either UA or NQWMI. Patients ($n = 3468$) were divided into three parallel groups and were randomized to one of the three following treatment regimens: (i) intravenous bolus of UFH (5000 IU) followed by an aPTT-adjusted infusion of UFH for 6 ± 2 d; (ii) an intravenous bolus of nadroparin 86 anti-Xa IU/kg, followed by subcutaneous injections of nadroparin 86 anti-Xa IU/kg for 6 ± 2 d; or (iii) an intravenous bolus of nadroparin 86 anti-Xa IU/kg, followed by subcutaneous injections of nadroparin 86 anti-Xa IU/kg 2× daily for 14 d. The composite primary outcome used in the study was that of cardiac death, MI, refractory angina, or recurrence of UA at d 14. With regard to the primary outcome, no statistically significant effects were recorded between the three treatment regimens, with a RRR of 3.9% (Fig. 2). Additionally, there were no significant intergroup differences with respect to secondary endpoints. However, with respect to major hemorrhage, there was a statistically significant increased risk in the 14-d nadroparin group compared with the UFH group (3.5 vs 1.6%, p = 0.0035). From the study findings, it was concluded that, although it may be easier to administer, nadroparin given over 6 ± 2 d offers similar efficacy and safety in the treatment of acute UA or NQWMI to UFH. However, prolonged treatment with nadroparin, over 14 d, provides no additional clinical benefits, but does increase the risk of hemorrhage.

Differences in the pharmacokinetics, pharmacodynamics and efficacy of different LMWHs clearly exist. A prospective study of 438 patients with UA or NQWMI (Enoxaparin vs Tinzaparin in the Management of Unstable Coronary Artery Disease [EVET] study) compared the efficacy of enoxaparin with tinzaparin (55). Patients were randomized to receive either twice-daily subcutaneous injections of 100 UI/kg enoxaparin or once-daily 175 UI/kg tinzaparin for 7 d. Recurrence of UA was less frequent in the enoxaparin group than the tinzaparin group at 7 d (24 out of 220 vs 41 out of 218; p = 0.029), but no significant difference between the two groups were observed with respect to death, MI, or refractory angina at 7 d. At 30 d, the frequency of death and rehospitalization in each group was not significantly different, while the need for revascularization was significantly less in the enoxaparin group (36 out of 220 vs 57 out of 218; p = 0.019). This was achieved without the risk of bleeding complications increasing.

As so many patients with UA/NSTEMI also receive concomitant glycoprotein IIb/IIIa inhibitors (see Chapter 17 for further details), it is important that the safety of the two therapies when co-administered is investigated. Safety data on enoxaparin in combination with abciximab, tirofiban, and eptifibatide have been collected (56–58). In combination with tirofiban in UA/NSTEMI patients, a small pilot study (n = 55) showed that the combination of tirofiban and enoxaparin was safe and that co-administration of enoxaparin did not adversely affect the pharmacodynamics of tirofiban, when compared with UFH (57). A later study of 535 patients treated with both tirofiban and enoxaparin or tirofiban and UFH showed the combination of enoxaparin and tirofiban to be safe. Enoxaparin-treated patients had a low rate of major hemorrhage (0.2% for enoxaparin vs 0.5% for UFH), and a similar rate of clinical events was reported for both combinations (death or MI at d 30: 9.2% enoxaparin, 10% UFH) (58). A substudy of the Global Utilization of Streptokinase and Tissue Plasminogen Activator for Occluded Coronary Arteries (GUSTO) IV-ACS randomized trial (59) also revealed that treatment of high risk ACS patients with dalteparin for 5–7 d after starting either 24- or 48-h treatment with abciximab or placebo (315, 331, and 328 patients, respectively) does not increase the rate of major bleeding in any group, while an increased rate in minor bleeding was only seen in patients treated for 48 h with abciximab.

LMWH and Percutaneous Coronary Intervention

Two complementary registry studies evaluating the safety and usefulness of two specific dose regimens of enoxaparin with, and without, concomitant abciximab during percutaneous coronary intervention (PCI) have been reported by Kereiakes et al. (60). Patients undergoing PCI were enrolled in separate conducted by the National Investigators Collaborating on Enoxaparin (NICE) study groups (NICE 1 and NICE 4 studies). NICE 1 patients were treated with 1.0 mg/kg intravenous enoxaparin without abciximab, while NICE 4 patients received a reduced dose (0.75 mg/kg) intravenous enoxaparin combined with standard dose abciximab. The studies indicated that enoxaparin with or without abciximab provided safe and effective anticoagulation during PCI. A combina-

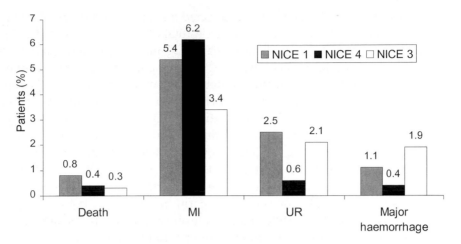

Fig. 3. Event rates for enoxaparin with or without glycoprotein IIb/IIIa antagonists in the NICE trials. NICE 1 patients received enoxaparin alone, NICE 4 patients received enoxaparin plus abciximab, while NICE 3 patients received enoxaparin plus either tirofiban, eptifibatide, or abciximab. Adapted from Kereiakes DJ, et al. J Invas Cardiol 2001;13:272–278.

tion of abciximab and reduced dose enoxaparin was associated with a low incidence of bleeding or ischemic events. Major and minor bleeding occurred in 1.1 and 6.2% of NICE 1 patients and 0.4 and 7.0% of NICE 4 patients, respectively, at 30 d post-PCI. There was a low incidence of thrombocytopenia with only 0.9 and 2.1% of NICE 1 and NICE 4 patients having a platelet count less than 100,000 at 30 d. The composite end point of death, MI, and urgent revascularization in-hospital (Fig. 3) and at 30 d post-PCI was 6.2 and 7.7% in NICE 1 patients and 6.5 and 6.8% in NICE 4 patients, respectively. Anticoagulant activity measured at 5 and 15 min post-enoxaparin bolus reflected values expected for 1.0 and 0.75 mg/kg enoxaparin treatment, while no differences occurred at 4 and 8 h. The conclusion from these studies is that enoxaparin (1.0 mg/kg) without abciximab, as well as enoxaparin (0.75 mg/kg) in combination with abciximab, provides safe and efficacious anticoagulation during PCI. Subsequently, the NICE-3 study was performed to assess the safety of subcutaneous enoxaparin in combination with eptifibatide, tirofiban, or abciximab, in patients who subsequently underwent PCI *(56)*. The study confirms the low risk of major bleeding (4.5%) found in the NICE 1 and 4 trials, and also demonstrated a low rate of clinical end points (death, MI, and urgent revascularization) of 4.5% for any glycoprotein IIb/IIIa inhibitor in combination with enoxaparin (Fig. 3). The Can Routine Ultrasound Influence Stent Expansion (CRUISE) study was also recently initiated to evaluate the safety and efficacy of either 0.75 mg/kg intravenous enoxaparin or 60 IU/kg intravenous UFH in combination with eptifibatide in patients undergoing nonemergency PCI with planned stent implantation. Bhatt et al. *(61)* recently presented results that showed that the risk of minor or major bleeding events was not significantly different between patients treated with a combination of eptifibatide and either enoxaparin (129 patients) or UFH (132 patients). They also reported that the efficacy of these combined therapies were not significantly different.

Although evidence has shown that UFH can be safely and effectively replaced in patients with UA or NQWMI by subcutaneous injections of LMWH, the optimal coagulation strategy for such patients when they require cardiac catheterization is not clear.

To address this issue, Collet et al. *(62)* conducted a study with the aim of evaluating a new anticoagulation strategy in these patients. A total of 451 patients with UA/NQWMI were treated for at least 48 h with twice-daily 1.0 mg/kg subcutaneous enoxaparin, cycled at 6 AM and 6 PM. From this group, 65% underwent coronary angiography within 8 h of the morning enoxaparin injection, followed by immediate PCI in 28% of patients. PCI was performed without any further UFH/LMWH treatment. Anti-Xa activity was 0.98 ± 0.03 IU/mL at the time of catheterization, >0.5 IU/mL in 97.6% of patients and did not relate to LMWH-to-catheterization time. At 30 d, the death and/or MI rate was 3.0% in the PCI group, 6.2% in the total population, and 10.8% in patients not undergoing catheterization. The bleeding rate at 30 d was 0.8% in the PCI group, which was comparable to that of patients not undergoing catheterization. They concluded that PCI conducted within 8 h of subcutaneous enoxaparin injection was both safe and efficacious. The early complications of PCI (abrupt closure and urgent revascularization) were prevented, and a low event rate at 1-mo follow-up was evident.

Differences in Efficacy Relating to Pharmacology

So far, only one LMWH has demonstrated superior results to UFH when treating UA. A meta-analysis of data from 5 major trials (ESSENCE, TIMI 11B, FRIC, FRISC, and FRAXIS) showed that enoxaparin gives better results than UFH for treating all groups of UA/NQWMI patients with regard to the composite end point of death, MI, and the need for revascularization, without increasing the risk of major bleeding *(63)*. The meta-analysis showed that neither dalteparin nor nadroparin were superior to UFH for treating ACS patients, although equivalence was demonstrated with dalteparin in the FRIC study *(48)*. Moreover, a direct comparison of the efficacy and safety of enoxaparin and tinzaparin in the EVET study *(55)* showed that enoxaparin is more effective in reducing both the incidence of recurrent angina at 7 d and the need for revascularization at 30 d in UA/NQWMI patients. This benefit is achieved without increasing bleeding complications. The multicenter, ARMADA study *(64)* evaluated the effects of enoxaparin, dalteparin, and UFH on von Willebrand factor and platelet activation (both predictors of adverse outcome) in UA/NQWMI patients. In agreement with earlier studies, enoxaparin and dalteparin blunted the rise of von Willebrand factor when compared with UFH, although the greater effect of enoxaparin on this factor was not confirmed. At 30 d, the incidences of clinical events were 13.0 and 18.8% for enoxaparin and dalteparin, respectively, compared to 27.7% for UFH. The study also showed that platelet GPIb/IX receptor (von Willebrand receptor) expression might also be associated with outcome in this patient group and that the highest GPIb/IX receptor expression was seen with enoxaparin. In addition, differential effects on tissue factor were also noted.

Montalescot et al. *(65)* have hypothesized that the control of von Willebrand factor, in light of its being a predictor of clinical outcome in UA, may relate to the effectiveness of anticoagulation, and that the degree of control may differ between the anticoagulants evaluated in UA. To test their hypothesis, they studied 154 patients with UA or NQWMI enrolled in a variety of clinical trials assessing anticoagulant treatments. In these studies, UFH, enoxaparin, and dalteparin were used to treat patients for a minimum of 48 h. Their findings confirmed that in patients with UA, a rise in von Willebrand factor over the initial 48 h is associated with impaired outcome at 30 d. They found that the early rise in von Willebrand factor seen in UA patients treated with UFH is less if treatment is undertaken with enoxaparin. However, such an early rise in von Willebrand factor was found to be minimally reduced by dalteparin. The authors concluded that this may be an explanation for the superiority noted with enoxaparin in clinical trials.

DIRECT THROMBIN INHIBITORS

Unlike UFH, direct thrombin inhibitors such as hirudin and bivalirudin do not require a cofactor to inhibit thrombin (66,67). The class prototype, hirudin, is a 65-amino-acid polypeptide derived from the medicinal leech (*Hirudo medicinalis*), that binds selectively to thrombin in a 1:1 fashion at 2 sites. The 72-amino-acid carboxy terminus binds to the fibrinogen recognition site of thrombin. The amino terminus binds to thrombin's catalytic site. This binding is not covalent but the dissociation rate is so slow that hirudin is essentially an irreversible inhibitor of thrombin. Importantly, it can bind and inactivate both free and bound thrombin. Additionally, PF4, vitronectin, or other plasma proteins do not inactivate it. Finally, direct thrombin inhibitors have a predictable and stable anticoagulant response (66–68).

The antithrombotic effects of hirudin have been demonstrated in animal models. Most notably in the pig model of deep arterial injury (68), where hirudin was a more effective inhibitor of both platelet deposition and thrombus formation than UFH at the site of arterial injury. Furthermore, hirudin completely eliminated macroscopic thrombus formation at an aPTT at least twice that of normal (68).

Given its mechanistic advantages, one might expect hirudin to result in better outcomes in ACS. The TIMI-5 (69) study investigated the efficacy of hirudin compared with UFH as an antithrombotic adjunct in patients with STE who were receiving thrombolytic therapy and aspirin. At 90 min, the primary end point of TIMI-3 flow at 90 min and 18–36 h was present in 62 and 49% of the hirudin and UFH groups, respectively ($p = 0.07$). At 18–36 h of therapy, the infarct related artery patency was significantly higher in the hirudin group (98 vs 89%, $p = 0.01$). Death or reinfarction occurred significantly less in the hirudin group (6.8 vs 16.7%, $p = 0.02$), while the total incidence of major hemorrhage was not significantly different, with 23.3% for UFH and 17.5% for hirudin.

In another angiographic study, 116 patients with UA and >60% stenosis of a culprit coronary artery or saphenous vein graft were randomized to receive either 1 of 2 doses of UFH or 1 of 4 doses of hirudin (70). After 72–120 h of therapy, patients treated with hirudin had significantly better calibre diameter and minimal cross-sectional area, reflecting thrombus dissolution or prevention of thrombus propagation. Additionally, there was a more consistent and stable elevation of the aPTT with hirudin along with a trend towards an improved composite end point of death, MI, and recurrent angina (14 vs 24%, $p = 0.14$). This data suggests that resolution of a coronary thrombus as judged by lesion severity might be associated with clinical benefit in UA/NQWMI patients.

The TIMI-7 investigators (71) also randomized UA patients, who were receiving daily aspirin, to 4 different doses of the direct thrombin inhibitor, Hirulog (bivalirudin), in a double-blind study. No differences were observed among the 4 groups of Hirulog dosing for the primary composite end point of death, nonfatal MI, rapid clinical deterioration, or recurrent angina at rest by 72 h. However, the secondary end point of death or nonfatal MI was 10% in the lowest dose group compared with 3.2% in the 3 combined higher dose groups at hospital discharge and persisting for 6 mo. The authors reasoned that the lowest dose could be used as a control group and concluded that Hirulog was effective in preventing adverse outcomes when used in addition to aspirin.

In the GUSTO IIb study *(72)*, 12,142 patients with chest pain associated with STE or depression or T-wave inversion were examined. Patients with STE received tPA, aspirin, and hirudin or UFH, while those without STE were administered aspirin and hirudin or UFH. The total risk of death or MI at 24 h was lower in the hirudin group than the UFH group (1.3 vs 2.1%, $p = 0.001$). However, this risk was not significantly different between the hirudin and UFH groups at 30 d (9.8 vs 8.9%, $p = 0.06$). When the UA/NSTEMI group was examined separately, there was no difference between hirudin and UFH therapy. There was also no difference in serious or life-threatening hemorrhage, although hirudin was associated with a higher incidence of moderate bleeding (8.8 vs 7.7%).

In summary, direct thrombin inhibitors have, thus far, failed to live up to their initial billing. One can theorize that although thrombin is an important antagonist of platelet activation, it represents only one pathway of platelet activation among nearly 100.

Oasis Trials

In a pilot study conducted by The Organisation to Assess Strategies for Ischemic Syndromes (OASIS) investigators *(73)*, low-dose hirudin (0.2 mg/kg bolus and infusion of 0.10 mg/kg/h) and medium-dose hirudin (0.4 mg/kg bolus and 0.15 mg/kg/h) were evaluated in conjunction with UFH. A total of 909 patients taking aspirin with UA or suspected MI without STE were randomly assigned UFH, low-dose hirudin, or medium-dose hirudin. At 7 d, the risk of cardiovascular death, MI, and refractory angina was significantly reduced in the medium-dose hirudin patient group.

The OASIS-2 *(74)* study involved 10,141 patients and assessed the superiority of medium-dose hirudin over UFH in preventing cardiovascular death, MI, and refractory angina. The primary outcome of cardiovascular death or new MI at 7 d was reached in 4.2% of patients in the UFH treatment group and 3.6% of patients in the hirudin group ($p = 0.077$). For the UFH treatment group, 6.7% of patients experienced cardiovascular death, new MI, or refractory angina at 7 d compared with 5.6% in the hirudin treatment group ($p = 0.0125$). This treatment effect was achieved in the first 72 h. Although there was a significant excess of major hemorrhage in the hirudin group (1.2 vs 0.7%, $p = 0.01$), there was not an excess of life-threatening strokes. It was concluded from the findings of OASIS-2 that hirudin is superior to UFH in preventing cardiovascular death, new MI, and refractory angina, and that it has an acceptable safety profile in patients with UA or NSTEMI. Furthermore, a combined analysis of the OASIS, OASIS-2, and GUSTO IIb studies indicated a 22% reduction in the relative risk of cardiovascular death or MI at 72 h, 17% reduction at 7 d, and 10% reduction at 35 d. Statistical significance was reached at 72 h and 7 d. It should be noted that in the OASIS II study, however, there was no significant difference between the incidence of death or MI in patients in the heparin- or hirudin-treated groups at 35 d. Additional studies of direct thrombin inhibitors are needed to establish benefits at 30 d or longer.

Bivalirudin

Kong et al. *(75)* performed a meta-analysis of six randomized trials to assess the effect of bivalirudin, a direct thrombin inhibitor, on 4 end points in patients with ACS: death, MI, major hemorrhage, and the composite of death or MI. The 6 randomized controlled trials of bivalirudin involved a total of 5674 patients; 4603 patients underwent elective percutaneous coronary revascularization and 1071 patients had ACS and received "medical" therapy only. A random-effects model was used for 4 trials, $n =$ 4973, comparing bivalirudin with UFH. In these trials, a significant reduction in the composite end point of death or MI was associated with bivalirudin at 30–50 days ($p =$ 0.02) or 14 fewer events/1000 patients treated. For the same trials, there was also a significant reduction in major hemorrhage ($p < 0.001$), or 58 fewer events/1000 patients treated. A similar analysis combined two dose-ranging trials, involving a total of 701 patients, comparing therapeutic (aPTT greater than 2× the control time) with subtherapeutic bivalirudin anticoagulation (aPTT less than 2× the control time). From this meta-analysis, it was concluded that bivalirudin is at least as efficacious as UFH with a superior safety profile. These benefits were further examined in the HERO-2 study *(76)*, in which 17,073 patients receiving aspirin and streptokinase were randomized to receive either UFH or bivalirudin. Data presented recently show a significant decrease in the composite end point death and MI, and nonfatal disabling stroke in the bivalirudin group compared with the UFH group (12.7 vs 13.8%, $p = 0.049$).

TRIM Study Group

The effect of three different doses of a thrombin inhibitor, inogatran, with UFH for unstable coronary disease was evaluated by the Thrombin Inhibition in Myocardial Ischemia (TRIM) study group *(77)*. In the study, 1209 patients admitted to the hospital with suspected UA or NQWMI were randomly assigned double-blind treatment with inogatran, a selective low-molecular-weight thrombin inhibitor, or UFH given as a bolus. Initial treatment was followed by a 3-d infusion with either a low, medium, or high dose of inogatran, or UFH. The primary composite end point was death, incidence of MI, refractory angina, or recurrent angina after 7 d. Secondary end points were as above after 3 and 30 d. Median activated aPTTs after 24 h were 36, 44, and 53 s for low-, medium-, and high-dose inogatran groups, respectively, compared with an aPTT of 54 s in the UFH group. At the end of the 3-d infusion period, patients receiving UFH had significantly fewer composite events than did inogatran-treated patients ($p = 0.01$). However, after 7 d, the event rate with respect to the primary outcome did not differ between the treatment groups. Death and MI occurred significantly less frequently in the UFH treatment group than in the three inogatran groups after 3 d ($p < 0.05$). After 7 d, although event rates continued to be lower in the UFH group, differences between groups were not statistically significant. Again, after 30 d, there were no significant differences in event rates between the four treatment groups. Within 7 d of treatment, major bleeding occurred in 1.1% of patients, with no differences between treatment groups. Therefore, during the study–drug infusion, none of the inogatran doses were better than UFH in preventing ischemic events. Nor was there a relationship between event rate and inogatran dosage. Consequently, despite a clear dose effect with respect to the prolongation of aPTT, this study did not indicate that inogatran's efficacy would improve at higher doses. Lastly, after withdrawal of UFH and inogatran treatment, event rates increased, suggesting a rebound effect.

ORAL DIRECT THROMBIN INHIBITORS

Oral thrombin inhibitors, such as megalatran, ximelagatran, and CI-1028, are currently being developed as potential agents for the prophylaxis and treatment of thrombosis. The first of the direct thrombin inhibitors to be used was hirudin; however, direct inhibitors with low molecular weights have since been developed (e.g., DuP 714, PPACK, efegatran), and these have an enhanced ability to inhibit clot-bound thrombin and the processes of thrombosis taking place at sites of arterial damage *(78,79)*. For many of the available oral direct thrombin inhibitors, suboptimal gastrointestinal absorption is an evident problem. H376/95 is a new oral direct thrombin inhibitor. It is a prodrug with two protective residues attached to the direct thrombin inhibitor megalatran. Gustafsson et al. *(80)* undertook a 3-part study comparing the intestinal absorption properties of melagatran on its own and in the H376/95 prodrug form, and also studied the affect of the prodrug on an experimental thrombosis model in rats. In the melagatran portion of the study, healthy male volunteers were given escalating single oral doses of the agent (57–200 mg) in an aqueous solution after an overnight fast. Four people were used at each dose level. In the prodrug study, healthy male volunteers were given escalating single oral doses between 5 and 98 mg, with 5 subjects at each dose level. By converting melagatran into the prodrug, the oral absorption of melagatran was between 2.7 and 5.5× higher than after oral administration of unaltered melagatran. It was concluded that, by using the prodrug principle in this way, melagatran becomes endowed with the pharmacokinetic properties necessary for oral administration without compromising the pharmacodynamic properties of the agent, thereby providing an oral direct thrombin inhibitor of use in a clinical setting. In the rat model, oral H 376/95 was found to be more effective in preventing thrombosis than was the LMWH, dalteparin.

Using a rat model, Mikulski et al. *(81)* assessed the effect of pretreatment with melagatran and inogatran for cerebral infarction. Ischemic stroke was induced in rats photochemically. A single oral dose of melagatran (30 μmol/kg) was found to significantly reduce the vol of the cortical infarct by 53% ($p < 0.05$) compared with control animals. Additionally, after administration of intravenous (6 μmol/kg) or oral (100 μmol/kg) inogatran, there was a decrease in cortical infarct vol of 83 and 19%, respectively, compared with controls. Therefore, the study demonstrated that experimental focal ischemic infarction, brought about by photochemically induced endothelial cell damage, can be significantly reduced with direct thrombin inhibitors given in oral form.

McClanahan et al. *(78)* have conducted a study with the objective of evaluating the efficacy of CI-1028, a direct thrombin inhibitor that is orally bioavailable, in a canine electrolytic injury model of venous and arterial thrombosis. Animals received either saline or CI-1028 in doses of 10, 15, 20, or 30 mg/kg. Maximum blood CI-1028 concentrations were generally achieved between 15 and 30 min of oral administration. The drug was found to increase time to occlusion (TTO). In the 20 mg/kg treatment group ($n = 8$), TTO was significantly longer than in controls both in arteries ($p = 0.05$) and in veins ($p < 0.05$). Likewise, at the 30 mg/kg dose ($n = 8$), TTO was significantly prolonged. Although surgical blood loss and template bleeding times had a tendency to increase in a dose-dependent fashion, this only reached statistical significance at the highest dose. Consistent with the agents' mechanism of action, dramatic changes in thrombin time were noted. Hardly any changes were detected in prothrombin time. Maximum aPTT and activated clotting time (ACT) were achieved at approx 30 min after administration, and they were in the region of 2- and 5-fold baseline values, respectively, at the 30 mg/kg dose. These findings demonstrate that CI-1028 provides a dose-dependent antithrombotic effect following oral administration in the canine model described.

WARFARIN

Mechanism of Action

Vitamin K, a cofactor required for the conversion of precursor proteins into active coagulation factors II, VII, IX, and X, is disrupted by warfarin. As a consequence, the vitamin K-dependent proteins exposed to warfarin during their synthesis are rendered dysfunctional. Where coagulation factors have already been completely synthesized prior to warfarin treatment, the drug has no effect. As a result, the coagulation factors that are fully established have to be depleted by way of normal catabolism before the beneficial effects of warfarin become apparent. Warfarin increases both prothrombin time and aPTT.

Studies with Warfarin

Despite the use of aspirin, the long-term risk of MI or death continues to be high in patients with UA. Consequently, additional treatments are constantly being considered. One candidate is warfarin.

In the Organization to Assess Strategies for Ischemic Syndromes (OASIS-2) substudy *(82)* warfarin anticoagulant therapy was compared with conventional therapy, for up to 5 mo, on the primary composite end point of cardiovascular death, MI, or stroke, and on the secondary composite end point of cardiovascular death, MI, stroke, and readmission to hospital for UA. Of the 10,141 patients entering the main trial, 3712 were randomized, 12–48 h later, to receive oral anticoagulant therapy ($n - 1848$) or standard therapy ($n = 1864$). Countries represented in the study were defined as being good or poor compliers (based on the use of oral anticoagulants at a rate of above or below 70% at 35 d). In the good-complier countries, both the primary and secondary composite outcomes were significantly reduced with oral anticoagulants compared with standard therapy (primary end point: 6.1 vs 8.9%, $p = 0.02$; secondary endpoint 11.9 vs 16.5%, $p = 0.005$). There were no significant differences in end points in the poor-complier countries. In the overall study, there was a significantly higher incidence of major bleeding, which was larger in the good-complier countries (relative risk 2.71) than in the poor-complier countries (relative risk 1.58). Additionally, in the good-complier countries, there were significant reductions in the number of cardiac catheterization procedures ($p = 0.004$) and reductions in revascularization procedures approached statistical significance ($p = 0.06$). Hence, considering participating countries according to their rate of compliance to anticoagulant therapy suggests that high compliance has the potential to lead to clinically significant reductions in major ischemic cardiovascular events.

In another study, conducted by Huynh et al. *(83)*, the potential benefit of secondary prevention with warfarin in patients with NSTE ACS and prior coronary artery bypass grafting (CABG) was investigated. In this double-blind trial, 135 patients with UA or NSTEMI, who had already undergone CABG, and were poor candidates for revascularization, were randomized to receive: (*i*) aspirin and placebo; (*ii*) warfarin and placebo; or (*iii*) aspirin and warfarin for 12 mo. A primary composite end point of death, MI, or UA requiring admission to hospital 1 yr after randomization was used in the study. This was reached in 14.6% of the patients in the warfarin alone group, 11.5% in the aspirin alone group, and in 11.3% in the combination therapy group ($p = 0.76$) Subgroup analysis by risk factors was unable to provide any indication that warfarin on its own, or in combination with aspirin, could be more beneficial than aspirin on its own. Additionally, in the two groups of patients receiving warfarin there was a greater frequency of bleeding.

In the ATACS trial *(84),* 214 UA/NSTEMI patients were randomized to receive either aspirin alone (162.5 mg daily) or a combination of aspirin (162.5 mg daily) plus UFH (aPTT, 2× control) followed by warfarin (internation normalized ration [INR], 2 to 3) as antithrombotic therapy. Therapy began within 9.5 ± 8.8 h of qualifying pain and continued for 12 wk. At 14 d, there was a significant decrease in the frequency of ischaemic events in the group treated with the combination therapy compared to the group treated with aspirin alone (10.5 vs 27%; $p = 0.004$). At 12 wk, however, there was a nonsignificant decrease in total ischemic events in the combination therapy group vs aspirin alone. From these results, Cohen et al. *(84)* concluded that the combination of antithrombotic therapy with aspirin plus anticoagulation with warfarin leads to a significant reduction in ischemic events in the early phase of UA.

In the recently presented Warfarin-Aspirin Reinfarction Study (WARIS)-II study, 3626 MI patients were randomized to treatment with aspirin 160 mg od, or warfarin INR 2.8–4.2, or both warfarin INR 2.0–2.5 and aspirin 75 mg once daily *(85).* Patients were followed-up for up to 4 yr. The combined warfarin and aspirin treatment was significantly more effective than aspirin alone at reducing death, nonfatal MI, and stroke. Warfarin treatment alone was also significantly more effective than aspirin alone, but to a lesser degree. One disadvantage of warfarin treatment was that major bleeding was 4× more common than with aspirin alone, but the overall bleeding rate in the study was relatively low.

SUMMARY

Advances in our understanding of coronary thrombosis made in the last 2 decades have led to the current standard of care for the treatment of NSTE ischemic syndromes becoming aspirin and UFH, or increasingly enoxaparin, which has been shown to have superior efficacy to UFH. The direct thrombin inhibitors, hirudin and bivalirudin, have shown variable results in patients with UA and NSTEMI, but some bleeding risks, and further studies are needed to clarify the usefulness of these therapies. However, even with these combination therapies, many patients go on to suffer MI or death. Advances in anticoagulant therapies, coupled with new antiplatelet therapies, will likely result in even greater reductions in adverse clinical outcomes for patients with NSTEMI.

REFERENCES

1. Fuster V, Badimon L, Cohen M, Ambrose J, Badimon J, Chesebro J. Insights into the pathogenesis of acute ischemic syndromes. Circulation 1988;77:1213–1220.
2. Fuster V, Stein B, Ambrose J, Badimon L, Badimon J, Chesebro J. Atherosclerotic plaque rupture and thrombosis: evolving concepts. Circulation 1990;82(Suppl. II):II-47–II-59.
3. Fuster V. Mechanisms leading to myocardial infarction: insights from studies of vascular biology. Circulation 1994;90:2126–2146.
4. Falk E, Shah P, Fuster V. Coronary plaque disruption. Circulation 1995;92:657–670.
5. Stein B, Fuster V, Halperin J, Chesebro J. Antithrombotic therapy in cardiac disease: an emerging approach based on pathogenesis and risk. Circulation 1989;80:1502–1513.
6. Theroux P, Lidon R. Unstable angina: pathogenesis, diagnosis, and treatment. Curr Probl Cardiol 1993; 18:157–231.
7. Cairns J, Lewis D Jr, Meade T, Sutton G, Theroux P. Antithrombotic agents in coronary artery disease. Chest 1995;108(Suppl.):380S–400S.

8. Grambow D, Topol E. Effect of maximal medical therapy on refractoriness of unstable angina pectoris. Am J Cardiol 1992;70:577–581.

9. DeWood M, Spores J, Notske R, et al. Prevalence of total coronary occlusion during the early hours of transmural myocardial infarction. N Engl J Med 1980;303:897–902.

10. Lewis H, Davis J, Archibald D, et al. Protective effects of aspirin against acute myocardial infarction and death in men with unstable angina. N Engl J Med 1983;309:396–403.

11. Cairns J, Gent M, Singer J, et al. Aspirin, sulfinpyrazone or both in unstable angina: results of a Canadian multicenter trial. N Engl J Med 1985;313:1369–1375.

12. The RISC Group. Risk of myocardial infarction and death during treatment with low dose aspirin and intravenous heparin in men with unstable coronary artery disease. Lancet 1990;336:827–830.

13. Balsano F, Rizzon P, Violi F, et al. Antiplatelet treatment with ticlopidine in unstable angina: a controlled, multicenter clinical trial. Circulation 1990;82:17–26.

14. The Clopidogrel in Unstable Angina to Prevent Recurrent Events Trial Investigators. Effects of clopidogrel in addition to aspirin in patients with acute coronary syndromes without ST-segment elevation. N Engl J Med 2001;345:494–502.

15. Oler A, Whooley M, Oler J, Grady D. Adding heparin to aspirin reduces the incidence of myocardial infarction and death in patients with unstable angina: a meta-analysis. JAMA 1996;276:811–815.

16. Eikelboom JW, Anand SS, Malmberg K, Weitz JI, Ginsberg JS, Yusuf S. Unfractionated heparin and low-molecular-weight heparin in acute coronary syndrome without ST elevation: a meta-analysis. Lancet 2000;355:1936–1942.

17. Cohen M, Antman EM, Murphey SA, Radley D. Mode and timing of treatment failure (recurrent ischemic events) after hospital admission for non-ST segment elevation acute coronary syndromes. Am Heart J 2002;143:63–69.

18. Hirsh J. Heparin. N Engl J Med 1991;324:1565–1574.

19. Yusuf S, Wittes J, Friedman L. Overview of results of randomized clinical trials in heart disease. I. Treatments following myocardial infarction. JAMA 1988;260:2088–2093.

20. Hennekens D, O'Donnell C, Ridker P. Current and future perspectives on antithrombotic therapy of acute myocardial infarction. Eur Heart J 1995;16(Suppl. D):2–9.

21. Telford A, Wilson C. Trial of heparin versus atenolol in prevention of myocardial infarction in intermediate coronary syndrome. Lancet 1981;1:1225–1228.

22. Theroux P, Ouimet H, McCans J, et al. Aspirin, heparin, or both to treat acute unstable angina. N Engl J Med 1988;319:1105–1111.

23. Theroux P, Waters D, Qui S, McCans J, deGuise P, Juneau M. Aspirin versus heparin to prevent myocardial infarction during the acute phase of unstable angina. Circulation 1993;88:2045–2048.

24. Neri Serneri G, Gensini G, Poggesi L, et al. Effect of heparin, aspirin, or alteplase in reduction of myocardial ischaemia in refractory unstable angina. Lancet 1990;335:615–618.

25. Neri Serneri GG, Modesti PA, Gensini GG, et al. Randomized comparison of subcutaneous heparin, intravenous heparin, and aspirin in unstable angina. Studio Epoorine Sottocutanea nell'Angina Instobile (SESAIR) Refrattorie Group. Lancet 1995;345:1201–1204.

26. Theroux P, Waters D, Lam J, Juneau M, McCans J. Reactivation of unstable angina after the discontinuation of heparin. N Engl J Med 1992;327:141–145.

27. Cohen M, Adams PC, Parry G, et al. Combination antithrombotic therapy in unstable rest angina and non-Q-wave infarction in nonprior aspirin users. Primary end points analysis from the ATACS trial. Antithrombotic therapy in acute coronary syndromes research group. Circulation 1994;89:81–88.

28. Holdright D, Patel D, Cunningham D, et al. Comparison of the effect of heparin and aspirin versus aspirin alone on transient myocardial ischemia and in-hospital prognosis in patients with unstable angina. J Am Coll Cardiol 1994;24:39–45.

29. Menon V, Berkowitz SD, Antman EM, Fuchs RM, Hochman JS. New heparin dosing recommendations for patients with acute coronary syndromes. Am J Med 2001;110:641–650.

30. Cohen M, Blaber R. Potential uses of a new class of low-molecular weight heparins in cardiovascular indications. Thromb Haemost 1996;22(Suppl. 2):25–27.

31. Samama M, Bara L, Gerotziafas G. Mechanisms for the antithrombotic activity in man of low molecular weight heparins. Haemostasis 1994;24:105–117.

32. Weitz JI. Low-molecular-weight heparins. N Engl J Med 1997;337:688–698.

33. Warkentin TE, Levine MN, Hirsh J, Horsewood P, Roberts RS, Gent M, Kelton JG. Heparin-induced thrombocytopenia in patients treated with low-molecular-weight heparin or unfractionated heparin. N Engl J Med 1995;332:1330–1335.

34. Planes A, Vochelle N, Mazzas F, et al. Prevention of postoperative venous thrombosis: a randomized trial comparing unfractionated heparin with low molecular weight heparin in patients undergoing total hip replacement. Thromb Haemost 1988;60:407–410.

35. Hull RD, Raskob GE, Pineo GF, et al. Subcutaneous low-molecular-weight heparin compared with intravenous heparin in the treatment of proximal-vein thrombosis. N Engl J Med 1992;326:975–982.

36. Lensing A, Prins M, Davidson B, Hirsh J. treatment of deep venous thrombosis with low molecular weight heparins: a meta-analysis. Arch Intern Med 1995;155:601–607.

37. Levine M, Gent M, Hirsh J, et al. A comparison of low-molecular-weight heparin administered primarily at home with unfractionated heparin administered in the hospital for proximal deep-vein thrombosis. N Engl J Med 1996:334:677–681.

38. Koopman M, Prandoni P, Piovella F, et al. Treatment of venous thrombosis with intravenous unfractionated heparin administered in the hospital as compared with subcutaneous low molecular weight heparin administered at home. N Engl J Med 1996;334:682–687.

39. Leizorovicz A, Simoneau G, Decousus H, Boissel J. Comparison of efficacy and safety of low molecular weight heparin in initial treatment of deep venous thrombosis: a meta-analysis. Br Med J 1994; 309:299–304.

40. Edmondson R, Cohen A, Das S, Wagner M, Kakkar V. Low molecular weight heparin versus aspirin and dipyridamole after femoropopliteal bypass grafting. Lancet 1994;344:914–918.

41. Kay R, Wong D, Yu Y, et al. Low molecular weight heparin for the treatment of acute ischemic stroke. N Engl J Med 1995;333:1588–1593.

42. Gurfinkel E, Manos E, Mejail R, et al. Low molecular weight heparin versus regular heparin or aspirin in the treatment of unstable angina and silent ischemia. J Am Coll Cardiol 1995;26:313–318.

43. Wallentin L, for the Fragmin During Instability in Coronary Artery Disease (FRISC) Group. Low molecular weight heparin during instability in coronary artery disease. Lancet 1996;347:561–568.

44. Klein W, Buchwald A, Hillis S, et al. Comparison of low molecular weight heparin with unfractionated heparin acutely and with placebo for 6 weeks in the management of unstable coronary artery disease: fragmin in unstable coronary artery disease study (FRIC). Circulation 1997;96:61–68.

45. Fragmin and Fast Revascularisation during InStability in Coronary artery disease (FRISC II) Investigators. Long-term low molecular-mass heparin in unstable coronary-artery disease: FRISC II prospective randomised multicentre study. Lancet 1999;354:701–707.

46. Cohen M, Demers C, Gurfinkel EP, et al. A comparison of low-molecular-weight heparin with unfractionated heparin for unstable coronary artery disease. N Engl J Med 1997;337:447–452.

47. Goodman SG, Cohen M, Bigonzi F, et al. Randomized trial of low molecular weight heparin (enoxaparin) versus unfractionated heparin for unstable coronary artery disease: one-year results of the ESSENCE Study. Efficacy and Safety of Subcutaneous Enoxaparin in Non-Q Wave Coronary Events. J Am Coll Cardiol 2000;36:693–698.

48. Montalescot G, Collet JP, Choussat R, Ankri A, Thomas D. A rise of troponin and/or von Willebrand factor over the first 48 h is associated with a poorer 1-year outcome in unstable angina patients. Int J Cardiol 2000;72:293–294.

49. Montalescot G, Collet JP, Lison L, et al. Effects of various anticoagulant treatments on von Willebrand factor release in unstable angina. J Am Coll Cardiol 2000;36:110–114.

50. Dose-ranging trial of enoxaparin for unstable angina: results of TIMI 11A. The Thrombolysis in Myocardial Infarction (TIMI) 11A Trial Investigators. J Am Coll Cardiol 1997;29:1474–1482.

51. Antman EM, McCabe CH, Gurfinkel EP, et al. Enoxaparin prevents death and cardiac ischemic events in unstable angina/non-Q-wave myocardial infarction. Results of the thrombolysis in myocardial infarction (TIMI) 11B trial. Circulation 1999;100:1593–1601.

52. Antman EM, Cohen M, Radley D, et al. Assessment of the treatment effect of enoxaparin for unstable angina/non-Q-wave myocardial infarction. TIMI 11B-ESSENCE meta-analysis. Circulation 1999;100: 1602–1608.

53. Antman EM, Cohen M, McCabe C, et al. Enoxaparin is superior to unfractionated heparin for preventing clinical events at 1-year followup of TIMI 11B and ESSENCE. Eur Heart J 2002;23:308–314.

54. Comparison of two treatment durations (6 days and 14 days) of a low molecular weight heparin wiht a 6-day treatment of unfractionated heparin in the initial management of unstable angina or non-Q wave myocardial infarction: FRAX.I.S. (FRAxiparine in Ischaemic Syndrome). Eur Heart J 1999;20: 1553–1562.

55. Michalis LK, Papamichail N, Katsouras CS, et al. Enoxaparin Versus Tinzaparin in the Management of Unstable Coronary Artery Disease (EVET Study) J Am Coll Cardiol 2001;37(Suppl. A):365A.

56. Cohen M, Theroux P, Weber S, et al. Combination therapy with tirofiban and enoxaparin in acute coronary syndromes. Int J Cardiol 1999;71:273–281.

57. Cohen M, et al. Anti-thrombotic combination using tirofiban and enoxaparin: the ACUTE II study. Circulation 2000;102:II-826.

58. Ferguson JJ, et al. The use of enoxaparin and IIb /IIIa antagonists in acute coronary syndromes—final results of the NICE-3 study. J Am Coll Cardiol 2001;37:365A.

59. The GUSTO IV-ACS Investigators. Effect of glycoprotein IIb/IIIa receptor blocker abciximab on outcome in patients with acute coronary syndromes without early coronary revascularisation: the GUSTO IV-ACS randomised trial. Lancet 2001;357:1915–1924.

60. Kereiakes DJ, Grines C, Fry E, et al. Enoxaparin and abciximab adjunctive pharmacotherapy during percutaneous coronary intervention. J Invasive Cardiol 2001;13:272–278.

61. Bhatt L, Lincoff AM, The CRUISE Investigators. Combined use of eptifibatide and enoxaparin in patients undergoing percutaneous coronary intervention: the results of the CRUISE trial [abstract]. Circulation 2001;104:II-384.

62. Collet JP, Montalescot G, Lison L, et al. Percutaneous coronary intervention after subcutaneous enoxaparin pretreatment in patients with unstable angina pectoris. Circulation 2001;103:658–663.

63. Cohen M. Low molecular weight heparins in the management of unstable angina/non-Q-wave myocardial infarction. Semin Thromb Hemost 1999;25(Suppl. 3):113 121.

64. Montalescot G, Drouet L. ARMADA study: a randomized comparison of enoxaparin, dalteparin and unfractionated heparin on markers of cell activation in patients with unstable angina Eur Heart J 2001;22;663.

65. Montalescot G, Collet JP, Lison L, et al. Effects of various anticoagulant treatments on von Willebrand factor release in unstable angina. J Am Coll Cardiol 2000;36(1):110–114.

66. Lidon R, Theroux P, Juneau M, Adelman B, Maraganore J. Initial experience with a direct antithrombin, hirulog, in unstable angina. anticoagulant, antithrombotic, and clinical effects. Circulation 1993;88:1495–1501.

67. Cannon C, Braunwald E. Hirudin: intial results in acute myocardial infarction, unstable angina and angioplasty. J Am Coll Cardiol 1995;25(Suppl. 7):30S–37S.

68. Heras M, Chesebro J, Webster M, et al. Hirudin, heparin, and placebo during deep arterial injury in the pig. The in vivo role of thrombin in platelet-mediated thrombosis. Circulation 1990;82:1476–1484.

69. Cannon C, McCabe C, Henry T, et al. A pilot trial of recombinant desulfatohirudin compared with heparin in conjunction with tissue-type plasminogen activator and aspirin for acute myocardial infarction: results of TIMI 5 trial. J Am Coll Cardiol 1994;23:993–1003.

70. Topol E, Fuster V, Harrington R, et al. Recombinant hirudin for unstable angina pectoris: a multicenter, randomized angiographic trial. Circulation 1994;89:1557–1566.

71. Fuchs J, Cannon C. Hirulog in the treatment of unstable angina. Results of the TIMI 7 trial. Circulation 1995;92:727–733.

72. The Global Use of Strategics to Open Occluded Coronary Arteries (GUSTO) IIb Investigators. A comparison of recombinant hirudin with heparin for the treatment of acute coronary syndromes. N Engl J Med 1996;33:775–782.

73. Organization to Assess Strategies for Ischemic Syndromes (OASIS) Investigators. Comparison of the effects of two doses of recombinant hirudin compared with heparin in patients with acute myocardial ischemia without ST elevation: a pilot study. Circulation 1997;96:769–777.

74. Organisation to Assess Strategies for Ischemic Syndromes (OASIS-2) Investigators. Effects of recombinant hirudin (lepirudin) compared with heparin on death, myocardial infarction, refractory angina, and revascularisation procedures in patients with acute myocardial ischaemia without ST elevation: a randomised trial. Lancet 1999;353:429–438.

75. Kong D, Topol E, Bittl J, et al. Clinical outcomes of bivalirudin for ischemic heart disease. Circulation 1999;100:2049–2053.

76. White HD. The HERO-2 trial. Presented at the European Society of Cardiology—XXIII Congress, 2001.

77. Thrombin inhibition in Myocardial Ischaemia (TRIM) study group. A low molecular weight, selective thrombin inhibitor, inogatran, vs. heparin, in unstable coronary artery disease in 1209 patients. A double-blind, randomized, dose-finding study. Eur Heart J 1997;18(9):1416–1425.

78. McClanahan T, Hicks G, Ignasiak D, et al. The antithrombotic effects of CI-1028, an orally bioavailable direct thrombin inhibitor, in a canine model of venous and arterial thrombosis. J Thromb Thrombolysis 2000;10:277–284.

79. Van Aken H, Bode C, Darius H, et al. Anticoagulation: the present and future. Clin Appl Thromb Hemost 2001;7:195–204.

80. Gustafsson D, Nystrom J, Carlsson S, et al. The direct thrombin inhibitor melagatran and its oral pro-drug H 376/95: intestinal absorption properties, biochemical and pharmacodynamic effects. Thromb Res 2001;101:171–181.

81. Mikulski A, Elg M, Gustafsson D. The effects of oral and intravenous direct thrombin inhibitors on the size of photochemically induced cortical infarction in rats. Thromb Res 2001;101:477–482.

82. The Organization to Assess Strategies for Ischemic Syndromes (OASIS) Investigators. Effects of long-term, moderate-intensity oral anticoagulation in addition to aspirin in unstable angina. J Am Coll Cardiol 2001;37:475–484.

83. Huynh T, Theroux P, Bogaty P, Nasmith J, Solymoss S. Aspirin, warfarin, or the combination for secondary prevention of coronary events in patients with acute coronary syndromes and prior coronary artery bypass surgery. Circulation 2001;103:3069–3074.

84. Cohen M, Adams PC, Parry G, et al. Combination antithrombotic therapy in unstable rest angina and non-Q-wave infarction in nonprior aspirin users: primary end points analysis from the ATACS trial. Circulation 1994;89:81–88.

85. Hurlen M, Smith P, Abdelnorr M, Erikssen J, Arnesen H. Effects of warfarin, aspirin and the two combined on mortality and thrombo-embolic morbidity after myocardial infarction. Presented at the 23rd Annual Meeting of the European Society of Cardiology, 2001.

17 Antiplatelet Therapy

Ian Conde-Pozzi, MD and
Neal S. Kleiman MD, FACC

CONTENTS

INTRODUCTION

The central importance of platelets in the pathogenesis of acute coronary syndromes (ACS) has increasingly been recognized over the past few years. Therefore in the last decade, a series of novel antiplatelet agents has been developed and our understanding of the role of the older agents has expanded as well. Platelets have intensively been studied not only for the elucidation of pathophysiologic mechanisms of disease, but also as central targets in the castrametation of therapeutic interventions in the field of thrombotic diseases. There is now overwhelming evidence that various classes of antiplatelet agents improve survival and reduce myocardial infarction in patients suffering an ACS (with or without ST-segment elevation) and in those undergoing percutaneous coronary intervention (PCI). This chapter will review the background, rationale, and data-driven evidence behind the applicability of the main antiplatelet classes of drugs approved for clinical use (aspirin, thienopyridines, and platelet glycoprotein [GP] IIb/IIIa antagonists) for the treatment of non-ST elevation ACS and highlight some of the most relevant aspects of their clinical use.

VASCULAR INJURY AND THROMBOSIS

Rupture or erosion of an atherosclerotic plaque with subsequent platelet aggregation and coronary artery thrombosis is a central pathophysiologic event across the entire

From: *Contemporary Cardiology: Management of Acute Coronary Syndromes, Second Edition*
Edited by: C. P. Cannon © Humana Press Inc., Totowa, NJ

spectrum of acute ACS *(1–3)*. As the plaque matures and increases in size, macrophages and foam cells preferentially infiltrate its shoulder regions *(4,5)* and are capable of releasing several enzymes and inflammatory mediators that play a crucial role in the degradation of the extracellular matrix and weakening of the fibrous cap *(6)*. In addition, contraction, bending, flexing and shear stress fluctuations of the cap during the cardiac cycle can weaken the plaque and render it prone to rupture *(1)*.

The resulting discontinuity in the fibrous cap leads to exposure of the highly thrombogenic fatty gruel contained within the plaque to flowing arterial blood *(7)*, with subsequent thrombosis on the luminal surface of the plaque. Endothelial denudation, exposure of subendothelial collagen and other matrix proteins, the initiation of the extrinsic pathway of coagulation by the high content of tissue factor (TF) present in the fatty gruel *(8)*, together with a turbulent flow around a swollen plaque, are all potent stimuli for platelet activation and thrombus formation. It is, therefore, not surprising that antiplatelet and antithrombin therapies are the cornerstones in the treatment of ACS.

PLATELET PATHOPHYSIOLOGY IN ARTERIAL THROMBOSIS

Platelets are the smallest of blood cells, with an average diameter of 1–2 μm and a mean cell volume of 5–6 fL, and have a life span of approx 7–10 d *(9)*, which apparently is not reduced in activated platelets *(10)*. The average platelet count is quite high, ranging from 140–440 × 10^9/L *(11)*. Therefore, even seemingly subtle changes related to the function and activation status of platelets may have a significant impact on physiologic or pathologic processes.

Platelets play a central role in the drama of hemostasis and serve as a fundamental link between the formation of platelet-rich thrombi and the activation of the coagulation cascade. In addition, although platelets have classically been viewed as only hemostatic in nature, there is a rapidly growing body of evidence indicating that platelets also play a role in effecting inflammatory responses, both directly and by modulating the activation of leukocytes. Therefore, antiplatelet therapy may well have a significant anti-inflammatory effect as well *(12,13)*.

A series of well orchestrated and punctually executed events must occur before an unactivated and circulating platelet reaches and adheres to a site of vascular injury or merges onto a developing thrombus. Although these events most probably occur in a more-or-less simultaneous fashion, they can be conceptually divided into the following phases: platelet adhesion, activation, granule secretion, and aggregation.

Platelet Adhesion

Whether it is spontaneous, as in the case of ACS, or iatrogenic, as in the case of percutaneous transluminal coronary angioplasty, platelet deposition occurs almost instantaneously after arterial injury *(14)*. After endothelial denudation, platelets translocate on the vessel wall by an interaction mediated by their constitutively expressed GP Ib-IX-V complex and von Willebrand Factor (vWf) affixed to the subendothelium *(15)*, and possibly also with newly expressed P-selectin on activated endothelial cells *(16)*. The GP Ib–vWF interaction is particularly important under conditions of increased shear stress *(17)*, such as those occurring in stenotic coronary artery lesions. It has also been proposed that vWF may form a bridge between exposed subendothelial collagen and GP Ib on platelets *(18)*, further facilitating the rolling of platelets. After this initial interaction,

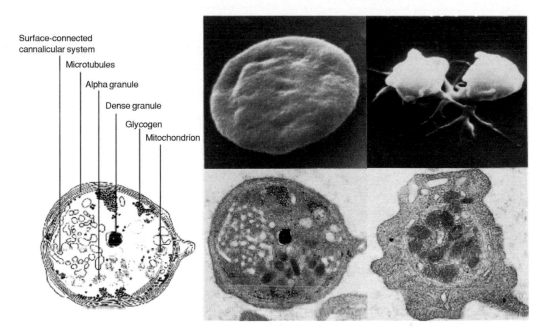

Fig. 1. Electron micrographs of resting and activated platelets. The top photographs are scanning electron micrographs of a resting, disc-shaped circulating platelet (upper left; ×20,000), and of two activated platelets, which have adopted a spherical form with the formation of long filopodia (upper right; ×10,000). The lower photographs are (from left to right), a schematic depiction of the cross-sectional view of a resting platelet, showing the subcellular platelet structures (bottom left); the actual electron micrograph of a resting platelet (bottom middle; ×21,000); and an electron micrograph of an activated platelet, showing the constriction of the microtubular ring around the centralized granules, with the formation of filopodia (bottom right; ×30,000). Reproduced with permission from: George JN. Hemostasis and Fibrinolyisis. In: Stein JH, et al, eds. Internal Medicine, 5th ed. Mosby, St. Louis, 1998:534–540.

platelets decelerate, become activated, and firmly adhere through integrins, most prominently $\alpha_{IIb}\beta_3$ (also known as GP IIb/IIIa) and $\alpha_2\beta_1$ (also known as GP Ia/IIa, one of many collagen receptors) *(15,18)*.

Platelet Activation

A myriad of platelet agonists, such as thrombin, adenosine diphosphate (ADP), thromboxane A_2 (TXA_2), platelet activating factor, and chemokines, are present in the thrombotic milieu and can induce platelet activation and aggregation. One of the first mechanisms that may activate platelets in the above-described model of platelet adhesion is the "outside-in" signaling through by ligated GP Ib *(19)* or collagen-induced activation through any of the platelet collagen receptors expressed on platelets (e.g., GP Ia/IIa and GP VI) *(18)*. Upon activation, platelets change from their normal round discoid shape to a compact spherical morphology with long dendritic prolongations called pseudopodia, which greatly facilitate their adhesion, aggregation and attachment to other cells *(20)* (Fig. 1).

During platelet activation, calcium currents are generated within the cells and bring about a change in shape and also induce the granule release reaction. These activated platelets adhere to the injured endothelial surface and flatten to form a platelet mono-

Table 1
Platelet Contents

Contents of Platelet Granules

1. a-granules
  Fibrinogen
  VWF
  GP IIb/IIIa
  P-selectin
  α_2-antitplasmin
  Plasminogen Activator Inhibitor-1 (PAI-1)
  Factor V
  Platelet Derived Growth Factor (PDGF)
  Platelet Factor 4
  Fibronectin
  Thromboglobulin
  Thrombospondin
  Albumin
  IgG
2. Dense granules
  ADP
  ATP
  Pyrophosphate
  Serotonin
  Calcium
  Magnesium
3. Lysozomes
  Lysozyme
4. Peroxisomes
  Catalase

layer to which other platelets or leukocytes can adhere. Additionally, and as part of the link between platelet-dependent hemostasis and strict coagulation, activated platelets undergo the so-called "flip-flop" reaction and provide an anionic phosphatidylserine-rich surface for the efficient assembly of a prothrombinase complex with consequent thrombin formation. Therefore, strategies aimed at interrupting platelet activation and aggregation may also result in decreased thrombin generation, both in vitro *(21)* and in vivo *(22)*.

Platelet Secretion

Because platelets are anucleate cells, it was long thought that they were incapable of any protein synthesis. However, it has recently been discovered that platelets, especially after thrombin stimulation, are indeed capable of translating constitutive mRNAs in their cytoplasm and of rapidly synthesizing interleukin (IL)-1β *(23)*, which may actively participate in thrombotic and inflammatory phenomena for extended periods of time. In addition, platelets contain potent pro-aggregatory mediators prepackaged in various granules (Table 1). α-Granules release a vast array of proteins, while dense granules contain several mediators that greatly amplify the activation and aggregation processes.

Some of the proteins contained within the α-granules are synthesized by the megakaryocyte and are subsequently passed on to platelets during their production in the bone marrow, while other proteins may simply enter the platelet by receptor-mediated endocytosis or fluid-phase pinocytosis (20).

Platelet Aggregation

Unlike the many receptors that intervene in platelet adhesion, GP IIb/IIIa seems to be the main receptor responsible for the final phases of platelet aggregation. The GP IIb/IIIa receptor (also denominated $\alpha_{IIb}\beta_3$ in the integrin nomenclature) is the most abundant receptor expressed on the platelet surface, with a density of about 70,000–90,000 receptors on the surface of a quiescent platelet, but which can be increased to more than 100,000 receptors per cell after platelet activation and translocation of an internal pool of GP IIb/IIIa located in α-granules (24). Like other members of the integrin superfamily, GP IIb/IIIa is a heterodimeric molecule with a large extracellular domain for cation ion-facilitated ligand binding, and short intracytoplasmic tails involved in "outside-in" signaling after its ligation (25) (Fig. 2). Several different molecules, such as vWf, fibrinogen, fibronectin, and vitronectin, serve as ligands to this receptor, nevertheless, fibrinogen appears to play the main role in the aggregation process (26). On the other hand, vWf is believed to be the principal ligand mediating shear-induced platelet aggregation (17,27). Two sequences are recognized by GP IIb/IIIa: (i) the RGD (Arg-Gly-Asp) sequence (28), which is present on several ligands including vWf, fibrinogen, and fibronectin; and (ii) the KQAGDV (Lys-Gln-Ala-Gly-Asp Val) sequence, which is only present in fibrinogen (29). In the resting state, GP IIb/IIIa has a low affinity for fibrinogen binding, however, platelet agonists functionally up-regulate this integrin via "inside-out" signaling, inducing conformational changes that lead to a binding-competent status (30) (Fig. 3). Therefore, during platelet activation, GP IIb/IIIa becomes receptive to ligand binding with the consequent formation of fibrinogen bridges between other GP IIb/IIIa receptors on platelets, thus forming platelet-rich thrombi (Fig. 4). In addition, fibrinogen may also form a bridge between activated GP IIb/IIIa on platelets and MAC-1 ($\alpha M\beta_2$ or CD11b/CD18) integrins expressed on leukocytes, thus forming platelet–leukocyte aggregates (31), which are likely to have an important role on inflammation linked to thrombosis.

ANTIPLATELET AGENTS

Aspirin

Aspirin has now been available for more than a century. The antiplatelet effect of aspirin is due to irreversible acetylation of the serine-529 residue, causing permanent inhibition of the cyclooxygenase enzyme (32). This action prevents the conversion of arachidonic acid to prostaglandin (PG) H_2, with the consequent inhibition of TXA_2, which promotes thrombosis through the amplification of platelet activation and aggregation, as well as by causing vasoconstriction. Aspirin, however, also blocks the synthesis of the platelet-inhibitory and vasodilator prostacyclin (PGI_2) in endothelial cells. In addition, a number of other roles for aspirin have since been proposed, including acetylation of other proteins, such as thrombin and fibrinogen, and 12-hydroxyeicosanotetraenoic acid (12-HETE) antagonism (33).

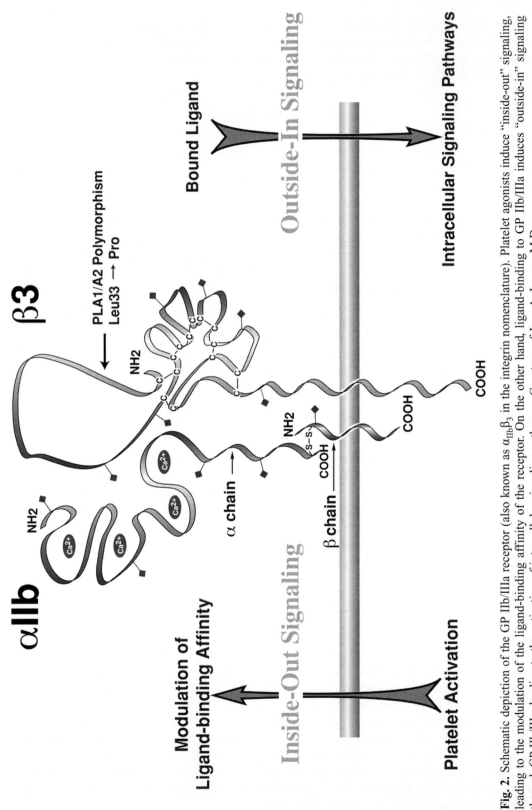

Fig. 2. Schematic depiction of the GP IIb/IIIa receptor (also known as $\alpha_{IIb}\beta_3$ in the integrin nomenclature). Platelet agonists induce "inside-out" signaling, leading to the modulation of the ligand-binding affinity of the receptor. On the other hand, ligand-binding to GP IIb/IIIa induces "outside-in" signaling through GP IIb/IIIa, leading to the activation of intracellular signaling pathways. Courtesy of Jose A. Lopez, M.D.

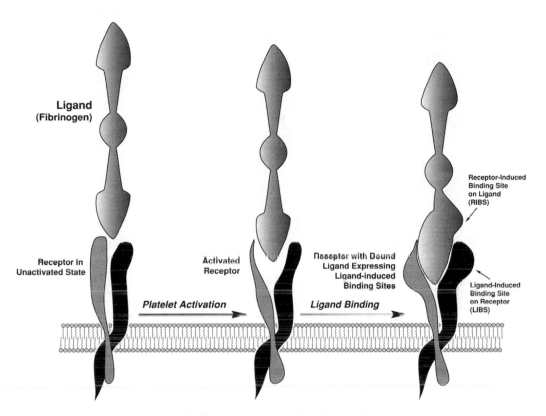

Fig. 3. Under resting conditions, GP IIb/IIIa has a low affinity for its ligands. After platelet activation, GP IIb/IIIa becomes receptive to ligand binding. As a result of outside in signaling induced by ligand binding, ligand-induced binding sites (LIBS) (neo-epitopes) are expressed on the receptor. In addition, receptor-induced binding sites (RIBS) on the ligand may also be expressed as a result of the interaction between the ligand and its receptor. Courtesy of Jose A. Lopez, M.D.

Although aspirin is a potent inhibitor of platelet aggregation induced by arachidonic acid, it is a relatively weak antiplatelet agent when platelets are stimulated by a number of other agonists including ADP and thrombin. Aspirin does not prevent α-granule release in response to platelet agonists and does not inhibit epinephrine-induced platelet aggregation *(34)*. Although aspirin blocked cyclic flow variations in a canine model of coronary stenosis and endothelial injury, this inhibition was overcome by the addition of epinephrine *(35)*. In spite of these observations, there is abundant evidence of the clear clinical efficacy of aspirin as an antiplatelet agent.

Aspirin is readily absorbed in the stomach and small intestine, with a systemic bioavailability approaching 50% for single doses in the range of 20–1300 mg *(36)*. Although salicylate levels in the portal vein increase within 5 min after aspirin ingestion, the time required to exert a clinically meaningful antiplatelet effect is not clear. In healthy volunteers, inhibition of arachidonic acid-induced platelet aggregation and TXA_2 production were demonstrated within 15 min after the ingestion of 81 mg of aspirin *(37)*. However, inhibition of thrombin-induced TXA_2 generation in clotting blood probably does not occur until approx 24 h after the ingestion of 75 mg of aspirin *(36)*.

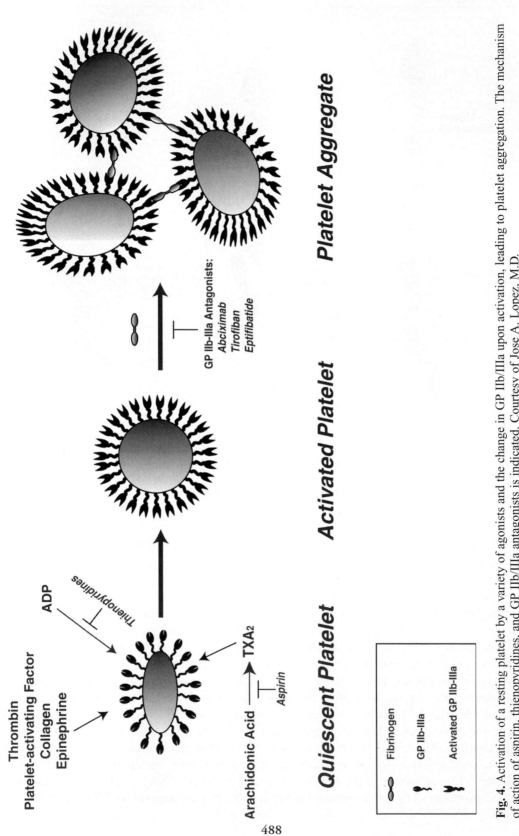

Fig. 4. Activation of a resting platelet by a variety of agonists and the change in GP IIb/IIIa upon activation, leading to platelet aggregation. The mechanism of action of aspirin, thienopyridines, and GP IIb/IIIa antagonists is indicated. Courtesy of Jose A. Lopez, M.D.

CLINICAL USES

The consistent and beneficial effects of aspirin have been documented in hundreds of thousands of patients suffering various manifestations of cardiovascular disease. In a meta-analysis of more than 75,000 patients with preexisting cardiovascular disease enrolled in several secondary prevention trials, aspirin reduced the combined end point of vascular death, myocardial infarction, and stroke by 27% in a highly significant way (38). More recently, in the Primary Prevention Project, low-dose aspirin (100 mg) reduced the risk of cardiovascular death by 44% among patients with at least one cardiovascular risk factor but with no known vascular disease, thus extending the indication of aspirin into a setting of primary prevention (39). Furthermore, in the Second International Study of Infarct Survival (ISIS-2) study, aspirin (162.5 mg) was as effective as streptokinase in reducing 5-wk vascular mortality in patients with suspected acute myocardial infarction (40). In consequence, because the ISIS-2

The benefits of aspirin in unstable angina pectoris have been clearly established by four major well-controlled clinical trials (Table 2). In the Veterans Administration Cooperative study (41), 1266 men were randomized to 324 mg of aspirin or placebo. At 3 mo, the combined risk of death or nonfatal myocardial infarction was reduced by 51% (10.1 vs 5%). This benefit was maintained at 12 mo with a 43% risk reduction of the combined end point, even though the study drugs were stopped 3 mo after enrollment. In the Canadian Multicenter Trial, 555 patients with unstable angina pectoris were randomized to receive aspirin, sulfinpyrazone, both, or placebo (42). At 2 yr, the risk reduction for the combined end point of cardiac death and nonfatal myocardial infarction, by intention-to-treat analysis, was 30%. An efficacy analysis for cardiac death alone showed a reduction of 70%. The Montreal Heart Institute study included 479 patients with unstable angina pectoris randomized to receive aspirin, heparin, both, or neither (43). Patients treated with aspirin had a risk reduction of 71% for in-hospital myocardial infarction. In the RISC study (44), 796 patients with unstable angina or non-Q wave myocardial infarction were randomized to aspirin, an intermittent bolus of heparin, both, or placebo. Risk reduction in the aspirin group was 57% at 5 d, 69% at 30 d, and 61% at 3 mo.

These observations have led to the firm recommendation that aspirin be administered to all patients as part of a primary and secondary prevention strategy for cardiovascular disease, to all patients undergoing PCI, and to all patients presenting with either a non-ST-elevation ACS or an acute myocardial infarction, unless they have a contraindication to its use.

ASPIRIN DOSE

The dose of aspirin required to achieve optimal clinical response remains controversial. The dose-response effect of aspirin on platelet aggregation and TXA_2 production is log-linear, but reaches a plateau at approx 80 mg (45). Lower doses can inhibit platelet aggregation without blocking the vascular production of vasodilating and anti-aggregatory prostaglandins, and also limit the frequency of gastrointestinal side effects (46,47). Therefore, theoretical reasons exist to favor low doses of aspirin vs higher doses. The meta-analysis performed by the Antiplatelet Trialists' Collaboration did not find lower aspirin doses (<350 mg) to be superior to higher doses in the prevention of cardiovascular events (38). A Dutch study involving 3131 patients with transient ischemic attacks compared the effects of aspirin 30 mg/d with 283 mg daily on the incidence of vascular death, stroke, or myocardial infarction. After a mean follow-up of 2.6 yr, there was no

Table 2

Major Trials of Aspirin, Heparin and Ticlopidine in Syndromes of Non-ST-Segment Elevation MI

Trial	No. of patients	Drugs studied	Follow-up	Death and nonfatal MI	P value	Risk reduction
VA coop.	1338	ASA 325 mg/d	3 mo	5 vs 10.1%	0.0005	51%
Canadian Multicenter	555	ASA 1300 mg/d	24 mo	8.6 vs 17%	0.008	51%
Montreal Heart Ins.	479	ASA 650 mg/d	6 d	3.3 vs 12%	0.01	72%
		Heparin, apt	6 d	1.2 vs 7%	<0.05	85%
RISC study	652	ASA 75 mg/d	30 days	4.3 vs 13.4%	0.0001	68%
		Heparin 14–20,000	30 d	3.4 vs 4.9%	NS	30%
Italian	652	Ticlopidine 500 mg/d	6 mo	7.6 vs 13.6%	0.009	53%
Montreal Heart Ins.	484	ASA vs heparin	5.3 d	3.7 vs 0.8%	0.035	88%
Telford et al	214	Heparin 30–40,000	7 d	3 vs 15%	<0.05	80%

ASA, acetylsalicylic acid (aspirin); MI, myocardial infarctions.

difference between the two groups in the incidence of the composite end point or its components (48). However, this issue was recently addressed by the Aspirin in Carotid Endarterectomy trial, which involved more than 2800 patients undergoing carotid endarterectomy (49). Patients randomly received either low-dose aspirin (81 or 325 mg) or high-dose aspirin (650 or 1300 mg) daily. The risk of death, myocardial infarction, or stroke were lower among patients who received either of the two lower doses of aspirin compared to the higher doses, both at 30 d (5.4 vs 7.0%, $p = 0.07$ [relative risk (RR) = 1.31]) and at 3 mo (6.2 vs 8.4%, $p = 0.03$ [RR = 1.34]). Therefore, this is the first direct evidence to support low doses of aspirin (81–325 mg daily). Given the weight of evidence against a dose-response effect of aspirin, in addition to apparent dose-related tolerability of aspirin therapy, as well as the theoretical concern about an imbalance between TXA_2 and PGI_2 production, it seems appropriate to favor the lower doses of aspirin shown to be effective for a given indication. In consequence, because the ISIS-2 trial conclusively established the efficacy of a 162 mg aspirin dose in patients with suspected myocardial infarction, it appears reasonable to administer 160–325 mg of aspirin to patients with non-ST-segment elevation ACS.

ASPIRIN RESISTANCE

About 5–40% of patients have been reported to manifest a new and vaguely defined entity called "aspirin resistance" (33,50–53). The wide range of reported frequencies of this condition possibly reflect the various definitions and methods and criteria that have been used to define it. Aspirin resistance has been variously defined in pharmacodynamic studies as failure of aspirin to prolong bleeding time or failure to reduce 12-HETE production (33); or failure of aspirin to reduce platelet aggregation by a certain percentage (depending on the agonist being used); or as having normal platelet aggregation despite aspirin therapy in newer platelet-function analyzers, such as the PFA-100 (53). The variability among these assays may be significant, and the findings have not been universally reproducible. Aspirin resistance has also been clinically defined as having a new cardiovascular event despite aspirin therapy. Thus, several problems may be encountered while trying to define this entity. In addition, it has also been proposed that more than being aspirin-resistant, some individuals may simply be more sensitive to a certain platelet agonist and, therefore, require higher aspirin doses to achieve a similar antiplatelet effect (54).

Regardless of how aspirin resistance is defined, it is apparent that a group of patients may not be deriving any benefit from aspirin therapy at the usual doses. Therefore, the question is whether aspirin resistance has an impact on the outcome of patients. Two studies have reported that aspirin resistance is clinically relevant. In one of these studies, patients who suffered a stroke were given 500 mg of aspirin $3\times$ daily. Based on the modified Wu and Hoak platelet function test, 40% of patients were found to be aspirin "non-responders." After a 2-yr follow-up period, aspirin nonresponders had a 20-fold higher rate of cardiovascular death, myocardial infarction, or recurrent stroke compared to aspirin responders (52). In a second study, compared to aspirin responders, patients who failed to fully respond to aspirin therapy had a greater frequency of vessel reocclusion after percutaneous transluminal ileofemoral angioplasty (55).

What the appropriate management of patients with aspirin resistance should be is currently somewhat speculative. Whether higher aspirin doses should be prescribed or aspirin should be substituted with a thienopyridine is not known. However, based on the findings of the Clopidogrel vs Aspirin in Patients at Risk of Ischaemic Events (CAPRIE) trial *(56)*, in which clopidogrel alone was at least as efficacious and safe compared to aspirin in patients with vascular disease, the substitution of aspirin for a thienopyridine (specifically clopidogrel) would seem sound.

LIMITATIONS AND ADVERSE EFFECTS OF ASPIRIN THERAPY

Side effects are seen infrequently with low-dose aspirin therapy and can easily be monitored. The major side effects of aspirin are gastrointestinal symptoms, which occur more frequent with higher aspirin doses *(49,57)* Gastrointestinal bleeding, however, appears to be equally likely to occur at any dose *(58)*. In a small number of patients (4%), particularly those with adult onset asthma, aspirin may cause bronchospasm and angioedema.

Concerns have been raised regarding a possible negative interaction between aspirin and angiotensin-converting enzyme (ACE) inhibitors. ACE inhibitors increase plasma levels of bradykinin, which is a potent stimulus for prostacyclin production, and may partly explain the favorable effects of this class of drugs. By blocking the cyclooxygenase enzyme, aspirin may also block prostacyclin production and blunt some of the effects of ACE inhibitors. Aspirin was seen to prevent several of the beneficial hemodynamic effects normally seen with ACE inhibitor therapy in patients with severe heart failure *(59)*. In addition, *post hoc* analyses of two large-scale multicenter trials suggested that aspirin attenuated the improved survival seen with ACE inhibitors in patients with moderate-to-severe heart failure *(60,61)*. In contradistinction, an analysis of more than 11,500 patients did not observe the purported negative interaction between aspirin and ACE inhibitors *(62)*. Because of the potential implications in the health of millions of patients taking both ACE inhibitors and aspirin, this issue will have to be directly addressed in a prospective fashion.

CLINICAL USE OF ASPIRIN IN PATIENTS WITH non-ST-ELEVATION ACS

Aspirin remains the cornerstone of anti-platelet therapy for patients with non-ST-elevation ACS. It should be administered as early as possible to all patients, unless there is history of severe intolerance. The American Heart Association/American College of Cardiology guidelines give a Class I recommendation for the administration of 162 mg to 325 mg of aspirin in the acute setting to patients (with no contraindications to aspirin) presenting with non-ST-segment elevation ACS, preferably chewing the first dose of a rapidly absorbable, nonenteric coated formulation to rapidly establish a high blood level; and thereafter, 75–160 mg of aspirin (enteric or nonenteric) per day, indefinitely. A thienopyridine, preferably clopidogrel, should be administered to patients who are unable to take aspirin because of hypersensitivity or severe gastrointestinal intolerance *(63)*.

Thienopyridines

ADP was identified more than 40 yr ago as a mediator derived from erythrocytes that could affect platelet adhesion and aggregation *(64)*. In fact, in the thrombotic milieu, ADP is released from erythrocytes that are lysed as they are subjected to high shear stress that may result from a severely stenotic lesion. In addition, ADP is present in platelet dense granules and is released upon activation, thus amplifying the aggregation and activation responses in both, an autocrine and paracrine fashion. ADP acts in synergy with other platelet agonists and potentiates most aggregation responses, even of weak agonists, such as serotonin, epinephrine *(65)*, or chemokines *(66)*. Thus, ADP is a necessary cofactor for the normal activation and aggregation of platelets. Further observations pointing to the central role of ADP in hemostasis is the profound impact ADP-removing enzymes have on platelet aggregation *(68)*, or the bleeding diatheses observed in patients with genetic defects of ADP receptors, or in those who have dense granules deficient in ADF *(68)*. Therefore, it is not surprising that platelet ADP receptors are potential targets for antithrombotic or pharmacologic interventions.

PLATELET ADP RECEPTORS

Transduction of the signal elicited by ADP involves a rise in free cytoplasmic calcium due to an influx of this cation from the extracellular medium, as well as the mobilization of the internal calcium stores and a concomitant inhibition of adenylyl cyclase *(68)*. Although, based on pharmacological studies, MacFarlane proposed in 1983 the existence of two distinct ADP receptors, one mediating platelet shape change and aggregation and the other the inhibition of adenylyl cyclase *(69)*, it was not until quite recently that the main platelet ADP receptors, which are essential in the normal aggregation process, were cloned and further characterized. These receptors can be divided into two groups: the G protein-coupled receptors, termed P2Y, and the ion-gated channel receptors termed P2X.

$P2Y_1$, a G protein-coupled receptor that activates Gq, was the first of the P2 (purinergic) receptors to be cloned *(70)*. Nevertheless, it soon became apparent that another ADP receptor was involved in ADP-induced platelet aggregation, as selective antagonists to $P2Y_1$ had no effect whatsoever on ADP-induced inhibition of platelet adenylyl cyclase, which is stimulated by anti-aggregatory mediators, such as prostacyclin or nitric oxide. Indeed, several groups nearly simultaneously published their observations showing that $P2Y_1$ is necessary but not sufficient for platelet aggregation *(71,72)*. Definitive evidence of the existence of an ADP receptor coupled to adenylyl cyclase inhibition came from studies using $P2Y_1$ knock-out mice, in which platelet shape change and aggregation in response to ADP were abolished, whereas adenylyl cyclase production of cyclic AMP was unaffected *(73)*.

The ADP receptor that remained to be identified was expected to also be of the purinoceptor P2Y superfamily, since ADP is known to activate the heterotrimeric Gi_2 protein. Depending on the author, this receptor was termed $P2Y_{ADP}$, $P2T_{AC}$, or P2cyc *(68)*. Very recently, this elusive receptor was cloned *(74)*. Sequence analysis identified the new receptor of the P2Y family and termed it $P2Y_{12}$. As expected, ADP stimulation of cells expressing only $P2Y_{12}$ led to adenylyl cyclase inhibition, a phenomenon reversed by treatment of these cells with selective $P2Y_{12}$ antagonists *(74,75)*. Even though $P2Y_{12}$ was very recently identified, this is the receptor targeted by the clinically used platelet ADP receptor antagonists, the thienopyridines: ticlopidine and clopidogrel.

The third ADP receptor expressed on platelets is $P2X_1$, an ATP-gated ion channel and a member of the ionotropic receptor superfamily involved in platelet shape-change upon stimulation *(76)*. This receptor is responsible for the rapid entry of calcium ions from the extracellular medium to the platelet upon ADP cell stimulation and is broadly expressed on a variety of tissues, specifically on excitable cells such as neurons and muscle cells. As opposed to the P2Y receptors, mice deficient in $P2X_1$ demonstrate no obvious hemostatic defects *(77)*. Future studies will define the precise role of this recep-

Table 3
Platelet Purinergic Receptors[a]

	$P2Y_1$	$P2Y_{12}$	$P2X_1$
ADP	Agonist.	Agonist.	True agonist or possible contamination of commercial sources of ADP with ATP.
ATP	Antagonist (receptor density-dependent effect?).	Antagonist (receptor density-dependent effect?).	Agonist.
Platelet function	Platelet shape change. Necessary but not sufficient for full ADP-induced aggregation. Transient aggregation.	Amplification of platelet granule secretion and aggregation. Platelet aggregation.	Shape change. Synergism with P2Y$_1$-induced Ca^{2+} responses.
Intracellular events	Intracellular Ca^{2+} mobilization.	Inhibition of adenylyl cyclase. Protein phosphorilation.	Fast Ca^{2+} entry into the cell after ATP/ADP stimulation.
Receptor	Coupled to Gq-protein.	Coupled to Gi-protein.	ATP-gated ion channel.
Expression profile	Widely distributed: platelets, heart, blood vessels, testis, prostate, ovaries.	Restricted to platelets, megakaryocytes and subregions of the brain.	Broadly expressed on excitable tissues, such as neurons, muscle cells and glial cells.
Chromosome	3	3	17
Blocked by thienopyridines	−	+	−

[a]Properties of the three main platelet ADP-receptors identified thus far.

tor in platelet function. Table 3 summarizes the key features of the three ADP receptors previously discussed.

Respective Roles of the ADP Receptors in Platelet Function

Based on a series of observations, it is believed that $P2Y_1$ is responsible for platelet shape change, which is an important event in platelet activation. In fact, $P2Y_1$ alone can trigger a clear but transient aggregation response, which is probably necessary during the initial phases of platelet aggregation. Nevertheless, this receptor is not sufficient for full platelet aggregation, and the $P2Y_{12}$ receptor appears to be responsible for the completion and amplification of platelet aggregation induced by ADP, as well as by other agonists. $P2Y_{12}$ plays a specific role in the activation of the GP IIb/IIIa receptor after ADP stimulation, and it also confers stability to the platelet macroaggregate (68).

In such a scenario, it appears that while $P2Y_1$ plays a specific role in the initial platelet activation response, characterized by shape change and formation of long filopodia, it is the $P2Y_{12}$ receptor that is involved in the amplification of platelet aggregation induced by other agonists such as thrombin, chemokines, epinephrine, or TXA_2. Therefore, there is a strong biological rationale behind the pharmacological antagonism of the ADP receptors.

Ticlopidine and Clopidogrel

Administration and Pharmacokinetics

Two thienopyridines are currently approved for clinical use in the United States. Ticlopidine was approved in 1991 and clopidogrel in 1998. These two compounds are only available in the oral form and share many features. They both have similar molecular structures, differing only in a carboxymethyl side group, which is present in clopidogrel but not in ticlopidine (78). Additionally, both of these drugs are prodrugs that lack any activity and must, therefore, undergo first-pass metabolism through the liver in order to become biologically active. Although food intake does not affect the absorption of ticlopidine or clopidogrel, it is recommended that the former be taken with food in order to minimize gastrointestinal symptoms. Antacids, on the other hand, decrease the absorption of ticlopidine. Both drugs attain peak plasma concentrations 1 to 2 h after administration, ticlopidine reaching them more rapidly than clopidogrel. However, the onset of action of the two thienopyridines differs. Platelet inhibition takes a few days to reach a plateau with either agent: from 3–5 d with ticlopidine, and from 4–7 d with clopidogrel. In order to accelerate platelet inhibition and rapidly achieve a therapeutic effect, ticlopidine and clopidogrel are commonly given with a first loading dose: 500 mg for ticlopidine and 300–600 mg for clopidogrel. When high (300–600 mg) loading doses of clopidogrel are administered orally, effects on markers of platelet activation (79), aggregation (80), and adhesion to a collagen surface (81) have been observed within 90 min of administration. After the initial bolus dose, 250 mg 2× daily of ticlopidine or 75 mg once daily of clopidogrel are administered. Because these two compounds irreversibly inhibit the platelet $P2Y_{12}$ receptor, their inhibitory effect lasts for the rest of the platelet's life span. Both, ticlopidine and clopidogrel have been evaluated in a wide range of clinical scenarios and have been similarly efficacious.

Secondary Prevention

In a meta-analysis of 39 randomized placebo-controlled trials involving more than 6500 patients with vascular disease, ticlopidine reduced the combined end point of vas-

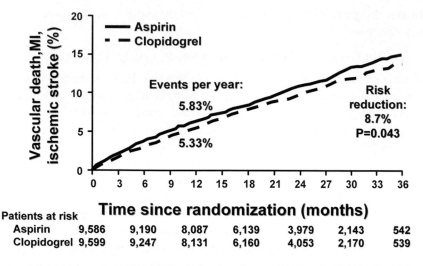

Fig. 5. Kaplan-Meier curve of the CAPRIE study showing an 8.7% reduction in the risk of death, hemorrhagic stroke, and nonfatal myocardial infarction (MI) with clopidogrel during 3 yr of follow-up *(56)*. Courtesy of Peter B. Berger, M.D. Reproduced with permission from: The CAPRIE Investigators. Lancet 1996;348:1329–1339.

cular death, myocardial infarction, and stroke by 33% *(38)*. When compared to aspirin, ticlopidine produced a 10% relative reduction in the combined end point of vascular death, myocardial infarction, and stroke among 3471 patients with prior stroke or transient ischemic attack, who had been enrolled in three randomized clinical trials *(38)*.

By far the largest study of thienopyridines has been the CAPRIE trial, which evaluated the efficacy of clopidogrel in the secondary prevention of cardiovascular events *(56)*. The trial involved 19,825 patients divided into three groups: (*i*) those with ischemic stroke within 1 wk to 6 mo; (*ii*) those suffering myocardial infarction in the previous 35 d before study entry; and (*iii*) those with peripheral vascular disease. Patients randomly received either aspirin (325 mg daily) or clopidogrel (75 mg daily). After a 3-yr follow-up period, patients receiving clopidogrel had a modest 8.7% (*p* = 0.043) risk reduction in the composite end point of vascular death, myocardial infarction, or ischemic stroke, consistent with the 10% risk reduction that had been previously seen in the ticlopidine meta-analysis for secondary prevention (Fig. 5). Clopidogrel was extremely well-tolerated and rarely led to its discontinuation because of side effects. In CAPRIE, patients with peripheral vascular disease derived particular benefit from clopidogrel, largely due to a reduction in the rate of myocardial infarction. Another subgroup analysis has recently showed that patients with prior cardiac surgery also derived particular benefit from clopidogrel compared to aspirin, with a 31% relative reduction in the composite end point of vascular death, myocardial infarction, stroke, or rehospitalization *(82)*.

ACS

The first evidence of thienopyridine efficacy in the management of patients with unstable angina came from the Studio della Ticlopidina nell' Angina Instabile (STAI) *(81)*. Patients received either conventional treatment (including β-blockers or calcium

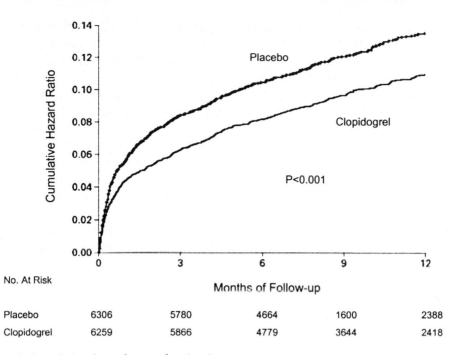

Fig. 6. Cumulative hazard rates for the first primary outcome of cardiovascular death, nonfatal myocardial infarction, or stroke during the 12 mo of the CURE trial *(84)*. Reproduced with permission from: The CURE Investigators. N Engl J Med 2001;345:494–502.

channel blockers, and nitrates), or the conventional treatment plus ticlopidine. Patients treated with ticlopidine had a 46% risk reduction in cardiovascular death and nonfatal myocardial infarction.

Definitive evidence supporting the use of a thienopyridine in the management of non-ST-elevation acute coronary syndromes comes from the recent Clopidogrel in Unstable Angina to Prevent Recurrent Events (CURE) Trial *(84)*. More than 12,500 patients presenting with an ACS (74.9% were diagnosed with unstable angina and 25.1% with suspected non-ST-elevation myocardial infarction) were randomly assigned to either aspirin (75–325 mg/d) plus clopidogrel (300 mg loading dose, plus 75 mg daily thereafter) or to aspirin plus placebo, in addition to the usual therapy. The primary end point of CURE was, as in CAPRIE, the combined end point of vascular death, myocardial infarction, or stroke. The mean follow-up period was 9 mo. The combination of clopidogrel and aspirin was associated with a significant reduction in the composite end point (9.3 vs 11.5%, RR 0.80, $p < 0.001$), largely influenced by a lower incidence of myocardial infarction (5.2 vs 6.7%, RR 0.77, $p < 0.001$), compared to aspirin plus placebo (Fig. 6). Combination therapy was associated with a reduced incidence of stroke (1.2 vs 1.4%, p = NS), but also associated with a significant increase in major bleeding (3.6 vs 2.7%, RR 1.38, p = 0.003) as well as minor bleeding (5.1 vs 2.4%, RR 2.12, $p < 0.001$). Within the first 24 h of treatment, the benefit of the clopidogrel plus aspirin regimen became evident and persisted thereafter; there was a relative risk reduction of 0.79 in the composite end point within the first 30 d and of 0.82 after 30 d.

In previous studies of ACS evaluating intravenous GP IIb/IIIa antagonists, benefit was observed primarily in high-risk patients (see below). In CURE, a comparable benefit was observed in both high-risk and low-risk patients, whether defined by troponin positivity (risk ratios of 0.81 and 0.79 for marker-positive and marker-negative patients, respectively) or by the presence of ST-segment changes (0.79 and 0.80 for those with and without ST-segment shifts, respectively). In addition, an observational substudy from CURE (the PCI-CURE study) showed that the dual antiplatelet regimen also reduced ischemic complications in patients who underwent PCI. In CURE, PCI was performed in 2,658 patients in a median of 10 d after they were randomized to clopidogrel or placebo. After the procedure, most patients received open-label thienopyridine for a mean of four weeks, after which the study drug was re-started for a mean follow-up of eight months. Compared to placebo, the combination of aspirin and clopidogrel reduced the relative risk of cardiovascular death, myocardial infarction or revascularization within 30 d by 30% (4.5 vs 6.4%, $p = 0.03$)*(85)*. Therefore, patients presenting with non-ST-segment elevation ACS and who undergo PCI should routinely receive clopidrogel in addition to aspirin. Nevertheless, because there was a lower proportion of patients with myocardial infarction or refractory ischemia in the clopidogrel group before the coronary intervention (12.1 vs 15.3%, $p = 0.008$), presumably as a result of the beneficial effects of clopidogrel at the time of the initial enrollment in CURE, concerns have been raised regarding the interpretation of PCI-CURE *(86)*.

LIMITATIONS AND ADVERSE EFFECTS OF TICLOPIDINE AND CLOPIDOGREL

There are a number of limitations in the use of thienopyridines, particularly in the case of ticlopidine. The slow onset of action is an unfavorable pharmacokinetic feature of thienopyridines. Loading doses may be used to speed up platelet inhibition, but toxicity limits the ease of administering large bolus doses, particularly in the case of ticlopidine. Indeed, as many as 20% of patients are forced to discontinue ticlopidine because of side effects, most commonly diarrhea, nausea, and skin rash. Neutropenia and thrombotic thrombocytopenic purpura (TTP) are probably the most severe adverse reactions attributed to ticlopidine, with an estimated incidence of about 3.3 and 0.02%, respectively. However, TTP, which usually occurs within the first month of therapy, can be fatal in up to 25–50% of cases. Because of these reactions, blood counts of patients being treated with ticlopidine must be frequently monitored. As opposed to ticlopidine, clopidogrel has demonstrated an excellent side effects profile, with an overall incidence of gastrointestinal symptoms (abdominal pain, gastritis, nausea, vomiting, or dyspepsia) lower than that seen in patients treated with aspirin. More importantly, in more than 3 million patients receiving clopidogrel, the incidence of TTP was comparable to that of the general population, and 100-fold lower than that reported in ticlopidine-treated patients *(87)*. In addition, no cases of clopidogrel-associated severe neutropenia have been reported. Another advantage of clopidogrel over ticlopidine is that it is about 70% cheaper.

In general terms, since clopidogrel appears to be as efficacious as ticlopidine but with a better safety and pharmacologic profile, the switch from ticlopidine to clopidogrel seems to be justified for the wide range of clinical settings in which these drugs have been tested *(88)*.

CLINICAL USE OF CLOPIDOGREL IN PATIENTS WITH NON-ST ELEVATION ACS

On the basis of the CURE trial, clopidogrel should be administered to patients presenting with an ACS. However, several points should be kept in mind regarding this trial. Only 4% of the CURE patients were enrolled in the United States, where an aggressive strategy, which includes early administration of intravenous GP IIb/IIIa antagonists and early angiography, with subsequent revascularization if deemed necessary, are commonly performed in patients with ACS. In fact, in the CURE trial, centers pursuing an invasive approach contemplating early angiography and revascularization were excluded from participation. Therefore the question remains as to what extent the CURE results are directly applicable to patients being managed in an aggressive manner. Furthermore, the early administration of clopidogrel in patients who require coronary bypass surgery during the initial hospitalization may well result in excess and potentially life-threatening perioperative bleeding. Unlike the intravenous GP IIb/IIIa antagonists, which either have a short (2–4 h) half-life or can be reversed by platelet transfusions, clopidogrel irreversibly inhibits ADP-induced platelet aggregation for the remaining platelet's life. Indeed, nonrandomized studies have reported significantly higher postoperative bleeding complication and re-operation rates because of bleeding in patients treated with a thienopyridine (10 vs 2% with no thienopyridine) (89,90). Therefore, clopidogrel should be withheld for at least 5–7 d in patients in whom elective coronary bypass surgery is planned. In hospitals where early (24–36 h of admission) diagnostic catheterization is commonly performed in patients with non-ST-segment elevation ACS, clopidogrel should be administered once it has been decided that coronary bypass surgery will not be scheduled within the next week or so. In case PCI is performed immediately following angiography, a loading dose (300-600 mg) of clopidogrel can be administered to a patient who is already on the catheterization table.

The current American Heart Association/American College of Cardiology guidelines recommend that patients presenting with non-ST-segment elevation ACS receive 300–600 g of clopidogrel as a loading dose, followed by 75 mg daily thereafter, in addition to aspirin, for at least 1 mo and up to 9 mo, regardless if PCI is planned. Whether clopidogrel should be stopped at 9 mo or continued for a longer period is not clear since the mean follow-up in CURE was 9 mo. This decision should be based on the individual patient's related risk factors. For example, diabetic patients, or those with diffuse coronary artery disease or in whom complete revascularization was not achieved, would probably benefit from prolonged dual antiplatelet therapy.

As with any antiplatelet drug, the increased bleeding risk associated with clopidogrel must be objectively balanced against the expected benefits of this therapy. In CURE, for every 1000 patients treated with clopidogrel, there were 21 fewer events pertaining to the first primary outcome (i.e., cardiovascular death, non-fatal myocardial infarctions, or stroke), in exchange for 10 excess major bleeding events (defined as substantially disabling bleeding, intraocular bleeding leading to loss of vision, or the need of a transfusion of at least two units of blood).

The Glycoprotein IIb/IIIa Antagonists

Because GP IIb/IIIa is indispensable for platelet aggregation, blockade of this integrin results in the inhibition of platelet aggregation irrespective of the platelet agonist or stimulus-response coupling pathway involved. GP IIb/IIIa antagonists are therefore the most powerful and specific inhibitors of platelet aggregation of the current antiplatelet armamentarium.

Table 4
Properties of Intravenous GP IIb/IIIa Antagonists

	Abciximab	Eptifibatide	Tirofiban	Lamifiban
Commercial name	ReoPro	Integrilin	Aggrastat	—
Supplier	Centocor/Eli Lilly	COR/Schering-Plough	Merck	Roche
Year of approval	1995	1998	1998	—
Structure	Antibody Fab fragment	Cyclic heptapeptide	Synthetic nonpeptide	Synthetic nonpeptide
Integrin selectivity	$\alpha_{IIb}\beta_3$ and $\alpha V\beta_3$	$\alpha_{IIb}\beta_3$ 0.83	$\alpha_{IIb}\beta_3$ <0.5	$\alpha_{IIb}\beta_3$ <0.5
Molecular weight (kDa)	48			
Plasma half-life	10–30 min	approx 2.5 h	approx 2 h	approx 2 h
Excretion	Unknown	approx 50% renal	40–70% renal	90% renal
Approved indications	PCI	NSTE ACS	NSTE ACS	Not approved
	Refractory unstable angina, if PCI is to be performed within 24 h			
Approved dose	PCI:	ACS:	ACS:	Not approved
	Bolus: 0.25 mg/kg	Bolus 180 µg/kg	0.4 µg/kg/min × 30 min,	
	Infusion: 0.125 µg/kg/min	Infusion: 2.0 µg/kg/min	then 0.1 µg/kg/min	
	(max 10 µg/min)	× 72–96 h	× 48–108 h	
	ACS + PCI (within 24 h)	PCI:		
	Same as above, for 12–24 h	Bolus: 135 µg/kg		
		Infusion 0.5 µg/kg/min		
		× 20–24 h		
		ESPRIT:		
		Bolus: 2x 180 µg/kg		
		(10 min apart), then		
		2.0 µg/k/min × 18–24 h		
Major clinical trials	EPIC, EPILOG, CAPTURE, EPISTENT, RAPPORT, ADMIRAL, CADILLAC, TARGET, GUSTO-IV, GUSTO-V	PURSUIT IMPACT-II	PRISM PRISM-PLUS RESOTRE TARGET	PARAGON A PARAGON B

NSTE, non-ST-segment elevation; PCI, percutaneous coronary intervention; ACS, acute coronary syndrome.

PHARMACOLOGY OF INTRAVENOUS GP IIB/IIIA ANTAGONISTS

Three intravenous GP IIb/IIIa antagonists have undergone extensive evaluation in several large-scale clinical trials in the settings of PCI and non-ST-segment elevation myocardial ischemia, and in pharmacologic-based reperfusion regimens for the treatment of acute myocardial infarction ("combination therapy") *(91)*. An additional GP IIb/IIIa antagonist, lamifiban, has also been evaluated in patients presenting with ACS, but is not approved for clinical use (Table 4).

ABCIXIMAB

Abciximab (ReoPro™) is the human–murine chimeric Fab fragment of the monoclonal antibody directed to GP IIb/IIIa, 7E3. Owing to its affinity for the β_3 (GP IIIa) subunit, abciximab also binds other β_3-containing integrins, most notably the vitronectin receptor $\alpha V \beta_3$, which is involved in cell adhesion, migration, and proliferation; however, the significance of this interaction remains unknown. After intravenous administration of the standard bolus dose of abciximab (0.25 mg/kg), approximately two-thirds of the drug rapidly binds to platelets and blocks approx 80% of the GP IIb/IIIa receptors, with a corresponding 80% inhibition of platelet aggregation in response to ADP (5–20 µM). Nevertheless, there is a fair amount of variability in the degree of platelet inhibition which is attained after a bolus dose, and even more so after the standard infusion (0.125 µg/kg/min) of abciximab *(92)*.

Free plasma levels of abciximab rapidly drop after administration. Internalization of abciximab in platelet α-granules has been documented *(93)* and may potentiate subsequent α-granule release *(94)*. Several in vivo and ex vivo studies show that once administered, abciximab is redistributed from platelet to platelet *(92)*. In fact, platelet-bound abciximab can be detected up to 3 wk after the initial administration, at a time when all of the platelets that were present during abciximab administration can be expected to have been removed from the circulation based on their 7–10 d life span. Low plasma levels of free, unbound abciximab allow rapid reversal of the drug's inhibitory effect by platelet transfusions. Nevertheless, because of abciximab's redistribution capacity, very large numbers of platelets may be needed in order to decrease GP IIb/IIIa blockade to under 50%, a level at which hemostasis should not longer be impaired.

EPTIFIBATIDE

Eptifibatide (Integrilin™) is a cyclic heptapeptide based on the KGD (Lys-Gly-Asp) sequence found in the venom of the southeastern pigmy rattlesnake, *Sisturus m. barbouri*. The molecular structure of the peptide derivative of this venom was modified by substitution of arginine for lysine (thus a KGD sequence), enhancing its specificity for GP IIb/IIIa, while cyclization of the amino acid sequence enhanced the anti-aggregatory potency of the compound *(95)*. Therefore, unlike abciximab, eptifibatide binds with high affinity and specificity to GP IIb/IIIa and does not cross-react with other integrins.

Renal clearance is thought to be the main elimination route of eptifibatide, which has a plasma half-life of approx 2.5 h. In contrast to abciximab, a very high number of unbound drug molecules, relative to the number of receptors, are attained after intravenous administration of eptifibatide. Therefore, platelet transfusions may not reverse eptifibatide's inhibitory effect, as the newly transfused platelets would most probably be rapidly inhibited by the unbound eptifibatide. In this regard, reversal of the antiplatelet

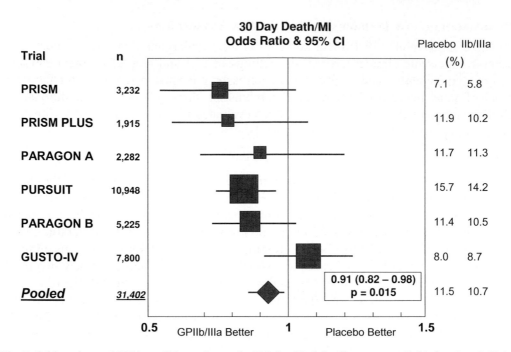

Fig. 7. Odds ratios and 95% confidence intervals (CI) for 30-d death or myocardial infarction (MI) in the six major trials of GP IIb/IIIa antagonists in non-ST-elevation ACS.

effect relies mainly on suspending the administration of the drug and waiting for at least 4 h for the drug to be cleared and for platelet aggregation to approx 50% of baseline levels *(92)*.

TIROFIBAN

Tirofiban (Aggrastat™) is a peptidomimetic agent with geometric, stereotactic, and charge characteristics similar to the RGD (Arg-Gly-Asp) sequence. It thus acts as a highly specific competitive antagonist of the GP IIb/IIIa receptor *(96)*. In a similar way to eptifibatide, after intravenous administration of tirofiban, the peak molecular concentration of the drug relative to the number of receptors is high; therefore, it is also unlikely that platelet transfusions are effective in reversing the antiplatelet effects of tirofiban. Again, similarly to eptifibatide, because of tirofiban's mean half-life of approx 2 h, reversal of the drug's antiplatelet effects relies on stopping the medication and waiting for approx 4 h to achieve approx 50% of the normal platelet aggregation *(92)*.

Clinical Trials of Intravenous GP IIb/IIIa Antagonists in Non-ST Elevation ACS

The role of intravenous GP IIb/IIIa antagonists in the treatment of non-ST-elevation ACS has been studied in six large prospective randomized trials involving approx 30,000 patients. Unlike the clear-cut positive results of the GP IIb/IIIa antagonists in the interventional arena, there has been considerable heterogeneity in the efficacy of these drugs in reducing cardiovascular events among patients presenting with non-ST-elevation ACS *(91)*. This heterogeneity may stem from several differences inherent to the ACS population. For example, as opposed to the "planned" vessel injury in patients undergoing elective PCI, patients with unstable angina or non-ST-elevation myocardial infarction present with spontaneously ruptured plaques and have ongoing coronary thrombosis. Therefore, maximal platelet inhibition cannot be afforded at the time of injury and onset of the ACS. In spite of these observations, the results of several clinical trials support the use of GP IIb/IIIa antagonists in patents suffering non-ST-elevation ACS (Fig. 7).

TRIAL DESIGNS

The Platelet Glycoprotein IIb/IIIa in Unstable Angina: Receptor Suppression Using Integrilin Therapy (PURSUIT) (97), Platelet Receptor Inhibition in Ischemic Syndrome Management in Patients Limited by Unstable Signs and Symptoms (PRISM-PLUS) (98), Platelet IIb/IIIa Antagonism for the Reduction of Acute Coronary Syndrome Events in a Global Organization Network (PARAGON) (99), and Platelet Receptor Inhibition in Ischemic Syndrome Management (PRISM) (100) trials, collectively known as the "4P's," are the basis for the use of GP IIb/IIIa antagonists for the treatment of ACS. Entry criteria were similar in these trials, although the PRISM study had a lower-risk population compared to the other trials. Indeed, 25% of patients enrolled in the PRISM study were diagnosed with non-Q wave myocardial infarction, compared to 45% in the higher risk populations enrolled in PRISM-PLUS and PURSUIT.

There were considerable differences between the trials regarding the therapeutic strategy to be followed. While PRISM and PARAGON focused primarily on the medical management of patients, discouraging early coronary catheterization and revascularization, PRISM-PLUS encouraged angiography and revascularization after an initial 48-h drug pretreatment period, maintaining drug therapy at the time of the procedure. PURSUIT, on the other hand, was a megatrial carried out in 28 countries and did not mandate any particular invasive or pharmacologic strategy apart from the study medication.

Regarding adjunctive pharmacotherapy, all patients received aspirin. Nevertheless, the use of heparin varied among the trials. In PURSUIT, heparin was encouraged during the active drug infusion, but was not protocol-mandated. Heparin co-administration to patients receiving GP IIb/IIIa inhibitor therapy was specifically tested in a randomized manner in the PRISM-PLUS and PARAGON-A studies. In the PRISM study, patients assigned to tirofiban did not receive adjunctive heparin. Table 5 summarizes the design of these four clinical trials.

The PARAGON-B trial enrolled 5225 high-risk patients with ischemic chest pain in the preceding 12 h, and either changes in the ST-segment or T wave, or positive cardiac enzymes (creatine kinase isoenzyme-cardiac muscle subunit [CK-MB] or troponins) (101). Patients were randomized to either lamifiban (500 mg iv bolus, followed by various infusion doses based on their estimated creatinine clearance over 72 h) or placebo for up to 120 h after any PCI.

The most recent of the GP IIb/IIIa antagonist in ACS trials is Global Use of Strategies to Open Occluded Arteries (GUSTO)-IV (102). Seven thousand eight hundred patients presenting with ischemic chest pain lasting more than 5 min in the preceding 24 h, and either positive troponins or at least 0.5 mm of ST-segment depression, randomly received either abciximab for 24 h, abciximab for 48 h, or a matching placebo. Abciximab was administered at the standard bolus and infusion doses. Early angiography and revascularization were strongly discouraged.

Table 5

Design of the Major Trials Evaluating GP IIb/IIIa Antagonists in ACS

Trial	Drug	n	Entry Criteria	Rx Duration	Heparin Use	Angiography and revascularization	Primary End Point
PRISM	Tirofiban	3232	Angina at rest or minimal exertion within 12 h, and either: Δ ECG or ↑ CPK-MB, or CAD history, or (+) stress test.	48 h	Control group.	Discouraged.	Death, MI, or refractory ischemia at 48 h.
PRISM-PLUS	Tirofiban	1915	Angina at rest or minimal exertion within 12 h, and either: Δ ECG or↑ CPK-MB.	48–96 h (96 h if PTCA).	Control group co-administered with tirofiban.	Encouraged after the 48-h drug infusion.	Death, MI, or refractory ischemia at 7 d.
PURSUIT	Eptifibatide	10,948	Angina at rest within 24 h, and either:Δ ECG or ↑ CPK-MB	Hospital discharge (96 h if PTCA).	Encouraged, but not randomized.	MD discretion.	Death or MI at 30 d.
PARAGON-A	Lamifiban	2282	Angina at rest within 12 h, and Δ EKG	72–120 h	Control group randomized.	MD discretion.	MD discretion.x30 d.
PARAGON-B	Lamifiban	5,225	Angina at rest within 12 hr + Δ ST or Δ T, or ↑ cardiac markers, or (+) troponins	72 h	Control group randomized	MD discretion (encouraged).	30 d all-cause mortality, MI, or severe recurrent ischemia.
GUSTO-IV	Abciximab	7,800	Angina for >5 min within 24 h and either: Δ ECG or ↑ troponin T or I, or >0.5mm transient _ST. LMWH substudy.	24–48 h	Control group Heparin co-administration with abciximab.	Encouraged.	Any-cause death, or MI at 30 d.

CPK-MB, creatine phosphokinase isoenzyme; CAD, coronary artery disease; PTCA, purcutaneous transluminal coronary angioplasty; MI, myocardial infarction; LMWH, low-molecular-weight heparin; MD, medical doctor; Δ, change.

Table 6

Short- and Medium-Term Clinical Outcomes of Patients Receiving GP IIb/IIIa Antagonists for ACS[a]

	48–96 h			30 d			6 mo		
	Death	MI	Death or MI	Death	MI	Death or MI	Death	MI	Death or MI
PRISM									
Heparin	0.4	1.4	1.4	3.6	4.3	7.1	—	—	—
Tirofiban	0.2	0.9	0.9	2.3	4.1	5.8	—	—	—
PRISM-PLUS									
Heparin	0.3	2.6	2.6	4.5	9.2	11.9	7.0	10.5	15.3
Tirofiban + heparin	0.1	0.9	0.9	3.6	6.6	8.7	6.9	8.3	12.3
PURSUIT									
Placebo	1.2	8.3	9.1	3.7	13.5	15.7	6.2	15.7	19.0
Eptifibatide	0.9	7.1	7.6	3.5	12.6	14.2	6.4	14.7	17.8
PARAGON-A									
Placebo	0.5	3.3	3.7	2.9	10.6	11.7	6.6	14.3	17.9
Lamifiban (low dose)	0.3	3.5	3.5	3.0	9.4	10.6	5.2	10.8	13.7
Lamifiban (high dose)	0.4	2.5	2.6	3.6	10.9	12.0	6.8	12.9	16.4
GUSTO-IV									
Placebo	0.3	1.3	1.5	3.9	3.9	5.1	8.0	—	—
Abciximab 24 h	0.7	1.3	1.9	1.9	3.4	5.6	8.2	—	—
Abciximab 48 h	0.9	1.4	2.2	2.2	4.3	5.9	9.1	—	—

[a]Short- and medium-term clinical outcomes from 5 major randomized trials of GP IIb/IIIa antagonists in the treatment of patients with non-ST-elevation ACS.
MI, myocardial infarction.
Modified from ref. 91.

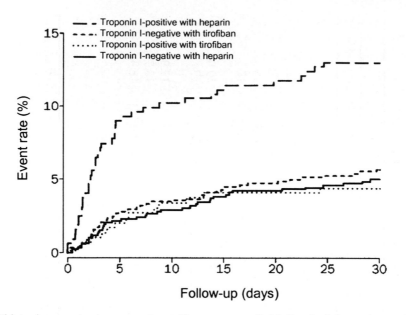

Fig. 8. Thirty-day event-rate curves (mortality or myocardial infarction) for patients with troponin-I concentrations higher or lower than 1.0 µg/mL. A reduction in death or myocardial infarction was observed in troponin I-positive patients who received tirofiban *(103)*. Reproduced with permission from: Heeschen C, Hamm CW, Goldman B, et al. Copyright by The Lancet Ltd, 1999.

TRIAL OUTCOMES

The net clinical benefit of GP IIb/IIIa antagonists in the treatment of non-ST-elevation myocardial ischemia has been shown in several trials, however, there has been a significant heterogeneity in their results (Table 6). In the PRISM study, patients who received tirofiban compared to heparin alone, had a reduced rate of the composite of death, new myocardial infarction, or refractory ischemia during the 48-h infusion period of the study drug (3.8 vs 5.6%, RR 0.67, $p = 0.01$), largely as a result of a reduction in recurrent ischemia. At 30 d, however, this difference was no longer significant ($p = 0.34$). A treatment effect at 30 d, however, was seen in PRISM-PLUS. Patients who received the combination of tirofiban and heparin had a reduced rate of 30-d mortality, myocardial infarction, refractory ischemia, or rehospitalization for unstable angina, compared to patients receiving heparin alone (18.5 vs 22.3%, RR 0.78, $p = 0.03$). Although this benefit was maintained at 6 mo, the 30-d composite end point did not quite reach the prespecified statistical significance of $p < 0.025$.

Although the PRISM population was low-risk, patient stratification based on positive troponin I or T levels revealed a number of interesting findings *(103)*. First, troponins identified patients at high risk for subsequent cardiovascular events, consistent with prior studies. Second, and most important of all, positive troponins served to identify patients who would benefit the most from tirofiban therapy. For example, 30-d death or myocardial infarction occurred in 13.0% of troponin I-positive patients, compared to 4.9% of troponin-negative patients ($p < 0.001$). Among troponin-positive patients, tirofiban reduced the risk of death and myocardial infarction by 75 ($p = 0.004$) and 63% ($p = 0.01$), respectively, whereas no treatment effect could be discerned among troponin-negative patients (Fig. 8).

Although the original design of PRISM-PLUS did contemplate a direct comparison between tirofiban only, heparin only, and a combination of tirofiban and heparin, such a comparison could not be completed, because the tirofiban-only arm was prematurely stopped when an interim analysis revealed an unexpected increase in death in this group, compared with the heparin-only arm. Although this observation could have resulted from the play of chance, as it was not statistically significant and was inconsistent with the results of the PRISM study, it raised the possibility of a prothrombotic effect of GP IIb/IIIa antagonism without adjunctive heparin use.

The multinational PURSUIT trial demonstrated a significant 1.5% absolute risk reduction in the occurrence of death or myocardial infarction as early as 96 h of initiating the study drug. The beneficial effects of eptifibatide among the high-risk PURSUIT population persisted at 7 d, 30 d, and at 6 mo follow-up, indicating that the treatment effect is durable. In addition to decreasing the incidence of myocardial infarction, eptifibatide was shown to reduce the size of the infarction.

In contrast to the clinical benefit observed in the other three trials, PARAGON-A did not show a reduction in 30-d death, myocardial infarction, or recurrent ischemia with either high dose or low dose lamifiban. However, after the initial 30-d period, the event-rate curves diverged, and by 6 mo there was a lower rate of death or myocardial infarction associated with the low dose of lamifiban plus heparin (odds ratio [OR] 0.66, $p = 0.025$, vs placebo + heparin). Retrospective analyses of PARAGON-A showed that optimal platelet inhibition and improved clinical outcomes among patients receiving lamifiban were attained when the plasma levels of the drug were between 18 and 42 ng/mL (104). As a result of this observation, the PARAGON-B trial studied the optimal dose of lamifiban based on renal function. All patients received aspirin and either unfractionated or low molecular weight heparin, in addition to placebo or lamifiban. Patients assigned to the active treatment group did not show an improved survival in terms of 30-d death or myocardial infarction (10.6% in the lamifiban group vs 11.5% in the placebo group, $p = 0.32$) (101). Interestingly, an 1160-patient troponin substudy found that patients who tested positive for troponin T had a 50% greater risk of dying, having myocardial infarction, or having severe recurrent ischemia within 30 d (the study's primary composite end point), compared to troponin-negative patients (105). In addition, only troponin-positive patients seemed to derive clinical benefit from lamifiban, reducing the risk of reaching the composite end point to almost the same as that of troponin-negative patients. Among troponin-positive patients, lamifiban reduced the primary composite from 19.4 to 11.0% ($p = 0.01$), while among troponin-negative patients, there was no significant treatment effect of lamifiban (11.2% for placebo vs 10.8% for lamifiban, $p = 0.86$). Thus, PARAGON-B confirmed that troponin positivity predicts a worse short-term clinical outcome and also identifies which patients are likely to benefit from GP IIb/IIIa blockade.

Although the CAPTURE trial strictly does not form part of the collection of trials that have studied GP IIb/IIIa antagonists in the medical management of patients with ACS, it is germane to the present discussion (106). In CAPTURE, more than 1200 patients with refractory unstable angina underwent angiography and were subsequently randomized to receive 18–24 h of either placebo or abciximab prior to planned angioplasty. Following angioplasty, the abciximab infusion was continued for an additional 1 h. The composite end point of death, myocardial infarction, or urgent revascularization at 30 d occurred significantly less frequently among patients receiving abciximab compared to placebo

(11.3 vs 15.9%, RR 0.64, $p = 0.01$). An angiographic analysis from this trial showed that abciximab promoted thrombus dissolution, consistent with the finding of reduced recurrent ischemia, as evidenced by continuous electrocardiographic monitoring. Abciximab not only decreased the number of events after the coronary intervention, but also prior to the procedure and as a result of the procedure per se (rate of myocardial infarction before PCI, 0.6 vs 2.1% [$p = 0.03$]; after PCI 2.6 vs 5.5% [$p = 0.009$]). Importantly, a subsequent analysis that stratified the CAPTURE patients according to their serum troponin T levels, found that the benefit of abciximab had been confined to patients with elevated troponin T levels *(107)*. Indeed, in this group of patients, abciximab reduced the risk of death or myocardial infarction at 6 mo by an impressive 68% ($p = 0.002$).

Based on the positive results of the CAPTURE trial, GUSTO-IV assessed the effect of a prolonged (24 or 48 h) infusion of abciximab in patients presenting within 24 h of the onset of a non-ST-elevation ACS. In contrast to the previous trials, GUSTO-IV showed no clinical benefit of GP IIb/IIIa blockade, compared to placebo. In fact, the 48-h infusion of abciximab consistently increased the incidence of death at 48 h (0.3% placebo vs 0.9% for 48-hr abciximab, OR 2.9, $p = 0.008$), at 7 d (1.8 vs 2.0% $p = 0.57$), and at 30 d (3.9 vs 4.3%, $p = 0.66$). The primary end point of death or myocardial infarction at 30 d was reached in 8.0, 8.2, and 9.1% in the placebo, 24-h abciximab, and 48-h abciximab groups, respectively. Furthermore, in contrast to the CAPTURE, PRISM, and PARAGON-B studies, in which troponin positivity identified high risk patients who derived particular benefit from GP IIb/IIIa therapy, a similar effect could not be discerned in GUSTO-IV *(102)*. The precise mechanisms explaining this phenomenon are currently unknown, however, several possibilities have been proposed. Compared to the other trials, GUSTO-IV may have enrolled lower risk patients. In addition, investigators knew that GUSTO-IV strongly discouraged early revascularization; this may have introduced a selection bias in which patients more likely to benefit from therapy were excluded. Other possibilities include platelet activation secondary to outside-in signaling through the GP IIb/IIIa integrin with a possible pro-inflammatory effect resulting from prolonged GP IIb/IIIa receptor occupancy *(25)*, and significant peak-through variations in platelet inhibition.

In spite of the negative results seen in GUSTO-IV, there is abundant evidence supporting the use of eptifibatide or tirofiban in the management of high risk patients presenting with non-ST-elevation ACS. In addition, the benefit of administering abciximab to high risk patients with refractory unstable angina, who are to undergo percutaneous coronary revascularization within 24 h, remains unchanged.

ROLE OF REVASCULARIZATION

The 4P trials clearly indicate an improvement in the clinical outcome of patients with an ACS who are treated with platelet GP IIb/IIIa antagonists. Nevertheless, these trials did not specifically evaluate the efficacy of GP IIb/IIIa antagonism in patients with ACS who subsequently underwent PCI. A meta-analysis of postrandomization observations from CAPTURE, PURSUIT, and PRISM-PLUS, however, provide evidence that GP IIb/IIIa antagonism not only reduces ischemic events during the infusion of the drug, but also significantly ameliorates ischemic complications resulting from PCI *(108)*. An overall 34% reduction in the composite of death or nonfatal myocardial infarction was found during medical management with GP IIb/IIIa antiplatelet therapy preceding PCI (2.5 vs 3.8%, OR 0.66), and an additional 41% reduction in PCI-related ischemic complications was noted among patients who received GP IIb/IIIa antagonists and who subsequently underwent PCI.

The recent Treat Angina with Aggrastat and Determine Cost of Therapy with an Invasive or Conservative Strategy, Thrombolysis in Myocardial Infarction (TACTICS-TIMI) 18 trial provided definitive evidence of the complementary roles of GP IIb/IIIa blockade and early PCI for the treatment of ACS *(109)*. In the TACTICS-TIMI 18 trial, 2220 patients presenting with non-ST-elevation ACS were treated with aspirin, tirofiban, and heparin, in addition to the usual management. Patients were subsequently randomized to either an invasive strategy, which included early (on average, 24 h after enrollment) catheterization and revascularization (if necessary), or to a conservative strategy of medical management, reserving coronary angiography to cases of recurrent or provokable ischemia. At 6 mo, the rate of the primary end point (consisting of death, myocardial infarction, or rehospitalization for an ACS) was reduced in patients managed according to the invasive strategy, compared to those being medically managed (15.9 vs 19.4%, p = 0.025). Additionally, TACTICS-TIMI 18 prospectively validated the notion that troponin-positive (i.e., high risk) patients derive an added benefit from an early invasive therapeutic strategy compared to those who do not have elevated troponin levels. Troponin T-positive (>0.01 ng/mL) patients randomized to the invasive strategy had a 45% relative reduction in the odds of reaching the primary end point, compared to lack of efficacy observed in troponin-negative patients ($p < 0.001$).

LIMITATIONS AND ADVERSE EFFECTS GP IIB/IIIA ANTAGONISTS

Platelet GP IIb/IIIa antagonists have been administered to tens of thousands of patients under a variety of settings and have consistently shown to have a very good safety profile.

Bleeding. Bleeding complications are the main concern regarding the safety of these agents. In the Evaluation of 7E3 for the Prevention of Ischemic Complications (EPIC) *(110)* trial, abciximab significantly increased the risk of major bleeding. Nevertheless, it was later determined that the non-weight-adjusted dose of heparin that had been used accounted for the excess bleeding events. In the subsequent Evaluation in Percutaneous Transluminal Coronary Angioplasty to Improve Long-Term Outcome with Abciximab GP IIb/IIIa blockade (EPILOG) and Evaluation of Platelet IIb/IIIa Inhibitor for Stent (EPISTENT) trials, in which weight-adjusted heparin doses had been in conjunction with early sheath removal, there was no excess in bleeding complications among patients being treated with abciximab *(111)*. Similarly, in the PRISM-PLUS study, tirofiban was associated with a slight but nonsignificant increase in major bleeding. In PRISM, tirofiban did not increase the risk of major bleeding. In the PURSUIT and Enhanced Suppression of the Platelet IIb/IIIa Receptor with Integrilin Therapy (ESPRIT) *(112)* trials, which used higher eptifibatide doses compared to Integrilin to Manage Platelet Aggregation to Prevent Coronary Thrombosis (IMPACT)-II *(113)*, there was a small but statistically significant increase in major bleeding. Importantly, in PURSUIT, patients who received eptifibatide and underwent coronary artery bypass surgery did not have additional bleeding complications compared to patients assigned to placebo. Additionally, it is reassuring that none of the GP IIb/IIIa antagonists have increased the risk of intracranial hemorrhage *(114)*.

Thrombocytopenia. Abciximab has been reported to cause both, pseudothrombocytopenia and true thrombocytopenia. In patients receiving abciximab and who develop thrombocytopenia, EDTA-induced pseudothrombocytopenia should always be considered and ruled-out by directly examining a peripheral blood smear for the presence of platelet aggregates, as the automated platelet counters do not normally distinguish this entity from true thrombocytopenia (115). In addition, EDTA-dependent pseudothrombocytopenia does not constitute an indication to stop abciximab therapy. Another condition that must be considered and ruled-out is heparin-induced thrombocytopenia, as patients receiving abciximab also frequently receive heparin.

True abciximab-induced profound thrombocytopenia (platelet count $<20,000/\mu L$) occurs in about 0.3–1.0% of patients (115). In these patients, a significant decrease in their platelet count can normally be detected within the first hours after drug administration, therefore it is essential that a platelet count be obtained within 2–4 h after initiating abciximab. Most patients with severe thrombocytopenia respond well to platelet transfusions, and their platelet count usually recovers within 5 d, but may take over a wk to do so.

The mechanisms of abciximab-induced thrombocytopenia are unknown, but may include the presence of an antibody to a neoepitope expressed after abciximab binding to GP IIb/IIIa, or abciximab-induced platelet activation with subsequent platelet sequestration from the circulation. At the moment, available data lend support to an immune-mediated mechanism for abciximab-induced thrombocytopenia, as high titer antibodies are detected in the plasma of patients after they have been treated with abciximab.

Additional concerns have been raised as approx 6% of patients who receive abciximab develop human antichimeric antibodies (HACA), however, these antibodies do not appear to affect the in vitro platelet inhibition by abciximab. Importantly, the ReoPro Readministration Registry (116), which included 500 patients who received abciximab for a second time, reported: (i) a high clinical success rate; (ii) no cases of hypersensitivity, bleeding, or death; and (iii) an incidence of thrombocytopenia comparable to patients receiving abciximab for the first time. A shift in the incidence of thrombocytopenia, from mild to profound thrombocytopenia, however, was observed. There were also several cases of delayed (0.8%) (approx 6 d after hospital discharge) and recurrent thrombocytopenia (0.8%), the latter occurring despite platelet transfusions. It is therefore recommended that clinicians obtain a second platelet count 24 h after the readministration of abciximab, and that they maintain a high index of suspicion for the delayed development of abciximab-induced thrombocytopenia. Although there have been no reports of immune reactions associated with either tirofiban or eptifibatide, decreased platelet counts occasionally occur (100).

MONITORING PLATELET FUNCTION

As with any form of pharmacologic therapy, there is a significant inter-individual variability in the response to GP IIb/IIIa antagonists. Differences in platelet size and counts, activation status, number of GP IIb/IIIa receptors expressed per platelet, splenic size, renal function, and platelet GP IIb/IIIa genetic polymorphisms, can all influence the pharmacological response to a given GP IIb/IIIa antagonist. Furthermore, these asseverations are not merely theoretical, as a significant intra- and interindividual variability in platelet inhibition has been documented in patients and healthy subjects receiving antiplatelet therapy (117). To assess these differences, a number of assays for analyzing platelet function have been developed and range from the well-validated turbidometric aggregometry method, to modern platelet function analyzers such as the PFA-100 and the rapid PFA (RPFA), which are both available for clinical use.

Several studies have evaluated the pharmacokinetic and pharmacodynamic properties of the intravenous GP IIb/IIIa antagonists, however, the GOLD trial is the largest and the first study to correlate platelet function in patients receiving GP IIb/IIIa antagonists with clinical outcomes *(118)*. The GOLD trial monitored platelet function using the RPFA device in 485 patients who underwent PCI and received GP IIb/IIIa antagonist therapy: abciximab (84%), tirofiban (9%), and eptifibatide (7%). Patients who achieved >95% platelet inhibition within 10 min, had a 6.4% event rate of major adverse cardiac events, compared to 14.4% of patients who attained <95% inhibition ($p = 0.006$). At 8 h, patients who had >70% inhibition, had lower event rates than those who achieved <70% platelet inhibition (8.1 vs 25%, $p = 0.009$). The GOLD study confirms important interindividual variations in platelet inhibition after GP IIb/IIIa blockade therapy and also reveals that a significant proportion of patients do not reach optimal platelet inhibition. The question, however, remains as to whether clinical events can be reduced by adjusting the dose of GP IIb/IIIa antagonist to an optimal antiplatelet effect.

Clinical Use of Intravenous GP IIb/IIIa Antagonists in Patients with Non-ST Elevation ACS

Data from the PRISM, PRISM-PLUS, and PURSUIT studies favor the use of tirofiban or eptifibatide in patients with non-ST-elevation ACS, particularly among high-risk patients with positive troponins, or in patients undergoing adjunctive PCI.

However, unlike the decision to administer GP IIb/IIIa antagonists to patients undergoing elective PCI, the administration of this form of antiplatelet therapy to patients presenting with ACS is less straightforward. Indeed, the diagnosis of unstable angina remains largely clinical. Furthermore, the diagnosis of non-ST-elevation myocardial infarction is frequently made retrospectively, based upon the examination of enzymatic markers of myocardial necrosis. Therefore, GP IIb/IIIa antagonist therapy is commonly initiated in an "empiric" way in this group of patients, in spite of the observation that the benefit of this therapy seems to be somewhat confined to high-risk unstable angina patients particularly to those with elevated troponin levels and to those who proceed to PCI. A meta-analysis of the six trials shown in Table 5 and Fig. 7 indicates hat GP IIb/IIIa antagonist therapy is associated with a 9% relative (or 1% absolute) reduction in the odds of death or myocardial infarction at 30 d *(119)*. Subgroup analyses of this study suggest that patients with elevated troponins or who undergo PCI, are those who derive most benefit from GP IIb/IIIa blockade.

Putting these data in context with the TACTICS trial, patients presenting within the first few h (<3 h) after the onset of the non-ST-elevation ACS, in whom troponin elevation would not be detected yet, should probably receive intravenous GP IIb/IIIa antagonists (tirofiban or eptifibatide) and undergo early coronary catheterization and revascularization if deemed appropriate. If, however, a patient is found to not have an elevated troponin level 12 h or more after the onset of symptoms, a noninvasive approach would seem adequate. If GP IIb/IIIa antagonists were to be administered to a patient with these characteristics, benefit from this form of therapy would not be expected to be significant.

One concern of the "up-front" or empiric administration of GP IIb/IIIa therapy is that patients with ACS may require coronary artery bypass grafting (CABG) surgery. A sub-

Table 7
High Risk Features in Patients with Non-ST-Elevation ACS

	High Risk
Feature	*At least 1 of the following must be present:*
History	Accelerating tempo of ischemic symptoms In preceding 48 h
Character of pain	Prolonged, ongoing (>20 min) rest pain.
Clinical findings	Pulmonary edema, most likely due to ischemia.
	New or worsening mitral regurgitation murmur.
	S_3 or new/worsening rales.
	Hypotension, bradycardia, tachycardia.
	Age >75 yr
ECG	Angina at rest with transient ST-segment changes >0.5 mV.
	Bundle-branch block, new or presumed new.
	Sustained ventricular tachycardia.
Cardiac markers	Elevated.

Adapted from ref. *63*.

analysis of PURSUIT has shown that eptifibatide is not only safe, but also significantly improves the outcome of patients undergoing CABG *(120)*. Once the decision to perform CABG surgery has been made in patients receiving either tirofiban or eptifibatide, the drug infusion should be stopped, and at least 4 h must pass in order to reverse the antiplatelet effect. In patients with ACS who receive abciximab because of a planned PCI within the next 24 h, but who for some reason or another proceed to CABG surgery, the medication should be stopped and platelets may need to be transfused.

A critical issue regarding GP IIb/IIIa antagonists in patients with ACS is the role of concomitant heparin therapy, however, this point has been difficult to determine from the results of the above-discussed trials. While in PRISM heparin was directly compared with tirofiban, the combination of tirofiban plus heparin was not examined. Conversely, although in PRISM-PLUS one of the treatment arms was tirofiban plus heparin and the control group received heparin only, the tirofiban-only arm was stopped prematurely because of an increase in mortality. In the PURSUIT trial, investigators were encouraged to use concomitant heparin, however, this was not done in a standardized fashion. PARAGON-A was the only trial to specifically test the interaction between heparin and GP IIb/IIIa blockade because of its 2 × 2 factorial design, in which patients randomized to lamifiban were further randomized to receive either heparin or no heparin. Although there were no differences in outcome between the groups at 30 d, the combination of low-dose lamifiban with heparin had a lower rate of death or myocardial infarction compared to the other groups at 6 mo, and a lower mortality at 1 yr. Although this study would provide direct evidence supporting the concomitant use of both classes of agents, it was not adequately powered to establish differences between the two groups.

The most recent American Heart Association/American College of Cardiology guidelines for the treatment of non-ST-elevation ACS give a class I recommendation for the administration of a GP IIb/IIIa antagonist, in conjunction with aspirin and heparin, to patients in whom catheterization and PCI are planned. If, however, clopidogrel has already been adminstered to these patients, the recommendation to administer a GP

IIb/IIIa antagonist is class IIa, meaning that the weight of evidence favors the selected treatment, although there may be divergent opinions in this matter. Also given as a class IIa recommendation is the administration of tirofiban or eptifibatide, in addition to aspirin and heparin (either unfractionated or low-molecular weight) to patients *with* continuing ischemia or with other high-risk features (Table 7) and in whom an invasive approach is *not* planned. The general opinion is that the benefit of tirofiban or eptifibatide in low-risk ACS patients who do not have continuing ischemia and in whom PCI is not planned, would not outweigh the associated risks.

ACKNOWLEDGMENT

The authors would like to thank José A. López, M.D. (Department of Thrombosis Research, Baylor College of Medicine, Houston, TX) for having generously contributed to this chapter with Figs. 2, 3, and 4.

REFERENCES

1. Zaman AG, Helft G, Worthley SG, Badimon JJ. The role of plaque rupture and thrombosis in coronary artery disease. Atherosclerosis 2000;149:251–266.
2. Forrester JS. Role of plaque rupture in acute coronary syndromes. Am J Cardiol 2000;86:15J–23J.
3. Fuster V, Badimon L, Badimon JJ, Chesebro JH. The pathogenesis of coronary artery disease and the acute coronary syndromes (1). N Engl J Med 1992;326:242–250.
4. Richardson PD, Davies MJ, Born GV. Influence of plaque configuration and stress distribution on fissuring of coronary atherosclerotic plaques. Lancet 1989;2:941–944.
5. Poston RN, Haskard DO, Coucher JR, Gall NP, Johnson Tidey RR. Expression of intercellular adhesion molecule-1 in atherosclerotic plaques. Am J Pathol 1992;140:665–673.
6. Libby P. Molecular bases of the acute coronary syndromes. Circulation 1995; 91(11):2844–2850
7. Davies MJ, Richardson PD, Woolf N, Katz DR, Mann J. Risk of thrombosis in human atherosclerotic plaques: role of extracellular lipid, macrophage, and smooth muscle cell content. Br Heart J 1993;69: 377–381.
8. Fernandez-Ortiz A, Badimon JJ, Falk E, et al. Characterization of the relative thrombogenicity of atherosclerotic plaque components: implications for consequences of plaque rupture. J Am Coll Cardiol 1994;23:1562–1569.
9. Kamath S, Blann AD, Lip GY. Platelet activation: assessment and quantification. Eur Heart J 2001; 22:1561–1571.
10. Michelson AD, Barnard MR, Hechtman HB, et al. In vivo tracking of platelets: circulating degranulated platelets rapidly lose surface P-selectin but continue to circulate and function. Proc Natl Acad Sci USA 1996;93:11877–11882.
11. Mast A. Barnes-Jewish Hospital Laboratory Reference Values. In: Carey CF, Lee HH, Woeltje KF eds. The Washington Manual of Medical Therapeutics. Lippincott-Raven, Philadelphia, 1998, pp. 527–533.
12. Lincoff AM, Kereiakes DJ, Mascelli MA, et al. Abciximab suppresses the rise in levels of circulating inflammatory markers after percutaneous coronary revascularization. Circulation 2001;104:163–167.
13. Chew DP, Bhatt DL, Robbins MA, et al. Effect of clopidogrel added to aspirin before percutaneous coronary intervention on the risk associated with C-reactive protein. Am J Cardiol 2001;88:672–674.
14. Gawaz M, Neumann FJ, Ott I, Schiessler A, Schomig A. Platelet function in acute myocardial infarction treated with direct angioplasty. Circulation 1996;93:229–237.
15. Savage B, Saldivar E, Ruggeri ZM. Initiation of platelet adhesion by arrest onto fibrinogen or translocation on von Willebrand factor. Cell 1996;84:289–297.
16. Romo GM, Dong JF, Schade AJ, et al. The glycoprotein Ib-IX-V complex is a platelet counterreceptor for P-selectin. J Exp Med 1999;190:803–814.
17. Alevriadou BR, Moake JL, Turner NA, et al. Real-time analysis of shear-dependent thrombus formation and its blockade by inhibitors of von Willebrand factor binding to platelets. Blood 1993;81: 1263–1276.
18. Clemetson KJ, Clemetson JM. Platelet collagen receptors. Thromb Haemost 2001;86:189–197.

19. Andrews RK, Shen Y, Gardiner EE, Dong JF, Lopez JA, Berndt MC. The glycoprotein Ib-IX-V complex in platelet adhesion and signaling. Thromb Haemost 1999;82:357–364.

20. George JN. Platelets. Lancet 2000;355:1531–1539.

21. Reverter JC, Beguin S, Kessels H, Kumar R, Hemker HC, Coller BS. Inhibition of platelet-mediated, tissue factor-induced thrombin generation by the mouse/human chimeric 7E3 antibody. Potential implications for the effect of c7E3 Fab treatment on acute thrombosis and "clinical restenosis". J Clin Invest 1996;98:863–874.

22. Moliterno DJ, Califf RM, Aguirre FV, et al. Effect of platelet glycoprotein IIb/IIIa integrin blockade on activated clotting time during percutaneous transluminal coronary angioplasty or directional atherectomy (the EPIC trial). Evaluation of c7E3 Fab in the Prevention of Ischemic Complications trial. Am J Cardiol 1995;75:559–562.

23. Lindemann S, Tolley ND, Dixon DA, et al. Activated platelets mediate inflammatory signaling by regulated interleukin 1beta synthesis. J Cell Biol 2001;154:485–490.

24. Wagner CL, Mascelli MA, Neblock DS, Weisman HF, Coller BS, Jordan RE. Analysis of GPIIb/IIIa receptor number by quantification of 7E3 binding to human platelets. Blood 1996;88:907–914.

25. Du XP, Plow EF, Frelinger AL, III, O'Toole TE, Loftus JC, Ginsberg MH. Ligands "activate" integrin alpha IIb beta 3 (platelet GPIIb-IIIa). Cell 1991;65:409–416.

26. Phillips DR, Charo IF, Parise LV, Fitzgerald LA. The platelet membrane glycoprotein IIb-IIIa complex. Blood 1988;71:831–843.

27. Niiya K, Hodson E, Bader R, et al. Increased surface expression of the membrane glycoprotein IIb/IIIa complex induced by platelet activation. Relationship to the binding of fibrinogen and platelet aggregation. Blood 1987;70:475–483.

28. Pierschbacher MD, Ruoslahti E. Cell attachment activity of fibronectin can be duplicated by small synthetic fragments of the molecule. Nature 1984;309:30–33.

29. Kloczewiak M, Timmons S, Hawiger J. Recognition site for the platelet receptor is present on the 15-residue carboxy-terminal fragment of the gamma chain of human fibrinogen and is not involved in the fibrin polymerization reaction. Thromb Res 1983;29:249–255.

30. Shattil SJ, Ginsberg MH. Integrin signaling in vascular biology. J Clin Invest 1997;(Suppl. 100): S91–S95.

31. Weber C, Springer TA. Neutrophil accumulation on activated, surface-adherent platelets in flow is mediated by interaction of Mac-1 with fibrinogen bound to alphaIIbbeta3 and stimulated by platelet-activating factor. J Clin Invest 1997;100:2085–2093.

32. Patrono C. Aspirin as an antiplatelet drug. N Engl J Med 1994;330:1287–1294.

33. Buchanan MR, Brister SJ. Individual variation in the effects of ASA on platelet function: implications for the use of ASA clinically. Can J Cardiol 1995;11:221–227.

34. Rinder CS, Student LA, Bonan JL, Rinder HM, Smith BR. Aspirin does not inhibit adenosine diphosphate-induced platelet alpha- granule release. Blood 1993;82:505–512.

35. Folts JD, Crowell EB Jr, Rowe GG. Platelet aggregation in partially obstructed vessels and its elimination with aspirin. Circulation 1976;54:365–370.

36. Pedersen AK, FitzGerald GA. Dose-related kinetics of aspirin. Presystemic acetylation of platelet cyclooxygenase. N Engl J Med 1984;311:1206–1211.

37. Dabaghi SF, Kamat SG, Payne J, et al. Effects of low-dose aspirin on in vitro platelet aggregation in the early minutes after ingestion in normal subjects. Am J Cardiol 1994;74:720–723.

38. Collaborative overview of randomised trials of antiplatelet therapy—I: prevention of death, myocardial infarction, and stroke by prolonged antiplatelet therapy in various categories of patients. Antiplatelet Trialists' Collaboration. BMJ 1994;308:81–106.

39. Low-dose aspirin and vitamin E in people at cardiovascular risk: a randomised trial in general practice. Collaborative Group of the Primary Prevention Project. Lancet 2001;357:89–95.

40. Randomised trial of intravenous streptokinase, oral aspirin, both, or neither among 17,187 cases of suspected acute myocardial infarction: ISIS-2. ISIS-2 (Second International Study of Infarct Survival) Collaborative Group. Lancet 1988;2:349–360.

41. Lewis HD Jr, Davis JW, Archibald DG, et al. Protective effects of aspirin against acute myocardial infarction and death in men with unstable angina. Results of a Veterans Administration Cooperative Study. N Engl J Med 1983;309:396–403.

42. Cairns JA, Gent M, Singer J, et al. Aspirin, sulfinpyrazone, or both in unstable angina. Results of a Canadian multicenter trial. N Engl J Med 1985;313:1369–1375.

43. Theroux P, Ouimet H, McCans J, et al. Aspirin, heparin, or both to treat acute unstable angina. N Engl J Med 1988;319:1105–1111.

44. Risk of myocardial infarction and death during treatment with low dose aspirin and intravenous heparin in men with unstable coronary artery disease. The RISC Group. Lancet 1990;336:827–830.

45. De Caterina R, Giannessi D, Bernini W, et al. Selective inhibition of thromboxane-related platelet function by low- dose aspirin in patients after myocardial infarction. Am J Cardiol 1985;55:589–590.

46. Weksler BB, Pett SB, Alonso D, et al. Differential inhibition by aspirin of vascular and platelet prostaglandin synthesis in atherosclerotic patients. N Engl J Med 1983;308:800–805.

47. Clarke RJ, Mayo G, Price P, FitzGerald GA. Suppression of thromboxane A_2 but not of systemic prostacyclin by controlled-release aspirin. N Engl J Med 1991;325:1137–1141.

48. A comparison of two doses of aspirin (30 mg vs 283 mg a day) in patients after a transient ischemic attack or minor ischemic stroke. The Dutch TIA Trial Study Group. N Engl J Med 1991;325:1261–1266

49. Taylor DW, Barnett HJ, Haynes RB, Ferguson GG, Sackett DL, Thorpe KE et al. Low-dose and high-dose acetylsalicylic acid for patients undergoing carotid endarterectomy: a randomised controlled trial. ASA and Carotid Endarterectomy (ACE) Trial Collaborators. Lancet 1999;353:2179–2184.

50. Helgason CM, Tortorice KL, Winkler SR, Penney DW, Schuler JJ, McClelland TJ et al. Aspirin response and failure in cerebral infarction. Stroke 1993;24:345–350.

51. Helgason CM, Bolin KM, Hoff JA, Winkler SR, Mangat A, Tortorice KL et al. Development of aspirin resistance in persons with previous ischemic stroke. Stroke 1994;25:2331–2336.

52. Grotemeyer KH, Scharafinski HW, Husstedt IW. Two-year follow-up of aspirin responder and aspirin non responder. A pilot-study including 180 post-stroke patients. Thromb Res 1993;71:397–403.

53. Gum PA, Kottke-Marchant K, Poggio ED, Gurm H, Welsh PA, Brooks L et al. Profile and prevalence of aspirin resistance in patients with cardiovascular disease. Am J Cardiol 2001;88:230–235.

54. Kawasaki T, Ozeki Y, Igawa T, Kambayashi J. Increased platelet sensitivity to collagen in individuals resistant to low-dose aspirin. Stroke 2000;31:591–595.

55. Mueller MR, Salat A, Stangl P, Murabito M, Pulaki S, Boehm D et al. Variable platelet response to low-dose ASA and the risk of limb deterioration in patients submitted to peripheral arterial angioplasty. Thromb Haemost 1997;78:1003–1007.

56. A randomised, blinded, trial of clopidogrel versus aspirin in patients at risk of ischaemic events (CAPRIE). CAPRIE Steering Committee. Lancet 1996;348:1329–1339.

57. UK-TIA Study Group. United Kingdom transient ischaemic attack (UK TIA) aspirin trial: interim results. British Medical Journal Clinical Research Ed. 1994[1998], 316–320. 1994. Ref Type: Journal (Full)

58. Derry S, Loke YK. Risk of gastrointestinal haemorrhage with long term use of aspirin: meta-analysis. BMJ 2000;321:1183–1187.

59. Hall D, Zeitler H, Rudolph W. Counteraction of the vasodilator effects of enalapril by aspirin in severe heart failure. J Am Coll Cardiol 1992;20:1549–1555.

60. Nguyen KN, Aursnes I, Kjekshus J. Interaction between enalapril and aspirin on mortality after acute myocardial infarction: subgroup analysis of the Cooperative New Scandinavian Enalapril Survival Study II (CONSENSUS II). Am J Cardiol 1997;79:115–119.

61. Al Khadra AS, Salem DN, Rand WM, Udelson JE, Smith JJ, Konstam MA. Antiplatelet agents and survival: a cohort analysis from the Studies of Left Ventricular Dysfunction (SOLVD) trial. J Am Coll Cardiol 1998;31:419–425.

62. Leor J, Reicher-Reiss H, Goldbourt U, Boyko V, Gottlieb S, Battler A et al. Aspirin and mortality in patients treated with angiotensin-converting enzyme inhibitors: a cohort study of 11,575 patients with coronary artery disease. J Am Coll Cardiol 1999;33:1920–1925.

63 Braunwald E, Antman EM, Beasley JW, et al. ACC/AHA 2002 guideline update for the management of patients with unstable angina and non-ST-segment elevation myocardial infarction: a report of the American College of Cardiology/American Heart Association Task Force on Practice Guidelines (Committee on the Management of Patients with Unstable Angina). 2002. Available at http://www.acc.org/clinical/guidelines/unstable/unstable.pdf.

64. Gaarder A, Jonsen L, Laland S, Hellem A, Owren PA. Adenosine diphosphate in red cells as a factor in the adhesiveness of human blood platelets. Nature 192, 531–532. 1961. Ref Type: Generic

65. Lanza F, Beretz A, Stierle A, Hanau D, Kubina M, Cazenave JP. Epinephrine potentiates human platelet activation but is not an aggregating agent. Am J Physiol 1988;255(6 Pt 2):H1276–H1288.

66. Clemetson KJ, Clemetson JM, Proudfoot AE, Power CA, Baggiolini M, Wells TN. Functional expression of CCR1, CCR3, CCR4, and CXCR4 chemokine receptors on human platelets. Blood 2000;96: 4046–4054.

67. Enjyoji K, Sevigny J, Lin Y, Frenette PS, Christie PD, Esch JS et al. Targeted disruption of cd39/ATP diphosphohydrolase results in disordered hemostasis and thromboregulation. Nat Med 1999;5: 1010–1017.
68. Gachet C. ADP receptors of platelets and their inhibition. Thromb Haemost 2001;86:222–232.
69. Macfarlane DE, Srivastava PC, Mills DC. 2-Methylthioadenosine[beta-32P]diphosphate. An agonist and radioligand for the receptor that inhibits the accumulation of cyclic AMP in intact blood platelets. J Clin Invest 1983;71:420–428.
70. Leon C, Vial C, Cazenave JP, Gachet C. Cloning and sequencing of a human cDNA encoding endothelial P2Y1 purinoceptor. Gene 1996;171:295–297.
71. Hechler B, Leon C, Vial C, Vigne P, Frelin C, Cazenave JP et al. The P2Y1 receptor is necessary for adenosine 5'-diphosphate-induced platelet aggregation. Blood 1998;92:152–159.
72. Savi P, Beauverger P, Labouret C, Delfaud M, Salel V, Kaghad M et al. Role of P2Y1 purinoceptor in ADP-induced platelet activation. FEBS Lett 1998;422:291–295.
73. Leon C, Hechler B, Freund M, Eckly A, Vial C, Ohlmann P et al. Defective platelet aggregation and increased resistance to thrombosis in purinergic P2Y(1) receptor-null mice. J Clin Invest 1999;104: 1731–1737.
74. Hollopeter G, Jantzen HM, Vincent D, Li G, England L, Ramakrishnan V et al. Identification of the platelet ADP receptor targeted by antithrombotic drugs. Nature 2001;409:202–207.
75. Foster CJ, Prosser DM, Agans JM, Zhai Y, Smith MD, Lachowicz JE et al. Molecular identification and characterization of the platelet ADP receptor targeted by thienopyridine antithrombotic drugs. J Clin Invest 2001;107:1591–1598.
76. Rolf MG, Brearley CA, Mahaut-Smith MP. Platelet shape change evoked by selective activation of P2X1 purinoceptors with alpha, beta-methylene ATP. Thromb Haemost 2001;85:303–308
77. MacKenzie AB, Mahaut-Smith MP, Sage SO. Activation of receptor-operated cation channels via P2X1 not P2T purinoceptors in human platelets. J Biol Chem 1996;271:2879–2881.
78. Solet DJ, Zacharski LR, Plehn JF. The role of adenosine 5'-diphosphate receptor blockade in patients with cardiovascular disease. Am J Med 2001;111:45–53.
79. Helft G, Osende JI, Worthley SG, Zaman AG, Rodriguez OJ, Lev EI et al. Acute antithrombotic effect of a front-loaded regimen of clopidogrel in patients with atherosclerosis on aspirin. Arterioscler Thromb Vasc Biol 2000;20:2316–2321.
80. Muller I, Seyfarth M, Rudiger S, Wolf B, Pogatsa-Murray G, Schomig A et al. Effect of a high loading dose of clopidogrel on platelet function in patients undergoing coronary stent placement. Heart 2001;85:92–93.
81. Cadroy Y, Bossavy JP, Thalamas C, Sagnard L, Sakariassen K, Boneu B. Early potent antithrombotic effect with combined aspirin and a loading dose of clopidogrel on experimental arterial thrombogenesis in humans. Circulation 2000;101:2823–2828.
82. Bhatt DL, Chew DP, Hirsch AT, Ringleb PA, Hacke W, Topol EJ. Superiority of clopidogrel versus aspirin in patients with prior cardiac surgery. Circulation 2001;103:363–368.
83. Balsano F, Rizzon P, Violi F, Scrutinio D, Cimminiello C, Aguglia F et al. Antiplatelet treatment with ticlopidine in unstable angina. A controlled multicenter clinical trial. The Studio della Ticlopidina nell'Angina Instabile Group. Circulation 1990;82:17–26.
84. Yusuf S, Zhao F, Mehta SR, Chrolavicius S, Tognoni G, Fox KK. Effects of clopidogrel in addition to aspirin in patients with acute coronary syndromes without ST-segment elevation. N Engl J Med 2001; 345:494–502.
85. Mehta SR, Yusuf S, Peters RJ, Bertrand ME, Lewis BS, Natarajan MK et al. Effects of pretreatment with clopidogrel and aspirin followed by long-term therapy in patients undergoing percutaneous coronary intervention: the PCI-CURE study. Lancet 2001;358:527–533.
86. Stables RH. Clopidogrel in invasive management of non-ST-elevation ACS. Lancet 2001;358: 520–521.
87. Bennett CL, Connors JM, Carwile JM, Moake JL, Bell WR, Tarantolo SR et al. Thrombotic thrombocytopenic purpura associated with clopidogrel. N Engl J Med 2000;342:1773–1777.
88. Berger PB. Clopidogrel instead of ticlopidine after coronary stent placement: is the switch justified? Am Heart J 2000;140:354–358.
89. Swarup V, Oh C, Richard EN. Risk of post-operative hemorrhage associated with ticlopidine or clopidogrel use prior to coronary artetry bypass grafting. Circulation 102(II), 648A. 2000. Ref Type: Abstract
90. Hongo R, Ley J, Yee R. Impact of preoperative clopidogrel in coronary artery bypass grafting. Circulation 102(II). 2000. Ref Type: Abstract

91. Jeffrey Lefkovits EJT. Intravenous Glycoprotein IIb/IIIa Receptor Inhibitor Agents in Ischemic Heart Disease. In: Eric J.Topol, editor. Acute Coronary Syndromes. New York: Marcel Dekker, 2001, pp. 419–451.

92. Coller BS. Anti-GPIIb/IIIa drugs: current strategies and future directions. Thromb Haemost 2001;86: 427–443.

93. Nurden P, Poujol C, Durrieu-Jais C, Winckler J, Combrie R, Macchi L et al. Labeling of the internal pool of GP IIb-IIIa in platelets by c7E3 Fab fragments (abciximab): flow and endocytic mechanisms contribute to the transport. Blood 1999;93:1622–1633.

94. Schneider DJ, Taatjes DJ, Sobel BE. Paradoxical inhibition of fibrinogen binding and potentiation of alpha-granule release by specific types of inhibitors of glycoprotein IIb- IIIa. Cardiovasc Res 2000;45: 437–446.

95. Scarborough RM, Naughton MA, Teng W, Rose JW, Phillips DR, Nannizzi L et al. Design of potent and specific integrin antagonists. Peptide antagonists with high specificity for glycoprotein IIb-IIIa. J Biol Chem 1993;268:1066–1073.

96. Barrett JS, Murphy G, Peerlinck K, De L, I, Gould RJ, Panebianco D et al. Pharmacokinetics and pharmacodynamics of MK-383, a selective non- peptide platelet glycoprotein-IIb/IIIa receptor antagonist, in healthy men. Clin Pharmacol Ther 1994;56:377–388.

97. Inhibition of platelet glycoprotein IIb/IIIa with eptifibatide in patients with acute coronary syndromes. The PURSUIT Trial Investigators. Platelet Glycoprotein IIb/IIIa in Unstable Angina. Receptor Suppression Using Integrilin Therapy. N Engl J Med 1998;339:436–443.

98. Inhibition of the platelet glycoprotein IIb/IIIa receptor with tirofiban in unstable angina and non-Q-wave myocardial infarction. Platelet Receptor Inhibition in Ischemic Syndrome Management in Patients Limited by Unstable Signs and Symptoms (PRISM-PLUS) Study Investigators. N Engl J Med 1998;338:1488–1497.

99. International, randomized, controlled trial of lamifiban (a platelet glycoprotein IIb/IIIa inhibitor), heparin, or both in unstable angina. The PARAGON Investigators. Platelet IIb/IIIa Antagonism for the Reduction of Acute coronary syndrome events in a Global Organization Network. Circulation 1998; 97:2386–2395.

100. A comparison of aspirin plus tirofiban with aspirin plus heparin for unstable angina. Platelet Receptor Inhibition in Ischemic Syndrome Management (PRISM) Study Investigators. N Engl J Med 1998; 338.1498–1505.

101. Kleiman NS, Califf RM. Results from late-breaking clinical trials sessions at ACCIS 2000 and ACC 2000. American College of Cardiology. J Am Coll Cardiol 2000;36:310 325.

102. Simoons ML. Effect of glycoprotein IIb/IIIa receptor blocker abciximab on outcome in patients with acute coronary syndromes without early coronary revascularisation: the GUSTO IV-ACS randomised trial. Lancet 2001;357:1915–1924.

103. Heeschen C, Hamm CW, Goldmann B, Deu A, Langenbrink L, White HD. Troponin concentrations for stratification of patients with acute coronary syndromes in relation to therapeutic efficacy of tirofiban. PRISM Study Investigators. Platelet Receptor Inhibition in Ischemic Syndrome Management. Lancet 1999;354:1757–1762.

104. Moliterno DJ. Patient-specific dosing of IIb/IIIa antagonists during acute coronary syndromes: rationale and design of the PARAGON B study. The PARAGON B International Steering Committee. Am Heart J 2000;139:563–566.

105. Newby LK, Ohman EM, Christenson RH, Moliterno DJ, Harrington RA, White HD et al. Benefit of glycoprotein IIb/IIIa inhibition in patients with acute coronary syndromes and troponin t-positive status: the paragon-B troponin T substudy. Circulation 2001;103:2891–2896.

106. Randomised placebo-controlled trial of abciximab before and during coronary intervention in refractory unstable angina: the CAPTURE Study. Lancet 1997;349:1429–1435.

107. Hamm CW, Heeschen C, Goldmann B, Vahanian A, Adgey J, Miguel CM et al. Benefit of abciximab in patients with refractory unstable angina in relation to serum troponin T levels. c7E3 Fab Antiplatelet Therapy in Unstable Refractory Angina (CAPTURE) Study Investigators. N Engl J Med 1999;340: 1623–1629.

108. Boersma E, Akkerhuis KM, Theroux P, Califf RM, Topol EJ, Simoons ML. Platelet glycoprotein IIb/IIIa receptor inhibition in non-ST-elevation acute coronary syndromes: early benefit during medical treatment only, with additional protection during percutaneous coronary intervention. Circulation 1999;100:2045–2048.

109. Cannon CP, Weintraub WS, Demopoulos LA, Vicari R, Frey MJ, Lakkis N et al. Comparison of early invasive and conservative strategies in patients with unstable coronary syndromes treated with the glycoprotein IIb/IIIa inhibitor tirofiban. N Engl J Med 2001;344:1879–1887.

110. Use of a monoclonal antibody directed against the platelet glycoprotein IIb/IIIa receptor in high-risk coronary angioplasty. The EPIC Investigation. N Engl J Med 1994;330:956–961.

111. Tcheng JE. Glycoprotein IIb/IIIa receptor inhibitors: putting the EPIC, IMPACT II, RESTORE, and EPILOG trials into perspective. Am J Cardiol 1996;78:35–40.

112. O'Shea JC, Hafley GE, Greenberg S, Hasselblad V, Lorenz TJ, Kitt MM et al. Platelet glycoprotein IIb/IIIa integrin blockade with eptifibatide in coronary stent intervention: the ESPRIT trial: a randomized controlled trial. JAMA 2001;285:2468–2473.

113. Randomised placebo-controlled trial of effect of eptifibatide on complications of percutaneous coronary intervention: IMPACT-II. Integrilin to Minimise Platelet Aggregation and Coronary Thrombosis-II. Lancet 1997;349:1422–1428.

114. Blankenship JC. Bleeding complications of glycoprotein IIb-IIIa receptor inhibitors. Am Heart J 1999; 138(4 Pt 2):287–296.

115. Berkowitz SD, Sane DC, Sigmon KN, Shavender JH, Harrington RA, Tcheng JE et al. Occurrence and clinical significance of thrombocytopenia in a population undergoing high-risk percutaneous coronary revascularization. Evaluation of c7E3 for the Prevention of Ischemic Complications (EPIC) Study Group. J Am Coll Cardiol 1998;32:311–319.

116. Tcheng JE, Kereiakes DJ, Lincoff AM, George BS, Kleiman NS, Sane DC et al. Abciximab readministration: results of the ReoPro Readministration Registry. Circulation 2001;104:870–875.

117. Steinhubl SR, Kottke-Marchant K, Moliterno DJ, Rosenthal ML, Godfrey NK, Coller BS et al. Attainment and maintenance of platelet inhibition through standard dosing of abciximab in diabetic and nondiabetic patients undergoing percutaneous coronary intervention. Circulation 1999;100:1977–1982.

118. Steinhubl SR, Talley JD, Braden GA, Tcheng JE, Casterella PJ, Moliterno DJ et al. Point-of-care measured platelet inhibition correlates with a reduced risk of an adverse cardiac event after percutaneous coronary intervention: results of the GOLD (AU-Assessing Ultegra) multicenter study. Circulation 2001;103:2572–2578.

119. Boersma E, Harrington RA, Moliterno DJ, et al. Platelet glycoprotein IIb/IIIa inhibitors in acute coronary syndromes: a meta-analysis of all major randomised clinical trials. Lancet 2002;359(9302): 189–198.

120. Marso SP, Bhatt DL, Roe MT, Houghtaling PL, Labinaz M, Kleiman NS et al. Enhanced efficacy of eptifibatide administration in patients with acute coronary syndrome requiring in-hospital coronary artery bypass grafting. PURSUIT Investigators. Circulation 2000;102:2952–2958.

18 Thrombolytics and Invasive vs Conservative Strategies in Unstable Angina

Ali Moustapha MD *and*
H. Vernon Anderson MD

CONTENTS

INTRODUCTION

Acute coronary syndromes represent a clinical spectrum that extends all the way from unstable angina presenting with a transient episode of chest pain, to non-ST-elevation myocardial infarction (MI) with more prolonged chest pain and biochemical evidence of MI, to ST-elevation MI with more extensive myocardial damage and formation of Q waves on the surface electrocardiogram (ECG), and finally to sudden cardiac death. Pathophysiologic correlations include minor plaque ulceration and transient thrombus formation in unstable angina, more extensive thrombosis in non-Q wave MI, and complete occlusion in ST-elevation MI and sudden death. Despite initially promising small studies, a large randomized trial showed that thrombolytic therapy is not beneficial and may even be harmful in unstable angina and non-ST-elevation MI. Several trials have compared conservative vs early invasive strategies in unstable angina and non-ST-elevation MI. Results of these trials were conflicting, and most antedated the use of platelet glycoprotein (GP) IIb/IIIa receptor inhibitors and coronary stenting. Risk stratification models, based on simple clinical and laboratory parameters, potentially might allow identification of high risk patients who will benefit the most from an early invasive approach and those with lower risk, in which early conservative management may be more appropriate.

From: *Contemporary Cardiology: Management of Acute Coronary Syndromes, Second Edition*
Edited by: C. P. Cannon © Humana Press Inc., Totowa, NJ

PATHOPHYSIOLOGY OF ACUTE CORONARY SYNDROMES

Plaque rupture with thrombus formation is the primary pathophysiologic mechanism behind acute coronary syndromes *(1–5)*. This process is complex and starts with exposure of subendothelial constituents like collagen, von Willebrand factor, fibronectin, and vitronectin. These elements are recognized by platelet surface receptor glycoprotein Ib and lead to platelet activation and adhesion to the vessel wall. Activated platelets release from their α-granules substances such as thromboxane A_2, thrombin, adenosine diphosphate, and serotonin. These are vasoconstrictor substances, and they cause a physiological obstruction superimposed on the mechanical disruption. More important, they lead to further platelet activation and aggregation. The final common pathway of platelet aggregation involves activation of the GP IIb/IIIa surface receptors, which cross-link platelets via fibrinogen bridges. Aggregated platelets facilitate the conversion of prothrombin to thrombin, and this leads to increased thrombin formation, which in turn is a potent agonist for further platelet activation. Finally, the thrombus is stabilized by thrombin-mediated conversion of fibrinogen to fibrin.

Angioscopy studies have confirmed these findings and demonstrated intracoronary thrombus or complex plaques in 90–100% of patients presenting with unstable angina *(6,7)* Angiography studies, on the other hand, are limited by a low sensitivity for detecting intracoronary thrombus and have revealed its presence in only about 30–40% of patients *(8,9)*. Moreover, the demonstration of improved clinical outcomes with the administration of aspirin and heparin has provided indirect evidence that coronary thrombosis plays a central role in acute coronary syndromes *(10,11)*.

THROMBOLYTIC THERAPY FOR ACUTE CORONARY SYNDROMES

Because of the high incidence and detrimental role of intracoronary thrombus in acute coronary syndromes, much attention has been focused on the potential use of thrombolytic agents to improve outcomes. Several randomized trials *(12–25)* were undertaken in the late 1980s and early 1990s to assess the effect of thrombolytic therapy on angiographic and clinical outcomes in patients with unstable angina and non-ST-elevation MI. These studies involved relatively small numbers of patients and used a variety of thrombolytic agents including tissue-type plasminogen activator, streptokinase, or urokinase. The findings of these studies were not consistent, and most, but not all, showed angiographic and clinical benefits (Table 1). Because of their small size and the conflicting results, no definitive conclusions could be reached about the efficacy of thrombolytic therapy in unstable angina and non-ST-elevation MI.

The Thrombolysis in Myocardial Infarction (TIMI) III trial was the first large randomized, placebo-controlled trial that used a 2×2 factorial design to compare tissue-type plasminogen activator and placebo, and conservative vs early invasive strategies in unstable angina and non-ST-elevation MI. A total of 1473 patients presenting within 24 h of ischemic chest discomfort were randomized to either tissue-type plasminogen activator or placebo. All patients received aspirin, intravenous heparin, β-blockers, calcium channel blockers, and nitrates. The angiographic results of a subgroup were published in the TIMI IIIA analysis *(26)*; among 306 patients who underwent angiography at baseline and at 18–48 h, treatment with tissue-type plasminogen activator did not influence either improvement in the caliber of the culprit lesion (by ≥10% reduction) or improve-

Table 1
**Small Randomized Trials of Thrombolytic Therapy Compared to Placebo
in Acute Coronary Syndromes**

Trial (reference	Year	N	Thrombolytic agent	Results
Neri Serneri et al. *(12)*	1990	97	tPA	Mild reduction in angina within 24 h only.
Ardissino et al. *(13)*	1990	24	tPA	Reduction in recurrent ischemia.
Chaudhary et al. *(14)*	1992	50	tPA	Reduction in recurrent ischemia and revascularization.
Gold et al. *(15)*	1987	24	tPA	Reduction in angina.
Romeo et al. *(16)*	1995	67	tPA	Reduction in recurrent ischemia and acute MI.
Topol et al. *(17)*	1988	40	tPA	Reduction in need for PTCA.
Williams et al. *(18)*	1990	67	tPA	Mild improvement in coronary stenosis.
Freeman et al. *(19)*	1992	70	tPA	Reduction in coronary thrombi but not on clinical events.
van den Brand et al. *(20)*	1991	36	tPA	No effect.
Saran et al. *(21)*	1990	48	SK	Reduction in recurrent ischemia, acute MI, and mortality.
Chatterjee et al. *(22)*	1993	100	SK	Reduction in recurrent ischemia, acute MI, and revascularization.
White et al. *(23)*	1995	112	SK	No effect.
Schreiber et al. *(24)*	1989	25	UK	Reduction in early progression of ischemia and MI.
Sansa et al. *(25)*	1991	43	UK	No effect.

tPA, tissue-type plasminogen activator; SK, streptokinase; UK, urokinase; MI, myocardial infarction; PTCA, percutaneous transluminal coronary angioplasty.

ment in flow by at least two TIMI flow grades. However, in patients with angiographically documented thrombus, and in those with non-ST-elevation MI, treatment with tissue-type plasminogen activator appeared to improve the angiographic end points.

The 6-wk *(27)* and 1-yr *(28)* clinical outcomes of the entire cohort were reported in the TIMI IIIB study. At 6 wk, patients had worse outcomes if they had received tissue-type plasminogen activator, with a combined incidence of death and MI of 8.2 vs 6.2% for placebo ($p = 0.05$). At 1 yr, the incidence of death and MI was similar in both groups (12.4 vs 10.6%, $p - 0.24$) (Fig. 1). Subgroup analysis of patients with true unstable angina demonstrated an excess of death or MI at 6 wk with tissue-type plasminogen activator, while in patients with non-ST-elevation MI at entry, no differences were seen between tissue-type plasminogen activator and placebo at both 6 wk and 1 yr.

The role of adjunctive intracoronary thrombolytic therapy with angioplasty in unstable angina and non-ST-elevation MI was studied in the Thrombolysis and Angioplasty in Unstable Angina (TAUSA) trial *(29,30)*. Similar to the TIMI III trial, treatment with the thrombolytic agent urokinase increased the incidence of acute closure and the combined end point of recurrent ischemia, infarction, or emergency coronary artery bypass grafting (CABG) (Table 2).

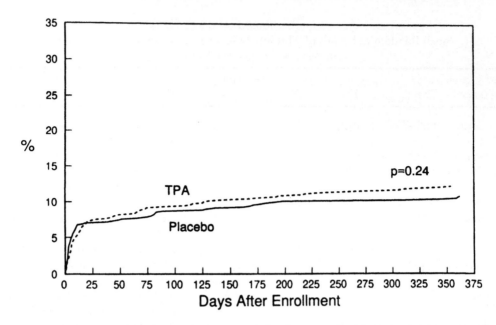

Fig. 1. Cumulative rates of death or MI in the tPA and placebo groups in TIMI IIIB trial. Reproduced with permission from Anderson et al. One year results of the thrombolysis in myocardial infarction (TIMI) IIIB clinical trial. J Am Coll Cardiol 1995;26:1643–1650. tPA, tissue-type plasminogen activator.

Table 2
Clinical End Points in the TAUSA Trial Demonstrating Worse Clinical Outcome with the Use of Intracoronary Urokinase in Conjunction with Angioplasty in Patients with Unstable Angina[a]

End point	Urokinase [No. (%)]	Placebo [No. (%)]	p value
Recurrent ischemia	23 (9.9)	8 (3.4)	0.005
(Re)infarction	6 (2.6)	5 (2.1)	NS
CABG	12 (5.2)	5 (2.1)	0.09
Recurrent ischemia, MI, or CABG	30 (12.9)	15 (6.3)	0.018

[a]CABG, coronary artery bypass grafting; MI, myocardial infarction.

In conclusion, both the TIMI III and TAUSA trials showed that intravenous thrombolytic therapy, alone or when given prior to angioplasty, is not beneficial and may even be harmful in patients with unstable angina or non-Q wave MI. It is unclear why, despite the central role of intracoronary thrombus, thrombolytic therapy is beneficial in acute ST-elevation MI but not in unstable angina or non-ST-elevation MI. Some studies have suggested that thrombi associated with unstable angina and non-ST-elevation MI are usually platelet rich, contain little thrombin, and are therefore resistant to thrombolytic effects *(7)*. Patients with ST-elevation MI, on the other hand, have more mature erythrocyte-rich thrombi containing abundant thrombin, which are more susceptible to lysis by thrombolytic agents *(31)*. In addition, it is well established that thrombolytic agents do exert a paradoxical platelet-activating effect, which might potentially exacerbate thrombus formation and lead to a worse prognosis in patients with unstable angina and non-ST-elevation MI.

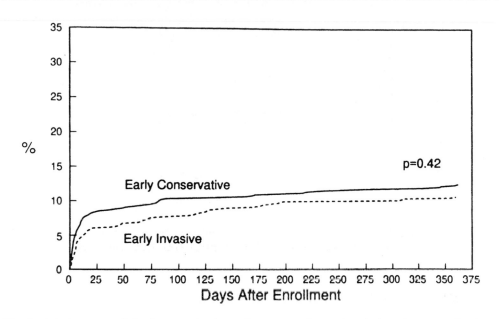

Fig. 2. Relative rates of death or MI in the early conservative and early invasive strategies in TIMI IIIB trial. Reproduced with permission from Anderson et al. One year results of the thrombolysis in myocardial infarction (TIMI) IIIB clinical trial. J Am Coll Cardiol 1995,26.1643–1650.

if they had postinfarct angina, $\geq$2 mm ST depression on exercise stress test, and $\geq$2 distribution area defects or increased lung uptake on thallium stress test. All patients received aspirin and diltiazem. Nitrates, angiotensin-converting enzymes (ACEs) inhibitors, β-blockers, heparin and thrombolytics were permitted.

After a mean follow-up of 23 mo, 96% of patients in the invasive arm and 48% in the conservative arm had undergone coronary angiography, and 44 and 33% underwent revascularization respectively. A total of 152 primary end point events (26.9% of patients) occurred in the invasive arm compared to 138 events (29.9% of patients) in the conservative arm ($p = 0.35$, Fig. 3). However, during the first yr, there was a significantly higher incidence of both the primary end point and death in the invasive arm (111 vs 85 events, $p = 0.05$ for the primary end point, and 58 vs 36, $p = 0.024$ for death) (Fig. 4). This difference was largely related to excess in-hospital mortality (21 vs 6 patients, $p = 0.007$). Further analysis revealed that 11 of 21 deaths occurred after CABG, and no deaths were reported after angioplasty.

Important limitations of this trial include marked delays in angiography (2 d) and revascularization (8 d) in the invasive group. In addition, angioplasty or CABG was performed in only 44% of patients in the invasive group, and the use of angioplasty was actually more frequent in the conservative group (33 vs 22%). Finally, patients included in the VANQWISH trial were labeled as "moderate risk." High-risk patients that would benefit mostly from an early invasive approach, such as those with postinfarct angina, congestive heart failure or persistent left bundle-branch block, were excluded from the study.

Despite those limitations, the investigators of this study concluded that patients with non-Q wave MI do not benefit from routine, early invasive management consisting of coronary angiography and revascularization, and that a conservative, ischemia-guided initial approach is both safe and effective.

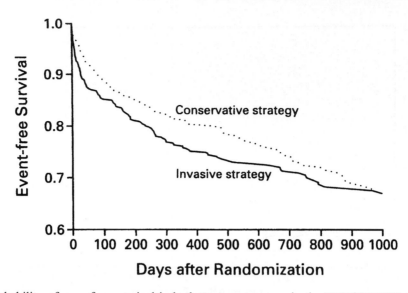

Fig. 3. Probability of even-free survival in both treatment groups in the VANQWUISH trial during 12–44 mo of follow-up. Reproduced with permission from Boden et al. Outcomes in patients with acute non-Q-wave myocardial infarction randomly assigned to an invasive as compared with a conservative management strategy. Veterans Affairs Non-Q-Wave Infarction Strategies in Hospital (VANQWISH) trial investigators. N Engl J Med 1998;338:1785–1792.

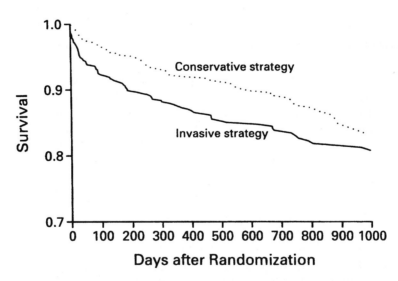

Fig. 4. Probability of survival in both treatment groups in the VANQWUISH trial during 12–44 mo of follow-up. Reproduced with permission from Boden et al. Outcomes in patients with acute non-Q-wave myocardial infarction randomly assigned to an invasive as compared with a conservative management strategy. Veterans Affairs Non-Q-Wave Infarction Strategies in Hospital (VANQWISH) trial investigators. N Engl J Med 1998;338:1785–1792.

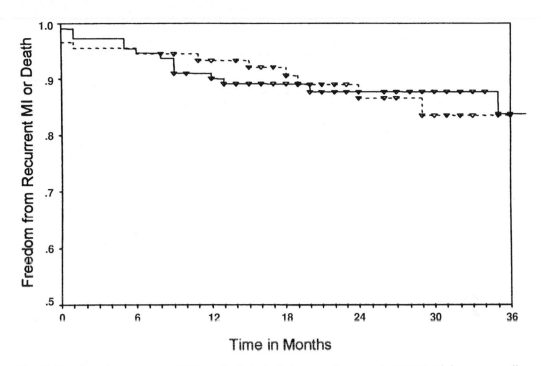

Fig. 5. Freedom from recurrent MI or death in both treatment groups in MATE trial over a median follow-up of 21 mo. Reproduced with permission from McCullough et al. A prospective randomized trial of triage angiography in acute coronary syndromes ineligible for thrombolytic therapy. Results of the medicine versus angiography in thrombolytic exclusion trial (MATE) trial. J Am Coll Cardiol 1998;32:596–605.

MATE Trial

This small randomized trial *(36)* evaluated the outcomes of 201 patients with acute coronary syndromes ineligible for thrombolytic therapy. Patients were randomized to early triage angiography and subsequent therapies based on the angiogram vs conventional medical therapy consisting of aspirin, intravenous heparin, nitroglycerin, β-blockers, and analgesics. Sixty-four patients (58%) in the triage angiography group and 33 patients (37%) in the medical group received revascularization ($p = 0.004$). At hospital discharge, the primary end point of recurrent ischemic events or death occurred in 14 patients (13%) in the triage angiography vs 31 patients (34%) in the conservative group (45% risk reduction, 95% confidence interval [CI]: 27–59%, $p = 0.0002$). Long-term follow-up at a median of 21 mo revealed, however, no significant differences in the end points of late revascularization, recurrent MI or all-cause mortality (Fig. 5).

FRISC II Trial

The FRISC II trial *(37,38)* was the first trial comparing early invasive and early conservative strategies in the stenting era. This was a large randomized placebo-controlled trial that used a 2 × 2 factorial design to compare dalteparin vs placebo, and early conservative vs early invasive strategy in patients with unstable angina and non-ST-elevation MI. A total of 2457 patients (median age = 66 yr, 70% men) were recruited. All of them received aspirin, β-blockers, nitrates, and dalteparin for 5 d. Thereafter, patients were ran-

Table 4
End Points after 12 mo in Invasive and Non-invasive Groups

	Patients assessed		Patients with endpoint			p
Endpoint	Invasive group	Noninvasive group	Invasive group	Noninvasive group	Risk ratio (95% CI)	
Death and/ or MI	1219	1234	127 (10.4%)*	174 (14.1%)	0.74 (0.60-0.92)	0.005
MI	1219	1234	105 (8.6%)	143 (11.6%)	0.74 (0.59-0.94)	0.015
Death	1222	1234	27 (2.2%)	48 (3.9%)	0.57 (0.36-090)	0.016

MI = myocardial infarction.
*Six (0.5%) of these events occurred before the randomized revascularisation procedure.
Adapted from Wallentin et al. Outcomes at one year after an invasive compared with a non-invasive strategy in unstable coronary artery disease. The FRISC II invasive randomized trial. FRISC II Investigators Fast Revascularization during Instability in Coronary artery disease. Lancet 2000;356–16 (ref. 38)

domized to an invasive approach (coronary angiography within 2–7 d) or to a conservative strategy. In addition, patients were randomized to dalteparin or placebo for 3 mo. After 6 mo, 78% of patients in the invasive arm had undergone revascularization vs 43% in the conservative arm. Of those who underwent percutaneous revascularization, 60% were stented. At 1 yr (Table 4), patients randomized to the invasive arm had lower rates of death (2.2 vs 3.9%, risk ratio 0.57 [95% CI: 0.36–0.90], $p = 0.016$), MI (8.6 vs 11.6%, risk ratio 0.74 [0.59–0.94], $p = 0.015$), death or MI (10.4 vs 14.1%, risk ratio 0.74 [0.60–0.92], $p = 0.005$). They also had less hospital readmission (37 vs 57%, risk ratio 0.67 [0.62–0.72]), and target vessel revascularization (7.5 vs 31%, risk ratio 0.24 [0.20–0.30], $p < 0.01$). In other words, after 1 yr in 100 patients, an invasive strategy saved 1.7 lives, prevented 2.0 nonfatal MIs and 20 readmissions, and provided earlier and better symptom relief at the cost of 15 more patients with CABG and 21 more with PTCA.

In summary, based on the FRISC II trial, the investigators concluded that an early invasive approach should be the preferred strategy in most patients with unstable coronary artery disease who have signs of ischemia on electrocardiography or raised biochemical markers of myocardial damage.

TACTICS-TIMI 18

This trial (39) has the greatest relevance to current practice, since it involved the use of stenting and the GP IIb/IIIa platelet inhibitor tirofiban. A total of 2220 patients with unstable angina or non-ST-elevation MI were included. All patients had one of the following: ischemic EKG changes, elevated cardiac markers, or history of coronary artery disease. All patients received aspirin, heparin, and tirofiban. Patients in the invasive arm underwent coronary angiography within 4–48 h (mean of 24 h), and were revascularized if indicated. Patients in the conservative arm underwent cardiac catheterization only with refractory angina, a positive stress test, new MI or rehospitalization for unstable angina, or hemodynamic instability. At 6-mo follow-up, coronary angiography had been performed in 97% of patients in the invasive arm and 51% in the conservative arm. Revascularization had been performed in 61 and 44%, respectively. The primary end point of

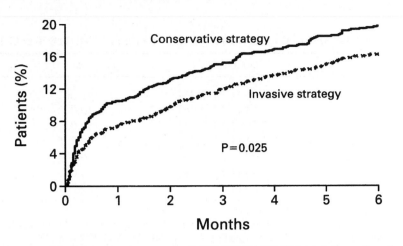

Fig. 6. Outcomes of both treatment groups in the TACTICS-TIMI18 trial. Reproduced with permission from Cannon et al. TACTICS (Treat Angina with Aggrastat and Determine Cost of Therapy with an Invasive or Conservative Strategy). Thrombolysis in Myocardial Infarction 18 Investigators. Comparison of early invasive and conservative strategies in patients with unstable coronary syndromes treated with the glycoprotein IIb/IIIa inhibitor tirofiban. N Engl J Med 2001;344:1879–1887.

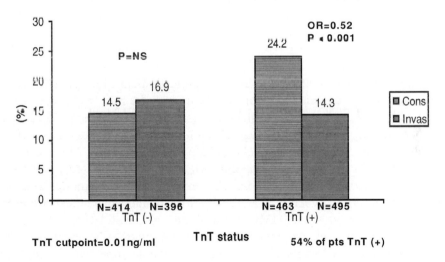

Fig. 7. Outcomes of invasive and conservative strategies in TACTICS-TIMI 18 according to troponin T level.

death, MI, or rehospitalization for acute coronary syndrome occurred significantly less often in the invasive arm (15.9 vs 19.4%, $p = 0.025$) (Fig. 6). In addition, death or MI alone was also significantly reduced by an invasive strategy (7.3 vs 9.5%, $p < 0.05$). One important finding of TACTICS-TIMI 18 is the verification of the "troponin hypothesis", whereby patients with elevated baseline troponin T levels achieved the greatest benefit from an early invasive strategy (14.3 vs 24.2%, $p < 0.001$) (Fig. 7). Thus, in the current era of GP IIb/IIIa inhibitors and stents, it appears that an invasive strategy is beneficial in patients with unstable angina or non-ST-elevation MI. The greatest benefit seems to be achieved in high risk patients with elevated troponin T levels and ischemic ECG changes.

Table 5
Independent Predictors of Cardiac Adverse Events at 14 d in TIMI 11B Test Cohort

Risk factor	OR [95% CI]	p
Age ≥65 yr	1.75 [1.35–2.25]	<0.001
≥3 CAD risk factors	1.54 [1.16–2.06]	0.003
Prior stenosis >50%	1.70 [1.30–2.21]	<0.001
ST deviation	1.51 [1.13–2.02]	0.005
≥2 anginal events <24 h	1.53 [1.20–1.96]	0.001
ASA in last 7 d	1.74 [1.17–2.59]	0.006
Elevated cardiac markers	1.56 [1.21–1.99]	<0.001

CAD, coronary artery disease; ASA, aspirin.
Adapted from Antman et al. The TIMI risk score for unstable angina/non-ST elevation MI: a method for prognostication and therapeutic decision making. JAMA 2000;284:835–842 (ref. 46).

RISK STRATIFICATION IN ACUTE CORONARY SYNDROMES

A possible explanation of the conflicting results in the above trials is the fact that patients with unstable angina and non-ST-elevation wave MI present with a wide spectrum of clinical risk for death and cardiac ischemic events. Ideally, one ought to be able to identify high risk patients who might benefit mostly from an aggressive invasive approach, and those with lower risk where conservative management might be more appropriate.

Several analyses have been performed attempting to identify prognostic risk factors in patients with unstable angina and non-ST-elevation wave MI. Traditional risk factors associated with worse outcomes have included increased age, accelerated or rest angina, associated pulmonary edema, mitral regurgitation murmur or S3 sound, ischemic ECG changes, elevated creatinine kinase levels, and a positive stress test. More recently identified risk factors include elevated troponin (40–42), fibrinogen (43), and C-reactive protein levels (44,45). The most comprehensive risk assessment model to date is the TIMI risk score proposed by Antman at al. (46). In that analysis, the test cohort was the unfractionated heparin group in TIMI 11B trial and the 3 validation cohorts were the unfractionated heparin group from the Efficacy and Safety of Subcutaneous Enoxaparin in Non-Q Wave Coronary Events (ESSENCE) trial and both enoxaparin groups from the TIMI 11B and ESSENCE trials. The TIMI risk score was derived by selection of independent prognostic factors using multivariate logistic regression, and the numbers of factors present were added to categorize patients into risk strata. The seven TIMI risk score predictor variables were: age ≥65 yr, ≥3 risk factors for coronary artery disease, prior coronary stenosis >50%, ST-segment deviation on ECG on presentation, ≥2 anginal events in less than 24 h, use of aspirin in prior 7 d, and elevated serum markers (Table 5). Events rates increased significantly as the TIMI risk score increased, and ranged from 4.7%, when none or one risk factor is present, to 40.9%, when 6 or 7 risk factors are present (Fig. 8). The prognostic value of this model was confirmed in the unfractionated heparin group from the ESSENCE trial, both enoxaparin groups from the TIMI 11B and ESSENCE trials, and the Platelet Receptor Inhibition in Ischemic Syndrome Management in Patients Limited by Unstable Signs and Symptoms (PRISM-PLUS) and TACTICS-TIMI 18 trials (Figs. 9a,b).

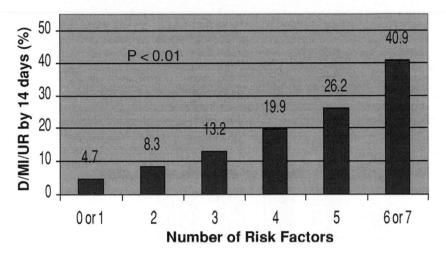

Fig. 8. Risk of cardiac adverse events at 14 d in relation to number of TIMI risk factors. Reproduced with permission from Antman et al. The TIMI risk score for unstable angina/non-ST elevation MI: a method for prognostication and therapeutic decision making. JAMA 2000;284:835–842.

Having established those risk factors, investigators have attempted to identify those patients who would fail medical therapy, or conversely, those who would benefit most from an early invasive approach. Stone et al. *(47)* studied the 733 patients enrolled in the conservative arm in the TIMI IIIB database and found that baseline characteristics predictive of failure of medical therapy included rest angina with ST-segment depression, prior treatment with aspirin or heparin, history of prior angina, older age, and family history of premature coronary artery disease. The incidence of developing a clinical event ranged from 8% if none of the risk factors were present, to 63% if all are present. Using the TIMI risk score model in the TACTICS-TIMI 18 trial (Fig. 9b), an invasive approach was most beneficial when the TIMI risk score was 5–7 (OR = 0.55, 95% CI: 0.33–0.91). When the TIMI risk score is 0–2, on the other hand, early invasive or conservative approaches were similar.

Based on these studies, it seems that patients with unstable angina or non-ST-elevation MI who are at higher risk are likely to benefit the most from an early invasive approach. In lower risk patients, both approaches yield similar outcomes but a conservative approach might be more cost-effective. Further studies will help clarify these points.

CONCLUSION

Plaque rupture with subsequent thrombus formation is the central mechanism behind acute coronary syndromes. Clinical manifestations depend mainly on the extent of thrombosis and degree of coronary flow obstruction. In unstable angina, only minor plaque ulceration and transient thrombus formation occur, while more extensive thrombosis happens in non-ST-elevation MI and sudden death. Despite initial promising results, a large randomized trial showed that thrombolytic therapy is not beneficial, and may even be harmful in unstable angina and non-ST-elevation MI. Possible explanations include the predominance of platelet-rich rather than fibrin-rich thrombi, and paradoxical activation of platelet by thrombolytics. Initial trials comparing early invasive and conservative strategies in the management of acute coronary syndromes yielded conflicting

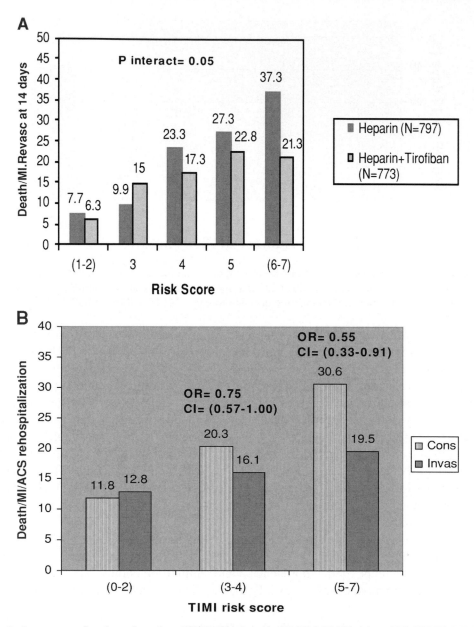

Fig. 9. Outcomes of patients based on TIMI risk score in PRISM PLUS **(a)** and TACTICS-TIMI 18 **(b)** trials.

results. In the modern era of stenting and glycoprotein IIb/IIIa receptor blockers, an early invasive strategy seems to be more effective, especially in high-risk patients. Low risk patients may benefit more from a conservative strategy.

REFERENCES

1. Constantinides P. Plaque fissuring in human coronary thrombosis. J Atheroscler Res 1966;6:1–6.
2. Davies MJ, Thomas AC. Plaque fissuring-the cause of acute myocardial infarction, sudden cardiac death, and crescendo angina. Br Heart J 1985;53:363–373.

3. Falk E. Plaque rupture with severe pre-existing stenosis precipitating coronary thrombosis. Characteristics of coronary atherosclerotic plaques underlying fatal occlusive thrombi. Br Heart J 1983;50: 127–134.

4. Fuster V, Badimon L, Badimon JJ, Chesebro JH. The pathogenesis of coronary artery disease and the acute coronary syndromes. N Engl J Med 1992;326:242–250.

5. Libby P. Molecular bases of the acute coronary syndromes. Circulation 1995;91:2844–2850.

6. Sherman CT, Litvack F, Grundfest W, et al. Coronary angioscopy in patients with unstable angina pectoris. N Engl J Med 1986;315:913–919.

7. Mizuno K, Satomura K, Miyamoto A, et al. Angioscopic evaluation of coronary-artery thrombi in acute coronary syndromes. N Engl J Med 1992;326:287–291.

8. Capone G, Wolfe NM, Meyer B, Meister SG. Frequency of intracoronary filling defects by angiography in angina pectoris at rest. Am J Cardiol 1985;56:403–406.

9. Vetrovec GW, Cowley MJ, Overton H, Richardson DW. Intracoronary thrombus in syndromes of unstable myocardial ischemia. Am Heart J 1981;102:1202–1208.

10. Theroux P, Ouimet II, McCans J, et al. Aspirin, heparin, or both to treat acute unstable angina. N Engl J Med 1988;319:1105–1111.

11. Cairns JA, Gent M, Singer J, et al. Aspirin, sulfinpyrazone, or both in unstable angina. Results of a Canadian multicenter trial. N Engl J Med 1985;313:1369–1375.

12. Neri Serneri GC, Gensini GF, Poggesi L, et al. Effect of heparin, aspirin, or alteplase in reduction of myocardial ischaemia in refractory unstable angina. Lancet 1990;335:615–618.

13. Ardissino D, Barberis P, De Servi S, et al. Recombinant tissue-type plasminogen activator followed by heparin compared with heparin alone for refractory unstable angina pectoris. Am J Cardiol 1990;66: 910–914.

14. Chaudhary II, Crozier I, Hamer A, Foy S, Shirlaw T, Ikram H. Tissue plasminogen activator using a rapid-infusion low-dose regimen for unstable angina. Am J Cardiol 1992;69:173–175.

15. Gold HK, Johns JA, Leinbach RC, et al. A randomized, blinded, placebo-controlled trial of recombinant human tissue-type plasminogen activator in patients with unstable angina pectoris. Circulation 1987;75:1192–1199.

16. Romeo F, Rosano GM, Martuscelli E, et al. Effectiveness of prolonged low-dose recombinant tissue-type plasminogen activator for refractory unstable angina. J Am Coll Cardiol 1995;25:1295–1299.

17. Topol EJ, Nicklas JM, Kander NH, et al. Coronary revascularization after intravenous tissue plasminogen activator for unstable angina pectoris: results of a randomized, double-blind, placebo-controlled trial. Am J Cardiol 1988;62:368–371.

18. Williams DO, Topol EJ, Califf RM, et al. Intravenous recombinant tissue-type plasminogen activator in patients with unstable angina pectoris. Circulation 1990;82:376–383.

19. Freeman R, Langer A, Wilson RF, Morgan CD, Armstrong PW. Thrombolysis in unstable angina. Circulation 1992;85:150–157.

20. van den Brand M, van Zijl A, Geuskens R, de Feyter J, Serruys PW, Simoons ML. Tissue plasminogen activator in refractory unstable angina. A randomized double-blind placebo-controlled trial in patients with refractory unstable angina and subsequent angioplasty. Eur Heart J 1991;12:1208–1214.

21. Saran RK, Bhandari K, Narain VS, et al. Intravenous streptokinase in the management of a subset of patients with unstable angina: a randomized controlled trial. Int J Cardiol 1990:28:209–213.

22. Chatterjee SS, Bhattacharya R, Das Biswas A, et al. Intravenous thrombolytic therapy in unstable angina. Indian Heart J 1993;45:103–108.

23. White HD, French JK, Norris RM, Williams BF, Hart HH, Cross BC. Effects of streptokinase in patients presenting within 6 hours of prolonged chest pain with ST segment depression. Br Heart J 1995; 73:500–505.

24. Schreiber TL, Macina G, McNulty A, et al. Urokinase plus heparin versus aspirin in unstable angina and non-Q-wave myocardial infarction. Am J Cardiol 1989;64:840–844.

25. Sansa M, Cernigliaro C, Campi A, Simonetti I. Effects of urokinase and heparin on minimal cross-sectional area of the culprit narrowing in unstable angina pectoris. Am J Cardiol 1991;68:451–456.

26. The TIMI IIIA investigators. Early effects of tissue-type plasminogen activator added to conventional therapy on the culprit coronary lesion in patients presenting with ischemic cardiac pain at rest: results of the Thrombolysis in Myocardial Infarction (TIMI IIIA) trial. Circulation 1993;87:38–52.

27. The TIMI IIIB investigators. Effects of tissue plasminogen activator and a comparison of early invasive and conservative strategies in unstable angina and non-Q-wave myocardial infarction: results of the TIMI IIIB trial. Circulation 1994;89:1545–1556.

28. Anderson HV, Cannon CP, Stone PH, et al. One year results of the thrombolysis in myocardial infarction (TIMI) IIIB clinical trial. J Am Coll Cardiol 1995;26:1643–1650.

29. Ambrose JA, Almeida OD, Sharma SK, et al. Adjunctive thrombolytic therapy during angioplasty for ischemic rest angina: results of the TAUSA trial. Circulation 1994;90:69–77.

30. Mehran R, Ambrose JA, Bongu RM, et al. Angioplasty of complex lesions in ischemic rest angina: results of the TAUSA trial. J Am Coll Cardiol 1995;26:961–966.

31. Jang IK, Gold HK, Ziskind AA, et al. Differential sensitivity of erythrocyte-rich and platelet-rich arterial thrombi to lysis with recombinant tissue-type plasminogen activator: a possible explanation for resistance to coronary thrombolysis. Circulation 1989;79:920–928.

32. Zaret BL, Wackers FJ. Nuclear cardiology. N Engl J Med 1993;329:775–783;855–863.

33. Conti RC. Unstable angina: costs of conservative and invasive strategies using TIMI IIIB as a model. Clin Cardiol 1995;8:187–188.

34. Ferry DR, O'Rourke RA, Blaustein AS, et al. Design and baseline characteristics of the Veterans Affairs Non-Q-Wave Infarction Strategies In-Hospital (VANQWISH) trial. VANQWISH trial Research Investigators. J Am Coll Cardiol 1998; 31:312–320.

35. Boden WE, O'Rourke RA, Crawford MH, et al. Outcomes in patients with acute non-Q-wave myocardial infarction randomly assigned to an invasive as compared with a conservative management strategy. Veterans Affairs Non-Q-Wave Infarction Strategies in Hospital (VANQWISH) trial investigators. N Engl J Med 1998;338:1785–1792.

36. McCullough PA, O'Neill WW, Graham M, et al. A prospective randomized trial of triage angiography in acute coronary syndromes ineligible for thrombolytic therapy. Results of the medicine versus angiography in thrombolytic exclusion trial (MATE) trial. J Am Coll Cardiol 1998;32:596–605.

37. FRISC II Investigators. Invasive compared with non-invasive treatment in unstable coronary-artery disease: FRISC II prospective randomized multicentre study. Fragmin and fast Revascularization during Instability in Coronary artery disease investigators. Lancet 1999;354:708–715.

38. Wallentin L, Lagerqvist B, Husted S, Kontny F, Stahle E, Swahn E. Outcomes at one year after an invasive compared with a non-invasive strategy in unstable coronary-artery disease. The FRISC II invasive randomized trial. FRISC II Investigators. Fast Revascularization during Instability in Coronary artery disease. Lancet 2000;356:9–16.

39. Cannon CP, Weintraub WS, Demopoulos LA, et al. TACTICS (Treat Angina with Aggrastat and Determine Cost of Therapy with an Invasive or Conservative Strategy). Thrombolysis in Myocardial Infarction 18 Investigators. Comparison of early invasive and conservative strategies in patients with unstable coronary syndromes treated with the glycoprotein IIb/IIIa inhibitor tirofiban. N Engl J Med 2001;344:1879–1887.

40. Galvani M, Ottani F, Ferrini D, et al. Prognostic influence of elevated values of cardiac troponin I in patients with unstable angina. Circulation 1997; 95:2053–2059.

41. Lindahl B, Andren B, Ohlsson J, Venge P, Wallentin L. Risk stratification in unstable coronary artery disease. Additive value of troponin T determinations and pre-discharge exercise tests. FRISK Study Group. Eur Heart J 1997;18:762–770.

42. Lindahl B, Venge P, Wallentin L. Relation between troponin T and the risk of subsequent cardiac events in unstable coronary artery disease. The FRISC Study Group. Circulation 1996;93:1651–1657.

43. Becker RC, Cannon CP, Bovill EG, et al. Prognostic value of plasma fibrinogen concentration in patients with unstable angina and non-Q-wave myocardial infarction (TIMI IIIB trial). Am J Cardiol 1996;78:142–147.

44. Haverkate F, Thompson SG, Pyke SD, Gallimore JR, Pepys MB. Production of C-reactive protein and risk of coronary events in stable and unstable angina. European Concerted Action on Thrombosis and Disabilities Angina Pectoris Study Group. Lancet 1997;349:462–466.

45. Morrow DA, Rifai N, Antman EM, et al. C-reactive protein is a potent predictor of mortality independently of and in combination with troponin T in acute coronary syndromes A TIMI 11A substudy. Thrombolysis In Myocardial Infarction. J Am Coll Cardiol 1998;31:1460–1465.

46. Antman EM, Cohen M, Bernink PJ, et al. The TIMI risk score for unstable angina/non-ST elevation MI: A method for prognostication and therapeutic decision making. JAMA 2000;284:835-842.

47. Stone PH, Thompson B, Zaret BL, et al. Factors associated with failure of medical therapy in patients with unstable angina and non-Q-wave myocardial infarction. A TIMI IIIB database study. Eur Heart J 1999;20:1084–1093.

19

Current Device Strategies in the Management of Acute Coronary Syndromes

Kanwar P. Singh, MD and
C. Michael Gibson, MS, MD

INTRODUCTION

Early head-to-head trials suggested no advantage of an early invasive approach to an early conservative approach in patients with acute coronary syndromes (ACS) *(1–3)*. In part, the limitations to conventional percutaneous transluminal coronary intervention (PTCA) were due to dissection and attendant abrupt vessel closure, as well as frequent adverse clinical events: 5% incidence of myocardial infarction (MI), 2–3% risk of emergent coronary artery bypass graft (CABG) surgery, and 30–50% rate of late restenosis. Since these early trials, significant advances have been made in the understanding of the underlying pathologic processes that have historically limited PTCA. For example, a great deal of attention has focused on the development of new device strategies that diminish the degree of endothelial trauma and arterial wall inflammation. Major advances in adjuvant medications, including the judicious use of potent antiplatelet (thienopyridines and glycoprotein [Gp] IIb/IIIa antagonists) agents have dramatically decreased the rates of both early and late complications. Technological advances include stents (medicating and coated), directional coronary atherectomy, rotational atherectomy, laser atherectomy, cutting balloons, brachytherapy, and intravascular ultrasound. Together, the advances in medications and technology have greatly improved outcomes and have lead to the re-examination of the conclusion that medical therapy is preferred

From: *Contemporary Cardiology: Management of Acute Coronary Syndromes, Second Edition*
Edited by: C. P. Cannon © Humana Press Inc., Totowa, NJ

(4). The dramatic increase in available techniques has driven interventional cardiologists to take a lesion-specific approach to therapy, and in this context, the term percutaneous coronary intervention (PCI) has been adopted to reflect conventional PTCA and its alternatives. This chapter will summarize: (*i*) current techniques employed in PCI; (*ii*) coronary stents, including the techniques to treat in-stent restenosis; (*iii*) new pharmacologic approaches to ACS; and (*iv*) future directions in device strategies for the management of ACS.

GENERAL MECHANISMS OF ACTION OF NEW DEVICES

The mechanism by which percutaneous devices enlarge obstructed coronary arteries can be classified using two basic categories: dilating devices and tissue removal (atherectomy) devices. Dilating devices expand coronary arteries, displacing the obstructing plaque or thrombus radially to create an expanded arterial lumen diameter. These devices generally use balloon dilation to provide the force for radial displacement. Examples include conventional angioplasty balloons, heated balloons, cutting balloons, and balloon-expandable stents. Atherectomy devices work by removing the obstructing plaque or thrombus, thus expanding the arterial lumen diameter by "debulking" the lesion. Although the predominant mechanism of action with these devices is debulking the lesion, they also dilate the lesion via "Dottering" (i.e., lumen dilation that accompanies the insertion of a rigid body). Atherectomy devices may be further divided into ablative lasers, which remove plaque via tissue vaporization, and the mechanical atherectomy devices. Directional coronary atherectomy and transluminal extraction catheters are examples of devices that collect plaque into an isolated chamber that can be removed from the body. Rotational atherectomy, on the other hand, ablates plaque into debris smaller than red blood corpuscles (2–5 μm in diameter), which ultimately passes through the coronary microcirculation and then is cleared by the reticuloendothelial system.

MEASURING SUCCESS

In order to compare outcomes in PCI across device strategies, it is necessary to use a common vocabulary. Outcomes in percutaneous coronary interventions are categorized in three ways: angiographic success, procedural success, and clinical success. Angiographic success refers to the achievement of a residual stenosis diameter less than 50% in the presence of Thrombolysis in Myocardial Infarction (TIMI) grade 3 flow as defined by the TIMI Trial *(5)*. In the modern era of scaffolding technology such as stents, an additional term, optimal angiographic result, was created to describe the achievement of a postprocedural minimum stenosis diameter of less than 20%. Procedural success requires that angiographic success be coupled to the absence of specific complications during hospitalization (MI, emergent CABG, death). In order to standardize the definition of periprocedural MI, the current American College of Cardiology/American Heart Association (ACC/AHA) Guidelines for Percutaneous Coronary Intervention recommend creatine kinase isoenzyme-cardiac muscle subunit (CK-MB) isoenzyme values threefold higher than the upper limit of normal and do not include the routine use of cardiac troponins or CK *(6)*. Achievement of clinical success requires relief of patients' symptoms, in addition to angiographic and procedural success benchmarks, and is divided into short-term and long-term. Short-term clinical success is achieved if a patient's symptoms are relieved after recovery from the procedure, whereas long-term success requires that relief be durable at 6 mo

CURRENT TECHNIQUES IN PCI

Conventional Angioplasty

Although balloon catheters are used as adjunctive devices in most modern-era interventional therapies, they stand alone in conventional PTCA. The technical design of conventional PTCA equipment has evolved considerably in the last several years. Improvements include more supportive and flexible guiding catheters, more trackable and flexible guide wires, and improved crossing profiles of balloon catheters. These technical improvements have led to a 92% procedural success rate, and less than a 1% rate of periprocedural mortality and emergency CABG *(7)*.

Most luminal improvement following conventional PTCA results from plaque redistribution and overstretching of the vessel rather than plaque compression. Overstretching frequently results in elastic recoil following balloon deflation, often leaving behind a stretched vessel with some residual stenosis *(8)*. Recent studies have shown that larger postprocedural lumen diameters are associated with less restenosis or larger lumens at 6-mo follow-up. This observation has come to be known as "bigger is better" *(9)*. However, this benefit in late outcomes must be carefully weighed against the acute risk of coronary dissection and abrupt closure if oversized balloons are used *(10)*. By reducing and even eliminating elastic recoil, new device strategies such as stenting and directional atherectomy can provide lower postprocedural residual stenoses (0–10%), which are associated with a lower rate of restenosis. Fortunately, achieving a larger lumen diameter with new device strategies does not carry the same risk of dissection and abrupt closure as conventional PTCA.

Laser Angioplasty

Light amplification by stimulated emission of radiation (LASER) angioplasty utilizes highly organized light emitted from optical fibers at the catheter tip to destroy obstructing atherosclerotic tissue. The two types of systems currently available are the excimer laser coronary angioplasty (ELCA), which emits light with wavelength 308 nm, and the holmium yttrium-aluminum-garnet (Ho:YAG), which emits light with wavelength 2100 nm. The specific effects on atherosclerotic tissue (vaporization, direct molecular breakdown, or ejection of debris) depend on the source of energy used. Laser angioplasty requires adjunctive balloon angioplasty to achieve an optimal angiographic result in greater than 90% of cases *(11)*, giving rise to the term "laser-facilitated angioplasty." The New Approaches to Coronary Intervention (NACI) registry of 1000 lesions in 887 patients reported a high procedural success rate (84%) and low rates of death (1.2%), Q wave MI (0.7%), and CABG surgery (4.5%) with ELCA (12). Three randomized controlled trials have been performed using laser angioplasty. In the Laser Angioplasty vs Angioplasty (LAVA) trial *(13)*, 215 patients were randomized to PTCA or laser-facilitated angioplasty. Compared to conventional PTCA, excimer laser-facilitated angioplasty resulted in a more complicated hospital course, including a significantly higher rate of nonfatal MI (4.3 vs 0%, $p = 0.04$) without immediate or long-term clinical benefits. In the Excimer Laser Rotablator and Balloon Angioplasty for the treatment of Complex Lesions (ERBAC) trial *(14)*, 620 patients with complex lesions were randomized to rheolytic, excimer laser-facilitated, or PTCA therapy. In this trial, there was an increased risk for target vessel revascularization in the ELCA group (46 vs 32% for PTCA, $p = 0.013$), though rates of procedural success were similar. Finally, the Amsterdam–Rotterdam (AMRO) trial *(15)* randomized 308 patients with stable coronary artery disease (CAD) and complex lesions with length >10 mm to laser-facilitated or stand-alone balloon angioplasty. Angiographic and procedural success rates were similar, but there was a trend towards an increase in restenosis at 6 mo with laser (51.6 vs 41.3%, $p = 0.13$).

The technique of laser-facilitated angioplasty is primarily used to treat complex lesions (i.e., diffuse, ostial, and vein-graft lesions) not suited for conventional PTCA and stenting, and it is relatively contraindicated with heavily calcified and tortuous vessels. Failure to achieve large residual lumen diameters without adjunctive PTCA is a significant limitation of ELCA. Dissection is the major complication associated with this procedure, although it usually does not result in acute vessel closure, and has been reduced by the use of saline solution flush techniques during the procedure *(16)*. Special training required in laser safety for operators and cardiac catheterization laboratory personnel also limits its use.

Mechanical Atherectomy and Thrombectomy

To overcome some of the limitations previously described for conventional PTCA, coronary atherectomy was developed as a method of excising or ablating atherosclerotic tissue by using directional, rotational, and extractional devices. Thrombectomy can be achieved by the installation of intracoronary thrombolytic or by rheolysis.

DIRECTIONAL CORONARY ATHERECTOMY

Directional coronary atherectomy (DCA) enlarges the stenotic coronary lumen primarily by cutting and extracting the atherosclerotic tissue, and secondarily via the Dottering effect. The catheter is designed with a 9-mm-long cutting window that is open 120° in its cross-sectional dimension. The cutting surface is apposed to atherosclerotic tissue by inflation of a contralateral balloon. Rotation of the catheter at 2500 rpm carves out an arc of tissue, which is then isolated in a storage chamber. Progressive inflation pressures are used to appose the catheter and atheroma, and the catheter's position is serially rotated to face the circumference of lesions.

Whereas initial single-center experiences reported DCA to be a highly effective interventional therapy *(17)*, subsequent randomized-controlled trials of DCA vs conventional PTCA, such as the Coronary Angioplasty Versus Excisional Atherectomy Trial (CAVEAT-I) *(18)*, the Canadian Coronary Atherectomy Trial (CCAT) *(19)* in native coronary lesions, and CAVEAT-II *(20)* in saphenous vein graft lesions, did not show a significant reduction in angiographic restenosis rates for DCA, although there was a trend favoring DCA over conventional PTCA in the CAVEAT-I trial (50 vs 57%, $p = 0.06$) (Table 1). The 1-yr follow-up in CAVEAT-I showed a higher mortality rate in patients treated with DCA than in patients treated with conventional PTCA (2.2 vs 0.6%, $p = 0.035$), however, these results are confounded by noncardiac deaths *(21)*. Because routine balloon postdilation was discouraged in these trials, the postprocedural residual stenosis was $>25\%$, a value similar to that of conventional PTCA. Indeed, a multivariate analysis of CAVEAT-1 angiographic data showed the postprocedural lumen diameter to be the most significant determinant of angiographic restenosis, regardless of the

Table 1
Results from Randomized Trials Comparing PTCA with DCA

OUTCOME	CAVEAT (18) PTCA n = 500	DCA n = 512	C-CAT (168) PTCA n = 136	DCA n = 138	BOAT(23) PTCA n = 492	DCA n = 497	CAVEAT-II (20) PTCA n = 156	DCA n = 149
Angiographic success (%)	80	89[a]	91	98	NR	NR	79.0	89.2[a]
Procedural success (%)	76	82	88	94	87	93[a]	NR	NR
Early complications (%) (death, MI, CABG)	5	11[a]	6	5	3.6	2.0	12.2	20.1
Restenosis (%)	57	50	43	46	39.8	31.4[a]	50.5	45.6
Late complications (%) (death, MI, TLR)	42.4	38.7	29	29	24.8	21.1[b]	44.3	40.3

MI, myocardial infarction; CABG, coronary artery bypass graft; TLR, target lesion revascularization; NR, not reported
[a]$p < 0.05$
[b]death, MI, target vessel revascularization.

device used (22). The high rate of restenosis associated with DCA in these trials was attributed to the 25% residual stenoses that were not treated with routine postdilation following DCA. Thus, the goal of more recent trials has been to perform "optimal" atherectomy, in which case the postprocedure lumen diameter is made as large as possible and the residual stenosis minimized (<10%). Two atherectomy trials, the Balloon vs Optimal Atherectomy Trial (BOAT) (23) and the Optimal Atherectomy Restenosis Study (OARS) (24), tested DCA followed by adjunctive low-pressure balloon dilation. High procedural success rates 97–98% and low rates of major in-hospital complications (death, Q wave MI, CABG surgery) (2.1–3.5%) were achieved in DCA patients with adjunctive PTCA (23,24). In addition, final diameter stenosis was reduced to less than 10% in both trials after adjunctive PTCA. The BOAT study also confirmed a 21% relative reduction in the 6-mo angiographic restenosis rate for DCA with adjunctive PTCA over PTCA alone (31.4 vs 39.8%, $p = 0.01$), thereby confirming that "bigger is better" (23). Because an increased postprocedural lumen diameter is such a significant correlate of reduced restenosis rates, conventional PTCA has become a common adjunct to successful but suboptimal (>10% residual stenosis) DCA procedures when the risk of additional atherectomy cuts seem to be substantial.

DCA has been associated with an increased risk of significant CK-MB leak. However, it is not clear that low levels of myocardial necrosis portend poorer prognoses in this subset of patients (25). Moreover, the use of adjunctive abciximab (a Gp IIb/IIIa antagonist) can reduce the incidence of periprocedural non-Q wave MI by over 50% (26). DCA provides a unique opportunity to essentially "biopsy" the lesion. This has demonstrated that the risk of restenosis following DCA may be influenced by other factors, such as prior cytomegalovirus infection (27). At present, DCA is indicated as an alternative to PTCA in de novo lesions in vessels >3 mm, bifurcation lesions, ostial lesions, and for the treatment of in-stent restenosis (ISR).

ROTATIONAL ATHERECTOMY

Rotational atherectomy (RA) is a treatment technique that utilizes a diamond-studded burr spinning at speeds from 140,000–200,000 rpm to ablate atherosclerotic tissue in coronary arteries. This technique operates under the principle of differential cutting, whereby the less compliant diseased calcified tissue is preferentially abraded in preference to the more compliant nondiseased vascular tissue. The abrasive nature of lesion debulking leads to distal embolization of plaque microparticles, which are approx 2–5 μm in size (i.e., smaller than a red blood cell) and generally pass through microcirculation, and are eventually cleared by the reticuloendothelial system. Occasionally, when these microparticles are liberated to the distal microvasculature in large concentrations, they can cause myocardial ischemia or even infarction. Indeed, the no-reflow phenomenon is more frequent in RA (7.7%) than PTCA procedures (0.3%) *(28)*. As a result of this risk, RA of the right coronary artery is typically done with a temporary pacing wire in place, as A-V block and bradycardia are significant risks of right coronary artery manipulation. To combat the effects of no-reflow during RA procedures, intracoronary vasodilators such as nitrates and calcium channel blockers are routinely administered, therefore adequate vol status must be maintained. Recent evidence demonstrates that slower speeds *(29)* and the use of adjunctive Gp IIb/IIIa antagonists *(30)* decrease platelet activation and aggregation and decreases the risk of no-reflow.

Intravascular ultrasound (IVUS) studies of rotational atherectomy have shown that improvement in lumen diameter is primarily due to selective removal of calcified plaque, with minimal stretching of the vessel *(31)*. Due to the small diameter of available burrs, however, low-pressure adjunctive balloon PTCA is required in most rotational atherectomy cases *(32)*.

In the ERBAC trial *(14)*, rotational atherectomy was compared to conventional PTCA in complex lesions. Rotational atherectomy had a higher procedural success rate (91 vs 80%, $p < 0.001$), a lower residual percent diameter stenosis (31 vs 36%, $p < 0.05$), a similar restenosis rate (62 vs 54%, $p = NS$), but a higher repeat revascularization rate at 6 mo (46 vs 35%, $p = 0.04$) compared to conventional PTCA. A report from a 709 patient multicenter rotational atherectomy registry showed a high rate of procedural success (95%) and low rates of death (0.8%), Q wave MI (0.9%), non-Q wave MI (3.8%), and emergency CABG surgery (1.7%) *(33)*. There was a somewhat lower 6-mo angiographic restenosis rate (38%) in 527 patients available for repeat angiography in this registry compared with that reported in the ERBAC study *(33)*.

A pooled analysis of 5250 patients undergoing rotational atherectomy shows a 93.7% (4920 out of 5250) rate of procedural success, a 0.6% (32 out of 5035) mortality rate, a 1.6% (83 out of 5035) rate of CABG surgery, a 1.4% (72 out of 5035) rate of Q wave MI, and 6.8% (276 out of 4033) rate of non-Q wave MI *(32–42)* (Table 2). The rate of restenosis was 42% (697 out of 1657) at follow-up, a rate similar to that of conventional PTCA. Although there are observational data suggesting clinical benefits from RA in certain lesion subsets, there have been no multicenter randomized trials demonstrating its superiority over conventional PTCA.

Research into optimal rotational atherectomy strategies is ongoing. The Study to Determine Rotablator System and Transluminal Angioplasty Strategy (STRATAS) trial *(43)* was performed to evaluate an "aggressive" strategy ($n = 249$) with burr/artery ratio >0.70 alone or with low-pressure adjunctive balloon ≤1 atmosphere vs the "routine"

Table 2
Pooled Data from Early Studies of Rotational Atherectomy

Study	Patient number	Procedural success (%)	Mortality (%)	CABG (%)	Q wave MI (%)	Non-Q wave MI (%)	Restenosis (% patients)
Dietz 1991	106	73	0.0	1.9	0.0	4.7	42
Barrione 1993	166	95	1.8	0.0	0.6	8.4	—
Gilmore 1993	143	92	0.9	2.8	0.9	2.8	—
Guerin 1993	67	93	0.0	1.6	1.6	6.6	—
Stertzer 1993	346	94	0.0	1.0	2.6	—	37
Ellis 1994	400	90	0.3	0.9	2.2	5.7	—
Safian 1994	116	95	1.0	1.9	4.8	2.9	51
Vandormael 1994	215	91	—	—	—	—	62
Warth 1994	874	95	0.8	1.7	0.9	3.8	38
MacIsaac 1995	2161	95	0.8	2.0	0.7	8.8	—
Stertzer 1995	656	96	0.5	1.4	3.4	—	—
Total experience	5250	93.7% (4920 out of 5250)	0.6% (32 out of 5035)	1.6% (83 out of 5035)	1.4% (72 out of 5035)	6.8% (276 out of 4033)	42% (697 out of 1657)

Procedural success is defined as a residual stenosis <50% with no incidence of death, Q wave MI, or emergency CABG.

All complications (mortality, CABG surgery, Q wave MI, non-Q wave MI) are in hospital.

strategy (n = 248) with burr/artery ratio < or = to 0.70 with balloon inflation ≥4 atmosphere. Initial and 6-mo follow-up clinical and angiographic results were similar, but multivariate analysis showed that left anterior descending location (odds ratio 1.67, p = 0,02) and operator-reported excessive speed decreases of >5000 rpm (odds ratio 1.74, p = 0.01) were independent predictors of restenosis. Similarly, the Coronary Angioplasty versus Rotablator Atherectomy Trial (CARAT) (44) was performed to evaluate whether a lesion-debulking strategy, accomplished with large burr/artery ratios (>0.7) conferred any advantage over a lesion-modifying strategy with smaller burr/artery ratios (<0.7). Angiographic success rates were similar, but larger burr/artery ratios were associated with more frequent serious angiographic complications when compared to smaller burr/artery ratios (12.7% vs 5.1%, p = 0.05).

Rotational atherectomy can be an effective technique in those lesions with angiographic characteristics predictive of low success rates following conventional PTCA. These include calcified lesions, ostial lesions, in-stent restenosis, and possibly total occlusions.

TRANSLUMINAL EXTRACTION CATHETER

Transluminal extraction catheter (TEC) atherectomy enlarges the arterial lumen by cutting, aspirating, and removing thrombus, plaque, and other obstructing debris. In contrast to the discrete tissue fragments retrieved by DCA, TEC results in a slurry of blood and debris. The difficulty associated with treating highly thrombotic native coronary or saphenous vein graft lesions, distal thromboembolism (DTE), and the "no reflow" phenomenon with conventional PTCA prompted the development of the TEC device and the Angiojet rheolytic thrombectomy catheter. The NACI registry has reported on the largest cohort of patients treated with this device. These results show a low device success rate (48%), but an acceptable procedural success rate with adjunctive PTCA (87%) *(45)*. As a result of the small size (≤2.5 mm) of the TEC cutters and a limited ability to aspirate, this procedure is associated with inadequate lumen enlargement when used as a "stand-alone" device *(45)*. Follow-up reports from NACI have demonstrated that the multivariate predictors of DTE with TEC are noncardiac disease, stand-alone TEC, thrombus, and larger vessel size *(46)*. The rate of DTE is 8.3% in this registry of high-risk patients, and it carries a high in-hospital mortality rate (18.5%).

RHEOLYTIC THERAPY

The Angiojet rheolytic thrombectomy system is a novel treatment technique that employs the Bernoulli principle in vacuum-extracting thrombus. The catheter has a stainless-steel tip that houses three jets that propel saline proximally into an effluent port system. The saline rushes past a circumferential opening (0.5 mm in width) in the catheter tip creating a relative vacuum that aspirates blood and thrombus adjacent to the tip into the effluent chamber. As thrombus enters the catheter, it is mechanically broken down by the action of the saline and flushed out of the body. Typically, the catheter is passed multiple times, until no further obstructing thrombus is seen, or no further improvements are made with additional passes.

Pilot studies of the Angiojet were encouraging, with significant reductions in thrombus burden, and high degrees of procedural and clinical success, notably in a relatively high-risk patient population with acute ischemic syndromes *(47)*. Subsequent randomized comparative trials have demonstrated its relative safety and efficacy in comparison to the intracoronary administration of the thrombolytic medications urokinase *(48)*. A recent trial of patients with acute MI demonstrated that the angiographic success was 93.8% with the use of adjunctive measures in 95% of cases (67% stent, 26% balloon alone, 1% RA, 1% DCA) *(49)*. Procedural success was 87.5%, with an in-hospital mortality of 7.1%. Of note, bradycardia occurred in 52% of patients, requiring atropine, temporary pacemaker, or both in up to 31% of cases. The results of this trial are remarkable in light of the nonexclusion of patients with cardiogenic shock. Sixteen percent of patients met clinical criteria for shock at time of enrollment, a factor that has portended a very poor outcome in previous trials of acute MI *(50)*. Thirty-day outcomes were excellent: no further MIs or deaths occurred, and freedom from major adverse cardiac event rate was 92.9%, reflecting the initial mortality of 7.1%.

The present indications for rheolytic thrombectomy therapy are the presence of moderate or severe thrombus in native vessels or saphenous vein grafts larger than 2.0 mm prior to the performance of definitive therapy with stent, PTCA, or other PCI for myocardial ischemia.

IVUS

IVUS is a catheter-based technique that provides cross-sectional tomographic images of coronary vessels from wall to luminal surface. It is generally performed by motorized endoluminal pullback at a rate of 0.5 mm/s. Its greatest utility has been in its contribution to the understanding of the pathophysiologic processes of coronary artery disease in terms of restenosis *(51)*, in-stent restenosis *(52)*, optimal balloon dilation *(53)*, and stent deployment *(54)*. IVUS studies have demonstrated that even optimal angiographic appearance belies potential residual plaque appearance, which can be improved with IVUS-guided angioplasty. IVUS is not routinely recommended, but emerging evidence suggests that it should be used in certain scenarios: (*i*) to document optimal stent deployment in long and complex lesions; (*ii*) determination of nature of in-stent restenosis for therapy optimization; (*iii*) evaluation of coronary obstruction not easily visualized by conventional angiography; (*iv*) assessment of suboptimal result after PCI; and (*v*) management of coronary artery disease after transplantation *(6)*.

CORONARY STENTING

Coronary stents are fenestrated tubes expanded by balloon dilation to scaffold disrupted atherosclerotic tissue within the culprit vessel, maintain the expanded lumen diameter by supporting stretched diseased segments, and minimize contact between blood and thrombogenic subintimal tissue. Stent implantation reduces elastic recoil and medial dissection, both of which contribute to the high rates of abrupt closure and restenosis associated with conventional PTCA *(55–57)*.

Stents differ in composition (metallic or nonmetallic), thickness, architectural design (slotted tube versus coiled wire), and mode of implantation (self-expanding or balloon expandable). To date, almost all stents have been made from either stainless steel or tantalum. Ideally, a stent should consist of nonthrombogenic material, sufficient flexibility for passage through tortuous vessels, great radial strength, minimal metal surface area, and sufficient radiopacity for fluoroscopic visualization. Although it has been difficult to develop a single stent with all of these properties, excellent designs have emerged.

Stenting procedures continue to grow in number, and this is partly due to the impressive early and late angiographic and clinical results achieved to date. The results from stenting are so impressive compared to PTCA that clinicians feel compelled to maximize their use. However, patients included in randomized stent trials were subject to specific inclusion and exclusion criteria, which may not be strictly held in common practice. Interestingly, one study revealed that only 20% of patients who received stents would have met criteria for inclusion into trials that have demonstrated their benefit *(58)*.

De Novo Lesions

Coronary stent implantation was originally assessed in the treatment of focal *de novo* lesions in large native coronary arteries. Early trials such as Belgium and Netherlands Stent Trial (BENESTENT) *(55)* and Stress Restenosis Study Investigation (STRESS) *(56)* measured the safety and efficacy of stents vs PTCA for stable CAD. These trials both demonstrated that stents conferred significant advantages in angiographic restenosis rates, and trends towards decreased target vessel revascularization (TVR), and adverse clinical events (death, MI, CABG, TVR) at 6 mo. The Stents and Radiation Trial (START) trial *(59)* included patients with both stable and unstable angina and demonstrated similar results of decreased restenosis, and though death and MI rates were similar, the effects on restenosis were durable at 4 yr.

Restenotic Lesions

Stent use for restenotic lesions in native vessels previously treated with PTCA was evaluated in the Restenosis Stent Trial (REST) *(60)*. Patients (383) with restenosis were randomized to repeat angioplasty or stent placement. Angiographic follow-up revealed that restenosis was less frequent in the stent group vs the PTCA group (18 vs 32%, $p = 0.03$), as was target lesion revascularization (TLR) (10 vs 27%, $p = 0.001$).

Vein Grafts

Recurrent restenoses of saphenous vein grafts (SVG) are a common occurrence despite good angiographic results with angioplasty. Stent use was tested in focal SVG lesions in the Saphenous Vein Graft De Novo (SAVED) trial *(61)* in an attempt to achieve a decreased rate of recurrent restenosis. Patients (220) with new SVG lesions were randomized to PTCA or stent therapy. Stenting not only achieved better initial angiographic results (92 vs 69% angiographic success rate), but also carried an improved rate of freedom from adverse events (73 vs 58%, $p = 0.03$). Interestingly, there was only a trend towards improvement in restenosis rate associated with stenting vs PTCA (37 vs 46%, p = NS). A separate large, multicenter investigation of 589 patients with SVG lesions experienced a 29.7% restenosis rate at 6 mo, lower than historical controls of PTCA *(62)*.

Chronic Coronary Occlusions

Chronic coronary occlusions are particularly difficult to treat with PTCA in light of the high rate of procedural failure and recurrence. Three randomized controlled trials have investigated the utility of stents in this setting. The Stenting in Chronic Coronary Occlusion (SICCO) trial *(63)* randomized 119 patients with angiographically successful PTCA to adjunctive stent or no further interventional procedure. The stent group had less restenosis at 6-mo angiography compared with the PTCA alone group (34 vs 72%, $p = 0.001$). Long-term follow-up (mean 33 ± 6 mo) demonstrated that the stent group suffered fewer cardiac events (cardiovascular death, lesion-related acute MI, TLR, or angiographic demonstration of recurrent reocclusion) (24 vs 59%, $p = 0.002$) *(64)*. The Groupo Italiano per lo Studio sullo Stent nelle Occlusioni Coronariche (GISSOC) trial *(65)* has a similar design with 110 patients. Angiographic follow-up at 9 mo demonstrated larger mean diameters, less reocclusion, less recurrent ischemia, less TLR, and, notably, less restenosis (32 vs 68%, $p < 0.001$). The Total Occlusion Study of Canada (TOSCA) *(66)* trial randomized 410 patients to PTCA vs PTCA and stent after passing the guidewire (crossover rate 10%). Maintenance of TIMI 3 grade flow (the primary end point) was significantly higher in the stent group (89.1 vs 80.5%, $p = 0.024$). The stent group also had a lower restenosis rate (55 vs 70%, $p < 0.01$), and less TVR (8.4 vs 15.4%, $p = 0.03$).

Other Indications

In addition, there is observational data suggesting benefits of stent deployment in aorto-ostial lesions *(67)*, left main lesions *(68)*, bifurcation lesions *(69)*, residual stenoses, and mild dissections following conventional PTCA.

"Bail-Out" Stenting

Maintaining the patency of severely injured vessels by means of mechanical scaffolding was one of the first roles envisioned for intracoronary stenting. Although techniques such as prolonged balloon inflations *(70)*, directional atherectomy *(71)*, and

Table 3
Results of Large Series Bail-out Stenting Studies

	Schomig (P-S Stent)	Palmaz-Schatz NACI Registry	Gianturco-Roubin Multicenter	Wiktor European Stent Study	Total Experience
Patient number	339	107	518	69	1033
Indication of acute closure (%)	15	19	32	30	25
Angiographic success (%)	96.5	99	92.9	92.6	94.7
Procedural success (%)	87.2	78	87.3	76.6	85.6
Death[a] (%)	1.8	4.9	2.2	2.9	2.4
MI[a] (%)	5.6	17.6	5.5	NR	6.9
CABG[a] (%)	9.1[c]	3.9	7.3	14.5[c]	8.2
Stent thrombosis[a] (%)	7.0	NR	8.7	15.6	8.5
Repeat PTCA[b] (%)	16.1	6.5	8.5	21.0	12.4
Restenosis rate[b] (%)	30	NR	39	27	35

Adapted from ref. 78

Procedural success was defined as angiographic success (stent deployed and <50% residual stenosis) with no inhospital death, MI, or CABG surgery. Procedural success is recorded as the percentage of patients with angiographic success, since not all studies reported the procedural outcome of patients without angiographic success.

[a]All early adverse events were assessed in-hospital except for the Schomig study, which assessed early adverse event within 4 wk.

[b]6-Mo follow-up data.

[a]In 26 patients (8% with successful stent deployment) from the Schomig study, and 5 patients (7.8%) from the Wiktor European Stent study, stenting was performed prior to early nonemergency CABG surgery due to uncertainty regarding subacute thrombosis risk and the extent of myocardium at risk.

NR, not reported.

intracoronary thrombolytic infusion *(72)* were effective at times, MI and/or death were frequent sequelae of acute vessel closure prior to the introduction of coronary stenting. Indeed, the 1985/1986 National Heart Lung and Blood Institute (NHLBI) registry showed that following acute vessel closure, 5% of patients died in hospital, 32% were sent for CABG surgery, and 42% sustained MI *(73)*. Several small, randomized trials have shown stenting to be an effective "bail-out" technique in cases of post-PTCA acute vessel closure, which can be caused by coronary dissection, spasm, or thrombus *(74–76)*. A pooled analysis of "bail-out" stenting in 1033 patients (25% presenting with acute vessel closure) reported a procedural success rate of 85.6%, a mortality rate of 2.4%, an emergency CABG rate of 8.2%, an acute MI rate of 6.9%, and a stent thrombosis rate of 8.5% *(74–78)* (Table 3). Given the apparent benefits from prior historical NHLBI data, a randomized trial testing the efficacy of "bail-out" stenting seems highly unlikely. The frequency of stent use as a "bail-out" technique has declined as primary stenting of "off label" indications has increased. However, it continues to be an accepted back-up measure for those lesions that are best managed initially by PTCA.

Subacute Thrombosis after Coronary Stenting

A major limitation of coronary stenting in early trials was the risk of subacute thrombosis, which occurred in up to 8% of cases, and generally eventuated in MI or death *(55,56,79,80)*. Because subacute thrombosis generally occurs late, at 2–14 d postintervention, it is a more feared complication than abrupt closure immediately following conventional PTCA, which generally occurs while the patient is still in the cardiac catheterization laboratory. Initial efforts involving intensive anticoagulation regimens of aspirin, dipyridamole, dextran, and heparin during stent deployment and warfarin postprocedure, failed to prevent subacute thrombosis and caused significant bleeding complications.

IVUS studies have shown that subacute thrombosis appears to arise primarily at sites of poorly supported plaque. Despite the angiographic appearance of complete stent expansion, it was observed that many stents were inadequately deployed by traditional balloon inflation pressures (6–8 atmospheres) and had poor apposition to the arterial wall *(81)*. Repeat balloon inflations using higher pressures (16–20 atmospheres) were observed to result in larger lumen diameters with complete apposition of the stent struts, thereby reducing subacute thrombosis even in patients not receiving systemic long-term coumarin anticoagulation therapy *(58)*. Although IVUS imaging was initially used regularly to assess adequacy of stent expansion, subsequent reports have suggested that it is not routinely needed if high-pressure balloon inflations are used *(82)*.

In the Intracoronary Stenting and Antithrombotic Regimen (ISAR) trial *(83)*, 517 patients who underwent successful stenting were randomized to antithrombotic therapy with antiplatelet therapy (aspirin + ticlopidine) or anticoagulation therapy (aspirin + phenprocoumon). At 30 d, the antiplatelet group experienced 75% fewer cardiac events, including fewer MIs (1.6 vs 6.2%, $p = 0.02$), and importantly, no bleeding events. Similarly, the Stent Anticoagulation Regimen Study (STARS) *(84)*, a randomized trial evaluating elective Palmaz-Schatz stenting in patients treated with aspirin, aspirin and coumadin, or aspirin and ticlopidine, showed 2.9, 2.4, and 0.6% rates of stent thrombosis, respectively, at 30 d ($p < 0.05$). Thus, inhibition of platelet activation is a more effective way of limiting subacute thrombosis than inhibition of the coagulation cascade. As a result of adjunctive high-pressure balloon inflations and antiplatelet therapy, the rate of subacute thrombosis is now less than 2%. A pooled analysis of 8176 patients from 33 studies evaluating coronary stenting using aspirin and ticlopidine in the absence of acute MI shows a 1.5% rate of subacute thrombosis, a 0.8% mortality rate, a 1.1% rate of MI, and a 0.5% rate of emergency CABG surgery *(53,82–112)* (Table 4). Newer stent designs, such as heparin-coated stents *(113)*, may further reduce rates of subacute thrombosis as a result of coating the thrombogenic metallic surface with antithrombotic agents or biological conduits like veins or biodegradable materials (i.e., either endogenous materials like fibrin or exogenous materials like a polymer). Urgent PCI is the preferred method of treating subacute thrombosis, particularly if a technical problem is discovered upon review of the initial deployment (inadequate coverage of dissection, inadequate expansion, outflow obstruction, etc.), and CABG surgery is usually performed in refractory cases. In the case of unavailability of cardiac catheterization laboratory facilities, or anticipated delays in PCI, intravenous thrombolysis is the accepted alternative *(114)*.

Table 4
Pooled Analysis of Stenting Using Aspirin and Ticlopidine in the Absence of Acute MI

Study	Patient number	Stent	Subacute Sthrombosis (%)	Mortality) (%)	MI (%)	CABG (%)
Jordan 1994 (63)	132	PSS	0	—	—	—
Wong 1994 (64)	28	PSS	0	0	0	0
Colombo 1994 (65)	50	Wiktor	2.2	—	—	—
Elias 1994 (66)	79	Wiktor	1.3	0	0	0
Hall 1994 (67)	44	GRS	0	—	—	—
Aubry 1994 (68)	643	All	2.5	3.7	3.7	1.3
Morice 1995 (69)	1250	All	1.7	0.7	0.6	0.4
Morice 1995 (70)	397	All	1.5	1	0.3	1
Morice 1995 (71)	246	All	1.2	0.4	0	0.8
La Blanche 1995 (72)	98	All	0	2	4	3
Barragan 1995 (59)	208	PSS, GRS	0.5	1	1	0.5
Colombo 1995 (58)	60	GRS	0	1	—	4
Wong 1995(73)	33	PSS	0	0	0	0
Fajadet 1995 (74)	119	PSS	0	0.8	—	—
Blassini 1995 (75)	60	PSS	0	0	0	0
Reifart 1995 (76)	98	GRS	—	1	0	1
Hall 1995 (77)	68	GRS	3	1.5		
Hasse 1995 (78)	46	PSS	0	0	0	0
Goods 1995(79)	152	GRS	0.7	0	0	0.7
Belli 1995 (80)	88	—	0	0	0	0
Morice 1995 (81)	1156	All	1.6	0.3	2.7	0.3
Caravalho 1995 (82)	87	GRS	1.1	0	0	0
Hall 1996 (83)	123	All	0.8	0	0.8	0
Lefevre 1996 (84)	245	All	2	3	1.6	0
Morice 1996 (85)	260	PSS	1.2	—	1.9	0.4
Goods 1996 (86)	296	GRS	0.7	0.3	—	0.7
Marco 1996 (87)	18	GRS-II	0	0	0	0
Elias 1996 (88)	240	Wiktor	3.6	1.2	—	1.2
Elias 1996 (88)	182	Wiktor	1	1	—	0
Schomig 1996 (89)	257	PSS	0.8	0.4	0.8	0
Leon 1996 (61)	244	PSS	0.6	—	—	—
Moussa 1997 (90)	1042	All	1.9	—	—	—
Nakamura 1997 (59)	127	All	3.1	—	3.1	0.8
Total Experience	8176	—	1.5% (n = 121)	0.8% (n = 63)	1.1% (n = 86)	0.5% (n = 38)

GRS, Gianturco-Roubin Stent; PSS, Palmaz-Schatz Stent.
All event rates (mortality, MI, CABG) are in-hospital.

The limitations to antiplatelet therapy with ticlopidine are the frequent occurrence of side effects: gastrointestinal upset (up to 20%); rash (up to 15%); liver enzyme abnormalities (though cholestatic hepatitis is rare), and neutropenia and bone marrow toxicity (1%, reversible). Clopidogrel, a new thienopyridine medication, has been shown to be as effective as ticlopidine, and far better tolerated (114–116). The pharmacokinetics of clopidogrel has been studied; a loading dose of 300 mg, followed by 75 mg daily, results in effective platelet inhibition 4 to 5 d sooner than both without the loading dose and regular 250 mg 2× daily ticlopidine dosing regimens *(115)*.

Primary Stenting in Acute MI

By reducing residual stenoses, relieving intraluminal obstruction and sealing dissection planes created by PTCA, primary stenting may provide additional short- and long-term benefits in acute MI. Despite initial concerns of stent thrombosis in the setting of acute MI, experiences with primary stenting have revealed favorable results thus far. A pooled analysis of 1357 patients from 20 nonrandomized studies of primary stenting shows a mortality rate of 2.4%, a reinfarction rate of 1.1%, an emergency CABG rate of 1.3%, and a stent thrombosis rate of 1.5% (using ticlopidine) of patients *(117)*. In the Stent- Primary Angioplasty in Myocardial Infarction (Stent-PAMI) trial *(118)*, 900 patients who had acute MI (defined as 1 mm ST-segment elevation in two contiguous lead, or if electrocardiogram [ECG] nondiagnostic, objective evidence in the cardiac catheterization laboratory of high-grade stenosis, and wall-motion abnormality), with stentable lesions were randomized to PTCA (15% crossover rate) or Palmaz-Schatz heparin-coated stents. The primary combined end point (death, MI, CVA, TVR at 6 mo) occurred less in the stent group than in the PTCA group (12.6 vs 20.1%, $p < 0.01$), though the difference was entirely accounted for by the decrease in TVR. Stented patients also had less angina (11.3 vs 16.9%, $p = 0,02$), less TVR (7.7 vs 17.0%, $p < 0.001$), and less restenosis (20.3 vs 33.5%) at 6-mo follow-up angiography. There was no difference in mortality rates, except among patients with a closed artery at presentation in which the mortality was higher among stented patients.

Limitations of Coronary Stenting

The preprocedural arterial lumen size remains a major issue in stenting procedures. A meta-analysis of the Benestent-I and STRESS-I/II trials showed that arteries less than 2.6 mm and greater than 3.4 mm in diameter (the smallest and largest quintiles treated) did not have better restenosis rates than arteries treated with conventional PTCA *(119)*. A pooled analysis of quantitative angiographic data from the TIMI 4 and TIMI 10 trials shows that 69% of patients presenting with acute MI had a proximal reference segment diameter (PRSD) > 2.75 mm, and 56% had a PRSD > 3.0 mm *(117)*. Despite recent advances in stenting techniques, the fact that smaller vessels may derive reduced benefits from coronary stenting due to greater risks of subacute thrombosis and intimal hyperplasia remains a significant challenge in coronary stenting.

Another challenge associated with stenting involves the treatment of in-stent restenosis. Although balloon angioplasty is the most common method of treating in-stent restenosis and is associated with a greater than 90% procedural success rate, it has been observed to have a high rate of restenosis (54%) *(120)*. This is perhaps because balloon angioplasty of in-stent restenosis works by compressing and extruding the intimal tissue rather than by expanding the stent.

Although the stenting of highly thrombotic lesions is generally avoided, in a small trial stents were placed in 86 thrombus-containing lesions in patients with ACS. Despite this, there was a low rate of subacute thrombosis (1%) and restenosis (33%) *(121)*. In addition to the risk of subacute thrombosis, other potential limitations of stenting include side branch occlusion, stent embolization, and inadequate access to more distal disease and significant side branches post-stent-implantation, the occasional inability to deliver a stent to the target lesion, and the potential for the wire to become entrapped in stents while recrossing. The impact of stenting on subsequent bypass procedures is unknown.

Many new stent designs currently under investigation include welded tubular stents, integrated flexible-coil stents, interlocking coil-strut stents, self-expanding stents, and radiation-emitting stents. Although it is unlikely that any single design will be suitable for all patients, diversity in composition and structure are likely to offer the interventionalist a wide variety of options in the future.

Restenosis and In-Stent Restenosis

New insights into the pathophysiology of restenosis have emerged concurrently with developments in coronary stenting. Early animal studies suggested that intimal proliferation after arterial injury is the predominant cause of restenosis. As a result, several clinical trials tested the effect of various antiproliferative agents on coronary restenosis. These trials, however, showed no significant beneficial effect in preventing restenosis *(122)*.

The results of several recent studies have challenged the theory that intimal proliferation is the sole or predominant mechanism of restenosis following conventional PTCA. For instance, molecular studies using immunohistochemical labeling of proliferating cell nuclear antigens in human atherectomy specimens, revealed minimal evidence of cellular proliferation in both primary as well as restenotic lesions following conventional PTCA *(123)*. In addition, serial IVUS imaging studies have shown intimal proliferation to be a minor contributor (30%) to late diameter loss and have demonstrated that shrinkage of the dilated segment (measured as a reduction in the cross-sectional area of the vessel subtended by the external elastic lamina) is a major contributor to lumen loss following conventional PTCA *(124)*. With respect to in-stent restenosis, serial IVUS studies have demonstrated that neo-intimal proliferation, through the stent struts, accounts for almost all of the late diameter loss, with almost no evidence of vessel shrinkage or stent collapse *(125)*. Three large randomized trials comparing stenting (using Palmaz-Schatz stents) with conventional PTCA for the treatment of focal *de novo* native vessel lesions including the Benestent-I and Benestent-II *(55,169)* and the STRESS-I *(56)* studies, revealed larger acute lumen diameters and a 25–30% relative reduction in the rate of restenosis after stenting compared with conventional PTCA (Table 5). Thus, coronary stenting is associated with reduced restenosis rates because it maintains expanded lumen diameters and prevents pathologic remodeling.

Although current stenting techniques have reduced restenosis, they have not eliminated it. Recently, much attention has been focused on stent designs with better scaffolding properties that may be able to minimize intimal injury and prevent subsequent restenosis. The rate of restenosis at 6 mo using aspirin (without ticlopidine) with the ACS multilink stent (West European Stent Trial [WEST]-II trial) was lower (10%) than that when using the Palmaz-Schatz stent (Multicenter Ultrasound Stenting in Coronaries trial [MUSIC]) (13%), despite the inclusion of smaller vessels and a greater number of patients with unstable angina in the WEST-II trial *(126)*. Brachytherapy, the use of local radiation, has emerged as a viable option for the prevention of recurrent ISR, and

Table 5
Multicenter Randomized Trials Comparing Conventional PTCA with Stenting

Outcome	STRESS (23)		BENESTENT-I (24)		BENESTENT-II (169)	
	PTCA n = 202	Stent n = 205	PTCA n = 257	Stent n = 259	PTCA n = 410	Stent n = 413
Angiographic success (%)	92.6	99.5[a]	98.1	96.9	99	99
Procedural success (%)	89.6	96.1[a]	92.7	91.1	95	96
Early complications (%) (death, Q-wave MI, CABG)	7.9	5.9	6.2	6.9	5.1	3.9
Late complications (death, Q-wave MI, TVR)	23.8	19.5	30	20[a]	19.3	12.8[a]
Restenosis	42.1	31.6[a]	32	22[a]	31	16[a]
Bleeding complications	4.0	7.3	NR	NR	1.0	1.2

MI, myocardial infarction; CABG, coronary artery bypass graft; NR, not reported.
[a]$p < 0.05$.

trials with medicating stents coated with substances such as paclitaxel and sirolimus are underway.

BRACHYTHERAPY

Brachytherapy prevents restenosis by decreasing intimal hyperplasia and cellular proliferation within treated segments of atherosclerotic coronary arteries. In November 2000, the Food and Drug Administration (FDA) approved two sources of radiation for the prevention of recurrent ISR. The first utilizes γ radiation (photons) emitted from an iridium-192 source; the second utilizes β radiation (electrons) emitted from yttrium-90 or phosphorous-32 sources. Radiation is delivered via a "ribbon", which is temporarily introduced into the coronary artery by a catheter-based delivery. Radioactive stents are presently being studied as an alternative delivery system.

γ Radiation has been studied in three randomized controlled trials (127–129). The protocols of these trials involved recruitment of patients with optimal angiographic results after combinations of PTCA, RA, ELCA, and DCA for ISR, randomization to either adjunctive γ radiation or placebo, and routine post-PCI care with thienopyridines (clopidogrel or ticlopidine) and aspirin. Gp IIb/IIIa inhibitors were contraindicated. The SCRIPPS Coronary Radiation to Inhibit Proliferation Post Stenting (SCRIPPS) trial (127) recruited patients with restenoses of any kind, whereas the Washington Radiation for In-Stent Restenosis Trial (WRIST) (128) and the GAMMA-ONE (129) trials targeted only patients with ISR. GAMMA-ONE was the only multicenter trial. Results from each trial were compelling. Restenosis rates were decreased by 42–68%, and TLR rates were decreased by 43–73%. Important caveats to these results were found, however. Although composite end points including death, MI, TLR, CABG, and thrombosis were improved, the difference was almost entirely accounted for by the decrease in TLR, a variable likely influenced by the protocol-driven follow-up angiography (130). Furthermore, in WRIST, there was an increase in TVR (7.6%) and TLR (9.3%) in mo

6–12 in the treatment group, suggestive of the possibility that radiation delayed the recurrence ISR rather than prevented it. There was also a trend towards the increase in late thrombotic events in the treatment group (9.2 vs 3.5% at 12 mo, p = NS). In GAMMA-ONE, late thromboses were also more common in the irradiated group (5.3 vs 0.7%, p = 0.07). All events occurred in patients who had received new stents at the time of irradiation and had discontinued thienopyridine therapy for more than 1 mo. The conclusion of the authors of the GAMMA-ONE trial was that γ radiation would not be a viable option for the subset of patient who had received a new stent in the context of treatment for ISR, until the issue of late thrombosis was resolved.

Following this study, the Washington Radiation for In-Stent Restenosis Trial plus 6 mo of clopidogrel (WRIST-PLUS) trial treated 120 patients with ISR with intracoronary γ radiation, but extended clopidogrel therapy to 6 mo. Repeat stenting was discouraged but allowed (28.3% received new stents) *(131)*. The primary end point of this study was the occurrence of late thrombosis, as well as the combined end point of death, MI, and TLR at 6 mo. Control groups were historical from the WRIST study. Outcomes for WRIST-PLUS were similar to the placebo arms of the historical controls, and better than the irradiated results of the controls, in terms of late total occlusion and late thrombosis. This important finding indicates that a strategy of reduced new stent placement and long-term clopidogrel therapy effectively removed all of the increased late thrombotic side-effects of γ radiation. Notably, the FDA advises against the use of new stents with γ radiation, but recommends 1 yr of antiplatelet therapy in that context *(132)*.

β Radiation confers several practical advantages over γ radiation: decreased radiation exposure to patient, medical personnel, and environment; decreased procedure time; and obviated need for catheterization laboratory redesign. The Beta Energy Restenosis Trial (BERT) was a pilot trial that treated 21 patients with β radiation from a Sr/Y^{90} source and found no in-hospital or 30-d morbidity or mortality *(133)*. Restenosis rate was lower than expected at 15%, and late loss index was also low. This motivated three random-ized-controlled trials (RCTs): Stents and Radiation Therapy (START) *(134)*; Prolifera-tion Reduction with Vascular Energy Trial (PREVENT) *(135)*; and BETA-WRIST *(136)*. START was the largest of the three, randomizing 476 patients to β radiation or placebo. Stent use was discouraged and only occurred in 21% of cases. Thienopyridine therapy was administered for 90 d. In 8 mo of follow-up, no late thromboses occurred, and restenosis rate was 14% in the treatment group vs 41% in the placebo group. A recent dose-finding study was performed in patients with *de novo* lesions *(137)*. The largest dose given (18 gy) was found to actually increase luminal size on angiographic follow-up, and the overall restenosis rate across doses was 16%. As the authors note, a randomized clinical trial comparing a strategy of stentless PCI plus radiation vs PCI with stent for the prevention of restenosis is needed.

MEDICATED STENTS

Stent-based delivery systems for medication appear to be a viable option for local medication to prevent restenosis *(138)*. Animal models suggested that antimitotic agents might be beneficial in decreasing the proliferative and hyperplastic response to endothe-lial damage *(139)*. At present, only sirolimus (Rapamune)-coated stents have had any human experience in the U.S. Sirolimus' FDA-approved indication is as an immune-modulator to prevent rejection in patients with renal transplants. Mechanistically, it binds to an intracellular protein and up-regulates p27, leading to cell-cycle arrest. It has been shown to inhibit human smooth muscle cell proliferation in vitro *(140)*. In a pilot trial, 30 patients with angina pectoris were randomized to receive fast-release or slow release sirolimus-coated stents, and were studied with IVUS immediately postprocedure and at 4 mo. Patients took daily aspirin and clopidogrel for 60 d. Clinical follow-up was also performed at 8 mo. Angiographic results were impressive: intimal hyperplasia was 10.7% by IVUS *(141)* compared to historic IVUS controls of 19–48%, and there was essentially no late lumen loss or edge-effect. At 8 mo, there were no clinical events (MI, death, TLR, TVR, cerebrovascular accident [CVA], stent thromboses). The effects were seen with both formulations.

Paclitaxel, the antineoplastic agent used in certain malignancies such as breast, has a different mechanism of action. It binds microtubules and polymerizes them, making them unstable, thereby arresting the cell cycle. Elegant animal models have demonstrated that stents eluting paclitaxel are promising in their ability to prevent neointimal hyperplasia and proliferation *(139)*. Their impact on human coronary arteries is yet to be determined.

PHOTOPHORESIS

Photophoresis is an immunomodulatory treatment, in which patients are phlebotomized, and their blood is separated into leukocyte-poor blood, which is returned to the patient, and leukocyte-rich plasma, which is exposed to uv light in the presence of a photo-activated substance such as methoxsalen, which covalently binds DNA, cell surface molecules, and cytoplasmic components in the exposed leukocytes prior to being returned to the patient. Reinfused, the T-cell response is modulated. A small pilot RCT of methoxsalen photophoresis in the prevention of restenosis was recently reported *(142)*. Seventy-eight patients being treated with single-vessel angioplasty were randomized to photophoresis or control. Patients were followed clinically for 6 mo including routine exercise treadmill testing (ETT). Clinical restenosis rates were significantly lower in the treatment group compared to the control group (8 vs 27%, $p = 0.04$).

PHARMACOTHERAPEUTIC STRATEGIES DURING PCI

Combined aspirin and heparin is the most frequently used antiplatelet–antithrombotic therapy during coronary angioplasty to achieve and maintain activated clotting times (ACT) greater than 200 s. Because thrombin is generated during PTCA and potentially activates platelets, direct thrombin inhibitors (hirudin and hirulog) were developed as agents that could potentially inhibit platelet activation.

Despite these theoretical benefits, several multicenter trials have been unable to demonstrate that hirudin is a superior antithrombotic agent compared to heparin *(143–148)*. Although hirudin has greater potential to reduce thrombin activity by inhibiting both fluid-phase and clot-bound thrombin, heparin has greater potential to inhibit earlier steps in the coagulation cascade. The net result may be an equal decrement in thrombus deposition within the culprit vessel. Although not significantly more efficacious than heparin, direct thrombin inhibitors may be safer than heparin.

Whereas there are multiple pathways for platelet activation, a single receptor (the Gp IIb/IIIa receptor) on the platelet surface mediates the final common pathway of platelet aggregation. By preventing the platelet Gp IIb/IIIa receptor from binding fibrinogen to cross-link platelets, Gp IIb/IIIa inhibitors exert potent effects during interventional procedures. There are three approved intravenous Gp IIb/IIIa antagonists presently available for use during PCI: abciximab (Reopro); eptifibatide (Integrilin); and tirofiban (Aggrastat). Each has a distinct biochemical profile, and trials of these drugs have shown varying effects. These medications have been tested in a variety of contexts including unstable angina, non-ST-segment elevation MI, ST-segment elevation MI, and PCI.

Abciximab

Abciximab is the Fab fragment of a human–mouse chimeric antibody directed against the Gp IIb/IIIa receptor. It has a high affinity for the receptor, and has a biological half-life of 8–12 h. It is cleared by the reticuloendothelial system and, therefore, is not affected by renal or hepatic dysfunction. Its activity is reversed by drug discontinuation and platelet transfusion. It is approved for use in primary PCI and refractory unstable angina with planned PCI within 24 h, but not in the routine medical management of patients with ACS.

PCI

Abciximab was evaluated in the Evaluation of Abciximab for the Prevention of Ischemic Complications (EPIC) trial *(149)*, a randomized controlled trial of 2099 patients undergoing high-risk PTCA or directional atherectomy. The results showed a 35% reduction in clinical events (freedom from death, nonfatal MI, and urgent intervention) at 30 d for patients treated with an abciximab bolus and a 12-h infusion (8.3% events) vs placebo (12.8% events) ($p < 0.01$). The reduction of clinical events in the abciximab bolus and infusion group remained evident at 6 mo (23%, $p = 0.001$) and at 3 yr (13%, $p = 0.009$) *(150)*. These long-term results favoring abciximab were largely driven by a reduced need for repeat revascularization, not by death or reinfarction. While it has been claimed that the drug reduced the incidence of "clinical restenosis," the true rate of angiographic restenosis in patients treated with abciximab, however, was not determined in this trial. Major bleeding complications were twice as frequent in the abciximab bolus and infusion group (14%) than in the placebo group (7%, $p = 0.001$) *(149)*. The risk of excessive bleeding with abciximab tended to be greater in patients with higher ACT levels, lower body weights, and higher doses of heparin *(149)*. Given this bleeding risk, lower doses of weight-adjusted heparin were used in the Evaluation in PTCA to Improve Long-Term Outcome with Abciximab Gp IIb/IIIa receptor blockade (EPILOG) trial. This randomized prospective multicenter placebo-controlled trial of 2792 patients undergoing elective PTCA evaluated lower doses of weight-adjusted heparin. The results again revealed favorable outcomes with abciximab, with no significant increase in bleeding complications *(151)*. At 30 d, abciximab again significantly reduced the incidence of the composite end point (acute MI, urgent revascularization, or death) (5.2% in the abciximab and low-dose heparin group vs 11.7% in the placebo and standard-dose heparin group, $p < 0.0001$), but this did not come at the expense of excess bleeding (2.0 vs 3.1% for placebo, $p = NS$) *(151)*. In the c7E3 Fab Antiplatelet Therapy in Unstable Refractory Angina (CAPTURE) trial *(152)*, 1265 patients with refractory unstable angina and a culprit lesion amenable to angioplasty were randomized to abciximab therapy (18–24 h pre-PCI and 1 h post-PCI or placebo. The abciximab group had a 29% reduction in the combined end point of death, MI, TLR in 30 d, though this benefit was not durable at 6 mo.

ACS

In CAPTURE, abciximab was beneficial to patients as pre-PCI therapy. Its role as an initial medical therapy for patients not planned to undergo early PCI for ACS was investigated in the Global Use of Strategies to Open Occluded Arteries (GUSTO) IV-Acute Coronary Syndromes Trial *(153)*. Seven thousand eight hundred patients with ACS were randomized to abciximab bolus plus 24-h infusion, bolus plus 48-h infusion, or placebo, in addition to standard therapy with aspirin and heparins. The primary end point of death or MI at 30 d was not significantly different across groups (8.0 placebo vs 8.2% 24-h infusion vs 9.1% 48-h infusion). Interestingly, this lack of benefit was seen across subgroups, including those with positive cardiac troponins (a group that has seen the most benefit in other Gp IIb/IIIa trials).

ST-Segment Elevation MI

Abciximab was found to reduce combined end points of death, MI, and TVR in by 48% at 30 d in the Reopro in Acute Myocardial Infarction and Primary PTCA Organization and Randomized Trial (RAPPORT) trial *(154)*, in which 483 patients were randomized to abciximab or placebo prior to primary angioplasty for acute MI. Abciximab also reduced that combined end point by 52% at 30 d in the ISAR-2 trial *(155)*, in which 401 patients were randomized to abciximab or placebo prior to primary stenting for acute MI, and by 47% at 30 d in the Abciximab before Direct Angioplasty and Stenting in Myocardial Infarction Regarding Acute and Long-Term Follow-up (ADMIRAL) trial involving 300 randomized patients *(156)*. Abciximab has also been beneficial in small angiographic trials following thrombolytic administration *(157,158)*.

Eptifibatide

Eptifibatide is a cyclic heptapeptide with low affinity and high specificity for Gp IIb/IIIa receptors. It is 50% renally cleared, and therefore, its dose must be altered in patients with renal dysfunction, and it should be avoided in patients with renal failure. Its biological half-life is approx 2.5 h, and its activity is best reversed by discontinuation of infusion. The role of platelet transfusion in reversal is unclear. Its use is approved for use in both ACS and PCI.

PCI

In the Integrilin to Manage Platelet Aggregation to prevent Coronary Thrombosis (IMPACT) II trial of 4010 patients undergoing PTCA, the 30-d clinical event rate (death, acute MI, or repeat PTCA) tended to be lower in patients treated with a low-dose bolus and infusion of eptifibatide than in the placebo group (9.2 vs 11.4%, $p = 0.06$), with no significant increase in bleeding complications *(159)*. The benefits were especially evident in patients undergoing elective procedures. In patients treated with high-dose bolus followed by infusions of eptifibatide, there was no significant reduction in the 30-d clinical event rate. In the recently reported Enhanced Suppression of the Platelet IIb/IIIa Receptor with Integrilin Therapy (ESPRIT) trial *(160)*, eptifibatide was administered in a double-bolus with infusion fashion to prevent the potential dip in platelet inhibition at 10–15 min that had occurred in previous evaluations. Two thousand sixty-four patients who were undergoing scheduled PCI with stents in native arteries were randomized to receive eptifibatide or placebo in addition to standard therapy with aspirin and heparin and post-PCI thienopyridine. The critical findings of this study are that eptifibatide did not significantly decrease any of several categories of angiographic complications, though at 48 h, the relative rate of death or MI was reduced by 43% ($p = 0.0017$). Interestingly, eptifibatide appeared to decrease the relative risk of MI most in patients in whom there were no angiographic complications (relative risk ratio 43%, $p = 0.03$).

ACS

In the large Platelet Glycoprotein IIb/IIIa in Unstable Angina: Receptor Suppression Using Integrilin Therapy (PURSUIT) trial (161), 10,948 patients with ACS were randomized to a 72-h infusion of eptifibatide or placebo in addition to standard therapy with aspirin and heparin. Patients were permitted to go to the cardiac catheterization laboratory at the discretion of the attending physician (11.2%). Overall, eptifibatide therapy was associated with a significant decrease in the composite end point of death or MI at 30 d (14.2 vs 15.7%, $p = 0.04$). This advantage was most apparent in the subgroup that underwent PCI within the first 72 h, but those that did not undergo PCI still had a statistically significant benefit to therapy.

ST-Segment Elevation MI

Eptifibatide has been studied in two trials of ST-segment elevation MI with thrombolytic medications, but it has not been studied in the primary PCI for MI setting. The IMPACT-AMI trial (162) was a dual-phase dose-ranging and RCT combining eptifibatide and alteplase. In the dose-ranging portion, the highest dose of eptifibatide used demonstrated improved patency rates, but the RCT failed to reproduce the benefit. Preliminary results of the Integrilin and Reduced Dose Thrombolytic in Acute Myocardial Infarction (INTRO AMI) trial (163), have reported promising TIMI grade 3 flow rates with decreased dose eptifibatide and alteplase.

Tirofiban

Tirofiban is a synthetic nonpeptide with high specificity and low affinity for the Gp IIb/IIIa receptor. Its biologic half-life is approx 2 h, and is best reversed by discontinuation. Platelet transfusion may also be helpful in reversal of drug effect. It is renally cleared to varying degrees (40–70%), so similar it eptifibatide, its dose must be decreased in patients with renal dysfunction, and its use should be avoided in patients with renal failure. Tirofiban is approved for use in ACS.

PCI

In the Randomized Efficacy Study of Tirofiban for Outcomes and Restenosis (RESTORE) trial (164) of 2139 patients, there was a 38% relative reduction (5.4 vs 8.7% in the placebo group, $p = 0.005$) of the composite end point (death, acute MI, repeat revascularization, or stent placement) at 2 d, and a 27% relative reduction at 7 d ($p = 0.02$) in patients treated with tirofiban, with no significant increase in bleeding complications. At 30 d and 6 mo, the 3% difference in absolute event rates was unchanged, and the reduction in the event rates tended to be significant. When the end point was constructed to be consistent with that in other trials (i.e., urgent revascularization rather than repeat revascularization), a significant difference in event rates was maintained (8.0 vs 10.5% for placebo, $p = 0.05$). The RESTORE study has the only angiographic substudy to evaluate the risk of restenosis following Gp IIbIIIa inhibition, and there was no significant difference in the rate of restenosis between treated and control patients (165).

ACS

Tirofiban has been evaluated in two trials of ACS. The Platelet Receptor Inhibition In Ischemic Syndrome Management (PRISM) trial *(166)* randomized 3232 patients with ACS to tirofiban or heparin infusions for 48 h in addition to aspirin. The primary end point (composite of death, MI, or refractory ischemia during the infusion) was significantly less frequently observed in the tirofiban group than in the heparin group (3.8 vs 5.6%, $p = 0.01$), although this was entirely accounted for by the decrease in refractory ischemia (3.5 vs 5.3%, $p = 0.01$). Neither death, nor MI, nor combined death or MI was reduced by the administration of tirofiban. Interestingly, there were no beneficial effects attributable to tirofiban at 7 d, but at 30 d, a reduced rate of death had become statistically significant (2.3% tirofiban vs 3.6% heparin, $p = 0.02$). The Platelet Receptor Inhibition in Ischemic Syndrome Management in Patients Limited by Unstable Signs and Symptoms (PRISM-PLUS) trial *(167)* randomized 1915 patients with ACS to tirofiban, heparin, or combination tirofiban and heparin. All patients received aspirin therapy. The tirofiban-alone group was terminated prematurely due to excessive deaths at 7 d. The primary end point (composite death, MI, refractory ischemia within 7 d) was lower among the combination therapy group than the heparin-alone group (12.9 vs 17.9%, $p = 0.03$). These results were noted at 48 h, and were durable at 30 d and 6 mo. Refractory ischemia was durably decreased in the combination therapy group at 48 h, 7 d, 30 d and 6 mo. MI was decreased at 7 d, but was not durable to 30 d and 6 mo.

ST-Segment Elevation MI

There are presently no trials reported that support the use of tirofiban in acute ST-segment elevation MI.

A pooled analysis of 11,040 patients in trials of Gp IIb/IIIa inhibitors during interventional procedures shows lower 30-d (7.8 vs 11.4%, $p < 0.001$) and 6-mo (26.2 vs 29.6%, $p = 0.001$) event rates, but a higher rate of bleeding complications (5.9 vs 4.3%, $p = 0.001$) for Gp IIb/IIIA inhibitors when compared with placebo (Table 6). Several orally bioavailable synthetic inhibitors of Gp IIb/IIIa have been developed and tested, but results have been disappointing. No oral Gp IIb/IIIa inhibitor has any accepted indication at this time.

FUTURE DIRECTIONS

The remarkable development of new devices for coronary revascularization over the last decade has led to considerable expansion in the number of patients treatable using interventional procedures, and improvements in short- and long-term outcomes. Indications and methods of use for the current devices will continue to be expanded and refined, with randomized trials playing a major role. Newer technologies directed at limiting or even eliminating in-stent restenosis are one of the major focuses at this time. To this end, site-specific drug-delivery systems such as medicating stents that prevent restenosis and in-stent restenosis are a very active area of development. In addition, experimental technologies like intravascular magnetic resonance imaging may make their way into the clinical realm to allow more precise guidance of interventional devices, and optimal plaque ablation and remodeling while limiting arterial injury. Finally, an increased understanding of vascular biology, thrombosis, and restenosis will hopefully lead to pharmacological therapies designed to ameliorate adverse thrombotic, proliferative, and remodeling responses.

Table 6
Trials of GpIIb/IIIa Inhibitors during Interventional Procedures

Trial	Patients	30-day Composite Endpoint[a]			30-day Major Bleeding			6-month Composite Endpoint[f]		
		Drug (%)	Placebo (%)	p-Value	Drug (%)	Placebo (%)	p-Value	Drug (%)	Placebo (%)	p-Value
EPIC[a]	2,099	8.3	12.8	0.008	14.0	6.6	0.001	27.0	35.1	0.001
EPILOG[b]	2,792	5.2	11.7	<0.001	2.0	3.1	0.19	22.8	25.8	0.07
IMPACT-II[c]	4,010	9.2	11.4	0.06	4.8	5.1	NS	30.1	31.5	NS
RESTORE[d]	2,139	10.3	12.2	0.16	5.3	3.7	0.09	24.1	27.1	0.11
Total Experience	11,040	8.4 (341/4063)	11.9 (479/4033)	<0.001	5.9 (240/4063)	4.3 (175/4033)	0.001	26.2 (1057/4029)	29.6 (1183/3999)	0.001

[a]c7E3 bolus and infusion vs. placebo in high-risk PTCA/DCA

[b]c7E3 with low-dose heparin vs. placebo in elective PTCA/DCA

[c]Integrelin (low-dose bolus and infusion) in elective and high-risk PTCA/DCA except elective stents (randomized group)

[d]Tirofiban bolus and infusion vs. placebo in high-risk PTCA/DCA

[e]Death, MI, or urgent revascularization

[f]Death, MI, or repeat revascularization

RRR = relative risk reduction

REFERENCES

1. Boden WE, O'Rourke RA, Crawford MH, et al. Outcomes in patients with acute non-Q-wave myocardial infarction randomly assigned to an invasive as compared with a conservative management strategy. Veterans Affairs Non-Q-Wave Infarction Strategies in Hospital (VANQWISH) Trial Investigators. N Engl J Med 1998;338:1785–1792.

2. Fragmin and Fast Revascularisation during Instability in Coronary artery disease Investigators. Invasive compared with non-invasive treatment in unstable coronary-artery disease: FRISC II prospective randomised multicentre study. Lancet 1999;354:708–715.

3. Thrombolysis in Myocardial Ischemia Study Group. Effects of tissue plasminogen activator and a comparison of early invasive and conservative strategies in unstable angina and non-Q-wave myocardial infarction. Circulation 1994;89:1545–1556.

4. Cannon CP, Weintraub WS, Demopoulos LA, et al. Comparison of early invasive and conservative strategies in patients with unstable coronary syndromes treated with the glycoprotein IIb/IIIa inhibitor tirofiban. N Engl J Med 2001;344:1879–1887.

5. The TIMI Study Group. The Thrombolysis in Myocardial Infarction (TIMI) Trial. N Engl J Med 1985; 312:932–936.

6. Smith SC Jr, Dove JT, Jacobs AK, et al. ACC/AHA guidelines for percutaneous coronary intervention: a report of the American College of Cardiology/American Heart Association task force on practice guidelines (Committee to revise the 1993 guidelines for percutaneous transluminal coronary angioplasty). J Am Coll Cardiol 2001;37:2215–2239.

7. Ryan TJ, Bauman WB, Kennedy JW, et al. Guidelines for percutaneous transluminal coronary angioplasty: a report of the ACC/AHA task force. J Am Coll Cardiol 1993;22:2033.

8. Rozenman Y, Gilon D, Welber S, Sapoznikov D, Gotsman MS. Clinical and angiographic predictors of immediate recoil after successful coronary angioplasty and relation to late restenosis. Am J Cardiol 1993;72:1020.

9. Kuntz RE, Gibson CM, Nobuyoshi M, Baim DS. Generalized model of restenosis after conventional balloon angioplasty, stenting and directional atherectomy. J Am Coll Cardiol 1993;21:15–25.

10. Roubin GS, Douglas JS, King SB, Lin SF, et al. Influence of balloon size on initial success, acute complications, and restenosis after percutaneous transluminal coronary angioplasty: a prospective randomized study. Circulation 1988;78:557–565.

11. Baumbach A, Bittl JA, Fleck E, et al. Acute complications of excimer laser coronary angioplasty: a detailed analysis of multicenter results. Coinvestigators of the U.S. and European Percutaneous Excimer Laser Coronary Angioplasty (PELCA) Registries. J Am Coll Cardiol 1994;23:1305–1313.

12. Holmes DR, Mehta S, George CJ, et al. Excimer laser coronary angioplasty: The New Approaches to Coronary Intervention (NACI) Experience. Am J Cardiol 1997;80:99K–105K.

13. Stone GW, de Marchena E, Dageforde D, et al. Prospective, randomized, multicenter comparison of laser-facilitated balloon angioplasty versus stand-alone balloon angioplasty in patients with obstructive coronary artery disease. The Laser Angioplasty Versus Angioplasty (LAVA) Trial Investigators. J Am Coll Cardiol 1997;30:1714–1721.

14. Reifart N, Vandormael M, Krajcar M, et al. Randomized comparison of angioplasty of complex coronary lesions at a single center. Excimer Laser, Rotational Atherectomy, and Balloon Angioplasty Comparison (ERBAC) Study. Circulation 1997;96:91–98.

15. Appelman YE, Piek JJ, Strikwerda S, et al. Randomised trial of excimer laser angioplasty versus balloon angioplasty for treatment of obstructive coronary artery disease. Lancet. 1996;347:79–84.

16. Deckelbaum LI, Natarajan MK, Bittl JA, et al. Effect of intracoronary saline infusion on dissection during excimer laser coronary angioplasty: a randomized trial. The percutaneous excimer laser coronary angioplasty (PELCA) investigators. J Am Coll Cardiol 1995;26:1264–1269.

17. Safian RD, Gelbfish JS, Erny RE, Schnitt SJ, Schmidt DA, Baim DS. Coronary atherectomy. Clinical, angiographic, and histological findings and observations regarding potential mechanisms. Circulation 1990;82:69–79.

18. Topol EJ, Leya F, Pinkerton CA, et al. A comparison of directional atherectomy with coronary angioplasty in patients with coronary artery disease. The CAVEAT Study Group. N Engl J Med 1993;329: 221–227.

19. Adelman AG, Cohen EA, Kimball BP, et al. A comparison of directional atherectomy with balloon angioplasty for lesions of the left anterior descending artery. N Engl J Med 1993;329:228.

20. Holmes DR, Topol EJ, Califf RM, et al. A multicenter, randomized trial of coronary angioplasty versus directional atherectomy for patients with saphenous vein graft lesions: CAVEAT-II Investigators. Circulation 1995;91:1966–1974.

21. Elliott JM, Berdan LJ, Holmes DR, et al. One-year follow-up in the coronary angioplasty versus excisional atherectomy trial (CAVEAT-I). Circulation 1995;91:2158.

22. Lincoff A, Keeler G, Debowey D, Topol E. Is clinical site variability an important determinant of outcome following percutaneous revascularization with new technology? Insights from CAVEAT. Circulation 1993;88(Suppl. I):I-653.

23. Baim DS, Cutlip DE, Sharma SK, et al. Final results of the balloon versus optimal atherectomy trial (BOAT). Circulation 1998;97:322–331.

24. Leon M, Kuntz R, Popma J, et al. Acute angiographic, intravascular ultrasound and clinical results of directional atherectomy in the optimal atherectomy restenosis study. J Am Coll Cardiol 1995;25:137A.

25. Kini A, Marmur JD, Kini S, et al. Creatine kinase-MB elevation after coronary intervention correlates with diffuse atherosclerosis, and low-to-medium level elevation has a benign clinical course: implications for early discharge after coronary intervention. J Am Coll Cardiol 1999;34:663–671.

26. Ghaffari S, Kereiakes DJ, Lincoff AM, et al. Platelet glycoprotein IIb/IIIa receptor blockade with abciximab reduces ischemic complications in patients undergoing directional coronary atherectomy. EPILOG Investigators. Evaluation of PTCA to Improve Long-term Outcome by c7E3 GP IIb/IIIa Receptor Blockade. Am J Cardiol 1998;82:7–12.

27. Zhou YF, Leon MB, Waclawiw MA. Association between prior cytomegalovirus infection and the risk of restenosis after coronary atherectomy. N Engl J Med 1996;335:624–627.

28. Weyrens FJ, Mooney J, Lesser J, Mooney MR. Intracoronary diltiazem for microvascular spasm after interventional therapy. Am J Cardiol 1995;75:849–850.

29. Reisman M, Shuman BJ, Dillard D, et al. Analysis of low-speed rotational atherectomy for the reduction of platelet aggregation. Cathet Cardiovasc Diagn 1998;45:208–214.

30. Williams MS, Coller BS, Vaananen HJ, Scudder LE, Sharma SK, Marmur JD. Activation of platelets in platelet-rich plasma by rotablation is speed-dependent and can be inhibited by abciximab (c7E3 Fab; ReoPro). Circulation 1998;98:742–748.

31. Kovach JA, Mintz GS, Pichard AD, et al. Sequential intravascular ultrasound characterization of the mechanisms of rotational atherectomy and adjunct balloon angioplasty. J Am Coll Cardiol 1993;22:1024.

32. Ellis SG, Popma JJ, Buchbinder M, et al. Relation of clinical presentation, stenosis morphology, and operator technique to the procedural results of rotational atherectomy and rotational atherectomy facilitated angioplasty. Circulation 1994;89:882–892.

33. Appelman YE, Piek JJ, Strikwerda S, et al. Randomised trial of excimer laser angioplasty versus balloon angioplasty for treatment of obstructive coronary artery disease. Lancet 1996;347:79–84.

34. Warth DC, Leon MB, O'Neill W, Zacca N, Polissar N, Buchbinder M. Rotational atherectomy multicenter registry: acute results, complications and six month angiographic follow-up in 709 patients. J Am Coll Cardiol 1994;24:641.

35. Dietz UR, Erbel R. Angiographic and histologic findings in high frequency rotational ablation in coronary arteries in vitro. Zeitschrift fur Kardiologie 1991;80:222–229.

36. Borrione M, Hall P, Almagor Y, et al. Treatment of simple and complex coronary stenosis using rotational ablation followed by low-pressure balloon angioplasty. Cath Cardiovasc Diagn 1993;30:131–137.

37. Gilmore PS, Bass TA, Conetta DA, et al. Single site experience with high-speed coronary rotational atherectomy. Clin Cardiol 1993;16:311–316.

38. Guerin Y, Rahal S, Desnos M, et al. Coronary angioplasty combining rotational atherectomy and balloon dilatation. Results in 67 complex stenoses. Arch Mal du Coeur 1993;86:1535–1541

39. Stertzer SH, Rosenblum J, Shaw RE, et al. Coronary rotational ablation: initial experience in 302 procedures. J Am Coll Cardiol 1993;21:287–295.

40. Safian RD, Niazi KA, Strzelecki M, et al. Detailed angiographic analysis of high-speed mechanical rotational atherectomy in human coronary arteries. Circulation 1993;88:961–968.

41. MacIsaac AI, Bass TA, Buchbinder M, et al. High speed rotational atherectomy: outcome in calcified and non-calcified coronary artery lesions. J Am Coll Cardiol 1995;26:531–536.

42. Stertzer SH, Pomerantsev EV, Fitzgerald PJ, et al. Effects of technique modification on immediate results of high speed rotational atherectomy in 710 procedures on 656 patients. Cathet Cardiovasc Diagn 1995;36:304–310.

43. Whitlow PL, Bass TA, Kipperman RM, et al. Results of the study to determine rotablator and transluminal angioplasty strategy (STRATAS). Am J Cardiol 2001;87:699–705.
44. Safian RD, Feldman T, Muller DW, et al. Coronary angioplasty and Rotablator atherectomy trial (CARAT): immediate and late results of a prospective multicenter randomized trial. Catheter Cardiovasc Interv 2001;53:213–220.
45. Sketch MH, Davidson CJ, Yeh W, et al. Predictors of acute and long-term outcome with transluminal extraction catheter atherectomy: The new approaches to coronary intervention (NACI) registry. Am J Cardiol 1997;80:68K–77K.
46. Moses JW, Moussa I, Popma JJ, Sketch MH Jr, Yeh W. Risk of distal embolization and infarction with transluminal extraction atherectomy in saphenous vein grafts and native coronary arteries. NACI Investigators. New Approaches to Coronary Interventions. Catheter Cardiovasc Interv 1999;47: 149–154.
47. Nakagawa Y, Matsuo S, Kimura T, et al. Thrombectomy with AngioJet catheter in native coronary arteries for patients with acute or recent myocardial infarction. Am J Cardiol 1999;83:994–999.
48. Cohen DJ, Ramee S, Baim DS, et al. Economic assessment of rheolytic thrombectomy versus intracoronary urokinase for treatment of extensive intracoronary thrombus: results from a randomized clinical trial. Am Heart J 2001;142:648–656.
49. Silva JA, Ramee SR, Cohen DJ, et al. Rheolytic thrombectomy during percutaneous revascularization for acute myocardial infarction: experience with the AngioJet catheter. Am Heart J 2001;141:353–359.
50. Hochman JS, Sleeper LA, White HD, et al. Should We Emergently Revascularize Occluded Coronaries for Cardiogenic Shock. One-year survival following early revascularization for cardiogenic shock. JAMA 2001;285:190–192.
51. Kinlay S. What has intravascular ultrasound taught us about plaque biology? Curr Atheroscler Rep 2001;3:260–266.
52. Radke PW, Klues HG, Haager PK, et al. Mechanisms of acute lumen gain and recurrent restenosis after rotational atherectomy of diffuse in-stent restenosis: a quantitative angiographic and intravascular ultrasound study. J Am Coll Cardiol 1999;34:33–39.
53. Colombo A, Hall P, Nakamura S, et al. Intracoronary stenting without anticoagulation accomplished with intravascular ultrasound guidance. Circulation 1995;91:1676–1688.
54. Fitzgerald PJ, Oshima A, Hayase M, et al. Final results of the Can Routine Ultrasound Influence Stent Expansion (CRUISE) study. Circulation 2000 Aug 1;102:523–530.
55. Serruys PW, de Jaegere P, Kiemeneji F, et al. A comparison of balloon-expandable stent implantation with balloon angioplasty in patients with coronary artery disease. Benestent Study Group. N Engl J Med 1994;331:489–495.
56. Fischman DL, Leon MB, Baim DS, et al. A randomized comparison of coronary stent placement and balloon angioplasty in the treatment of coronary artery disease. Stent Restenosis Study Investigators. N Engl J Med 1994;331:496–501.
57. Nobuyoshi M, Kimura T, Nosaka H, et al. Restenosis after successful percutaneous transluminal coronary angioplasty: serial angiographic follow up of 229 patients. J Am Coll Cardiol 1988;12:616–623.
58. Sawada Y, Nokasa H, Kimura T, et al. Initial and six months outcomes of Palmaz-Schatz stent implantations: STRESS-BENESTENT equivalent vs non-equivalent lesions [abstract]. J Am Coll Cardiol 1996;27:252.
59. Betriu A, Masotti M, Serra A, et al. Randomized comparison of coronary stent implantation and balloon angioplasty in the treatment of de novo coronary artery lesions (START): a four-year follow-up. J Am Coll Cardiol 1999;34:1498–1506.
60. Erbel R, Haude M, Hopp HW, et al. Restenosis Stent Study: randomized trial comparing stenting and balloon angioplasty for treatment of restenosis after balloon angioplasty. J Am Coll Cardiol 1996;27: 139A.
61. Douglas JS, Savage MP, Bailey SR, et al. Randomized trial of coronary stent and balloon angioplasty in the treatment of saphenous vein graft stenoses. J Am Coll Cardiol 1996;27:178A.
62. Wong SC, Baim DS, Schatz RA, et al. Immediate results and late outcomes after stent implantation in saphenous vein graft lesions: the multicenter U.S. Palmaz-Schatz stent experience. The Palmaz-Schatz Stent Study Group. J Am Coll Cardiol 1995;26:704–712.
63. Sirnes PA, Golf S, Myreng Y, et al. Stenting in Chronic Coronary Occlusion (SICCO): a randomized, controlled trial of adding stent implantation after successful angioplasty. J Am Coll Cardiol 1996;28: 1444–1451.

64. Sirnes PA, Golf S, Myreng Y, et al. Sustained benefit of stenting chronic coronary occlusion: long-term clinical follow-up of the Stenting in Chronic Coronary Occlusion (SICCO) study. J Am Coll Cardiol 1998;32:305–310.

65. Rubartelli P, Niccoli L, Verna E, et al. Stent implantation versus balloon angioplasty in chronic coronary occlusions: results from the GISSOC trial. Gruppo Italiano di Studio sullo Stent nelle Occlusioni Coronariche. J Am Coll Cardiol 1998;32:90–96.

66. Buller CE, Dzavik V, Carere RG, et al. Primary stenting versus balloon angioplasty in occluded coronary arteries: the Total Occlusion Study of Canada (TOSCA). Circulation 1999;100:236–242.

67. Zampieri P, Colombo A, Almagor Y, Maiello L, Finci L. Results of coronary stenting of ostial lesions. Am J Cardiol 1994;73:901–903.

68. Fajadet J, Brunel P, Jordan C, Cassagneau B, Marco J. Is stenting of left main coronary artery a reasonable procedure. Circulation 1995;92(Suppl. I):I-74.

69. Colombo A, Maiello L, Itoh A, et al. Coronary stenting of bifurcation lesions: immediate and follow-up results. J Am Coll Cardiol 1996;27(Suppl. A):277A.

70. Kuntz RE, Piana R, Pomerantz RM, et al. Changing incidence and management of abrupt closure following coronary intervention in the new device era. Cathet Cardiovasc Diagn 1992;27:183–190.

71. Webb JG, Dodek AA, Allard M, Carere R, Marsh I. "Salvage atherectomy" for discrete arterial dissections resulting from balloon angioplasty. Can J Cardiol 1992;8:481–486.

72. Schieman G, Cohen BM, Kozina J, et al. Intracoronary urokinase for intracoronary thrombus accumulation complicating percutaneous transluminal coronary angioplasty in acute coronary syndromes. Circulation 1990;82:2052–2060.

73. Detre KM, Holmes DR Jr, Holubkov R, et al. Incidence and consequences of periprocedural occlusion. The 1985-86 National Heart, Lung and Blood Institute Percutaneous Transluminal Coronary Angioplasty Registry. Circulation 1990;82:739–750.

74. Schomig A, Kastrati A, Mudra H, et al. Four year experience with Palmaz-Schatz stenting in coronary angioplasty complicated by dissection with threatened or present vessel closure. Circulation 1994;90:2716–2724.

75. Carroza JP, George CJ, Curry C. Palmaz-Schatz stenting for non-elective indications: Report from the New Approaches to Coronary Intervention (NACI) registry. Circulation 1995;92(Suppl. I):I-86.

76. George BS, Voorhees WD, Roubin GS, et al. Multicenter investigation of coronary stenting to treat acute or threatened closure after percutaneous transluminal coronary angioplasty: clinical and angiographic outcomes. J Am Coll Cardiol 1993;22:135–143.

77. Vrolix M, Piessens J. Usefulness of the Wiktor stent for treatment of threatened or acute closure complicating coronary angioplasty. The European Wiktor Stent Study Group. Am J Cardiol 1994;73:737–741.

78. Cohen EA, Schwartz L. Coronary artery stenting: indications and cost implications. Prog Cardiovasc Dis 1996;39:83–110.

79. Mak KH, Belli G, Ellis SG, Moliterno DJ. Subacute stent thrombosis evolving issues and current concepts. J Am Coll Cardiol 1996;27:494–503.

80. Bittl JA. Subacute stent occlusion: thrombus horribilis. J Am Coll Cardiol 1996;28:368–370.

81. Mudra H, Klauss V, Blasini R, et al. Ultrasound guidance of Palmaz-Schatz intracoronary stenting with a combined intravascular ultrasound balloon catheter. Circulation 1994;90:1252.

82. Nakamura S, Hall P, Gaglione A, et al. High pressure assisted coronary stent implantation accomplished without intravascular ultrasound guidance and subsequent anti-coagulation. J Am Coll Cardiol 1997;29:21–27.

83. Schomig A, Neumann FJ, Kastrati A, et al. A randomized comparison of antiplatelet and anticoagulant therapy after the placement of coronary-artery stents. N Engl J Med. 1996;334:1084–1089.

84. Leon MB, Baim DS, Gordon P, et al. Clinical and angiographic results from the stent anticoagulation regimen study (STARS). Circulation 1996;94:I-685.

85. Jordan C, Carvalho H, Fajadet J, Cassagneau B, Robert G, Marco J. Reduction of acute thrombosis rate after coronary stenting using a new anticoagulant protocol. Circulation 1994;90:I-125.

86. Wong SC, Popma J, Mintz G, et al. Preliminary results from the Reduced Anticoagulation in Saphenous vein grafts Stent Trial (RAVES). Circulation 1994;90:I-125.

87. Colombo A, Nakamura S, Hall P, Maiello L, Blengino S, Martini G. A prospective study of Wiktor coronary stent implantation treated only with antiplatelet therapy. Circulation 1994;90:I-124.

88. Elias J, Monassier JP, Puel J, et al. Medtronic Wiktor stent implantation without coumadin: Hospital outcome. Circulation 1994;90:I-124.

89. Hall P, Colombo A, Nakamura S, et al. A prospective study of Gianturco Roubin stent implantation without subsequent anticoagulation. Circulation 1994;90:I-124.

90. Aubry P, Royer T, Spaulding C, et al. Coronary stenting without coumadin. Phase II and III, the bail out group. Circulation 1994;90:I-124.

91. Morice MC. Advances in post-stenting medication protocol. J Interv Cardiol 1995;7:32A–v35A.

92. Morice MC, Bourdonnec C, Lefevre T, et al. Coronary stenting without coumadin. Phase III. Circulation 1994;90:I-125.

93. Morice MC, Zemour G, Benveniste E, et al. Intracoronary stenting without coumadin. One month results of a French multicenter study. Cathet Cardiovasc Diagn 1995;35:1–7.

94. Lablanche JM, Grollier G, Danchin N, et al. Full antiplatelet therapy without anticoagulation after coronary stenting. J Am Coll Cardiol 1995;25:181A.

95. Wong C, Popma J, Chuang Y, et al. Economic impact of reduced anticoagulation after saphenous vein graft stent placement. J Am Coll Cardiol 1995;25:80A.

96. Fajadet J, Jordan C, Carvalho H, et al. Percutaneous transradial coronary stenting without coumadin can reduce vascular access complications and hospital stay. J Am Coll Cardiol 1995;25:182A.

97. Blasini R, Mudra H, Schuhlen H, et al. Intravascular ultrasound guided optimized emergency coronary Palmaz-Schatz stent placement without post-procedural systemic anti-coagulation. J Am Coll Cardiol 1995:25:197A.

98. Reifart N, Haase J, Vandormael M, et al. Gianturco-Roubin Stent Acute Closure Evaluation (GRACE): thirty-day outcomes compared to drug regimen. Circulation 1995;92:I-409.

99. Hall P, Colombo A, Itoh A, et al. Gianturco-Roubin stent implantation in small vessels without anti-coagulation. Circulation 1995;92:I-795.

100. Haase H, Reifart N, Baier T, et al. Bail-out stenting (Palmaz-Schatz) without anti-coagulation. Circulation 1995;92:I-795.

101. Goods C, Al-Shaibi K, Iyer S, et al. Flexible coil coronary stenting without anti-coagulation or intravascular ultrasound: a prospective observational study. Circulation 1995;92:I-795.

102. Belli G, Whitlow P, Gross L, et al. Intracoronary stenting without oral anti-coagulation: The Cleveland Clinic Registry. Circulation 1995;92:I-796.

103. Morice M, Breton C, Bunouf P, et al. Coronary stenting without anti-coagulant, without intravascular ultrasound. Results of the French Registry. Circulation 1995;92:I-796.

104. Carvalho H, Fajadet J, Jordan C, et al. A lower rate of complications after Gianturco-Roubin coronary stenting using a new anti-platelet and anti-coagulant protocol. Circulation 1994;90:I-125.

105. Hall P, Nakamura S, Maiello L, et al. A randomized comparison of combined ticlopidine and aspirin therapy versus aspirin therapy alone after successful intravascular ultrasound guided stent implantation. Circulation 1996;93:215–222.

106. Lefevre T, Morice M, Labrunie B, et al. Coronary stenting in elderly patients. Results from the stent without coumadin French Registry. J Am Coll Cardiol 1996;27:252A.

107. Morice M, Valelx B, Marco J, et al. Preliminary results of the MUST trial, major clinical events during the first month. J Am Coll Cardiol 1996;27:137A.

108. Goods C, Al-Shaibi K, Negus B, et al. Is ticlopidine a necessary component of anti-platelet regimens following coronary artery stenting. J Am Coll Cardiol 1996;27:137A.

109. Elias J, Monassier J, Carrie D, et al. Final results of the phase II, III, IV, and V of Medtronic Wiktor stent implantation without coumadin. J Am Coll Cardiol 1996;27:15A.

110. Walter H, Neumann FJ, Richardt G, et al. Antiplatelet vs anticoagulation treatment after intracoronary Palmaz-Schatz stent placement in acute myocardial infarction. A prospective randomized trial. J Am Coll Cardiol 1996;27:279A.

111. Moussa I, DiMario C, Reimers B, Akiyama T, Tobis J, Colombo A. Subacute stent thrombosis in the era of intravascular ultrasound guided coronary stenting without anti-coagulation: frequency, predictors, and clinical outcome. J Am Coll Cardiol 1997;29:6–12.

112. Serruys PW, Emanuelsson H, van der Giessen W, et al. Heparin coated Palmaz-Schatz stents in human coronary arteries: Early outcome of the Benestent II pilot trial. Circulation 1996;93:412–422.

113. Haude M, Erbel R, Issa H, et al. Subacute thrombotic complications after intracoronary implantation of Palmaz-Schatz stents. Am Heart J. 1993;126:15–22.

114. Bertrand ME, Rupprecht HJ, Urban P, et al. Double-blind study of the safety of clopidogrel with and without a loading dose in combination with aspirin compared with ticlopidine in combination with aspirin after coronary stenting: the clopidogrel aspirin stent international cooperative study (CLASSICS). Circulation. 2000;102:624–629.

115. Berger PB, Bell MR, Rihal CS, et al. Clopidogrel versus ticlopidine after intracoronary stent placement. J Am Coll Cardiol 1999;34:1891–1894.

116. Moussa I, Oetgen M, Roubin G, et al. Effectiveness of clopidogrel and aspirin versus ticlopidine and aspirin in preventing stent thrombosis after coronary stent implantation. Circulation. 1999;99: 2364–2366.

117. Gibson M, Marble S, Rizzo M, et al. Pooled analysis of primary stenting in acute MI in 1,357 patients. Circulation 1997;96:I-340.

118. Grines CL, Cox DA, Stone GW, et al. Coronary angioplasty with or without stent implantation for acute myocardial infarction. Stent Primary Angioplasty in Myocardial Infarction Study Group. N Engl J Med 1999;341:1949–1956.

119. Azar AJ, Detre K, Goldberg S, Kiemeneij F, Leon MB, Serruys PW. A meta-analysis on the clinical and angiographic outcomes of stents versus PTCA in the different coronary vessel sizes in the Benestent-I and the STRESS-I/II trials. Circulation 1995;92:I-475.

120. Baim DS, Levine MJ, Leon MB, et al. Management of restenosis within Palmaz-Schatz coronary stent (the U S Multicenter Experience). The US Palmaz-Schatz Stent Investigators. Am J Cardiol 1993;71:364–366.

121. Alfonso F, Rodriguez P, Phillips P, et al. Clinical and angiographic implications of coronary stenting in thrombus containing lesions. J Am Coll Cardiol 1997;29:725–733.

122. Curier JW, Faxon DP. Restenosis after PTCA: have we been aiming at the wrong target ? J Am Coll Cardiol 1995;25:516–520.

123. O'Brien ER, Alpers CE, Stewart DK, et al. Proliferation in primary and restenotic coronary atherectomy tissue: implications for anti-proliferative therapy. Circ Res 1993;73:223–231.

124. Mintz GS, Popma JJ, Pichard AD, et al. Intravascular ultrasound predictors of restenosis after percutaneous transluminal coronary angioplasty. J Am Coll Cardiol 1996;27:1678–1687.

125. Dussaillant GR, Mintz GS, Pichard AD, et al. Small stent size and intimal hyperplasia contribute to restenosis: a volumetric intravascular ultrasound analysis. J Am Coll Cardiol 1995;26:720–724.

126. Alexander W. Low restenosis with aspirin only after stenting. No difference in stent designs. Int Med World Report 1997;Dec:10.

127. Malhotra S, Teirstein PS. The SCRIPPS trial   catheter-based radiotherapy to inhibit coronary restenosis. J Invasive Cardiol 2000;12:330–332.

128. Waksman R, White RL, Chan RC, et al. Intracoronary gamma-radiation therapy after angioplasty inhibits recurrence in patients with in-stent restenosis. Circulation 2000;101:2165–2171.

129. Leon MB, Teirstein PS, Moses JW, et al. Localized intracoronary gamma-radiation therapy to inhibit the recurrence of restenosis after stenting. N Engl J Med 2001,344:250–256.

130. Topol EJ, Nissen SE. Our preoccupation with coronary luminology. The dissociation between clinical and angiographic findings in ischemic heart disease. Circulation. 1995;92:2333–2342.

131. Waksman R, Ajani AE, White RL, et al. Prolonged antiplatelet therapy to prevent late thrombosis after intracoronary gamma radiation in patients with in-stent restenosis: Washington Radiation for In-Stent Restenosis Trial plus 6 months of clopidogrel (WRIST PLUS). Circulation. 2001;103: 2332–2335.

132. Sapirstein W, Zuckerman B, Dillard J. FDA approval of coronary-artery brachytherapy. N Engl J Med 2001;344:297–299.

133. King SB III, Williams DO, Chougule P, et al. Endovascular beta-radiation to reduce restenosis after coronary balloon angioplasty: results of the beta energy restenosis trial (BERT). Circulation 1998;97: 2025–2030.

134. Summary of safety and effectiveness data: the Novoste Beta-Cath. Norcrosse, Ga.:Novoste. (See http://www.fda.gov/cdrh/pma/pmanov00.html).

135. Raizner AE, Oesterle SN, Waksman R, et al. Inhibition of restenosis with beta-emitting radiotherapy: Report of the Proliferation Reduction with Vascular Energy Trial (PREVENT). Circulation 2000;102: 951–958.

136. Waksman R, Bhargava B, White L, et al. Intracoronary beta-radiation therapy inhibits recurrence of in-stent restenosis. Circulation 2000;101:1895–1898.

137. Verin V, Popowski Y, de Bruyne B, et al. Endoluminal beta-radiation therapy for the prevention of coronary restenosis after balloon angioplasty. The Dose-Finding Study Group. N Engl J Med. 2001;344: 243–249.

138. Lincoff AM, Topol EJ, Ellis SG. Local drug delivery for the prevention of restenosis: fact, fancy, and future. Circulation 1994;90:2070–2084.

139. Drachman DE, Edelman ER, Seifert P, et al. Neointimal thickening after stent delivery of paclitaxel: change in composition and arrest of growth over six months. J Am Coll Cardiol. 2000;36:2325–2332.

140. Poon M, Marx SO, Gallo R, et al. Rapamycin inhibits vascular smooth muscle cell migration. J Clin Invest 1996;98:2277–2283.

141. Sousa JE, Costa MA, Abizaid A, et al. Lack of neointimal proliferation after implantation of sirolimus-coated stents in human coronary arteries: a quantitative coronary angiography and three-dimensional intravascular ultrasound study. Circulation 2001;103:192–195.

142. Bisaccia E, Klainer AS, Gonzalez J, et al. Feasibility of photopheresis to reduce the occurrence of restenosis after percutaneous transluminal coronary angioplasty: a clinical pilot study. Am Heart J 2001;142:461–465.

143. Rigel DF, Olson RW, Lappe RW. Comparison of hirudin and heparin as adjuncts to streptokinase thrombolysis in a canine model of coronary thrombolysis. Circulation 1993;72:1091–1102.

144. Cannon CP, McCabe CH, Henry TD, et al. A pilot trial of recombinant desulfatohirudin with heparin in conjunction with tissue type plasminogen activator and aspirin for acute myocardial infarction: Results of the Thrombolysis in Myocardial Infarction (TIMI) 5 Trial. J Am Coll Cardiol 1994;23: 993–1003.

145. Antman EM, for the TIMI 9A Investigators. Hirudin in acute myocardial infarction: Safety report from the Thrombolysis and Thrombin Inhibition in Myocardial Infarction (TIMI) 9A trial. Circulation 1994; 90:1624–1630.

146. The Global Use of Strategies to Open Occluded Coronary Arteries (GUSTO) IIA Investigators. A randomized trial of intravenous heparin vs recombinant hirudin for acute coronary syndromes. Circulation 1994;90:1631–1637.

147. Ferguson JJ. Meeting highlights: AHA 68th Scientific Sessions, "TIMI 9B": Heparin vs hirudin as adjunctive therapy for thrombolysis in acute myocardial infarction. Circulation 1996;93:843.

148. Armstrong P, Granger C, Califf R, Van der Werf F, Topol E. GUSTO 2B trial. American College of Cardiology, Orlando, 1996.

149. The EPIC Investigators. Use of monoclonal antibody directed against the platelet glycoprotein IIb/IIIa receptor in high risk angioplasty. N Engl J Med 1994;330:956–961.

150. Topol EJ, Ferguson JJ, Weisman HF, et al. Long-term protection from myocardial ischemic events in a randomized trial of brief integrin β_3 blockade with percutaneous coronary intervention. J Am Med Assoc 1997;278:479–484.

151. Lincoff AM, for the EPILOG Investigators. Platelet glycoprotein IIbIIIa receptor blockade and low-dose heparin during percutaneous coronary revascularization. N Engl J Med 1997;336:1689–1696.

152. Hamm CW, Heeschen C, Goldmann B, et al. Benefit of abciximab in patients with refractory unstable angina in relation to serum troponin T levels. c7E3 Fab Antiplatelet Therapy in Unstable Refractory Angina (CAPTURE) Study Investigators. N Engl J Med 1999;340:1623–1629.

153. Simoons ML, GUSTO IV-ACS Investigators. Effect of glycoprotein IIb/IIIa receptor blocker abciximab on outcome in patients with acute coronary syndromes without early coronary revascularisation: the GUSTO IV-ACS randomised trial. Lancet 2001;357:1915–1924.

154. Brener SJ, Barr LA, Burchenal JE, Wolski KE, Effron MB, Topol EJ. Effect of abciximab on the pattern of reperfusion in patients with acute myocardial infarction treated with primary angioplasty. RAPPORT investigators. ReoPro And Primary PTCA Organization and Randomized Trial. Am J Cardiol 1999;84:728–730,

155. Neumann FJ, Kastrati A, Schmitt C, et al. Effect of glycoprotein IIb/IIIa receptor blockade with abciximab on clinical and angiographic restenosis rate after the placement of coronary stents following acute myocardial infarction. J Am Coll Cardiol 2000;35:915–921.

156. Montalescot G, Barragan P, Wittenberg O, et al. Platelet glycoprotein IIb/IIIa inhibition with coronary stenting for acute myocardial infarction. N Engl J Med 2001;344:1895–1903.

157. de Lemos JA, Gibson CM, Antman EM, et al. Abciximab and early adjunctive percutaneous coronary intervention are associated with improved ST-segment resolution after thrombolysis: observations from the TIMI 14 Trial. Am Heart J 2001;141:592–598.

158. Herrmann HC, Moliterno DJ, Ohman EM, et al. Facilitation of early percutaneous coronary intervention after reteplase with or without abciximab in acute myocardial infarction: results from the SPEED (GUSTO-4 Pilot) Trial. J Am Coll Cardiol 2000;36:1489–1496.

159. The IMPACT Investigators. Randomized placebo controlled trial of the effect of eptifibatide on complications of percutaneous coronary intervention: IMPACT-II. Lancet 1997;349:1422–1428.

160. Blankenship JC, Tasissa G, O'Shea JC, et al. Effect of glycoprotein IIb/IIIa receptor inhibition on angiographic complications during percutaneous coronary intervention in the ESPRIT trial. J Am Coll Cardiol 2001;38:653–658.

161. Peterson JG, Topol EJ, Roe MT, et al.Prognostic importance of concomitant heparin with eptifibatide in acute coronary syndromes. PURSUIT Investigators. Platelet glycoprotein IIb/IIIa in unstable angina: receptor suppression using integrilin therapy. Am J Cardiol 2001;87:532–536.

162. Ohman EM, Kleiman NS, Gacioch G, et al. Combined accelerated tissue-plasminogen activator and platelet glycoprotein IIb/IIIa integrin receptor blockade with Integrilin in acute myocardial infarction. Results of a randomized, placebo-controlled, dose-ranging trial. IMPACT-AMI Investigators. Circulation 1997;95:846–854.

163. INTRO-AMI. Data on file. COR Therapeutics, Inc.

164. King SB III, for the RESTORE Investigators. Effects of platelet glycoprotein IIB/IIIa blockade with tirofiban on adverse cardiac events in patients with unstable angina or acute myocardial infarction undergoing coronary angioplasty. Circulation 1997;96:1445–1453.

165. Gibson CM, Rizzo MJ, McLean C, et al. The TIMI Frame Count & Restenosis: Faster is Better. J Am Coll Cardiol 1997;29:201A.

166. Study Investigators. A comparison of aspirin plus tirofiban with aspirin plus heparin for unstable angina. Platelet Receptor Inhibition in Ischemic Syndrome Management (PRISM). N Engl J Med 1998;338:1498–1505.

167 Study Investigators. Inhibition of the platelet glycoprotein IIb/IIIa receptor with tirofiban in unstable angina and non-Q-wave myocardial infarction. Platelet Receptor Inhibition in Ischemic Syndrome Management in Patients Limited by Unstable Signs and Symptoms (PRISM PLUS). N Engl J Med 1998;338:1488–1497.

168. Adelman AG, Cohen EA, Kimball BP, et al. A comparison of directional atherectomy with balloon angioplasty for lesions of the left anterior descending coronary artery. N Eng J Med 1993;329: 228–233.

169. Serruys PW, van Hout B, Bonnier H, et al. Randomised comparison of implantation of heparin-coated stents with balloon angioplasty in selected patients with coronary artery disease (Benestent–II). Lancet 1998;352:673–681.

V SPECIAL ASPECTS OF ACUTE CORONARY SYNDROMES

20 Women and Acute Coronary Syndromes

Jane A. Leopold, MD and Alice K. Jacobs, MD

CONTENTS

INTRODUCTION

Cardiovascular disease remains the leading cause of death in women in the United States, and the rate of decline remains less than that observed for men *(1)*. Owing to an increased awareness of these statistics, and a focus on women's health issues in general, there has been an intense interest in women with heart disease. Accordingly, gender differences in the presentation, evaluation, access to care, management, and acute- and long-term outcomes of women with acute coronary syndromes continue to be evaluated. Therefore, the goal of this chapter is to review briefly the epidemiology, risk factors, clinical presentation and evaluation of women with acute coronary syndromes, discuss gender differences in patients treated with medical therapy and coronary revascularization procedures, and highlight issues specific to women with unstable angina, myocardial infarction, and cardiogenic shock.

EPIDEMIOLOGY

The incidence of coronary heart disease increases with age in women, although the clinical presentation of the disease lags 10 yr behind that in men, and by 20 yr for more serious clinical events such as myocardial infarction and sudden death. While the life-

From: *Contemporary Cardiology: Management of Acute Coronary Syndromes, Second Edition*
Edited by: C. P. Cannon © Humana Press Inc., Totowa, NJ

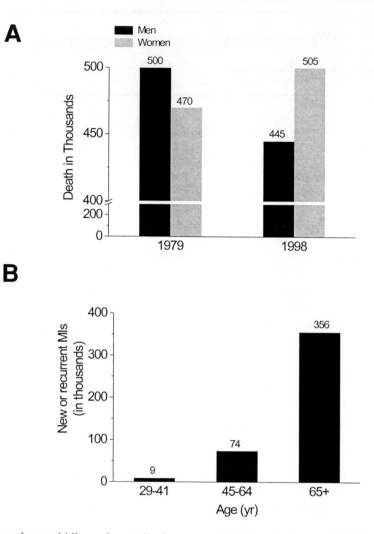

Fig. 1. Cardiovascular morbidity and mortality in women. **(A)** There has been a significant decline in cardiovascular mortality for men from 1979–1998, yet an increase in women for the same time period. **(B)** Women age 65 yr or older are more likely to have a myocardial infarction than younger women (*1*). MIs, myocardial infarctions; yr, years.

time risk of developing coronary heart disease after age 40 is 49% for men and only 32% for women, women are more likely to experience significant morbidity and mortality associated with an acute coronary syndrome (*1*). Interestingly, while mortality rates have declined over time for men, they have increased for women (Fig. 1). In part, because women have myocardial infarctions at older ages than men, they are more likely to die following the event, and mortality usually occurs within a few weeks (Fig. 1). In fact, 38% of women, compared to 25% of men, will die within 1 yr after having an initial recognized myocardial infarction, and by 6 yr after the index event, 35% of women will have a second acute coronary syndrome compared to only 18% of men (*1*). African-American women are at particularly high risk for adverse outcomes associated with acute coronary syndromes as evidenced by mortality data from 1998 that revealed that deaths from cardiovascular disease occurred in 400.7/1000 for black females compared to 294.9/1000 for white females (1).

Cardiovascular disease has been recognized as the leading cause of morbidity and mortality in women since the early 1900s, accounting for the death of 53% of women compared to 47% of men in the United States in 1998. Recent data from the Nurses' Health Study revealed a 31% decrease in coronary artery disease incidence in this cohort of women from the 2-yr period 1980–1982 to the 2-yr period 1992–1994; however, the rates of decline have been slower in women compared to men and the risk of death, reinfarction, and congestive heart failure following a nonfatal myocardial infarction remained higher in women than in men (1,2).

RISK FACTORS

The traditional and well-studied risk factors for coronary heart disease in men, namely, hypertension, diabetes mellitus, hypercholesterolemia, cigarette smoking, a family history of premature atherosclerotic vascular disease, and obesity appear to be operative in women as well; however, in the presence of any of these risk factors, the incidence of coronary heart disease is higher in men than in women (3). For example, although the incidence of coronary heart disease is higher among men than among women with systolic hypertension, the relative risk of coronary heart disease (in comparison with a gender-matched population without hypertension) is the same in women and men. Furthermore, women have a higher incidence of hypertensive heart disease and common causes of hypertension, such as renovascular hypertension due to fibromuscular dysplasia, are more common in women than in men (4,5).

Women with diabetes mellitus have twice the risk of myocardial infarction as nondiabetic women and the same risk of a myocardial infarction as a nondiabetic male of the same age (3). In addition, the increased risk associated with diabetes appears to be synergistic with gender. In one study, cardiovascular mortality rates were 3–7× higher in diabetic women than nondiabetic women, as compared to 2–4× higher in diabetic men than in nondiabetic men (6).

Interestingly, gender differences have been noted in cardiovascular risk attributed to hypercholesterolemia. In fact, decreased high-density lipoprotein (HDL) levels are a stronger predictor of risk in women than in men (7,8), and elevated low-density lipoprotein (LDL) levels, a strong predictor of atherosclerotic heart disease in men, do not constitute as strong a risk factor for coronary artery disease as low HDL levels in women who do not have established clinical coronary disease (9,10). Elevated triglyceride levels also appear to be an independent predictor of coronary disease in older women, and there is evidence to suggest that lipoprotein(a) [Lp(a)] is strongly associated with coronary artery disease in younger women (9,11).

It is noteworthy that cigarette smoking remains the leading cause of preventable coronary heart disease in women and that over 50% of myocardial infarctions occurring among middle-aged women are attributable to tobacco use (12). The magnitude of increased risk, a two- to four-fold increase compared to nonsmokers, is similar in women and men, occurs with even minimal exposure, and is related to the number of cigarettes smoked (13). Moreover, the risk of coronary heart disease begins to decline within months and reaches the level of nonsmokers 3–5 yr after smoking cessation. Although the prevalence of current tobacco use is similar in women and men with acute

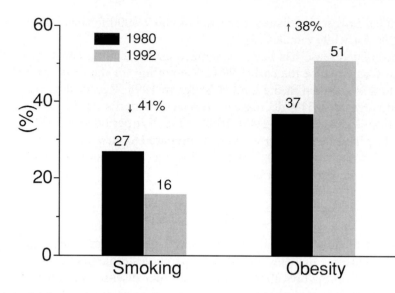

Fig. 2. Trends in risk factors for coronary artery disease. Rates of cigarette smoking have decreased from 1980–1992 in women; however, obesity and lack of regular exercise have increased significantly *(2)*.

coronary syndromes undergoing revascularization procedures, the prevalence of former smoking is higher in men and reflects reports documenting a slower decline in smoking cessation rates in women (Fig. 2) *(14)*. For women over the age of 35 yr who use oral contraceptives, there is a synergistic effect with tobacco use to increase the risk of atherothrombotic coronary artery disease *(15)*. These unfavorable smoking patterns in women, particularly among young women, have widespread clinical implications.

Obesity and sedentary lifestyle contribute to increased risk of coronary artery disease in women (Fig. 2). In fact, one-third of adult women are classified as obese, and up to 60% of women report no regular physical activity. Central, or abdominal, obesity has been identified as a significant coronary disease risk factor for women, and studies suggest women who participate in a regular exercise program have a 50% risk reduction compared to sedentary women *(12)*.

CLINICAL PRESENTATION

Whereas almost two-thirds of men with coronary heart disease present with myocardial infarction or sudden death as the initial manifestation of disease, over 50% of women may have angina pectoris as their first symptom (Fig. 3) *(16)*, yet establishing the diagnosis of ischemic heart disease in women remains problematic. This is, in part, due to the relatively high prevalence in women of chest pain in the absence of significant epicardial coronary artery stenoses.

To address this issue, several studies have examined the predictive value of chest pain utilizing angiographic assessment of coronary anatomy and determined that there is a poor correlation between chest pain symptoms and angiographic evidence of coronary disease *(17)*. At best, a clinical history of angina correlated with angiographic disease only one-half of the time in women. Even when unstable symptoms were present, the correlation was no better than 59%. The best correlation occurred in women thought not

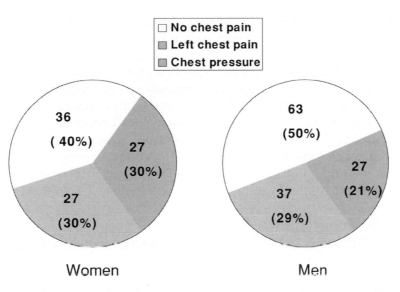

Fig. 3. Clinical presentation differs between women and men. Women who present for evaluation of an acute coronary syndrome complain of chest pain or pressure more frequently than men, and, in fact, 60% of women compared to 50% of men report chest pain symptoms on initial presentation *(20)*.

to have angina by history in which coronary artery disease was absent 95% of the time. Some added predictive value occurred when women were stratified by presence of coronary heart disease risk factors. For example, significant coronary artery disease was found in 55% of women with two or more risk factors, but only 7% of women with fewer than two risk factors *(18)*.

One of the initial studies to recognize the diagnostic value of chest pain in women was the Coronary Artery Surgery Study (CASS) *(19)*. In this study, definite angina, probable angina, probably not angina, and definitely not angina were carefully defined. Over 20,000 patients, of whom 4000 were women, were prospectively enrolled in this study, and all underwent coronary angiography to define coronary disease prevalence. Significant coronary disease, defined as at least 70% coronary artery stenosis, was found in 72% of the women with definite angina and 36% of the women with probable angina. The other two categories, probably not angina and definitely not angina, were combined under a category of nonspecific chest pain, and only 6% of the women so classified had significant coronary artery disease. In men, a similar classification resulted in significantly different prevalence rates of 93, 66, and 14%, respectively *(19)*.

Therefore, chest pain in women is neither sensitive nor specific in predicting the presence of underlying coronary artery disease. The highest sensitivity is found in women presenting with symptoms of typical angina pectoris, whereas the highest specificity is found in women presenting with nonspecific symptoms of chest pain.

In fact, women with acute coronary syndromes often present with symptom patterns that differ from their male counterparts. In a recent study of patients presenting to the emergency department, who subsequently had the diagnosis of acute coronary syndrome confirmed during hospitalization, chest pain was the most frequently reported symptom in both men and women; however, women were more likely than men to present with mid-back pain, nausea and/or vomiting, dyspnea, palpitations, and indigestion

(20,21). Similarly, in patients presenting with an acute myocardial infarction, men were significantly less likely to complain of neck pain, back pain, jaw pain, and nausea, than women *(22)*.

The magnitude and frequency of anginal-type chest pain, as well as nonspecific chest pain, in the absence of significant epicardial coronary stenoses is of practical importance but remains largely unexplained. This phenomenon has been attributed to mitral valve prolapse, vasospastic angina, and microvascular endothelial dysfunction *(23)*. Reduction of circulating estrogen following menopause is associated with profound impairment of endothelial vasodilator function and has been suggested to contribute to chest pain syndromes *(24)*. In fact, recent studies demonstrate that coronary microvascular dysfunction is present in approximately one-half of women who present with chest pain in the absence of obstructive epicardial coronary disease and cannot be predicted by risk factors for atherosclerosis and hormone levels *(25)*.

In women, studies of the control of blood flow in angiographically normal coronary vessels suggest that endothelial vasomotor dysfunction may mediate myocardial ischemia by contributing to pathologic coronary constriction or failure to dilate appropriately under conditions of increased demand *(26)*. This phenomenon was demonstrated by measuring coronary vasodilator reserve in patients with chest pain but angiographically normal coronary arteries using a doppler-tipped flow wire. Interestingly, there was a trend for a higher coronary vasodilatory reserve in men compared to women *(27)*.

Therefore, endothelial microvascular dysfunction may play a more important role in the production of ischemia in women than in men, and coronary angiography alone may fail to diagnose the etiology of chest pain. These observations suggest further, that in the setting of chest pain and angiographically normal or insignificant epicardial coronary artery disease, hemodynamic analysis of the coronary vasculature may be warranted.

NONINVASIVE EVALUATION

In women with acute coronary syndromes, in whom symptoms stabilize or in whom the diagnosis of coronary artery disease is uncertain, noninvasive testing is usually performed. In general, noninvasive evaluation of coronary artery disease in women is less accurate than in men, owing primarily to the lower prevalence of disease in women. The most widely employed and best studied diagnostic modality is the exercise treadmill test *(28)*, and it is predictably problematic in women due to a lower prevalence of coronary artery disease in premenopausal women, a higher prevalence of mitral valve prolapse and hyperventilation-induced ST-segment depression, a higher incidence of hypertensive heart disease, and limited ability to exercise to an adequate heart rate response. In contrast to what is observed in men, resting ST-T wave abnormalities on an electrocardiogram in women do not predict exercise stress test outcome independent of other clinical risk factors of coronary disease (Fig. 4) *(29)*.

Myocardial perfusion imaging with thallium has improved the diagnostic accuracy of noninvasive stress testing and increased sensitivity to 84–90% and specificity to 75–87% in women, but the diagnostic accuracy may be reduced in patients who are obese or have large breasts. Accuracy may be improved further with technetium-99m (Tc-99m) sestamibi, which has a similar sensitivity (85–90%) to thallium, while the specificity of Tc-

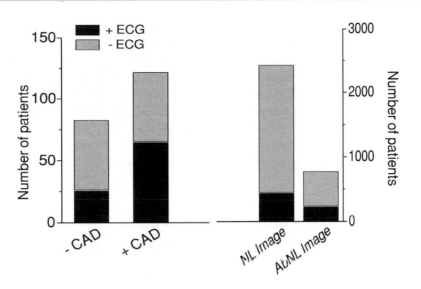

Fig. 4. Results of exercise electrocardiogram utilizing coronary angiography and myocardial perfusion imaging as a reference standard in women. In 3213 women evaluated by exercise ECG stress testing, sensitivity remains low whether myocardial perfusion imaging or coronary angiography is used as the reference standard. ECG, electrocardiogram; CAD, coronary artery disease; NL image, normal myocardial perfusion image; AbNL image, abnormal myocardial perfusion image *(31)*.

99m is higher (84–94%) than that of thallium (71%) *(30)*. A study of 8671 patients (3213 women, 5458 men) who underwent exercise treadmill stress testing with myocardial perfusion imaging confirmed that more women than men had a false-positive test, while the false-negative rate was significantly lower in women than men. Compared with men, women had lower test sensitivity and positive predictive value, but higher test specificity, negative predictive value, and accuracy. In patients with a false-negative exercise electrocardiogram, "high-risk" scans were less prevalent in women *(31)*.

Diagnostic noninvasive stress testing has an improved accuracy when multiple risk parameters, including ST deviation, chest pain, and exercise time, are included in the test interpretation. For women, a low-risk Duke treadmill score is associated with a 97% 5-yr survival, with 80% of these patients having no evidence of epicardial coronary artery disease at angiography. Multivessel disease is confirmed in 70% of women with a high-risk treadmill score; however, owing to early intervention is associated with a 90% 5-yr survival rate. For tests performed with nuclear imaging, 3-yr cardiac survival ranged from 99 to 85% for 0 to 3 vascular territories with perfusion abnormalities, respectively *(32)*.

Exercise echocardiography appears promising in women and is more specific than exercise electrocardiography *(33)*. Stress echocardiography is reported to have a high sensitivity (86%) and specificity (86%), but often examiners stop the test before detecting less severe areas of damage *(30)*. Similarly, the presence of a new echocardiographic wall motion abnormality following dobutamine administration has been found to be a highly specific manifestation of ischemia, even in women *(34)*. The sensitivity of dobutamine stress echocardiography is as good as what is reported for exercise treadmill stress testing, while the specificity and accuracy are increased significantly *(35)*. The prognostic significance of stress echocardiography was evaluated in 135 women with a high probability of coronary artery disease. In women with a high pretest likelihood of coronary heart disease, a negative stress echocardiography exam identified a subgroup of women who were at low risk of cardiac events and, therefore, were not recommended for further invasive investigation, while a positive stress echocardiography exam identified a subgroup of women at increased risk for subsequent cardiac events *(36)*. Furthermore, three-dimensional imaging with magnetic resonance imaging, positron emission tomography, and electronic beam computed tomography are under active investigation in women *(37)*, yet recent studies demonstrate that presently, the diagnostic accuracy of electron beam computed tomography reveals a sensitivity of 88% and a specificity of only 49% *(32)*.

MEDICAL THERAPY
Antiplatelet Agents

The role of adjunctive pharmacologic therapy in the treatment of patients with acute myocardial infarction has been well studied, although data on gender differences in response to treatment are limited. In general, results of trials performed predominantly in men and therefore, treatment recommendations, have been extrapolated to women. It should be noted, however, that women with a high baseline risk profile have the most to gain from risk reduction therapy.

Although few studies addressed the efficacy of aspirin for primary prevention in women, a meta-analysis of randomized trials of aspirin therapy revealed a 25% reduction in the risk of subsequent cardiovascular events in both women and men with vascular disease *(38)*. Further review revealed that only one-third of postmenopausal women with cardiovascular disease were taking daily aspirin, and, the majority of these women were doing so for primary prevention *(39)*. In the Second National Registry of Myocardial Infarction (NRMI 2), women were less likely to receive aspirin both on hospital admission and at discharge than their male counterparts *(40)*.

Recently, inhibitors of the glycoprotein IIb/IIIa receptor, a receptor on the platelet surface that mediates platelet aggregation, have been developed and, in clinical trials, have demonstrated efficacy in the initial medical stabilization of patients with acute coronary syndromes and as an adjunct to percutaneous revascularization procedures *(41)*. As it has also been suggested that there is a gender-based difference in platelet function and women are believed to have hyperreactive platelets, it therefore follows that they should experience a greater benefit from these platelet inhibitors *(42)*.

To evaluate the role of glycoprotein IIb/IIIa receptor antagonists in the medical management of acute coronary syndromes, the Platelet Receptor Inhibition in Ischemic Syndrome Management in Patients Limited by Unstable Signs and Symptoms (PRISM-PLUS) trial randomized 1915 patients with acute coronary syndromes to tirofiban or placebo and demonstrated a 32% reduction in the composite endpoint of death, myocardial infarction, refractory ischemia or rehospitalization for recurrent ischemia, at 7 d, a 22% reduction at 30 d, and a 19% decrease at 6 mo in patients treated with tirofiban. Women treated with tirofiban had a 30% reduction in events at 7 d, which was similar to the 27% reduction observed in men *(43)*. Interestingly, these benefits for women were not as readily recognized in the Platelet Glycoprotein IIb/IIIa in Unstable Angina: Receptor Suppression Using Integrilin Therapy (PURSUIT) trial. This study randomized 10,948 patients to eptifibatide or placebo treatment groups. Treatment with eptifi-

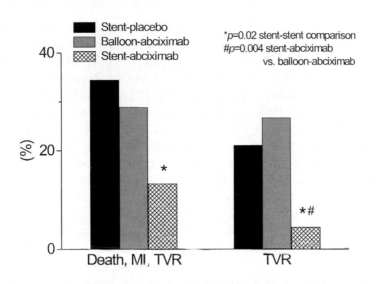

Fig. 5. Diabetic women benefit from glycoprotein IIb/IIIa antagonism. Women with diabetes in the EPISTENT trial who were treated with abciximab and coronary stent placement demonstrated a significant reduction in adverse outcomes at 1 yr compared to women treated with placebo or the combination of balloon angioplasty and abciximab. MI, myocardial infarction; TVR, target vessel revascularization *(48).*

batide was associated with a significant reduction in the incidence of death or myocardial infarction. Treatment effect consistently favored eptifibatide in all major subgroups except women (odds ratio for women, 1.10; 95% confidence interval [CI]: 0.91–1.34); however, there was a geographic disparity in outcomes and among both men and women in North America, there was a benefit associated with treatment with eptifibatide (incidence of the composite end point: among men, 16.2% in the placebo group vs 12.4% in the eptifibatide group, $p = 0.006$; among women, 12.9 vs 10.6%, respectively, $p = 0.19$) *(44).*

In women treated with abciximab in the Evaluation of 7E3 for the Prevention of Ischemia Complications (EPIC), Evaluation in Percutaneous Transluminal Coronary Angioplasty to Improve Long-Term Outcome with Abciximab GP IIb/IIIa blockage (EPILOG), and Evaluation of Platelet IIb/IIIa Inhibitor for Stent (EPISTENT) trials, there was a significant reduction in mortality, myocardial infarction, or urgent revascularization at 30 d (12.7 to 6.5%, $p < 0.001$). This decrease in major adverse cardiac events was evident at 6 mo (16.0 vs 9.9%, $p < 0.001$), and at 1 yr there was a reduction in mortality from 4 to 2.5% *(45).* In the EPISTENT trial, women treated with abciximab who underwent balloon angioplasty fared better than if a stent was placed without abciximab therapy (5.1 vs 11.7% event rate, $p < 0.021$), in contrast to what was observed in men *(46).* At 1-yr follow-up, stent placement with adjunctive abciximab therapy resulted in a lower mortality rate than either stenting or abciximab alone (placebo plus stent, 2.4%, abciximab plus percutaneous transluminal coronary angioplasty PTCA, 2.1%, abciximab plus stent, 1.0%) *(47).*

Of note, diabetic women, a high-risk subset of women, appeared to benefit significantly from abciximab administration (Fig. 5). While there were no differences in outcome noted at 30-d or 6-mo, at 1 yr there was a marked mortality benefit as well as a reduction in myocardial infarction and target vessel revascularization in women treated with abciximab who had a stent placed or underwent balloon angioplasty (13.3 vs 28.9 vs 34.5%, $p = 0.02$ for stent–stent comparison and $p = 0.09$ for stent–abciximab and balloon–abciximab comparison). This benefit was mostly driven by a decline in target vessel revascularization rates, which were significantly reduced from 21.1% in stent–placebo and 26.7% in balloon–abciximab to 4.5% in stent–abciximab, ($p = 0.02$ for stent–stent comparison and $p = 0.004$ for stent–abciximab and balloon–abciximab comparison) (48). Major hemorrhagic events were not significantly different between women treated with placebo or abciximab, but there was an increase in minor bleeding events (4.7 vs 6.7%). Female gender, abciximab use, and age >70 yr were independent predictors of an increased risk of hemorrhagic complications (48).

Women treated with eptifibatide as an adjunct to percutaneous revascularization procedures had a significant reduction in the rate of death, myocardial infarction, urgent revascularization, or bailout stent placement from 11.6 to 9.1% $p = 0.04$, which was gender-independent and not associated with a significant increase in bleeding (49). To extend these observations to contemporary percutaneous revascularization, the ESPRIT trial evaluated the safety of eptifibatide with stent implantation. The ESPRIT trial demonstrated a 37% relative reduction in the primary composite end point of death, myocardial infarction, and urgent target vessel revascularization at 48 h and a 36% relative reduction at 30 d with continued benefit observed at 6 mo. Subgroup analysis revealed that women treated with eptifibatide had a 58% relative reduction in events compared with women treated with placebo (50).

Lipid Lowering Agents

Although the U.S. National Cholesterol Education Program (NCEP) guidelines recommend an LDL cholesterol goal of less than 100 mg/dL for men and women with documented coronary heart disease, the Heart Estrogen/Progestin Replacement Study (HERS) trial of postmenopausal women with atherosclerotic coronary artery disease revealed that only 47% of women were taking lipid-lowering medication, and LDL cholesterol was above target in 91% of the study group. In fact, only 33% of women with LDL cholesterol >160 mg/dL were receiving lipid lowering therapy (51). To address this issue, the Women's Atorvastatin Trial on Cholesterol (WATCH) aggressively treated women and importantly demonstrated that 87% of women with 2 or more coronary artery disease risk factors and 80% of women with documented coronary heart disease treated with atorvastatin reached their LDL cholesterol goal (52).

Studies of cholesterol-lowering agents for primary prevention of coronary heart disease that included women were underpowered to detect absolute decreases in mortality; however, the Air Force/Texas Coronary Atherosclerosis Prevention Study (AFCAPS/TexCAPS) revealed that after an average of 5.2 yr follow-up, the risk of a first major acute coronary event was reduced in both men and women with a decrease in relative risk of 46% in women (53).

The Scandinavian Simvastatin Survival Study was a trial of simvastatin therapy for secondary prevention of coronary heart disease that enrolled 3617 men and 827 women with angina or a prior myocardial infarction. At a median follow-up of 5.4 yr, simvastatin therapy achieved a 37.4% reduction of LDL cholesterol in women resulting in a 49% decrease in the need for percutaneous or surgical revascularization procedures. In contrast to what was observed in men, women did not experience a significant reduc-

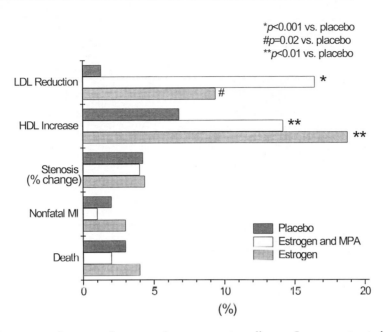

Fig. 6. Hormone replacement therapy and coronary artery disease. In women treated with estrogen or a combination of estrogen and medroxyprogestin (MPA), there was a reduction in LDL cholesterol and an increase in HDL cholesterol; however, this improvement in lipid profile did not translate into a regression of coronary artery disease at angiography, nor did it lead to a significant reduction in clinical events. LDL, low-density lipoprotein cholesterol; HDL, high-density lipoprotein cholesterol; MI, myocardial infarction *(60)*.

tion in cardiovascular or all-cause mortality. One potential explanation for these results is that women who participated in the study were more likely to have angina as the entry criteria to the study than men (37 vs 17%), and, therefore, may not have had significant epicardial coronary artery disease *(54)*. Similarly, in the Cholesterol and Recurrent Events (CARE) trial, 3583 men and 576 postmenopausal women with a history of myocardial infarction and elevated LDL cholesterol were randomized to pravastatin or placebo, and, at 5-yr follow-up, the reduction of risk of cardiovascular death in women treated with pravastatin was twice that seen in men (43 vs 21%). In addition, women had a greater reduction in nonfatal myocardial infarction than men (51 vs 15%) and a 56% decrease in stroke *(55)*.

Hormone Replacement Therapy

Postmenopausal hormone replacement therapy has been suggested to reduce cardiovascular morbidity by up to 56% in healthy women who take estrogen compared to women who have never taken hormone replacement medications *(56)*; however, these observations from small clinical trials may overestimate the actual cardiovascular benefits derived from hormone replacement therapy (Fig. 6). Theoretically, estrogen supplementation may reduce coronary events by improving cholesterol profiles, promoting endothelium-derived vasodilation, and by serving as an antioxidant *(12,57–59)*. Despite these potential therapeutic benefits, the HERS trial failed to demonstrate the therapeutic efficacy of estrogen replacement therapy compared to placebo with respect to coronary heart disease, nonfatal myocardial infarction, or mortality at 5 yr follow-up *(60)*. In fact,

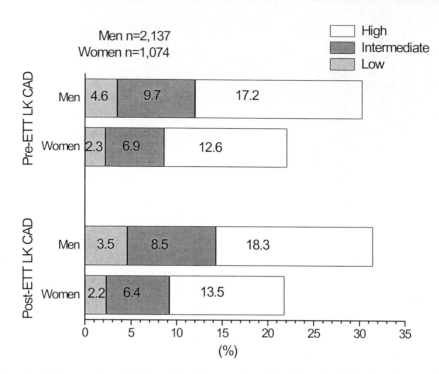

Fig. 7. Gender differences in referral patterns for cardiac catheterization following diagnostic stress testing. Men are more likely to be referred for coronary angiography than women early after exercise nuclear stress testing. This was most pronounced in patients with a high pre- and posttest likelihood of coronary disease. High, Intermediate, Low, refers to likelihood of coronary artery disease; Pre-ETT LK CAD, pretest likelihood of coronary artery disease; Post-ETT LK CAD, posttest likelihood of coronary artery disease *(64)*.

hormone replacement therapy was associated with a three-fold increase in venous thromboembolic events, a 3- to 8-fold increase in lifetime risk of developing endometrial cancer, and an increase in gallbladder disease *(60,61)*. The Estrogen Replacement and Atherosclerosis (ERA) Study utilized quantitative coronary angiography to confirm these findings. Women were treated with hormone replacement therapy or placebo and underwent cardiac catheterization. After 3 yr of follow-up the mean change in lumen diameter was not significantly different between treatment groups *(62)*. These trials, therefore, form the basis for the current American Heart Association/American College of Cardiology (AHA/ACC) recommendation that hormone replacement therapy does not play a role in the primary prevention of coronary heart disease; however, for women who presently take estrogen compounds, there is no benefit to discontinue this therapy *(63)*.

GENDER DIFFERENCES IN REFERRAL PATTERNS

Several early studies suggested that a gender-related difference in the referral rate for coronary angiography existed, despite the availability of noninvasive stress testing to risk-stratify patients (Fig. 7) *(64)*. After an abnormal nuclear stress test, women were less likely than men to be referred for coronary angiography *(65)* even when the pretest suspicion of coronary artery disease was high *(66)*. Women were referred for additional studies with less frequency than men following a similar abnormal stress test (38 vs 62.3%) despite follow-up evidence that demonstrated that women with a positive stress test were at increased risk for coronary events compared to men (14.3 vs 6.0%) *(23,66)*. In fact, women were also only half as likely as men to undergo cardiac catheterization before presenting with a myocardial infarction, even after reporting chest pain symptoms and functional disability from angina *(67)*. It has been suggested that this delay in the referral for diagnostic coronary angiography may contribute to the higher morbidity and mortality in women with documented coronary disease as compared to men.

Other factors that have been cited to account for the observed gender differences in the referral rate for coronary angiography include the physician's awareness of the prevalence of coronary heart disease in women, the sensitivity and specificity of noninvasive stress testing, the presence of comorbid conditions that may influence the decision for revascularization if disease is confirmed, gender differences in risks and benefits of coronary revascularization, and the patients' enthusiasm to proceed with cardiac catheterization *(68,69)*. Interestingly, when 174 patients who presented for stress testing were questioned with respect to willingness to undergo an invasive study, women were much more likely to accept the recommendation for cardiac catheterization than men (OR 7.1; 95% CI: 1.1, 45.3) *(70)*.

It has also been suggested that any perceived gender bias in referral patterns may actually reflect an inappropriate overutilization of cardiac catheterization in men at low risk for coronary disease as opposed to an underutilization of the procedure in women *(71,72)*. To evaluate this possibility, the records of 1335 patients who underwent coronary angiography were reviewed. Angiography that was deemed inappropriate was not gender-specific, and the rate of catheterization deemed inappropriate was not significantly different between women and men (5 and 4%, respectively) *(73)*.

Recently, the role of gender bias with respect to referral patterns for coronary angiography has been disputed. In one series of patients with chest pain who underwent exercise stress testing, the adjusted referral rates for cardiac catheterization for women were similar to men *(74)* and, even more surprising was the observation that physicians tended to overestimate, rather than underestimate, the probability of coronary disease in women *(74)*. Similarly, review of patients undergoing nuclear stress testing revealed that even though women were more likely to have normal perfusion studies than their male counterparts (70.9 vs 50.5%, $p < 0.05$), women with abnormal images were equally referred for diagnostic cardiac catheterization and that the presence of reversible and persistent defects, not gender, was the only independent predictor of referral for angiography *(75)*. In the setting of severe ischemia documented by stress testing, women were actually referred for angiography more frequently than men *(64)*. These seemingly contradictory observations regarding referral patterns for coronary angiography illustrate the growing awareness of the incidence and prevalence of coronary artery disease in women as well as the overall increased availability of coronary angiography in the community.

The observed absence of gender bias in referral for angiography may not be a universal phenomenon. In Austria, a country with a state-run health system and free access to high-technology medicine with no age limits, a recent analysis of 476 patients revealed that there is a significant delay for women to undergo cardiac catheterization compared to men. For patients undergoing cardiac catheterization, 4.5% of women reported recent onset of symptoms compared to 13.7% of men, chest pain of less than 1 yr duration for 27.1% of women and 34% of men, but greater than 1 yr for 68.4% of women compared to 52.3% of men. Prior to cardiac catheterization women were more likely to receive a trial of medical therapy (87.1 vs 78.8%), but fewer women than men had been referred to a cardiologist and, at the time of coronary angiography, a greater percentage of women were New York Heart Association (NYHA) class III–IV *(76)*.

The existence of gender bias in referral patterns for coronary angiography in women following myocardial infarction also remains controversial. As the role of cardiac catheterization in patients who have had a myocardial infarction is to determine the extent and severity of disease prior to revascularization procedures, there should not be any difference in the rate of angiography based on gender amongst postinfarction patients. Yet historically it has been shown that women hospitalized with a myocardial infarction were 15–28% less likely to undergo cardiac catheterization than men *(77)*. This finding was confirmed in the Myocardial Infarction and Triage and Intervention (MITI) Registry, where cardiac catheterization was utilized less frequently in women following myocardial infarction than in men *(78)*. In fact, even in women with a class I or IIa indication for coronary angiography as determined by the ACC/AHA guidelines, cardiac catheterization was less likely to be performed *(79)*. In contrast to these observations, review of a series of 2473 patients admitted with acute myocardial infarction revealed that after adjustment for age, there was no gender bias in the rate of referral for coronary angiography *(80)*. Furthermore, in 439 patients admitted with an acute myocardial infarction, angiography rates were nearly identical in women and men, and the only predictors of cardiac catheterization following myocardial infarction were ACC/AHA class of indications and age *(81)*.

CORONARY REVASCULARIZATION

There are numerous and remarkably consistent gender-based differences in clinical characteristics and acute and long-term outcome in patients with acute coronary syndromes requiring percutaneous or surgical revascularization procedures. As expected, women are older than men and have a baseline clinical and angiographic profile that confers higher procedural risk for adverse outcome *(82)*. Despite these unfavorable pre-procedure characteristics, more advanced comorbid disease and complex coronary anatomy, the outcome of women who undergo coronary revascularization procedures continues to improve *(83)*.

Baseline Clinical and Angiographic Characteristics

Gender differences in patients with coronary heart disease undergoing surgical (Table 1) *(84–88)* or percutaneous (Table 2) *(89–93)* revascularization procedures have been extremely consistent in virtually all published reports. Women who undergo revascularization procedures are older and have a higher prevalence of hypertension, diabetes, and hypercholesterolemia than men. Fewer women have had a prior myocardial infarction, and the prevalence of left ventricular dysfunction is lower in women than in men. In addition, women have a higher incidence of comorbid disease, and fewer women are considered to be ideal candidates for surgical revascularization in comparison with men.

Large-scale studies of patients undergoing coronary revascularization have also consistently shown that women have a significantly higher incidence of congestive heart failure than men *(94)*. As women are reported to have an overall higher left ventricular ejection fraction than men owing to a history of fewer previous myocardial infarctions,

Table 1
Gender Differences in Baseline Clinical Characteristics in Patients
Undergoing Coronary Bypass Surgery[a]

Authors (reference)	Sex	No.	Mean age (yr)	HTN (%)	DM (%)	CHF (%)	USAP (%)	EF (%)
Capdeville et al. (86)	W	61	68	79	44	28		47
	M	126	65[b]	67	33	17[c]		45
Aldea et al. (85)	W	523	68	82	42	23	55	49
	M	1220	64[d]	74[d]	27[d]	18[d]	48[d]	48
Abramov et al. (84)	W	932	65	60	31	7	47	
	M	3891	62[d]	45[d]	22[d]	3[d]	33[d]	
Williams et al. (88)	W	5395	68		24			47
	M	13,797	64[d]		37[d]			49[d]
Edwards et al. (87)	W	97,153		70	37	16	63	
	M	247,760			59[d]	25[d]	11[d]	57[d]

[a]Abbreviations: HTN, hypertension; DM, diabetes mellitus; CHF, congestive heart failure; USAP, unstable angina pectoris; EF, ejection fraction.
[b]$p < 0.05$.
[c]$p < 0.005$.
[d]$p < 0.001$.

Table 2
Gender Differences in Baseline Clinical Characteristics in Patients
Undergoing Percutaneous Coronary Interventions[a]

Authors (reference)	Sex	No.	Mean age (yr)	HTN (%)	DM (%)	↑Chol (%)	Prior MI (%)	CHF (%)	USAP (%)
Mehilli et al. (90)	W	1001	69	75	27	57	33		40
	M	3263	63[b]	68[b]	19[b]	47[b]	37[c]		38
Alfonso et al. (89)	W	158	66	65	34	59	38	4	72
	M	823	59[b]	42[b]	16[b]	49[c]	47[c]	4	72
Peterson et al. (91)	W	35,571	66	59	30		34	10	33
	M	74,137	62[b]	48[b]	20[b]		40[b]	6[b]	30[b]
Robertson et al. (92)	W	975	66	64	28	62	41	17	70
	M	1880	62[b]	49[b]	20[b]	56[b]	48[b]	10[b]	59[b]
Welty et al. (93)	W	2101	67	41	36	46	38	7	63
	M	3888	61[b]	31[b]	22[b]	44	41	4[b]	55[b]

[a]Abbreviations: HTN, hypertension; DM, diabetes mellitus; (Chol, hypercholerolemia; MI, myocardial infarction; CHF, congestive heart failure; USAP, unstable angina pectoris.
[b]$p < 0.001$.
[c]$p < 0.05$.

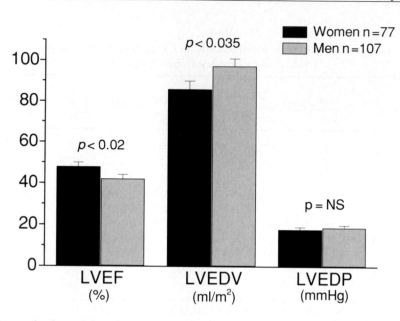

Fig. 8. Congestive heart failure in women with coronary artery disease. Although there is an increased prevalence of congestive heart failure in women compared to men, women have a higher left ventricular ejection fraction and a lower left ventricular end-diastolic volume suggesting that diastolic dysfunction contributes significantly to congestive heart failure symptoms in women. LVEF, left ventricular ejection fraction; LVEDV, left ventricular end-diastolic volume; LVEDP, left-ventricular end-diastolic pressure *(95)*.

this "gender paradox" has been explained by the presence of diastolic dysfunction and the finding of a steep left ventricular pressure–volume relationship in women in comparison to men (Fig. 8) *(95)*. Whether ischemia in women is due to diastolic dysfunction is unclear, but the latter may partially explain the increased occurrence of unstable symptoms despite a lower incidence of multivessel coronary disease in women compared to men.

Despite gender-related differences in referral patterns for the use of diagnostic cardiac catheterization, at catheterization, women have been shown to have the same or less angiographic evidence for coronary artery disease than men despite reporting more functional disability in terms of anginal chest pain. In fact, women undergoing coronary revascularization are more likely to have severe angina (Canadian class III or IV) and unstable symptoms than men *(96,97)*. One explanation for this finding is a gender-related difference in the pathophysiology of the ruptured plaque *(98,99)*.

Women who are found to have significant epicardial coronary stenoses at cardiac catheterization present with the same degree of coronary artery disease in comparison to men with respect to severity and distribution of lesions *(100,101)*, including the prevalence of left main and three-vessel disease *(73)*. In fact, over a 16-yr period, there was no significant gender difference observed with respect to extent and localization of coronary lesions in patients with angiographically documented coronary artery disease. Of note, there was a significant shift from the diagnosis of multivessel disease toward single-vessel disease in both men and women indicating that, over time, diagnostic car-

Table 3
Gender Differences in Operative Mortality in Patients Undergoing
Coronary Artery Bypass Surgery[a]

Authors (reference)	Sex	Patients No.	Mortality (%)	MI (%)	CVA/TIA
Capdeville et al. *(86)*	W	61	0.8	1.6	0
	M	126	3.3	0	1.6
Abramov et al. *(84)*	W	932	2.7	4.5	2.4
	M	3891	1.8	3.1[b]	1.8
Aldea et al. *(85)*	W	523	1.5	0.6	1.1
	M	1220	1.0	0.6	0.4
Williams et al. *(88)*	W	5395	3.5	1.0	1.6
	M	13,797	2.1[c]	0.6[d]	1.3

[a]Abbreviations: MI, myocardial infarction; CVA, cerebrovascular accident, TIA, transient ischemic attack.
[b]$p < 0.05$.
[c]$p < 0.001$.
[d]$p < 0.004$.

diac catheterization had become utilized with increasing frequency in a wider subset of patients earlier in the course of their disease.

Acute Outcome

Improvements in myocardial protection and advances in surgical techniques have allowed surgical revascularization procedures to be offered to a larger subset of women with symptomatic coronary heart disease. Despite these advances, gender differences in in-hospital mortality following coronary artery bypass surgery have persisted and have been notably consistent during the past 20 yr (Table 3). Specifically, in-hospital mortality is approx 2.5-fold higher in women in comparison with men, is only partially explained by older age and a higher risk profile in women *(102,103)*, and has been attributed to more urgent or emergency procedures owing to unstable symptoms as well as greater technical difficulty in operating in women *(102)*. Small coronary vessel diameter has been associated with increased mortality, and several studies have reported that when body surface area (a surrogate for vessel size) is considered, female gender is no longer an independent predictor of in-hospital mortality *(104)*. Congestive heart failure has been shown to be independently associated with mortality *(105)*, particularly in women, as well as excess hemorrhagic complications.

These observations have been confirmed in a recent retrospective study of 4823 patients, including 932 (19.3%) women, undergoing coronary artery bypass surgery that revealed significant gender-based differences in morbidity and mortality. Compared to men, women who underwent coronary artery bypass surgery were older, had a smaller mean body surface area, and a higher prevalence of diabetes, hypertension, peripheral vascular disease, congestive heart failure, history of percutaneous revascularization procedures, and NYHA class III or IV angina. Women were more likely to require urgent surgery with an increased frequency of preoperative intra-aortic balloon pump usage. Women had fewer bypass grafts constructed than men and were less likely to have inter-

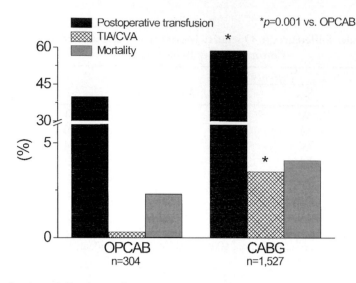

Fig. 9. Complications following "off-pump" surgical revascularization. In a series of women deemed appropriate for "off-pump" surgical revascularization, postoperative complications were significantly decreased as compared to women who underwent traditional surgical revascularization procedures. OPCAB, "off-pump" coronary artery bypass; CABG, coronary artery bypass grafting; TIA/CVA, transient ischemic attack/cerebrovascular accident *(107)*.

nal mammary artery grafting, multiple arterial conduits, or coronary endarterectomy performed at the time of surgery. The early mortality rate in women in this series was 2.7 vs 1.8% in men ($p = 0.09$), and women were found to be more prone to perioperative myocardial infarction (4.5 vs 3.1% $p < 0.05$). Interestingly, after adjustment for other risk factors, female gender was not an independent predictor of early mortality, but was a weak independent predictor for the composite end point of death, perioperative myocardial infarction, intra-aortic balloon pump placement, or cerebrovascular accident (8.55 vs 5.9%; odds ratio, 1.30; 95% CI: 0.99–1.68; $p = 0.05$). Recurrent anginal symptoms were more frequent in female patients (15.2 ± 4.0% vs 8.5 ± 2.0% at 60 mo, $p = 0.001$) but did not result in an increase in repeat percutaneous or surgical revascularization procedures *(106)*.

Surgical myocardial revascularization in women has increasingly been performed utilizing an off-pump (without cardiopulmonary bypass) technique (Fig. 9). In a series of patients deemed appropriate for off-pump revascularization procedures, the mortality for women was lower compared to their on-pump counterparts, despite an older age and higher incidence of diabetes. In fact, the mortality rate for women operated on without cardiopulmonary bypass dropped to the mortality rate typically seen in men. This was associated with a shorter length of stay and a lower incidence of transient ischemic attacks, cerebrovascular accidents, postoperative bleeding complications, and blood transfusions; however, these favorable outcomes in women may reflect patient selection and require further study *(107)*.

Historically, women undergoing coronary angioplasty had a lower procedural success rate than men *(108)*; however, recent reports have demonstrated similar angiographic outcome and rates of periprocedural myocardial infarction and emergency coronary bypass surgery (Table 4) *(97,105)*. Yet, in-hospital mortality is significantly higher in

Table 4
Gender Differences in Acute Outcome in Patients Undergoing
Percutaneous Coronary Interventions[a]

Authors (reference)	Patients		Angiographic success	Death (%)	Nonfatal MI (%)	TVR (%)	CABG (%)
	Sex	No.					
Mehilli et al. (90)	W	1001		1.7	1.4	3.2	0.9
	M	3263		0.8[b]	1.0	2.2	0.7
Alfonso et al. (89)	W	182	89	6	6	1	
	M	947	94[b]	2[b]	3	0	
Peterson et al. (91)	W	35,571	92	1.8	1.5	4.8	
	M	74,137	90[c]	1[c]	1.2[c]	4.4[c]	
Robertson et al. (92)	W	975	86	1.4	6.7		3.3
	M	1880	89[c]	1.1	5.2		1.9[c]
Welty et al. (93)	W	2092			1.2	0	0.4
	M	3878		0.5[b]	0.3		0.2

[a]Abbreviations: MI, myocardial infarction; TVR, target vessel revascularization; CABG, coronary
artery bypass grafting.
[b]$p < 0.05$
[c]$p < 0.005$

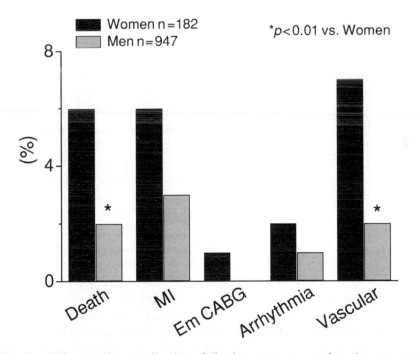

Fig. 10. Gender differences in complications following coronary stenting. As compared to men,
women who had coronary stents placed between 1990–1997 had an increased risk of adverse outcome
following the procedure. MI, myocardial infarction; Em CABG, emergent coronary artery bypass
grafting (89).

women, and an independent effect of gender on acute mortality following coronary angioplasty persists despite adjustment for differences in baseline clinical and angiographic characteristics (Fig. 10) (96,97). There is no single explanation for this increase in mortality, but it has been hypothesized that women poorly tolerate periods of transient ischemia during percutaneous revascularization procedures (109), and a higher incidence of periprocedural congestive heart failure and pulmonary edema has been reported (105). In fact, congestive heart failure has been shown to be a gender-independent predictor of mortality in both women and men undergoing coronary angioplasty (96,97).

Furthermore, during angioplasty, women mount different autonomic and hemodynamic responses to abrupt coronary occlusion than men. In a series of 140 men and 65 women undergoing single vessel percutaneous revascularization, total occlusion of a coronary artery was associated with more pronounced ST-segment changes and chest pain in women compared to men. This was associated with a higher incidence of significant bradycardia (31 vs 13%) or increase in heart rate variability (25 vs 11%) accompanied by a drop in systemic blood pressure (110).

In the New Approaches to Coronary Intervention (NACI) Registry, women undergoing percutaneous revascularization procedures with new devices were older and had more recent onset of severe or unstable chest pain than their male counterparts. Despite this adverse clinical profile, procedural success rates with respect to final percent diameter stenosis and Thrombolysis in Myocardial Ischemia (TIMI) flow grade was similar between women and men; however, women were more likely to experience procedure related complications, including coronary dissection, vascular access repair, hypotension, and transfusion, than men (92). There was no significant gender-based difference in the rate of in-hospital death, Q wave myocardial infarction, and emergent coronary bypass surgery, and gender was not an independent predictor of major adverse cardiac events. In the Bypass Angioplasty Revascularization Investigation (BARI) registry, women undergoing balloon angioplasty had similar rates of in-hospital mortality, myocardial infarction, and emergency coronary bypass surgery as men, although women had a higher incidence of periprocedural congestive heart failure and pulmonary edema (105).

To assess the influence of gender on coronary artery stent placement, 158 consecutive women undergoing coronary stenting were compared with 823 consecutive men. Women who underwent stent placement were found to have a higher in-hospital mortality, and female gender was independently associated with procedural complications (relative risk 2.4, 95% CI: 1.2–4.8) (89). Interestingly, the increased risk of death or nonfatal myocardial infarction occurred only during the first 30 d after stent placement. The combined rate of death or myocardial infarction was 3.1% for women compared to 1.8% for men, and the multivariate-adjusted hazard ratio (HR) for women was 2.02 (95% CI: 1.27–3.19) (90). Therefore, stents have not fulfilled their promise to rid of the gender difference in outcomes in patients treated with percutaneous coronary intervention.

Long-Term Outcome

Following hospitalization for coronary bypass surgery, long-term mortality and event-free survival are similar in women and men. In fact, after adjusting for advanced age and a higher risk profile in women, female gender has been shown to be an independent predictor of improved survival (105), and actuarial survival at 5 yr was greater in women then men ($93.1 \pm 1.7\%$ vs $90.0 \pm 1.0\%$). After adjustment for other risk factors, female gender was found to be predictive of late survival (risk ratio, 0.40; 95% CI: 0.16–0.74; $p < 0.005$) *(106)*.

Reports of gender differences in long-term outcome in patients treated with percutaneous coronary intervention reveal that at 1-yr follow-up, more women than men reported an improvement in their anginal symptoms (70 vs 62%) and fewer women required repeat target vessel revascularization (32 vs 36%) *(92)*. In fact, the benefits of percutaneous revascularization in women are realized up to 5 yr following the procedure as demonstrated in the BARI trial. At an average of 5.4 yr, follow-up mortality rates were similar between these high-risk women and men (12.8 vs 12.0%, respectively), and after adjustment for baseline characteristics, women had a significantly lower risk of death *(105)*. In the stent era, similar long-term outcomes have been observed, and at 1 yr, the outcome was similar for both men and women *(111)*.

SPECIFIC SYNDROMES

Unstable Angina

Women and men who present with unstable angina have different coronary heart disease risk factors and clinical symptoms, yet have a similar rate of revascularization procedure utilization and mortality rates. One prospective registry followed 4305 men and 2847 women with unstable angina who were admitted to coronary care units in King County, Washington, between 1988 and 1994. Women were older and had a higher incidence of hypertensive heart disease and congestive heart failure than men, but had lower rates of tobacco use, previous myocardial infarction, and prior percutaneous intervention *(112)*. Women were less likely to receive Agency for Health Care Policy Research (AHCPR) recommended pharmacologic treatment, diagnostic cardiac catheterization, and percutaneous or surgical coronary revascularization procedures than their male counterparts *(113)*. Although women were more likely to require rehospitalization for recurrent symptoms than men, early and late mortality rates were similar after adjustment for age *(112)*. By contrast, other studies have demonstrated a significant increase in mortality for women who present with unstable angina compared to men. In fact, women who present with unstable angina have in-hospital mortality rates that are reported to be up to $3\times$ higher (9.3 vs 3.0%) than what is observed for men, accounting for a relative risk of 3.07. In logistic regression models, the association between gender and mortality was not significantly altered when corrected for age, ST-segment electrocardiogram changes, and coronary heart disease risk factors *(114)*.

Interestingly, following an emergency department visit for the first presentation of unstable angina, women were less likely than men to undergo noninvasive and invasive diagnostic tests, and conversely, male sex was associated with a 24% increase in the use of cardiac procedures. Despite this utilization of resources, men had an increased risk of major adverse cardiac events compared to women *(115)*.

Myocardial Infarction

PROGNOSIS

Women have a worse prognosis following acute myocardial infarction than men, both prior to *(116)* and following the advent of thrombolytic therapy *(117)*. In the Framingham Study cohort, the initial fatality rate was 44% in women and 27% in men, and dur-

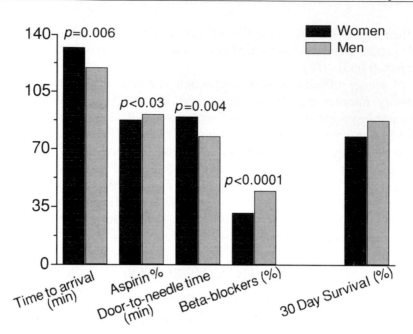

Fig. 11. Gender differences in the initial treatment for myocardial infarction. Women with an acute myocardial infarction take longer to seek medical attention compared to men. Once at the emergency room, they are less likely to receive aspirin and β-blockers and take longer to start thrombolytic therapy *(120)*.

ing the first 5 yr following the index event, women had an average annual rate of rein-farction of 9.6% in comparison with 2.9% in men *(116)*. In the Multicenter Investiga-tion of the Limitation of Infarct Size (MILIS) study, in-hospital mortality was 13% in women as compared to 7% in men, and cumulative mortality at 48 mo was 36% in women vs 21% in men *(118,119)*.

The extent to which this increased risk can be attributed to differences in treatment is not well defined; however, review of 1737 patients admitted to a cardiac intensive care unit with an acute myocardial infarction (Fig. 11) revealed that women took longer to seek medical treatment, were less likely to receive aspirin acutely (87.8 vs 91.3%, $p <$ 0.03), and had longer door-to-needle times (90 min [range 60–143.5 min] compared to 78 min [range 50–131 min], $p = 0.004$) for men. This resulted in an estimated survival at 30 d of only 78.4% (range 74.4–81.9%) for women compared to 88.0% (range 86.1 to 89.7%) for men. Increased risk of an adverse outcome persisted in this cohort of women even after adjustment for age, racial group, and diabetes (HR 1.52; 95% CI: 1.15–2.01). Estimated 30-d survival free of reinfarction and unstable angina was also lower for women than for men (75% [range 71–79%] vs 86% [range 84–88%]). Inter-estingly, at 12 mo, there was no observed gender-based differences in the influence of treatment variables on the differential risks for women and men *(120)*.

These observations were supported by data from data from the Cooperative Cardio-vascular Project that reviewed records from 138,956 Medicare beneficiaries (49% of them women) who had an acute myocardial infarction in 1994 or 1995. Women in all age groups were less likely to be recommended for diagnostic catheterization than men, and this difference was especially pronounced among women 85 yr of age or older.

Women were somewhat less likely than men to receive thrombolytic agents within 60 min (adjusted relative risk, 0.93; 95% CI: 0.90–0.96) or aspirin within 24 h after arrival at the hospital (adjusted relative risk, 0.96; 95% CI: 0.95–0.97), yet were equally likely to receive β-blockers (adjusted relative risk, 0.99; 95% CI: 0.95–1.03). Despite less aggressive treatment of women compared to men during the early management of acute myocardial infarction, 30-d mortality rates in this study were similar (121).

The prognosis for women following acute myocardial infarction in the thrombolytic era remains controversial. Women admitted during the first 6 h of an acute myocardial infarction, treated with thrombolytic agents or primary or rescue angioplasty, were more likely to be older (57 vs 67 yr, $p < 0.001$), with a greater incidence of hypertension and contraindications to thrombolytic therapy (28.5 vs 42.5%, $p = 0.02$) than men. Regardless of strategy, when equivalent rates of successful reperfusion of the infarct-related artery were achieved, women had a significantly higher in-hospital mortality compared to men (18.7 vs 7.2%, $p = 0.001$) (122). These observations were confirmed in a study that demonstrated that women treated with thrombolytic agents reach similar 90-min patency rates and regional ventricular function as men; however, these benefits did not influence 30-d mortality rates, which remained higher for women (13.1 vs 4.8%, $p < 0.0001$) (123).

It has been suggested that women have a worse outcome than men following acute myocardial infarction due to differences in recommendation and utilization of diagnostic coronary angiography and, therefore, revascularization, as part of the treatment plan. In the Atherosclerosis Risk in Communities (ARIC) study, women were less likely than men to undergo coronary angiography whether treated at a community or tertiary hospital (124). In contrast to these observations, a recent single center experience demonstrated that age-adjusted rates of coronary angiography following acute myocardial infarction were similar between women and men (125).

ST-Elevation Myocardial Infarction

THROMBOLYTIC THERAPY

While aggressive reperfusion therapy with pharmacologic agents has been shown to reduce in-hospital mortality by as much as 25–30%, women are more likely to have a contraindication to thrombolysis and, therefore, not receive thrombolytic therapy (122). This observation was confirmed in a series of 1059 patients who presented with an acute myocardial infarction, which revealed that women were less likely to receive thrombolytic agents than men (126). Moreover, it has been shown that only 55% of eligible women compared with 78% of eligible men receive tissue plasminogen activator. In contrast to these observations, a recent retrospective review of women age 50 yr or younger, who presented with an acute myocardial infarction, determined that 94% of women met eligibility criteria for thrombolytic agents, and 91% of these women were treated with drug. The most common reasons for withholding thrombolytic agents were nondiagnostic electrocardiogram and late presentation (>12 h after symptom onset) to the emergency department (127).

Once administered, thrombolytic agents have similar efficacy in women and men as demonstrated by 90-min infarct-related artery patency rates (39 vs 38%), reocclusion rates (8.7 vs 5.1%), and left ventricular ejection fraction and regional ventricular function, which has been reported to be similar in women and men, although women have more recurrent ischemia (21.4 vs 17.0%). Despite these similarities, the 30-d mortality rate was 13.1% in women vs 4.8% in men ($p \leq 0.0001$), and after adjustment for other clinical and angiographic variables, gender remained an independent predictor of 30-d mortality *(123)*.

In a meta-analysis of the Fibrinolytic Therapy Trialists' Collaboration Group, which included all randomized clinical trials that compared thrombolytic agents with a placebo or control group, the absolute benefit of thrombolytic therapy with regard to 35-d mortality was 2.2% in female patients compared to 1.9% in male patients. In addition, female gender and low body weight were identified as independent risk factors for cerebrovascular and hemorrhagic complications associated with thrombolytic therapy *(128)*. Furthermore, the Assessment of the Safety and Efficacy of a New Thrombolytic (ASSENT-2) study revealed a trend toward lower total stroke rate and 30-d mortality in female patients over 75 yr of age treated with tenecteplase than in those treated with alteplase. These observations suggest that female patients, especially over 75 yr of age, will probably benefit greatly from a thrombolytic agent with a weight-based dosing regimen *(128)*.

The Global Utilization of Streptokinase and Tissue Plasminogen Activator for Occluded Coronary Arteries (GUSTO-I) trial database evaluated 41,021 patients with suspected acute myocardial infarction and demonstrated a significant gender difference with respect to the unadjusted 1-yr mortality rate for the initial GUSTO-I population and 30-d survivors. For the initial population, when adjusted for age, women had a significantly worse outcome than men (odds ratio = 1.4, 95%, CI: 1.3–1.5, $p < 0.001$). Interestingly, for the 30-d survivors, adjustment based on age alone explained the 1-yr mortality difference (risk ratio = 0.96, 95% CI: 0.85–1.07, $p = 0.441$) between men and women *(129)*.

Treatment of young women with thrombolytic therapy was previously thought to be problematic owing to the increased risk of hemorrhage associated with active menstruation. Although studies have suggested that there may be an increase in the risk of moderate bleeding in menstruating patients treated with thrombolytic agents, the GUSTO-I study revealed that the mortality reduction associated with thrombolytic therapy for acute myocardial infarction should not be withheld because of active menstruation *(130)*.

PRIMARY ANGIOPLASTY

Percutaneous revascularization strategies to restore coronary artery patency during acute myocardial infarction in the absence of prior thrombolytic therapy, or primary angioplasty, results in a higher infarct-related coronary artery patency rate *(131)*, smaller enzymatic infarct size, increased preservation of left ventricular function, and improved clinical outcome compared to thrombolytic therapy *(131–133)*. A pooled analysis of early clinical trials of primary angioplasty revealed a 44% mortality reduction during hospitalization (OR 0.56, CI: 0.53–0.94) and a 9% mortality reduction at 1 yr *(134)*. Yet, despite the observed survival benefit, women are more likely to refuse catheterization as a therapeutic modality for acute myocardial infarction. Of the 2.4% of patients who reported that they were likely to refuse primary angioplasty, a significant proportion were older women with a history of prior myocardial infarction *(135)*.

Women who present with acute myocardial infarction who undergo primary angioplasty comprise a higher risk patient population compared to men. This was demonstrated in The Primary Angioplasty in Myocardial Infarction (PAMI) trial, which compared primary angioplasty with tissue-type plasminogen activator, and revealed that women were older (65.7 vs 57.7 yr, $p < 0.0001$) and had a higher incidence of diabetes (19 vs 10%, $p < 0.03$), hypertension (54 vs 39%, $p < 0.005$), and a history of congestive heart failure (5 vs 0%, $p = 0.002$) compared to men. Women were more likely to present later after symptom onset than their male counterparts (229 vs 174 min, $p = 0.0004$), and in-hospital mortality for women was 3.3-fold higher than men (9.3 vs 2.8%, $p = 0.0005$) (131,136). In the subset of women who were assigned to the angiography arm of the study, women were less likely than men to undergo percutaneous revascularization procedures owing to a higher prevalence of surgical disease or the presence of a noncritical stenosis. In women that did undergo angioplasty, the in-hospital mortality rate was similar to men (4.0 vs 2.1%), and percutaneous revascularization and younger age were independent predictors of in-hospital survival in women. Importantly, cerebrovascular hemorrhage occurred in 5.3% of women treated with a thrombolytic agent compared with 0.7% men ($p = 0.037$), while there was no increase in hemorrhagic events, regardless of gender, with primary angioplasty. These observations suggest that primary angioplasty improves survival in women, such that it is comparable to men, and reduces the risk of hemorrhagic stroke that is associated with thrombolytic therapy (136,137).

Women with acute myocardial infarction tend to have a worse prognosis then men because they present much later after symptom onset. To examine the influence of late presentation on the efficacy of primary angioplasty, a study of 496 patients with acute myocardial infarction who underwent primary angioplasty specifically assessed outcome in patients who were treated between 6 and 24 h. Patients who presented late were more often female, underwent primary angioplasty procedures with a lower success rate compared to patients with early presentation, resulting in a greater deterioration of left ventricular function. Patients who did undergo a successful revascularization procedure were more likely to have reocclusion of the infarct-related artery, repeat myocardial infarction, and a significantly higher mortality rate at 6 mo (138).

As coronary stents are increasingly utilized in primary revascularization procedures, the Stent-PAMI trial compared coronary stent implantation with balloon angioplasty for the treatment of acute myocardial infarction. At 6-mo follow-up, the combined primary end point of death, reinfarction, cerebrovascular accident, or target-vessel revascularization for ischemia, was reached by fewer patients in the stent group than in the angioplasty group (12.6 vs 20.1%, $p < 0.01$) (139). Women in this trial were older (66 ± 12 vs 58 ± 12 yr, $p < 0.0001$), had a higher incidence of hypertension, hypercholesterolemia, diabetes, and smaller size infarct-related artery at angiography compared to men. Even though TIMI grade 3 flow was restored in a greater percentage of women than men (94 vs 90.0%, $p = 0.07$), by 6 mo, women had increased rates of death (7.9 vs 2.0%, $p = 0.0002$), reinfarction (6.4 vs 2.7%, $p = 0.01$), and stroke (2.0 vs 0.3%, $p = 0.01$), with similar rates of late target vessel revascularization. These data have been confirmed in other studies (140) and demonstrate that women undergoing percutaneous revascularization in the stent era remain at high risk for adverse events (142).

Non-ST-Segment Elevation Myocardial Infarction

Few studies have specifically addressed the influence of gender differences on the outcome of patients who present with non-ST-segment elevation myocardial infarction undergoing percutaneous coronary revascularization procedures. Women who present with non-ST-segment elevation myocardial infarction that undergo angioplasty are consistently older, and have an increased incidence of hypertension with a preserved left ventricular ejection fraction when compared men. In one study, 941 women who underwent coronary angioplasty had a similar success, in-hospital mortality, and emergency coronary artery bypass surgery rate as men and overall survival during a mean follow-up period of 4 yr was comparable. Although women were more likely to experience severe angina than men, women were less likely to undergo coronary artery bypass grafting during this time *(141)*.

Women with unstable angina or non-Q wave myocardial infarction enrolled in the TIMI-IIIB trial were older with a higher prevalence of diabetes and hypertension, and were more likely to be given a trial of medical therapy compared to men. Although women were less likely to have significant epicardial coronary artery disease at cardiac catheterization, the 42-d rate of death and myocardial infarction was similar *(142)*. These findings were confirmed in the Global Unstable Angina Registry and Treatment Evaluation (GUARANTEE) Registry. At cardiac catheterization, women had less severe epicardial coronary artery stenoses and were more likely than men to have insignificant coronary artery disease (25 vs 14%, $p = 0.0001$) *(143)*.

A recent series evaluated outcome in 101 women who presented with non-Q wave infarction and underwent percutaneous revascularization during that hospitalization. Procedural success rates were similar for women and men, although women were less likely to undergo multivessel intervention. In-hospital adverse cardiac events were similar between men and women, although there was a trend towards a higher in-hospital death rate in women (4 vs 1%, $p = 0.058$), and at 1-yr follow-up, women had a significantly worse survival rate than men (89 vs 95%, $p < 0.04$) *(144)*.

Cardiogenic Shock

Cardiogenic shock complicates acute myocardial infarction in 5–15% of patients *(145)* and is recognized clinically as systemic hypotension resulting in end-organ hypoperfusion in the presence of elevated cardiac filling pressures. The subset of patients who present with or develop cardiogenic shock are more likely to be women, tend to be older, have more coronary artery disease risk factors, and are more likely to have had a prior myocardial infarction or surgical revascularization *(146)*.

To evaluate the role of coronary revascularization strategies in the treatment of cardiogenic shock, the SHOCK (Should we emergently revascularize Occluded Coronary arteries for cardiogenic shocK) trial was conducted *(147,148)*. This multicenter trial randomized 302 patients who presented with acute myocardial infarction and cardiogenic shock due to left ventricular dysfunction confirmed by both clinical and hemodynamic criteria. Approximately 37% of women were assigned to undergo revascularization and 27% to medical therapy. While there was no significant difference in 30-d mortality between treatment groups (46.7 vs 56.0%), by 6 mo, there was a survival benefit for patients who underwent percutaneous or surgical revascularization procedures. Interestingly, age ≥75 yr was found to be an independent predictor of increased morbidity and mortality for patients that underwent angioplasty or coronary artery bypass grafting at both 30 d and 6 mo *(148)*. As women who present with acute myocardial infarction and cardiogenic shock are often older, these observations suggest that coronary revascularization procedures may not improve mortality, and in fact, may predict a worse outcome in this cohort.

Importantly, a total of 1492 patients were screened for the SHOCK trial, and 1107 were deemed ineligible and entered into a registry. Women accounted for approx 40% of Registry patients and were more likely to be in cardiogenic shock due to isolated right ventricular shock *(149)*, acute severe mitral regurgitation *(150)*, or ventricular septal rupture *(151)*, than from predominant left ventricular failure. Women entered in the Registry had a higher incidence of diabetes and 2- or 3-vessel disease, yet the combined percutaneous and surgical revascularization rate for these women was lower than that for nondiabetic patients with single vessel disease *(152)*.

CONCLUSIONS

In patients with coronary heart disease, numerous and consistent gender differences in presentation, evaluation, treatment strategies, and outcome of treatment with thrombolytic therapy, percutaneous revascularization procedures, and coronary artery bypass surgery have been well documented. Women with acute coronary syndromes are older, with more high-risk clinical and angiographic factors and comorbid disease than men, and undergo treatment at increased risk for an adverse outcome. Many of the observed gender differences in acute and long-term outcome can be attributed to the older age and higher clinical risk profile in women. Despite these unfavorable features, recent studies suggest that the outcome in women is improving, and in particular, percutaneous and surgical revascularization procedures are effective treatment strategies in women.

REFERENCES

1. American Heart Association. 2001 Heart and Stroke Statistical Update. American Heart Association, Dallas, 2001.
2. Hu FB, Stampfer MJ, Manson JE, et al. Trends in the incidence of coronary heart disease and changes in diet and lifestyle in women. N Engl J Med 2000;343:530–537.
3. Castelli WP. Cardiovascular disease in women. Am J Obstet Gynecol 1988;158:1553–1567.
4. Kannel WB. Hypertension, hypertrophy, and the occurrence of cardiovascular disease. Am J Med Sci 1991;302:199 204.
5. Komanoff AR-NC, Woo B. Women's health. In: Braunwald EIK, et al. ed. Harrison's Principles of Internal Medicine. 14th ed. McGraw Hill, New York, 1998, pp. 21–24.
6. Mosca L, Grundy SM, Judelson D, et al. Guide to Preventive Cardiology for Women. AHA/ACC Scientific Statement Consensus panel statement. Circulation 1999;99:2480–2484.
7. Miller VT. Lipids, lipoproteins, women and cardiovascular disease. Atherosclerosis 1994;108(Suppl.): S73–S82.
8. Braunwald E. Cardiovascular disease in women. In: EB, ed. Heart Disease: A Textbook of Cardiovascular Medicine. 5th ed. W.B. Saunders, Philadelphia, 1997, pp. 1704–1714.
9. Bass KM, Newschaffer CJ, Klag MJ, Bush TL. Plasma lipoprotein levels as predictors of cardiovascular death in women. Arch Intern Med 1993;153:2209–2216.
10. Walsh JM, Grady D. Treatment of hyperlipidemia in women. JAMA 1995;274:1152–1158.
11. Orth-Gomer K, Mittleman MA, Schenck-Gustafsson K, et al. Lipoprotein(a) as a determinant of coronary heart disease in young women. Circulation 1997;95:329–334.
12. Mosca L, Manson JE, Sutherland SE, Langer RD, Manolio T, Barrett-Connor E. Cardiovascular disease in women: a statement for healthcare professionals from the American Heart Association. Writing Group. Circulation 1997;96:2468–2482.
13. Rich-Edwards JW, Manson JE, Hennekens CH, Buring JE. The primary prevention of coronary heart disease in women. N Engl J Med 1995;332:1758–1766.

14. Anonymous. Surveillance for selected tobacco use behaviors—United States, 1900–1994. MMWR 1994;43:1–43.
15. Jneid H, Thacker HL. Coronary artery disease in women: different, often undertreated. Cleve Clin J Med 2001;68:441–448.
16. Lerner DJ, Kannel WB. Patterns of coronary heart disease morbidity and mortality in the sexes: a 26-year follow-up of the Framingham population. Am Heart J 1986;111:383–390.
17. Welch CC, Proudfit WL, Sheldon WC. Coronary arteriographic findings in 1,000 women under age 50. Am J Cardiol 1975;35:211–215.
18. Waters DD, Halphen C, Theroux P, David PR, Mizgala HF. Coronary artery disease in young women: clinical and angiographic features and correlation with risk factors. Am J Cardiol 1978;42:41–47.
19. Chaitman BR, Bourassa MG, Davis K, et al. Angiographic prevalence of high-risk coronary artery disease in patient subsets (CASS). Circulation 1981;64:360–367.
20. Milner KA, Funk M, Richards S, Wilmes RM, Vaccarino V, Krumholz HM. Gender differences in symptom presentation associated with coronary heart disease. Am J Cardiol 1999;84:396–399.
21. Goldberg R, Goff D, Cooper L, et al. Age and sex differences in presentation of symptoms among patients with acute coronary disease: the REACT Trial. Rapid Early Action for Coronary Treatment. Coron Artery Dis 2000;11:399–407.
22. Goldberg RJ, O'Donnell C, Yarzebski J, Bigelow C, Savageau J, Gore JM. Sex differences in symptom presentation associated with acute myocardial infarction: a population-based perspective. Am Heart J 1998;136:189–195.
23. Douglas PS, Ginsburg GS. The evaluation of chest pain in women. N Engl J Med 1996;334:1311–1315.
24. Reis SE, Gloth ST, Blumenthal RS, et al. Ethinyl estradiol acutely attenuates abnormal coronary vasomotor responses to acetylcholine in postmenopausal women. Circulation 1994;89:52–60.
25. Reis SE, Holubkov R, Conrad Smith AJ, et al. Coronary microvascular dysfunction is highly prevalent in women with chest pain in the absence of coronary artery disease: results from the NHLBI WISE study. Am Heart J 2001;141:735–741.
26. Reddy KG, Nair RN, Sheehan HM, Hodgson JM. Evidence that selective endothelial dysfunction may occur in the absence of angiographic or ultrasound atherosclerosis in patients with risk factors for atherosclerosis. J Am Coll Cardiol 1994;23:833–843.
27. Kern MJ, Bach RG, Mechem CJ, et al. Variations in normal coronary vasodilatory reserve stratified by artery, gender, heart transplantation and coronary artery disease. J Am Coll Cardiol 1996;28:1154–1160.
28. Weiner DA, Ryan TJ, McCabe CH, et al. Exercise stress testing. Correlations among history of angina, ST-segment response and prevalence of coronary-artery disease in the Coronary Artery Aurgery Study (CASS). N Engl J Med 1979;301:230–235.
29. Elhendy A, van Domburg RT, Bax JJ, Roelandt JR. Gender differences in the relation between ST-T-wave abnormalities at baseline electrocardiogram and stress myocardial perfusion abnormalities in patients with suspected coronary artery disease. Am J Cardiol 1999;84:865–869.
30. Judelson DR. Examining the Gender Bias in Evaluating Coronary Disease in Women. Medscape Womens Health 1997;2:5.
31. Miller TD, Roger VL, Milavetz JJ, et al. Assessment of the exercise electrocardiogram in women versus men using tomographic myocardial perfusion imaging as the reference standard. Am J Cardiol 2001;87:868–873.
32. Shaw LJ, Hachamovitch R, Redberg RF. Current evidence on diagnostic testing in women with suspected coronary artery disease: choosing the appropriate test. Cardiol Rev 2000;8:65–74.
33. Marwick T. Current status of stress echocardiography in the diagnosis of coronary artery disease. Cleve Clin J Med 1995;62:227–234.
34. Baptista J, Arnese M, Roelandt JR, et al. Quantitative coronary angiography in the estimation of the functional significance of coronary stenosis: correlations with dobutamine-atropine stress test. J Am Coll Cardiol 1994;23:1434–1439.
35. Ho YL, Wu CC, Huang PJ, et al. Assessment of coronary artery disease in women by dobutamine stress echocardiography: comparison with stress thallium-201 single-photon emission computed tomography and exercise electrocardiography. Am Heart J 1998;135:655–662.
36. Davar JI, Roberts EB, Coghlan JG, Evans TR, Lipkin DP. Prognostic value of stress echocardiography in women with high (> or = 80%) probability of coronary artery disease. Postgrad Med J 2001;77:573–577.

37. Patterson RE, Churchwell KB, Eisner RL. Diagnosis of coronary artery disease in women: roles of three dimensional imaging with magnetic resonance or positron emission tomography. Am J Card Imaging 1996;10:78–88.

38. Collaborative overview of randomised trials of antiplatelet therapy—II: maintenance of vascular graft or arterial patency by antiplatelet therapy. Antiplatelet Trialists' Collaboration. BMJ 1994;308:159–168.

39. Lawlor DA, Bedford C, Taylor M, Ebrahim S. Aspirin use for the prevention of cardiovascular disease: the British Women's Heart and Health Study. Br J Gen Pract 2001;51:743–745.

40. Becker RC, Burns M, Gore JM, Lambrew C, French W, Rogers WJ. Early and pre-discharge aspirin administration among patients with acute myocardial infarction: current clinical practice and trends in the United States. J Thromb Thrombolysis 2000;9:207–215.

41. Kong DF, Califf RM, Miller DP, et al. Clinical outcomes of therapeutic agents that block the platelet glycoprotein IIb/IIIa integrin in ischemic heart disease [see comments]. Circulation 1998;98:2829–2835.

42. Goldschmidt-Clermont PJ, Schulman SP, Bray PF, et al. Refining the treatment of women with unstable angina—a randomized, double-blind, comparative safety and efficacy evaluation of Integrelin versus aspirin in the management of unstable angina. Clin Cardiol 1996;19:869–874.

43. Inhibition of the platelet glycoprotein IIb/IIIa receptor with tirofiban in unstable angina and non-Q-wave myocardial infarction. Platelet Receptor Inhibition in Ischemic Syndrome Management in Patients Limited by Unstable Signs and Symptoms (PRISM PLUS) Study Investigators. N Engl J Med 1998;338:1488–1497.

44. Inhibition of platelet glycoprotein IIb/IIIa with eptifibatide in patients with acute coronary syndromes. The PURSUIT Trial Investigators. Platelet Glycoprotein IIb/IIIa in Unstable Angina: Receptor Suppression Using Integrilin Therapy. N Engl J Med 1998;339:436–443.

45. Cho L, Topol EJ, Balog C, et al. Clinical benefit of glycoprotein IIb/IIIa blockade with Abciximab is independent of gender: pooled analysis from EPIC, EPILOG and EPISTENT trials. Evaluation of 7E3 for the Prevention of Ischemic Complications. Evaluation in Percutaneous Transluminal Coronary Angioplasty to Improve Long-Term Outcome with Abciximab GP IIb/IIIa blockade. Evaluation of Platelet IIb/IIIa Inhibitor for Stent. J Am Coll Cardiol 2000;36:381–386.

46. Randomised placebo-controlled and balloon-angioplasty-controlled trial to assess safety of coronary stenting with use of platelet glycoprotein-IIb/IIIa blockade. The EPISTENT Investigators. Evaluation of Platelet IIb/IIIa Inhibitor for Stenting [see comments]. Lancet 1998;352:87–92.

47. Topol EJ, Mark DB, Lincoff AM, et al. Outcomes at 1 year and economic implications of platelet glycoprotein IIb/IIIa blockade in patients undergoing coronary stenting: results from a multicentre randomised trial. EPISTENT Investigators. Evaluation of Platelet IIb/IIIa Inhibitor for Stenting [see comments] [published erratum appears in Lancet 2000 Mar 25;355(9209):1104]. Lancet 1999;354:2019–2024.

48. Cho L, Marso SP, Bhatt DL, Topol EJ. Optimizing percutaneous coronary revascularization in diabetic women: analysis from the EPISTENT trial [In Process Citation]. J Womens Health Gend Based Med 2000;9:741–746.

49. Randomised placebo-controlled trial of effect of eptifibatide on complications of percutaneous coronary intervention: IMPACT-II. Integrilin to Minimise Platelet Aggregation and Coronary Thrombosis-II [see comments]. Lancet 1997;349:1422–1428.

50. Kleiman NS, Califf RM. Results from late-breaking clinical trials sessions at ACCIS 2000 and ACC 2000. American College of Cardiology. J Am Coll Cardiol 2000;36:310–325.

51. Schrott HG, Bittner V, Vittinghoff E, Herrington DM, Hulley S. Adherence to National Cholesterol Education Program Treatment goals in postmenopausal women with heart disease. The Heart and Estrogen/Progestin Replacement Study (HERS). The HERS Research Group. Jama 1997;277:1281–1286.

52. McPherson RGJJ, Angus C, Murray P. The Women's Atorvastatin Trial on Cholesterol (WATCH): frequency of achieving NCEP-II target LDL-C levels in women with and without established CVD. 71st European Atherosclerosis Society Congress and Satellite Symposia. Athens, Greece, 1999.

53. Downs JR, Clearfield M, Weis S, et al. Primary prevention of acute coronary events with lovastatin in men and women with average cholesterol levels: results of AFCAPS/TexCAPS. Air Force/Texas Coronary Atherosclerosis Prevention Study. JAMA 1998;279:1615–1622.

54. Miettinen TA, Pyorala K, Olsson AG, et al. Cholesterol-lowering therapy in women and elderly patients with myocardial infarction or angina pectoris: findings from the Scandinavian Simvastatin Survival Study (4S). Circulation 1997;96:4211–4218.

55. Lewis SJ, Sacks FM, Mitchell JS, et al. Effect of pravastatin on cardiovascular events in women after myocardial infarction: the cholesterol and recurrent events (CARE) trial. J Am Coll Cardiol 1998;32: 140–146.

56. Stampfer MJ, Colditz GA. Estrogen replacement therapy and coronary heart disease: a quantitative assessment of the epidemiologic evidence. Prev Med 1991;20:47–63.

57. Gilligan DM, Badar DM, Panza JA, Quyyumi AA, Cannon RO 3rd. Acute vascular effects of estrogen in postmenopausal women. Circulation 1994;90:786–791.

58. Gilligan DM, Quyyumi AA, Cannon RO 3rd. Effects of physiological levels of estrogen on coronary vasomotor function in postmenopausal women. Circulation 1994;89:2545–2551.

59. Welty FK. Who Should Receive Hormone Replacement Therapy? J Thromb Thrombolysis 1996;3: 13–21.

60. Hulley S, Grady D, Bush T, et al. Randomized trial of estrogen plus progestin for secondary prevention of coronary heart disease in postmenopausal women. Heart and Estrogen/progestin Replacement Study (HERS) Research Group. JAMA 1998;280:605–613.

61. Folsom AR, Mink PJ, Sellers TA, Hong CP, Zheng W, Potter JD. Hormonal replacement therapy and morbidity and mortality in a prospective study of postmenopausal women. Am J Public Health 1995;85:1128–1132.

62. Herrington DM, Reboussin DM, Klein KP, et al. The estrogen replacement and atherosclerosis (ERA) study: study design and baseline characteristics of the cohort. Control Clin Trials 2000;21:257–285.

63. Ryan TJ, Antman EM, Brooks NH, et al. 1999 update: ACC/AHA guidelines for the management of patients with acute myocardial infarction. A report of the American College of Cardiology/American Heart Association Task Force on Practice Guidelines (Committee on Management of Acute Myocardial Infarction). J Am Coll Cardiol 1999;34:890–911.

64. Hachamovitch R, Berman DS, Kiat H, et al. Gender-related differences in clinical management after exercise nuclear testing. J Am Coll Cardiol 1995;26:1457–1464.

65. Tobin JN, Wassertheil-Smoller S, Wexler JP, et al. Sex bias in considering coronary bypass surgery. Ann Intern Med 1987;107:19–25.

66. Shaw LJ, Miller DD, Romeis JC, Kargl D, Younis LT, Chaitman BR. Gender differences in the noninvasive evaluation and management of patients with suspected coronary artery disease. Ann Intern Med 1994;120:559–566.

67. Steingart RM, Packer M, Hamm P, et al. Sex differences in the management of coronary artery disease. Survival and Ventricular Enlargement Investigators [see comments]. N Engl J Med 1991;325: 226–230.

68. Holdright DR, Fox KM. Characterization and identification of women with angina pectoris [published erratum appears in Eur Heart J 1996 Sep;17(9):1452]. Eur Heart J 1996;17:510–517.

69. Bell MR. Are there gender differences or issues related to angiographic imaging of the coronary arteries? Am J Card Imaging 1996;10:44–53.

70. Saha S, Stettin GD, Redberg RF. Gender and willingness to undergo invasive cardiac procedures. J Gen Intern Med 1999;14:122–125.

71. Bickell NA, Pieper KS, Lee KL, et al. Referral patterns for coronary artery disease treatment: gender bias or good clinical judgment? [see comments]. Ann Intern Med 1992;116:791–797.

72. Laskey WK. Gender differences in the management of coronary artery disease: bias or good clinical judgement? [editorial; comment]. Ann Intern Med 1992;116:869–871.

73. Bernstein SJ, Hilborne LH, Leape LL, Park RE, Brook RH. The appropriateness of use of cardiovascular procedures in women and men. Arch Intern Med 1994;154:2759–2765.

74. Mark DB, Shaw LK, DeLong ER, Califf RM, Pryor DB. Absence of sex bias in the referral of patients for cardiac catheterization [see comments]. N Engl J Med 1994;330:1101–1106.

75. Roeters van Lennep JE, Borm JJ, Zwinderman AH, Pauwels EK, Bruschke AV, van der Wall EE. No gender bias in referral for coronary angiography after myocardial perfusion scintigraphy with technetium-99m tetrofosmin. J Nucl Cardiol 1999;6:596–604.

76. Hochleitner M. Coronary heart disease: sexual bias in referral for coronary angiogram. How does it work in a state-run health system? J Womens Health Gend Based Med 2000;9:29–34.

77. Ayanian JZ, Epstein AM. Differences in the use of procedures between women and men hospitalized for coronary heart disease [see comments]. N Engl J Med 1991;325:221–225.

78. Maynard C, Litwin PE, Martin JS, Weaver WD. Gender differences in the treatment and outcome of acute myocardial infarction. Results from the Myocardial Infarction Triage and Intervention Registry. Arch Intern Med 1992;152:972–976.

79. Wong CC, Froelicher ES, Bacchetti P, et al. Influence of gender on cardiovascular mortality in acute myocardial infarction patients with high indication for coronary angiography. Circulation 1997;96:II-51–II-57.

80. Krumholz HM, Douglas PS, Lauer MS, Pasternak RC. Selection of patients for coronary angiography and coronary revascularization early after myocardial infarction: is there evidence for a gender bias? [see comments]. Ann Intern Med 1992;116:785–790.

81. Kilaru PK, Kelly RF, Calvin JE, Parrillo JE. Utilization of coronary angiography and revascularization after acute myocardial infarction in men and women risk stratified by the American College of Cardiology/American Heart Association guidelines. J Am Coll Cardiol 2000;35:974–979.

82. Philippides GJ, Jacobs AK. Coronary angioplasty and surgical revascularization: emerging concepts. Cardiology 1995;86:324–338.

83. Jacobs AK, Kelsey SF, Yeh W, et al. Documentation of decline in morbidity in women undergoing coronary angioplasty (a report from the 1993-94 NHLBI Percutaneous Transluminal Coronary Angioplasty Registry). National Heart, Lung, and Blood Institute. Am J Cardiol 1997;80:979–984.

84. Abramov D, Tamariz MG, Sever JY, et al. The influence of gender on the outcome of coronary artery bypass surgery. Ann Thorac Surg 2000;70:800–806.

85. Aldea GS, Gaudiani JM, Shapira OM, et al. Effect of gender on postoperative outcomes and hospital stays after coronary artery bypass grafting. Ann Thorac Surg 1999;67:1097–1103.

86. Capdeville M, Chamogeogarkis T, Lee JH. Effect of gender on outcomes of beating heart operations. Ann Thorac Surg 2001;72:S1022–S1025.

87. Edwards FH, Carey JS, Grover FL, Bero JW, Hartz RS. Impact of gender on coronary bypass operative mortality. Ann Thorac Surg 1998;66:125–131.

88. Williams MR, Choudhri AF, Morales DL, Helman DN, Oz MC. Gender differences in patients undergoing coronary artery bypass surgery, from a mandatory statewide database. J Gend Specif Med 2000; 3:41–48.

89. Alfonso F, Hernandez R, Banuelos C, et al. Initial results and long-term clinical and angiographic outcome of coronary stenting in women. Am J Cardiol 2000;86:1380–1383.

90. Mehilli J, Kastrati A, Dirschinger J, Bollwein H, Neumann FJ, Schomig A. Differences in prognostic factors and outcomes between women and men undergoing coronary artery stenting. JAMA 2000;284: 1799–1805.

91. Peterson ED, Lansky AJ, Kramer J, Anstrom K, Lanzilotta MJ. Effect of gender on the outcomes of contemporary percutaneous coronary intervention. Am J Cardiol 2001;88:359–364.

92. Robertson T, Kennard ED, Mehta S, et al. Influence of gender on in-hospital clinical and angiographic outcomes and on one-year follow-up in the New Approaches to Coronary Intervention (NACI) registry. Am J Cardiol 1997;80:26K–39K.

93. Welty FK, Lewis SM, Kowalker W, Shubrooks SJ Jr. Reasons for higher in-hospital mortality >24 hours after percutaneous transluminal coronary angioplasty in women compared with men. Am J Cardiol 2001;88:473–477.

94. Davis KB, Chaitman B, Ryan T, Bittner V, Kennedy JW. Comparison of 15-year survival for men and women after initial medical or surgical treatment for coronary artery disease: a CASS registry study. Coronary Artery Surgery Study. J Am Coll Cardiol 1995;25:1000–1009.

95. Mendes LA, Davidoff R, Cupples LA, Ryan TJ, Jacobs AK. Congestive heart failure in patients with coronary artery disease: the gender paradox. Am Heart J 1997;134:207–212.

96. Malenka DJ, O'Connor GT, Quinton H, et al. Differences in outcomes between women and men associated with percutaneous transluminal coronary angioplasty. A regional prospective study of 13,061 procedures. Northern New England Cardiovascular Disease Study Group. Circulation 1996;94:II99–II104.

97. Kelsey SF, James M, Holubkov AL, Holubkov R, Cowley MJ, Detre KM. Results of percutaneous transluminal coronary angioplasty in women. 1985–1986 National Heart, Lung, and Blood Institute's Coronary Angioplasty Registry [see comments]. Circulation 1993;87:720–727.

98. Davies MJ. The composition of coronary-artery plaques [editorial; comment]. N Engl J Med 1997;336: 1312–1314.

99. Mautner SL, Lin F, Mautner GC, Roberts WC. Comparison in women versus men of composition of atherosclerotic plaques in native coronary arteries and in saphenous veins used as aortocoronary conduits. J Am Coll Cardiol 1993;21:1312–1318.

100. Sullivan AK, Holdright DR, Wright CA, Sparrow JL, Cunningham D, Fox KM. Chest pain in women: clinical, investigative, and prognostic features. BMJ 1994;308:883–886.

101. Jong P, Mohammed S, Sternberg L. Sex differences in the features of coronary artery disease of patients undergoing coronary angiography [published erratum appears in Can J Cardiol 1996 Sep;12(9):781]. Can J Cardiol 1996;12:671–677.

102. O'Connor GT, Morton JR, Diehl MJ, et al. Differences between men and women in hospital mortality associated with coronary artery bypass graft surgery. The Northern New England Cardiovascular Disease Study Group. Circulation 1993;88:2104–2110.

103. Weintraub WS, Wenger NK, Jones EL, Craver JM, Guyton RA. Changing clinical characteristics of coronary surgery patients. Differences between men and women. Circulation 1993;88:II79–II86.

104. Christakis GT, Weisel RD, Buth KJ, et al. Is body size the cause for poor outcomes of coronary artery bypass operations in women? J Thorac Cardiovasc Surg 1995;110:1344–1358.

105. Jacobs AK, Kelsey SF, Brooks MM, et al. Better outcome for women compared with men undergoing coronary revascularization: a report from the bypass angioplasty revascularization investigation (BARI) [see comments]. Circulation 1998;98:1279–1285.

106. Abramov D, Tamariz MG, Fremes SE, et al. Trends in coronary artery bypass surgery results: a recent, 9-year study. Ann Thorac Surg 2000;70:84–90.

107. Petro KR, Dullum MK, Garcia JM, et al. Minimally invasive coronary revascularization in women: a safe approach for a high-risk group. Heart Surg Forum 2000;3:41–46.

108. Cowley MJ, Mullin SM, Kelsey SF, et al. Sex differences in early and long-term results of coronary angioplasty in the NHLBI PTCA Registry. Circulation 1985;71:90–97.

109. Greenberg MA, Mueller HS. Why the excess mortality in women after PTCA? [editorial; comment]. Circulation 1993;87:1030–1032.

110. Airaksinen KE, Ikaheimo MJ, Linnaluoto M, Tahvanainen KU, Huikuri HV. Gender difference in autonomic and hemodynamic reactions to abrupt coronary occlusion. J Am Coll Cardiol 1998;31:301–306.

111. Mehilli J, Kastrati A, Dirschinger J, Bollwein H, Neumann FJ, Schomig A. Differences in prognostic factors and outcomes between women and men undergoing coronary artery stenting. JAMA 2000;284: 1799–1805.

112. Kim C, Schaaf CH, Maynard C, Every NR. Unstable angina in the myocardial infarction triage and intervention registry (MITI): short- and long-term outcomes in men and women. Am Heart J 2001; 141:73–77.

113. Scirica BM, Moliterno DJ, Every NR, et al. Differences between men and women in the management of unstable angina pectoris (The GUARANTEE Registry). The GUARANTEE Investigators. Am J Cardiol 1999;84:1145–1150.

114. Passos LC, Lopes AA, Costa U, Lobo N, Rabelo Junior A. Difference in the in-hospital mortality of unstable angina pectoris between men and women. Arq Bras Cardiol 1999;72:669–676.

115. Roger VL, Farkouh ME, Weston SA, et al. Sex differences in evaluation and outcome of unstable angina. JAMA 2000;283:646–652.

116. Kannel WB, Sorlie P, McNamara PM. Prognosis after initial myocardial infarction: the Framingham study. Am J Cardiol 1979;44:53–59.

117. Becker RC, Terrin M, Ross R, et al. Comparison of clinical outcomes for women and men after acute myocardial infarction. The Thrombolysis in Myocardial Infarction Investigators. Ann Intern Med 1994;120:638–645.

118. Tofler GH, Stone PH, Muller JE, Braunwald E. Mortality for women after acute myocardial infarction: MILIS Study Group. Am J Cardiol 1989;64:256.

119. Tofler GH, Stone PH, Muller JE, et al. Effects of gender and race on prognosis after myocardial infarction: adverse prognosis for women, particularly black women. J Am Coll Cardiol 1987;9:473–482.

120. Barakat K, Wilkinson P, Suliman A, Ranjadayalan K, Timmis A. Acute myocardial infarction in women: contribution of treatment variables to adverse outcome. Am Heart J 2000;140:740–746.

121. Gan SC, Beaver SK, Houck PM, MacLehose RF, Lawson HW, Chan L. Treatment of acute myocardial infarction and 30-day mortality among women and men. N Engl J Med 2000;343:8–15.

122. Cariou A, Himbert D, Golmard JL, et al. Sex-related differences in eligibility for reperfusion therapy and in-hospital outcome after acute myocardial infarction. Eur Heart J 1997;18:1583–1589.

123. Woodfield SL, Lundergan CF, Reiner JS, et al. Gender and acute myocardial infarction: is there a different response to thrombolysis? J Am Coll Cardiol 1997;29:35–42.

124. Weitzman S, Cooper L, Chambless L, et al. Gender, racial, and geographic differences in the performance of cardiac diagnostic and therapeutic procedures for hospitalized acute myocardial infarction in four states. Am J Cardiol 1997;79:722–726.

125. Hendricks AS, Goodman B, Stein JH, Carnes M. Gender differences in acute myocardial infarction: the University of Wisconsin experience. WMJ 1999;98:30–36.

126. Mahon NG, McKenna CJ, Codd MB, O'Rorke C, McCann HA, Sugrue DD. Gender differences in the management and outcome of acute myocardial infarction in unselected patients in the thrombolytic era. Am J Cardiol 2000;85:921–926.

127. Garg S, Nashed AH, Roche LM. Fibrinolytic therapy in young women with acute myocardial infarction. Ann Emerg Med 1999;33:646–651.

128. Vermeer F. Thrombolytic therapy in patients of female gender. Thromb Res 2001;103(Suppl. 1): S101–S104.

129. Moen EK, Asher CR, Miller DP, et al. Long-term follow-up of gender-specific outcomes after thrombolytic therapy for acute myocardial infarction from the GUSTO-I trial. Global Utilization of Streptokinase and Tissue Plasminogen Activator for Occluded Coronary Arteries. J Womens Health 1997; 6:285–293.

130. Karnash SL, Granger CB, White HD, Woodlief LH, Topol EJ, Califf RM. Treating menstruating women with thrombolytic therapy: insights from the global utilization of streptokinase and tissue plasminogen activator for occluded coronary arteries (GUSTO-I) trial. J Am Coll Cardiol 1995;26:1651–1656.

131. Grines CL, Browne KF, Marco J, et al. A comparison of immediate angioplasty with thrombolytic therapy for acute myocardial infarction. The Primary Angioplasty in Myocardial Infarction Study Group [see comments]. N Engl J Med 1993;328:673–679.

132. Zijlstra F, de Boer MJ, Hoorntje JC, Reiffers S, Reiber JH, Suryapranata H. A comparison of immediate coronary angioplasty with intravenous streptokinase in acute myocardial infarction [see comments]. N Engl J Med 1993;328:680–684.

133. Weaver WD, Simes RJ, Betriu A, et al. Comparison of primary coronary angioplasty and intravenous thrombolytic therapy for acute myocardial infarction: a quantitative review [see comments] [published erratum appears in JAMA 1998 Jun 17;279(23):1876]. JAMA 1997,278.2093–2098.

134. Michels KB, Yusuf S. Does PTCA in acute myocardial infarction affect mortality and reinfarction rates? A quantitative overview (meta-analysis) of the randomized clinical trials [see comments]. Circulation 1995;91:476–485.

135. Rathore SS, Weinfurt KP, Oetgen WJ, Gersh BJ, Schulman KA. Refusal of catheterization during acute myocardial infarction: influence of patient characteristics. J Am Coll Cardiol 1999;33:356A.

136. Stone GW, Grines CL, Browne KF, et al. Predictors of in-hospital and 6-month outcome after acute myocardial infarction in the reperfusion era. the Primary Angioplasty in Myocardial Infarction (PAMI) trail. J Am Coll Cardiol 1995;25:370–377.

137. Stone GW, Grines CL, Browne KF, et al. Influence of acute myocardial infarction location on in-hospital and late outcome after primary percutaneous transluminal coronary angioplasty versus tissue plasminogen activator therapy. Am J Cardiol 1996;78:19–25.

138. van't Hof AW, Liem A, Suryapranata H, Hoorntje JC, de Boer MJ, Zijlstra F. Clinical presentation and outcome of patients with early, intermediate and late reperfusion therapy by primary coronary angioplasty for acute myocardial infarction. Eur Heart J 1998;19:118–123.

139. Grines CL, Cox DA, Stone GW, et al. Coronary angioplasty with or without stent implantation for acute myocardial infarction. Stent Primary Angioplasty in Myocardial Infarction Study Group [see comments]. N Engl J Med 1999;341:1949–1956.

140. Antoniucci D, Valenti R, Moschi G, et al. Sex-based differences in clinical and angiographic outcomes after primary angioplasty or stenting for acute myocardial infarction. Am J Cardiol 2001;87: 289–293.

141. Keelan ET, Nunez BD, Grill DE, Berger PB, Holmes DR Jr, Bell MR. Comparison of immediate and long-term outcome of coronary angioplasty performed for unstable angina and rest pain in men and women [see comments]. Mayo Clin Proc 1997;72:5–12.

142. Hochman JS, McCabe CH, Stone PH, et al. Outcome and profile of women and men presenting with acute coronary syndromes: a report from TIMI IIIB. TIMI Investigators. Thrombolysis in Myocardial Infarction. J Am Coll Cardiol 1997;30:141–148.

143. Scirica BM, Moliterno DJ, Every NR, et al. Differences between men and women in the management of unstable angina pectoris (The GUARANTEE Registry). The GUARANTEE Investigators. Am J Cardiol 1999;84:1145–1150.

144. Gowda MS, Vacek JL, Hallas D. Gender-related risk factors and outcomes for non-Q wave myocardial infarction patients receiving in-hospital PTCA. J Invasive Cardiol 1999;11:121–126.

145. Wong SC, Sanborn T, Sleeper LA, et al. Angiographic findings and clinical correlates in patients with cardiogenic shock complicating acute myocardial infarction: a report from the SHOCK Trial Registry. SHould we emergently revascularize Occluded Coronaries for cardiogenic shocK? J Am Coll Cardiol 2000;36:1077–1083.

146. Berger PB, Tuttle RH, Holmes DR Jr, et al. One-year survival among patients with acute myocardial infarction complicated by cardiogenic shock, and its relation to early revascularization: results from the GUSTO-I trial. Circulation 1999;99:873–878.

147. Hochman JS, Sleeper LA, Godfrey E, et al. SHould we emergently revascularize Occluded Coronaries for cardiogenic shocK: an international randomized trial of emergency PTCA/CABG-trial design. The SHOCK Trial Study Group. Am Heart J 1999;137:313–321.

148. Hochman JS, Sleeper LA, Webb JG, et al. Early revascularization in acute myocardial infarction complicated by cardiogenic shock. SHOCK Investigators. Should We Emergently Revascularize Occluded Coronaries for Cardiogenic Shock [see comments]. N Engl J Med 1999;341:625–634.

149. Hochman JS, Buller CE, Sleeper LA, et al. Cardiogenic shock complicating acute myocardial infarction—etiologies, management and outcome: a report from the SHOCK Trial Registry. SHould we emergently revascularize Occluded Coronaries for cardiogenic shocK? J Am Coll Cardiol 2000;36: 1063–1070.

150. Thompson CR, Buller CE, Sleeper LA, et al. Cardiogenic shock due to acute severe mitral regurgitation complicating acute myocardial infarction: a report from the SHOCK Trial Registry. Should we use emergently revascularize Occluded Coronaries in cardiogenic shocK? J Am Coll Cardiol 2000;36: 1104–1109.

151. Menon V, White H, LeJemtel T, Webb JG, Sleeper LA, Hochman JS. The clinical profile of patients with suspected cardiogenic shock due to predominant left ventricular failure: a report from the SHOCK Trial Registry. SHould we emergently revascularize Occluded Coronaries in cardiogenic shocK? J Am Coll Cardiol 2000;36:1071–1076.

152. Shindler DM, Palmeri ST, Antonelli TA, et al. Diabetes mellitus in cardiogenic shock complicating acute myocardial infarction: a report from the SHOCK Trial Registry. SHould we emergently revascularize Occluded Coronaries for cardiogenic shocK? J Am Coll Cardiol 2000;36:1097–1103.

21

The Modern Strategy for Cardiogenic Shock

Gary E. Lane, MD *and*
David R. Holmes Jr., MD

CONTENTS

INTRODUCTION

Although emergency cardiac care resources are oriented toward rapid implementation of reperfusion therapy with resultant myocardial salvage and improvement in survival, cardiogenic shock remains the leading cause of death among hospitalized patients with acute myocardial infarction (Fig. 1) *(1–5)*.

In the past several years important information has emerged from analysis of patients with cardiogenic shock in thrombolytic therapy trials and through prospective registries of patients with infarction. The role of reperfusion therapy in cardiogenic shock has been further clarified with the publication of the important Should We Emergently Revascularize Occluded Coronaries for Cardiogenic Shock (SHOCK) trial *(6)*.

This review will discuss the modern concepts and controversies regarding the management of cardiogenic shock occurring as a result of myocardial damage in the setting of acute myocardial infarction.

From: *Contemporary Cardiology: Management of Acute Coronary Syndromes, Second Edition*
Edited by: C. P. Cannon © Humana Press Inc., Totowa, NJ

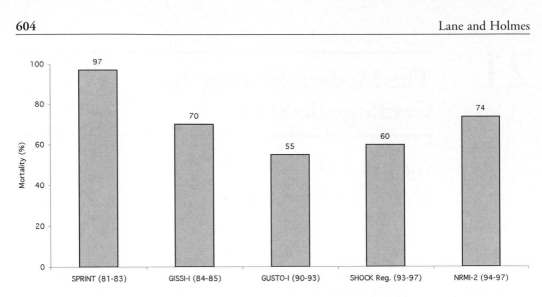

Fig. 1. Hospital mortality rates from trials/registries over the past 2 decades *(1–5)*.

DEFINITION AND RECOGNITION

Circulatory shock describes a state of tissue hypoperfusion. In the setting of an acute ischemic event (usually myocardial infarction) the "shock" state may arise from cardiogenic or noncardiogenic mechanisms. Noncardiogenic causes occurring in the setting of myocardial infarction include adverse effects of pharmacologic agents such as nitrates, angiotensin-converting enzyme inhibitors, and other vasodilator drugs. Hypotension may also arise during the infusion of thrombolytic agents such as streptokinase. Hemorrhagic shock may occur secondary to gastrointestinal or occult retroperitoneal bleeding as most patients receive anticoagulant and/or thrombolytic agents. Massive pulmonary emboli can result in circulatory shock. A tension pneumothorax may result from mechanical ventilation or after cardiac arrest. Hypovolemia should always be considered as a result of diaphoresis, vomiting, and overdiuresis. Sepsis can result in a shock state in patients with other comorbid illnesses.

Cardiogenic etiologies of shock may occur in the setting of myocardial infarction independent of myocardial damage. Tachyarrhythmias such as ventricular tachycardia and rapid atrial fibrillation require prompt correction in the setting of hypotension. Hypotension may not only arise from direct effects of thrombolytic agents but have also resulted from hemopericardium with tamponade without identifiable rupture *(7)*. Ascending aortic dissection can lead to the complex of pericardial tamponade and myocardial infarction. Associated cardiac conditions such as significant aortic stenosis, may importantly contribute to the development of shock. Excessive vagal tone can result in hypotension in the early phase of infarction commonly in association with bradycardia although isolated hypotension can occur from this accentuated cardiac reflex *(8)*.

Direct myocardial damage may lead to a heterogeneous group of derangements resulting in circulatory shock. Pump failure from extensive left ventricular damage is the primary cause of cardiogenic shock. Mechanical defects as a direct result of myocardial injury occur less commonly and include papillary muscle dysfunction/rupture, ventricular septal defect, and free wall myocardial rupture with tamponade. Right ventricular infarction with an accompanying left ventricular infarction may also lead to shock.

Clinical recognition of circulatory shock includes identifying manifestations of a low cardiac output such cyanosis, cool extremities, altered mental status, and oliguria in the setting of hypotension. These findings with concomitant pulmonary edema establish relatively confirmatory evidence for cardiogenic shock. However, hemodynamic monitoring allows diagnostic confirmation and can guide management decisions. The hemodynamic manifestations of cardiogenic shock include a systolic blood pressure <90 mmHg (or >30 mmHg below basal levels), an elevated pulmonary capillary wedge pressure >15 mmHg, and a reduced cardiac index <2.2 L/min/m^2 .

EPIDEMIOLOGY

Examination of several investigations elucidates the circumstances of cardiogenic shock. The incidence of cardiogenic shock was reported in 1954 to occur in 19.7% of 816 patients admitted with acute myocardial infarction (9). Killip and Kimball described shock in 19% of 250 patients seen in a single cardiac care unit (CCU) over a 2-yr period (10). Later information derived from trials conducted before the reperfusion era identified an incidence of 6.4% in the Secondary Prevention Reinfarction Israeli Nifedipine Trial (SPRINT) registry (1) and 6.5% in the Multicenter Investigation of the Limitation Infarct Size (MILIS) trial (11). The long-term population-based Worcester Heart Attack Study determined the incidence of cardiogenic shock during 11 1-yr periods between 1975–1997 (12). The overall incidence average 7.1%. After adjustment for potentially confounding risk factors, there was no significant change in the proportion of patients with shock over the study period. Of the 426,253 patients reported in the second National Registry of Myocardial Infarction (NRMI) registry the incidence of cardiogenic shock averaged 6.2% with only a slight decline noted between 1994 (6.6%) and 1997 (6.0%) (5).

Several trials of thrombolytic therapy have reported this complication. Shock was identified in 7% in International Study of Infarct Survival (ISIS)-3 and 7.2% of the Global Utilization of Streptokinase and Tissue Plasminogen Activator for Occluded Coronary Arteries (GUSTO)-I trial patients (3,13). In contrast, shock was reported in 5.2% of patients enrolled in GUSTO-III, which compared tissue-type plasminogen activator (tPA) to recombinant plasminogen activator (rPA) and 4.0% in the Anglo-Scandinavian Study of Early Thrombolysis (ASSENT-2) trial which compared tPA against tenecteplase (TNK) (14,15).

There is considerable reported variability in the temporal onset of shock in the course of infarction. This is significantly influenced by the study conditions. In the era preceding widespread use of reperfusion therapy, cardiogenic shock was reported on presentation in 4.5% among 2931 patients in the MILIS trial (7.1% developed shock during hospitalization) (11). In the SPRINT registry 2.6% (24% of shock patients) of 3465 patiets admitted in Killip class I developed shock at an average of 4 ± 4 (median 2) d after admission (1). In contrast, cardiogenic shock occurred after admission (most within 48 h) in 89% of 2972 patients in the GUSTO-I trial (3). However, early shock may be underestimated in thrombolytic trials due to entry criteria, difficulties with informed consent in critically ill patients, and physician bias regarding management strategy.

In the Israeli Thrombolytic Survey Group 56% of 254 patients presented in cardiogenic shock (16). Of the 26,280 patients with cardiogenic shock reported in the NRMI-2 registry 28% presented with shock on admission (5).

Table 1
Temporal Onset of Shock and Mortality Related to Culprit Vessel in Shock Registry *(17,18)*

Infarct related vessel	MI onset → shock (median hours)	Hospital mortality (%)
Left main	1.7	78.6
Right coronay artery	3.5	37.4
Left circumflex	3.9	42.4
Left anterior descending	11	42.3
Saphenous vein graft	10.9	69.7

MI, myocardial infarction.

In the SHOCK trial registry shock due to left ventricular failure developed at a median of 6.2 h after infarction symptom onset and at median 4.6 h after hospital admission *(17)*. In this registry (45% were transferred from outside hospitals), 9% were in shock on arrival, and shock developed within 6 h in 46% and by 24 h in 74%. The significant proportion of patients developing shock after admission emphasizes the value of early identification and intervention in an attempt to impact the ominous prognosis.

The classification of patients into pre- or postadmission shock does reveal important differences in the anatomy and pathophysiology of shock development. In the SHOCK registry early shock was more often associated with multilead ST-elevation and multiple electrocardiogram (ECG) infarct locations *(17)*. The median time to onset of shock was shortest in those with a culprit left main coronary occlusion (1.7 h), which was significantly shorter than with other locations (Table 1) *(17,18)*. Furthermore, the mortality was higher (62.6 vs 53.6%) with early (<24 h) vs late (>24 h) shock, however almost half of the patients were transferred form other institutions. In contrast, the 30-d mortality of patients classified as preadmission shock was lower (69 vs 87%) than those developing shock after hospital admission in the Israeli Thrombolytic Survey Group *(16)*.

Mechanical complications of infarction account for shock in a minority of patients. The distribution of causes of shock in the SHOCK registry are depicted in Fig. 2 *(4)*. Women had a significantly higher incidence of mechanical complications *(19)*. Although mechanical complications occur in a distinct minority of patients, they must be excluded in the early management of patients with shock.

THE PATHOPHYSIOLOGY OF CARDIOGENIC
SHOCK FROM MYOCARDIAL INFARCTION

A comprehensive understanding of the pathophysiologic characteristics and events of cardiogenic shock must be attained to impact the discouraging outcome of patients with this entity. The assiduous hemodynamic decline involves several interactive processes.

Early (initial 60 min) in the course of infarction autonomic disturbances have a predominant influence on a patient's hemodynamic status. As reported by Webb et al. *(8)* sympathetic overactivity (tachycardia and hypertension) occurred in 36% of patients (monitored within 30–60 min of infarction onset). However, the majority (55%) exhibited bradyarrhythmias and/or hypotension. This is a manifestation of the Bezold-Jarish reflex *(20)*, which is expressed commonly during acute inferior-posterior infarction

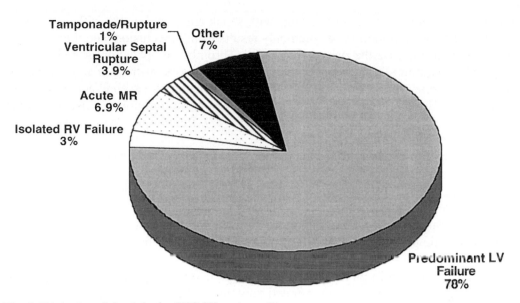

Fig. 2. Etiologies of shock in the SHOCK registry *(4)*.

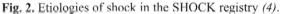

(77%). Webb and colleagues also noted vagal effects in 32% of anterior infarctions. The likely mechanism of this response involves a mechanical stimulus of vagal afferents probably from systolic bulging of ischemic myocardium which results in vasodilation and bradycardia with additional inhibition of the arterial baroreflex *(8,20,21)*.

An intravascular volume deficit has been recognized in up to 20% of patients with cardiogenic shock *(22)*. This would be characterized as a Killip or hemodynamic class III state. Relative hypovolemia is most commonly encountered in the setting of right ventricular infarction. It has been shown that left ventricular performance is optimal during infarction with a pulmonary capillary wedge pressure of 14–18 mmHg *(23)*. Although vol infusion can restore class I status to some patients initially categorized in class III, the majority do not appreciably improve reflecting evidence of primary cardiac compromise *(24)*. In the SHOCK trial registry, 31% of patients presenting with shock did not exhibit signs of pulmonary congestion by radiographic or physical examination. Notably, the 28% of patients with clinical hypoperfusion without pulmonary congestion had a mean pulmonary capillary wedge pressure of 21.5 ± 6.7 mmHg vs 24.3 ± 8.1 mmHg in patients with hypoperfusion and pulmonary congestion. The hospital mortality in each of these groups was high at 70 and 60%, respectively *(25)*.

The early development of cardiogenic shock in the course of infarction most commonly results from the loss of a large amount of myocardium. Autopsy studies have demonstrated that shock typically occurs after damage to ≥35–40% of left ventricular muscle *(26–28)*. This may result from occlusion at a perilous site within a single coronary artery supplying a large region of myocardium or from cumulative damage after previous infarction. The elimination of the collateral function of an infarct-related artery could significantly enhance the destructive effect of a single vessel occlusion.

Later in the course, extension of infarct damage may occur as a result of multiple mechanisms. Infarct extension or reinfarction identified by enzyme elevation was reported in 23.3% of patients developing cardiogenic shock by the MILIS study group, compared with 7.4% of patients without shock ($p < 0.001$) *(11)*. In the GUSTO-I trial, reinfarction occurred in 11% of patients with shock compared to 3% without shock (p < 0.001) (3). Reinfarction most commonly results from reocclusion, and this event has been shown to increase the risk of shock (29). Thrombus propagation or embolization might also result in reinfarction. Passive collapse and vasoconstriction at a second site within the coronary circulation can also result in ischemia or a second acute infarction (30). In the SHOCK registry, recurrent ischemia was more common in those with shock of late onset (>24 h) (38 vs 13.2%, p < 0.001) (17). Reinfarction was seen equally in early and late shock (8.2 and 8.3%).

Extension of infarction into the border zone in a subepicardial or lateral direction has been documented pathologically in the majority of patients with cardiogenic shock in some series (26,27). Factors which could adversely extend infarction into the border zone include impaired collateral flow, increased myocardial oxygen consumption by sympathetic activation or inotropic agents, changes in the balance of arterial driving pressure (aortic pressure—left ventricular diastolic pressure) from hypotension or congestive failure, and the possibility of reperfusion injury.

The phenomenon of reperfusion injury remains controversial (31–33). Investigation in experimental models has demonstrated pathologic evidence for progression to irreversible injury of viable myocardium in reperfused infarct zones and reduction of infarct size with agents that modify reperfusion injury. However, data are lacking to corroborate the importance of this phenomenon in a clinical situation. In fact, the GUSTO-I trial demonstration that rapid achievement of thrombolysis in myocardial infarction (TIMI) grade 3 flow by thrombolysis results in the lowest mortality would suggest that reperfusion injury is unlikely to have an important effect on outcome (34).

The pathologic picture of cardiogenic shock is characterized by progressive myocardial necrosis with an irregular extension of infarction not only into the border zone, but with focal regions of necrosis throughout both the left and right ventricles (26,27). This latter form of extension is a reflection of the hemodynamic state as it can be seen with other etiologies of circulatory shock.

Hypotension leads to ongoing myocardial injury. This progressive myocardial necrosis is confirmed by observation of a persistent elevation of creatine kinase isoenzyme-cardiac muscle subunit (CK-MB) (35). Left ventricular function is further impaired by the inefficiency of infarct zone expansion leading to increased wall stress (36). This progressive cardiac dysfunction leads to a "vicious cycle" of hypotension, declining coronary perfusion, and deteriorating left ventricular function culminating in an irreversible shock state. This shock state is potentiated by maladaptive compensatory mechanisms including sympathetic stimulation, fluid retention, and vasoconstriction. Lactic acidosis further impairs myocardial function.

In addition to ischemia-induced myocardial necrosis, recent data suggests a role for apoptosis in myocyte cell death during myocardial infarction. This process appears to predominate in areas of acutely distended myocardium remote form the infarct area or in the border zone in myocytes that are not rescued (37,38).

As stated earlier in this section, shock typically occurs when ≥35–40% of the left ventricular muscle is involved. There is not a threshold level of damage for defining patients with cardiogenic shock. A series of 16 patients with final infarct sizes of >40% of the left ventricle quantitated by Technetium-99m sestamibi tomography reported a 94% survival with development of cardiogenic shock in only one patient (39).

The variable neurohumoral response to left ventricular dysfuntion has often been implicated to explain the discrepancies in the clinical manifestations of similar size infarctions. However, the function of myocardium remote from the infarct region plays a pivotal role in hemodynamic response and has been recognized to be of considerable prognostic importance *(40)*. Normally the noninfarct segments become hyperkinetic. An absence of hyperkinesis or asynergy of noninfarcted regions identify patients at high risk for early mortality *(41)*. Diffuse hypokinesis has been recognized as a distinguishing feature for the development of cardiogenic shock in patients with similar size infarctions by echocardiography *(42)*.

The corollary of abnormal remote myocardial function is multivessel coronary artery disease. In two autopsy series of patients dying from cardiogenic shock, 2 or 3 vessel disease (>75% obstruction) was identified in all patients *(42,43)*. The left anterior descending artery is predominantly involved. Angiographic studies have reported left main and/or multivessel disease in 60 90% of patients with cardiogenic shock *(18,42,44–48)*. The SHOCK registry reported multivessel disease in 77% (2 vessel disease, 21%; 3 vessel disease, 56%) with significant (≥50%) left main disease in 16.2% of patients with ventricular failure *(18)*. The left anterior descending is the predominant culprit vessel in patients with left ventricular power failure (Fig. 3).

A canine model of myocardial infarction simulating the presence of single or multi-vessel disease illustrates the devastating effect of additional coronary obstructive disease remote from the infarct artery. Beyersdorf et al. *(49)* demonstrated that, although animals with isolated left anterior descending occlusion exhibited a 100% 6-h survival of the acute infarction, those with a coexistent 50% left circumflex stenosis suffered a 57% mortality from cardiogenic shock or intractable ventricular fibrillation.

Shock can also result from distinct cardiac structural damage with a less extensive left ventricular infarction. Right ventricular infarction can be detected in 40–50% of patients with left ventricular inferior infarction. A deficit of right ventricular pump function from proximal occlusion of the right coronary artery leads to a decline in left ventricular preload as the principle mechanism of the shock state seen in approx 10% of patients with inferior wall infarction. The right ventricle dilates, and the pericardium further constrains left ventricular filling, resulting in hemodynamic parameters similar to pericardial constriction (diastolic equalization, right ventricle dip/plateau pressure configuration and ventricular interdependence). Abnormal interventricular septal function shifts toward the left ventricle in diastole contributing to the low-output state *(50)*. Significant left ventricular damage is common with a clinically evident right ventricular infarction *(51)*.

Rupture of the ventricular free wall, interventricular septum, and papillary muscle represent the major mechanical complications of myocardial infarction. These complications result from necrosis of critical cardiac structures and share a similar pathophysiological substrate. They have been commonly associated with a first myocardial infarction *(52–56)*. The infarction is usually small to moderate in size in patients with free wall or papillary muscle rupture *(28,52)*. The majority of studies have reported less extensive coronary artery disease in patients with these complications compared to other patients with infarction *(52,54,55,57)*. It has been proposed that patients with more severe coronary artery disease and left ventricular dysfunction cannot generate sufficient contractile stress to produce cardiac rupture. Infarct expansion has been demonstrated to be a harbinger of myocardial rupture *(58)*.

Left Ventricular Failure

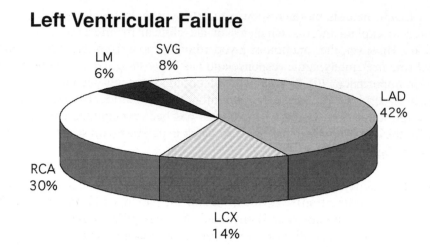

Mechanical Complications

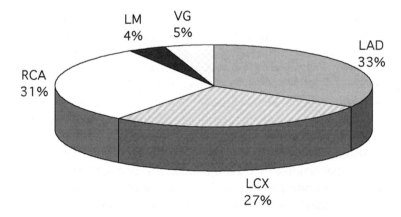

Fig. 3. The culprit vessel distribution in patients with ventricular failure and mechanical complication etiologies of cardiogenic shock in the SHOCK Trial registry. (LAD = left anterior descending; LCX, left circumflex; RCA, right coronary artery; LM, left main.

Controversy remains over the possible accentuation of cardiac rupture by thrombolytic therapy *(59)*. Honan et al. *(60)* reporting a meta-analysis of clinical trials suggested that while early thrombolysis decreases the risk of cardiac rupture, late therapy may enhance this potential complication. However, Late Assessment of Thrombolytic Efficacy (LATE) trial results did not show an increased risk of rupture in patients treated >12 h from onset, but thrombolysis did accelerate the time to rupture *(61)*. In a report from the NRMI participants, data suggested that thrombolysis accelerated myocardial rupture typically within 24–48 h *(62)*. Furthermore, the median time from myocardial infarction onset to diagnosis of interventricular septal rupture was 1 d in the GUSTO-I trial *(63)*. Significantly, it has been shown that patients with cardiac rupture almost uniformly exhibit ineffective perfusion of the infarct artery *(64)*.

Rupture of the free wall of the left ventricle can occur with left and, less commonly, right ventricular infarction *(28,65)*. Rupture usually results from a transmural infarction

(28). Free wall rupture is often a sudden catastrophic event culminating in electro-mechanical dissociation and death. However a subacute presentation (approx 20%) man-ifested as hypotension, and right heart failure has been recognized perhaps representing an initial small hemopericadial accumulation *(66,67).* Patients may exhibit a transient episode of hypotension and bradycardia portending death in minutes to days.

The reported distribution of infarct location with an acute ventricular septal defect has been variable although more recent reports suggest a predominance of inferior wall involvement *(68–70).* A simple direct perforation or complex serpentine tracts may com-municate between the two ventricles. The hemodynamic derangement is usually more substantial with inferior infarction reflecting associated right ventricular involvement and ineffective compensation for the shunt volume *(71).*

The complexity of the mitral valve apparatus and the subendocardial location of the papillary muscle blood supply explains the occurrence of papillary muscle dysfuntion during infarction. Cardiogenic shock occurs commonly in patients with partial or com-plete rupture of one of the papillary muscles *(52,72).* The posteromedial papillary mus-cle is more frequently involved because of the single vessel blood supply from the posterior descending branch of the right or left circumflex coronary artery. The antero-lateral muscle has a dual blood supply from the left anterior descending and left cir-cumflex arteries *(73).*

It can appreciated that patients with preexisting severe valvular heart disease may have little reserve available to tolerate a large myocardial infarction, and like patients with previous infarction, they will be at higher risk for cardiogenic shock. Additionally, there have been several recent descriptions of patients presenting with an acute anteroapical infarction with compensatory hyperdynamic function of the preserved basal segments resulting in systolic anterior motion of the mitral valve leading to car-diogenic shock from left ventricular outflow tract obstruction *(74–76).* These patients have presented with a systolic murmur and shock in the setting of an acute infarction, often with only a small enzyme elevation. Recognition of this syndrome must be con-sidered as common treatments for shock, including inotropic agents and afterload reduc-tion including intra-aortic balloon counterpulsation, may lead to further clinical deterioration. Effective therapeutic measures include β-blockade and utilization of α-agonists *(74).*

Finally, it should be recognized that peripheral vasodilation may be seen in the seen in the terminal phase of shock from any cause. This could be manifest as a lower than expected systemic vascular resistance and a poor response to vasoconstrictor agents. Several mechanisms may play a role in this failure of vascular smooth cell contraction including activation of K_{ATP} channels by lactic acidosis, unregulated nitric oxide syn-thesis, and depletion of vasopressin stores *(77).*

PREDICTIVE INDICATORS OF CARDIOGENIC SHOCK

Recognition of the predictive indicators of cardiogenic shock may allow implemen-tation of strategies that could impact on the disappointing survival of these patients (Table 2) .

Historical characteristics have been defined that are predictive of cardiogenic shock. Patients who develop shock are typically older *(1,3,5,11,12,78).* In the GUSTO-I trial, it was recognized that, for each decade increase in age, the risk of developing shock rose

Table 2
Predictive Indicators of Cardiogenic Shock

Historical features:
  Age >65 yr
  Female gender
  Previous infarction
  Known multivessel coronary disease
  Previous angina or other vascular disease
Physical examiniation:
  Sinus tachycardia
  Clinical hemodynamic status class III-IV
  Agitation, abnormal mental status
Clinical events:
  Reinfarction
  Hypotension
Laboratory findings:
  Hyperglycemia (>180 mg%)
  Increased blood lactate
  CK-MB >160 IU/L
Cardiac testing:
  Bundle branch block on ECG
  LVEF < 0.35
  Remote asynergy
  Wall motion index
  Coronary artery jeopardy score

LVEF, left ventricular ejection fraction.

47% *(79)*. A relative preponderance of women has been identified compared to the overall population of patients hospitalized with myocardial infarction *(1,5,12,78)*. A previous infarction enhances the risk of cardiogenic shock as documented in several studies *(3,5,11,12)*. Patients with shock are more likely to have a history of angina, stroke, or peripheral vascular disease *(5,11)*.

A diagnosis of diabetes mellitus increases the likelihood of cardiogenic shock *(3,5,11,12)*. Notably, the presence of diabetes mellitus did not increase risk in the SPRINT trial, but an admission glucose of >180 mg% was predictive of shock particularly in nondiabetics *(1)*. An enhanced activation of stress-related compensatory mechanisms (release of catecholamines, cortisol, etc.) in patients destined for shock may explain this finding *(80)*. Elevation of blood lactate levels have also preceded the manifestations of cardiogenic shock *(81)*.

Considering the pathophysiology of cardiogenic shock, the clinician should embrace certain clues from examination of the patient to lower the threshold for the diagnosis of shock. Evaluation of every hypotensive event should lead to consideration of a cardiogenic etiology. Sinus tachycardia has been recognized as a significant risk factor for early death *(82)*. Abnormal mental status, agitation, and cool extremities should lead to further clarification of the hemodynamic status *(24,83)*. The survival of patients with myocardial infarction have been categorized by clinical and hemodynamic subsets. Patients may be stratified in class IV (hypoperfusion and pulmonary congestion) without blood pressure criteria for a diagnosis of cardiogenic shock. These patients with "nonhypotensive shock" were identified in the SHOCK registry and were more likely to have an anterior infarction. A higher systemic vascular resistance was noted in this group, and although hospital mortality was somewhat better compared to classic hypotensive shock (43 vs 66%, $p = 0.001$), many patients later developed circulatory collapse (84). Patients in class III (isolated hypoperfusion) often do not respond to volume expansion and are also likely in an early phase of cardiogenic shock (24).

Events occurring during the course of infarction should alert the clinician to the potential for hemodynamic deterioration. The principle predictive event for cardiogenic shock is represented by recurrent infarction. Infarct extension or reinfarction was detected in a significantly greater proportion of patients with than without shock in both the MILIS (23.3 vs 7.4%, $p < 0.001$) and GUSTO-I trials (11 vs 3%, $p < 0.001$) (3,11).

Some studies have identified significant elevation of cardiac enzyme levels (CK-MB > 160 IU/L, lactate dehydrogenase [LDH] > 4× normal) reflecting infarct size as risk factors for cardiogenic shock (1,11). However, enzyme determinations may be confounded by timing, the early peak of reperfusion, and reinfarction. Patients with bundle-branch block are more likely to develop cardiogenic shock (85). Determination of acute global left ventricular function by contrast ventriculography, radionuclide angiography, and echocardiography has been demonstrated to have predictive value for mortality and complications such as cardiogenic shock (40,86–88). An ejection fraction of <0.35 was an independent predictive variable for cardiogenic shock occurring after admission in the MILIS trial (11). The presence of remote asynergy and/or the absence of regional hyperkinesia has important prognostic implications regarding mortality and cardiogenic shock (11). Quantitation of regional function by echocardiography has been utilized as a predictive instrument for cardiogenic shock. Gibson et al. (89) showed that calculation of a wall motion index in Killip class I or II patients was highly predictive of later hemo-dynamic deterioration. A discriminate equation was developed from their data (1.44 [Killip class] + 2.11 [wall motion index]) with a result of ≥6.04 predicting 78% of patients with cardiogenic shock.

Multivessel disease is a common component of cardiogenic shock. Knowledge of coronary anatomy from previous or acute coronary angiography may allow foresight into the potential for the development of shock. In theory, utilization of a coronary artery jeopardy score could predict hemodynamic deterioration as utilized for prediction of cardiogenic shock in patients undergoing elective angioplasty (90).

Multivariate analysis utilizing logistic regression of patients in the SPRINT registry and the MILIS trial identified several predictive variables that allowed assignment of a probability for the development of cardiogenic shock with additive accumulation of each variable. The MILIS study distinguished the variables of age >65 yr, admission left ventricular ejection fraction <0.35, CK-MB >160 IU/L, diabetes mellitus, and previous infarction with a probability of developing cardiogenic shock at 18% with 3 variables and 54% with 5 variables (11). In a similar fashion, the SPRINT registry defined age, female gender, history of angina, stroke, or peripheral vascular disease, peak LDH >4× normal, and admission glucose >180 mg% with the probability of shock at 20% for 4 risk factors and 35% for all 6 risk factors (1). A scoring system based primarily on age and physical findings on presentation has been derived from the GUSTO-I trial that accurately predicts the risk of shock (validated in the GUSTO-III cohort) after thrombolytic therapy (Table 3) (79). A similar prediction algorithm for shock in patients with non-ST-elevation acute

Table 3
Table 3
Prediction Algorithm for Cardiogenic Shock with ST-Elevation Infarction *(79)*

Predictive factor	*Points*	*Predictive factor*	*Points*		
Age		**HR**			
20	6	40	3		
30	12	60	0	**Sum Predictive Factor Pts.**	
40	19	80	8	Age + BW + MI location +	
50	25	100	14	Msc. RF + Treatment +	
60	31	120	17	HR + SBP + DBP +	
70	37	140	19	Killip class	
80	43	160	22		
90	49	180	24		
		200	27		
Body weight (kg.)		220	29		
40	19	240	32		
60	17	260	34		
80	15				
100	12	**Systolic BP (mmHg)**			**Shock**
120	10	80	59	**Total points**	**probability (%)**
140	8	100	49	92	1
160	6	120	39	103	2
180	4	140	32	110	3
200	2	160	27	114	4
220	0	180	23	118	5
		200	18	130	10
MI location		220	14	137	15
Anterior	8	240	9	142	20
Inferior	1	260	5	146	25
Other	0	280	0	149	30
				152	35
Misc. risk factors		**Diastolic BP (mmHg)**		155	40
Previous MI	5	40	4	158	45
Previous CABG	6	60	5	160	50
No previous PTCA	6	80	7		
Female	3	100	9		
Hypertension	2	120	11		
USA residence	2	140	13		
		160	15		
Treatment		180	16		
tPa	0	200	18		
Streptokinase IV	5				
Streptokinase SQ	6	**Killip class**			
		I	0		
		II	9		
		III	17		

HR, heart rate; MI, myocardial infarction; CABG, coronary artery bypass graft; PTCA, percutaneous transluminal coronary angioplasty; IV, intravenous; SQ, subcutaneous; BP, blood pressure.

coronary syndromes was determined from the Platelet Glycoprotein IIb/IIIa in Unstable Angina: Receptor Suppression Using Integrilin Therapy (PURSUIT) Trial data *(91)*.

CLINICAL ASSESSMENT

A decline in blood pressure should prompt search for correlative findings to confirm a diagnosis of circulatory shock. This includes assessment of vital signs, peripheral perfusion, mentation, and urine output. A consideration of noncardiogenic causes of shock should be entertained and directly proceed with appropriate diagnostic testing.

Physical examination should be directed toward assessment of volume status with attention to pulse volume, jugular veins, and perfusion. Cardiac examination must focus on a search for signs of tamponade, aortic dissection, or pulmonary embolus. Auscultation of a murmur should lead to consideration of severe mitral regurgitation or a ventricular septal defect. Occasionally the murmur from these defects may be unimpressive or absent *(92)*. As described above, dynamic left ventricular outflow tract obstruction should also be considered in the setting of shock, anterior infarction, and a systolic murmur *(74)*.

A portable chest X-ray will support the diagnosis of pulmonary edema, tamponade, emboli, or dissection. Laboratory studies should include determinations of hemoglobin, platelets, electrolytes, glucose, markers of myocardial injury, and lactate.

Electrocardiography will aid in the assessment of acute hemodynamic deterioration. Most patients with cardiogenic shock will demonstrate ECG findings of an acute transmural infarction with ST-elevation or new left bundle-branch block. In patients with shock due to left ventricular failure, the infarction is most commonly in an anterior distribution (50–80% in recent series) *(3,4,11,93)*. ST-elevation in aVR lead is characteristic of shock due to left main coronary artery occlusion *(94)*.

A non-ST-elevation infarction is present in 14–36% of recent series of shock due to left ventricular power failure. A left circumflex coronary artery occlusion should be considered as the etiology shock in these patients *(11,93,95)*. ECG is also a necessary component in the evaluation of patients developing shock after admission in view of the common association of reinfarction.

Echocardiography is a vital tool in the evaluation of patients with cardiogenic shock. The technique allows rapid quantitation of global ventricular function and assessment of regional wall motion *(89,96)*. In patients with left ventricular failure, echocardiography reveals a significant systolic dysfunction (mean left ventricular ejection fraction 0.31 ± 11 in the SHOCK trial), extensive regional wall motion abnormalities, and commonly demonstrate a restrictive filling pattern by Doppler *(97,98)*. Mechanical complications can be accurately diagnosed in an expedient manner *(99)*. Right ventricular infarction can be confirmed as a significant contributor to shock. Two-dimensional and doppler echocardiographic studies can identify the site of ventricular septal rupture and allow shunt quantification *(100)*. Echocardiography is essential for the diagnosis of free wall rupture and associated cardiac tamponade *(67)*. Papillary muscle rupture can also be detected *(101,102)*. Transesophageal echocardiography may be necessary in patients on mechanical ventilators and can more accurately quantitate mitral regurgitation *(103)*.

Hemodynamic monitoring is usually required to manage patients with cardiogenic shock. Right heart catheterization with a balloon floatation catheter can confirm the hemodynamic diagnosis and greatly aid in monitoring the effectiveness of therapy

(83,104). This technique is usually combined with arterial pressure monitoring especially when administering vasoactive pharmacology. By sampling oxygen saturations, a ventricular septal defect can be detected and severe mitral regurgitation may be suggested by detection of giant "V" waves in the wedge position. The characteristic hemodynamic findings of right ventricular infarction include a disproportionate elevation of right heart filling pressures with normal or only mildly elevated left heart filling pressure (RA/PCW > 0.80) *(105).* Tamponade can be established with the presence of a pericardial effusion and differentiated from the "constrictive" physiology of a right ventricular infarction *(50).*

The hazards of pulmonary artery catheterization have been implicated in the adverse outcome of critically ill patients *(106).* However, such monitoring continues to be utilized in the majority of patients with cardiogenic shock (68% in SHOCK registry) *(107).* Cardiogenic shock remains a Class I indication for right heart hemodynamic monitoring according to American College of Cardiology/American Heart Association (ACC/AHA) guidelines *(108).* The inaccuracy of clinical assessment and, in particular, the underestimation of pulmonary wedge pressure has been previously emphasized *(25).* Notably in observational studies examining the use of pulmonary artery catheterization in acute myocardial infarction, the mortality of subset patients with cardiogenic shock was not adversely affected by this intervention *(109).* A recent analysis from the SHOCK registry noted an association of more aggressive therapy, lower mortality and no harm from pulmonary artery catheterization *(107).* The multifaceted benefits of hemodynamic monitoring warrant its application in these critically ill patients.

THEURAPEUTIC MEASURES
General Measures

The principal therapeutic goals in cardiogenic shock associated with myocardial infarction include restoration of an adequate cardiac output and mitigation of myocardial injury and its effect on organ function.

While the patient is being evaluated, it is essential to begin therapeutic measures to reverse circulatory shock. A cautious trial of volume expansion is warranted unless the patient exhibits clear signs of pulmonary edema. Oxygenation should be assessed and hypoxia must be rapidly corrected by supplemental oxygen and, if necessary, mechanical ventilation to reduce myocardial oxygen demand. The majority of patients require mechanical ventilation (76% in the SHOCK registry) *(110).* Prompt treatment of arrhythmias (including DC cardioversion and temporary pacing) may lead to considerable hemodynamic improvement.

Attention to multiorgan function is an important component of intensive treatment of the shock syndrome. One fifth of patients in the SHOCK trial had suspected sepsis, and nearly 60% had a confirmed infectious etiology (pulmonary 54%, invasive lines 30%) *(111).*

Pharmacologic

In Griffith and colleagues' original 1954 description of a large series of patients with cardiogenic shock, the use of sympathomimetic agonists provided encouraging evidence for effective medical therapy *(9).* There is little evidence that vasopressor therapy improves the survival of these patients, yet it remains a critical component for early stabilization and ongoing hemodynamic support *(112).* The principal pharmacologic agents utilized are compared in Table 4.

Table 4
Inotropic Agents

Agent	Mechanism/ receptor action	Dose	Cardiovascular effects					Comments
			HR	BP	C.O.	SVR	PCW	
Dopamine	DA at 2–5 µg/kg/min β1, NE release at 5–10 µg/kg/min alpha at >10 µg/kg.min	2–30 µg/kg/min	↑	↑	↑	0–↑	↑	50% of action secondary to NE release. Stimulation of dopamine receptors leads to increased renal and splanchnic blood flow.
Dobutamine	β1, β2	2–30 µg/kg/min	+	0	↑	↓–0	↓–0	Racemic mixture of (+) and (–) isomers. Renal perfusion is increased by elevated cardiac output.
Norepinephrine	α, β1	0.5–80 µg/min	↓–0	↑	↓–0	↑	0–↑	Potent vasoconstrictor.
Epinephrine	α, β1, β2	0.005–0.5 µg/kg/min	↑	↑	↑	↓	↑	Potent renal vasoconstrictor. Epinephrine induced hypokalemia may accentuate potential for arrhythmias.
Amrinone	Phosphodiesterase inhibitor increases cAMP enhancing contractility and vasodilation.	0.75 mg/kg then 5–10 µg/kg/min	0–↑	0–↓	↑	↓	↓	Half-life = 2–6 h Thrombocytopenia:2–4%.
Milrinone	Same as amrinone.	50 µg/kg then 0.25–1.0 µg/kg/min	0–↑	0–↓	↑	↓	↓	Half-life = 0.5–2 h. Thrombocytopenia rare.

C.O. cardiac output; SVR systemic vascular resistance; PCW pulmonary capillary wedge pressure; DA Dopamine.

These agents increase cardiac contractility and enhance cardiac performance but often at the expense of an elevated myocardial oxygen demand. The sympathomimetic drugs have a similar rapid onset (<5 min) and peak effect (15 min) with a half-life of 1.5–2.5 min *(113)*. Proarrhythmic actions are the most serious side effect. The pharmacodynamics of these drugs must be considered including the logarithmic increase in concentration necessary to produce linear increases in effect, the development of tolerance due to receptor desensitization and the complex interaction of individual agents upon the adrenergic receptor subtypes *(114)*. The balance of inotropic, chronotropic, and vasoactive effects of each drug are optimally applied with accurate information regarding the patient's hemodynamic status.

Dopamine is usually the initial drug utilized in treating patients with cardiogenic shock. It is effective in increasing arterial pressure and raising cardiac output providing a necessary initial step in the patient with significant hypotension. The effectiveness of dopamine diminishes after 24 h, not only from receptor down-regulation, but also from depletion of norepinephrine stores *(115)*. Dobutamine's β-effects increase cardiac output, reduce vascular resistance and pulmonary capillary wedge pressure, but without alteration in arterial pressure *(116)*. Norepinephrine is usually reserved for patients with very severe hypotension or those who fail to respond to other inotropic agents. It can effectively improve coronary perfusion by increasing arterial pressure *(117)*. Epinephrine is a potent inotropic agent but use may be limited by tachycardia and ventricular arrhythmias *(114)*. Phenylephrine is an α-1 vasoconstictor agent that should be reserved for shock with a loss of vascular tone. It is contraindicated for patients with a systemic vascular resistance of >1200 dynes · s/cm^{-5} *(118)*. The phosphodiesterase inhibitors amrinone and milrinone have positive inotropic and significant vasodilator actions producing a rise in cardiac output, a fall in left ventricular filling pressure, with minimal effect on myocardial oxygen demand. However there is a risk of significant hypotension with these agents, and they possess a long half-life *(119)*.

By combining agents therapy may achieve the advantages of modest inotropic doses while minimizing the risk of side effects. Dopamine and dobutamine have often been utilized together to optimize the benefits of each drug. Both drugs infused at a rate of 7.5 µg/kg/min have been shown to achieve a more ideal hemodynamic state than higher doses of either drug alone in patients with cardiogenic shock *(120)*. Other drugs can also be utilized in combination, such as norepinephrine and low-dose dopamine, to maintain arterial pressure and renal perfusion. The addition of a phophodiesterase inhibitor may further improve cardiac output in patients on sympathomimetic drugs. Vasodilators, such as nitroprusside, may be used cautiously in patients with an adequate arterial pressure but a low cardiac output. Diuretics are utilized in an ongoing fashion to optimize left ventricular filling pressures. A vigilant attention to the patient's status is critical to avoid wide variations in hemodynamic parameters that may lead excessive drug doses, proarrhythmia, and catastrophic deterioration.

The loss of vascular tone in the late phases of all types of shock has been noted *(77)*. Vasopressin has been utilized in shock associated with refractory cardiac arrest *(121)*. A nitrous oxide synthetase inhibitor, L-NMMA has been infused in patients with "refractory cardiogenic shock," leading to a significant increase in mean arterial pressure (+43%) although a transient drop in cardiac output was noted that rose after 5 h *(122)*. A small (n = 22) randomized trial demonstrated a favorable effect on hemodynamic status and survival *(123)*.

Other innovative pharmacological advances may be proven effective in the future. The incremental benefits of limiting reperfusion injury may prove substantial in cardiogenic shock. Several methods have been examined to impede oxygen-free radical damage utilizing oxygen radical scavengers, adenosine, and neutrophil inhibitors (antibodies to adhesion receptors or selectin blockade) (32,33,124,125).

Myocardial metabolism is not only altered within the infarct zone, but also in remote regions with or without ongoing ischemia (49,126). "Substrate" infusions of glutamate/aspartate, glucose-insulin-potassium, coenzyme Q_{10} and 2-mercato-propionyl-glycine have restored remote myocardial function in an experimental model of cardiogenic shock (127). Carnitine may protect myocardial metabolism in ischemia (128). A survival of 78% was reported for 27 patients receiving high doses of intravenous L-carnitine (129). Meta-analysis of trials evaluating the use of glucose-insulin-potassium in myocardial infarction have suggested a benefit, for applying these citric acid cycle-repleting techniques to patients with cardiogenic shock (130–132). Ongoing clinical investigation will examine the benefits of these approaches.

Mechanical Support of the Circulation

INTRA-AORTIC BALLOON COUNTERPULSATION

Intra-aortic balloon counterpulsation has been utilized to treat patients with cardiogenic shock for the past 30 yr. Experimental augmentation of coronary diastolic flow was described by Kantrowitz and Kantrowitz in 1953 (133). The application of this principle was reported by Claus and colleagues (134) utilizing a device that cycled blood in the aorta. The gas-driven balloon displacement pump introduced in clinically by Kantrowitz et al. in 1968 (135) has persisted as an essential adjunct in the therapy of patients with cardiogenic shock.

By inflating the balloon catheter during diastole coronary perfusion pressure increases, and the collapse of the balloon with the onset of systole results in a decline in left ventricular afterload. Hemodynamic effects in cardiogenic shock include a reduction systolic aortic pressure and a rise in diastolic aortic pressure, with no change in mean aortic pressure (136). Cardiac output improves and heart rate decreases. The reduction in afterload is beneficial to patients with mechanical complications (mitral regurgitation and ventricular septal defect) (137). Overall, there is a decline in myocardial oxygen demand with a reduction in diastolic left ventricular pressure and volume (138,139). Coronary sinus lactate levels are decreased with counterpulsation indicating a beneficial effect on myocardial energetics (136,140).

Counterpulsation increases coronary driving pressure with a resultant rise in coronary blood flow (138,140). Although there is controversy regarding the efficacy of this technique to increase flow beyond a coronary obstruction, variations in experimental preparations or clinical conditions along with differences in coronary flow measurements may account for these discrepancies (138,141,142). In theory, regional perfusion may be enhanced to remote myocardium through a subcritical compliant stenosis or via collateral circulation (30,138,143). Counterpulsation alone has not been shown to decrease infarct size in acute infarction (144), but theoretically, may minimize the "piecemeal" extension of necrosis induced by the shock state.

The use of the intra-aortic balloon pump will result in hemodynamic stabilization of >75% of patients with medically refractory cardiogenic shock (136,145,146). Despite these benefits, the intra-aortic balloon pump appears to be underutilized in

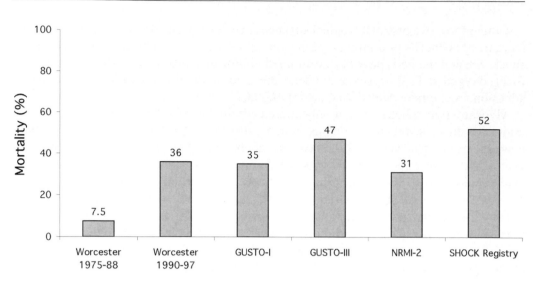

Fig. 4. The utilization of intra-aortic balloon counterpulsation in several investigations of patients with cardiogenic shock *(12,14,147–149)*.

patients with cardiogenic shock, although the proportion appears to be increasing (Fig. 4) *(12,14,147–149)*.

Although counterpulsation is an ACC/AHA Class I recommendation for cardiogenic shock *(108)*, the independent effect of this support on survival in remains controversial. Early studies noted a persistent high mortality rate of patients treated with shock. For example, a cooperative trial of 87 patients reported a 77% hospital mortality in 1969 *(136)*. Other investigation also suggested little survival benefit despite the marked clinical improvement *(150)*. In most studies, counterpulsation was often applied many hours after shock had developed and nearly always after a failure of intense vasopressor support.

In the modern era of infarct reperfusion therapy, interventional procedures (thrombolysis, angioplasty, bypass surgery) are often combined with counterpulsation. Observational studies have demonstrated an association with a lower hospital mortality in patients receiving balloon pump support *(151)*. However, patients treated with balloon pump support are often younger with fewer comorbidities *(148,149)*. The combination with emergency coronary bypass surgery has been used to treat patients with cardiogenic shock successfully for three decades *(152–154)*. Clear discrimination of a unique benefit for counterpulsation is more complex with these common coexistent treatment variables.

The utilization of intra-aortic balloon pump support and thrombolysis appears to have a unique synergistic effect (*see* Thrombolysis section below). A favorable trend on 30-d and 1-yr mortality was noted with early counterpulsation in the GUSTO-I trial *(155)*. Combined analysis of the GUSTO-I and GUSTO-III shock patients demonstrated an improved 30-d survival with balloon pump support (45 vs 58%, $p = 0.001$) regardless of patient age *(156)*. Evaluation of 5563 shock patients who received thrombolysis in the NRMI-2 database revealed a significant reduction in mortality for patients undergoing counterpulsation (49 vs 67%) *(148)*. This positive effect of balloon pump support on mortality reduction for shock patients treated with thrombolysis was also evident in the SHOCK registry (47 vs 63%, $p < 0.0001$) *(149)*.

In contrast to the relatively defined benefit for counterpulsation with thrombolysis, the survival advantage in combination with primary angioplasty is less apparent. No survival improvement was seen in the SHOCK registry, and a higher mortality (47 vs 42%, $p < .01$) was noted in the NRMI-2 registry *(148,149)*. This may reflect a more favorable clinical status of patients undergoing primary angioplasty without balloon pump support. Furthermore, the intra-aortic balloon pump improves the safety of cardiac catheterization and primary angioplasty during cardiogenic shock. Brodie et al. noted fewer adverse catheterization laboratory events in patients with cardiogenic shock (14.5 vs 35.1%, $p = 0.009$) in patients undergoing counterpulsation before intervention *(157)*.

The hazards of intra-aortic balloon counterpulsation must be considered. Major complications (10–20%) are primarily related to limb ischemia or hemorrhage requiring surgery and/or transfusion *(158)*. Other major complications include death (<1%), thromboembolism, aortic dissection, sepsis, cholesterol embolization, stroke, and limb loss. Female gender, peripheral vascular disease, diabetes mellitus and body surface area are predictors of complications *(158–160)*. Intra-aortic balloon pump complications are not more frequent in shock patients *(161)*.

Intra-aortic balloon counterpulsation remains an important adjunct for the support of patients with cardiogenic shock. The relative benefit of balloon pump support is uncertain. Although randomized investigation is needed, it remains difficult to conduct in these critically ill patients. Notably, the less than expected benefit of revascularization in the SHOCK trial has been attributed to the uniform aggressive supportive therapy utilized, which included balloon counterpulsation (86% in both treatment arms) *(6)*.

OTHER MECHANICAL SUPPORT DEVICES

Although adequate circulation can be restored in many patients by intra-aortic balloon counterpulsation, approx 25% will fail to improve and a stable cardiac rhythm is necessary for continued effectiveness *(136)*. Several innovative techniques have been introduced to extend hemodynamic support to even the most critically ill patients. These methods have been utilized to allow time for recovery of ischemic border zone myocardium or favorable remodeling processes *(162)* and provide an opportunity for corrective procedures, such as revascularization or as bridge therapy prior to transplantation.

The ideal mechanical support device should maintain an adequate cardiac output, improve coronary perfusion, and decrease myocardial oxygen consumption while allowing rapid, uncomplicated, safe implementation. While no device fulfills all of these criteria, several have effectively supported critically ill patients.

Peripheral cardiopulmonary bypass has been used to support patients in cardiogenic shock *(163–167)*. The main components of the percutaneous cardiopulmonary bypass support (PCPS) include, a centrifugal nonocclusive pump, hollow-fiber membrane oxygenator, and a heat exchanger. Femoral arterial and venous access is obtained via 18–20 French cannulas. The PCPS can achieve flow rates of up to 6 L/min. This technique can be rapidly instituted in the catheterization laboratory or at the bedside and can be applied to patients in cardiac arrest.

PCPS has been utilized primarily to support patients undergoing elective high risk angioplasty. In these patients bypass support results in a reduction of left ventricular afterload and left ventricular systolic volume with no change in mean arterial pressure (summation of a fall in systolic and rise in diastolic pressure). However, there is deterioration of regional myocardial function in areas supplied by stenotic vessels *(168)*.

Other limitations include difficult application with significant peripheral vascular disease and inadequate ventricular unloading (169). Complications of PCPS are principally related to hemorrhage at the access sites. A time limitation of 6–8 h has been recommended with PCPS due to an increased risk of metabolic abnormalities, hemolysis, and disseminated intravascular coagulation. However, success has been reported with more prolonged (29 ± 26 h) use of this device in cardiogenic shock when combined with revascularization (166). Other forms of extracorpeal membrane oxygenation support have been reported (169).

Shawl and colleagues reported institution of bypass within 30–180 min of shock onset (4.4 h from infarct onset) in 8 patients, with 100% survival in all 7 patients who underwent revascularization at 8 mo (163). Other small series have also reported success with this technique (166,167,170).

The Hemopump support device consists of a continuous flow pump based on an Archimedes screw principle, contained within a 14 or 21 French catheter. The pump rotates at 27,600–45,000 rpm propelling blood from a vent within the left ventricle to the aorta. The larger device allows flow rates up to 3.5 L/min, whereas the smaller percutaneously inserted 14F device is limited to rates of 1.7–2.2 L/min (171–173). The Hemopump has been shown to effect significant ventricular unloading, while improving regional function to ischemic and reperfused myocardium (174,175). The device can be utilized for several d. Its use is also limited by peripheral vascular disease and is contraindicated with significant aortic vascular or aortic valve disease. Complications are primarily related to thrombocytopenia requiring platelet transfusion (7%), thromboembolism (9.6%), and ventricular arrhythmias (27%) (176).

In a series of 11 patients with cardiogenic shock, there was a significant rise in mean arterial pressure and a fall in left ventricular end-diastolic pressure. Four of the 11 patients survived despite performance of revascularization procedures in 10 out of 11 patients (177). This device is no longer available in the United States.

A variety of ventricular assist devices have been utilized to support patients in cardiogenic shock. Biventricular support is usually not necessary in this setting (178). These devices provide sufficient hemodynamic support and can unload the left ventricle potentially reducing infarct size (178–180). Long-term support can be achieved, but a thoracotomy is usually required. Other less invasive (including percutaneous application) assist devices have been introduced utilizing inflow from the left atrium, via a transseptal catheter, with return to an arterial cannula (181–183). However, experience is limited.

These devices provide a considerable increment in circulatory support compared to the intra-aortic balloon pump and can sustain prolonged survival, provided they are implemented before shock-induced irreversible organ damage. Despite left ventricular unloading and, theoretically, an opportunity for myocardial healing (184) and recovery, only a few patients have undergone device explantation unless utilized as a bridge to transplantation (178,185). This latter approach has been utilized successfully in several series (178,185–188).

Reperfusion and Survival in Cardiogenic Shock

The myocardial salvage and survival benefits of achieving a patent infarct artery have established the importance of reperfusion therapy for myocardial infarction (2,189,190). This concept remains at the foundation of modern therapy for acute myocardial infarc-

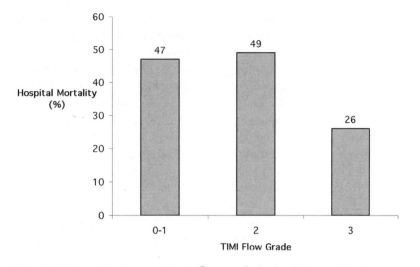

Fig. 5. Relationship between TIMI flow grade in the infarct-related vessel and hospital mortality in the SHOCK registry *(18)*.

tion A critical link was established between early attainment of complete (TIMI 3 flow) infarct artery patency and survival by the GUSTO-1 angiographic substudy *(191)*. Intuitively, one would predict a similar salutary connection between early patency and survival in cardiogenic shock. In a series of 200 patients with cardiogenic shock, the mortality rate in patients with patent infarct arteries was 33 vs 75% with closed arteries *(93)*. Recent data from the SHOCK registry verified the relationship between complete infarct artery patency and survival (Fig. 5) *(18)*. The strong association between infarct artery patency and outcome highlights a meaningful achievable target in the progress toward improving the survival of cardiogenic shock.

Recent large population studies have demonstrated improving survival of patients with shock. In the Worcester Heart Attack Study, mortality fell from 70 85% between 1975 1990 to 50–60% in 1995–1997. This was associated with a substantial increase intra-aortic balloon counterpulsation (5 → 42%), thrombolysis (0 → 25%), angioplasty (0 → 29%), and coronary bypass surgery (0 → 14%) *(12)*. In a similar fashion, patients surviving shock were more likely to undergo revascularization procedures in the NRMI-2 registry *(5)*. A comparable benefit from more extensive use of interventions, including revascularization, has been postulated to explain the lower mortality for patients in the GUSTO-I trial with shock hospitalized in the U.S. compared with other countries *(192)*. Despite this evidence and recent trial data *(6)*, there remains skepticism (primarily due to concerns about selection bias) regarding the advantage of reperfusion therapy in patients with cardiogenic shock *(193)*.

Thrombolysis

The mortality reduction by thrombolytic therapy for acute myocardial infarction led to hopeful speculation that these agents favorably influence the survival of the subgroup with cardiogenic shock. It appears that thrombolysis does reduce the incidence of cardiogenic shock. In the Anglo-Scandinavian Study of Early Thrombolysis (ASSET)-1 trial, the incidence was reduced from 5.1 to 3.8% ($p < 0.05$) with tPA *(190)*. Shock (onset >24 h after admission) was also decreased with treatment in the anistreplase (APSAC) multicenter trial from 9.5 to 3.2% ($p = 0.03$) *(194)*.

An analysis of 94 thrombolytic trials involving 81,005 patients with myocardial infarction noted that 22% included patients with cardiogenic shock *(195)*. Only 3 trials performed subgroup analysis on this complication and one trial reported data comparing thrombolysis with a control group. The Gruppo Italiano per lo Studio della Streptochinasi nell'Infarto Miocardico (GISSI) trial reported data regarding the effect of intravenous streptokinase on patients with defined cardiogenic shock, and no benefit on hospital survival was identified with treatment (n = 280, mortality: streptokinase 69.9%, untreated 70.1% p = NS) *(2)*. However, both the APSAC Intervention Mortality Study (AIMS) and the ISIS-2 (streptokinase) trials reported a survival benefit for treatment with these agents in patients with hypotension with a 33 and 23% reduction in mortality, respectively *(189,196)*. Likewise, the Fibrinolytic Therapy Trialist analysis noted that the absolute benefits of thrombolysis are largest in patients with evidence of hemodynamic impairment identified by hypotension, defined by a systolic blood pressure <100 mmHg (60 lives saved/1000 patients treated) or the combination of hypotension and tachycardia, heart rate (HR) >100 beats/min (bpm) (73 lives saved/1000 patients treated) *(197)*. Nevertheless, the mortality of the relatively small number of patients with shock or hypotension remained high in the major thrombolytic therapy trials.

The equivocal or marginal benefit apparent in these trials may reflect the diminished efficacy of thrombolysis in cardiogenic shock. A reperfusion rate of 44% was reported for 44 cardiogenic shock patients receiving intracoronary streptokinase in the Society for Cardiac Angiography's registry compared to an overall reperfusion rate of 71% *(198)*. Bengston et al. reported similar results with a patent infarct artery found in 48% (33 out of 69) of patients receiving intravenous thrombolysis *(93)*. The effectiveness of thrombolysis is determined by complex mechanical, hemodynamic, and metabolic factors. For example, acidosis can impair the transformation of plasminogen to plasmin decreasing the efficacy of thrombolytic agents in circulatory shock *(199)*.

The reduction of coronary perfusion pressure occurring with cardiogenic shock interferes with the delivery of plasminogen and plasminogen activators to the thrombus *(200)*. Experimental data with magnetic resonance imaging have demonstrated enhanced lysis with pressure-induced permeation of whole blood thrombi *(201)*. Both norepinephrine infusion and intra-aortic balloon counterpulsation have been shown to augment coronary thrombolysis in intact animal models *(202–204)*. This principle of pressure-dependent thrombolysis has been extended to the clinical setting. Garber et al. *(205)* reported successful thrombolysis (tPA) in cardiogenic shock patients who responded to dopamine or norepinephrine with a rise in mean arterial pressure (64–102 mmHg, 6 of 8 patients treated). A small retrospective community hospital series has demonstrated an improved survival of patients who underwent combined thrombolysis and counterpulsation compared with either treatment alone (n = 36; combined 40%, intra-aortic balloon pump 10%, thrombolysis 6%, p = 0.04), all without angioplasty or surgery *(206)*. This combined strategy may play an important role in hospitals without revascularization facilities by stabilizing patients and facilitating their transfer to tertiary centers *(207)*. The synergistic benefits of intra-aortic balloon counterpulsation and thrombolysis have been previously detailed (*see* Intra-aortic Balloon Counterpulsation section).

Differences have been noted in the relative efficacy of thrombolytic agents in cardiogenic shock. Patients receiving accelerated tPA were less likely to develop cardiogenic shock in the GUSTO-I trial (5.5%) compared to those treated with streptokinase (6.9%) ($p < 0.001$) (3). However, there was a trend for a lower 30-d mortality in those who developed shock and were treated with streptokinase and subcutaneous heparin compared with tPA (51 vs 57%, $p = 0.061$). A similar advantage for streptokinase was noted in the International Study Group (208). The mortality of patients with shock treated with retaplase is equivalent to tPA therapy (209).

The exclusion criteria and selection bias present in most trials of thrombolytic therapy have led to an incomplete understanding of its role in treating patients with cardiogenic shock. Patients who experience successful reperfusion of the infarct artery with thrombolysis will likely attain a survival benefit. The hospital mortality was reduced overall in patients treated with thrombolysis in the SHOCK registry (54 vs 63%, $p = 0.05$) (149) and as noted, survival was further enhanced with balloon pump support. Thrombolysis especially when combined with intra-aortic balloon counterpulsation is an important initial treatment modality at hospitals without revascularization capabilities.

Coronary Angioplasty

Reperfusion of an occluded infarct artery by primary angioplasty offers several advantages over thrombolytic therapy. These include superior reperfusion efficacy, near-elimination of the risk of intracranial hemorrhage, and reduction of recurrent ischemia and/or infarction (210). There are also benefits to this reperfusion method in the elderly, patients with prior bypass surgery, and in those who are ineligible for thrombolysis. Meta-analysis of randomized controlled trials has shown an advantage for primary angioplasty over thrombolysis with a reduction in mortality, reinfarction, and stroke (211). The reduced effectiveness of thrombolysis in cardiogenic shock has led to a presumed superiority of primary angioplasty as a reperfusion modality.

A review of nonrepetitive patient series (Table 5) (44,45,47,48,93,212–229) examining balloon angioplasty in cardiogenic shock demonstrates considerable improvement in the hemodynamic parameters of patients undergoing successful angioplasty, with a reduction in left ventricular filling pressure and a rise in cardiac output (214,217,219,230–232). A significant increase in left ventricular ejection fraction has also been reported (223,231,233).

Although, superior to thrombolytic therapy, reperfusion efficacy in cardiogenic shock is decreased compared to the >90–95% success reported in the overall patient population undergoing primary angioplasty (210). For example, in the SHOCK registry, angioplasty was successful (defined as TIMI flow grade 2 or 3 with a residual stenosis <50%) in 75% with <TIMI grade 3 flow in 18% (223).

Examination of these series (Table 5) suggests that survival is enhanced by angioplasty. These studies consistently demonstrate a lower mortality for patients undergoing successful angioplasty compared with historical controls, concurrent patients who do not undergo angioplasty, or fail the procedure. There are concerns regarding selection bias in these reports. Patients who are more critically ill or die prior to attempted revascularization may be excluded. A lower risk group may be selected for angiography. In both the GUSTO-I trial and SHOCK registry, patients who underwent catheterization without revascularization had an improved survival over those who did not undergo invasive evaluation (3,234). Consecutive application of angioplasty in a series (n = 25)

Table 5
Angioplasty and Cardiogenic Shock

Series reference	N	Age	Thrombolysis (%)	Reperfusion (%)	Time (h)	Mortality (%)				MVD (%)	Yr	Stent Support (%)
						Hosp/ 30d	Successful RP	Unsuccessful RP	Long Term			
O'Neill (212)	27	—	41	88	17[a]	30	25	67	—	—	Pre-1985	0
Lee (47)	69	58	29	71	4.7[b]	45	31	80	45% at 24 m	60	1982–1985	0
Shani (214)	9	59	0	67	2.3[a]	33	—	—	38% at 10 m	—	Pre-1986	0
Heuser (215)	10	—	0	60	—	40	17	75	—	—	Pre-1986	0
Laramie (216)	39	64	0	86	3.9[a]	41	—	—	32% at 24 m	87	1981–1987	0
Hibbard (45)	45	63	29	6	6[a]	44	29	71	56% at 27 m	58	1982–1989	0
Yamamoto (217)	26	67	23	62	3.5[a]	62	44	90	69% at 12 m	53	1985–1990	0
Moosvi (48)	38	63	25	76	33[b]	44	38	78	—	66	1985–1990	0
Gacioch (218)	48	59	46	73	24[b]	55	39	93	64% at 12 m	—	1985–1990	0
Eltchaninoff (44)	33	65	21	76	23[a]	36	24	75	48% at 12 m	67	1986–1990	0
Bengston (93)	50	66	36	85	2.8[b]	43	38	71	—	—	1987–1988	0
Morrison (219)	17	—	0	71	—	53	25	100	—	65	1988–1994	0
Himbert (220)	21	67	14	86	4.5[a]	70	72	66	84% at 17 m	68	1989–1993	0
Emmerich (221)	16	53	0	100	2.9[a]	19	19	—	19% at 14 m	69	1990–1994	0
Urban (222)	27	66	34	85	—	67	62	—	77% at 12 m	83	1982–1996	13
Webb (223)	276	64	—	75	3.3[b]	46	33	86	—	78	1993–1997	24
Yip (224)	42	62	—	83	4.7[a]	31	—	—	—	26	1993–2000	0
Perez-Castellano (225)	65	67	—	72	—	70	62	94	—	72	1994–1997	50
Zeymer (226)	390	64	—	78	4.1[a]	52	40	83	—	65	1994–1998	0
Calton (227)	18	53	0	79	1.8[b]	28	21	50	—	45	1995–1997	0
Antoniucci (228)	66	65	0	94	3.3[b]	26	21	100	29 at 6 m	67	1995–1997	47
Ajani (229)	46	64	0	63	3.8[a]	37	—	—	40 at 2 m	35	1995–1999	35

Time Interval:
[a]MI symptoms—angioplasty.
[b]Shock—angioplasty.
RP, reperfusion; MVD, Multivessel disease.

reported by Himbert et al. *(220)* demonstrated a mortality of 81% in patients with a successful procedure. However, a more contemporary report of 66 consecutive patients reported by Antoniucci and colleagues *(228)* demonstrated a procedure success rate of 94% and a hospital mortality of 26% with early shock (within 1 h of admission) undergoing stent (47%) supported angioplasty.

In the SHOCK registry, patients who underwent angioplasty had a lower hospital mortality rate than medically treated patients (46.4 vs 78%, $p < 0.001$). The mortality rate did correlate with reperfusion efficacy (33% with TIMI grade 3 flow, 50% with TIMI grade 2 flow, and 86% with TIMI 0–1 grade flow) *(223)*.

MODERN ADVANCES IN TRANSLUMINAL REVASCULARIZATION

Stents have ascended to a predominant role in transluminal revascularization. Although the impact was delayed by early concerns regarding implantation of stents in the thrombotic mileau of an acute infarct artery, stenting evolved from a bailout procedure to routine application to patients undergoing primary catheter-based reperfusion. Randomized trials comparing primary stenting with angioplasty in acute infarction have consistently demonstrated a reduction in recurrent ischemia and reinfarction *(210)*. However, in the Stent Primary Angioplasty in Myocardial Infarction (Stent-PAMI) trial, the final TIMI 3 flow rate was lower in the stent group (93 vs 89%, $p = 0.0006$) with a trend for a higher 6-mo mortality (4.3 vs 2.8%, $p = 0.06$) *(235)*. These limitations were not seen in the Controlled Abciximab and Device to Lower-Late Angioplasty Complications (CADILLAC) trial with an overall significant reduction in 6 mo Major Adverse Cardiac Events (MACE) in the stent group (10.4 vs 18.4%, $p < 0.001$) and no evidence of reduced TIMI grade 3 flow or survival with stent implantation *(236)*.

In cardiogenic shock, initial utilization of stent support after balloon angioplasty for suboptimal results or complications (dissection) has enhanced reperfusion success *(228,237)*. Several reports suggest that this improved efficacy may translate into a survival benefit *(238–241)*. In the SHOCK trial, stent use was associated with improved procedure success in the early revascularization group (92 vs 76%, $p = 0.045$) and success was correlated with reduced 30-d mortality (38 vs 79%, $p = 0.003$) *(242)*.

Glycoprotein IIb/IIIa inhibitors have been clearly established as important adjuncts for transluminal revascularization principally by reducing ischemic events *(243)*. However, the use of IIb/IIIa inhibition with catheter-based reperfusion therapy for acute ST-elevation infarction remains controversial *(244)*. Trial data are somewhat discordant in regards to the advantage of the addition of abciximab over primary stenting alone *(236,245)*. Analysis of two prospective databases of patients with cardiogenic shock determined a benefit for patients undergoing primary angioplasty and a synergistic advantage with the use of stents *(241,246)*.

Although directional and transluminal extraction atherectomy devices have been utilized as primary reperfusion modalities in acute myocardial infarction, superiority over balloon angioplasty and stenting has not been demonstrated *(247,248)*. However, extensive thrombus burden may be present in some infarct arteries (particularly large [>4.0 mm] right coronary arteries) and result in reduced procedure success, the no reflow phenomenon, and decreased survival *(224)*. Recently, successful thrombus removal utilizing the AngioJet rheolytic thrombectomy device has been reported during acute infarction and in the setting of cardiogenic shock *(249,250)*. Future investigation of this and other thrombectomy devices may validate the effectiveness of this approach.

Table 6
Coronary Artery Bypass Surgery and Cardiogenic Shock

Series reference	N	Age	Time	Hospital Mort. (%)	Year
Johnson (255)	5	58	2.5–12[a]	40	1962–1974
Mundth (256)	22	51	>24	40	1968–1972
Keon (257)	21	—	7.8[b]	67	1970–1974
Mills (258)	10	50	<24–48[a]	0	1971–1974
Miller (259)	10	55	36–144[b]	40	Pre-1974
O'Rourke (251)	6	54	74[a]	67	1971–1972
Cascade (260)	7	57	4–24[b]	29	1971–1974
Bardet (146)	4	54	24–40[b]	50	1972–1974
Ehrich (261)	3	51	>24[b]	67	1972–1974
Willerson (152)	3	46	48[b]	67	Pre-1975
Dewood (153)	19	52	—	42	1973–1978
Nunley (330)	14	58	—	14	1974–1981
Subramanian (262)	20	55	—	45	1976–1978
Hines (263)	7	—	276[b]	14	1976–1980
Phillips (264)	34	51	8[a]	24	1975–1982
Connolly (265)	14	66	230[a]	28	1982–1984
Laks (266)	50	—	103[a]	30	1981–1986
Guyton (267)	9	63	6.7[a]	22	1983–1986
Sergeant (268)	89	61	2.8[a]	21	1971–1992
Allen (269)	66	59	6.3[a]	9	1986–1991
Donatelli (270)	8	65	2.2[b]	50	1994–1995
Edep (271)	185	70	—	23	1994
Webb (223)	109	64	—	34	1993–1997

Time Interval:
[a] MI symptoms—surgery.
[b] Shock—surgery.

Coronary Artery Bypass Surgery

The introduction of the intra-aortic balloon pump brought considerable immediate hemodynamic improvement to patients in cardiogenic shock. However, the challenge of balloon pump-dependent patients and the realization of limited survival benefits led to early use of cardiac surgery. Patients were commonly operated on >24–48 h after the onset of shock, but mortality rates of less than 60% were encouraging (46,251,252). Infarctectomy or aneurysmectomy (sometimes performed without revascularization) was often combined with bypass grafting. The benefits of myocardial resection have not been proven, and this is now rarely performed (253,254).

The reports (Table 6) of patients undergoing coronary artery bypass surgery for cardiogenic shock share many of the same drawbacks (primariy related to selection bias) as noted with angioplasty series (146,152,153,223,251,255–272,330).

Dewood and colleagues (153) emphasized the importance of early revascularization in achieving successful results of bypass surgery. In their series, patients operated on within 16 h of infarction onset had a significantly lower mortality than those operated on later (25 vs 71%, $p < 0.03$). If revascularization is delayed, and there is evidence for mulitorgan failure, mortality rates are high (254,266). Patients undergoing bypass surgery for cardiogenic shock may have a relatively high rate of postoperative complications *(267)*.

The results of coronary bypass surgery in cardiogenic shock have improved over the past 3 decades. Although better patient selection may play a role, the necessity of early and complete revascularization has been recognized. Advances in surgical practice have evolved that have led to impressive results in some series. There has been considerable progress in techniques of myocardial protection utilizing blood-based cardioplegia solutions, sometimes substrate-enriched (amino acids, oxygen, glucose), and implemented through novel methods of administration (continuous, retrograde). These techniques continue to evolve. The strategy of revascularization may depend on the timing of surgery proceeding with the infarct artery in early evolving infarction and revascularizing critical "remote" vessels initially when surgery occurs later in the course. Controversy remains regarding the choice of conduits (mammary artery or vein grafts) with some utilizing double grafting techniques to the left anterior descending artery *(126,273)*. A few patients have been reported to undergo bypass surgery without cardiopulmonary bypass support ("off-pump") in the setting of cardiogenic shock *(274)*.

Perhaps the most compelling results have been reported by Allen et al. *(269)* in a multicenter study reporting a 9% mortality for 66 patients in cardiogenic shock undergoing controlled surgical reperfusion, including vented cardiopulmonary bypass and warm amino acid-enriched blood cardioplegia. Although the investigators emphasize the benefits of prolonged controlled surgical reperfusion in minimizing reperfusion injury *(126,269)*, the surgical advantage allowing early complete revascularization of remote ischemic myocardium is likely the predominant influence explaining these results.

Of 2972 patients with cardiogenic shock in the GUSTO-I trial, 11.4% underwent coronary bypass surgery with an average 30-d mortality of 29% *(3)*. In the SHOCK registry, 109 patients underwent bypass surgery as primary therapy for shock secondary to left ventricular failure with a hospital mortality of 23.9% *(223)*. An analysis of hospital admissions with cardiogenic shock in California during 1994 revealed that 185 patients underwent coronary bypass surgery with a hospital mortality of 23.4% *(271,272)*. In reviewing the breadth of recent studies involving reperfusion therapy of cardiogenic shock in myocardial infarction, coronary bypass surgery has shown the most favorable overall results. Concern remains regarding the nonrandomized nature of these studies and the selection process that occurs before the patient reaches the operating room, yet this procedure remains a vital approach in patients with left main or multivessel disease and in patients with concomitant mechanical complications of the infarction.

The Essential Role of Revascularization in Cardiogenic Shock

Although the reperfusion paradigm is at the foundation of modern therapy of acute myocardial infarction, there is persistent debate over the influence of revascularization on the outcome of patients with cardiogenic shock *(193,275)*.

Analysis of several prospective databases support a role for revascularization therapy. The association of improving survival and more aggressive treatment strategies, including revascularization, was noted in both the Worcester Heart Attack Study and the NRMI-2 registry (*see* Reperfusion and Survival in Cardiogenic Shock section) *(5,12)*. A similar fall in hospital mortality (71 to 60%) from 1992–1997 was accompanied by an increase in the proportion of patients undergoing revascularization (34 to 51%) in the SHOCK Registry *(276)*. The California analysis (n = 1122) of cardiogenic shock admis-

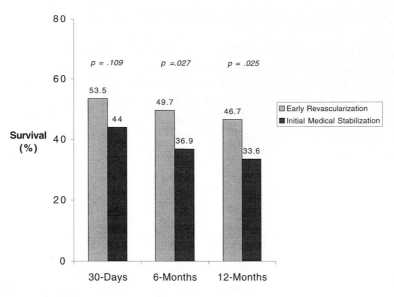

Fig. 6. The temporal relation to survival for patients randomized in the SHOCK trial by treatment strategy *(6,280)*.

sions in 1994 recognized revascularization independently reducing the odds of death by 80% *(272)*. Mortality (n = 837) was also independently decreased by revascularization therapy (62.5 vs 84.3%, *p* = 0.001) in the Maximal Individual Therapy of Acute Myocardial Infarction (MITRA) study *(277)*. In the GUSTO-I trial, the 30-d mortality was reduced among patients undergoing angioplasty and/or bypass surgery (38 vs 62%, *p* = 0.001), although revascularization patients were younger with less prior infarction and shorter thrombolytic reperfusion times *(278)*. However, in multivariate logistic regression analysis, an invasive revascularization strategy was independently associated with reduction in 30-d and 1-yr mortality *(278,279)*.

Only two randomized trials of urgent revascularization therapy have been conducted. The Swiss Multicenter trial of Angioplasty for Shock (SMASH) enrolled only 55 patients because of insufficient recruitment *(222)*. The reduction in 30-d mortality noted for the invasive group 69 vs 78%) was not significant.

The SHOCK trial deserves special attention *(6)*. Patients with shock due to predominantly left ventricular dysfunction (ST-elevation or new left bundle-branch block) were enrolled. Notably, 55% were transferred from other hospitals with a median time to randomization equaling 11 h. Over the recruitment period (1993–1998), 302 patients were randomly assigned to an early revascularization strategy (angioplasty [55%] or bypass surgery [38%]) within 6 h of randomization (median = 1.4 h). Thrombolytic therapy (63%) was recommended in the medical stabilization group, and delayed (≥54 h) revascularization (angioplasty [14%], bypass surgery [11%]) was recommended if clinically appropriate. Intra-aortic balloon support was recommended (86% in both groups).

At 30 d, the survival advantage (primary end point) observed with early revascularization did not achieve statistical significance. However, a significant benefit was noted at 6 mo and 1 yr (Fig. 6) *(6,280)*. This benefit appeared to be limited to patients <75 yr of age.

Although the treatment difference in the primary end point did not achieve statistical significance, the trial was somewhat underpowered, and the aggressive treatment

Table 7
ACC/AHA Guidelines[a] for Emergency Revascularization for
Acute Myocardial Infarction with Cardiogenic Shock

Primary percutaneous interventions (PCI)
  Class I
    In patients who are within 36 h of an acute ST-elevation/Q wave or new LBBB MI who
    develop cardiogenic shock, are <75 yr old, and in whom revascularization can be per-
    fromed within 18 h of the onset of shock.
PCI after thromblysis
  Class IIa
    Cardiogenic shock or hemodynamic instability.
Emergency coronary bypass surgery
  Class I
    1. Failed angioplasty with persistent pain or hemodynamic instability.
    2. At the time of surgical repair of postinfarction ventricular septal defect.
  Class Iia
    Cardiogenic shock with coronary anatomy suitable for surgery.

[a]1999 revision *(108)*.
PCI, percutaneous coronary intervention; LBBB, left bundle-branch block, MI, myocardial infarction.

(thrombolysis and balloon counterpulsation) in the medical stabilization group may
have mitigated the apparent benefits. The SHOCK registry confirmed similar benefits
for an early revascularization strategy *(4)*.

The experimental and clinical importance of multivessel disease in the pathophysiol
ogy of cardiogenic shock has been established *(42,43,49)*. In some studies, multivessel
disease and incomplete revascularization have been related to mortality *(224,228)*. In
the SHOCK trial, angioplasty was recommended for patients with 1 or 2 vessel disease
and bypass surgery for severe triple vessel or left main disease *(281)*. In both the
SHOCK trial and registry, mortality was increased in patients undergoing angioplasty
with triple vessel disease *(223,282)*. There has been little investigation regarding the role
of multivessel angioplasty in the setting of cardiogenic shock, although utilization of
stents may allow safer application of this strategy.

Although controversy remains, available evidence supports the application of early
revascularization procedures to patients with cardiogenic shock secondary to left ventricular failure (Table 7) *(108)*.

Special Clinical Situations

RIGHT VENTRICULAR INFARCTION

In the SHOCK registry, the prognosis of patients with shock due to primarily left ventricular or right ventricular shock was similar (61 vs 54%) *(283)*.

The initial management of patients with shock from right ventricular infarction
involves administration of volume to augment right ventricular function and maintain
adequate left ventricular preload. Venous dilatation with drugs such as nitroglycerin
must be avoided. Volume loading alone may not optimize hemodynamic parameters.
This may result from accentuated right ventricular distension and adverse ventricular
interdependence effects. The use of inotropic agents, such as dobutamine, have been
reported to increase the cardiac output in this situation *(284)*.

Maintenance of right atrial contraction is important and may require AV sequential pacing or cardioversion of arrhythmias. Intra-aortic balloon counterpulsation should be employed with persistent hypotension, especially in the presence of multivessel coronary artery disease. Percutaneous cardiopulmonary bypass, right ventricular assist devices, and pulmonary artery counterpulsation have also been utilized *(50)*.

Revascularization therapy has been shown to improve the hemodynamic status and outcome of patients with right ventricular infarction *(283,285,286)*. Bowers et al. *(285)* reported a series of 53 patients with acute right ventricular infarction who underwent primary angioplasty. In patients with successful complete reperfusion of the right main coronary artery and major right ventricular branches, marked improvement in right ventricular function occurred. Unsuccessful reperfusion resulted in more frequent hypotension and low cardiac output (83 vs 12%, $p = 0.002$) and a higher mortality (58 vs 2%, $p = 0.001$) than in those with successful reperfusion.

ACUTE ISCHEMIC SYNDROMES WITHOUT ST-ELEVATION

In two large trials evaluating patients with non-ST-elevation acute coronary syndromes, cardiogenic shock developed 2.5% of patients *(91,287)*. In both the SHOCK registry and GUSTO IIb trial, patients developing shock without ST-elevation were older and had more frequent comorbid factors, including more prior infarction, congestive heart failure, and bypass surgery compared to shock patients with ST-elevation *(95,287)*. The onset of shock in the GUSTO-IIb trial was significantly later (76.2 vs 9.6 h, $p < 0.001$) in patients without ST-elevation *(287)*.

Although mechanical causes of shock are uncommon in this setting, the pathogenesis of this syndrome is heterogeneous. Compared with ST-elevation infarction, recurrent ischemia and reinfarction are more common. Triple vessel disease is significantly more likely. The left circumflex coronary artery is more frequently identified as the culprit artery *(95,287)*. It is known that total occlusion of the left circumflex artery may occur without ST-elevation on a standard 12-lead ECG *(288)*.

Despite typically smaller infarctions in patients with shock secondary to non-ST-elevation infarction, the outcome is similar to patients with ST-elevation. In the SHOCK registry, hospital mortality occurred in 62.5% with non-ST-elevation compared with 60.4% of ST-elevation infarction *(95)*. The 30-d mortality of patients without ST-elevation in the GUSTO-IIb trial was actually higher than with ST-elevation (72.5 vs 63%, $p = 0.05$) *(287)*.

The role of revascularization for patients with shock secondary to non-ST-elevation syndromes remains uncertain *(95)*. In the PURSUIT trial, the 30-d mortality was lower in patients who received eptifibatide (58.2 vs 73.5%, $p = 0.02$) *(91)*.

THE ELDERLY

Approximately 85% of deaths from myocardial infarction occur in patients ≥65 yr *(289)*. The senescent cardiovascular system has a reduced capacity to compensate for myocardial injury sustained during infarction *(290,291)*. In the GUSTO-I trial, older age is the variable most strongly predictive of the development of shock and 30-d mortality with shock *(79,292)*.

The advantage of primary angioplasty over thrombolysis is magnified in the elderly *(293)*. However, in the SHOCK trial patients ≥75 yr in the early revascularization group had a higher mortality at 30 d compared to those assigned to medical stabilization (53 vs 75%) *(6)*. Echocardiographic data accumulated during the trial suggested that elderly patients in this small cohort (n = 56) had a significant excess of low ejection fractions and remote zone hypokinesis at randomization compared to younger patients *(294)*. In contrast, in the SHOCK registry, there was an apparent survival benefit for those aged ≥75 yr who were clinically selected for early revascularization *(4,295)*.

A decline in hospital fatality rate was noted for elderly patients (>65 yr) over time in the Worcester Heart Attack Study. Early revascularization was an independent predictor of hospital survival *(296)*. The excess mortality and complex comorbid status in the elderly patient with cardiogenic shock impedes definition of the expected advantages of revascularization. Further investigation is necessary to refine selection for therapy in this high risk group.

PRIOR CORONARY BYPASS SURGERY

Patients presenting with infarction and previous coronary bypass surgery are older and have more extensive coronary artery disease, worse left ventricular function, and more associated comorbidities *(297,298)*. In the GUSTO-I trial, patients with prior CABG exhibited a higher 30-d mortality (10.7 vs 6.7%, $p < 0.001$) and more cardiogenic shock (9 vs 5.8%, $p < 0.001$) *(299)*. Although angioplasty was performed on equivalent proportion of patients with (26.5 vs 29.6%) and without prior bypass surgery in the SHOCK registry, very few patients in the latter group underwent repeat bypass surgery *(300)*. There was a reduction in mortality associated with revascularization in the prior bypass surgery group (56.5 vs 84.45, $p = 0.018$) similar to those without prior surgery (44 vs 80%, $p < 0.001$). Revascularization should be considered for cardiogenic shock in patients with prior coronary bypass surgery.

THE LEFT MAIN SHOCK SYNDROME

As one might expect, the extensive myocardial insult resulting from left main coronary artery occlusion is characterized commonly by a dramatic presentation and a substantial hemodynamic derangement. The timing of shock onset and mortality related to the culprit infarct vessel is depicted in Table 1 *(17,18)*. The rapid onset of shock is associated with widespread ST-elevation, especially associated with ST-elevation in a VR *(94)*.

Quigley et al. *(301)* reported a 94% mortality for the "left main shock syndrome" (acute anterior infarction, severe left main stenosis, and cardiogenic shock) and suggested that conservative therapy may be indicated in this subset. Although infarction and shock arising from left main obstruction is often a catastrophic event, several reports have demonstrated survival with an aggressive approach including emergency catheterization and revascularization with either surgery and/or transluminal revascularization *(302–304)*.

Shock and Mechanical Complications of Myocardial Infarction

VENTRICULAR SEPTAL RUPTURE

Cardiogenic shock associated with rupture of the interventricular septum is a highly lethal event. In the shock registry (n = 55) the hospital mortality was 87% *(69)*. Risk factors for this complication include advanced age, female gender, hypertension, and lack of previous infarction *(63,69)*.

Intra-aortic balloon counterpulsation may stabilize the patients' hemodynamic status *(137)*, but the potential for sudden decompensation remains *(305)*. Previous data suggested a lower operative mortality when surgery was delayed. However, a deadly selection process occurs with a substantial proportion of patients unable to survive until a late operation. Early surgical repair is a necessary strategy. Very few patients in cardiogenic shock survive without surgery *(57,69,305)*. In the SHOCK registry, mortality was reduced with surgery (81 vs 96%) *(69)*. Other surgical reports suggest better outcome *(306,307)*, but preoperative cardiogenic shock is a predictor of operative mortality *(308,309)*. Patients with inferior infarction and posterior septal rupture have an increased mortality due to more complex defects and extensive right ventricular involvement *(63,69,71)*. Recently, successful closure of postinfarction septal defects has been reported with transcatheter septal occluder devices *(310–313)*. Future trials will clarify the role of these devices in the management of this lethal complication *(314)*.

PAPILLARY MUSCLE DYSFUNCTION OR RUPTURE

Acute severe mitral regurgitation resulting in shock during myocardial infarction is also likely to resultant in death without prompt surgical intervention *(315–317)*. In the SHOCK registry, patients with this complication were more likely female (52 vs 37%, $p < 0.004$) and were less likely to exhibit ST-elevation (41 vs 63%, $p < 0.001$) compared to shock due to left ventricular failure *(318)*. Shock developed at a median of 12.8 h after onset of the infarction.

As with septal rupture, intense medical therapy and balloon pump support may stabilize the patient, but the prognosis is poor without surgical intervention *(137)*. Again, surgical delay often leads to rapid clinical deterioration and death. Early surgery is recommended *(319)*. Several series have documented success with this approach *(92,320)*. In the SHOCK registry, mortality was lower with early (16.6 h) surgery *(318)*. Valve repair without replacement was possible in 6 out of 42 patients. A few patients with papillary muscle dysfunction have been treated successfully with angioplasty *(321,322)*. However, this approach must be taken cautiously. Tcheng et al. reported higher mortality with angioplasty compared with medical or surgical treatment *(323)*. In the SHOCK registry 9 patients were treated with angioplasty and 6 died *(318)*.

FREE WALL RUPTURE

Free wall rupture of the left or right ventricle is commonly a fatal event. Risk factors include advanced age, female gender, hypertension, and less prior infarction *(60,324,325)*.

Patients identified by electromechanical dissociation requiring ongoing cardiopulmonary resuscitation have rarely survived, although a few successful surgical cases have been reported *(253)*. Surgical results in subacute rupture are more favorable (50% survival) *(67,326,327)*. Hemodynamic improvement may occur through the maneuvers of volume administration, inotropic agents, and pericardiocentesis, allowing stabilization for transfer to the operating room. Medical management of selected patients with left ventricular free wall rupture has been reported by Figueras and colleagues *(328)*. Survivors (15 out of 19) were successfully treated with intravenous volume and dobutamine and survived with subsequent bedrest and β-blocker administration. A method utilizing pericardiocentesis, followed by injection of "fibrin glue" (composed of fibrinogen, Factor XIII, and aprotinin) in the pericardial space, has also been reported to successfully

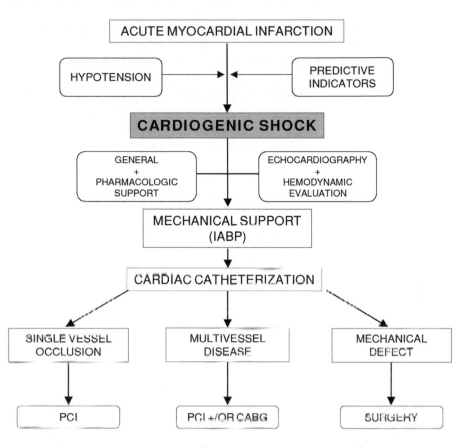

Fig. 7. The modern strategic approach to cardiogenic shock. IABP, intra-aortic balloon pump; CABG, coronary artery bypass graft surgery; PCI, percutaneous coronary intervention.

treat this complication *(329)*. Thus, survival is possible through cautious medical management in some patients who recover from the initial tamponade.

In the SHOCK registry, 28 patients (2.7%) presented in shock with free wall rupture or tamponade *(327)*. Nearly all (27 out of 28) patients were treated with surgical repair (*n* = 21, 38% survival) or pericardiocentesis (*n* = 6, 50% survival). Rapid diagnosis with echocardiography in patients with shock is an essential component in the management of patients with free wall rupture.

CARDIOGENIC SHOCK: THE MODERN STRATEGIC APPROACH

The management of patients with cardiogenic shock mandates a rapid decision process and efficient delivery of care (Fig. 7). Assessment of the predictive indicators of shock should accentuate the goal of myocardial salvage in patients at risk. Early reperfusion and immediate intervention in treating recurrent ischemia may curtail myocardial injury, thereby decreasing the possibility of left ventricular power failure. Early meticulous management of hypotension or heart failure may prevent progression.

In patients with established shock, diagnostic evaluation and supportive therapy should proceed as parallel processes. Hemodynamic evaluation, echocardiography, and vasopressor therapy should be enacted promptly. Available data supports a strategy of early cardiac catheterization and revascularization. Thrombolytic therapy and balloon counterpulsation should be instituted in patients who present with shock to hospitals without revascularization facilities. Transfer to a revascularization center should follow. Single vessel obstruction can usually be approached with coronary angioplasty. Correlation of coronary anatomy and regional left ventricular function may aid decisions regarding revascularization of patients with multivessel disease. Urgent surgery should follow in patients identified with mechanical complications.

CONCLUSIONS

Cardiogenic shock is the primary cause of hospital death after myocardial infarction. Several conditions must be distinguished from left ventricular power failure as the etiology of hypotension accompanying myocardial infarction. Multivessel coronary artery disease effects abnormal function of regions remote from the infarct segment and plays a major role in the pathophysiology of cardiogenic shock.

Aggressive management of cardiogenic shock includes concomitant diagnostic and therapeutic measures. Identification of predictive indicators may allow early preventative actions. Pharmacologic and mechanical supportive maneuvers are necessary adjuncts. In patients with ventricular septal defect or papillary muscle rupture, early operative correction is necessary to impact the poor overall outcome of these mechanical defects.

The survival benefit of early infarct artery reperfusion in acute myocardial infarction appears to extend to the subset with cardiogenic shock. Transluminal revascularization and coronary artery bypass surgery appear to be superior to thrombolytic therapy in effecting infarct artery patency in this hemodynamic subset.

Despite increased understanding and therapeutic promise, cardiogenic shock remains an ominous diagnosis. The revascularization strategy for cardiogenic shock will continue to evolve. The role of metabolic myocardial support, mitigation of reperfusion injury, and newer circulatory support devices must also be clarified.

REFERENCES

1. Leor J, Goldbourt U, Reicher-Reiss H, Kaplinsky E, Behar S. Cardiogenic shock complicating acute myocardial infarction in patients without heart failure on admission: incidence, risk factors, and outcome. SPRINT Study Group. Am J Med 1993;94:265–273.
2. Gruppo Italiano per lo Studio della Streptochinasi nell'Infarto Miocardico (GISSI). Effectiveness of intravenous thrombolytic treatment in acute myocardial infarction. Lancet 1986;1:397–402.
3. Holmes DR Jr, Bates ER, Kleiman NS, et al. Contemporary reperfusion therapy for cardiogenic shock: the GUSTO-I trial experience. The GUSTO-I Investigators. Global Utilization of Streptokinase and Tissue Plasminogen Activator for Occluded Coronary Arteries. J Am Coll Cardiol 1995;26:668–674.
4. Hochman JS, Buller CE, Sleeper LA, et al. Cardiogenic shock complicating acute myocardial infarction—etiologies, management and outcome: a report from the SHOCK Trial Registry. SHould we emergently revascularize Occluded Coronaries for cardiogenic shocK? J Am Coll Cardiol 2000;36: 1063–1070.
5. Goldberg RJ, Gore JM, Thompson CA, Gurwitz JH. Recent magnitude of and temporal trends (1994-1997) in the incidence and hospital death rates of cardiogenic shock complicating acute myocardial infarction: the second national registry of myocardial infarction. Am Heart J 2001;141:65–72.
6. Hochman JS, Sleeper LA, Webb JG, et al. Early revascularization in acute myocardial infarction complicated by cardiogenic shock. SHOCK Investigators. Should We Emergently Revascularize Occluded Coronaries for Cardiogenic Shock. N Engl J Med 1999;341:625–634.

7. Renkin J, Carlier M, De Man P, Al Shwafi K, Van de Werf F, Col J. Cardiogenic shock developing within 48 hours after thrombolysis for acute anterior myocardial infarction may be related to hemorrhagic cardiac tamponade without rupture. J Am Coll Cardiol 1997;29:14A.

8. Webb SW, Adgey AA, Pantridge JF. Autonomic disturbance at onset of acute myocardial infarction. Br Med J 1972;3:89–92.

9. Griffith GC, Wallace WB, Cochran B, Nerlich WE, Frasher WG. The treatment of shock associated with myocardial infarction. Circulation 1954;9:527–532.

10. Killip T, Kimball JT. Treatment of myocardial infarction in a coronary care unit: a two year experience with 250 patients. Am J Cardiol 1967;20:457–464.

11. Hands ME, Rutherford JD, Muller JE, et al. The in-hospital development of cardiogenic shock after myocardial infarction: incidence, predictors of occurrence, outcome and prognostic factors. The MILIS Study Group. J Am Coll Cardiol 1989;14:40–48.

12. Goldberg RJ, Samad NA, Yarzebski J, Gurwitz J, Bigelow C, Gore JM. Temporal trends in cardiogenic shock complicating acute myocardial infarction. N Engl J Med 1999;340:1162–1168.

13. ISIS-3 (Third International Study of Infarct Survival) Collaborative Group. ISIS-3: a randomised comparison of streptokinase vs tissue plasminogen activator vs anistreplase and of aspirin plus heparin vs aspirin alone among 41,299 cases of suspected acute myocardial infarction. Lancet 1992;339: 753–770.

14. Menon V, Hochman JS, Stebbins A, et al. Lack of progress in cardiogenic shock: lessons from the GUSTO trials. Eur Heart J 2000;21:1928–1936.

15. Single bolus tenecteplase compared with front-loaded alteplase in acute myocardial infarction: the ASSENT-2 double-blind randomised trial. Assessment of the Safety and Efficacy of a New Thrombolytic Investigators. Lancet 1999;354:716–722.

16. Barbash IM, Hasdai D, Behar S, et al. Usefulness of pre- versus postadmission cardiogenic shock during acute myocardial infarction in predicting survival. Am J Cardiol 2001;87:1200–1203.

17. Webb JG, Sleeper LA, Buller CE, et al. Implications of the timing of onset of cardiogenic shock after acute myocardial infarction: a report from the SHOCK Trial Registry. SHould we emergently revascularize Occluded Coronaries for cardiogenic shocK? J Am Coll Cardiol 2000;36:1084–1090.

18. Wong SC, Sanborn T, Sleeper LA, et al. Angiographic findings and clinical correlates in patients with cardiogenic shock complicating acute myocardial infarction: a report from the SHOCK Trial Registry. SHould we emergently revascularize Occluded Coronaries for cardiogenic shocK? J Am Coll Cardiol 2000;36:1077–1083.

19. Wong SC, Sleeper LA, Monrad ES, et al. Absence of gender differences in clinical outcomes in patients with cardiogenic shock complicating acute myocardial infarction. A report from the SHOCK Trial Registry. J Am Coll Cardiol 2001;38:1395–1401.

20. von Bezold A, Hirt L. Uber die physiologischen Wirkungen des esigsauren veratrins. Untersuchungen aus dem physiologischen laboratorium Wuzberg 1867;75–156.

21. Mark AL. The Bezold-Jarisch reflex revisted: clinical implications of inhibitory reflexes originating in the heart. J Am Coll Cardiol 1983;1:90–102.

22. Allen HN, Danzig R, Swan HJC. Incidence and significance of relative hypovolemia as a cause of shock associated with acute myocardial infarction. Circulation 1967;36:II-50.

23. Crexells C, Chatterjee K, Forrester JS, Dikshit K, Swan HJC. Optimal level filling pressure in the left side of the heart in acute myocardial infarction. N Engl J Med 1973;289:1263–1266.

24. Forrester JS, Diamond GA, Swan HJC. Correlative classification of clinical and hemodynamic function after acute myocardial infarction. Am J Cardiol 1977;39:137–145.

25. Menon V, White H, LeJemtel T, Webb JG, Sleeper LA, Hochman JS. The clinical profile of patients with suspected cardiogenic shock due to predominant left ventricular failure: a report from the SHOCK Trial Registry. SHould we emergently revascularize Occluded Coronaries in cardiogenic shocK? J Am Coll Cardiol 2000;36:1071–1076.

26. Alonso DR, Scheidt S, Post M, Killip T. Pathophysiology of cardiogenic shock. Quantification of myocardial necrosis, clinical, pathologic and electrocardiographic correlations. Circulation 1973;48: 588–596.

27. Page DL, Caulfield JB, Kastor JA, DeSanctis RW, Sanders CA. Myocardial changes associated with cardiogenic shock. N Engl J Med 1971;285:133–137.

28. Saffitz JE, Fredrickson RC, Roberts WC. Relation of size of transmural acute myocardial infarct to mode of death, interval between infarction and death and frequency of coronary arterial thrombus. Am J Cardiol 1986;57:1249–1254.

29. Ohman EM, Califf RM, Topol EJ, et al. Consequences of reocclusion after successful reperfusion therapy in acute myocardial infarction. TAMI Study Group [see comments]. Circulation 1990;82: 781–791.

30. Santamore WP, Yelton BW Jr, Ogilby JD. Dynamics of coronary occlusion in the pathogenesis of myocardial infarction. J Am Coll Cardiol 1991;18:1397–1405.

31. Farb A, Kolodgie FD, Jenkins M, Virmani R. Myocardial infarct extension during reperfusion after coronary artery occlusion: pathologic evidence. J Am Coll Cardiol 1993;21:1245–1253.

32. Kloner RA. Does reperfusion injury exist in humans? J Am Coll Cardiol 1993;21:537–545.

33. Reimer KA, Vander Heide RS, Richard VJ. Reperfusion in acute myocardial infarction: effect of timing and modulating factors in experimental models. Am J Cardiol 1993;72:13G–21G.

34. Kleiman NS, White HD, Ohman EM, et al. Mortality within 24 hours of thrombolysis for myocardial infarction: the importance of early reperfusion. Circulation 1994;90:2658–2665.

35. Gutovitz AL, Sobel BE, Roberts R. Progressive nature of myocardial injury in selected patients with cardiogenic shock. Am J Cardiol 1978;41:469–475.

36. Eaton LW, Weiss JL, Bulkley BH, Garrison JB, Weisfeldt ML. Regional cardiac dilatation after acute myocardial infarction: recognition by two-dimensional echocardiography. N Engl J Med 1979;300: 57–62.

37. Bartling B, Holtz J, Darmer D. Contribution of myocyte apoptosis to myocardial infarction? Basic Res Cardiol 1998;93:71–84.

38. Olivetti G, Quaini F, Sala R, et al. Acute myocardial infarction in humans is associated with activation of programmed myocyte cell death in the surviving portion of the heart. J Mol Cell Cardiol 1996;28: 2005–2016.

39. McCallister BD Jr, Christian TF, Gersh BJ, Gibbons RJ. Prognosis of myocardial infarctions involving more than 40% of the left ventricle after acute reperfusion therapy. Circulation 1993;88:1470–1475.

40. Grines CL, Topol EJ, Califf RM, et al. Prognostic implications and predictors of enhanced regional wall motion of the noninfarct zone after thrombolysis and angioplasty therapy of acute myocardial infarction. Circulation 1989;80:245–253.

41. Jaarsma W, Visser CA, Eenige Van J, et al. Prognostic implications of regional hyperkinesia and remote asynergy of noninfarcted myocardium. Am J Cardiol 1986;58:394–398.

42. Widimsky P, Gregor P, Cervenka V, et al. Severe diffuse hypokinesis of the remote myocardium—the main cause of cardiogenic shock? An echocardiographic study of 75 patients with extremely large myocardial infarctions. Cor Vasa 1988;30:27–34.

43. Wackers FJ, Lie KI, Becker AE, Durrer D, Wellens HJ. Coronary artery disease in patients dying from cardiogenic shock or congestive heart failure in the setting of acute myocardial infarction. Br Heart J 1976;38:906–910.

44. Eltchaninoff H, Simpfendorfer C, Franco I, Raymond RE, Casale PN, Whitlow PL. Early and 1-year survival rates in acute myocardial infarction complicated by cardiogenic shock: a retrospective study comparing coronary angioplasty with medical treatment. Am Heart J 1995;130:459–464.

45. Hibbard MD, Holmes DR Jr, Bailey KR, Reeder GS, Bresnahan JF, Gersh BJ. Percutaneous transluminal coronary angioplasty in patients with cardiogenic shock [see comments]. J Am Coll Cardiol 1992;19:639–646.

46. Leinbach RC, Gold HK, Dinsmore RE, et al. The role of angiography in cardiogenic shock. Circulation 1973;48:(Suppl. 3):95–98.

47. Lee L, Erbel R, Brown TM, Laufer N, Meyer J, O'Neill WW. Multicenter registry of angioplasty therapy of cardiogenic shock: initial and long-term survival. J Am Coll Cardiol 1991;17:599–603.

48. Moosvi AR, Khaja F, Villanueva L, Gheorghiade M, Douthat L, Goldstein S. Early revascularization improves survival in cardiogenic shock complicating acute myocardial infarction [see comments]. J Am Coll Cardiol 1992;19:907–914.

49. Beyersdorf F, Acar C, Buckberg GD, et al. Studies on prolonged acute regional ischemia. III. Early natural history of simulated single and multivessel disease with emphasis on remote myocardium. J Thorac Cardiovasc Surg 1989;98:368–380.

50. Chatterjee K. Pathogenesis of low output in right ventricular myocardial infarction. Chest 1992;102: 590S–595S.

51. Gewirtz H, Gold HK, Fallon JT, Pasternak RC, Leinbach RC. Role of right ventricular infarction in cardiogenic shock associated with inferior myocardial infarction. Br Heart J 1979;42:719–725.

52. Barbour DJ, Roberts WC. Rupture of a left ventricular papillary muscle during acute myocardial infarction: analysis of 22 necropsy patients. J Am Coll Cardiol 1986;8:558–565.

53. Figueras J, Curos A, Cortadellas J, Sans M, Soler-Soler J. Relevance of electrocardiographic findings, heart failure, and infarct site in assessing risk and timing of left ventricular free wall rupture during acute myocardial infarction. Am J Cardiol 1995;76:543–547.

54. Mann JM, Roberts WC. Acquired ventricular septal defect during acute myocardial infarction: analysis of 38 unoperated necropsy patients and comparison with 50 unoperated necropsy patients without rupture. Am J Cardiol 1988;62:8–19.

55. Mann JM, Roberts WC. Rupture of the left ventricular free wall during acute myocardial infarction: analysis of 138 necropsy patients and comparison with 50 necropsy patients with acute myocardial infarction without rupture. Am J Cardiol 1988;62:847–859.

56. Roberts WC, Ronan JA, Harvey WP. Rupture of left ventricular free wall (LVFW) or ventricular septum (VS) secondary to acute myocardial infarction (AMI): an occurrence virtually limited to the first transmural AMI in a hypertensive individual. Am J Cardiol 1975;35:166.

57. Lemery R, Smith HC, Giuliani ER, Gersh BJ. Prognosis in rupture of the ventricular septum after acute myocardial infarction and role of early surgical intervention. Am J Cardiol 1992;70:147–151.

58. Schuster EH, Bulkley BH. Expansion of transmural myocardial infarction: a pathophysiologic factor in cardiac rupture. Circulation 1979;60:1532–1538.

59. Massel DR. How sound is the evidence that thrombolysis increases the risk of cardiac rupture? Br Heart J 1993;69:284–287.

60. Honan MB, Harrell FE Jr, Reimer KA, et al. Cardiac rupture, mortality and the timing of thrombolytic therapy: a meta-analysis [see comments]. J Am Coll Cardiol 1990;16:359–367.

61. Becker RC, Charlesworth A, Wilcox RG, et al. Cardiac rupture associated with thrombolytic therapy: impact of time to treatment in the Late Assessment of Thrombolytic Efficacy (LATE) study. J Am Coll Cardiol 1995;25:1063–1068.

62. Becker RC, Gore JM, Lambrew C, et al. A composite view of cardiac rupture in the United States national registry of myocardial infarction. J Am Coll Cardiol 1996;27:1321–1326.

63. Crenshaw BS, Granger CB, Birnbaum Y, et al. Risk factors, angiographic patterns, and outcomes in patients with ventricular septal defect complicating acute myocardial infarction. GUSTO-I (Global Utilization of Streptokinase and TPA for Occluded Coronary Arteries) Trial Investigators. Circulation 2000;101:27–32.

64. Cheriex EC, de Swart H, Dijkman LW, et al. Myocardial rupture after myocardial infarction is related to the perfusion status of the infarct-related coronary artery. Am Heart J 1995;129:644–650.

65. Bates RJ, Berler S, Resnekov L, Anagnostopoulos CE. Cardiac rupture: challenge in diagnosis and management. Am J Cardiol 1977;40:429–437.

66. Oliva PB, Hammill SC, Edwards WD. Cardiac rupture, a clinically predictable complication of acute myocardial infarction: report of 70 cases with clinicopathologic correlations [see comments]. J Am Coll Cardiol 1993;22:720–726.

67. Lopez-Sendon J, Gonzalez A, Lopez De Sa E, et al. Diagnosis of subacute ventricular wall rupture after acute myocardial infarction: sensitivity and specificity of clinical, hemodynamic and echocardiographic criteria. J Am Coll Cardiol 1992;19:1145–1153.

68. Vlodaver Z, Edwards JE. Rupture of ventricular septum or papillary muscle complicating myocardial infarction. Circulation 1977;55:815–822.

69. Menon V, Webb JG, Hillis LD, et al. Outcome and profile of ventricular septal rupture with cardiogenic shock after myocardial infarction: a report from the SHOCK Trial Registry. SHould we emergently revascularize Occluded Coronaries in cardiogenic shocK? J Am Coll Cardiol 2000;36:1110–1106.

70. Chaux A, Blanche C, Matloff JM, DeRobertis MA, Miyamoto A. Postinfarction ventricular septal defect. Semin Thorac Cardiovasc Surg 1998;10:93–99.

71. Moore CA, Nygaard TW, Kaiser DL, Cooper AA, Gibson RS. Postinfarction ventricular septal rupture: the importance of location of infarction and right ventricular function in determining survival. Circulation 1986;74:45–55.

72. Kishon Y, Oh JK, Schaff HV, Mullany CJ, Tajik AJ, Gersh BJ. Mital valve operation in postinfarction rupture of a papillary muscle: immediate results and long-term follow-up of 22 patients. Mayo Clin Proc 1992;67:1023–1030.

73. Estes EH, Dalton FM, Entman ML, Dixon HBI, Hackel DB. The anatomy and blood supply of the papillary muscles of the left ventricle. Am Heart J 1966;71:356–362.

74. Haley JH, Sinak LJ, Tajik AJ, Ommen SR, Oh JK. Dynamic left ventricular outflow tract obstruction in acute coronary syndromes: an important cause of new systolic murmur and cardiogenic shock. Mayo Clin Proc 1999;74:901–906.

75. Armstrong WF, Marcovitz PA. Dynamic left ventricular outflow tract obstruction as a complication of acute myocardial infarction. Am Heart J 1996;131:827–830.

76. Joffe, II, Riley MF, Katz SE, Ginsburg GS, Douglas PS. Acquired dynamic left ventricular outflow tract obstruction complicating acute anterior myocardial infarction: serial echocardiographic and clinical evaluation. J Am Soc Echocardiogr 1997;10:717–721.

77. Landry DW, Oliver JA. The pathogenesis of vasodilatory shock. N Engl J Med 2001;345:588–595.

78. Scheidt S, Ascheim R, Killip Td. Shock after acute myocardial infarction. A clinical and hemodynamic profile. Am J Cardiol 1970;26:556–564.

79. Hasdai D, Califf RM, Thompson TD, et al. Predictors of cardiogenic shock after thrombolytic therapy for acute myocardial infarction. J Am Coll Cardiol 2000;35:136–143.

80. Bellodi G, Manicardi V, Malavasi V, et al. Hyperglycemia and prognosis of acute myocardial infarction in patients without diabetes mellitus. Am J Cardiol 1989;64:885–888.

81. Mavric Z, Zaputovic L, Zagar D, Matana A, Smokvina D. Usefulness of blood lactate as a predictor of shock development in acute myocardial infarction [published erratum appears in Am J Cardiol 1991 Apr 15;67(9):912]. Am J Cardiol 1991;67:565–568.

82. Lee KL, Woodlief LH, Topol EJ, et al. Predictors of 30-day mortality in the era of reperfusion for acute myocardial infarction: results of a trial of 41,021 patients. Circulation 1995;91:1659–1668.

83. Forrester JS, Diamond G, Chatterjee K, Swan HJC. Medical therapy of acute myocardial infarction by application of hemodynamic subsets (first of two parts). N Engl J Med 1976;295:1354–1362.

84. Menon V, Slater JN, White HD, Sleeper LA, Cocke T, Hochman JS. Acute myocardial infarction complicated by systemic hypoperfusion without hypotension: report of the SHOCK trial registry. Am J Med 2000;108:374–380.

85. Sgarbossa EB, Pinski SL, Topol EJ, et al. Acute myocardial infarction and complete bundle branch block at hospital admission: clinical characteristics and outcome in the thrombolytic era. GUSTO-I Investigators. Global Utilization of Streptokinase and t-PA [tissue-type plasminogen activator] for Occluded Coronary Arteries. J Am Coll Cardiol 1998;31:105–110.

86. Abrams DS, Starling MR, Crawford MH, O'Rourke RA. Value of noninvasive techniques for predicting early complications in patients with clinical class II acute myocardial infarction. J Am Coll Cardiol 1983;2:818–825.

87. Ong L, Green S, Reiser P, Morrison J. Early prediction of mortality in patients with acute myocardial infarction: a prospective study of clinical and radionuclide risk factors. Am J Cardiol 1986;57:33–38.

88. Shah PK, Maddahi J, Staniloff HM, et al. Variable spectrum and prognostic implications of left and right ventricular ejection fractions in patients with and without clinical heart failure after acute myocardial infarction. Am J Cardiol 1986;58:387–393.

89. Gibson RS, Bishop HL, Stamm RB, Crampton RS, Beller GA, Martin RP. Value of early two dimensional echocardiography in patients with acute myocardial infarction. Am J Cardiol 1982;49: 1110–1119.

90. Ellis SG, Myler RK, King SB III, et al. Causes and correlates of death after unsupported coronary angioplasty: implications for use of angioplasty and advanced support techniques in high-risk settings. Am J Cardiol 1991;68:1447–1451.

91. Hasdai D, Harrington RA, Hochman JS, et al. Platelet glycoprotein IIb/IIIa blockade and outcome of cardiogenic shock complicating acute coronary syndromes without persistent ST-segment elevation. J Am Coll Cardiol 2000;36:685–692.

92. Nishimura RA, Schaff HV, Gersh BJ, Holmes DR Jr, Tajik AJ. Early repair of mechanical complications after acute myocardial infarction. JAMA 1986;256:47–50.

93. Bengtson JR, Kaplan AJ, Pieper KS, et al. Prognosis in cardiogenic shock after acute myocardial infarction in the interventional era. J Am Coll Cardiol 1992;20:1482–1489.

94. Hori T, Kurosawa T, Yoshida M, Yamazoe M, Aizawa Y, Izumi T. Factors predicting mortality in patients after myocardial infarction caused by left main coronary artery occlusion: significance of ST segment elevation in both aVR and aVL leads. Jpn Heart J 2000;41:571–581.

95. Jacobs AK, French JK, Col J, et al. Cardiogenic shock with non-ST-segment elevation myocardial infarction: a report from the SHOCK Trial Registry. SHould we emergently revascularize Occluded coronaries for Cardiogenic shocK? J Am Coll Cardiol 2000;36:1091–1096.

96. Nishimura RA, Tajik AJ, Shub C, Miller FA Jr, Ilstrup DM, Harrison CE. Role of two-dimensional echocardiography in the prediction of in-hospital complications after acute myocardial infarction. J Am Coll Cardiol 1984;4:1080–1087.

97. Picard MH, Davidoff R, Mendes L, et al. Echocardiographic findings of shock complicating acute MI and the effects of early revascularization on LV structure and function: the SHOCK trial. J Am Coll Cardiol 1999;33:399A.
98. Chow C, Davidoff R, Mendes L, et al. Early echo-doppler findings in shock complicating acute MI. J Am Coll Cardiol 2000;35:228A.
99. Buda AJ. The role of echocardiography in the evaluation of mechanical complications of acute myocardial infarction. Circulation 1991;84:I-109–I-121.
100. Helmcke F, Mahan F, Nanda NC, et al. Two-dimensional echocardiography and doppler color flow mapping in the diagnosis and prognosis of ventricular septal rupture. Circulation 1990;81:1775–1783.
101. Nishimura RA, Shub C, Tajik AJ. Two-dimensionsl echocardiographic diagnosis of partial papillary muscle rupture. Br Heart J 1982;48:598–600.
102. Erbel R, Schweizer P, Bardos P, Meyer J. Two-dimensional diagnosis of papillary muscle rupture. Chest 1981;79:595–598.
103. Zotz RJ, Dohmen G, Genth S, Erbel R, Dieterich HA, Meyer J. Transthoracic and transesophageal echocardiography to diagnose ventricular septal rupture: importance of right heart infarction. Coronary Artery Disease 1993;4:911–917.
104. Forrester JS, Diamond G, Chatterjee K, Swan HJC. Medical therapy of acute myocardial infarction by application of hemodynamic subsets (second of two parts). N Engl J Med 1976;295:1404–1413.
105. Lopez-Sendon J, Coma-Canella I, Gamallo C. Sensitivity and specificity of hemodynamic criteria in the diagnosis of acute right ventricular infarction. Circulation 1981;64:515–525.
106. Connors AF Jr, Speroff T, Dawson NV, et al. The effectiveness of right heart catheterization in the initial care of critically ill patients. SUPPORT Investigators. JAMA 1996;276:889–897.
107. Menon V, Sleeper LA, Fincke R, Hochman JS. Outcomes with pulmonary artery catheterization in cardiogenic shock. J Am Coll Cardiol 1998;31:397A.
108. Ryan TJ, Antman EM, Brooks NH, et al. 1999 update: ACC/AHA Guidelines for the Management of Patients With Acute Myocardial Infarction: Executive Summary and Recommendations: A report of the American College of Cardiology/American Heart Association Task Force on Practice Guidelines (Committee on Management of Acute Myocardial Infarction). Circulation 1999;100:1016–1030.
109. Dalen JE, Bone RC. Is it time to pull the pulmonary artery catheter? JAMA 1996;276:916–918.
110. Shindler DM, Palmeri ST, Antonelli TA, et al. Diabetes mellitus in cardiogenic shock complicating acute myocardial infarction: a report from the SHOCK Trial Registry. SHould we emergently revascularize Occluded Coronaries for cardiogenic shocK? J Am Coll Cardiol 2000;36:1097–1103.
111. Kohsaka S, Menon V, Lange M. High incidence of suspected sepsis complicating shock following acute myocardial infarction. Circulation 2001;104:11–483.
112. Holzer J, Karliner JS, O'Rourke RA, Pitt W, Ross J Jr. Effectiveness of dopamine in patients with cardiogenic shock. American Journal of Cardiology 1973;32:79–84.
113. McGhie AI, Goldstein RA. Pathogenisis and management of acute heart failure and cardiogenic shock: role of inotropic therapy. Chest 1992;102:626S–632S.
114. Zaritsky AL. Catecholamines, inotropic medications, and vasopressor agents. In: Chernow B, ed. The Pharmacologic Approach to the Critically Ill Patient. 3rd ed. Williams & Wilkins, Baltimore, 1994, pp. 387–404.
115. Maekawa K, Liang C-S, Hood WBJ. Comparison of dobutamine and dopamine in acute myocardial infarction. Circulation 1983;67:750–759.
116. Sonnenblick EH, Frishman WH, LeJemtel TH. Dobutamine: a new synthetic cardioactive sympathetic amine. N Engl J Med 1979;300:17–22.
117. Mueller H, Ayres SM, Gregory JJ, Gianelli S, Grace WJ. Hemodynamics, coronary blood flow, and myocardial metabolism in cornary shock; response to L-norepinephrine and isoproterenol. J Clin Invest 1970;49:1885–1902.
118. Gregory JS, Bonfiglio MF, Dasta JF, Reilley TE, Townsend MC, Flancbaum L. Experience with phenylephrine as a component of the pharmacologic support of septic shock. Crit Care Med 1991;19:1395–1400.
119. Kelly RA, Smith TW. Pharmacologic Treatment of Heart Failure. In: Hardman JG, Limbird LE, eds. Goodman & Gilman's The Phamacologic Basis of Therapeutics. 9th ed. McGraw-Hill New York, 1996, pp. 809–838.
120. Richard C, Ricome JL, Rimailho A, Bottineau G, Auzepy P. Combined hemodynamic effects of dopamine and dobutamine in cardiogenic shock. Circulation 1983;67:620–626.

121. Lindner KH, Prengel AW, Brinkmann A, Strohmenger HU, Lindner IM, Lurie KG. Vasopressin administration in refractory cardiac arrest. Ann Intern Med 1996;124:1061–1064.

122. Cotter G, Kaluski E, Blatt A, et al. L-NMMA (a nitric oxide synthase inhibitor) is effective in the treatment of cardiogenic shock. Circulation 2000;101:1358–1361.

123. Cotter G, Kaluski E, Milovanov O, et al. LINCS: L-NMMA in cardiogenic shock: preliminary results from a prospective randomized study. Circulation 2001;104:II-483.

124. Ma XL, Tsao PS, Lefer AM. Antibody to CD-18 exerts endothelial and cardiac protective effects in myocardial ischemia and reperfusion. J Clin Invest 1991;88:1237–1243.

125. Silver MJ, Sutton JM, Hook S, et al. Adjunctive selectin blockade successfully reduces infarct size beyond thrombolysis in the electrolytic canine coronary artery model. Circulation 1995;92:492–499.

126. Beyersdorf F, Buckberg GD. Myocardial protection in patients with acute myocardial infarction and cardiogenic shock. Semin Thorac Cardiovasc Surg 1993;5:151–161.

127. Beyersdorf F, Acar C, Buckberg GD, et al. Studies on prolonged acute regional ischemia. V. Metabolic support of remote myocardium during left ventricular power failure. J Thorac Cardiovasc Surg 1989; 98:567–579.

128. Lango R, Smolenski RT, Narkiewicz M, Suchorzewska J, Lysiak-Szydlowska W. Influence of L-carnitine and its derivatives on myocardial metabolism and function in ischemic heart disease and during cardiopulmonary bypass. Cardiovasc Res 2001;51:21–29.

129. Corbucci GG, Loche F. L-carnitine in cardiogenic shock therapy: pharmacodynamic aspects and clinical data. Int J Clin Pharmacol Res 1993;13:87–91.

130. Diaz R, Paolasso EA, Piegas LS, et al. Metabolic modulation of acute myocardial infarction. The ECLA (Estudios Cardiologicos Latinoamerica) Collaborative Group. Circulation 1998;98:2227–2234.

131. Fath-Ordoubadi F, Beatt KJ. Glucose-insulin-potassium therapy for treatment of acute myocardial infarction: an overview of randomized placebo-controlled trials. Circulation 1997;96:1152–1156.

132. Taegtmeyer H. Metabolic support for the postischemic heart. Lancet 1995;345:1552–1555.

133. Kantrowitz A, Kantrowitz A. Experimental augmentation of coronary flow by retardation of arterial pressure pulse. Surgery 1953;34:678–687.

134. Claus RH, Birtwell WC, Albertal G, et al. Assisted circulation. I. The arterial counterpulsator. J Thorac Cardiovasc Surg 1961;41:447–458.

135. Kantrowitz A, Tjonneland S, Freed PS, Phillips SJ, Butner AN, Sherman JL. Initial clinical experience with balloon pumping in cardiogenic shock. JAMA 1968;203:135–140.

136. Scheidt S, Wilner G, Mueller H, et al. Intra-aortic balloon counterpulsation in cardiogenic shock. Report of a co-operative clinical trial. N Engl J Med 1973;288:979–984.

137. Gold HK, Leinbach RC, Sanders CA, Buckley MJ, Mundth ED, Austen WG. Intraaortic balloon pumping for ventricular septal defect or mitral regurgitation complicating acute myocardial infarction. Circulation 1973;47:1191–1196.

138. Kern MJ, Aguirre FV, Tatineni S, et al. Enhanced coronary blood flow velocity during intraaortic balloon counterpulsation in critically ill patients. J Am Coll Cardiol 1993;21:359–368.

139. Weber KT, Janicki JS. Intraaortic balloon counterpulsation: a review of physiologic principles, clinical results, and device safety. Ann Thorac Surg 1974;17:602–620.

140. Mueller H, Ayres SM, Conklin EF, et al. The effects of intra-aortic conterpulsation on cardiac performance and metabolism in shock associated with acute myocardial infarction. J Clin Invest 1971; 50:1885–1900.

141. Kimura A, Toyota E, Lu S, et al. Effects of intraaortic balloon pumping on septal arterial blood flow velocity waveform during severe left main coronary artery stenosis [see comments]. J Am Coll Cardiol 1996;27:810–816.

142. Hutchison SJ, Thaker KB, Chandraratna PA. Effects of intraaortic balloon counterpulsation on flow velocity in stenotic left main coronary arteries from transesophageal echocardiography. Am J Cardiol 1994;74:1063–1065.

143. Flynn MS, Kern MJ, Donohue TJ, Aguirre FV, Bach RG, Caracciolo EA. Alterations of coronary collateral blood flow velocity during intraaortic balloon pumping. Am J Cardiol 1993;71:1451–1455.

144. Flaherty JT, Becker LC, Weiss JL, et al. Results of a randomized prospective trial of intraaortic balloon counterpulsation and intravenous nitroglycerin in patients with acute myocardial infarction. J Am Coll Cardiol 1985;6:434–446.

145. Moulopoulos S, Stamatelopoulos S, Petrou P. Intraaortic balloon assistance in intractable cardiogenic shock. Eur Heart J 1986;7:396–403.

146. Bardet J, Masquet C, Kahn JC, et al. Clinical and hemodynamic results of intraortic balloon counterpulsation and surgery for cardiogenic shock. Am Heart J 1977;93:280–288.

147. Goldberg RJ, Gore JM, Alpert JS, et al. Cardiogenic shock after acute myocardial infarction. Incidence and mortality from a community-wide perspective, 1975 to 1988 [see comments]. N Engl J Med 1991; 325:1117–1122.

148. Barron HV, Every NR, Parsons LS, et al. The use of intra-aortic balloon counterpulsation in patients with cardiogenic shock complicating acute myocardial infarction: data from the National Registry of Myocardial Infarction 2. Am Heart J 2001;141:933–939.

149. Sanborn TA, Sleeper LA, Bates ER, et al. Impact of thrombolysis, intra-aortic balloon pump counterpulsation, and their combination in cardiogenic shock complicating acute myocardial infarction: a report from the SHOCK Trial Registry. SHould we emergently revascularize Occluded Coronaries for cardiogenic shocK? J Am Coll Cardiol 2000;36:1123–1129.

150. O'Rourke MF, Norris RM, Campbell TJ, Chang VP, Sammel NL. Randomized controlled trial of intraaortic balloon counterpulsation in early myocardial infarction with acute heart failure. Am J Cardiol 1981;47:815–820.

151. Ohman EM, Hochman JS. Aortic counterpulsation in acute myocardial infarction: physiologically important but does the patient benefit? Am Heart J 2001;141:889–892.

152. Willerson JT, Curry GC, Watson JT, et al. Intraaortic balloon counterpulsation in patients in cardiogenic shock, medically refractory left ventricular failure and/or recurrent ventricular tachycardia. Am J Med 1975;58:183–191.

153. DeWood MA, Notske RN, Hensley GR, et al. Intraaortic balloon counterpulsation with and without reperfusion for myocardial infarction shock. Circulation 1980;61:1105–1112.

154. Dunkman WB, Leinbach RC, Buckley MJ, et al. Clinical and hemodynamic results of intraaortic balloon pumping and surgery for cardiogenic shock. Circulation 1972;46:465–477.

155. Anderson RD, Ohman EM, Holmes DR Jr, et al. Use of intraaortic balloon counterpulsation in patients presenting with cardiogenic shock: observations from the GUSTO-I Study. Global Utilization of Streptokinase and TPA for Occluded Coronary Arteries. J Am Coll Cardiol 1997;30:708–715.

156. Hudson MP, Granger CB, Stebbins A, et al. Cardiogenic shock survival and use of intraaortic balloon counterpulsation: results from the GUSTO I and III trials. Circulation 1999,100.I-370.

157. Brodie BR, Stuckey TD, Hansen C, Muncy D. Intra-aortic balloon counterpulsation before primary percutaneous transluminal coronary angioplasty reduces catheterization laboratory events in high-risk patients with acute myocardial infarction. Am J Cardiol 1999;84:18–23.

158. Cohen M, Dawson MS, Kopistansky C, McBride R. Sex and other predictors of intra-aortic balloon counterpulsation- related complications: prospective study of 1119 consecutive patients. Am Heart J 2000;139:282–287.

159. Eltchaninoff H, Dimas AP, Whitlow PL. Complications associated with percutaneous placement and use of intraaortic balloon counterpulsation. Am J Cardiol 1993;71:328–332.

160. Patel JJ, Kopisyansky C, Boston B, Kuretu ML, McBride R, Cohen M. Prospective evaluation of complications associated with percutaneous intraaortic balloon counterpulsation. Am J Cardiol 1995;76: 1205–1207.

161. Ferguson JJ, Cohen M, Miller MF, et al. Intra-aortic balloon counterpulsation in patients with cardiogenic shock: the BENCHMARK registry experience. J Am Coll Cardiol 2000;35:197A.

162. McKay RG, Pfeffer MA, Pasternak RC, et al. Left ventricular remodeling after myocardial infarction: a corollary to infarct expansion. Circulation 1986;74:693–702.

163. Shawl FA, Domanski MJ, Hernandez TJ, Punja S. Emergency percutaneous cardiopulmonary bypass support in cardiogenic shock from acute myocardial infarction. Am J Cardiol 1989;64:967–970.

164. Shawl FA, Baxley WA. Role of percutaneous cardiopulmonary bypass and other support devices in interventional cardiology. Cardiol Clin 1994;12:543–557.

165. Yuda S, Nonogi H, Itoh T, et al. Survival using percutaneous cardiopulmonary support after acute myocardial infarction due to occlusion of the left main coronary artery—a report of two cases. Jpn Circ J 1998;62:779–782.

166. Jaski BE, Lingle RJ, Overlie P, et al. Long-term survival with use of percutaneous extracorporeal life support in patients presenting with acute myocardial infarction and cardiovascular collapse. ASAIO J 1999;45:615–618.

167. Aiba T, Nonogi H, Itoh T, et al. Appropriate indications for the use of a percutaneous cardiopulmonary support system in cases with cardiogenic shock complicating acute myocardial infarction. Jpn Circ J 2001;65:145–149.

168. Pavlides GS, Hauser AM, Stack RK, et al. Effect of peripheral cardiopulmonary bypass on left ventricular size, afterload and myocardial function during elective supported coronary angioplasty. J Am Coll Cardiol 1991;18:499–505.

169. Pagani FD, Lynch W, Swaniker F, et al. Extracorporeal life support to left ventricular assist device bridge to heart transplant: A strategy to optimize survival and resource utilization. Circulation 1999; 100:II206–II210.

170. Kurose M, Okamoto K, Sato T, Kukita I, Taki K, Goto H. Emergency and long-term extracorporeal life support following acute myocardial infarction: rescue from severe cardiogenic shock related to stunned myocardium. Clin Cardiol 1994;17:552–557.

171. Wampler RK, Frazier OH, Lansing AM, et al. Treatment of cardiogenic shock with the Hemopump left ventricular assist device. Ann Thorac Surg 1991;52:506–513.

172. Scholz KH, Dubois-Rande JL, Urban P, et al. Clinical experience with the percutaneous hemopump during high-risk coronary angioplasty. Am J Cardiol 1998;82:1107–1110, A6.

173. Sweeney MS. The Hemopump in 1997: a clinical, political, and marketing evolution. Ann Thorac Surg 1999;68:761–763.

174. Smalling RW, Cassidy DB, Barrett R, Lachterman B, Felli P, Amirian J. Improved regional myocardial blood flow, left ventricular unloading, and infarct salvage using an axial-flow, transvalvular left ventricular assist device. A comparison with intra-aortic balloon counterpulsation and reperfusion alone in a canine infarction model. Circulation 1992;85:1152–1159.

175. Merhige ME, Smalling RW, Cassidy D, et al. Effect of the hemopump left ventricular assist device on regional myocardial perfusion and function. Reduction of ischemia during coronary occlusion. Circulation 1989;80:III158–III166.

176. Aroesty JM, Shawl FA. Circulatory assist devices. In: Baim DS, Grossman W, eds. Cardiac Catheterization, Angiography, and Intervention. 5th ed. William & Wilkins, Baltimore, 1996, pp. 421–479.

177. Smalling RW, Sweeney M, Lachterman B, et al. Transvalvular left ventricular assistance in cardiogenic shock secondary to acute myocardial infarction. Evidence for recovery from near fatal myocardial stunning. J Am Coll Cardiol 1994;23:637–644.

178. Park SJ, Nguyen DQ, Bank AJ, Ormaza S, Bolman RM III. Left ventricular assist device bridge therapy for acute myocardial infarction. Ann Thorac Surg 2000;69:1146–1151.

179. Zumbro GL, Kitchens WR, Shearer G, Harville G, Bailey L, Galloway RF. Mechanical assistance for cardiogenic shock following cardiac surgery, myocardial infarction, and cardiac transplantation. Ann Thorac Surg 1987;44:11–13.

180. Moritz A, Wolner E. Circulatory support with shock due to acute myocardial infarction. Ann Thorac Surg 1993;55:238–244.

181. Edmunds LH Jr, Herrmann HC, DiSesa VJ, Ratcliffe MB, Bavaria JE, McCarthy DM. Left ventricular assist without thoracotomy: clinical experience with the Dennis method. Ann Thorac Surg 1994;57: 880–885.

182. Satoh H, Kobayashi T, Nakano S, et al. Percutaneous left ventricular assist system using a modification of the Dennis method: initial clinical evaluation and results. Surg Today 1995;25:883–890.

183. Thiele H, Lauer B, Boudroit E, Hambrecht R, Cohen HA, Schuler G. Reversal of cardiogenic shock by left atrial-to-femoral arterial bypass assistance. Circulation 2001;104:2917–2922.

184. Young JB. Healing the heart with ventricular assist device therapy: mechanisms of cardiac recovery. Ann Thorac Surg 2001;71:S210–S219.

185. Chen JM, DeRose JJ, Slater JP, et al. Improved survival rates support left ventricular assist device implantation early after myocardial infarction. J Am Coll Cardiol 1999;33:1903–1908.

186. Hill JD, Farrar DJ, Hershon JJ, et al. Use of a prosthetic ventricle as a bridge to cardiac transplantation for postinfarction cardiogenic shock. N Engl J Med 1986;314:626–628.

187. Hendry PJ, Masters RG, Mussivand TV, et al. Circulatory support for cardiogenic shock due to acute myocardial infarction: a Canadian experience. Can J Cardiol 1999;15:1090–1094.

188. Tayarra W, Starling RC, Young JB, et al. Improved survival following acute myocardial infarction complicated by cardiogenic shock with LVAD/transplant support: a study comparing aggressive intervention with conservative treatment. J Am Coll Cardiol 2000;35:229A.

189. ISIS-2 (Second International Study of Infarct Survival) Collaborative Group. Randomised trial of intravenous streptokinase, oral aspirin, both, or neither among 17,187 cases of suspected acute myocardial infarction: ISIS-2. Lancet 1988;2:349–360.

190. Wilcox RG, von der Lippe G, Olsson CG, Jensen G, Skene AM, Hampton JR. Trial of tissue plasminogen activator for mortality reduction in acute myocardial infarction. Anglo-Scandinavian Study of Early Thrombolysis (ASSET). Lancet 1988;2:525–530.

191. The effects of tissue plasminogen activator, streptokinase, or both on coronary artery patency, ventricular function, and survival after acute myocardial infarction. N Engl J Med 1993;329: 1615–1622.

192. Holmes DR Jr, Califf RM, Van de Werf F, et al. Difference in countries' use of resources and clinical outcome for patients with cardiogenic shock after myocardial infarction: results from the GUSTO trial. Lancet 1997;349:75–78.

193. Williams SG, Wright DJ, Tan LB. Management of cardiogenic shock complicating acute myocardial infarction: towards evidence based medical practice. Heart 2000;83:621–626.

194. Meinertz T, Kasper W, Schumacher M, Just H. The German multicenter trial of anisoylated plasminogen streptokinase activator complex versus heparin for acute myocardial infarction. Am J Cardiol 1988;62:347–351.

195. Col NF, Gurwitz JH, Alpert JS, Goldberg RJ. Frequency of inclusion of patients with cardiogenic shock in trials of thrombolytic therapy. Am J Cardiol 1994;73:149–157.

196. AIMS Trial Study Group. Long-term effects of intravenous anistreplase in acute myocardial infarction: final report of the AIMS study. Lancet 1990;335:427–431.

197. Fibrinolytic Therapy Trialists. Indications for fibrinolytic therapy in suspected acute myocardial infarction: collaborative overview of early mortality and major morbidity results from all randomised trials of more than 1000 patients. Fibrinolytic Therapy Trialists' (FTT) Collaborative Group. Lancet 1994; 343:311–322.

198. Kennedy JW, Gensini GG, Timmis GC, Maynard C. Acute myocardial infarction treated with intracoronary streptokinase: a report of the Society for Cardiac Angiography. Am J Cardiol 1985;55: 871–877.

199. Becker RC. Hemodynamic, mechanical, and metabolic determinants of thrombolytic efficacy: a theoretic framework for assessing the limitations of thrombolysis in patients with cardiogenic shock [editorial]. Am Heart J 1993;125:919–929.

200. Zidansek A, Blinc A. The influence of transport parameters and enzyme kinetics of the fibrinolytic system on thrombolysis: mathematical modelling of two idealised cases. Thromb Haemost 1991;65: 553 559.

201. Blinc A, Planinsic G, Keber D, et al. Dependence of blood clot lysis on the mode of transport of urokinase into the clot—a magnetic resonance imaging study in vitro. Thromb Haemost 1991;65:549–552.

202. Prewitt RM, Gu S, Garber PJ, Ducas J. Marked systemic hypotension depresses coronary thrombolysis induced by intracoronary administration of recombinant tissue-type plasminogen activator. J Am Coll Cardiol 1992;20:1626–1633.

203. Prewitt RM, Gu S, Schick U, Ducas J. Intraaortic balloon counterpulsation enhances coronary thrombolysis induced by intravenous administration of a thrombolytic agent. J Am Coll Cardiol 1994;23: 794–798.

204. Gurbel PA, Anderson RD, MacCord CS, et al. Arterial diastolic pressure augmentation by intra-aortic balloon counterpulsation enhances the onset of coronary artery reperfusion by thrombolytic therapy. Circulation 1994;89:361–365.

205. Garber PJ, Mathieson AL, Ducas J, Patton JN, Geddes JS, Prewitt RM. Thrombolytic therapy in cardiogenic shock: effect of increased aortic pressure and rapid tPA administration. Can J Cardiol 1995; 11:30–36.

206. Stomel RJ, Rasak M, Bates ER. Treatment strategies for acute myocardial infarction complicated by cardiogenic shock in a community hospital. Chest 1994;105:997–1002.

207. Kovack PJ, Rasak MA, Bates ER, Ohman EM, Stomel RJ. Thrombolysis plus aortic counterpulsation: improved survival in patients who present to community hospitals with cardiogenic shock. J Am Coll Cardiol 1997;29:1454–1458.

208. The International Study Group. In-hospital mortality and clinical course of 20,891 patients with suspected acute myocardial infarction randomised between alteplase and streptokinase with or without heparin. Lancet 1990;336:71–75.

209. Hasdai D, Holmes DR Jr, Topol EJ, et al. Frequency and clinical outcome of cardiogenic shock during acute myocardial infarction among patients receiving reteplase or alteplase. Results from GUSTO-III. Global Use of Strategies to Open Occluded Coronary Arteries. Eur Heart J 1999;20:128–135.

210. Lane GE, Holmes DR. The essential role of percutaneous interventions in the management of acute coronary syndromes. In: Pifarre R, Scanlon PJ, eds. Evidence-Based Management of the Acute Coronary Syndrome. Hanley & Belfus, Philadelphia, 2001, pp. 293–340.

211. Weaver WD, Simes RJ, Betriu A, et al. Comparison of primary coronary angioplasty and intravenous thrombolytic therapy for acute myocardial infarction: a quantitative review. JAMA 1997;278: 2093–2098.

212. O'Neill W, Erbel R, Laufer N, et al. Coronary angioplasty therapy of cardiogenic shock complicating acute myocardial infarction. Circulation 1985;72:III-309.

213. O'Neill WW. Angioplasty therapy of cardiogenic shock: are randomized trials necessary? [editorial; comment]. J Am Coll Cardiol 1992;19:915–917.

214. Shani J, Rivera M, Greengart A, Hollander G, Kaplan P, Lichstein E. Percutaneous transluminal coronary angioplasty in cardiogenic shock. J Am Coll Cardiol 1986;7:149A.

215. Heuser RR, Maddoux GL, Goss JE, Ramo BW, Raff GL, Shadoff N. Coronary angioplasty in the treatment of cardiogenic shock: the therapy of choice. J Am Coll Cardiol 1986;7:219A.

216. Laramee LA, Rutherford BD, Ligon RW, McConahay DR, Hartzler GO. Coronary angioplasty for cardiogenic shock following myocardial infarction. Circulation 1988;78:II-634.

217. Yamamoto H, Hayashi Y, Oka Y, et al. Efficacy of percutaneous transluminal coronary angioplasty in patients with acute myocardial infarction complicated by cardiogenic shock. Jpn Circ J 1992;56: 815–821.

218. Gacioch GM, Ellis SG, Lee L, et al. Cardiogenic shock complicating acute myocardial infarction: the use of coronary angioplasty and the integration of the new support devices into patient management [see comments]. J Am Coll Cardiol 1992;19:647–653.

219. Morrison D, Crowley ST, Bies R, Barbiere CC. Systolic blood pressure response to percutaneous transluminal coronary angioplasty for cardiogenic shock. Am J Cardiol 1995;76:313–314.

220. Himbert D, Juliard JM, Steg PG, Karrillon GJ, Aumont MC, Gourgon R. Limits of reperfusion therapy for immediate cardiogenic shock complicating acute myocardial infarction. Am J Cardiol 1994; 74:492–494.

221. Emmerich K, Ulbricht LJ, Probst H, et al. Cardiogenic shock in acute myocardial infarction. Improving survival rates by primary coronary angioplasty. Zeitschrift fur Kardiologie 1995;84:25–42.

222. Urban P, Stauffer JC, Bleed D, et al. A randomized evaluation of early revascularization to treat shock complicating acute myocardial infarction. The (Swiss) Multicenter Trial of Angioplasty for Shock-(S)MASH. Eur Heart J 1999;20:1030–1038.

223. Webb JG, Sanborn TA, Sleeper LA, et al. Percutaneous coronary intervention for cardiogenic shock in the SHOCK Trial Registry. Am Heart J 2001;141:964–970.

224. Yip HK, Wu CJ, Chang HW, et al. Comparison of impact of primary percutaneous transluminal coronary angioplasty and primary stenting on short-term mortality in patients with cardiogenic shock and evaluation of prognostic determinants. Am J Cardiol 2001;87:1184–1188.

225. Perez-Castellano N, Garcia E, Serrano JA, et al. Efficacy of invasive strategy for the management of acute myocardial infarction complicated by cardiogenic shock. Am J Cardiol 1999;83:989–993.

226. Zeymer U, Vogt A, Niederer W, et al. Primay PTCA with and without stent implantation in 671 patients with acute myocardial infarction complicated by cardiogenic shock. Results of the ALKK primary PTCA registry. J Am Coll Cardiol 2000;35:363A.

227. Calton R, Jaison TM, David T. Primary angioplasty for cardiogenic shock complicating acute myocardial infarction. Indian Heart J 1999;51:47–54.

228. Antoniucci D, Valenti R, Santoro GM, et al. Systematic direct angioplasty and stent-supported direct angioplasty therapy for cardiogenic shock complicating acute myocardial infarction: in-hospital and long-term survival. J Am Coll Cardiol 1998;31:294–300.

229. Ajani AE, Maruff P, Warren R, et al. Impact of early percutaneous coronary intervention on short- and long- term outcomes in patients with cardiogenic shock after acute myocardial infarction. Am J Cardiol 2001;87:633–635.

230. Seydoux C, Goy JJ, Beuret P, et al. Effectiveness of percutaneous transluminal coronary angioplasty in cardiogenic shock during acute myocardial infarction. Am J Cardiol 1992;69:968–969.

231. Verna E, Repetto S, Boscarini M, Ghezzi I, Binaghi G. Emergency coronary angioplasty in patients with severe left ventricular dysfunction or cardiogenic shock after acute myocardial infarction. Eur Heart J 1989;10:958–966.

232. Lee L, Bates ER, Pitt B, Walton JA, Laufer N, O'Neill WW. Percutaneous transluminal coronary angioplasty improves survival in acute myocardial infarction complicated by cardiogenic shock. Circulation 1988;78:1345–1351.

233. Iwamori K, Sakata K, Kurihara H, Yoshino H, Ishikawa K. Emergent angioplasty prevents left ventricular dilation in patients with acute anterior wall myocardial infarction and cardiogenic shock. Clin Cardiol 2000;23:743–750.

234. Hochman JS, Boland J, Sleeper LA, et al. Current spectrum of cardiogenic shock and effect of early revascularization on mortality. Results of an International Registry. SHOCK Registry Investigators [see comments]. Circulation 1995;91:873–881.

235. Grines CL, Cox DA, Stone GW, et al. Coronary angioplasty with or without stent implantation for acute myocardial infarction. Stent Primary Angioplasty in Myocardial Infarction Study Group. N Engl J Med 1999;341:1949–1956.

236. Stone GW, Grines CL, Cox DA, et al. A prospective, multicenter, international randomized trial comparing four reperfusion strategies in acute myocardial infarction: principal report of the controlled abciximab and device investigation to lower late angioplasty complications (CADILLAC) trial. J Am Coll Cardiol 2001;37:342A.

237. Webb JG, Carere RG, Hilton JD, et al. Usefulness of coronary stenting for cardiogenic shock. Am J Cardiol 1997;79:81–84.

238. Silva JA, Nunez E, Vivekananthan K, et al. Cardiogenic shock complicating acute myocardial infarction: a comparison of primary angioplasty versus primary stenting in in-hospital outcomes. J Am Coll Cardiol 1999;33:368A.

239. Nakagawa Y, Hamasaki N, Kimura T, Nosake H, Nobuyoshi M. Stent implantation in acute myocardial infarction is more beneficial in patients with cardiogenic shock than those without. J Am Coll Cardiol 1998;31:232A.

240. Lefevre T, Morice MC, Karrillon GJ, et al. Coronary stenting in acute myocardial infarction with cardiogenic shock. J Am Coll Cardiol 1998;31:95A.

241. Chan AW, Chew DP, Bhatt DL, Moliterno DJ, Ellis SG. Sustained mortality benefit from combination of stents and abciximab for cardiogenic shock complicating acute MI: experience from an 8-year registry. Circulation 2001;104:II-386.

242. Webb JG, Sanborn T, Carere RG, et al. Coronary stenting in the SHOCK trial. Circulation 1999;100:I-87.

243. Smith SC Jr, Dove JT, Jacobs AK, et al. ACC/AHA guidelines for percutaneous coronary interventions (revision of 1993 PTCA guidelines). J Am Coll Cardiol 2001;37:2215–2239.

244. Santoro GM, Bolognese L. Coronary stenting and platelet glycoprotein IIb/IIIa receptor blockade in acute myocardial infarction. Am Heart J 2001;141:S26–S35.

245. Brener SJ, Barr LA, Burchenal JE, et al. Randomized, placebo-controlled trial of platelet glycoprotein IIb/IIIa blockade with primary angioplasty for acute myocardial infarction. ReoPro and Primary PTCA Organization and Randomized Trial (RAPPORT) Investigators. Circulation 1998;98:734–741.

246. Girl S, Klernan J, Mitchel JF, et al. Synergistic interaction between intracoronary stenting and IIb/IIIa inhibition for improving clinical outcomes in primary angioplasty for cardiogenic shock. Circulation 1999;100:I-380.

247. Kaplan BM, Larkin T, Safian RD, et al. Prospective study of extraction atherectomy in patients with acute myocardial infarction. Am J Cardiol 1996;78:383–388.

248. Kurisu S, Sato H, Tateishi H, et al. Usefulness of directional coronary atherectomy in patients with acute anterior myocardial infarction. Am J Cardiol 1997;79:1392–1394.

249. Silva JA, Ramee SR, Cohen DJ, et al. Rheolytic thrombectomy during percutaneous revascularization for acute myocardial infarction: experience with the AngioJet catheter. Am Heart J 2001;141:353–359.

250. Lee DP, Lo S, Herity NA, Ward M, Yeung AC. Utility of mechanical rheolysis as an adjunct to rescue angioplasty and platelet inhibition in acute myocardial infarction and cardiogenic shock; a case report. Cathet Cardiovasc Intervent 2001;52:220–225.

251. O'Rourke MF, Sammel N, Chang VP. Arterial counterpulsation in severe refractory heart failure complicating acute myocardial infarction. Br Heart J 1979;41:308–316.

252. Sanders CA, Buckley MJ, Leinbach RC, Mundth ED, Austen WG. Mechanical circulatory assistance. Current status and experience with combining circulatory assistance, emergency coronary angiography, and acute myocardial revascularization. Circulation 1972;45:1292–1313.

253. Bolooki H. Emergency cardiac procedures in patients in cardiogenic shock due to complications of coronary artery disease. Circulation 1989;79:I137–I148.

254. Pennington DG. Emergency management of cardiogenic shock. Circulation 1989;79:I149–I151.

255. Johnson SA, Scanlon PJ, Loeb HS, Moran JM, Pifarre R, Gunnar RM. Treatment of cardiogenic shock in myocardial infarction by intraaortic balloon counterpulsation surgery. Am J Med 1977;62:687–692.

256. Mundth ED, Buckley MJ, Leinbach RC, Gold HK, Daggett WM, Austen WG. Surgical intervention for the complications of acute myocardial ischemia. Ann Surg 1973;178:379–390.

257. Keon WJ. Surgical reperfusion of acute myocardial infarction. Can J Cardiol 1985;1:8–15.

258. Mills NL, Ochsner JL, Bower PJ, Patton RM, Moore CB. Coronary artery bypass for acute myocardial infarction. South Med J 1975;68:1475–1480.

259. Miller MG, Hedley-White J, Weintraub RM, Restall DS, Alexander M. Surgery for cardiogenic shock. Lancet 1974;2:1342–1345.

260. Cascade PN, Wajszczuk WJ, Rubenfire M, Pursel SE, Kantrowitz A. Patient selection for cardiac surgery in left ventricular power failure. Arch Surg 1975;110:1363–1367.

261. Ehrich DA, Biddle TL, Kronenberg MW, Yu PN. The hemodynamic response to intra-aortic balloon counterpulsation in patients with cardiogenic shock complicating acute myocardial infarction. Am Heart J 1977;93:274–279.

262. Subramanian VA, Roberts AJ, Zema MJ, et al. Cardiogenic shock following acute myocardial infarction; late functional results after emergency cardiac surgery. NY State J Med 1980;80:947–952.

263. Hines GL, Mohtashemi M. Delayed operative intervention in cardiogenic shock after myocardial infarction. Ann Thorac Surg 1982;33:132–138.

264. Phillips SJ, Zeff RH, Skinner JR, Toon RS, Grignon A, Kongtahworn C. Reperfusion protocol and results in 738 patients with evolving myocardial infarction. Ann Thorac Surg 1986;41:119–125.

265. Connolly MW, Gelbfish JS, Rose DM, et al. Early coronary artery bypass grafting for complicated acute myocardial infarction. J Cardiovasc Surg 1988;29:375–382.

266. Laks H, Rosenkranz E, Buckberg GD. Surgical treatment of cardiogenic shock after myocardial infarction. Circulation 1986;74:III11–III16.

267. Guyton RA, Arcidi JM Jr, Langford DA, Morris DC, Liberman HA, Hatcher CR Jr. Emergency coronary bypass for cardiogenic shock. Circulation 1987;76:V22–V27.

268. Sergeant P, Blackstone E, Meyns B. Early and late outcome after CABG in patients with evolving myocardial infarction. Eur J Cardio-Thoracic Surg 1997;11:848–855.

269. Allen BS, Buckberg GD, Fontan FM, et al. Superiority of controlled surgical reperfusion versus percutaneous transluminal coronary angioplasty in acute coronary occlusion. J Thorac Cardiovasc Surg 1993;105:864–884.

270. Donatelli F, Benussi S, Triggiani M, Guarracino F, Marchetto G, Grossi A. Surgical treatment for life-threatening acute myocardial infarction: a prospective protocol. Eur J Cardio-Thoracic Surg 1997;11:228–233.

271. Edep ME, Barber E, Brown DL. Cardiogenic shock complicating acute myocardial infarction in California: effect of invasive procedures on mortality. J Am Coll Cardiol 1998;31:398A.

272. Edep ME, Brown DL. Effect of early revascularization on mortality from cardiogenic shock complicating acute myocardial infarction in California. Am J Cardiol 2000;85:1185–1188.

273. Sekela ME. Cardiac surgical procedures following myocardial infarction. Cardiol Clin 1995;13:449–457.

274. Mohr R, Moshkovitch Y, Shapira I, Amir G, Hod H, Gurevitch J. Coronary artery bypass without cardiopulmonary bypass for patients with acute myocardial infarction. J Thorac Cardiovasc Surg 1999;118:50–56.

275. Marber MS, Redwood SR. The management of cardiogenic shock: can anything be learnt from registries? Eur Heart J 2001;22:444–445.

276. Carnendran L, Abboud R, Sleeper LA, et al. Trends in cardiogenic shock: report from the SHOCK Study. The SHould we emergently revascularize Occluded Coronaries for cardiogenic shocK? Eur Heart J 2001;22:472–478.

277. Gitt AK, Schiele R, Seidl K, Glunz HG, Limbourg P, Senges J. Influence of recanalisation therapy on prognosis of cardiogenic shock in acute myocardial infarction in unselected patients of the MITRA-study. J Am Coll Cardiol 1999;33:375A.

278. Berger PB, Holmes DR Jr, Stebbins AL, Bates ER, Califf RM, Topol EJ. Impact of an aggressive invasive catheterization and revascularization strategy on mortality in patients with cardiogenic shock in the Global Utilization of Streptokinase and Tissue Plasminogen Activator for Occluded Coronary Arteries (GUSTO-I) trial. An observational study. Circulation 1997;96:122–127.

279. Berger PB, Tuttle RH, Holmes DR Jr, et al. One-year survival among patients with acute myocardial infarction complicated by cardiogenic shock, and its relation to early revascularization: results from the GUSTO-I trial. Circulation 1999;99:873–878.

280. Hochman JS, Sleeper LA, White HD, et al. One-year survival following early revascularization for cardiogenic shock. JAMA 2001;285:190–192.
281. Hochman JS, Sleeper LA, Godfrey E, et al. SHould we emergently revascularize Occluded Coronaries for cardiogenic shocK: an international randomized trial of emergency PTCA/CABG-trial design. The SHOCK Trial Study Group. Am Heart J 1999;137:313–321.
282. White HD, Stewart JT, Aylward P, et al. Angioplasty versus surgery for cardiogenic shock: results from the SHOCK trial. Circulation 1999;100:I-370.
283. Jacobs AK, Leopold JA, Modur S, et al. Right ventricular infarction complicated by cardiogenic shock: observations and implications. the NHLBI SHOCK registy. J Am Coll Cardiol 2000;35:385A.
284. Dell'Italia LJ, Starling MR, Blumhardt R, Lasher JC, O'Rourke RA. Comparative effects of volume loading, dobutamine, and nitroprusside in patients with predominant right ventricular infarction. Circulation 1985;72:1327–1335.
285. Bowers TR, O'Neill WW, Grines C, Pica MC, Safian RD, Goldstein JA. Effect of reperfusion on biventricular function and survival after right ventricular infarction. N Engl J Med 1998;338:933–940.
286. Lederman RJ, Hagan PG, Knight BP, Eitzman DT, Ohman EM, Bates E. Cardiogenic shock complicating right ventricular myocardial infarction: outcome after percutaneous revasvcularization. J Am Coll Cardiol 1999;33:367A.
287. Holmes DR Jr, Berger PB, Hochman JS, et al. Cardiogenic shock in patients with acute ischemic syndromes with and without ST-segment elevation. Circulation 1999;100:2067–2073.
288. Boden WE, Kleiger RE, Gibson RS, et al. Electrocardiographic evolution of posterior acute myocardial infarction: importance of early precordial ST-segment depression. Am J Cardiol 1987;59:782–787.
289. Biostatistical Fact Sheet. Older americans and cardiovascular diseases. American Heart Association, 1998.
290. Wei JY. Age and the cardiovascular system. N Engl J Med 1992;327:1735–1739.
291. Olivetti G, Melissari M, Capasso JM, Anversa P. Cardiomyopathy of the aging human heart. Myocyte loss and reactive cellular hypertrophy. Circ Res 1991;68:1560–1568
292. Hasdai D, Holmes DR Jr, Califf RM, et al. Cardiogenic shock complicating acute myocardial infarction: predictors of death. GUSTO Investigators. Global Utilization of Streptokinase and Tissue-Plasminogen Activator for Occluded Coronary Arteries. Am Heart J 1999;138:21–31
293. Lane GE, Holmes DR Jr. Primary angioplasty for acute myocardial infarction in the elderly. Coron Artery Dis 2000;11:305–313.
294. Januzzi JL, Davidoff R, Mendes L, et al. Explaining the relationship between age, cardiogenic shock and outcomes: echocardiographic observations from the SHOCK trial. J Am Coll Cardiol 2000;35:219A.
295. Dzavik V, Sleeper LA, Hosat S, Cocke T, LeJemtel T, Hochman JS. Effect of age on treatment and outcome of patients in cardiogenic shock. Eur Heart J 1998;19:28.
296. Dauerman HL, Goldberg RJ, Malinski M, Yarzebski J, Lessard D, Gore JM. Outcomes and early revascularization for patients >/=65 years of age with cardiogenic shock. Am J Cardiol 2001;87:844–848.
297. Stone GW, Brodie BR, Griffin JJ, et al. Clinical and angiographic outcomes in patients with previous coronary artery bypass graft surgery treated with primary balloon angioplasty for acute myocardial infarction. Second Primary Angioplasty in Myocardial Infarction Trial (PAMI-2) Investigators. J Am Coll Cardiol 2000;35:605–611.
298. Suwaidi JA, Velianou JL, Berger PB, et al. Primary PTCA in patients with acute myocardial infarction and prior coronary artery bypass grafting. J Am Coll Cardiol 2000;35:19A.
299. Labinaz M, Sketch MH Jr, Ellis SG, et al. Outcome of acute ST-segment elevation myocardial infarction in patients with prior coronary artery bypass surgery receiving thrombolytic therapy. Am Heart J 2001;141:469–477.
300. Aylward PE, Knight JL, White HD, Sleeper LA, Hochman JS, Lejemtel TH. Cardiogenic shock in patients with prior coronary artery bypass surgery: a report from the SHOCK trial registry. Circulation 1997;96:I-453.
301. Quigley RL, Milano CA, Smith LR, White WD, Rankin JS, Glower DD. Prognosis and management of anterolateral myocardial infarction in patients with severe left main disease and cardiogenic shock. The left main shock syndrome. Circulation 1993;88:II65–II70.
302. Yip HK, Wu CJ, Chen MC, et al. Effect of primary angioplasty on total or subtotal left main occlusion: analysis of incidence, clinical features, outcomes, and prognostic determinants. Chest 2001;120:1212–1217.

303. Tomioka H, Watanabe S, Hayashi K, Okada O, Minami M. Prognosis and management in patients with left main shock syndrome—emergency PTCA following CABG. Jpn J Thorac Cardiovasc Surg 1998;46:1253–1259.

304. Hsu RB, Chien CY, Wang SS, Chu SH. Surgical revascularization for acute total occlusion of left main coronary artery. Tex Heart Inst J 2000;27:299–301.

305. Radford MJ, Johnson RA, Daggett WMJ. Ventricular septal rupture: a review of clinical and physiologic features and an analysis of survival. Circulation 1981;64:545–553.

306. Komeda M, Fremes SE, David TE. Surgical repair of postinfarction ventricular septal defect. Circulation 1990;82:IV243–IV247.

307. Skillington PD, Davies RH, Luff AJ, et al. Surgical treatment for infarct-related ventricular septal defects. Improved early results combined with analysis of late functional status. J Thorac Cardiovasc Surg 1990;99:798–808.

308. Deja MA, Szostek J, Widenka K, et al. Post infarction ventricular septal defect—can we do better? Eur J Cardiothorac Surg 2000;18:194–201.

309. Cummings RG, Califf R, Jones RN, Reimer KA, Kong YH, Lowe JE. Correlates of survival in patients with postinfarction ventricular septal defect. Ann Thorac Surg 1989;47:824–830.

310. Pienvichit P, Piemonte TC. Percutaneous closure of postmyocardial infarction ventricular septal defect with the CardioSEAL septal occluder implant. Catheter Cardiovasc Interv 2001;54:490–494.

311. Pesonen E, Thilen U, Sandstrom S, et al. Transcatheter closure of post-infarction ventricular septal defect with the Amplatzer Septal Occluder device. Scand Cardiovasc J 2000;34:446–448.

312. Lee EM, Roberts DH, Walsh KP. Transcatheter closure of a residual postmyocardial infarction ventricular septal defect with the Amplatzer septal occluder. Heart 1998;80:522–524.

313. Mullasari AS, Umesan CV, Krishnan U, Srinivasan S, Ravikumar M, Raghuraman H. Transcatheter closure of post-myocardial infarction ventricular septal defect with Amplatzer septal occluder. Catheter Cardiovasc Interv 2001;54:484–487.

314. Waight DJ, Hijazi ZM. Post-myocardial infarction ventricular septal defect: a medical and surgical challenge. Catheter Cardiovasc Interv 2001;54:488–489.

315. Vlodaver Z, Edwards JE. Rupture of ventricular septum or papillary muscle complicating myocardial infarction. Circulation 1977;55:815–822.

316. Wei JY, Hutchins GM, Bulkley BH. Papillary muscle rupture in fatal acute myocardial infarction: a potentially treatable form of cardiogenic shock. Ann Intern Med 1979;90:149–152.

317. Nishimura RA, Schaff HV, Shub C, Gersh BJ, Edwards WD, Tajik AJ. Papillary muscle rupture complicating acute myocardial infarction: analysis of 17 patients. Am J Cardiol 1983;51:373–377.

318. Thompson CR, Buller CE, Sleeper LA, et al. Cardiogenic shock due to acute severe mitral regurgitation complicating acute myocardial infarction: a report from the SHOCK Trial Registry. SHould we use emergently revascularize Occluded Coronaries in cardiogenic shocK? J Am Coll Cardiol 2000;36:1104–1109.

319. Nishimura RA, Gersh BJ, Schaff HV. The case for an aggressive surgical approach to papillary muscle rupture following myocardial infarction: "From paradise lost to paradise regained". Heart 2000;83:611–613.

320. Kishon Y, Oh JK, Schaff HV, Mullany CJ, Tajik AJ, Gersh BJ. Mitral valve operation in postinfarction rupture of a papillary muscle: immediate results and long-term follow-up of 22 patients. Mayo Clin Proc 1992;67:1023–1030.

321. Shawl FA, Forman MB, Punja S, Goldbaum TS. Emergent coronary angioplasty in the treatment of acute ischemic mitral regurgitation: long-term results in five cases. J Am Coll Cardiol 1989;14:986–991.

322. Heuser RR, Maddoux GL, Goss JE, Ramo BW, Raff GL, Shadoff N. Coronary angioplasty for acute mitral regurgitation due to myocardial infarction. A nonsurgical treatment preserving mitral valve integrity. Ann Intern Med 1987;107:852–855.

323. Tcheng JE, Jackman JD Jr, Nelson CL, et al. Outcome of patients sustaining acute ischemic mitral regurgitation during myocardial infarction. Ann Intern Med 1992;117:18–24.

324. Shapira I, Isakov A, Burke M, Almog C. Cardiac rupture in patients with acute myocardial infarction. Chest 1987;92:219–223.

325. Rokos IC, Thompson SL, Guigliano RP. Risk factors for cardiac rupture in the modern era of new reperfusion regimens for acute myocardial infarction. Circulation 2001;104:II-482.

326. Reardon MJ, Carr CL, Diamond A, et al. Ischemic left ventricular free wall rupture: prediction, diagnosis, and treatment. Ann Thorac Surg 1997;64:1509–1513.

327. Slater J, Brown RJ, Antonelli TA, et al. Cardiogenic shock due to cardiac free-wall rupture or tamponade after acute myocardial infarction: a report from the SHOCK Trial Registry. Should we emergently revascularize occluded coronaries for cardiogenic shock? J Am Coll Cardiol 2000;36:1117–1122.
328. Figueras J, Cortadellas J, Evangelista A, Soler-Soler J. Medical management of selected patients with left ventricular free wall rupture during acute myocardial infarction. J Am Coll Cardiol 1997;29:512–518.
329. Murata H, Masuo M, Yoshimoto H, et al. Oozing type cardiac rupture repaired with percutaneous injection of fibrin-glue into the pericardial space: case report. Jpn Circ J 2000;64:312–315.
330. Nunley, DL, Grunkemeier, GL, Teply, JF, et al. Coronary bypass operation following acute complicated myocardial infarction. J Thorac Cardiovasc Surg 1983;85:485–491.

22
Myocardial Infarction in the Younger Patient

James C. Fang, MD *and Jorge Plutzky,* MD

CONTENTS

INTRODUCTION

Coronary atherosclerosis in younger patients is quite common *(1,2)*, and early evidence of this disease appears to be present in many, if not most, Americans by the age of 30 *(3)*. Autopsy studies on casualties of both war and other trauma reveal early signs of atherosclerosis in up to 70% of individuals 30 yr old or younger, with significant flow-limiting stenoses in 10% *(4)*. Recent intravascular ultrasound studies (IVUS) from cardiac transplant recipients also confirm these reports. In these studies, where the average donor age was 33.4 ± 13.2 yr, a remarkable 51.9% of the donor coronary arteries demonstrated IVUS evidence of atheroma when these arteries were examined soon after transplantation. Furthermore, in patients under the age of 20, an astonishing 17% had evidence of disease *(5)*.

Although atherosclerosis may be present early, the clinical manifestations of coronary artery disease (CAD) in young patients—myocardial infarction (MI) and angina pectoris—are less frequent *(6)*. Yet these manifestations may provide the only opportunity to intervene in this potentially lethal disease. There are other reasons to study these patients in greater depth. First, the number of patients experiencing MI at the age of 45 or less is not insignificant: approx 125,000 patients/yr or 5% of all MIs in the United States *(7)*. Second, there are unique etiologies to consider more closely in evaluating these patients *(8)*. Third, we may be able to learn a great deal about the CAD process

From: *Contemporary Cardiology: Management of Acute Coronary Syndromes, Second Edition*
Edited by: C. P. Cannon © Humana Press Inc., Totowa, NJ

itself by studying its manifestations in younger patients, such as insight regarding novel risk factors and biologic variables that may be applicable to all patients. In fact, the younger MI patient may afford the possibility of observing CAD without other confounding variables and comorbid conditions. Finally, management of younger survivors of MI may present a particular challenge to the physician given the potential number of years ahead in which risk reduction, anti-atherosclerotic, anti-anginal, and/or anti-congestive heart failure (CHF) efforts must be maintained. This chapter will review the unique pathologic and clinical features regarding premature CAD, and then consider additional risk factors that clinicians may want to consider evaluating when treating the younger patient who has suffered an MI. The study of these issues is limited by both the lack of consolidated data in this population and by the differences in definitions as to what constitutes a young patient. In general, we will define this group of patients as individuals 45 yr of age or younger, although we will consider data from studies that set somewhat different standards for "premature" CAD.

ETIOLOGIC CONSIDERATIONS IN THE YOUNGER MI PATIENT

It is important distinguish between nonatherosclerotic and atherosclerotic mechanisms of MI in the younger patient (8). Although it is tempting to consider more unusual reasons for the acute infarct in the young patient, the process is more often due to typical atherosclerosis stemming from traditional risk factors (9). Nevertheless, it is also true that the nonatherosclerotic and more unusual risk factors are found disproportionately more often among younger MI patients (10). This may be due in part to selection bias, with physicians more inclined to look for unusual etiologies in the younger patient.

NONATHEROSCLEROTIC MECHANISMS OF ACUTE MI
IN THE YOUNGER PATIENT

Any process that blocks coronary artery blood flow may lead to infarction (11). In addition, focal areas of myocardial damage can occur independent of a change in the vascular supply to that area. An extensive list of nonatherosclerotic causes have been reported in studies and case reports in the medical literature; this group has been summarized in Table 1. Although all these causes have been reported to cause MI, not all have been reported *per se* in the younger patient. A select few will be discussed here with the reader directed to other sources and reviews for more details.

Coronary artery spasm (CAS), also known as variant or Prinzmetal's angina, can account for MI in the absence of obvious atherosclerosis (12). First described in 1959, CAS is defined by an abrupt decrease in the diameter of an epicardial artery due to vasoconstriction. The classical description is of symptoms that occur at rest, unrelated to exertion (8). Subsequent studies have shown electrocardiogram (ECG) abnormalities consistent with acute injury, as well as responsiveness to nitroglycerin. Prolonged vasospasm can lead to frank infarction. There is a suggestion of coincident atherosclerosis contributing to the tendency for spasm, as well as worsening what is otherwise an excellent prognosis (89–97% 5-yr survival). Vasospasm probably reflects a diffuse abnormality in endothelial function that some have reported in patients with a family history of premature CAD, as well as younger individuals before the onset of clinically evident atherosclerosis (13). CAS is important to consider in the younger MI patient,

Table 1
Nonatherosclerotic Causes of MI

Aortic disease
  Aortic stenosis
  Aortic insufficiency
  Aortic dissection extending to coronary arteries
Toxicity
  Carbon monoxide poisoning
  Cocaine
Hematological abnormalities
  Polycythemia vera
  Thrombocytosis
  Disseminated intravascular coagulation
Trauma
  Myocardial contusion
  Coronary artery laceration
  Coronary artery abnormalities
  Coronary artery dissection
Coronary artery spasm (Prinzmetal's Angina)
Coronary anomalies
  Anomalous coronaries
  Arteriovenous (AV) fistula
  Aneurysm
Emboli to the coronary artery
Myocardial processes
  Focal myocarditis
  Metabolic or intimal proliferative diseases
Inherited metabolic syndromes/mucopolysaccharidose
  Fabry disease
  Amyloidosis
  Juvenile initimal sclerosis
  Intimal hyperplasia (contraceptive steroids or post-partum state)
  Cerebrotendinous Xanthomathomatosis
  Pseudoxanthoma elasticum sitosterolemia
  Werner's syndrome
Miscellaneous
  Progeria
Idiopathic MI with normal coronary arteriogram

given the frequency of normal-appearing arteriograms at the time of catheterization in young MI victims *(14)*. CAS is one potential explanation for an "evanescent" cessation in coronary blood flow. In the catheterization laboratory, CAS can be investigated through the administration of various intracoronary pharmacologic agents (ergonovine, acetylcholine, methacholine, epinephrine, histamine) or application of certain techniques (cold pressor test, hyperventilation). Management of CAS may include nitrates and/or calcium channel blockers as well as an avoidance of β-blockers out of concern for unopposed α stimulation.

CAS may be one mechanism of MI in cocaine abuse, another cause of nonathero-sclerotic MI that is seen disproportionately in the young *(15)*. As a hyperadrenergic stimulus, cocaine can precipitate CAS while also increasing myocardial oxygen demand through increased blood pressure and heart rate. Of note, patients may present many h after the cocaine use, perhaps due to the effects of active metabolites such as benzoyiergonovine *(16)*. Cocaine is also atherogenic, increases platelet aggregation, and is associated with endocarditis with embolic infarcts when abused intravenously. Routine toxicology screen for cocaine use is warranted in young patients presenting with acute MI or chest pain in the absence of other known major predisposing factors. Coronary angiography is normal in one-third of cocaine-related infarcts with the majority of the remaining angiograms demonstrating some degree of thrombus or CAD *(17)*.

Coronary emboli are another nonatherosclerotic cause of MI in the young *(11)*. Arterial thrombi can occur as a complication of infective endocarditis, paradoxical emboli through a patent foramen ovale, hypercoagulable states, and atrial myxomas. In general, such occurrences in the coronary circulation appear to be rare. Coronary artery anomalies may also cause ischemia, infarction, and/or sudden cardiac death due to compression by surrounding structures *(18)*. For example, origin of the left coronary artery from the right or noncoronary aortic sinus of Valsalva can be associated with sudden cardiac death, particularly when the artery runs between aortic and pulmonary artery roots. Finally, deep myocardial bridges and spontaneous coronary dissections should be considered when atherosclerosis is not evident.

ATHEROSCLEROTIC MECHANISMS OF ACUTE MI IN THE YOUNGER PATIENT

General Issues

Although it is important to consider nonatherosclerotic etiologies for acute MI in the young, most infarctions are likely due to typical atherosclerosis, since traditional risk factors are common in these patients. Genest and colleagues reviewed patients less than 60 yr of age who underwent admission for MI to the cardiac intensive care unit and found that most of these patients had known risk factors for CAD *(19)*. Other data support these findings. For example, increasing number of traditional risk factors in a young patient predicts more extensive CAD *(6)*. The most common risk factors are smoking *(20)*, dyslipidemia *(21)*, and a family history of CAD *(22)*. Hypertension and diabetes are less correlated with MI in the young patient, perhaps reflecting the long-term toll these processes take on the vasculature *(23)*.

There may be several reasons why one patient with multiple, but common, risk factors experiences an MI at an earlier age than another patient. It may result from the particular severity of a given known risk factor, the combination of multiple known risk factors, an underlying genotype, which has amplified the pathologic response, or a combination of the above. In addition, young patients with atherosclerosis may place higher demands on the myocardium due to increased exertion. The cases, which receive extensive attention, are often those that occur in the world class athlete *(24)*.

In considering traditional risk factors, cigarette smoking is at the top of list. Several studies have estimated that between 60–90% of young patients experiencing an MI are smokers *(25–27)*. The Pathologic Determinants of Atherosclerosis in the Young (PDAY) study has found a correlation between raised atherosclerotic lesions in the right coronary artery and abdominal aorta of young men, 15–34 yr of age who died of violent causes, and their thiocyanate levels a marker of cigarette smoke *(28,29)*. Thrombolysis in Myocardial Infarction (TIMI) studies have also suggested that cigarette smoking is associated with infarction at a younger age and is more often associated with thrombosis of a less critical lesion, thus implicating plaque rupture *(30)*. More recent work has suggested the importance of counseling high risk patients to avoid passive smoke inhalation. Certainly not all smokers develop premature clinical atherosclerosis, suggesting a "two hit" process with some patients being more susceptible to smoking's toxic vascular effects. Regardless, cigarette smoking remains an obvious target for the physician who hopes to subtract a powerful factor from contributing to a patient's risk.

Another reason why one patient may develop CAD before another is the presence of either undefined, or not yet confirmed, risk factors. Although statistically, most premature CAD does result from traditional risk factors, emerging risk factors have also been disproportionately associated with the younger patient *(19,31)*. As mentioned earlier, this may stem from increased attention to these other risk factors in the younger MI patient. For example, hyperinsulinemia appears to have an epidemiologic and biologic evidence to support its role in premature atherogenesis *(32)*. In a Canadian study of monogenic insulin resistance, the presence of the homozygous mutation increased the risk of needing bypass surgery from 1 in 7350 to 1 in 3.75 in women ages 35–54 yr *(33)*. These emerging risk factors may not be solely associated with premature CAD, but relevant to CAD in general. Clinicians should consider screening for these risk factors in any patient who suffers an MI in the absence of other obvious risk factors.

It has been suggested that the patient who has an MI before the age of 45 has an approx 50% chance of having some form of an inherited genetic disorder *(22,34)*. The possibilities for the nature of this disorder are considerable and reflect much of our new insight into vascular biology. A detailed review of these disorders is beyond the scope of this chapter although the broad nature of some of these disorders can be considered.

Lipoprotein(a)

One study of acute MI in 102 young men revealed lipoprotein(a) [Lp (a)] excess was the most common abnormality found (18.6%), with other familial disorders declining from there (Table 2) *(19,35)*. Other studies have suggested a similar correlation between Lp(a) and CAD *(36,37)*, although no such correlation was noted in the Physicians' Health Study *(38)*. Lp(a) is a particularly intriguing molecule, since basic science work has suggested a plausible mechanism to support its association with CAD *(39)*. Lp(a) consists of a low-density lipoprotein (LDL)-like apolipoprotein B particle linked to an apolipoprotein(a) [apo(a)] moiety *(40)*. Lp(a) is known to be deposited directly in the arterial wall where it may incite pathological reactions contributing to atherosclerosis. In addition, the apo(a) moiety bears considerable homology to plasminogen, thus creating a decoy for plasminogen activator, resulting in competitive inhibition of fibrinolysis and a putative hypercoagulable state. Lp(a) thus represents a potential intersection between lipoproteins and the coagulation system. Lp(a) may be of particular importance in explaining the striking increased incidence of premature atherosclerosis among young Asian Indians, in spite of their typical vegetarian diets *(41,42)*. Treatment of Lp(a) excess is difficult. No significant Lp (a) lowering is achieved with most medications that lower LDL, although there have been reports of lowering with niacin *(43)*.

Table 2
Frequency of Lipoprotein Abnormalities in Men with Premature Coronary Heart Disease

	Controls (n = 901)	Cases (n = 321)	
		Not Adjusted	Adjusted[a]
HDL-c < 10th%	10%	46%	36%
Apo A-I < 10th%	10%	37%	36%
Apo B > 90th%	10%	24%	36%
Triglycerides > 90th%	10%	26%	26%
LDL-c > 90th%	10%	12%	22%
Lipoprotein(a) > 90th%	10%	16%	16%

[a]Significantly different than controls ($p < 0.01$).
HDL-c, high-density lipoprotein cholesterol; LDL-c, low-density lipoprotein cholesterol.
Adapted with permission.

HDL

Most clinicians who care for MI patients will eventually encounter one young patient, usually a male, with premature CAD, whose sole lipid abnormality is a significantly low high-density lipoprotein (HDL) level *(44)*. Often, such patients will have low LDL levels, suggesting that LDL is not the major culprit lipoprotein. Most likely, such patients have hypoalphalipoproteinemia, an inherited lipid disorder *(45)*. The inverse relationship between HDL levels and CAD has been well established. What is less clear is the ease with which we can significantly change someone's HDL levels, or if such a change in HDL levels will alter their clinical course *(46)*. A major limitation has been, in part, due to the lack of medications that can significantly change HDL levels significantly. Diet and exercise, in particular lowering the body mass index, can raise HDL levels. Niacin is probably the most effective drug for raising HDL levels, perhaps as much as 10–15% in patients who can tolerate its side effects *(47)*. Niacin can be administered successfully if carefully managed by the physician. Manufacturers of new preparations of niacin given once in the evening report fewer side effects, although clinical experience continues to emerge. Although modest alcohol intake can raise HDL levels, many physicians feel uncomfortable endorsing such a practice. In patients with low HDL who are on β-blockers, one should consider using a β-blocker with intrinsic sympathomimetic activity (ISA), given the evidence that those with ISA tend to not lower HDL as much. This consideration should be balanced against the proven efficacy of more conventional β-blockers in post-MI survival trials, and therefore, clinical judgement will be needed on a case-by-case basis *(47)*.

However, more modest changes in HDL may also be beneficial. In the now landmark Veterans Affairs (VA) HDL Cholesterol Intervention Trial (VA-HIT), 2531 veterans with known CAD and HDL <40, LDL <140, and triglycerides <300 were randomized in a double-blinded placebo-controlled trial of gemfibrozil (1200 mg/d). After a median follow-up of 5.1 yr, the primary end point of nonfatal MI and death from coronary causes was decreased by 22%. The striking finding was the modest 6% increase of HDL from 32 to 34 mg/dL *(48)*. LDL did not change (113 mg/dL), but triglycerides fell 31% from 160 to 115 mg/dL. Gemfibrozil was well tolerated; dyspepsia was the only side effect more common in the active treatment arm. Statin use was reportedly low, although not specified. Whether these findings are a class effect remains to be determined, but other earlier studies with fibrates have suggested that their benefit may, in fact, be due to an HDL effect *(49,50)*.

One should also be alert to the potential for improving HDL levels by lowering triglyceride levels. Diet (especially the high carbohydrate diet so often taken by those on low fat regimens), exercise, and treatment of secondary factors (diabetes, nephrotic syndrome, thyroid disorders) can lower triglyceride levels *(51,52)*. More recent studies, for example Airforce/Texas Coronary Atherosclerosis Prevention Study (AFCAPS), in which patients could not be enrolled if HDL levels were too high, raise the question of treating isolated low HDL by lowering the LDL level further *(53,54)*. In that study, statin therapy appeared to "neutralize" the effects of the low HDL *(55)*. The potential impact of therapeutic agents that could raise HDL levels to the same extent, ease, and tolerability as statins are anxiously awaited given their potential benefit, especially among these younger patients with isolated low HDL certainly the benefits seen from niacin likely derive in large part from its HDL effects. One cannot ignore evidence that suggests that MIs, regardless of age, are rare in patients with hyperalphalipoproteinemia, a protective genetic mutation in which HDL levels are often above 100 mg/dL *(56)*. One can easily imagine the potential impact of a pharmacologic agent that might be able to induce such levels.

Interestingly, familial hypercholesterolemia (FH), a disease strongly associated with a predisposition to premature CAD, represented only 3% of the premature infarct population in the ICY study cited above. This percentage would be expected to change in other populations where FH is a well described common problem, e.g., French Canadians.

In addition to inherited lipid disorders, we continue to learn more about the interactive nature of modest levels of dyslipidemia. Recent work has suggested that the combination of elevated LDL, lower HDL, and elevated triglycerides ("syndrome X") may be particularly atherogenic. The exact reasons for this remain unclear, but may involve small dense LDL, the low HDL, an effect of triglycerides themselves, or underlying insulin resistance. Interestingly, some studies, such as the post hoc analysis of the Helsinki Heart Study and more recently the Paris Prospective Study, suggest that the elevated triglyceride level confers increased risk even among patients with the same LDL/HDL ratio *(57)*.

Also of note is the frequency with which no known familial lipid disorder is found in genetic studies of young MI survivors *(19)*. Certainly, this is a reflection of how much we have yet to learn about the variables that contribute to atherosclerosis, in particular those that extend beyond lipids and lipoproteins. Table 3 lists many of the nontraditional risk factors currently under intensive investigation in basic science laboratories and in clinical trials.

Homocysteine

Homocysteine is one such example of an emerging risk factor that may play a role in premature atherosclerosis *(58,59)*. The suggestion that homocysteine might be atherogenic stemmed from the recognition that congenital homozygous homocystinuria, a disease fatal in early childhood, included premature vascular disease as part of its phenotype *(60)*. Subsequent studies have suggested that the genetically determined elevation in homocysteine levels may contribute to CAD and other types of vascular dis-

Table 3
Nontraditional/Emerging Risk Factors for Atherosclerosis/Premature Vascular Disease

Lp(a)
Homocysteine levels
Insulin levels
Fibrinogen levels
DHEA-s
LDL particle size (small, dense, LDL, Pattern B)
Oxidized LDL levels
Decreases HDL2 subfractions

ease *(61)*. A basis for this interaction has been suggested by in vitro studies demonstrating damage to endothelial cells, perhaps through oxidation, as well as stimulation of smooth muscle cell proliferation, inhibition of endothelial cell nitric oxide production, and increased endothelial cell production of thrombomodulin *(62)*. In vivo primate studies suggest vascular lesions can be induced by infusion of homocysteine. The incidence of homocystinuria, an autosomal recessive disorder, has been estimated at 1: 200,000, while heterozygosity is placed at 1:100 *(63)*.

Several epidemiologic studies have supported an association of hyperhomocystinemia with MI, peripheral vascular disease (PVD), and cardiovascular disease (CVD), as well as a "concentration-dependent" effect, even within normal ranges. In the Physician Health Study, homocysteine levels in the upper 5% of men 40–84 yr of age were associated with a 3.1 relative risk increase of MI compared to those with the lowest levels of homocysteine *(64,65)*. Similar prospective associations were seen in the Tromso study *(66)*. Furthermore, lowering plasma homocysteine levels appears to beneficial. In a study of another paradigm for accelerated atherosclerosis, postangioplasty restenosis, the use of vitamin B12, pyridoxine, and folate decreased the amount of angiographic restenosis (39.9 $\pm$ 20.3% vs 48.2 $\pm$ 28.3%, $p = 0.01$, the rate of restenosis (19.6 vs 37.6%, $p = 0.01$), and the clinical need for revascularization (10.8 vs 22.3%, $p = 0.047$), while concomitantly lowering plasma homocysteine levels (11.1 $\pm$ 4.3 to 7.2 $\pm$ 2.4 µmol/L, $p < 0.001$) *(67)*.

The relationship between homocysteine and CAD in the younger MI patient has not been fully explored. In attempting to establish the relationship between homocysteine and vascular disease, most studies have set age cutoffs around 50 yr of age. Nevertheless, a Framingham angiographic study of 170 men (mean age 50 yr) with CAD suggested that homocysteine was an independent risk factor *(58)*. In contrast, other studies have failed to demonstrate a clear association between homocysteine levels and premature CAD. Kang and colleagues could not demonstrate a difference between homocysteine levels in patients with CAD who were less than 40 yr of age and case controls *(68)*. There was a significant difference in homocysteine levels between case and control groups among older patients. This age-dependent phenomenon may be related to the lack of dietary B vitamins and folate intake within older populations. The use and study of homocysteine in clinical practice has been limited by the different methods to measure homocysteine levels (random level vs methione loading), the existing overlap between normal levels and abnormal levels of homocysteine, and the ease of treatment with oral folate, leading some clinicians to simply have patients take folate supplementation empirically.

Fibrinogen

Fibrinogen rremains under extensive evaluation for its role in atherosclerosis and, to a more limited extent, in premature CAD *(22,69)*. Multiple studies have suggested a relationship between fibrinogen levels and CAD/MI *(69)*. This association is biologically plausible given the presumed effects of increased fibrinogen levels on coagulation and blood viscosity. Framingham data (1315 patients) suggest that fibrinogen levels increase with age, and the incidence of CAD becomes significantly greater when baseline levels of fibrinogen exceeded 3.1 g/L. Five of the published fibrinogen studies have included patients less than 45 yr of age, yet evidence that fibrinogen contributes to the development of premature CAD remains inconclusive *(70)*. Hamsten et al. reported the largest group although in a retrospective case-controlled study *(71)*. In this setting, elevated fibrinogen was among the best markers of ischemic heart disease in the 148 patients less than 45 yr of age. Perhaps fibrinogen as a risk factor has received less attention due to our inability to modify its levels. Thus far, only alcohol use and estrogen therapy in women have been suggested to decrease its levels.

Other Novel Factors

The thrombospondin family of proteins has also been recently implicated from studies employing state-of-the-art genomics technology. These proteins are important in angiogenesis, vascular healing, cell adhesion, and anticoagulation and serve as ligands for specific receptors, such as oxidized LDL and integrins. At the Cleveland Clinic, investigators recently identified three single nucleotide polymorphisms in the thrombospondin gene in a survey of more than 50,000 genetic polymorphisms involving 398 families with a history of premature CAD in a case-controlled study. Thrombospondin was one of 62 candidate genes, which were selected on the basis of their roles in vascular biology, lipidology, and hemostasis. The investigators go on to speculate that the polymorphisms in this gene family may be responsible for the accelerated atherosclerosis in these patients *(72)*. Other nontraditional risk factors and biologic variables for both vascular disease and premature vascular disease are being examined, as well including dehydroepiandrosterone sulfate (DHEA-s), iron, and c-reactive protein *(65)*.

CLINICAL FEATURES AND PATTERNS OF CAD IN THE YOUNGER PATIENT

The younger patient with a MI typically has less extensive CAD, with fewer numbers of lesions, as well as stenoses that tend to be less severe *(25)*. Negus and colleagues found that the majority of angiograms in post-MI patients less than 40 yr of age had a stenosis in a single vessel, most often the left anterior descending artery *(63)*. Similar result were reported by Wolfe and Vacek in catheterizations in 35 patients less than 35 yr of age from the US Air Force: high rates of single vessel left anterior descending artery (LAD) disease, with more frequent total occlusions as compared to a group of 100 patients over 55 yr *(73)*. It is also not unusual to find no evidence for significant flow-limiting lesions at cardiac catheterization of the younger MI survivor. In the Coronary Artery Surgery Study (CASS) database, 504 young adults with MI underwent angiograms, with 16% of men and 21% of women having normal coronary arteries *(74)*. Some of the possible etiologies for MI in these patients have been discussed previously. In addition, particularly in this age group, one should be reminded that the early stages of atherosclerosis move in an abluminal direction, thereby preserving the dimensions of the lumen despite the presence of significant atherosclerosis within the vessel wall. Such "young" lesions may well be more prone to rupture, thus explaining recent evidence that the majority of MIs occur at the site of modest stenoses, typically no greater than 70% *(75–77)*. Cardiac catheterization in fact only reveals the nature of the lumen, thus limiting its value in the study of premature atherosclerosis. Intravascular ultrasound and ultrafast computerized tomography (CT) have been suggested as alternatives in these settings because of their ability to image the vascular wall.

Beyond the anatomic distribution of the CAD, the younger patient is more likely to experience an infarct as opposed to angina pectoris. This observation is also suggestive of plaque rupture as a primary mechanism for infarction in these patients as opposed to increasing degrees of stenoses where supply ultimately is outstripped by demand. Pathologic studies support such hypotheses, even if currently limited to studies with few patients. Dollar and coworkers analyzed the atherosclerotic plaques in the coronaries of 8 women who had MIs before the age of 40 and compared them to 37 adults over 45 yr *(78)*. These young women tended to have more foam cells and less dense fibrous tissue, both of which are markers of more unstable plaques. Corrado et al. from Italy also found similar results in 200 consecutive Italian patients less than 35 yr who died suddenly: one-quarter had acute thrombosis superimposed upon a lipid rich core *(79)*.

Only the CASS study has addressed left ventricular function in young patients with MI *(74)*. There was no significant difference in overall left ventricular function as compared to older patients with MI. This finding is consistent with previous observations that younger patients tend to have less extensive multivessel CAD. Perhaps these younger patients had less time to develop collateral circulation. Interestingly, despite the preservation in ventricular function in the younger patients, they tended to have less heart failure.

CONCLUSION

The frequency of atherosclerosis and its consequences, such as MI in a younger population, highlights the need for risk reduction efforts in a primary care primary prevention setting. Even beyond primary prevention in the adult, this problem also raise issues regarding screening and treatment in pediatric populations *(80–82)*. Currently, we are facing an on-going struggle to ensure that adults are appropriately screened and treated for established risk factors. Studies suggest that the majority of events in the younger population are greatly influenced by remediable risk factors like cigarette smoking, hypertension, and common forms of dyslipidemia for which effective interventions exist *(83)*. The issues surrounding these younger patients with atherosclerosis offer support for the National Cholesterol Education Panel's recommendation that all Americans over the age of 21 yr should know their lipid profile. An important advance relevant to premature atherosclerosis is the growing recognition of the artificial and potentially misleading nature of distinguishing between primary and secondary prevention *(84)*. In the new guidelines, patients without prior history of CAD are treated aggressively if their 10-yr risk warrants it, independent of prior history. One such example of a high risk population is diabetic patients, all of whom should be treated to secondary prevention levels *(84)*. Although contrarian views have previously argued against this approach out of concern for inducing unnecessary treatment too early in a patient's life, this concern seems incorrectly placed, especially in the face of lipid-lowering benefits in patients at lower and lower degrees of risk. All too many patients will die from their first MI, obviating any opportunity for their benefiting from the many cardiovascular therapies now available. This places a clearcut challenge at the feet of primary care physicians to recognize risk and intervene before that first event. For others, the loss of ventricular function will leave them incapacitated to various extents. Beyond this, it is difficult to estimate the loss and impact to a family, to individual productivity, or to society in general when a patient suffers an MI. Such events are all the more unfortunate to the extent they may have been preventable. These issues are perhaps even more dramatic when the patient has not yet reached mid-life. The ability to identify risk and intervene in whatever way is appropriate in altering known risk factors, while continuing to understand emerging ones, remains among the few options we have available against a complex, variable, and recurrent disease.

Careful study of MI in the younger patient will certainly yield further insight into the atherosclerotic process, with implications for both this population as well as other patients with vascular disease. For now, a common sense approach to these patients would include consideration of screening and treating nontraditional risk factors when MI occurs in the absence of other established significant risk factors, particularly when there is a clear family history for premature CAD. Similarly, older patients with CAD without obvious risk factors can also be considered for screening for these other emerging risk factors. Clearly, physicians must not pass up the opportunity to mitigate those established risk factors for which we have proven interventions, especially in the younger patient who may be facing the challenge of surviving 30–40 more yr if he is to meet the life expectancy of his peers. For now, physicians will be left to their own clinical judgement regarding young MI patients in terms of several issues. Should one use empiric folate treatment for homocysteine levels? Is there further benefit from even greater reductions in LDL levels beyond <100 mg/dL? Do the potential pleiotropic benefits of statins argue that all patients should be on these agents? What is the incremental benefit-to-risk reduction when adding second agents targeting HDL and triglycerides to existing statin treatment? Hopefully, study of this young post-MI population will offer us some answers to these questions, if not insight into the basic biologic mechanisms at work in atherosclerosis.

REFERENCES

1. Yater W, Traum AH, Brown WB, Fitzgerald RP, Geisler MA, Wilcox BB. Coronary artery disease in men eighteen to thirty-nine years of age: report of eight hundred sixty-six cases, four hundred fifty with necropsy examinations. Am Heart J 1948;36:334–337.
2. National Health and Nutrition Examination Survey 1976–1980 (NHANES II). 1980.
3. Enos W, Holmes RH, Beyer J. Coronary disease among United States soldiers killed in action in Korea. JAMA 1953;152:1090.
4. Lamm G. The epidemiology of acute myocardial infarction in young age groups. In: Roskamm H. ed. Myocardial Infarction at Young Age. Springer-Verlag, Heidelberg, 1981, pp. 5–10.
5. Tuzcu EM, Kapadia SR, Tutar E, et al. High prevalence of coronary atherosclerosis in asymptomatic teenagers and young adults: evidence from intravascular ultrasound. Circulation 2001;103:2705–2710.
6. Uhl GS, Farrel PW. Risk factors and natural history. In: Roskamm H. ed. Myocardial Infarction at Young Age. Springer-Verlag, Heidelberg, 1981, pp. 29–44.
7. Chen L, Chester M, Kaski JC. Clinical factors and angiographic features associated with premature coronary artery disease. Chest 1995;108:364–369.

8. Antman EM, Braunwald E. Acute myocardial infarction. In: Braunwald E. ed. Heart Disease. W.B. Saunders, Philadelphia, 1997, pp. 1184–1288.

9. Hamsten A. Myocardial infarction at a young age: mechanisms and management. Vasc Med Rev 1991; 2:45–60.

10. Hamsten A, de Faire U. Risk factors for coronary artery disease in families of young men with myocardial infarction. Am J Cardiol 1987;59:14–19.

11. Waller BF, Fry ET, Hermiller JB, Peters T, Slack JD. Nonatherosclerotic causes of coronary artery narrowing—Part III. Clin Cardiol 1996;19:656–661.

12. Maseri AB, L'Abbatte G and A. Coronary vasopasm as a possible cause of myocardial infarction. N Eng J Med 1978;299:1271–1277.

13. Schachinger V, Britten MB, Elsner M, Walter DH, Scharrer I, Zeiher AM. A positive family history of premature coronary artery disease is associated with impaired endothelium-dependent coronary blood flow regulation. Circulation 1999;100:1502–1508.

14. Hamsten A, Walldius G, Szamosi A, Dahlen G, de Faire U. Relationship of angiographically defined coronary artery disease to serum lipoproteins and apolipoproteins in young survivors of myocardial infarction. Circulation 1986;73:1097–1110.

15. Pitts WR, Lange RA, Cigarroa JE, Hillis LD. Cocaine-induced myocardial ischemia and infarction: pathophysiology, recognition, and management. Prog Cardiovasc Dis 1997;40:65–76.

16. Hollander JE. Cocaine-associated myocardial infarction. J R Soc Med 1996;89:443–447.

17. Boghdadi MS, Henning RJ. Cocaine: pathophysiology and clinical toxicology. Heart Lung 1997;26: 466–485.

18. Friedman W. Congenital heart disease in infancy and childhood. In: Braunwald E. ed. Heart Disease. W.B. Saunders, Philadelphia, 1997.

19. Genest JJ, McNamara JR, Salem DN, Schaefer EJ. Prevalence of risk factors in men with premature coronary artery disease. Am J Cardiol 1991;67:1185–1189.

20. PDAY Study Group. Relationship of atherosclerosis in young men to serum lippoprotein cholesterol concentrations and smoking. JAMA 1990;264:3018–3024.

21. Klag MJ, Ford DE, Mead LA, et al. Serum cholesterol in young men and subsequent cardiovascular disease [see comments]. N Engl J Med 1993;328:313–318.

22. Genest J Jr, Cohn JS. Clustering of cardiovascular risk factors: targeting high- risk individuals. Am J Cardiol 1995;76:8A–20A.

23. Plutzky J. Emerging concepts in metabolic abnormalities associated with coronary artery disease. Curr Opin Cardiol 2000;15:416–421.

24. Franklin, BA, Fletcher GF, Gordon NF, Noakes TD, Ades PA, Balady GJ. Cardiovascular evaluation of the athlete. Issues regarding performance, screening and sudden cardiac death. Sports Med 1997;24: 97–119.

25. Chen L, Chester M, Kaski JC. Clinical factors and angiographic features associated with premature coronary artery disease. Chest 1995;108:364–369.

26. Baseline risk factors and their association with outcome in the West of Scotland Coronary Prevention Study. The West of Scotland Coronary Prevention Study Group. Am J Cardiol 1997;79:756–762.

27. McGill HC Jr, McMahan CA, Malcom GT, Oalmann MC, Strong JP. Effects of serum lipoproteins and smoking on atherosclerosis in young men and women. The PDAY Research Group. Pathobiological Determinants of Atherosclerosis in Youth. Arterioscler Thromb Vasc Biol 1997;17:95–106.

28. Strong JP, Malcom GT, Oalmann MC. Environmental and genetic risk factors in early human atherogenesis: lessons from the PDAY study. Pathobiological Determinants of Atherosclerosis in Youth. Pathol Int 1995;45:403–408.

29. Strong JP, Malcom GT, Oalmann MC, Wissler RW. The PDAY Study: natural history, risk factors, and pathobiology. Pathobiological Determinants of Atherosclerosis in Youth. Ann NY Acad Sci 1997;811: 226–237.

30. Zahger D, Cercek B, Cannon CP, et al. How do smokers differ from nonsmokers in their response to thrombolysis? (the TIMI-4 trial) [see comments]. Am J Cardiol 1995;75:232–236.

31. Beigel Y, George J, Leibovici L, Mattityahu A, Sclarovsky S, Blieden L. Coronary risk factors in children of parents with premature coronary artery disease. Acta Paediatr 1993;82:162–165.

32. Despres JP, Lamarche B, Mauriege P, Cantin B, Lupien PJ, Dagenais GR. Risk factors for ischaemic heart disease: is it time to measure insulin? Eur Heart J 1996;17:1453–1454.

33. Hegele RA. Premature atherosclerosis associated with monogenic insulin resistance. Circulation 2001; 103:2225–2229.

34. Kontula K, Ehnholm C. Regulatory mutations in human lipoprotein disorders and atherosclerosis. Curr Opin Lipidol 1996;7:64–68.
35. Fortmann SP, Marcovina SM. Lipoprotein(a), a clinically elusive lipoprotein particle [editorial; comment]. Circulation 1997;95:295–296.
36. Valentine RJ, Grayburn PA, Vega GL, Grundy SM. Lp(a) lipoprotein is an independent, discriminating risk factor for premature peripheral atherosclerosis among white men. Arch Intern Med 1994; 154:801–806.
37. Wilcken DE, Wang XL, Greenwood J, Lynch J. Lipoprotein(a) and apolipoproteins B and A-1 in children and coronary vascular events in their grandparents [see comments]. J Pediatr 1993;123:519–526.
38. Ridker PM, Hennekens CH. A prospective study of lipoprotein(a) and the risk of myocardial infarction. JAMA 1993;270:2195–2199.
39. White AL, Lanford RE. Biosynthesis and metabolism of lipoprotein (a). Curr Opin Lipidol 1995;6: 75–80.
40. Scanu AM. Structural and functional polymorphism of lipoprotein(a): biological and clinical implications. Clin Chem 1995;41:170–172.
41. Shaukat N, de Bono DP, Jones DR. Like father like son? Sons of patients of European or Indian origin with coronary artery disease reflect their parents' risk factor patterns. Br Heart J 1995;74:318–323.
42. Enas EA, Dhawan J, Petkar S. Coronary artery disease in Asian Indians: lessons learnt and the role of lipoprotein(a). Indian Heart J 1997;49:25–34.
43. Angelin B. Therapy for lowering lipoprotein (a) levels. Curr Opin Lipidol 1997;8:337–341.
44. Calabresi L, Franceschini G. High density lipoprotein and coronary heart disease: insights from mutations leading to low high density lipoprotein. Curr Opin Lipidol 1997;8:219–224.
45. Vega GL, Grundy SM. Hypoalphalipoproteinemia (low high density lipoprotein) as a risk factor for coronary heart disease. Curr Opin Lipidol 1996;7:209–216.
46. Kwiterovich PO Jr. Diagnosis and management of familial dyslipoproteinemia in children and adolescents. Pediatr Clin North Am 1990;37:1489–1523.
47. Schaefer EJ. Familial lipoprotein disorders and premature coronary artery disease. Med Clin North Am 1994;78:21–39.
48. Rubins HB, Robins SJ, Collins D, et al. Gemfibrozil for the secondary prevention of coronary heart disease in men with low levels of high-density lipoprotein cholesterol. Veterans Affairs High-Density Lipoprotein Cholesterol Intervention Trial Study Group. N Engl J Med 1999;341:410–418.
49. De Man FH, Cabezas MC, Van Barlingen HH, Erkelens DW, de Bruin TW. Triglyceride-rich lipoproteins in non-insulin-dependent diabetes mellitus: post-prandial metabolism and relation to premature atherosclerosis. Eur J Clin Invest 1996;26:89–108.
50. de Faire U, Ericsson, CG, Grip L, Nilsson J, Svane B, Hamsten A. Secondary preventive potential of lipid-lowering drugs. The Bezafibrate Coronary Atherosclerosis Intervention Trial (BECAIT). Eur Heart J 1996;17(Suppl. F):37–42.
51. Austin MA, Hokanson JE. Epidemiology of triglycerides, small dense low-density lipoprotein, and lipoprotein(a) as risk factors for coronary heart disease. Med Clin North Am 1994;78:99–115.
52. Avogaro P, Ghiselli G, Soldan S, Bittolo Bon G. Relationship of triglycerides and HDL cholesterol in hypertriglyceridemia. Atherosclerosis 1992;92:79–86.
53. Downs JR, Clearfield M, Weis S, et al. Primary prevention of acute coronary events with lovastatin in men and women with average cholesterol levels: results of AFCAPS/TexCAPS. Air Force/Texas Coronary Atherosclerosis Prevention Study. JAMA 1998;279:1615–1622.
54. Clearfield M, Whitney EJ, Weis S, et al. Air Force/Texas Coronary Atherosclerosis Prevention Study (AFCAPS/TexCAPS): baseline characteristics and comparison with USA population. J Cardiovasc Risk 2000;7:125–133.
55. Gotto AM Jr, Whitney E, Stein EA, et al. Relation between baseline and on-treatment lipid parameters and first acute major coronary events in the Air Force/Texas Coronary Atherosclerosis Prevention Study (AFCAPS/TexCAPS). Circulation 2000;101:477–484.
56. Assmann G, von Eckardstein A, Funke H. High density lipoproteins, reverse transport of cholesterol, and coronary artery disease. Insights from mutations. Circulation 1993;87:III28–III34.
57. Fontbonne AM, Eschwege EM. Insulin and cardiovascular disease: Paris Prospective Study. Diabetes Care 1991;14:461–469.
58. Genest JJ Jr, McNamara JR, Salem DN, Wilson PW, Schaefer EJ, Malinow MR. Plasma homocyst(e)ine levels in men with premature coronary artery disease. J Am Coll Cardiol 1990;16: 1114–1119.

59. Gallagher PM, Meleady R, Shields DC, et al. Homocysteine and risk of premature coronary heart disease. Evidence for a common gene mutation. Circulation 1996;94:2154–2158.
60. Fowler B. Disorders of homocysteine metabolism. J Inherit Metab Dis 1997;20:270–285.
61. Boers GH. Hyperhomocysteinemia as a risk factor for arterial and venous disease. A review of evidence and relevance. Thromb Haemost 1997;78:520–522.
62. Duell PB, Malinow MR. Homocyst(e)ine: an important risk factor for atherosclerotic vascular disease. Curr Opin Lipidol 1997;8:28–34.
63. Selhub J, Jacques PF, Bostom AG, et al. Association between plasma homocysteine concentrations and extracranial carotid artery stenosis. N Engl J Med 1995;332:286–291.
64. Christen WG, Ridker PM. Blood levels of homocysteine and atherosclerotic vascular disease. Curr Atheroscler Rep 2000;2:194–199.
65. Ridker PM, Stampfer MJ, Rifai N. Novel risk factors for systemic atherosclerosis: a comparison of C-reactive protein, fibrinogen, homocysteine, lipoprotein(a), and standard cholesterol screening as predictors of peripheral arterial disease. JAMA 2001;285:2481–2485.
66. Arnesen E, Refsum H, Bonaa KH, Ueland PM, Forde OH, Nordrehaug JE. Serum total homocysteine and coronary heart disease. Int J Epidemiol 1995;24:704–709.
67. Schnyder G, Roffi M, Pin R, et al. Decreased rate of coronary restenosis after lowering of plasma homocysteine levels. N Engl J Med 2001;345:1593–1600.
68. Kang SS, Wong PWK, Malinow MR. Hyperhomocyst(e)inemia as a risk factor for occlusive vascular disease. Ann Rev Nutr 1992;12:279–298.
69. Rallidis LS, Papageorgakis NH, Megalou AA, Anagnostou ED, Chatzidimitriou GI, Tsitouris GK. Fibrinogen in the offspring of men with premature coronary artery disease. Eur Heart J 1995;16:1814–1818.
70. Holvoet P, Collen D. Thrombosis and atherosclerosis. Curr Opin Lipidol 1997;8:320–328.
71. Hamsten A, Blomback M, Wiman B, et al. Haemostatic function in myocardial infarction. Br Heart J 1986;55:58–66.
72. Topol EJ, McCarthy J, Gabriel S, et al. Single nucleotide polymorphisms in multiple novel thrombospondin genes may be associated with familial premature myocardial infarction. Circulation 2001;104:2641–2644.
73. Wolfe J, Vacek ML. Myocardial infarction in the young: angiographic features and risk factor analysis of patients with MI at or before the age of 35. Chest 1994;94:926–930.
74. Zimmerman FH, Cameron A, Fisher LD, Ng G. Myocardial infarction in young adults: angiographic characterization, risk factors and prognosis (Coronary Artery Surgery Study Registry). J Am Coll Cardiol 1995;26:654–661.
75. Ambrose JA, Tannenbaum MA, Alexopoulos D, et al. Angiographic progression of coronary artery disease and the development of myocardial infarction. J Am Coll Cardiol 1988;12:56–62.
76. Topol EJ, Nissen SE. Our preoccupation with coronary luminology. The dissociation between clinical and angiographic findings in ischemic heart disease [see comments]. Circulation 1995;92:2333–2342.
77. Libby P. Current concepts of the pathogenesis of the acute coronary syndromes. Circulation 2001; 104:365–372.
78. Dollar AL, Kragel AH, Fernicola DJ, Waclawiw MA, Roberts WC. Composition of atherosclerotic plaques in coronary arteries in women less than 40 years of age with fatal coronary artery disease and implications for plaque reversibility. Am J Cardiol 1991;67:1223–1227.
79. Corrado D, Thiene G, Pennelli N. Sudden death as the first manifestation of coronary artery disease in young people (less than or equal to 35 years). Eur Heart J 1988;9(Suppl. N):139–144.
80. Berenson GS, Srinivasan SR, Nicklas TA, Johnson CC. Prevention of adult heart disease beginning in the pediatric age. Cardiovasc Clin 1990;20:21–45.
81. Starc TJ, Belamarich PF, Shea S, et al. Family history fails to identify many children with severe hypercholesterolemia. Am J Dis Child 1991;145:61–64.
82. Muhonen LE, Burns TL, Nelson RP, Lauer RM. Coronary risk factors in adolescents related to their knowledge of familial coronary heart disease and hypercholesterolemia: the Muscatine Study. Pediatrics 1994;93:444–451.
83. Zehr KJ, Lee PC, Poston RS, Gillinov AM, Greene PS, Cameron DE. Two decades of coronary artery bypass graft surgery in young adults. Circulation 1994;90:II133–II139.
84. Executive Summary of The Third Report of The National Cholesterol Education Program (NCEP) Expert Panel on Detection, Evaluation, And Treatment of High Blood Cholesterol In Adults (Adult Treatment Panel III). JAMA. 2001;285:2486–2497.

23 Cholesterol Lowering

Terje R. Pedersen, MD, PhD *and*
Serena Tonstad, MD, PhD

CONTENTS

SERUM LIPIDS AND CORONARY HEART DISEASE

The evidence that cholesterol plays the central role in the atherosclerotic process is derived from all disciplines of medical research, ranging from molecular biology to randomized clinical trials. The epidemiologic proof is particularly strong and consistent. Coronary heart disease (CHD) is rare in populations with low serum cholesterol levels *(1,2)* comparisons of countries with varying incidence of CHD, there is a strong positive correlation between serum cholesterol levels and the risk of CHD events *(3)* countries experiencing an increase in mortality from CHD, a preceding substantial rise in serum cholesterol levels has been observed *(4)*. In Finland, where the mortality from CHD has been the highest in the world, the recent decline in mortality has been preceded by a decline in population serum cholesterol levels *(5)*. In epidemiological surveys within Western societies, serum cholesterol is a strong risk factor for CHD *(6,7)*. A raised level of low-density lipoprotein (LDL) constitutes the main cause of coronary atherosclerosis *(8)*, in particular small dense LDL *(9)*. In addition, strong evidence indicates that low levels of serum high-density lipoprotein (HDL) cholesterol and high levels of serum triglycerides are independent risk factors for CHD *(7,10,11)*. The combination of

From: *Contemporary Cardiology: Management of Acute Coronary Syndromes, Second Edition*
Edited by: C. P. Cannon © Humana Press Inc., Totowa, NJ

borderline high-risk LDL cholesterol, raised triglycerides, small LDL particles, and low HDL cholesterol has been labeled as the atherogenic lipoprotein phenotype (12), or atherogenic dyslipidemia (13), and is the central feature of the metabolic syndrome. The other components of this syndrome include central obesity, hypertension, insulin resistance, and a procoagulant state. Further evidence has identified another apolipoprotein B-containing particle, intermediate-density lipoprotein (IDL), as atherogenic (14–17). High serum triglyceride levels may reflect high levels of the triglyceride-rich lipoprotein particles very-low-density lipoprotein (VLDL) and IDL.

Observational research indicates a linear relationship between population levels of serum cholesterol and CHD, with a 20% increase in risk of CHD for each 10% increase in serum cholesterol (18). This dose-response effect occurs at any level of cholesterol, in both men and women (1). Because CHD is almost entirely absent in societies with very low serum cholesterol levels, even though smoking and hypertension are prevalent, elevated serum cholesterol seems to be a prerequisite for development of coronary atherosclerosis. On the other hand, risk factors like cigarette smoking and hypertension are not a prerequisite for atherosclerosis in individuals with genetically elevated serum LDL cholesterol (familial hypercholesterolemia). Such risk factors can, however, strongly enhance the rate of transport of LDL through the arterial wall (19) by enhancing its atherogenic modification (20–23).

In patients with established CHD, serum cholesterol has not been among the strongest predictors of subsequent risk, because myocardial damage from atherosclerosis and thrombosis tends to dominate (24). Still, serum cholesterol stands out as a significant risk factor in patients surviving acute myocardial infarction (25).

ANTI-ATHEROSCLEROTIC MECHANISMS OF CHOLESTEROL LOWERING

The complexity of the pathogenesis of atherosclerosis makes it difficult to understand what parts of the process are most influenced by cholesterol lowering. Moreover, the effects of lipid lowering are difficult to study in humans. Atherosclerosis results from an interaction between blood and vessel wall. Components of importance are of a genetic, immunological, inflammatory, particle kinetic, cell kinetic, proliferative, synthetic, degenerative, cytotoxic, and mechanical nature, including blood pressure and flow pattern (21,26). The diseased vessel wall tends to activate the coagulation system and platelets to form thrombi that may further enhance the process of atherosclerosis. Plasma lipoproteins seem to be involved in the entire spectrum of the process, e.g., LDL seems to have a direct, receptor-independent augmentative effect on platelet reactivity (27). Much focus has been put on the formation of foam cells and the resulting core of lipids that is found in many atherosclerotic plaques (28). Oxidized LDL particles have been believed to be pivotal for this process (20,29).

A number of studies have shown that unstable coronary atheromas often do not produce tight stenoses. It is the physical disruption of the plaque that ultimately leads to occlusive thrombi. Vulnerable plaques are characterized by a moderate to large lipid core, a large volume of macrophages, and a structurally weakened fibrous cap (30). Thus, plaque instability is predicted by its lipid-related features. The idea that marked reduction in serum LDL concentration would lead to a net flux of lipids out of the plaque core, which then stabilizes the plaque, has attracted much attention (26). Studies in non-human primates have demonstrated that such shrinkage takes place (31). Following sustained consumption of an atherogenic diet, there are substantial increases in coronary artery content of cholesterol. On return to a native vegetarian diet, lipid-laden macrophages disappear and core lipid volume diminishes. However, angiographic studies in humans reveal only small changes, indicating regression in coronary lesions with lipid-lowering treatment that do not account for the clinical benefits (32). Further studies in cholesterol-fed rabbits have demonstrated that newly formed plaques tend to accumulate inflammatory cells that express collagenolytic enzymes. After the rabbits are shifted to a low-cholesterol diet, or given a statin, the inflammatory cells almost disappear, levels of collagenolytic enzymes are markedly reduced, and in some studies, tissue factor diminishes (30,33).

In some cases of death from CHD and unstable coronary syndromes, plaque morphology does not include a lipid core, but signs of cell proliferation are present, as well as endothelial damage and inflammatory components (34–36). Lipid lowering may improve coronary endothelial function and vasomotor responses (37) decrease smooth muscle growth, and reduce proliferation of macrophages and lymphocytes in addition to its anti-inflammatory effects (38). However, it should be remembered that therapies shown to improve endothelium-dependent vasodilatation are not necessarily associated with reduced myocardial ischemia or cardiovascular risk. Estrogen therapy and α-tocopherol supplementation are cases in point (39). Moreover, effects of statins on smooth muscle cell proliferation appear to depend on the relative lipophilicity of the agent used. Pravastatin, which is the most hydrophilic of the currently available statins, has the least inhibitory effect on smooth muscle cell proliferation (40). However, both pravastatin and the more lipophilic statins lovastatin, simvastatin, and atorvastatin have demonstrated clinical benefits.

CHOLESTEROL AND DIET

Cholesterol levels are strongly related to consumption of dietary saturated fatty acids (41,42); high consumption of animal fat, in particular from milk (43), seems to explain much of the excess mortality from CHD in Western countries. Whereas energy from fat constitutes 35–45 % in countries with a high prevalence of CHD, a proportion of 15% and lower is typical in populations in which CHD is rare (44); the difference largely due to saturated fatty acids. Diets rich in monounsaturated fatty acids, such as olive oil, and polyunsaturated fatty acids, such as those found in plant seed oil, tend to reduce serum LDL cholesterol and increase HDL cholesterol (45). Such diets seem not to be atherogenic even when fat consumption constitutes 40% of energy, as exemplified by diets typical for Crete and other Mediterranean societies (45).

EFFECT OF DIETARY INTERVENTION

Substituting fish for red meat had no effect on CHD in three epidemiologic studies, but seemed protective against CHD in six epidemiologic and two case-control studies (46), and in one randomized-controlled trial in patients surviving myocardial infarction, the Diet and Reinfarction Trial (DART) (47). In the Chicago Western Electric Study, 430 deaths from CHD over 30 yr of follow-up were analyzed (46). In men consuming ≥35 g fish/d the relative risk of death from CHD was 0.62 (95% confidence interval: 0.40–0.94) compared with nonconsumers; also a significant ($p = 0.04$) graded relation between the relative risks and strata of fish consumption was seen. The protective components in fish have not yet been clearly defined; the n-3 long-chain polyunsaturated fatty acids may be effective, or it may simply be that less atherogenic nutrients are substituted for saturated fat. The St. Thomas Atherosclerosis Trial (STARS) randomized coronary patients to usual care, diet, or diet with cholestyramine *(48)*. Patients in whom disease progression occurred consumed 42 g/d of saturated fat, whereas those with regression consumed only 21 g/d.

Apart from DART, there have been few randomized clinical trials on dietary intervention following acute coronary syndromes, and all have been small. The first to show encouraging results was the study by Leren in 412 hypercholesterolemic men with a first myocardial infarction who were randomized to usual diet or advice to substitute vegetable oil for animal fats and avoid dietary cholesterol *(49)*. In the first 5 yr of follow-up, serum total cholesterol was reduced by 14% relative to the control group, from a mean baseline level of nearly 300 mg/dL. After 11 yr of follow-up, a significant 44% relative risk reduction in fatal myocardial infarction was found ($p = 0.004$) in the diet group, but CHD mortality was not statistically significantly different between the groups (diet 79 cases, control 94; $p = 0.097$).

The Lyon Heart Study randomized 605 patients younger than 70 yr with a first myocardial infarction to receive no dietary advice or to receive advice from a cardiologist and dietitian to adopt a Mediterranean-type diet: more bread, root and green vegetables, more fish, no day without fruit, less meat, and substitution of a margarine consisting of 48% oleic acid and enriched with α-linolenic acid (an n-3 fatty acid) for butter *(50)*. Interestingly, the advice did not result in any significant differences between the two groups in serum lipids and lipoprotein levels. Nevertheless, a significant ($p < 0.001$) reduction in the primary end points of cardiac death and nonfatal acute myocardial infarction was observed after a follow-up period of up to 5 yr (mean 27 mo) (Fig. 1). Unfortunately, the study was small, comprising only 41 primary end point events and has been criticized for premature termination and insufficient statistical power. When only fatal events are analyzed, the upper 95% confidence interval for the risk ratio is a less impressive 0.98 *(51)*. The basis for the reduction in sudden death may be due to an effect of n-3 fatty acids on arrhythmia threshold. Recently, the American Heart Association (AHA) issued their latest Dietary Guidelines that endorse the entire Mediterranean dietary pattern as exemplified in the Lyon study *(52)*. Specific recommendations include five or more fruit and vegetables/d, six or more servings of grain products/d, limited saturated fat to <7% of total energy, limited trans-fatty acids (e.g., cookies, crackers, commercially prepared fried foods, and some margarines), limited foods high in cholesterol, and substitution of unsaturated fatty acids from fish, vegetables, legumes, and nuts for saturated fatty acids.

A small secondary prevention trial used diet to reduce events after MI. The trial contrasted a diet with more fruit, vegetables, nuts, and grain products with the usual postmyocardial infarction diet. Significant changes were seen in weight loss, cardiovascular events, and total mortality *(53)*.

CURRENT DIET GUIDELINES: DO THEY WORK?

There is no general consensus on the most appropriate dietary advice for adults at high risk or with established CHD. The Expert Panel of the National Cholesterol Education Program (NECP) issued guidelines consisting of a two-step approach *(54)*: Step

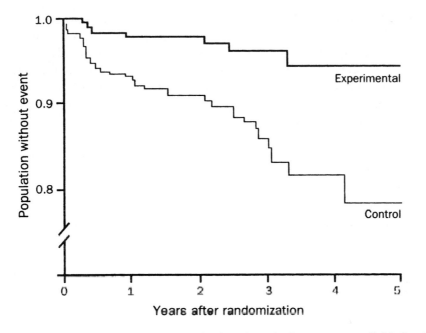

Fig. 1. Survival curves for combined cardiac death and nonfatal acute myocardial infarction in the Lyon Heart Study, comparing a Mediterranean-type diet with a conventional French diet. Reproduced with permission from ref. *50*.

1, 8–10% of energy from saturated fat, ≤30% of energy from total fat, and <300 mg of cholesterol/d; for Step 2, a further reduction of saturated fat to <7% and cholesterol to <200 mg/d. For patients with known CHD, the Step 2 diet was suggested. The guidelines of the European Atherosclerosis Society are essentially identical to the Step 1 diet *(55)*. In meta-analysis, the Step 1 and 2 diets caused a 12–16% reduction in LDL cholesterol and a 8% reduction in triglycerides, but also a 7% reduction in HDL cholesterol with the Step 2 diet *(56)*. Genetic differences exist in dietary response. For example, individuals with the atherogenic lipoprotein phenotype with small dense LDL particles respond with a reduction in apolipoprotein B and, hence, in LDL cholesterol, whereas those with a predominance of larger LDL particles respond with only modest reductions in LDL cholesterol and apolipoprotein B *(57)*.

Several arguments have been advanced to support the low-fat high-carbohydrate diets. Low-fat diets allow for easier weight loss and reduce postprandial lipemia. However, both compliance and the effect of the diet on triglycerides and HDL cholesterol have been a cause of concern. In hypercholesterolemic patients without elevated triglycerides, a low-fat diet may raise triglycerides *(58)*.

Recently, the guidelines of the NECP were updated *(59)*. The new guidelines suggest a multifaceted lifestyle approach including weight reduction and increased physical activity to reduce CHD risk. Reduction in saturated fat and cholesterol intakes to levels of the Step 2 diet is recommended, however, total fat is allowed to range from 25–35% of total energy. A higher intake of unsaturated fat (rather than saturated and trans-fatty acids) is suggested to help to reduce triglycerides and raise HDL cholesterol in persons with the metabolic syndrome. Other therapeutic options to enhance LDL cholesterol lowering include use of plant stanols/sterols (2 g/d) and increased viscous fiber (10–25 g/d).

Few randomized-controlled clinical trials have been carried out to establish the clinical benefit of these guidelines, in particular in middle-aged CHD patients. Since the consumption of dietary fat already has decreased in the Western populations during the last decades, the strategy of a Step 1 and 2 diet following a CHD event may produce relatively less clinical benefit than was possible before. In the Oslo Study a Step 1-type diet was tested in a randomized fashion among 1232 healthy men with high cholesterol levels; however, the participants were also given advice to stop smoking (60). It is therefore not clear what part of the observed 47% reduction of CHD events ($p = 0.028$) was due to the dietary advice. The authors estimated that the reduction in serum cholesterol accounted for about 60% of the reduction in events.

A recent review found six studies that compared the cholesterol-lowering effects of diet plus statin therapy with statin therapy alone (61). In each study, a diet low in total and saturated fat and in cholesterol was compared with a high-fat Western-style diet in hypercholesterolemic patients taking 10–40 mg/d of a statin. Five of these studies showed that a cholesterol-lowering diet had an independent and additive effect to statin treatment. Diet resulted in an additional 5–18.4% lowering of LDL cholesterol. Greater reductions in LDL cholesterol may require more extreme lifestyle changes. Very low fat diets that are high in complex carbohydrates and that are combined with exercise and/or meditation may cause substantial lowering of LDL cholesterol (62), even when added to statin therapy (63). It is likely that only a small minority of patients is willing and able to undergo such a turnabout of life.

FIBER AND SOY PROTEIN

Another dietary component that may have a favorable impact on serum lipids is dietary fiber, especially from cereals, dried beans, vegetables, and fruit, possibly due to decreased absorption of fatty acids and biliary cholesterol (64). Such diets may substantially lower blood pressure (65). A comprehensive meta-analysis suggested that 3 g soluble fiber from oats (three servings of oatmeal of 28 g each) decreases LDL cholesterol by 5 mg/dL. However, one randomized trial of men with CHD failed to demonstrate a benefit of increased fiber intake on recurrent infarction, possibly because the follow-up period was too short, only 2 yr (47). Consumption of 25–75 g/d of soy protein, rather than animal protein, has been shown to reduce LDL cholesterol by 13% in a meta-analysis (66).

ALCOHOL

Several epidemiological investigations have noted that regular moderate consumption of alcohol is associated with an increase in HDL cholesterol and a decreased mortality from CHD. In a study of 490,000 men and women, the rates of death from cardiovascular diseases were 30–40% lower among those reporting at least one drink daily than among abstainers (67). However, the drinking pattern may be important, as binge drinking of beer was associated with a six-fold increased risk of fatal myocardial infarction, in comparison with men drinking less than three bottles/session (68). In other investigations, the lowest mortality from CHD was seen in individuals drinking 2 to 3 U/d (69). Small amounts of alcohol taken regularly instead of the same amount taken 1 or 2 d/wk seem to result in greater benefit (70). Alcohol increases HDL-cholesterol subclasses that are protective of CHD; this effect is present whether the alcohol ingested is beer, wine, or liquor. About 50% of the inverse association between alcohol consumption and CHD death is explained by the HDL cholesterol level *(71)*. Red wine with meals reduces the propensity of LDL to undergo peroxidation *(72)*. Alcohol also has theoretically favorable effects on platelets and the coagulation-fibrinolytic system *(73)*. To date, however, no prospective randomized study has evaluated the feasibility and clinical and social consequences of advising abstainers and people who rarely taste alcohol to take up regular drinking to reduce the risk of CHD. Therefore, the putative effects of alcohol on CHD should be applied more to reassure moderate drinkers that their habits are not harmful than to encourage nondrinkers to drink.

DRUGS TO REDUCE CHOLESTEROL
Statins

A wide range of drugs affecting lipid metabolism has become available. They vary greatly in their mechanism of action and their potency in reducing LDL cholesterol and increasing HDL cholesterol. During the last decade, the hydroxy-methylglutaryl-CoA-reductase inhibitors, or statins, have become the most widely prescribed class of drugs because of their very low rate of side effects and greater effectiveness in reducing LDL cholesterol than other classes of drugs. Because they are the only class of drugs proved to reduce all-cause mortality, physicians without expert insight into lipid metabolism and pharmacology of the other classes of drugs are perfectly safe in using statins as the only lipid-lowering therapy.

Statins inhibit the rate-limiting step of mevalonate synthesis in the production of cholesterol, mainly in the liver. The number of LDL receptors on the liver cell membrane is, therefore, up-regulated to increase import of cholesterol from the blood to meet demand in the liver. As a consequence, the number of LDL particles in plasma is reduced. Ability to reduce LDL cholesterol concentrations, using the currently highest recommended dosages, ranges from 30–60% on average according to the following rank order: fluvastatin, pravastatin, lovastatin, simvastatin, and atorvastatin. Statins usually do not increase HDL cholesterol levels >10%, even at high dosages, but doubling of any statin dose typically produces another 6% decrease in LDL cholesterol. Usually triglycerides are reduced by 10%, but at higher dosages and in patients with hypertriglyceridemia, 30–45% reduction can be seen.

Statins have been found to induce a large number of direct, possibly beneficial effects on components in plasma and cells involved in the atherosclerotic and thrombotic process. These include inhibition of smooth muscle cell proliferation and migration *(74,75)*, inhibition of endogenous cholesterol synthesis in macrophages *(76)*, regulation of natural killer cell function *(77)*, and decreased platelet aggregation *(78)*, as well as numerous others. Several studies have focused on the antiinflammatory effects of statins. C-reactive protein, a nonspecific, acute-phase, inflammatory reactant, has been associated with coronary risk more extensively than other inflammatory markers of atherosclerosis. The first report that documented the effect of statin treatment on C-reactive protein levels involved a subgroup analysis of the Cholesterol and Recurrent Events (CARE) trial *(38)*. The reduction in coronary events with pravastatin treatment was much greater in patients with high levels of inflammatory markers (based on defined cut-off values) than in the rest of the subjects. Moreover, C-reactive protein levels increased in placebo-treated patients, but decreased in those that received pravastatin.

Other studies have demonstrated that reduction of C-reactive protein levels is a class effect of statins. Whether C-reactive protein is a marker or an actual mediator of athersclerosis has not been established, nor has it been determined whether lowering of C-reactive protein is a secondary effect related to lowering of LDL cholesterol. Thus, the clinical importance of these ancillary effects of statins, beyond reduction of LDL cholesterol, remains speculative at present.

Fibrates

Fibrates activate peroxisome proliferator-activated receptors (PPARs), which then induce the transcription of several genes that encode proteins controlling lipoprotein metabolism, including lipoprotein lipase and apolipoproteins A-I and A-II. Fibrates typically decrease serum triglycerides 30–40% or more in hypertriglyceridemia. HDL cholesterol is increased 10–20%. Adverse events are mostly gastrointestinal in nature and include increased incidence of gallstones. In a recent review, Bucher and coworkers found no statistically significant effects of fibrates on mortality, however, rates of non-coronary and total deaths tended to be higher in the fibrate than in the control groups *(79)*. Since this publication, reports from two additional major trials have appeared.

The Veterans Affairs Cooperative Studies Program High-Density Lipoprotein Intervention Trial (VA-HIT) was designed to assess if elevating HDL cholesterol in men with preexisting CHD and low HDL cholesterol levels and lowering triglycerides in men with normal or mildly increased triglycerides but with low LDL cholesterol levels at entry would reduce the incidence of nonfatal myocardial infarction or CHD death *(80)*. The 2531 men were randomized to gemfibrozil 1200 mg/d or placebo for 5 yr. The primary outcome variable of the combined incidence of CHD death and nonfatal MI was reduced 22% ($p < 0.006$). The study was not powered to achieve a significant reduction in total mortality, however, there was no apparent increase in non-CHD causes of death. Gemfibrozil treatment also resulted in a significant 59% reduction in transient ischemic attacks and a 65% decrease in carotid endarterectomy. In contrast to the major secondary prevention statin trials, the rates of revascularization and percutaneous transluminal coronary angioplasty or hospitalization for stable angina were not different between gemfibrozil and placebo. While LDL cholesterol levels were essentially unchanged, treatment with gemfibrozil led to moderate elevations in HDL cholesterol of 6% and reductions of 31% in triglycerides. A subsequent report suggested that the changes in remnant and smaller VLDL and IDL fractions were related to benefits in clinical end points. This report has revived interest in fibrates and suggests that modulating other lipoproteins than LDL cholesterol level may effectively prevent CHD.

These results contrast with those of the Bezafibrate Infarction Program (BIP) *(81)*, also a secondary prevention trial, but one that failed to demonstrate a beneficial effect of bezafibrate on CHD *(81)*. In this study, 1548 patients were assigned to bezafibrate and 1542 patients to placebo. Neither a 9.4% reduction in the primary end point or a 13% reduction in nonfatal myocardial infarction was statistically significant. However, in the subgroup of patients with baseline triglycerides >200 mg/dL, the cumulative probability of a primary end point was 39.5% lower ($p = 0.02$) in patients randomized to bezafibrate than in patients randomized to placebo. The confidence intervals for the VA-HIT comprise the BIP results, so the difference of outcome in the two studies could be due to chance *(82)*.

Additional data are available from the Diabetes Atherosclerosis Intervention Study (DAIS). In this trial, 418 men and women aged 40–65 yr with type-2 diabetes, under good glycemic control, were assigned to micronized fenofibrate (200 mg/d) or placebo for at least 3 yr. About half the patients had known CHD. The fenofibrate group showed a significantly smaller increase in percentage diameter stenosis by angiography than the placebo group. The trial was not powered to examine clinical end points, but these were fewer in the fenofibrate than the placebo group (38 vs 50) *(83)*.

Other Drugs

Niacin reduces the synthesis of VLDL by inhibiting the mobilization of free fatty acids from peripheral tissues reducing plasma triglyceride levels by about 30%. Niacin may also inhibit the conversion of VLDL into LDL and, thus, modestly reduce LDL cholesterol by 10–20%. Niacin generally is considered the most effective drug for raising HDL cholesterol levels, typically increasing levels by up to 30%, and reduces levels of lipoprotein(a). Niacin is a relatively inexpensive drug and has been shown to decrease myocardial infarction and stroke *(84)* and, in combination with resins, to prevent progression and cause regression of coronary atherosclerosis *(85)*. Although the use of niacin has been associated with several adverse effects, a once-nightly extended-release formulation has shown to cause minimal flushing and almost no hepatic toxicity *(86)*.

Resins bind to bile acids in the intestine, and the complex is not reabsorbed but excreted. This causes the liver to increase the synthesis of bile acids, and the subsequent increased demand for cholesterol induces the same effect as inhibition of cholesterol synthesis: an increase in the number of LDL receptors on the cell surface. This results in a reduction in plasma LDL cholesterol of up to 20% when cholestyramine or colestipol is used at dosages of 20–24 g daily. Adverse effects of gastrointestinal nature are frequent with high dosages. The resins offer no advantage over the statins, in either price or potency, and are today used mostly in combination with statins in patients with severe hypercholesterolemia. One disadvantage of resins is that triglyceride levels are sometimes increased, especially in hypertriglyceridemia. HDL cholesterol may increase by up to 10%. Treatment with resins has been shown to reduce coronary artery events *(87)*.

Fish oils with concentrated omega-3 polyunsaturated fatty acids decrease the production of VLDL, thus triglyceride levels decrease by up to 30–50% in hypertriglyceridemic patients. The Gruppo Italiano per lo Studio della Sopravvivenza nell'Infarto Miocardico (GISSI)-Prevenzione trial *(88)* randomly allocated 11,324 patients with recent myocardial infarction (≤3 mo) to four treatment groups: fish oil in the form of capsules containing about 1 g of eicosapentaenoic acid and docosahexaenoic acid in a 2:1 ratio, 300 mg vitamin E, fish oil and vitamin E combined, or no supplement. The trial had an open-label design and followed participants for 3.5 yr. In these patients, who were relatively low risk, fish oil supplements, but not vitamin E, reduced the combined primary end point of death, nonfatal myocardial infarction, and nonfatal stroke by 15% (95% confidence interval: 2–26%). All the benefit was due to the reduction of total mortality. This trial is the first to demonstrate that a pharmacological equivalent of a dietary component is capable of decreasing predefined end points of morbidity and mortality.

Hormone replacement therapy (HRT) with estrogen or the combination of estrogen and a progestin has been widely believed to be cardioprotective based on consistent reports from numerous observational studies. Estrogen typically produces a 10–15% reduction in LDL cholesterol and 10–25% increase in HDL cholesterol. In combination with most progestins, the effect on HDL cholesterol is attenuated. The effect on triglycerides is variable, and an increase may be observed, as well as a shift to smaller denser LDL particles.

The only randomized, placebo-controlled study with clinical end points in women with CHD, the Heart and Estrogen/Progestin Replacement Study (HERS), failed to show a benefit for CHD over the 4 yr of follow-up (89). HERS tested conjugated equine estrogen plus medroxyprogesterone in 2763 women with preexisting CHD and a mean age of 67 yr. Surprisingly, the study showed an excess of events in the hormone group during the first year after randomization. In line with the results from the HERS trial, the Effects of estrogen Replacement on the progression of coronary artery Atherosclerosis (ERA) study showed that initiation of HRT did not lead to an alteration in mean minimal coronary-artery diameter measured by coronary angiography (90). However, this study was not powered to study clinical end points. Likewise the Women's Health Initiative trial concluded that etrogen plus progestin use for an average of 5.2 y increased the risk of CHD and stroke in postmenopausal women (91). The AHA further suggested that the decision to continue or stop HRT in women with cardiovascular disease who have been undergoing long-term HRT should be based on established noncoronary benefits and risks and patient preference.

Plant sterols and their saturated derivatives the stanols are the naturally occurring equivalents of mammalian cholesterol. Plant sterols and stanols displace cholesterol from the micelles in the intestine, thus decreasing cholesterol absorption. These agents produce modest LDL cholesterol reductions even in the context of a healthy diet. A recent meta-analysis concluded that at daily intakes of 2 g plant sterols and stanols reduce LDL cholesterol levels by 9–14% with no effect on HDL cholesterol or triglycerides (92).

CHOLESTEROL LOWERING: THE ANGIOGRAPHIC EVIDENCE

Since 1984, the objective of a large number of clinical trials has been to investigate coronary vessel lumen morphology by angiography and the changes induced by long-term cholesterol lowering. (48,62,85,87,93–107). In most of these trials angiographic evidence of retardation of progression of atherosclerosis and prevention of new lesions were demonstrated with cholesterol lowering, almost regardless of what methods were used. However, even though these are often referred to as "regression" trials, signs of plaque shrinkage were much less convincing, and at best, the lumen diameter increased by a few percentage points or by a few hundred millimeters. Angiographic determination of the extent of atherosclerosis has inherent methodological problems, as compensatory remodeling of the vessel takes place over time (108), and plaques vulnerable to rupture and thrombosis are often invisible (109). It is often not possible to determine the difference between plaques and thrombi from an angiogram. Thrombi commonly undergo lysis or growth, and finally, local changes in vascular tone may be mistaken for atherosclerotic changes. Despite these pitfalls, the groups randomized to cholesterol lowering on average experienced regression in about one-fourth of lesions. A meta-analysis of 12 of these trials found that the relative risk of progression was 0.66 (95% confidence interval: 0.59–0.73) and of regression was 2.03 (95% confidence interval: 1.64–2.52) with cholesterol lowering (32).

In addition, trials have demonstrated retardation of intimal thickening of carotid arteries with cholesterol lowering using B-mode ultrasound (110–112).

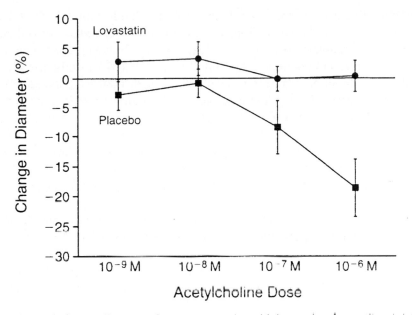

Fig. 2. Change in lumen diameter of coronary arteries with increasing doses of acetylcholine infusion after 6 mo of therapy with lovastatin or placebo. Reproduced with permission from ref. *37*.

ACUTE EFFECTS OF CHOLESTEROL LOWERING

In the angiographic regression studies, treatment duration was typically 2–4 yr before any morphological changes could be observed. In the Multicentre Anti-Atheroma Study (MAAS) trial, no significant difference between the two treatment groups was observed at the first angiography performed after 2 yr. Only after 4 yr of therapy did the difference become evident *(103)*. In the later statin studies with clinical end points, the time until significant differences appeared between the placebo and treated groups was about 14–18 mo, although a numerically small difference was present from mo 1 in the Scandinavian Simvastatin Survival Study (4S) and mo 6 in the West of Scotland Coronary Prevention Study (WOS). In all the secondary prevention statin studies, participants had experienced a coronary event several months earlier and had stabilized. If cholesterol lowering with statins has endothelial-relaxing or plaque-stabilizing effects, these effects may be clinically evident in the period immediately after an acute coronary syndrome has occurred. Several studies have examined this hypothesis.

A number of investigations have shown that physiological responses to cholesterol therapy can be observed early. Myocardial perfusion abnormalities improved after only 90 d of intensive cholesterol lowering, using dipyridamole and positron emission tomography imaging *(113)*. The pathological vasoconstrictory response of atherosclerotic coronary arteries to infusion of acetylcholine was blunted after 6 mo cholesterol lowering with lovastatin in one study *(37)* (Fig. 2), and after 12 mo with lovastatin in the combination with cholestyramine or probucol in another *(114)*. It was later shown that 1-mo therapy with simvastatin induced significant increases in the vasodilator response to acetylcholine in the forearm vasculature in hypercholesterolemic subjects *(115)*. Even a single LDL apheresis was shown to improve endothelium-dependent vasodilatation within minutes in hypercholesterolemic individuals *(116)*. Moreover, the Reduction of Cholesterol in Ischemia and Function of the Endothelium (RECIFE) study provided evidence that endothelial function can be improved by cholesterol lowering in patients with unstable coronary disease *(117)*. Flow-mediated vasodilation in the brachial artery improved in patients with acute coronary syndrome treated with pravastatin compared to placebo *(117)*. The abnormal vascular response is not only seen in patients with marked hypercholesterolemia. Even healthy individuals with LDL cholesterol levels well within the range considered as normal, had blunted responses to infusion of the endothelium-dependent vasodilator metacholine chloride, compared to those with low levels *(118)*.

Other studies have shown that in patients with stable coronary disease, platelet thrombus deposition measured in a perfusion flow chamber was more than twice as high in those with hypercholesterolemia compared with those with normal cholesterol levels *(119)*. After 2.4 mo of pravastatin treatment, cholesterol levels and platelet thrombus deposition were normalized. These observations have been replicated in subjects with high cholesterol levels but without coronary disease *(119)*.

Several studies have examined whether cholesterol lowering may have immediate clinical effects on hard end points. A prospective cohort study using data from the Swedish Register of Cardiac Intensive Care examined the effect of early initiation of statin treatment in patients with acute myocardial infarction on 1-yr mortality. The study compared 5528 patients who received statins at or before discharge to 14,071 patients who left the hospital without statin therapy *(120)*. After adjustment for confounding factors, early statin treatment was associated with a relative risk of 0.75 (95% confidence interval: 0.63–0.89) for 1-yr mortality. Preliminary reports from the Global Use of Strategies to Open Occluded coronary arteries (GUSTO-IIb) and Platelet Glycoprotein IIb/IIIa in Unstable Angina (PURSUIT) trials as well as the Orobifiban in Patients with Unstable Coronary Syndromes—Thrombolysis and Myocardial Infarction (OPUS-TIMI) trials showed that patients treated with lipid-lowering drugs showed a survival advantage already at 1 mo *(121)*. In all these observational studies, patients who were treated with lipid-lowering drugs were younger and healthier than patients who were not treated. This selection bias may account for the apparent benefit of statin treatment.

The Myocardial Ischemia Reduction and Aggressive Cholesterol Lowering (MIRACL) trial randomized 3086 patients who had experienced unstable angina or a non-Q wave myocardial infarction within 24–96 h after hospital admission to atorvastatin 80 mg/d or to placebo *(122)*. Patients for whom coronary revascularization was planned or who had a total cholesterol level >270 mg/dL were excluded. The primary end point of the trial was a composite that included nonfatal acute myocardial infarction, cardiac arrest, or symptomatic myocardial ischemia. The study treatment period lasted for 16 wk. A primary end point occurred in 228 patients (14.8%) in the atovastatin-treated group and 269 patients (17.4%) in the placebo group (a relative risk reduction of 16%; $p = 0.048$). The only component of the primary end point that attained statistical significance was a reduction in symptomatic myocardial ischemia. Additional studies of statins in acute coronary syndromes are ongoing.

Another study, the Atorvastatin Versus Revascularization Treatment (AVERT) trial, though not done in patients with acute coronary syndrome, included 341 patients who

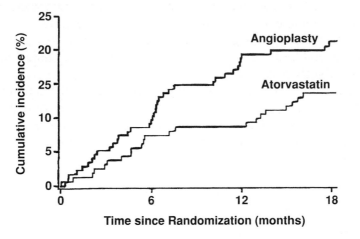

Fig. 3. Patient-by-patient effect of cholesterol lowering over 6 mo on the number of episodes of ischemic ST-segment depression in patients with coronary disease. Two of 20 in the placebo group vs 13 of 20 in the treatment group show resolution of ischemia. Reproduced with permission from ref. *123*.

were candidates for percutaneous revascularization (PTCA) *(123)*. Participants had stable CHD and a lesion in at least one vessel of ≥50%. Entry lipid levels included LDL cholesterol <115 mg/dL and triglycerides <500 mg/dL. Subjects were randomized to PTCA or to atorvastatin 80 mg/d and then followed for 18 mo. The PTCA group was not prevented from receiving lipid-lowering drugs, and 70% of this group did receive statin therapy. The atorvastatin group achieved a 46% reduction in LDL cholesterol compared with 18% in the PTCA group. Thus, in addition to examining the differences between PTCA and atorvastatin treatment, the study evaluated aggressive vs lipid lowering. The primary end point for ischemic events was 36% lower in the atorvastatin group (13 vs 21%) (Fig. 3). An adjustment penalty for interim analyses meant that this difference did not reach conventional statistical significance, however, the time taken to reach an ischemic event was statistically significantly longer in the atorvastatin-treated group ($p = 0.03$).

CLINICAL END POINT TRIALS OF CHOLESTEROL LOWERING DRUGS

Until 1994 over 25 randomized clinical trials of long-term cholesterol lowering drug therapy had reported mortality data *(18)*. The most important of these trials, involving patients with previous myocardial infarction as well as healthy hypercholesterolemic individuals, had used clofibrate, niacin, colestipol, cholestyramine, and gemfibrozil *(124–129)*. One trial used surgical therapy with ileal bypass *(97)*. However, no single trial had been able to demonstrate convincingly that all-cause mortality would be reduced with such therapies, even in high-risk populations such as patients with myocardial infarction. The focus on insignificant findings from these trials, suggesting increased risk of cancer, suicide, and violent deaths, as well as other hazards from cholesterol lowering created mistrust among the majority of physicians. Consequently, even if new powerful cholesterol-lowering drugs became available, they were rarely used, even in hypercholesterolemic patients with acute coronary syndromes. Since 1994, clinical practice has dramatically changed as new large-scale controlled trials using simvastatin, pravastatin, and lovastatin have demonstrated impressive clinical benefits with the long-term use of such drugs.

When considering trials of cholesterol-lowering therapy, the distinction between so-called primary and secondary prevention is artificial and should be avoided. None of the primary prevention trials were really primary in preventing atherosclerosis as they randomized middle-aged or elderly individuals and observed the rate of CHD events over a few years. At the time of randomization, it can be assumed that all patients developing a CHD event already had extensive coronary atherosclerotic lesions. Therefore, the primary and secondary preventive trials are only different with regard to the absolute risk of the study population.

The Statin Trials

The first study to demonstrate improved survival was the 4S trial *(130)*. This study randomized 4444 men and women, aged 35–70 yr, to long-term therapy with simvastatin or placebo in a double-blind fashion. Only patients with a fasting total cholesterol level of 212–309 mg/dL and triglyceride levels <221 mg/dL 2 mo after receiving dietary advice equivalent to the Step 1 diet of the NCEP guidelines *(54)* and the European Atherosclerosis Society guidelines *(55)* were included. The simvastatin dose was 20 mg daily and was titrated to 40 mg after 12 or 24 wk if serum total cholesterol exceeded 200 mg/dL, which was necessary in 37% of patients. This therapy led to a mean reduction of LDL cholesterol over the course of the study of 35% and of 10% in triglycerides, whereas HDL cholesterol increased by 8%. During the median follow-up of 5.4 yr (range of those surviving: 4.9–6.3), 256 patients (11.5%) died in the placebo group, vs 182 (8.2%) in the simvastatin group, a relative risk reduction of 30% (*p* = 0.0003) (Fig. 4). CHD mortality was reduced 42% relative to placebo, and fatal and nonfatal infarction and coronary deaths were reduced by 34%. In addition, coronary revascularization procedures (bypass surgery or angioplasty) were reduced by 37%. The difference between placebo and simvastatin groups with regard to coronary events was small in the first yr of therapy and reached clinical significance after approx 14 mo from randomization.

Three large studies with pravastatin were published in the next 3 yr. The first was WOS, done in 6595 men with LDL cholesterol levels in the range of 155–232 mg/dL, and using pravastatin 40 mg/d or placebo over a period of 5 yr *(131)*. Pravastatin lowered LDL cholesterol by 26%, leading to a relative risk reduction of 33% in the risk of CHD deaths, which resulted in a 22% reduction in all cause mortality (*p* = 0.051 when adjusted for baseline variables). Nonfatal myocardial infarction or death from CHD was reduced 31% (*p* < 0.001), and the need for coronary revascularisation was reduced 37% (*p* = 0.009).

The CARE study (Fig. 5) randomized 4159 men and women with previous myocardial infarction and LDL cholesterol levels of 115–174 mg/dL to placebo or pravastatin 40 mg daily for 5 yr *(132)*. In this study, pravastatin lowered LDL cholesterol by 28% relative to placebo, which was associated with a risk reduction of major coronary events by 24%. Coronary bypass surgery and angioplasty were performed in 26% fewer cases in the pravastatin group. The rates of death from CHD were low, and the 20% reduction

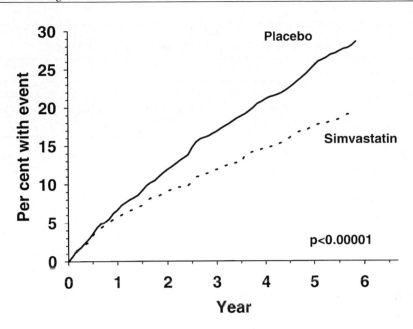

Fig. 4. Kaplan-Meier curves of the incidence of major coronary events: fatal CHD or nonfatal myocardial infarction in 4S.

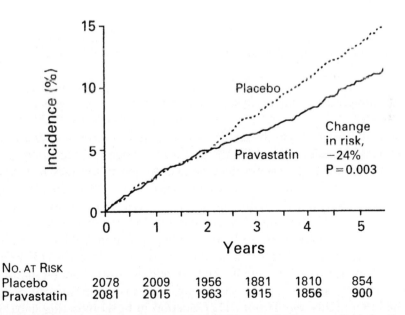

Fig. 5. Kaplan-Meier curves of the incidence of fatal CHD or nonfatal myocardial infarction, from the CARE study. Reproduced with permission from ref. *132*.

Table 1
Mortality and Morbidity in the 4S and in the CARE Study.

Event	4S		CARE	
	No. (%) of patients		No. (%) of patients	
	Placebo (n = 2223)	Simvastatin (n = 2221)	Placebo (n = 2078)	Pravastatin (n = 2081)
Coronary deaths	189 (8.5)	111 (5.0)	119 (5.7)	96 (4.6)
Other cardiovascular deaths	18	25	11	16
Death from cancer	35	33	45	49
Suicide, violence, trauma	7	6	4	8
Other deaths	7	7	15	11
Unclassified cause of death			2	0
All deaths	256 (11.5)	182 (8.2)	196 (9.4)	180 (8.6)
Nonfatal MI (definite)	270 (12.1)	164 (7.4)	173 (8.3)	135 (6.5)
Nonfatal MI (definite/probable)	418 (18.8)	279 (12.6)		
Death from CHD or nonfatal MI[a]	622 (28.0)	431 (19.4)	274 (13.2)	212 (10.2)
CABG or PTCA	383 (17.2)	252 (11.3)	391 (18.8)	294 (14.1)

[a]CABG, coronary artery bypass grafting; PTCA, percutaneous transluminal coronary angioplasty.
Numbers for 4S include definite and probable MI, as well as silent MI, diagnosed by annual ECG.

in the pravastatin group did not reach statistical significance. Although similar in size, the 4S and the CARE study differed in the risk of the study population (Table 1). This is not only explained by the fact that the CARE participants had lower cholesterol levels, but probably more so because 54% of the patients had undergone a recent coronary bypass surgery or angioplasty. In 4S, such patients were excluded, unless they had experienced a new infarction or recurrent angina following the procedure (8% of the patients).

The largest study with pravastatin was the Long-term Intervention with Pravastatin in Ischemic Disease (LIPID) study, which randomized 9014 men and women with previous acute coronary syndromes *(133)*. The study population had baseline total cholesterol levels in the range of 155–270 mg/dL, triglyceride levels <445 mg/dL, and a median LDL cholesterol of 150 mg/dL. The placebo-controlled double-blind study was stopped prematurely after 5 yr because of significant results in favor of pravastatin 40 mg/d, including a highly significant 24% reduction in CHD mortality and 23% reduction in all-cause mortality as well as similar percent reductions in coronary revascularisation procedures and major CHD events.

Finally, the Air Force/Texas Coronary Atherosclerosis Prevention Study (AFCAPS/ TexCAPS) study included 6605 men and women without clinical evidence of cardiovascular disease. LDL cholesterol levels were in the range of 180–264 mg/dL, HDL cholesterol levels were <50 mg/dL, and triglycerides <400 mg/dL *(134)*. This study used lovastatin 20–40 mg/d with the goal of lowering LDL cholesterol to <110 mg/dL. A 27% reduction in LDL cholesterol relative to placebo was achieved at yr 1. The primary end point of major coronary events, which included unstable angina pectoris, was reduced 36% ($p < 0.001$) with lovastatin, but the study was not powered to show reductions in coronary or total mortality.

Previous concerns in regard to an increase in the risk of noncardiovascular mortality have not been confirmed in the statin studies. Furthermore, the studies with most events showed a statistically significant 20–30 % reduction in the risk of cerebrovascular disease. The safety of long-term therapy with statins seems reassuring. Apart from a minimal risk of myopathy, no other serious adverse experiences have been seen in the long-term trials. The slight elevation of liver enzymes observed in a small proportion of patients has not been associated with increased incidence of clinical signs of liver disease *(135)*. A meta-analysis of the five published statin studies concluded that there was no association between statin use over a 5-yr period and the risk of fatal and nonfatal cancers *(136)*.

An additional important finding from the statin trials is the consistency of benefit observed across all major subgroups of patients that have been analyzed. This includes patients at the highest risk of major CHD events, like the elderly and patients with multiple risk factors, including cigarette smoking, hypertension, and diabetes. In 4S, the diabetic subpopulation had a 55% reduction in the risk of major coronary events ($p = 0.002$). Because the diabetic subgroup has a 2.5-fold higher risk than nondiabetics (almost half of the diabetic patients in the placebo group suffered a major event), the absolute risk reduction was formidable *(137)*.

These findings in subgroups from the five initial statin trials have recently been confirmed in the largest statin study to date, the Heart Protection Study (HPS), which was presented at the 2001 AHA meeting *(149)*. A total of 20,536 individuals were recruited to HPS, which was coordinated by the University of Oxford Clinical Trials Centre in the United Kingdom. The participants were at high risk of CHD, either because of established CHD, cerebrovascular disease, peripheral vascular disease, diabetes mellitus, or hypertension. The study compared simvastatin 40 mg/d, antioxidant vitamins (E, C, and β-carotene), the combination of simvastatin and vitamins or placebo. Patients were eligible for HPS with cholesterol levels >134 mg/dL provided that the patient's physician did not consider that lipid-lowering therapy was indicated (or contraindicated). The trial population was actively recruited so as to include substantial numbers of elderly people, women, people with below-average cholesterol levels, and people with diabetes without established CHD. The primary end points were all-cause mortality, CHD mortality, and non-CHD mortality. The HPS started recruitment in 1994. As the results of the 4S and following statin studies became available, increasing numbers of patients were given statins by their physicians, on the average 18% of the patients in the placebo group in the course of the study. Compliance in the simvastatin group was about 85%. These differences in compliance resulted in a diminishing difference in LDL cholesterol between the groups, from 46 mg/dL initially, to about 29 mg/dL by the end of the study. While vitamin supplementation had no effect on the primary end points, the preliminary results showed that simvastatin 40 mg/d reduced total CHD end points by 26%. Total mortality was reduced by 12% and CHD mortality by 17%. Death from ischemic stroke was reduced by 27% (all statistically significant results). These effects did not differ according to the category of preexisting disease (previous CHD, cerebrovascular disease, diabetes, peripheral vascular disease), in women or men, in those whose age was ≤ or >65 yr, and in those with baseline LDL cholesterol <100 mg/dL or ≥100 mg/dL.

Table 2
Major Randomized Clinical Trials of Cholesterol Lowering, Their Reduction in Total and LDL
Cholesterol with Therapy Relative to the Control Group, and the Relative Risk Reduction in
Coronary Mortality and Major Coronary Events

Study (reference)	Therapy	Reduction (%)		Risk Reduction (%)	
		Total cholesterol	LDL cholesterol	Coronary mortality	Major coronary events
CDP *(105)*	Clofibrate	7	?	13	9
WHO *(107)*	Clofibrate	9	?	11	20
CDP *(105)*	Niacin	10	?	2	13
LRC *(109)*	Cholestyramine	13	20	30	15
LIPID*(133)*	Pravastatin	20	24	24	23
WOS *(112)*	Pravastatin	20	26	33	31
CARE *(113)*	Pravastatin	20	28	20	24
POSCH *(78)*	Ilial bypass	23	38	37	35
4S *(111)*	Simvastatin	26	36	42	34

The results of the HPS confirm prospectively and in prespecified analyses previous subgroup observations made in the 4S study. In 4S, significant reductions in major CHD events were seen regardless of the baseline LDL cholesterol level, which ranged from 115–262 mg/dL *(138)*. In contrast, the CARE study found no benefits of cholesterol lowering in the subgroup with LDL cholesterol of 115–125 mg/dL *(132)*. This subgroup probably had too few end points to detect a benefit, as the 95% confidence interval ranged from a 23% reduction to a 38% increase in the relative risk. Table 2 shows the reduction in total and LDL cholesterol achieved in the largest trials and the resulting reductions in clinical end point. There is a clear trend that the more cholesterol is reduced, the greater is the reduction in events.

Cost-Effectiveness of Statins

Statins are regarded as relatively expensive drugs, in comparison with, e.g., antihypertensive therapy. However, health-economic calculations of data from the end point trial 4S speak in favor of wide application of this therapy in high-risk populations, such as patients with acute coronary syndromes. In a cost-minimization analysis based on prospectively collected data in 4S, the daily cost of simvastatin averaged U.S. $2.30 when U.S. costs were applied to the data. This cost was offset by 88% in the U.S. because of reduction in the use of healthcare resources, especially hospitalization for acute CHD and coronary revascularization procedures, making the effective cost of therapy only U.S. $0.28/d *(139)*. Cost-minimization analyses only quantify the direct economic impact of therapy and do not convert clinical benefits into financial terms (cost-benefit analysis) or into life-years saved (cost-effectiveness analysis).

In a cost-effectiveness analysis of the 4S data, using base costs in Sweden, the cost/life-yr saved was on average SEK 56,400 (approx U.S. $7700) *(140)*. The cost-effectiveness ratio is thus comparable with percutaneous angioplasty for severe or moderate angina and much more favorable than coronary artery bypass grafting in patients with three-vessel disease or treatment of mild hypertension *(141)*.

In a sensitivity analysis limited to direct cost, the cost/life-yr gained ranged from U.S. $3800 for a 70-yr-old man with CHD and total cholesterol of 309 mg/dL to U.S. $27,400 in a 35-yr-old female with 212 mg/dL in total cholesterol *(142)*. When healthcare costs in gained years are included in the analysis, the cost/life-yr saved is U.S. $10,400 in men and U.S. $16,800 in women. When both direct and indirect costs (such as increased labor production because of improved disease-free survival) are included in the analyses, reduction in the healthcare costs exceeded the cost of intervention in both men and women aged 35 yr. In patients aged 59 yr, cost/life-yr saved ranged from U.S. $1200 to U.S. $8600 according to sex and baseline total cholesterol level.

TREATMENT RECOMMENDATIONS

The AHA 1995 guidelines to reduce risk in patients with coronary and other vascular disease were updated in 2001 *(143)*. Again, as in 1995, the Consensus Panel statement was endorsed by the American College of Cardiology (ACC). The recommendations on lipid management are presented in Table 3. The primary goal of treatment remains attainment of an LDL cholesterol level <100 mg/dL, however, secondary goals have been modified. Secondary goals are now attaining non-HDL cholesterol levels <130 mg/dL if triglycerides are ≥200 mg/dL. These goals are slightly more ambitious than those suggested by the European Atherosclerosis Society, which recommends an LDL cholesterol level <115 mg/dL, however, cholesterol levels in European CHD patients are generally higher than in the U.S.

The guidelines of 2001 are likely to undergo modifications in the future as more evidence from clinical trials becomes available. Presently, the AHA guidelines are supported by reanalysis of 4S data and results of other more recent trials. In 4S, the relationship of LDL cholesterol levels achieved with simvastatin and the subsequent risk of major CHD events was almost linear down to levels well below 100 mg/dL *(144)*. In the Post Coronary Artery Bypass Graft Trial the strategy to reduce LDL cholesterol to less than 85 mg/dL was more beneficial in preventing death or angiographic deterioration of atherosclerosis than a strategy to obtain levels of 130–140 mg/dL. Meta-analysis of clinical trials shows that the more cholesterol is lowered, the greater the reduction in CHD events *(79)*. Trials of statins used in higher dosages show that some of them reduce elevated triglyceride levels as efficient as with fibrates and niacin, and therefore, it is likely that statins will dominate the field of risk prevention, even in hypertriglyceridemic patients *(145,146)*. Results of the VA-HIT study support use of fibrates in patients requiring additional therapy. Results of the HPS may move target LDL cholesterol levels even lower than at present.

In several major clinical trials, a period of dietary intervention of several mo preceded randomization to control or lipid lowering intervention. With the exception of the MIRACL trial, all trials were carried out in patients in stable condition with their most recent event having occurred several mo previously. Additional trials are in progress and should provide additional information on the effect of starting drug treatment before discharge in patients with acute coronary syndromes. At present, the AHA guidelines recommend that physicians should consider starting drug therapy on discharge *(147)*. Cholesterol lowering is now established beyond reasonable doubt as a fundamental part of risk reduction in patients with established CHD. Future challenges are not only to implement

Table 3

AHA/ACC Guide to Lipid Management for Patients with Coronary and Other Vascular Disease

Primary goal:

LDL < 100 mg/dL.

Start dietary therapy in all patients: (<7% saturated fat, <200 mg/d cholesterol) and promote physical activity and weight management. Encourage increased consumption of omega-3 fatty acids. Assess fasting lipid profile in all patients, and within 24 hr of hospitalization for those with an acute event. If patients are hospitalized, consider adding drug therapy on discharge. Add drug therapy according to the following guide:

LDL < 100 mg/dL (baseline or on-treatment). Further LDL-lowering therapy not required. Consider fibrate or niacin (if low HDL or high TG).	LDL 100–130 mg/dL (baseline or on-treatment). Therapeutic options: Intensify LDL-lowering therapy (statin or resina). Fibrate or niacin (if low HDL or high TG). Consider combined drug therapy (statin + fibrate or niacin) (if low HDL or high TG)	LDL ≥ 130 mg/dL (baseline or on-treatment). Intensify LDL-lowering therapy (statin or resina). Add or increase drug therapy with lifestyle therapies.

Secondary goal:

If TG ≥ 200 mg/dL,
    then non-HDL should be < 130 mg/dL.

If TG ≥ 150 mg/dL or HDL < 40 mg/dL:
    Emphasize weight management and physical activity. Advise smoking cessation.

If TG 200–499 mg/dL:
    Consider fibrate or niacin after LDL-lowering therapy[a].

If TG ≥ 500 mg/dL:
    Consider fibrate or niacin before LDL-lowering therapy.
    Consider omega-3 fatty acids as adjunct for high TG.

TG, triglycerides.

[a]The use of resin is relatively contraindicated when TG > 200 mg/dL.

treatment and reach goals but also to prevent discontinuation of therapy, as this may take place in a substantial number of patients *(148)*. Reduction of cost of statins will undoubtedly contribute to such improvement.

Key Points

- CHD is almost totally preventable with the right diet and nonsmoking.
- Dietary changes can improve prognosis, even in middle age.
- In Western societies, strict nonatherogenic diets are presently not generally accepted.
- Statins are the drug of choice in patients with acute coronary syndromes.
- Statins can lower the risk of CHD mortality by up to 42% in 5 to 6 yr.

REFERENCES

1. Chen Z, Peto R, Collins R, MacMahon S, Lu J, Li W. Serum cholesterol concentration and coronary heart disease in population with low cholesterol concentrations. BMJ 1991;303:276–282.

2. Robertson TL, Kato H, Grodon T, et al. Epidemiologic studies of coronary heart disease and stroke in Japanese men living in Japan, Hawaii and California. Incidence of myocardial infarction and death from coronary heart disease. Am J Cardiol 1977;39:239–243.

3. Keys A. Seven countries: A Multivariate Analysis of Health and Coronary Heart Disease. Harvard University Press, Harvard, Cambridge, MA, 1980.

4. Menotti A, Blackburn H, Kromhout D, et al. Changes in population cholesterol levels and coronary heart disease deaths in seven countries. Eur Heart J 1997;18:566–571.

5. Vartiainen E, Puska P, Pekkanen J, Tupmilehto J, Jousilahti P. Changes in risk factors explain changes in mortality from ischemic heart disease in Finland. BMJ 1994;309:23–27.

6. Martin MJ, Hulley SB, Browner WS, Kuller LH, Wentworth D. Serum cholesterol, blood pressure, and mortality: implications from a cohort of 361 662 men. Lancet 1986;2:933–936.

7. Castelli WP, Garrison RJ, Wilson PWF, Abbott RD, Kalousdian S, Kannel WB. Incidence of coronary heart disease and lipoprotein cholesterol levels. The Framingham Study. JAMA 1986;256:2835–2838.

8. Brown MS, Godstein JL. Heart attacks: gone with the century? Science 1996;272:629

9. Austin MA, Breslow JL, Hennekens CH, Buring BE, Willett WC, Krauss RM. Low density lipoprotein subclass patterns and risk of myocardial infarction. JAMA 1988;260:1917–1921.

10. Assman G, Schulte H. Relation of high-density lipoprtoein cholesterol and triglycerides to incidence of atherosclerotid coronary artery disease (the PROCAM experience) Am J Cardiol 1992;70:733–737.

11. Gaziano JM, Hennekens CH, O'Donnell CJ, Breslow JL, Buring JE. Fasting triglycerides, high-density lipoprotein, and risk of myocardial infarction. Circulation 1997;96:2520 2525.

12. Austin MA, King MC, Vranizan KM, Krauss RM. Atherogenic lipoprotein phenotype: a proposed genetic marker for coronary heart disease risk. Circulation 1990;82:495–506.

13. Grundy SM. Small LDL, atherogenic dyslipidemia, and the metabolic syndrome. Circulation 1997;95:1 4.

14. Tatami R, Mabuchi H, Ueda K, et al. Intermediate-density lipoprotein and cholesterol-rich very low density lipoprotein in angiographically determined coronary artery disease. Circulation 1981;64:1174–1184.

15. Rapp JH, Lespine A, Hamilton RL, et al. Triglyceride-rich lipoproteins isolated by selected-affinity anti-apolipoprotein B immunosorption from human atherosclerotic plaque. Arterioscler Thromb 1994;14:1767–1774.

16. Nordestgaard BG, Wootton R, Lewis B. Selective retention of VLDL, IDL, and LDL in the arterial intima of genetically hyperlipidemic rabbits in vivo: molecular size as a determinant of fractional loss from the intima-inner media. Thromb Vasc Biol 1995;15:534–542.

17. Hodis HN, Mack WJ, Dunn M, et al. Intermediate-density lipoproteins and progression of carotid arterial wall Intima-media thikness. Circulation 1997;95:2022–2026.

18. Law MR, Wald NJ, Thompson SG. By how much and how quickly does reduction in serum cholesterol concentration lower risk of ischaemic heart disease? BMJ 1994;308:367–372.

19. Nielsen NB. Transfer of low density lipoprotein into the arterial wall and the risk of atherosclerosis. Atherosclerosis 1996;123:1–15.

20. Steinberg D, Parthasarathy S, Carew TE, Khoo JC, Witztum JL. Beyond cholesterol: modifications of low-density lipoprotein that increase its atherogenecity. N Engl J Med 1989;233:227–232.

21. Libby P. Molecular bases of the acute coronary syndromes. Circulation 1995;91:2844–2850.

22. Cullen P, Schulte H, Assmann G. The Münster Heart Study (PROCAM): total mortality in middle-aged men is increased at low total and LDL cholesterol concentrations in smokers but not in non-smokers. Circulation 1997;96:2128–2136.

23. Miller ER, Apple LJ, Jiang L, Risby TH. Association between cigarette smoking and lipid peroxidation in a controlled feeding study. Circulation 1997;96:1097–1101.

24. Group Coronary Drug Project Research. Natural history of myocardial infarction in the Coronary Drug Project: long-term prognostic importance of serum lipid levels. Am J Cardiol 1978;42:489–.

25. Pekkanen J, Linn S, Heiss G, et al. Ten-year mortality from cardiovascular disease in relation to cholesterol level among men with and without preexisting cardiovascular disease. N Engl J Med 1990;322:1700–1707.

26. Falk E, Shah PK, Fuster V. Coronary plaque disruption. Circulation 1995;92:657–671.

27. Nofer J, Tepel M, Kehrel B, et al. Low-density lipoproteins inhibit the Na+/H+ antiport in muman platelets: a novel mechanism enhancing platelet activity in hypercholesterolemia. Circulation 1997;95: 1370–1377.

28. Davies MJ, Richardson PD, Woolf N, Katz DR, Mann J. Risk of thrombosis in human atherosclerotic plaques: role of extracellular lipid, macrophage, and smooth muscle cell content. Br Heart J 1993;69: 377–381.

29. Witzum JL. The oxidation hypothesis of atherosclerosis. Lancet 1994;344:793–795.

30. Libby P. Coronary artery injury and the biology of atherosclerosis: inflammation, thrombosis, and sta-bilization. Am J Cardiol 2000;86(Suppl.):3J–9J.

31. Wissler RW, Vesselinovitch D. Can atherosclerotic plaques regress? Anatomic and biochemical evi-dence from non-human animal models. Am J Cardiol 1990;65:33–40.

32. Thompson GR. Angiographic trials of lipid-lowering therapy: end of an era? Br Heart J 1995;74: 343–347.

33. Bustos C, Hernández-Presa MA, Ortego M, et al. HMB-CoA reductase inhibition by atorvastatin reduces neointimal inflammation in a rabbit model of atherosclerosis. J Am Coll Cardiol 1998;32: 2057–2064.

34. van der Wal AC, Becker AE, van der Loos CM, Das PK. The site of intimal rupture or erosion of throm-bosed coronary atherosclerotic plaques is characterized by an inflammatory process irrespective of the dominant plaque morphology. Circulation 1994;89:36–44.

35. Farb A, Burke AP, Tang AL, et al. Coronary plaque erosion without rupture into a lipid core. A fre-quent cause of coronary thrombosis in sudden coronary death. Circulation 1996;93:1354–1363.

36. Burke AP, Farb A, Malcom GT, Liang Y, Smialek J, Virmani R. Coronary risk factors and plaque mor-phology in men with coronary disease who died suddenly. N Engl J Med 1997;336:1276–1282.

37. Treasure CB, Klein JL, Weintraub WS, et al. Beneficial effects of cholesterol-lowering therapy on the coronary endothelium in patients with coronary artery disease. N Engl J Med 1995;332:481–487.

38. Ridker PM, Rifai N, Pfeffer MA, Sacks F, Braunwald E, for the Cholesterol and Recurrent Events (CARE) Investigators. Long-term effects of pravastatin on plasma concentrations of C-reactive pro-tein. Circulation 1999;100:230–235.

39. Cannon RO. Cardiovascular benefits of cholesterol lowering therapy: does improved endothelial vasodilator function matter? Circulation 2000;102:820–823.

40. Negre-Aminou P, van Vliet AK, van Erck M, van Thiel GC, van Leeuvwen RE, Cohen LH. Inhibition of proliferation of human smooth muscle cells by various HMG-CoA reductase inhibitors: compari-son with other human cell types. Biochim Biophys Acta 1997;1345:250–268.

41. Keys A, Anderson JT, Grande F. Serum cholesterol response to changes in the diet. IV. Particularily saturated fatty acids in the diet. Metabolism 1965;14:776–787.

42. Lewis B, Hammet F, Katan MB, et al. Towards an improved lipid-lowering diet: additive effects of changes in nutrient intake. Lancet 1981;2:1310–1313.

43. Artaud-Wild SM, Connor SL, Sexton G, Connor WE. Differences in coronary mortality can be explained by differences in cholesterol and saturated fat intakes in 40 countries but not in France and Finland. Circulation 1993;88:2771–2779.

44. Ueshima H, Iida M, Shimamoto T, et al. Dietary intake and serum total cholesterol level: their rela-tionship to different lifestyles in several Japanese populations. Circulation 1982;66:519–526.

45. Katan MB, Zock PL, Mensink RP. Dietary oils, serum lipoproteins, and coronary heart disease. Am J Clin Nutr 1995;61(Suppl.):1368S–1373S.

46. Daviglus ML, Stamler J, Orencia AJ, et al. Fish consumption and the 30-year risk of fatal myocardial infarction. N Engl J Med 1997;336:1046–1053.

47. Burr ML, Fehily AM, Gilbert JF, et al. Effects of changes in fat, fish, and fibre intakes on death and myocardial infarction. Diet and Reinfarction Trial (DART). Lancet 1989;2:757–761.

48. Watts GF, Lewis B, Brunt JN, et al. Effects on coronary artery disease of lipid-lowering diet, or diet plus cholestyramine, in the St Thomas' Atherosclerosis Regression Study (STARS). Lancet 1992;339: 563–569.

49. Leren P. The Oslo Diet Heart Study: eleven-year report. Circulation 1970;42:935–942.

50. de Lorgeril M, Renaud S, Mamelle N, et al. Mediterranean alpha-linolenic acid-rich diet in secondary prevention of coronary heart disease (see comments) (published erratum appears in Lancet 1995 Mar 18;345(8951):738). Lancet 1994;343:1454–1459.

51. McKeigue P. Diets for secondary prevention of coronary heart disease: can linolenic acid substitute for oily fish? Lancet 1994;343:1445.

52. AHA Dietary Guidelines, Revision 2000: a statement for health-care professionals from the Nutrition Committee of the American Heart Association. Circulation 2000;102:2296–2311.

53. Singh RB, Rastogi SS, Verma R, et al. Randomised controlled trial of cardioprotective diet in patients with recent acute myocardial infarction: results of one year follow up. BMJ 1992;304:1015–1019.

54. Expert Panel of the National Cholesterol Education Program (NECP). Report of the National Cholesterol Education Program Expert Panel on detection, evaluation, and treatment of high blood cholesterol in adults. Arch Intern Med 1988;148:36–69.

55. Study Group European Atherosclerosis Society. Strategies for the prevention of coronary heart disease: a policy statement of the European Atherosclerosis Society. Eur Heart J 1987;8:77–88.

56. Yu-Poth S, Zhao G, Etherton T, Naglak M, Jonnalagadda S, Kris-Etherton PM. Effects of the National Cholesterol Education Program's Step 1 and Step II dietary intervention programs on cardiovascular disease risk factors: a meta-analysis. Am J Clin Nutr 1999;69:632–646.

57. Dreon DM, Fernstrom HA, Miller B, Krauss RM. Low-density lipoprotein subclass patterns and lipoprotein response to a reduced-fat diet in men. FASEB J 1994;8:121–126.

58. Knopp RH, Walden CE, Retzlaff BM, et al. Long-term cholesterol lowering effects of 4 fat-restricted diets in hypercholesterolemic and combined hyperlipidemic men. JAMA 1997;278:1509–1515.

59. Expert Panel on Detection, Evaluation and Treatment of High Blood Cholesterol in Adults. Executive summary of the third report of the National Cholesterol Education Program (NECP) Expert Panel on detection, evaluation, and treatment of high blood cholesterol in adults (Adult Treatment Panel III). JAMA 2001;285:2486–2497.

60. Hjerman I, Velve Byre K, Holme I, Leren P. Effect of diet and smoking intervention on the incidence of coronary heart disease. Lancet 1981;2:1303–1310.

61. Clemmer KF, Binkoski AE, Coral SM, Zhao G, Kris-Etherton PM. Diet and drug therapy: a dynamic duo for reducing coronary heart disease risk. Curr Atheroscler Rep 2001;3:507–513.

62. Ornish D, Brown SE, Scherwitz LW, et al. Can lifestyle changes reverse atherosclerosis? Lancet 1990;336:129–133.

63. Barnard J, DiLauro S, Inkeles S. Effects of intensive diet and exercise intervention in patients taking cholesterol-lowering drugs. Am J Cardiol 1997;79:1112–1114.

64. Van Horn L. Fiber, lipids, and coronary heart disease. A statement for healthcare professionals from the Nutrition Committee, American Heart Assoociation. Circulation 1997;95.2701–2704.

65. Appel LJ, Moore TJ, Obarzanck E, et al. A clinical trial of the effects of dietary patterns on blood pressure. N Engl J Med 1997;336:1117–1124.

66. Anderson JW, Johnstone BM, Cook-Newell ME. Meta-analysis of the effects of soy protein intake on serum lipids. N Engl J Med 1995;333:276–282.

67. Thun MJ, Peto R, Lopez AD, et al. Alcohol consumption and mortality among middle-aged and elderly U.S. adults. N Engl J Med 1997;337:1705–1714.

68. Kauhanen J, Kaplan GA, Goldberg DE, Salonen JT. Beer binging and mortality: results from the Kuopio ischemic heart disease risk factor study, a prospective population based study. BMJ 1997;315:846–851.

69. Doll R, Pet R, Hall E, Wheatley K, Gray R. Mortality in relation to consumption of alcohol: 13 years' observation on male British doctors. BMJ 1994;309:911–918.

70. McElduff P, Dobson AJ. How much alcohol and how often? Population based case-control study of alcohol consumption and risk of a major coronary event. BMJ 1997;314:1159–1164.

71. Langer RD, Criqui MH, Reed DM. Lipoproteins and blood pressure as biological pathways for effect of moderate alcohol consumption on coronary heart disease. Circulation 1992;85:910–915.

72. Haskell WL, Camargo C, Williams PT, et al. The effect of cessation and resumption of moderate alcohol intake on serum high-density-lipoprotin subfractions: a controlled study. N Engl J Med 1984;310:805–810.

73. Renaud SC, Beswick AD, Fehily AM, Sharp PS, Elwood PC. Alcohol and platelet aggregation: the Caerphilly prospective heart disease study. Am J Clin Nutr 1992;55:1012–1017.

74. Corsini A, Pazzuconi F, Pfister P, Paoletti R, Sirtori C R. Inhibitor of proliferation of arterial smooth-muscle cells by fluvastatin. Lancet 1996;348:1584.

75. Hidaka Y, Eda T, Yonemoto M, Kamei T. Inhibiton of cultured vscular smooth muscle cell migration by simvastatin (MK-733). Atherosclerosis 1992;95:87–94.

76. Keidar S, Aviram M, Maor I, Oiknine J, Brook JG. Pravastatin inhibits cellular cholesterol synthesis and increases low densitiy lipoprotein receptor activitiy in macrophages: in vitro and in vivo studies. Br J Clin Pharmacol 1994;38:513–519.

77. McPherson R, Tsoukas C, Baines MG, et al. Effects of lovastatin on natural killer cell function and other immunological parameters in man. J Clin Immunol 1993;13:439–444.

78. Lacoste L, Lam JYT, Hung J, Letschacovski G, Solymoss CB, Water D. Hyperlipidemia and coronary disease: correction of the increased thrombogenic potential with cholesterol reduction. Circulation 1995;92:3127–3177.

79. Bucher HC, Griffith LE, Guyatt GH. systematic review on the risk and benefit of different cholesterol-lowering interventions. Arterioscler Thromb Vasc Biol 1999;19:187–195.

80. Rubins HB, Robins S, Collins, et al. Gemfibrozil for the secondary prevention of coronary heart disease in men with low levels of high-density lipoprotein cholesterol. N Engl J Med 1999;341: 410–418.

81. The BIP Study Group. Secondary prevention by raising HDL cholesterol and reducing triglycerides in patients with coronary artery disease. The Bezafibrate Infarction Prevention (BIP) Study. Circulation 2000;102:21–27.

82. Haffner SM. Secondary prevention of coronary heart disease. The role of fibric acids. Circulation 2000;102:2–4.

83. Anonymous. Effect of fenofibrate on progression of coronary-artery disease in type 2 diabetes: the Diabetes Atherosclerosis Intervention Study, a randomised study. Lancet 2001;357:905–910.

84. Canner PL, Berge KG, Wenger NK, et al. Fifteen year mortality in Coronary Drug Project Patients: long-term benefit with niacin. J Am Coll Cardiol 1986;8:1245–1255.

85. Blankenhorn DH, Nessim SA, Johnson RL, Sanmarco ME, Azen SP, Cashin-Hemphill L. Beneficial effects of combined colestipol.niacin therapy on coronary atherosclerosis and coronary venous bypass grafts. JAMA 987;257:3233–3240.

86. Knopp RH, Alagona P, Davidson M, et al. Equivalent efficacy of a time-release form of niacin (Niaspan) given once-a-night vs. plain niacin in the management of hyperlipidemia. Metabolism 1998;47: 1097–1104.

87. Levy RI, Brensike JF, Epstein ES, et al. The influence of changes in lipid values induced by cholestyramine and diet on progression of coronary arery disease: results of the NHBLI type II coronary intervention study. Circulation 1984.69:325–337.

88. GISSI-Prevenzione Investigators. Dietary supplementation with n-3 polyunsaturated fatty acids and vitamin E after myocardial infarction: results of the GISSI-Prevenzione trial. Lancet 1999;354: 447–455.

89. Hulley S, Grady D, Bush TL, et al. Randomized trial of estrogen plus progestin for secondary prevention of coronary heart disease in postmenopausal women. JAMA 1998;280:605–613.

90. Herrington DM, Reboussin DM, Brosnihan KB, et al. Effects of estrogen replacement on the progression of coronary artery atherosclerosis. N Engl J med 2000;343:522–529.

91. Writing Group for the Women's Health Initiative Investigators. Risks and benefits of estogen plus progestin in healthy postmenopausal women. JAMA 2002;288:321–333.

92. Law M. Plant sterol and stanol margarines and health. BMJ 2000;320:861–864.

93. Brensike JF, Levy RI, Kelsey SF, et al. Effects of therapy with cholestyramine on progression of coronary atherosclerosis: results of the NHBLI type II coronary intervention study. Circulation 1984;69: 313–324.

94. Arntzenius AC, Kromhout D, Barth JD, et al. Diet, lipoproteins, and the progression of coronary atherosclerosis. N Engl J Med 1995;312:805–811.

95. Brown G, Albers JJ, Fisher LD, et al. Regression of coronary artery disease as a result of intensive lipid-lowering therapy in men with high levels of apolipoprotein B (see comments). N Engl J Med 1990;323:1289–1298.

96. Cashin-Hemphill L, Mack WJ, Pogoda JM, Sanmarco M E, Azen S P, Blankenhorn D H. Beneficial effects of colestipol-niacin on coronary atherosclerosis. A 4-year follow-up. JAMA 1990;264:3013–3017.

97. Buchwald H, Varco RL, Matts JP, et al. Effect of partial ileal bypass on mortality and morbidity from coronary heart disease in patients with hypercholesterolemia—report of the Program on the Surgical Control of Hyperlipidemias (POSCH). N Engl J Med 1990;323:946–955.

 98. Kane JP, Malloy MJ, Ports TA, Phillips NR, Diehl JC, Havel RJ. Regression of coronary atherosclerosis during treatment of familial hypercholesterolemia with combined drug regimens (see comments). JAMA 1990;264:3007–3012.

 99. Schuler G, Hambrecht R, Schlierf G, et al. Regular physical exercise and low-fat diet: effects of progression of cornary artery disease. Circulation 1992;86:1–11.

100. Blankenhorn DH, Azen SP, Kramsch DM, et al. Coronary angiographic changes with lovastatin therapy. The Monitored Atherosclerosis Regression Study (MARS). The MARS Research Group (see comments). Ann Intern Med 1993;119:969–976.

101. Waters D, Higginson L, Gladstone P, et al. Effects of monotherapy with an HMG-CoA reductase inhibitor on the progression of coronary atherosclerosis as assessed by serial quantitative arteriography. The Canadian Coronary Atherosclerosis Intervention Trial. Circulation 1994;89:959–968.

102. Haskell WL, Alderman EL, Fair JM, et al. Effects of intensive multiple risk factor reduction on coronary atherosclerosis and clinical cardiac events in men and women with coronary artery disease: The Stanford Coronary Risk Intervention Project (SCRIP). Circulation 1994;89:975–990.

103. MAAS investigators. Effect of simvastatin on coronary atheroma: the Multicentre Anti-Atheroma Study (MAAS). Lancet 1994;344:633–638.

104. Sacks FM, Pasternak RC, Gibson CM, Rosner B, Stone PH, for the Havard Atherosclerosis Reversibility Project (HARP) Group. Effect of coronary atherosclerosis of decrease in plasma cholesterol concentrations in normocholesterolemic patients. Lancet 1994;344:1182–1186

105. Jukema JW, Bruschke AVG, van Boven AJ, et al. Effects of lipid lowering by pravastatin on progression and regression of coronary artery disease in symptomatic men with normal to moderately elevated serum cholesterol levels. The Regression Growth Evaluation Statin Study (REGRESS). Circulation 1995;91:2528–2540.

106. Bestehorn HP, Rensing UFE, Roskamm H, et al.The effect of simvastatin on progression of coronary artery disease: the multicenter coronary intervention study (CIS). Eur Heart J 1997;18:226–234.

107. Herd JA, Ballantyne CM, Farmer JA, et al. Effects of fluvastatin on coronary atherosclerosis in patients with mild to moderate cholesterol elevations (Lipoprotein and Coronary Atherosclerosis Study (LCAS)). Am J Cardiol 1997;80:278–286.

108. Glagov S, Weisenberg E, Zarins CK, Stankunavicius R, Kolettis GJ. Compensatory enlargement of human atherosclerotic coronary arteries. N Engl J Med 1987;316:1371–1375.

109. Petursson KK, Jonmundsson EH, Brekkan A, Hardarson T. Angiographic predictors of new coronary occlusions. Am Heart J 1985;129:515–520.

110. Furberg CD, Adams HP, Jr, Applegate WB, et al. Effect of lovastatin on early carotid atherosclerosis and cardiovascular events. Asymptomatic Carotid Artery Progression Study (ACAPS) Research Group (see comments). Circulation 1994;90:1679–1687.

111. Crouse JR, Byington RP, Bond MG, et al. Pravstatin, Lipids, and Atherosclerosis in the Carotid Arteries (PLAC-II): a clinical trial with atherosclerosis outcome. Am J Cardiol 1995;75:455–459.

112. Salonen R, Nyyssonen K, Porkkala E, et al. Kuopio Atherosclerosis Prevention Study (KAPS). A population-based primary preventive trial of the effect of LDL lowering on atherosclerotic progression in carotid and femoral arteries. Circulation 1995;92:1758–1764.

113. Gould KL, Martucci JP, Goldberg DI, et al. Short-term cholesterol lowering decreases size and severity of perfusion abnormalities by positron emission tomography after dipyridamole in patients with coronary artery disease. A potential noninvasive marker of healing coronary endothelium. Circulation 1994;89:1530–1538.

114. Anderson TJ, Meredith IT, Yeung AC, Frei B, Selwyn AP, Ganz P. The effect of cholesterol-lowering and antioxidant therapy on endothelium-dependent coronary vasomotion. N Engl J Med 1995;332:488–493.

115. O'Driscoll G, Green D, Taylor RR. Simvastatin, an HMG-coenzyme A reductase inhibitor, improves endothelial function within 1 month. Circulation 1997;95:1126–1131.

116. Tamai O, Matsuoka H, Itabe H, Wada Y, Kohno K, Imaizumi T. Single LDL-apheresis improves endothelium-dependent vasodilatation in hypercholesterolemic humans. Circulation 1997;95:76–82.

117. Dupuis J, Tardif JC, Cernacek P, Théroux P. Cholesterol reduction rapidly improves endothelial function after acute coronary syndromes. The RECIFE (Reduction of Cholesterol in Ischemia and Function of the Endothelium) Trial. Circulation 1999;99:3227–3233.

118. Steinberg HO, Bayazeed B, Hook G, Johnson A, Cronin J, Baron AD. Endothelial dysfunction is associated with cholesterol levels in the high normal range in humans. Circulation 1997;96:3287–3293.

119. LaCoste L, Lam JYT, Hung J, Letchacovski G, Solymoss CB, Waters D. Hyperlipidemia and coronary disease: correction of the increased thrombogenic potential with cholesterol reduction. Circulation 1995;92:3172–3177.

120. Stenestrand U, Wallentin L, for the Swedish Register of Cardiac Intensive Care (RIKS-HIA). Early statin treatment following acute myocardial infarction and 1-year survival. JAMA 2001;285: 430–436.

121. Waters DD. Early pharmacologic intervention and plaque stability in acute coronary syndromes. Am J Cardiol 2001;88(Suppl.):30K–36K.

122. Schwartz GG, Olsson AG, Ezekowitz MD, et al. Effects of atorvastatin on early recurrent ischemic events in acute coronary syndromes: the MIRACL study: a randomized controlled trial. JAMA 2001; 285:1711–1718.

123. Pitt B, Waters D, Brown WV, et al. Aggressive lipid-lowering therapy compared with angioplasty in stable coronary artery disease. N Engl J Med 1999;341:70–76.

124. Coronary Drug Project Research Group. Clofibrate and niacin in coronary heart disease. JAMA 1975; 231:360–381.

125. Carlson LA, Danielson M, Ekberg I, Klintemar B, Rosenhamer G. Reduction of myocardial rein-farction by the combined treatment with clofibrate and nicotinic acid. Atherosclerosis 1977;28: 81–86.

126. Committee of Principal Investigators. A co-operative trial in the primary prevention of ischemic heart disease using clofibrate. Br Heart J 1978;40:1069–1118.

127. Dorr AE, Gundersen K, Schneider JC, Spencer TW, Martin WB. Colestipol hydrochloride in hyperc-holesterolemic patients—effect on serum cholesterol and mortality. J Chron Dis 1978;31:5–14.

128. Lipid Research Clinics Program. The Lipid Research Clinics Coronary Primary Prevention Trial Results. JAMA 1984;251:351–374.

129. Frick MH, Elo O, Haapa K, et al. Helsinki Heart Study: Primary-Prevention Trial with Gemfibrozil in Middle-aged Men with Dyslipidemia (Safety of Treatment, Changes in Risk Factors, and Incidence of Coronary Heart Disease). N Engl J Med 1987;317:1237–1245.

130. Scandinavian Simvastatin Survival Study Group. Randomised trial of cholesterol lowering in 4444 patients with coronary heart disease: the Scandinavian Simvastatin Survival Study (4S). Lancet 1994; 344:1383–1389.

131. Shepherd J, Cobbe SM, Ford I, et al. Prevention of coronary heart disease with pravastatin in men with hypercholesterolemia. West of Scotland Coronary Prevention Study Group (see comments). N Engl J Med 1995;333:1301–1307.

132. Sacks FM, Pfeffer MA, Moye LA, et al. The effect of pravastatin on coronary events after myocardial infarction in patients with average cholesterol levels. N Engl J Med 1996;335:1001–1009.

133. The Long-Term Intervention with Pravastatin in Ischaemic Disease (LIPID) Study Group. Prevention of cardiovascular events and death with pravastatin in patients with coronary heart disease and a broad range of initial cholesterol levels. N Engl J Med 1998;339:1349–1357.

134. Downs JR, Clearfield M, Weis S, et al. Primary prevention of acute coronary events with lovastatin in men and women with average cholesterol levels: results of AFCAPS/TexCAPS Air Force/Texas Coro-nary Atherosclerosis Prevention Study. JAMA 1998;279:1615–1622.

135. Pedersen TR, Berg K, Cook TJ, et al. Safety and tolerability of cholesterol lowering with simvastatin during 5 years in the Scandinavian Simvastatin Survival Study. Arch Intern Med 1996;156:2085–2092.

136. Bjerre LM, LeLorier J. Do statins cause cancer? A meta-analysis of large randomized clinical trials. Am J Med 2001;110:716–723.

137. Pyörälä K, Pedersen TR, Kjekshus J, Faergeman O, Olsson AG, Thorgeirsson G. The Scandinavian Simvastatin Survival Study (4S) Group. Cholesterol lowering with simvastatin improves prognosis of diabetic patients with coronary heart disease. Diabetes Care 1997;20:614–620.

138. Scandinavian Simvastatin Survival Study Group. Baseline serum cholesterol and treatment effect in the Scandinavian Simvastatin Survival Study (4S). Lancet 1995;345:1274–1275.

139. Pedersen TR, Kjekshuh J, Berg K, et al. Cholesterol lowering and the use of healthcare resources. Results of the Scandinavian Simvastatin Survival Study. Circulation 1996;93:1796–1802.

140. Jonsson B, Johannesson M, Kjekshus J, et al. Cost-effectiveness of cholesterol lowering. Results from the Scandinavian Simvastatin Survival Study (4S). Eur Heart J 1996;17:1001–1007.

141. Tengs TO, Adams ME, Plsikin JS, et al. Five-hundred life-saving interventions and their cost-effec-tiveness. Risk Analysis 1995;15:369–390.

142. Johannesson M, Jönsson B, Kjekshus J, Olsson AG, Pedersen TR, Wedel H. Cost effectiveness of simvastatin treatment to lower cholesterol levels in patients with coronary heart disease. N Engl J Med 1997;336:332–336.
143. Smith SC, Blair SN, Bonow RO, et al. AHA/ACC guidelines for preventing heart attack and death in patients with atherosclerotic cardiovascular disease: 2001 update. A statement for healthcare professionals from the American Heart Association and the American College of Cardiology. Circulation 2001; 104:1577–1579.
144. Pedersen TR, Kjekshus J, Olsson AG, Cook TJ. 4S results support AHA guidelines to reduced LDL-cholesterol to less than 100 mg/dl in patients with CHD. Circulation:I-717.
145. Bakker-Arkema RG, Davidson MH, Goldstein RJ, et al. Efficacy and safety of a new HMG-CoA reductase inhibitor, atorvastatin, in patients with hypertriglyceridemia. JAMA 1996;275:128–133.
146. Davidson MH, Stein EA, Dujovne CA, et al. The efficacy and six-week tolerability of simvastatin 80 and 160 mg daily. Am J Cardiol 1997;79:38–42.
147. Grundy SM, Balady GJ, Criqui MH, et al. When to start cholesterol-lowering therapy in patients with coronary heart disease: a statement for healthcare professionals from the American Heart Association Task Force on Risk Reduction. Circulation 1997;95:1683–1685.
148. Andrade SE, Walker AM, Gottlieb LK, et al. Discontinuation of antihyperlipidemic drugs—do rates reported in clinical trials reflect rates in primary care settings? N Engl J Med 1995;332:1125–1131.
149. Heart Protection Study Collaborative Group. MRC/BHF Heart Protection Study of cholesterol lowering with simvastatin in 20,536 high-risk individuals: a randomised placebo-controlled trial. Lancet 2002;360:7–22.

24

"Secondary Prevention" of Myocardial Infarction

Jorge Plutzky, MD, FACC *and*
Roger S. Blumenthal, MD, FACC

CONTENTS

INTRODUCTION

According to data from the prethrombolytic era, a patient who survives a first myocardial infarction (MI) faces nearly an 80% chance of another cardiovascular disease (CVD) event within the next 5 yr *(1)*. More contemporary data indicate that within 6 yr of an MI, approx 20% of men and 35% of women will sustain another heart attack with similar percentages developing congestive heart failure (CHF) *(2)*. Thus, the diagnosis of an MI brings with it the high likelihood of recurrent cardiovascular events, compounding morbidity, and probable ultimate fatality. Viewed in this way, CVD is, in fact, much like many forms of cancer, although the reaction of many patients to those two diagnoses can be quite different. Perhaps this is related to antiquated notions, propagated at times by physicians, that mechanical cardiovascular therapies, such as bypass surgery and angioplasty, can "fix" the cardiovascular problem. The myriad of therapeutic options available to the cardiologist and their patients might further fuel such concepts. In reality, modern medicine might be better at "curing" some types of cancer than

From: *Contemporary Cardiology: Management of Acute Coronary Syndromes, Second Edition*
Edited by: C. P. Cannon © Humana Press Inc., Totowa, NJ

reversing advanced atherosclerosis. CVD patients suffer a chronic insidious disease that requires aggressive interventions to alter the complex process that led to its generation, propagation, and recurrence; steps untouched by acute mechanical treatments restoring patency or providing alternate paths of blood flow. Fortunately, the number of interventions, both medical and lifestyle, for so-called secondary prevention also continues to grow. Similarly, our understanding of atherogenesis and the development of acute coronary syndromes is also progressing, creating hope for the development of new, and perhaps more effective, therapeutic approaches. We are also left with the considerable challenge of applying those interventions known to reduce cardiovascular risk.

The need to use all interventions available for modifying risk factors and ameliorating the natural history of coronary artery disease (CAD) in the MI survivor is supported by epidemiologic and clinical trials data *(3,4)*. There is no higher risk group for future CVD events than the patient who has survived a heart attack or unstable angina *(5)*. Mortality rates post-MI are the greatest in the first year, but continue to be 2–5%/yr for men and women, depending on their age and left ventricular systolic function *(1,2)*. The simple presence of angina post-MI approximately doubles the risk of subsequent coronary heart disease mortality *(2,6)*. Issues regarding the secondary prevention of MI have been discussed throughout this book, as well as in thorough discussions in the literature *(3,7–9)*. As such, our aim is to provide a compendium of the interventions to consider in the post-MI patient.

The 27th Bethesda Conference, sponsored by the American College of Cardiology, carefully reviewed risk factors for atherosclerosis, organizing them into four categories: (*i*) interventions proven to lower CVD risk; (*ii*) likely to lower CVD risk; (*iii*) risk factors associated with increased risk that, if modified, might lower risk; and (*iv*) risk factors associated with CVD risk, but which cannot be modified (Table 1) *(10)*. Before discussing some of those therapies, it is important to discuss some issues of definition that arise when discussing the secondary prevention of MI.

More than 1 million first MIs will occur this year in the United States *(2)*. Although the survivors of these events are now technically candidates for "secondary prevention," there is little doubt that, in the majority of cases, in the days, weeks, months, and even years prior to that first MI, these patients already had considerable subclinical CAD. Given that at least one-quarter of those first MIs will prove fatal within 30 days, the need to intervene in high-risk patients, even in the absence of anginal symptoms is quite apparent. As such, there has been an appropriate movement away from using terms such as "primary" and "secondary" prevention based simply on the documentation of a prior MI. Instead, one can view patients as being on a spectrum of risk, independent of a preceding coronary event. In this way, one would consider patients without a history of MI, but with documented significant atherosclerosis in at least one vascular bed, as needing aggressive secondary prevention therapies. Such an approach is now adapted by the National Cholesterol Education Program (NCEP).

A similar argument can be made for the patient with diabetes mellitus *(11,12)*. The presence of this co-morbidity makes subclinical CAD so likely, that the American Diabetes Association and the NCEP Adult Treatment Panel (ATP) III have called for a "secondary prevention" approach to the management of all diabetic patients *(11)*. With this notion of a spectrum of risk, one must keep in mind those interventions specifically directed toward the infarcted myocardium, for example, β-blockers, antiplatelet agents, and angiotensin-converting enzyme (ACE) inhibitors, as opposed to those that reduce

Table 1
Risk Factor (RF) Intervention Categories for CVD

Category I: RF for which interventions are proven to lower CVD risk:
  Cigarette smoking
  LDL-C
  High saturated fat/cholesterol diet
  Left ventricular hypertrophy secondary to hypertension
  Thrombogenic factors
Category II: RF for which interventions are likely to lower CVD risk:
  Diabetes mellitus
  Physical inactivity
  HDL
  Triglycerides/small dense LDL
  Obesity
Category III: RF associated with increased risk that, if modified, might lower CVD risk:
  Psychosocial factors
  Lipoprotein (a)
  Homocysteine
  Oxidative stress
  No alcohol consumption
Category IV: RF associated with CVD risk, but cannot be modified:
  Age
  Male gender
  Family history of early onset CVD

Adapted from the 27th Bethesda Conference Report *(10)*.

long-term risk in general. As used here, the term secondary prevention refers to all patients at high risk for cardiac events because of the presence of known vascular disease, diabetes, or a confluence of risk factors that makes the 10 yr incidence of MI significantly high.

CHOLESTEROL LOWERING

One of the greatest accomplishments in modern medicine was the proving of the cholesterol hypothesis, which did not occur conclusively until 1994 with the publication of the Scandinavian Simvastatin Survival Study (4S) *(13)*. Although prior clinical trials had shown decreased cardiac events with lipid-lowering, no prior study had demonstrated a mortality benefit by decreasing cholesterol or LDL levels in patients with a prior history of MI. Given the side effects that often accompanied the older generation of lipid-lowering therapies (e.g. resins, niacin), many physicians were hesitant to routinely use these agents.

The 4S investigators performed a large randomized placebo-controlled study designed to investigate a primary end point of mortality benefit using simvastatin (20–40 mg to bring the total cholesterol <200 mg/dL) vs placebo. The subjects had a mean cholesterol of 261 mg/dL; 827 women numbered among the 4444 participants. Patients on active therapy experienced a 30% reduction in overall mortality (11.5 vs 8.2%) with a statistical significance of $p = 0.0003$. Subgroup analysis showed consistent benefit across subgroups of women, smokers, hypertensives, and the elderly *(14)*. Particularly striking in post hoc analysis was the benefit among diabetic patients with a risk reduction of 55% (*p* = 0.018) *(15)*. There was also a reduction in need for future revascularization procedures, with a 37% risk reduction (*p* < 0.00001). Beyond the clear-cut clinical benefit for patients, economic analysis reveals significant cost savings in the treated vs untreated groups *(11)*. Similar results have been reported in the other secondary prevention trials, using pravastatin in patients with CAD but with average or only mildly elevated cholesterol levels *(16,17)*.

The strength of these data has engendered obvious questions regarding the optimal LDL level in the post-MI patient. Restated, is there additional risk reduction achieved by reducing LDL levels from 100 mg/dL to approx 70 mg/dL? Previously, clues to the answer to this important question rested only in post hoc analyses from 4S and Cholesterol and Recurrent Events (CARE) trial. If one looks at patients with baseline LDL <125 mg/dL in CARE, no apparent benefit in terms of clinical events was seen with pravastatin therapy in this trial *(17,20)*. Is there a "floor" to the LDL level beyond which further lowering no longer accrues benefit to the patient? The CARE investigators also found, via post hoc analysis, that the absolute or percentage reduction in LDL had little relationship to subsequent coronary events in their study population of stable post-MI patients who had average cholesterol levels *(20)*. Similarly, the West of Scotland Coronary Prevention Study (WOSCOPS) investigators found that treatment benefit was not related to a patient's baseline LDL, and that there appeared to be no further benefit beyond an LDL-lowering of about 24%.

In contrast, the 4S investigators have reported that, in their patients (CAD patients with elevated cholesterol levels), CVD event reduction was related to the magnitude of LDL lowering. Now prospective data from the Oxford University-run Health Protection Study (HPS) can be added to these data as yet another statin trial likely to enter the pantheon of landmark statin trials. HPS addressed the effects of simvastatin 40 mg in patients with either a history of CAD, or at high risk for it on the basis of diabetes or other evident vascular disease among patients with LDL levels which, on average, were approx 80 mg/dL in the treatment group and approx 125 mg/dL in the placebo group *(21)*. In HPS, patients with vascular disease or diabetes had comparable major vascular event rate risk reductions of about 30% whether their baseline LDL-C was <100 mg/dL or >135 mg/dL *(21)*. In impressive fashion, HPS showed benefit across all subgroups and LDL levels. This issue will also be further considered in studies underway, such as Treat to New Targets (TNT), in which patients will achieve with atorvastatin either LDL levels of approx 100 mg/dL (atorvastatin 80 mg) or approx 70 mg/dL (atorvastatin 10 mg). A similar trial is underway with simvastatin. For now, given the excellent tolerability and safety of statins, the long-term risk for recurrent events in the MI survivor, as well as many years of evidence demonstrating the association between LDL and CVD risk, this more aggressive approach to treatment appears warranted. The ATP III recommends treating all patients with vascular disease or diabetes to an optimal LDL-C level of <100 mg/dL *(11)*.

The issue of LDL lowering for secondary prevention underscores several points raised earlier. The first is the relatively arbitrary distinction between what truly consists of secondary prevention vs primary prevention and the need for intervention in high-risk patients who have not yet experienced a first MI. The WOSCOPS demonstrated a

31% decrease in cardiac events in patients with high cholesterol and no prior MI *(18)*. The recommendation by the American Diabetes Association and the NCEP ATP III, that all diabetic patients begin lipid-lowering interventions if their LDL is >130 mg/dL independent of other risk factors, reflects this notion of cardiovascular risk as a continuous spectrum as opposed to discrete categories. Similarly, the NCEP ATP III recommends basing LDL intervention on the degree of risk. The statin trials also underscore the importance of modifying risk related to atherosclerosis in any vascular bed; both 4S, as part of post hoc analysis, and the CARE trial, as a primary end point, showed decreased stroke rates with statin therapy *(19)*. This has now also been suggested in HPS as well *(21a)*.

The potential benefit of lipid-lowering therapy in acute coronary syndromes rather than in stable CVD patients is now being examined. The Myocardial Ischemia Reduction with Aggressive Cholesterol Lowering (MIRACL) trial was designed to assess the benefits of aggressive lipid lowering immediately after an acute coronary event *(22)*. After just 16 wk, the composite primary end point of death, recurrent MI, cardiac arrest, or worsening angina with rehospitalization occurred in 14.8% of the atorvastatin group vs 17.4% of the placebo group (relative risk of 0.84, $p = 0.048$). The one component of the composite end point, which reached statistical significance, was recurrent symptomatic ischemia prompting rehospitalization (6.2 vs 8.4%, $p = 0.02$). Moreover, there are a number of ongoing trials designed to determine how low one should lower LDL-C in stable patients with documented atherosclerotic vascular disease *(23)*.

It is important that all CVD patients undergo lipid testing with aggressive dietary and medical treatment for any dyslipidemia that may be present. One should also remember that while the acute phase of an MI may change lipid levels, these effects will only lower LDL levels. As such, one can check the LDL level post-MI; if it is >100 mg/dL, one can begin at least a low dose of statin therapy with a safe assumption that the baseline LDL level prior to the cardiac event was only higher. If the LDL returns <100 mg/dL in the acute setting, it then becomes incumbent upon the physician to recheck levels later to see if treatment is warranted. Alternatively, the HPS findings suggest many patients with vascular disease or diabetes may benefit from statin therapy regardless of baseline lipid levels *(21a)*.

HYPERTENSION

Hypertension is defined as a blood pressure >140/90 mmHg, while normal BP is classified as <130/85 mmHg *(24)*. Hypertension affects about 50 million Americans, and it is a major independent risk factor for future CVD events. It contributes to left ventricular hypertrophy, it impairs vascular endothelial function, and it may increase the risk of plaque rupture due to increased hemodynamic shear stresses.

Most studies involving hypertension post-MI have suggested that persistently elevated blood pressure leads to higher reinfarction and mortality rates *(24,25)*. Many pharmacologic interventions routinely prescribed to CAD patients will lower blood pressure, for example, β-blockers or ACE inhibitors *(26)*. It appears that some of the benefits of these agents are related to factors other than improvement in blood pressure alone. Even when medication is employed for hypertension, dietary modification and exercise should be the cornerstones of therapy for all hypertensive CVD patients.

ASPIRIN

Unless contraindicated, essentially every post-MI patient should be taking an antiplatelet agent (e.g., aspirin or clopidogrel). Benefits have been demonstrated in acute MI in the ISIS-II trial, where the prompt use of aspirin was almost as effective as thrombolytic therapy in decreasing short-term mortality (23%) *(27)*. The utility of antiplatelet agents has also been shown in acute coronary syndromes in several studies, with doses ranging from 75 to 1300 mg/d *(28)*. The Antiplatelet Trialist Collaboration meta-analysis found reductions in cardiac events of about one-third *(29)*. Recently, the Clopidogrel in Unstable Angina to Prevent Recurrent Events (CURE) investigators found that adding clopidogrel to aspirin for an average of 9 mo decreased major events by 20% as compared to aspirin treatment alone *(30)*.

β-BLOCKERS

β-blockers appear to decrease the risk of recurrent cardiac events through effects on several mechanisms that might be contributing to myocardial ischemia: decreased oxygen consumption, and decreased blood pressure, and decreased ventricular arrhythmia *(31,32)*. Older trials, before thrombolytics, demonstrated the mortality benefit of β-blockers with a decreased incidence of sudden death (14% short-term mortality risk reduction suggested by meta-analysis) *(31,32)*. The use of high doses of nonselective β-blockers may be associated with modest adverse effects on the lipid profile, primarily in lowering high-density lipoprotein (HDL) *(33,34)*. There is some question regarding how long it is necessary to have CAD patients on β-blockers post-MI, but they are excellent choices for long-term blood control in CVD patients *(24)*.

ACE INHIBITORS

ACE inhibitors have been shown to have a mortality benefit post-MI *(26,35)*. The benefits, however, also include improved ventricular function, decreased symptoms and admissions for CHF, and less cardiovascular events in patients with left ventricular dysfunction, diabetes, or known vascular disease. In the Survival and Ventricular Enlargement (SAVE) trial, there was a 19% decrease in mortality among patients on ACE inhibitors. Currently, the general recommendation is for the initiation of ACE inhibitors within 1 to 2 d post-MI. The Heart Outcomes Prevention Evaluation (HOPE) trial suggests that ACE inhibitors should be the standard of care in all patients with vascular disease or diabetes who have a systolic blood pressure >120 mmHg *(26)*.

HORMONE REPLACEMENT THERAPY

Estrogen has been reported to have significant vascular system benefits, with the assumption being that estrogen may explain the approx 10 yr lag phase in CAD events among women as compared to men *(37)*. As such, hormone replacement therapy (HRT) has received much scrutiny and study in both the literature and the media regarding its potential risks and benefits *(38)*. Unfortunately, the Heart Estrogen/Progestin Replacement Study (HERS) found no benefit of continuous combined conjugated equine estrogen and medroxyprogesterone acetate *(39)*. Similar findings were observed in the Woman's Health Initiative. The American Heart Association recently issued a statement summarizing the data regarding HRT and CVD and concluded that women should not take HRT for the sole purpose of trying to lower their risk of heart disease *(40)*.

EXERCISE AND REHABILITATION

Many physiologic benefits relevant to the cardiovascular system can be seen in response to exercise, whether within or independent of a rehabilitation program. A 22 trial meta-analysis (4600 patients) suggested that post-MI rehabilitation programs led to decreases in total mortality (20%), cardiovascular mortality (22%), and recurrent infarction (25%) *(41)*.

DIABETES–INSULIN RESISTANCE

Increasing attention has focused on the close relationship between diabetes and atheroslcerosis, a link that extends even to those patients with other forms of metabolic abnormalities, including impaired fasting glucose (IGT) and the insulin resistance syndrome (also known as the dysmetabolic syndrome) *(42)*. Diabetes mellitus is now recognized as a "risk equivalent" for CAD, which is an important concept adopted by the ATP III, with all diabetic patients treated to an LDL less than 100 mg/dL *(11,43,44)*. Consistent with this interest has been ongoing attention to the potential role of diabetic therapies on CAD. Although improved glucose control has been intently pursued in the past, more recent data from United Kingdom Prospective Diabetes Study (UKPDS) has found that tighter glycemic control and blood pressure treatment was associated with some degree of improved outcomes among diabetic patients *(45,46)*. Overall improvement in metabolic parameters, including better glycemic control, may also have indirect effects, for example, lowering triglycerides and raising HDL. Newer antidiabetic agents, such as thiazolidinediones, which may also have direct vascular effects that limit atherosclerosis or its complications, is an area of intent study *(47)*.

OTHER INTERVENTIONS

Considerable interest, especially on the part of patients has continued to focus on the potential benefits of vitamins, especially antioxidants like Vitamin E, in the prevention of recurrent cardiovascular events. In this regard, recent large clinical trials, including HOPE and the HPS, argue in a most definitive fashion that antioxidant vitamins, even in the theoretical optimal combination of Vitamin E and Vitamin C, fail to offer any protection against recurrent cardiovascular events *(1,44,48)*. The role of oxidation in atherosclerosis is well-supported and intriguing; it may simply be that the appropriate or effective antioxidant interventions have not yet been developed. Considerable interest has also focused on the use of folate as a means of treating vascular disease, especially when patients manifest elevated homocysteine levels. The extent of folate in typical diets has made such studies challenging, as has the overlapping nature of homocysteine levels among people with and without vascular disease. More recent work suggests folate therapy may offer some decrease in rates of restenosis *(49)*.

AN INTEGRATED APPROACH TO RISK REDUCTION
AMONG POST-MI PATIENTS

A comprehensive approach to the prevention of MI in high-risk patients must be tailored to the individual. A list of these approaches was developed by the National Institutes of Health (NIH) Consensus Conference and is adapted in Table 1. Given our inability to offer a "cure" for atherosclerosis, comprehensive risk factor modification strategies should be employed. Of course, such therapies only work when the physician

Table 2
The ABCs of CVD Risk Management (53,54)

A: Antiplatelet/anticoagulant agents (e.g., aspirin, clopidogrel, warfarin).
ACE inhibition (based on HOPE trial).
B: Blood pressure (normal <130/85 mmHg; <125/75 if >1 g proteinuria).
β-blockade (especially if post-MI, impaired ejection fraction, or inducible ischemia).
C: Cholesterol (optimal LDL is <100 mg/dL, normal triglycerides <150, HDL >40).
Cigarettes cessation (nicotine replacement, bupropion, counseling).
D: Diet/weight (normal body mass index [BMI] <25, decrease saturated fats, increase fruits,
vegetables, and soluble fiber).
Diabetes/glycemic control (normal fasting blood sugar is <110 mg/dL, normal HbA1C is
<7%).
E: Exercise (brisk activity 30 min/d most d of the wk, consider exercise stress test).
Education of patients and family members, provide emotional and psychosocial support.
Ejection Fraction (if low, consider ACE inhibitors/angiotensin receptors blocers [ARB],
β-blocker, digoxin, spironolactone).

---

implements them appropriately, and then does their best to ensure continued compliance *(50)*. Most studies to date suggest a poor performance on the part of physicians in using proven therapies in secondary prevention *(51)*. For example, best estimates suggest that only about a third of patients who have MIs will undergo appropriate screening and treatment for dyslipidemia *(52)*.

It remains part of our challenge to ensure that the proven ABCs of secondary prevention are put into practice (Table 2) *(53,54)*. In addition, we must remember that aggressive medical therapy and revascularization should be viewed as complementary strategies. All patients with vascular disease and diabetes should receive proven medical and lifestyle prescriptions to favorably alter the atherosclerotic process throughout the body. Revascularization without comprehensive risk factor modification is a suboptimal therapeutic strategy *(55,56)*.

REFERENCES

1. Schlant RC, Forman S, Stamler J, Canner PL. The natural history of coronary heart disease: prognostic factors after recovery from myocardial infarction in 2789 men. The 5-year findings of the coronary drug project. Circulation 1982;66:401–414.
2. American Heart Association. 2001 Heart and Stroke Statistical Update. American Heart Association, Dallas, 2001.
3. Outcomes in WHI Trial of Estrogen, Progestin. Writing Group for the Women's Health Initiative Investigators. JAMA 2002;288:321–333.
4. Holme I. Relationship between total mortality and cholesterol reduction as found by meta-regression analysis of randomized cholesterol- lowering trials. Control Clin Trials 1996;17:13–22.
5. Kannel WB, Castelli WP, Gordon T, McNamara PM. Serum cholesterol, lipoproteins, and the risk of coronary heart disease. The Framingham study. Ann Intern Med 1971;74:1–12.
6. Hilton TC, Chaitman BR. The prognosis in stable and unstable angina. Cardiol Clin 1991;9:27–38.
7. Rapaport E, Gheorghiade M. Pharmacologic therapies after myocardial infarction. Am J Med 1996; 101:4A61S–4A70S.
8. Grundy SM. Cholesterol management in patients with heart disease. Emphasizing secondary prevention to increase longevity. Postgrad Med 1997;102:81–90.
9. Brown BG, Zhao XQ, Bardsley J, Albers JJ. Secondary prevention of heart disease amongst patients with lipid abnormalities: practice and trends in the United States. J Intern Med 1997;241:283–294.

10. Furberg CD, Hennekens CH, Hulley SB, Manolio T, Psaty BM, Whelton PK. 27th Bethesda Conference: matching the intensity of risk factor management with the hazard for coronary disease events. Task Force 2. Clinical epidemiology: the conceptual basis for interpreting risk factors. J Am Coll Cardiol 1996;27:976–978.

11. Expert Panel on Detection, Evaluation, and Treatment of High Blood Cholesterol in Adults. Executive summary of the third report of the national cholesterol education program (NCEP) expert panel on detection, evaluation, and treatment of high blood cholesterol in adults (Adult Treatment Panel III). JAMA 2001;285:2486–2497.

12. Haffner, S. M. The Scandinavian Simvastatin Survival Study (4S) subgroup analysis of diabetic subjects: implications for the prevention of coronary heart disease [editorial; comment]. Diabetes Care 1997;20:469–471.

13. Scandanavian Simvastatin Survival Group. Randomised trial of cholesterol lowering in 4444 patients with coronary heart disease: the Scandinavian Simvastatin Survival Study (4S) [see comments]. Lancet 1994;344:1383–1389.

14. Kjekshus J, Pedersen TR. Reducing the risk of coronary events: evidence from the Scandinavian Simvastatin Survival Study (4S). Am J Cardiol 1995;76:64C–68C.

15. Pyorl K, Pedersen TR, Kjekshus J, Faergeman O, Olsson AG, Thorgeirsson G. Cholesterol lowering with simvastatin improves prognosis of diabetic patients with coronary heart disease. A subgroup analysis of the Scandinavian Simvastatin Survival Study (4S) [see comments]. Diabetes Care 1997;20: 614–620.

16. Tonkin AM. Management of the Long-Term Intervention with Pravastatin in Ischaemic Disease (LIPID) study after the Scandinavian Simvastatin Survival Study (4S). Am J Cardiol 1995;76: 107C–112C.

17 Sacks FM, Pfeffer MA, Moye LA, et al. The effect of pravastatin on coronary events after myocardial infarction in patients with average cholesterol levels. Cholesterol and Recurrent Events Trial investigators. N Engl J Med 1996;335:1001–1009.

18. Shepard J, Cobbe SM, Ford I, et al. Prevention of coronary heart disease with pravastatin in men with hypercholesterolemia. New Engl J Med 1995;333:1237–1245.

19. Hebert PR, Gaziano JM, Chan KS, Hennekens CH. Cholesterol lowering with statin drugs, risk of stroke, and total mortality. An overview of randomized trials. JAMA 1997;278:313 321.

20. Sacks FM, Moye LA, Davis BR, et al. Relationship between Plasma LDL Concentrations During Treatment With Pravastatin and Recurrent Coronary Events In the Cholesterol and Recurrent Events Trial. Circulation 1998;97;1446–1452.

21. MRC/BHF Heart Protection Study of antioxidant vitamin supplementation in 20,536 high-risk individuals: a randomised placebo-controlled trial. Lancet 2002;360(9326):23–33

21a. MRC/BHF Heart Protection Study of cholesterol lowering with simvastatin in 20,536 high-risk individuals: a randomized placebo-controlled trail. Lancet 2002;360(9326):7–22

22. Schwartz GG, Olsson AG, Ezekowitz MD, et al. Effects of atorvastatin on early recurrent ischemic events in acute coronary syndromes. JAMA 2001;285:1711–1718.

23. Blumenthal RS. Statins: effective antiatherosclerotic therapy. Am Heart J 2000;139:577–583.

24. The sixth report of the Joint National Committee on Prevention, Detection, Evaluation and Treatment of High Blood Pressure. Arch Intern Med 1997;157:2413–2446.

25. Kannel WB. Hypertension, hypertrophy, and the occurrence of cardiovascular disease. Am J Med Sci 1991;302:199–204.

26. The Heart Outcomes Prevention Evaluation Study Investigators. Effects of an angiotensin-converting enzyme inhibitor, ramipril, on cardiovascular events in high-risk patients. N Engl J Med 2000;342: 145–153.

27. Anonymous. Randomised trial of intravenous streptokinase, oral aspirin, both, or neither among 17,187 cases of suspected acute myocardial infarction: ISIS-2. ISIS-2 (Second International Study of Infarct Survival) Collaborative Group. Lancet 1988;2:349–360.

28. Yusuf S, Anand S, Avezum A Jr, Flather M, Coutinho M. Treatment for acute myocardial infarction. Overview of randomized clinical trials. Eur Heart J 1996;17(Suppl. F):16–29.

29. Antiplatelet Trialists Collaboration. Collaborative overview of randomised trials of antiplatelet therapy—I: prevention of death, myocardial infarction, and stroke by prolonged antiplatelet therapy in various categories of patients. Antiplatelet Trialists' Collaboration [see comments] [published erratum appears in BMJ 1994 Jun 11;308(6943):1540]. BMJ 1994;308:81–106.

30. The Clopidogrel in Unstable Angina to Prevent Recurrent Events Trial Investigators. Effects of clopidogrel in addition to aspirin in patients with acute coronary syndromes without ST-segment elevation. N Engl J Med 2001;345:494–502.

31. Anonymous. Randomised trial of intravenous atenolol among 16 027 cases of suspected acute myocardial infarction: ISIS-1. First International Study of Infarct Survival Collaborative Group. Lancet 1986;2:57–66.

32. Goldstein S. Beta-blocking drugs and coronary heart disease. Cardiovasc Drugs Ther 1997;11(Suppl. 1):219–225.

33. Suter PM, Vetter W. Metabolic effects of antihypertensive drugs. J Hypertens Suppl 1995;13:S11–S17.

34. Madu EC, Reddy RC, Madu AN, Anyaogu C, Harris T, Fraker TD Jr. Review: the effects of antihypertensive agents on serum lipids. Am J Med Sci 1996;312:76–84.

35. Latini R, Maggioni AP, Flather M, Sleight P, Tognoni G. ACE inhibitor use in patients with myocardial infarction. Summary of evidence from clinical trials. Circulation 1995;92:3132–3137.

36. Pfeffer MA, Greaves SC, Arnold JM, et al. Early versus delayed angiotensin-converting enzyme inhibition therapy in acute myocardial infarction. The healing and early afterload reducing therapy trial. Circulation 1997;95:2643–2651.

37. Stampfer MJ, Colditz GA, Willett WC, et al. Postmenopausal estrogen therapy and cardiovascular disease. Ten-year follow-up from the nurses' health study [see comments]. N Engl J Med 1991;325: 756–762.

38. Barrett-Connor E. The menopause, hormone replacement, and cardiovascular disease: the epidemiologic evidence. Maturitas 1996;23:227–234.

39. Hulley S, Grady D, Bush T, et al. Randomized trial of estrogen plus progestin for secondary prevention of coronary heart disease in postmenopausal women. Heart and Estrogen/Progestin Replacement Study (HERS) Research Group. JAMA 1998;280:605–613.

40. Mosca L, Collins P, Herrington DM, et al. AHA Scientific Statement: hormone replacement therapy and cardiovascular disease. A statement for healthcare professionals from the American Heart Association. Circulation 2001;104:499–503.

41. O'Connor GT, Buring JE, Yusuf S, et al. An overview of randomized trials after rehabilitation with exercise after myocardial infarction. Circulation 1989;80:234–244.

42. Plutzky J. Emerging concepts in metabolic abnormalities associated with coronary artery disease. Curr Opin Cardiol 2000;15:416–421.

43. Haffner SM, Lehto S, Ronnemaa T, Pyorala K, Laakso M. Mortality from coronary heart disease in subjects with type 2 diabetes and in nondiabetic subjects with and without prior myocardial infarction [see comments]. N Engl J Med 1998;339:229–234.

44. Yusuf S. Two decades of progress in preventing vascular disease. Lancet 2002;360(9326): 2–3.

45. Adler AI, Stratton IM, Neil HA, et al. Association of systolic blood pressure with macrovascular and microvascular complications of type 2 diabetes (UKPDS 36): prospective observational study. BMJ 2000;321:412–419.

46. Stratton IM, Adler AI, Neil HA, et al. Association of glycaemia with macrovascular and microvascular complications of type 2 diabetes (UKPDS 35): prospective observational study. BMJ 2000;321: 405–412.

47. Marx N, Libby P, Plutzky J. Peroxisome proliferator-activated receptors (PPARs) and their role in the vessel wall: possible mediators of cardiovascular risk? J Cardiovasc Risk 2001;8:203–210.

48. Lonn E, Yusuf S, Dzavik V, et al. Effects of ramipril and vitamin E on atherosclerosis: the study to evaluate carotid ultrasound changes in patients treated with ramipril and vitamin E (SECURE). Circulation 2001;103:919–925.

49. Schnyder G, Roffi M, Pin R, et al. Decreased rate of coronary restenosis after lowering of plasma homocysteine levels. N Engl J Med 2001;345:1593–1600.

50. Insull W. The problem of compliance to cholesterol altering therapy. J Intern Med 1997;241:317–325.

51. Qureshi A, Suri FK, Guterman LR, Hopkins N. Ineffective Secondary prevention in survivors of cardiovascular events in the US population. Report from the Third National Health and Nutrition Examination Survey. Arch Intern Med 2001;161:1621–1628.

52. Fonnarow GC, French WJ, Parsons LS, et al. Use of lipid lowering medication at discharge in patients with acute myocardial infarction: data from the National Registry of Myocardial Infarction 3. Circulation 2001;103:38–44.

53. Braunstein JB, Cheng A, Fakhry C, et al. ABCs of cardiovascular disease risk management. Cardiol Rev 2001;9:96–105.

54. Gibbons RJ, Chatterjee K, Daley J, et al. ACC/AHA/ACP-ASIM guidelines for the management of patients with chronic stable angina: a report of the American College of Cardiology/American Heart Association Task Force on Practice Guideline. J Am Coll Cardiol 1999;33:2092–2197.

55. Blumenthal RS, Cohn G, Schulman SP. Medical therapy versus coronary angioplasty in stable coronary artery disease: a critical review of the literature. J Am Coll Cardiol 2000;36:668–673.

56. Smith SC, Blair SN, Bonow RO, et al. AHA/ACC Guidelines for preventing heart attack and death in patients with atherosclerotic cardiovascular disease: 2001 update. J Am Coll Cardiol 2001;38: 1581–1583.

25 Cost and Cost-Effectiveness in Acute Coronary Syndromes

William S. Weintraub, MD

CONTENTS

OVERVIEW OF ACUTE CORONARY SYNDROMES

The high frequency and large amount of resources used in treating acute coronary syndromes (ACS) create a considerable economic burden. Coronary heart disease is the single largest cause of death in both men and women in industrialized societies, resulting in 459,841 deaths in the United States alone in 1998, which is one of every five deaths *(1)*. An estimated 1,100,000 Americans a year will have a new or recurrent coronary attack (myocardial infarction or sudden death due to coronary disease). Within 6 yr of a myocardial infarction, 18% of men and 35% of women with have a recurrent heart attack, 7% of men and 6% of women will suffer sudden death, and 22% of men and 46% of women will be disabled with heart failure. While about two-thirds of patients after a myocardial infarction do not make a complete recovery, 88% of those under age 65 return to work. A total of 1,263,000 men and 915,000 women diagnosed with coronary heart disease were discharged from hospitals in 1998. Between 1979 and 1998, these discharges increased 24.6% for men and 26.4% for women. Coronary heart disease is the leading cause of premature permanent disability in the U.S. labor force, accounting for 19% of disability allowances by the Social Security Administration. The total cost of coronary disease is estimated at $298.2 billion for 2001. Based on the a 6-mo cost of approx $20,000 from the Treat Angina with Aggrastat and Determine Cost of Therapy with an Invasive or Conservative Strategy—Thrombolysis in Myocardial Infarction (TACTICS-TIMI) 18 trial, the costs of ACS in the United States is in excess of 20 billion dollars annually. However, this is an underestimate as there can be continuing induced costs, both direct and indirect,

From: *Contemporary Cardiology: Management of Acute Coronary Syndromes, Second Edition*
Edited by: C. P. Cannon © Humana Press Inc., Totowa, NJ

Table 1
What is Different About the Economics of ACS?

Episode in a chronic disease rather than a procedure.
Clear starting point.
No clear stopping point.
Disease course may vary widely.
Management may vary widely.
Boundaries of what to include may be difficult.
Indirect costs may be substantial.
Health status may be affected significantly.

as patients become disabled and require more health care services over the ensuing months and years.

ACS represent an acute event that can have continuing costs, and thus differs from and is more complicated than a single form of therapy or diagnostic test (Table 1). When considering a new therapy for ACS, there is generally a clear starting point but often no clear stopping point (other than death). The natural history of ACS may vary substantially, as may management. The patient may be stable but then decompensate, resulting in a hospitalization and intensified therapy, presumably with a somewhat worse health state and associated costs. The goal of therapy is to return the patients to their baseline health state and maintain them there. Economic considerations should include direct cost as well as indirect costs, which may be substantial due to lost productivity. ACS may also have a considerable impact on how people feel (quality of life) and how they function (health status). A good design for an outcomes study in heart failure should take into account all of these possibilities.

BACKGROUND ON ECONOMIC ANALYSES

In an environment in which society cannot afford all possible medical services, all forms of care compete for resources based on effectiveness and cost. A comparison of cost between contending therapies can involve a simulation in which costs and outcome are estimated from nonrandomized comparisons and randomized controlled trials. Even within randomized trials, an economic analysis can range from a simulation to a very detailed component of the trial with extensive primary data collection. For any of these designs, the simplest type of economic study is a comparison of costs or a cost-minimization study. Such a study is useful when it is reasonable to assume that the two treatments offer similar outcomes.

When effectiveness cannot be assumed to be the same for competing therapies, there are three related forms of economic analyses that can be used to study the relationship of cost to outcome: cost-effectiveness, cost-utility, and cost-benefit. Cost-effectiveness analysis assumes that there is one overall measure of effectiveness, often survival *(2)*. This method breaks down when there are multiple measures of effectiveness. For instance, one form of therapy may increase the risk of death, but offers improved symptomatic status. This may, in principle, be addressed through cost-utility analysis, in which all measures of effectiveness are incorporated into one measure, utility *(2)*. A

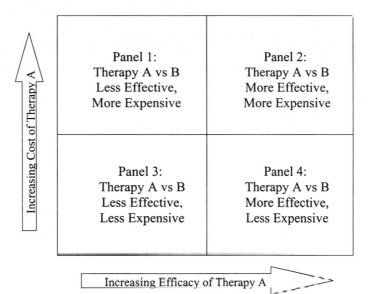

Fig. 1. Decision matrix.

third and somewhat less popular form of analysis is cost-benefit analysis, in which measures of both cost and effectiveness are reduced to dollars or other currency *(2)*.

We can begin to understand the approach of cost-effectiveness analysis by considering competing therapies, A and B, to treat the same condition (Fig. 1). In panel 1, therapy A is less effective but more expensive than therapy B. In this setting, B is said to dominate A. Similarly, in panel 4, A is more effective and less expensive than B. In this setting, A would dominate B. Commonly, however, the more effective therapy or test is also more expensive. Thus, in panel 2, A is more effective but also more expensive. Similarly, in panel 3, B is more effective but also more expensive. When a therapy is both more effective and more expensive than the competing therapy, cost-effectiveness analysis can help decision makers choose whether to allocate resources to the more effective service.

The perspective in these analyses can have an important impact on their structure and outcome. For instance, an analysis from a hospital's perspective might not include the long-term consequences of a particular clinical strategy, whereas this issue may be most important to the patient and the payer. The perspective of all of the various stakeholders may be viewed in aggregate as "society". To be most useful in serving societal goals, cost and cost-effectiveness analyses should be performed from a societal perspective, in which an attempt to measure all of the costs and measures of outcome associated with a particular treatment is made. These costs should include those incurred by the patient, the costs of medical resources that could have been used for other patients, and any loss of income that the patient sustained because of poor health, as well as the loss of income for those who may have provided informal care to the patient. Outcome should include events, quality of life, and survival. By looking at the sum of all of these costs in relation to outcome, a policy maker could decide, for example, whether the public good benefited more by allocating limited health care resources to preventive services or a new therapy for ACS.

Table 2
Nomenclature for Costs

Cost perspective:
    Provider, i.e., hospital or professional.
    Payer, i.e., insurance carrier.
    Patient.
Cost category:
    Direct costs.
    Indirect costs.
Accounting method:
    Top-down.
    Bottom-up.
Costs per service:
    Average cost.
    Marginal (incremental) cost.

DETERMINING COSTS

Nomenclature for Costs

Economists are more concerned with how society chooses to allocate limited resources rather than what something costs *per se (3)*. Cost may be used to sum resource use of several type, permitting an economic comparison of services with a common scale. Accounting methods are used to develop costs from resource use; a summary of accounting names is shown in Table 2.

Costs must be considered from one of several possible perspectives *(4)*. For hospitals, costs are their expenses related to providing a service. For payers, the cost is what the providers charge, plus their administrative expenses. In principle, cost studies often seek to determine societal costs, which can be used in cost-effectiveness analyses to gain the widest perspective. However, societal costs are never directly measurable, and thus combinations of cost proxies from one or several stakeholders, where measurable, are often used as estimates.

Costs are classified as direct or indirect *(5)*. Varying definitions of indirect costs may lead to uncertainty categorizing a particular cost. Theoretically, direct costs are those incurred by a stakeholder for a therapy or test, and indirect related costs are those incurred by other societal groups. More commonly, direct costs relate to the provision of medical care, while indirect costs are other societal costs.

Medical costs can also be divided into three components: in-hospital direct costs, follow-up direct costs, and indirect costs. Inpatient costs are comprised of hospital costs (e.g., room, laboratory testing, pharmacy, etc.) and physician professional billings. Follow-up direct costs include physician office visits, outpatient testing, medications, home health providers, and additional hospitalizations. In this setting, indirect costs reflect lost patient or business opportunity and may be referred to as productivity costs *(6)*.

A final way of thinking about costs is that direct costs are realistically linked to a particular service, while indirect costs are not. This type of indirect cost is also called overhead *(7)*.

The appropriate length of time over which to measure costs is dependent upon the procedures being studied and outcomes being measured. The cost of a hospitalization for ACS could be considered the initial hospitalization alone. Alternatively, the cost for a hospitalization for ACS could be considered to include the "induced" cost related to that hospitalization during a period of follow-up *(8)*.

Often in the United States, hospital provider costs are used as a proxy for societal costs. What a hospital charges for a service is not its cost *(9)*. Measuring hospital cost is difficult and has been approached by using what is called either top-down or bottom-up accounting *(10)*. Top-down costing involves dividing all the money spent on a hospitalization or procedures by the number of episodes of care of the particular type performed. In contrast, a bottom-up approach involves individually costing all resources used for a service, i.e., supplies, equipment depreciation and facilities, salaries, etc. All methods involve a set of assumptions and limitations. When considering the cost of a specific procedure using top-down costing, it must be assumed that costs in the department in which the procedure is provided can be separated from costs in other departments. There may also be variability within a department. Bottom-up methods also are limited by the ability to account for all resources consumed and to appropriately apply costs.

Another issue involved in measuring hospital costs is average vs marginal or incremental cost *(11)*. Average cost is calculated by dividing all costs for a therapy or test by the number of that particular type. In contrast, the marginal cost is the cost of the next similar procedure. Average costs include all resources used, including overhead, whose costs would not be decreased if not utilized. Marginal costing accepts fixed costs as a given and focuses only on variable costs or those additional resources consumed by each additional patient. Variable costs are analytically separated from fixed costs by establishing the perspective and time-frame as fixed. For instance, facilities' costs are commonly considered fixed, but how should marginal personnel costs be assigned? If an older test such as Swan Ganz catheters decreases as echocardiography becomes more common, how is the decrease in intensive care unit (ICU) nurse activity and increase in echocardiography technician activity reflected? Because of these difficulties, most cost and cost-effectiveness studies use average costs.

Cost Measurement

There is a detailed approach to top-down costing based on the UB92 summary of hospital charges, which is commonly used in the United States *(12)*. The UB92 is a uniform billing statement used by all third party carriers. The relationship between costs and charges, in the form of global specific cost to charge ratios, must be developed using American Hospital Association guidelines and then filed annually with Health Care Financing Administration (HCFA) in a Hospital Cost Report, which is in the public domain.

An alternative approach is to use bottom-up cost accounting and assign cost weights to each type of resource used *(13)*. The sum of resources times their cost weights yields total cost. However, the methods are sufficiently laborious that they are rarely used.

Another approach is to use a payer perspective *(14)*. In the United States, Medicare diagnosis-related group (DRG) reimbursement rates can be used to define cost. Similar methods are available in other countries. The use of DRGs to assign cost does not account for variation in cost within that DRG and may not even reflect average resource use.

To assess professional costs, it is not sufficient to consider only the primary physicians' fees alone, as other professionals provide services *(15,16)*. The goal must be to capture all of the professional services for an episode of care. In the United States, there has been an effort to rationalize physician payments by developing a set of scales for services *(17)*. This system, the resource-based relative value scale (RBRVS), was developed over time to try to assess the relative time, physical, and cognitive efforts associated with physician services *(17)*. Each service is assigned a number called the relative value unit (RVU). If the profile of physician services for a procedure or hospitalization is known, then RVUs for each service may be used to develop a proxy for the physician costs. The total RVUs may be converted to a dollar figure by a conversion factor from Medicare or private insurance carriers. Developing a profile of professional services is quite laborious and rarely undertaken. An alternative approach is to use published data in which professional services by DRG are estimated as a percent share of hospital costs *(18)*.

Determining the costs of outpatient services presents different challenges in assessing resource utilization, including direct and indirect medical costs. Direct costs include physician office visits, medications, procedures and testing, rehabilitation, nursing home stays, and home health services, as well as patient out of pocket expenses, including travel. Services can be assigned a cost using the Medicare Fee schedule as discussed above. Medication costs can be estimated from compiled prices by sampling pharmacies or using published wholesale pharmaceutical prices.

Indirect productivity costs include missed time from work by the patient or family members. In any case, it is not possible to directly measure all of the indirect costs. For instance, if an executive in a company has a myocardial infarction and is out of work for 6 wk, there may or may not be loss of pay, but the effect on the business cannot readily be determined. Indirect costs, if measured at all, are often confined to family loss of income, and the numbers must be examined with both interest and skepticism.

Inflation and Discounting

Costs in the future should be deflated by multiplying by a constant to convert from any one year to another, based on the medical inflation rate or the general inflation rate of the consumer price index (CPI) *(19)*. The medical inflation rate is generally larger than of the overall CPI and will give somewhat different figures. Future costs should also be discounted to reflect the opportunity costs of current dollars, i.e., future costs should be expressed at their present value *(20)*. For instance, if a policy maker were given the alternative of spending $1000 now or $1000 in 5 yr to treat a given condition and obtain the same outcome, the decision would always be the latter. Costs are generally discounted at a rate of 3–5%/yr *(20)*.

COMPARING COSTS TO OUTCOME

Determination of Patient Utility and Quality Adjusted Life Years

In the treatment of ACS, it is unusual for one measurement of outcome to be of sufficient clinical importance that all other outcome measures may be ignored in clinical decision making. While death generally overwhelms all other outcome measures in importance, these patients may also suffer from considerable disability. Thus, a therapy may be justified based on improved health status alone, even if not life saving. Improved health status should not be thought of as independent of a disease process.

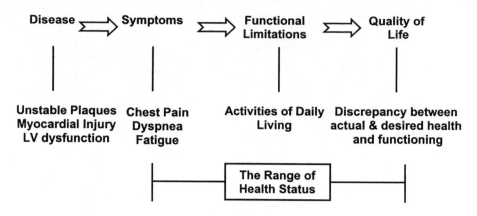

Fig. 2. Measures of health status and their relationship to disease status or severity.

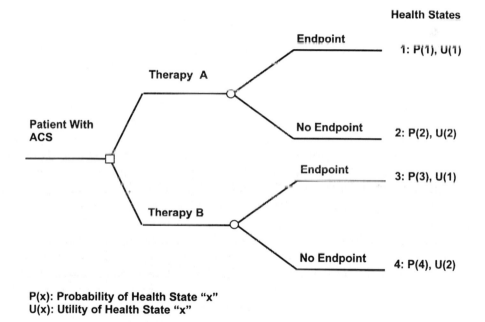

P(x): Probability of Health State "x"
U(x): Utility of Health State "x"

Fig. 3. Idealized decision tree for a decision on diagnostic strategy or therapeutic choice.

The relationship of health status to disease process, with a focus on ACS is shown in Fig. 2 *(21)*. Health status includes, symptoms, functional limitations, and the reaction to these limitations, which we may call quality of life. Decreased health status is dependent on the severity of the disease process. To incorporate health status measures into a cost-effectiveness analysis, an overall measure of health status is needed. In principle, this task may be accomplished through the determination of patient utility.

The utility of a therapy or test is the sum of benefits, both positive and negative, that accrues to a patient over time as the result of the procedure *(22)*. More technically, utility is a measure of patients' preferences for one health state over another. We may consider the assessment of utility beginning with a decision tree (Fig. 3), which takes a patient at a specific point and then considers, in principal, all possible events up to some

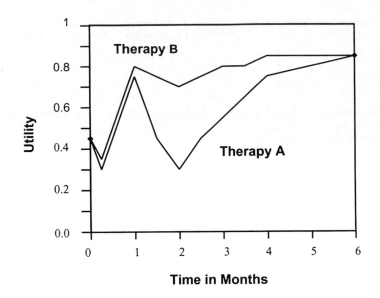

Fig. 4. Theoretical time course of utility for two different therapies for heart failure. With therapy A, there is a dip in utility followed by recovery, while for therapy B, utility gradually rises.

point in the future. In this model, nodes with squares represent choices, and nodes with circles represent chance events. In the simplified model shown, a single choice is made, and for each choice, there are two possible outcomes. Each outcome is called a health state. Each health state has a utility and a probability of occurrence. The utility of choice A in Fig. 3 is the sum of the utility of health state 1, times its probability plus the utility of health state 2, times its probability. Unlike this simplified model, for any one treatment, there may be multiple possible health states; it is generally difficult to determine the probability and utility health states.

Utility changes over time, corresponding to changes in health state. The utility of two alternative treatments after suffering an ACS are compared in Fig. 4. After initiating therapy A, the patient may feel well and utility rises. A recurrent symptomatic period between yr 1 and 2 causes utility to fall. With successful treatment, utility rises again. For therapy B, there is no episode of recurrent symptoms, and utility gradually rises. Ultimately, the patients get to the same point, but the patient who has the episode of recurrent heart failure suffers a period of decreased utility. Utility measurement reflects patient preference. One patient may dislike the disability of chest pain enough to be willing to undergo more aggressive therapy with revascularization. Another patient may dislike the difficulties involved with more aggressive care enough to be willing to put up with more functional limitation.

Utility may be measured indirectly using either a validated survey, such as the Health Utilities Index *(23)* or the EuroQol *(24)* or by directly assessing patient preference. The patient preference methods, Standard Gamble and Time Trade-off *(2)*, ask patients to directly evaluate their current state of health and then evaluate what they would give up or risk to achieve perfect health. The patient preference methods are probably superior to surveys because the evaluation of a patient's view of his/her own state of health is measured directly, but they are more difficult to administer. In the Time Trade-Off

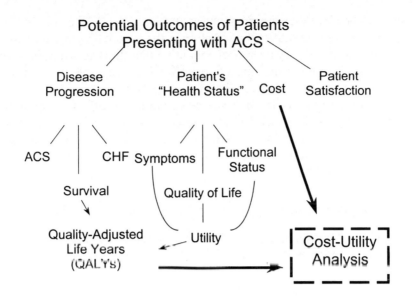

Fig. 5. Interrelationship between survival, utility, and cost to create a cost-utility analysis.

approach, patients weigh the fraction of expected survival they are willing to give up to live in perfect health. With the Standard Gamble, patients weigh what risk of death they are willing to take to live in perfect health. The Standard Gamble is probably superior because it includes the element of risk *(2)*.

Utility alone does not provide a final summary measure of outcome, because it does not include life expectancy. A summary measure can be created by combining utility and survival to obtain quality-adjusted life years (QALYs) (Fig. 5) *(21,25)*. Survival, as with cost presented above, is generally discounted, which means that patients value a year of survival at the present time more than a year of survival in the future. The "true" discount rate for survival is unknown. Values in the literature for the discount rate have varied from 2% to 10%, with 3% being the most popular, and it should be discounted at the same rate as cost *(20)*. Thus, with a discount rate of 3%, next year's survival is 3% less important than this year's survival. QALYs is the best summary measure of outcome in a cost-utility analysis because, it incorporates patient value, risk aversion, expected survival, and a discount rate.

Cost-Effectiveness and Cost-Utility Analysis

Cost-effectiveness is defined as the change in cost per unit increase in effectiveness. If the summary effectiveness measure is in QALYs, then the marginal or incremental cost-effectiveness of therapy or test A compared to therapy or test B is defined as: $COST_A - COST_B/QALYs_A - QALYs_B$. The cost-effectiveness ratio combines the three important outcome measures of utility, survival, and cost (Fig. 5).

Cost-effectiveness analysis involves multiple assumptions in measuring both cost and outcome, which introduces uncertainty or error. Uncertainty in clinical microeconomics is generally approached through sensitivity analysis. With sensitivity analysis, measurements in which there is uncertainty are varied between appropriate ranges, and the analysis is repeated. However, the appropriate ranges for the variables for sensitivity analysis may not be clear. Sensitivity analysis offers a sense of the stability of the cost-effectiveness ratio; in some studies the variation in the ratio with sensitivity analysis may be small, while in others it may be sufficiently large that the original point estimate may have little meaning. Therapies that appear cost-effective using only the central point estimate may not seem as cost-effective when the underlying assumptions are varied, or a ratio that was marginally cost-effective may seem quite cost-effective when the assumptions are varied; this may be especially true concerning the cost of a new therapy which may decline over time. In studies in which cost and effectiveness are directly measured, the variability of the cost-effectiveness ratio can be expressed with a 95% confidence interval (CI) determined by boot-strap analysis.

COST-EFFECTIVENESS OF THERAPY IN ACS

Clinical trials and subsequent economic evaluations have been carried out in most areas of medical decision making concerning ACS. These studies are discussed below and summarized in Table 3.

Coronary Care

Patients with an acute myocardial infarction, whether ST-segment elevation or not, often suffer life-threatening complications that require rapid high-level intervention. Consequently, the standard of care is generally to admit patients with an acute myocardial infarction to a coronary care unit. Admission to these units is costly and relatively few patients benefit from the units' advanced capabilities. The value of this triage for specific groups of patients can be illuminated through an economic analysis.

To address this issue, Tosteson and colleagues made use of clinical and resource utilization data from 12,139 emergency department patients who presented with acute chest pain *(26)*. They compared a coronary care unit with admission to an intermediate care facility with central electrocardiographic monitoring and personnel to detect and treat in-hospital complications. Information on the effectiveness of coronary care units is sparse, particularly in this setting of alternatives with some of the same capabilities. Based on data from the Multicenter Chest Pain Study, the authors estimated that mortality for patients with an acute myocardial infarction would be 15% higher for admission to an intermediate care unit compared with a coronary care unit *(27)*. Using this assumption, the value of admission to a coronary care unit varied depending on the age of the patient and the initial probability of an acute myocardial infarction. In 1992 dollars, for patients who were 55–64 yr old and had a 1% probability of infarction, admission to a coronary care unit had a cost-effectiveness ratio of $1.4 million/yr of life saved, while the same age patients with a 99% probability of an infarction had a cost-effectiveness ratio of $15,000/yr of life saved. The cost-effectiveness ratio was less than $75,000/yr of life saved if the probability of infarction exceeded 20%. The cost-effectiveness of coronary care units was less favorable for younger patients because of their lower underlying risk of a life-threatening complication.

Pharmacologic Reperfusion

With the advent of information about the efficacy of thrombolytic therapy for the treatment of patients with suspected acute myocardial infarction, interest turned to the economic value of this intervention. Since the two largest and earliest trials of

Table 3
Summary of Economic Studies in Acute Coronary Syndromes

Study (reference)	Intervention	Study basis (reference)	Study size	Study type	Cost and cost-effectiveness
Tosteson et al. (26)	Coronary care	Multicenter Chest Pain Study	12,139	Non-randomized	$15,000–1.4 million/yr of life saved, depending on patient characteristics.
Krumholz et al. (28)	Reperfusion	Literature	NA	Simulation	$21,200–$50,000/yr of life saved in elderly.
Mark et al. (33)	tPA vs streptokinase	GUSTO	41,021 survival 23,105 resource use	Partial simulation based on randomized trial	$13,410–$203,071/yr of life saved, depending on patient characteristics.
Kalish et al. (34)	tPA vs streptokinase	GUSTO	NA	Simulation based on randomized trial	Under $27,400 to over $1000/QALY depending on patient characteristics.
Reeder et al. (41)	PTCA vs tPA in ST-elevation MI	Clinical Trial	99	Based on randomized trial.	Inconclusive.
Stone et al. (42)	PTCA vs tPA in ST elevation MI	PAMI	358	Based on randomized trial	PTCA dominates.
Mark et al. (50)	Low-molecular-weight heparin	ESSENCE (49)	655	Based on randomized trial	LMWH dominates unfractionated heparin in non-Q MI.
Mark et al. (52)	GP IIb/IIIa in high risk PTCA	EPIC (51)	2038	Based on randomized trial	Cost saving for drug cost less than $1270.
Weintraub et al. (54)	GP IIb/IIIa in high risk PTCA	RESTORE (53)	1920	Based on randomized trial	Effective at no increased cost.
Weintraub (61)	Invasive strategy in UA/NSTEMI	TACTICS-TIMI 18	1722	Based on randomized trial	Effective at no increased cost.
Goldman et al. (63)	β-Blockade	Literature	NA	Simulation	$3,623–$23,457/yr of life saved, depending on level of risk.
Tsevat et al. (65)	ACE Inhibition	SAVE	2231	Simulation based on randomized trial	$3600–$60,800/QALY depending on level of risk.
McMurray et al. (66)	ACE inhibition	Literature	NA	Simulation based on randomized trial	1752–3110 British pounds/yr of life saved, depending on model characteristics.
Ades et al. (67)	Rehabilitation	Literature	NA	Simulation.	$4950/yr of life saved.

MI, myocardial infarction; LMWH, low-molecular-weight heparin; UA/NSTEMI, unstable angina non-ST-segment elevation myocardial infarction..

thrombolytic therapy used streptokinase, the early economic evaluations focused on this agent *(28–32)*.

A cost-effectiveness analysis published in 1992 examined the use of streptokinase compared with no treatment, since the two largest and earliest trials of thrombolytic therapy used streptokinase *(28)*. The investigators focused on the treatment of elderly patients with suspected acute myocardial infarction, a group for which there is less enthusiasm about using thrombolytic therapy. Based on data available from Gruppo Italiano per lo Studio della Streptochinasi nell' Infarto Myocardio (GISSI)-1 and Second International Study of Infarct Survival (ISIS-2), the relative benefit of thrombolytic therapy was assumed to be lower in elderly patients and the risk of thrombolytic therapy was higher, but the absolute risk after an acute myocardial infarction was much higher compared with younger patients. The smaller relative reduction in the higher risk associated with infarction offset the higher risk of complications. Thus, the decision analysis suggested that thrombolytic therapy was economically attractive over a broad range of assumptions about the risks and benefits. After considering the costs of the treatment, complications, and long-term health care of survivors, the authors estimated that the cost-effectiveness ratio of streptokinase compared with conventional medical therapy was $21,200/yr of life saved for an 80-yr-old patient. The authors calculated similar estimates for younger patients. Several studies have found similar results. One analysis has even suggested that thrombolytic therapy could be cost saving because of its impact on reducing rehospitalization *(32)*.

With the emergence of tissue-type plasminogen activator (tPA) as a more expensive and more effective alternative to streptokinase, studies addressed whether the incremental benefit was large enough to justify the incremental cost. The Global Utilization of Streptokinase and tPA for Occluded Coronary Arteries (GUSTO) trial investigators performed a substudy to address this issue specifically *(33)*. The investigators collected detailed information about resource consumption in a subgroup of the GUSTO subjects. They found that both treatment groups were similar in their use of resources in the year after enrollment. The treatment groups had a mean length of stay of 8 d, including an average of 3.5 d in the intensive care unit. During the initial hospitalization, the treatment groups had a similar rate of bypass surgery (13%) and angioplasty (31%). Overall, the 1-yr health costs, excluding the difference in the cost of the thrombolytic agent, were $24,990/patient treated with tPA and $24,575/patient treated with streptokinase. The major difference in the cost of the therapies was the cost of the drugs: $2750 for tPA and $320 for streptokinase. The primary analysis assumed no increase in costs for the tPA group after the first yr. Based on the GUSTO results and an estimate of the patients' life expectancy, the additional life expectancy per patient treated with tPA was estimated to be 0.14 yr. Based on these estimates, the authors concluded that the cost-effectiveness ratio of using tPA instead of streptokinase was $32,678/yr of life saved. This ratio varied considerably based on the infarction site and the age of the patient. In general, the younger and lower risk patients had higher cost-effectiveness ratios. For example, the cost-effectiveness ratio for tPA in a patient aged 40 yr or younger with an inferior infarction was $203,071/yr of life saved compared with $13,410/yr of life saved for a person aged 75 yr or older with an anterior infarction. An analysis conducted independent of the GUSTO trial reached similar conclusions *(34)*. Comparisons with other new agents await strong evidence of their superiority to tPA.

Pharmacologic Reperfusion Vs Primary Percutaneous Coronary Intervention

Mechanical approaches to reperfusion have been employed with increasing frequency. The clinical or economic advantage of primary angioplasty have been somewhat controversial (35–37). Several studies have suggested a substantial advantage of primary angioplasty (38–40). Economic analyses based on early studies suggested that primary angioplasty is associated with a reduction in mortality without increasing cost (41,42). In an early study by Reeder et al. (41) 99 patients with acute myocardial infarction presenting within 12 h after onset of symptoms were randomized to tPA or immediate angioplasty as the initial revascularization strategy. The primary outcome determinants were direct and indirect costs, including duration of hospital stay and return to work. No significant difference in cost between the two initial treatment strategies was noted. A trend was noted toward a briefer hospital stay and fewer late in-hospital procedures in patients treated initially with angioplasty. Other measures of indirect costs were not statistically different. The two strategies were considered to have similar cost-effectiveness.

In a larger and somewhat more recent study Stone et al. (42) evaluated the cost effectiveness of acute percutaneous coronary intervention (PCI) in the Primary Angioplasty in Myocardial Infarction (PAMI) trial. A total of 358 patients in the U.S. with acute myocardial infarction were randomized to tPA or primary percutaneous transluminal coronary angioplasty (PTCA). Compared with tPA, primary PTCA resulted in lower in-hospital mortality (2.3 vs 7.2%, $p = 0.03$), reinfarction (2.8 vs 7.2%, $p = 0.06$), recurrent ischemia (11.3 vs 28.7%, $p < 0.0001$), and stroke (0 vs 3.0%, $p = 0.02$), as well as shorter hospital stay (7.6 ± 3.3 d vs 8.4 ± 4.7 d, $p = 0.04$). Despite the initial costs of cardiac catheterization in all patients randomized to PTCA, total charges tended to be lower with PTCA ($27,653 ± $13,709 vs $30,227 ± $18,903, $p = 0.21$). At a mean follow-up time of 2.1 ± 0.7 yr, no major differences in postdischarge events or New York Heart Association functional class were present between PTCA and tPA-treated patients, suggesting, but not proving, similar late resource consumption. Compared with tPA, reperfusion by primary PTCA was felt to improve clinical outcomes with similar or reduced costs, suggesting a dominant strategy. However, the ability to generalize these results to the community setting where access to the catheterization laboratory may be limited has been less certain. Thus, additional studies of actual practice, however, have provided less impressive results associated with the use of primary angioplasty (37,43), making estimates of the effectiveness more difficult.

A fundamental problem in the area of reperfusion, both pharmacologic and mechanical is that the field is moving rapidly. Changes in costs and techniques require rapid access to recent data in order to develop relevant economic models. For example, stents, initially considered to be contraindicated in acute myocardial infarction because of concerns that they would incite thrombus formation, have become the standard for primary mechanical reperfusion therapy (44). As evidence of the efficacy of stents accumulates, there will be a need to examine their economic impact compared with balloon angioplasty and thrombolytic therapy. Also, as more rapid discharge protocols evolve for patients who receive reperfusion therapy, the balance of costs and effectiveness may shift (45).

Antithrombotic Agents

Aspirin reduces mortality and morbidity for patients with ACS. As a result of the marked benefit and the minimal cost of the therapy, no formal economic analysis of aspirin for the treatment of ACS has been published in the mainstream journals. The

ISIS-2 trial found that aspirin avoided 25 deaths for every 1000 patients with suspected acute myocardial infarction *(46)*. In addition, the 1 mo of aspirin therapy in ISIS-2 was associated with halving the risk of stroke or reinfarction. Aspirin avoided about 10 reinfarctions and 3 strokes for every 1000 patients treated. The avoidance of complications would likely translate into cost savings, leading aspirin to be considered a "strongly dominant" therapy.

Heparin for the treatment of acute myocardial infarction has also not been formally evaluated in an economic analysis, since it has not been shown to provide a strong benefit for acute myocardial infarction in the aspirin era *(47)*. In addition, while aspirin plus heparin is the standard of care for patients hospitalized with unstable angina, a meta-analysis of the unstable angina studies found only borderline significant results in favor of heparin *(48)*. Given the uncertainty about its effectiveness, heparin would only be a favored therapy if there were evidence that heparin reduces cost. No studies have revealed an economic advantage to heparin therapy in this setting.

New agents are emerging with increasing frequency. For example, low-molecular-weight heparin is emerging as an effective therapy for unstable angina *(49)*. The greater cost and benefit of this new treatment makes it ideal for economic analyses. Mark and colleagues performed an economic analysis for a subset of patients enrolled in the Efficacy and Safety of Subcutaneous Enoxaparin in Non-Q-Wave Coronary Events Study Group (ESSENCE) *(50)*. Patients treated with enoxaparin had lower resource use during the initial hospitalization, and this benefit persisted at 30 d, with a cumulative cost savings associated with enoxaparin of $1172 ($p = 0.04$). The investigators concluded that enoxaparin both improves important clinical outcomes and saves money relative to therapy with standard unfractionated heparin, making it a strongly dominant therapy.

Use of Glycoprotein IIb/IIIa Inhibitors in the Setting of High-Risk PCI

The use of the monoclonal antibody fragment abciximab inhibitor of the platelet receptor glycoprotein (GP) IIb/IIIa has become common in the setting of PCI, but especially so in patients undergoing PCI in the setting of ACS. Treatment of high risk patients undergoing coronary revascularization reduces the short-term risk of the composite of death, myocardial infarction or coronary revascularization *(51)*. An economic analysis of the Early Postmenopausal Intervention Cohort (EPIC) trial found that the use of this therapy for high-risk patients was associated with a cost savings of $622/patient during the initial hospitalization from reduced acute ischemic events *(52)*. During the 6-mo follow-up, the therapy decreased repeat hospitalization rates by 23% ($p = 0.004$) and repeat revascularization by 22% ($p = 0.04$), producing a mean $1270 savings/patient (exclusive of drug cost) ($p = 0.018$). If the cost of the drug were less than $1270, then the strategy would be effective and cost saving.

The Randomized Efficacy Study of Tirofiban for Outcomes and Restenosis (RESTORE) trial found that in patients undergoing coronary angioplasty for ACS, tirofiban protects against early adverse cardiac events related to abrupt closure *(53)*. A subsequent economic analysis reported that the use of tirofiban (including drug costs) was not associated with an increase in health care costs *(54)*.

Neither of these studies directly examined the use of these agents in patients with acute ischemic syndromes. TACTICS-TIMI 18 trial has specifically addressed this issue *(55)*.

Invasive vs Conservative Strategies in Non-ST-Segment Elevation ACS

The relative value of an invasive strategy with early catheterization and possible revascularization compared with a conservative strategy with exercise testing in patients with unstable angina or non-ST-segment elevation acute myocardial infarction has been studied in several clinical trials in the pre-stent, pre-GP IIb/IIIa blocker era, with equivocal results *(56–58)*. More recently the Fast Revascularization during Instability in Coronary Artery Disease (FRISC) trial, which included the use of coronary stents, showed a reduction in events at 6 mo with an invasive strategy. None of these trials included a prospective economic component.

An invasive vs a conservative strategy for non-ST-segment elevation ACS was studied in the TACTICS-TIMI 18 trial. TACTICS-TIMI 18 included the use of both intracoronary stents and the GP IIb/IIIa blocker aggrastat. It is also the first trial in this area with a formal cost and cost-effectiveness analysis built into the structure of the trial *(55,59)*. In TACTICS-TIMI 18, 2220 patients with unstable angina were randomized to an early invasive strategy with routine catheterization within 4–48 h and revascularization as appropriate, or to a more conservative ("selective invasive") strategy, with catheterization performed in the event of recurrent ischemia or a positive stress test *(60)*. The primary end point was a composite of death, myocardial infarction or rehospitalization for an ACS at 6 mo. The primary end point was reduced with the early invasive strategy compared to the conservative strategy, 15.9 vs 19.4%, odds ratio 0.78, 95% CI: 0.62–0.97, $p = 0.025$. The incidence of death or myocardial infarction at 6 mo was similarly reduced (7.3 vs 9.5%, respectively, OR 0.74, 95% CI: 0.54–1.00, $p = 0.0498$). Direct costs examined included those associated with: hospitalizations, emergency room visits, inpatient rehabilitation, nursing home stays, office visits and procedures, and cardiac-related medications *(61)*. Indirect costs resulting from lost productivity were estimated from work days missed and patient-reported work effectiveness levels according to employment classification. Total 6-mo costs did not differ significantly between the two treatment arms. Average total cost for the invasive arm was $20,616 vs $19,987 for the conservative arm. The 95% CI for the $629 difference (invasive minus conservative) was (–$1237, $2455). Mean cost of the initial hospitalization was significantly higher for the invasive arm ($14,660) than the conservative arm ($12,666); the 95% CI for the $1994 cost difference was ($610, $3288). However, mean 6-mo follow-up costs incurred postdischarge were significantly higher for the conservative arm: $7203 vs $6063, largely due to rehospitalizations. The –$1140 cost difference had an associated 95% CI of (–$2238–$36). In patients with unstable angina/non-ST-segment elevation myocardial infarction treated with the GPIIb IIIa inhibitor tirofiban, the clinical benefit of an early invasive strategy is achieved without an economically relevant increase in cost.

β-BLOCKER THERAPY

β-blocker therapy has been shown to reduce mortality following an acute myocardial infarction *(62)*. Goldman and colleagues conducted the most widely cited economic analysis of the costs and effectiveness of β-blocker therapy *(63)*. Using data from the literature, they estimated that β-blocker therapy produced a relative reduction in mortality of 25% in yr 1–3 after an infarction and a 7% reduction for yr 4–6. They evaluated the cost-effectiveness of the therapy under the assumption that the benefit did not persist after yr 6. Costs were calculated using 1987 dollars. The investigators stratified potential patients by their estimated mortality into low risk (1.5% in the first yr), medium risk (7.5% in the first yr), and high risk (13% in the first yr). The cost-effectiveness ratio was strongly associated with the underlying risk of the patient. For a 45-yr-old man with low risk, the cost-effectiveness ratio was $23,457, with medium risk was $5890, and with high risk was $3623.

Angiotensin-Converting Enzyme Inhibition

Several large randomized trials have demonstrated a reduction in acute myocardial infarction for patients with left ventricular dysfunction after an acute myocardial infarction who are treated with an angiotensin-converting enzyme (ACE) inhibitor *(64)*. Tsevat and colleagues *(65)* examined the cost-effectiveness of this intervention using resource utilization, survival, and health-related quality of life information from the Survival and Ventricular Enlargement (SAVE) trial, a randomized trial of captopril for survivors of a myocardial infarction with an ejection fraction of 40% or less. The investigators conservatively estimated that the benefit of captopril did not persist beyond 4 yr. The trial found that captopril improved survival at 3.5 yr by about 20%. Costs were calculated in 1991 dollars. The cost-effectiveness ranged from $60,800/quality-adjusted life year for 50-yr-old patients to $3600 for 80-yr-old patients. McMurray and colleagues also found that ACE inhibitors are an economically attractive intervention after myocardial infarction *(66)*.

Rehabilitation

In a decision analytic model, Ades et al. *(67)* studied the cost-effectiveness of cardiac rehabilitation to coordinate exercise training and secondary prevention after acute myocardial infarction. The cost-effectiveness of cardiac rehabilitation, in dollars/yr of life saved, was calculated by combining published results of randomized trials of cardiac rehabilitation on mortality rates, epidemiologic studies of long-term survival in the overall postinfarction population, and studies of patient charges for rehabilitation services and averted medical expenses for hospitalizations after rehabilitation. Cardiac rehabilitation participants had an incremental life expectancy of 0.202 yr. In 1988, the average cost of rehabilitation and exercise testing was $1485, partially offset by averted cardiac rehospitalizations of $850/patient. A cost-effectiveness value of $2130/yr of life saved was determined for the late 1980s, projected to a value of $4950/yr of life saved in 1995. A sensitivity analysis was conducted to support these findings.

SUMMARY

ACS remain a serious medical problem, which can be associated with death and disability on one hand, and considerable resource utilization on the other. The primary driver for choice of therapy must remain clinical efficacy. Once efficacy is established, cost-effectiveness analysis has an important role. Resources are limited, and responsible choices must be made. The methods involved in cost-effectiveness analysis are complicated, and data for the analysis are generally not fully optimal. Nonetheless, cost-effectiveness analysis offers the best method for helping society make rational medical decisions. Good therapy at a reasonable price for the treatment of ACS have generally proven to be cost-effective. Thus, most of the major therapies for ACS, including reperfusion, acute PCI, use of GP IIb/IIIa blockers, use of an invasive strategy in high risk patients, use of aspirin, β-blockers, and ACE inhibition are quite reasonably cost-effective.

REFERENCES

1. American Heart Association. 2001 Heart and Stroke Statistical Update. American Heart Association, Dallas, 2000.
2. Drummond MF, Stoddart GL, Torrance GW. Methods for the Economic Evaluation of Health Care Programmes. Oxford University Press, Oxford, 1990.
3. Schlander M. Rational resource allocation in the health care system, part 1—Why rationing may become inevitable. Medizinische Welt 1999;50:36–41.
4. Weintraub WS, Warner CD, Mauldin PD, et al. Economic winners and losers after introduction of an effective new therapy depend on the type of payment system. Am J Managed Care 1997;3:743–749.
5. Weintraub WS. Microeconomic methods in cardiovascular care. In: Talley JD, Mauldin PD, Becker ER eds. Cost-Effective Diagnosis and Treatment of Coronary Artery Disease. Williams & Wilkins, Baltimore, 1999, pp. 17–29.
6. Rothermich EA, Pathak DS. Productivity-cost controversies in cost-effectiveness analysis: review and research agenda. Clin Ther 1999;21:255–267.
7. Evans DB. Principles involved in costing. Med J Aust 1990;153:S10–S12.
8. Hlatky MA. Analysis of costs associated with CABG and PTCA. Ann Thorac Surg 1996;61:S30–S32.
9. Finkler SA. The distinction between costs and charges. Ann Intern Med 1982;96:102–109.
10. Finkler SA, Ward DM. Essentials of cost accounting for Health Care Organizations. 2nd edition. Aspen Publication, 1999, pp. 11–43.
11. Hlatky MA, Lipscomb J, Nelson C, et al. Resource use and cost of initial coronary revascularization: coronary angioplasty versus coronary bypass surgery. Circulation 1990;82(Suppl. IV):IV-208–IV-213.
12. Weintraub WS, Mauldin PD, Talley JD, et al. Determinants of hospital costs in acute myocardial infarction. Am J Managed Care 1996;2:977–986.
13. Lefebvre C, Van Der Perre T. Activity based costing. Acta Hospitalia 1994;34:5–16.
14. Coulam RF, Gaumer GL. Medicare's prospective payment system: a critical appraisal. Health Care Financ Rev 1991;13:45–77.
15. Becker ER, Mauldin PD, Culler SD, Kosinski AS, Weintraub WS, King SB III. Applying the Resource-Based Relative-Value Scale to the Emory Angioplasty vs Surgery Trial. Am J Cardiol 2000;85:685–691.
16. Becker ER, Mauldin PD, Bernadino ME. Using physician work RVUs to profile surgical packages: methods and results for kidney transplant surgery. Best Practi Benchmarking Healthc 1996;1:140–146.
17. Hsiao WC, Braun P, Yntema D, Becker ER. Estimating physicians' work for a resource-based relative value scale. N Engl J Med 1998;319:835–841.
18. Mitchell JB, Burge RT, Lee AJ, McCall NT. Per case prospective payment for episodes of hospital care. Final Report to HCFA for Master Contract No. 500-92-0020. Health Economics Research, Inc. Oct. 6, 1995.
19. Weintraub WS, Craver JM, Jones EL, et al. Improving cost and outcome of coronary surgery. Circulation 1998;98:23–28.
20. Gold MR, Siegel JE, Russell LB, et al. Cost-Effectiveness in Health and Medicine. Oxford University Press, New York, 1996.
21. Spertus JA, Tooley J, Poston C, et al. Expanding the outcomes in clinical trials of heart failure: the quality of life and economic components of EPHESUS (Eplerenone's neuroHormonal Efficacy and Survival Study). Am Heart J 2002;143:636–642.
22. Alchian A. The meaning of utility measurement. Am Econ Review 1953;43:26–50.
23. Feeny DH, Torrance GW, Furlong WJ. Health utilities index. In: Spilker B, ed. Quality of Life and Pharmacoeconomics in Clinical Trials. Lippincott-Raven Press, Philadelphia, 1996, pp. 239–252.
24. Cook TA, O'Regan M, Galland RB. Quality of life following percutaneous transluminal angioplasty for claudication. Eur J Vasc Endovasc Surg 1996;11:191–194.
25. Loomes G, McKenzie L. The use of QALYs in health care decision making. Soc Sci Med 1989;28: 299–308.

26. Tosteson AN, Goldman L, Udvarhelyi IS, Lee TH. Cost-effectiveness of a coronary care unit versus an intermediate care unit for emergency department patients with chest pain. Circulation 1996;94: 143–150.

27. Beamer AD, Lee TH, Cook EF, et al. Diagnostic implications for myocardial ischemia of the circadian variation of the onset of chest pain. Am J Cardiol 1987;60:998–1002.

28. Krumholz HM, Pasternak RC, Weinstein MC, et al. Cost effectiveness of thrombolytic therapy with streptokinase in elderly patients with suspected acute myocardial infarction. N Engl J Med 1992;327: 7–13.

29. Laffel GL, Fineberg HV, Braunwald E. A cost-effectiveness model for coronary thrombolysis/reperfusion therapy. J Am Coll Cardiol 1987;5(Suppl. B):79B–90B.

30. Simoons ML, Vos J, Martens LL. Cost-utility analysis of thrombolytic therapy. Eur Heart J 1991;12:694–699.

31. Midgette AS, Wong JB, Beshansky JR, Porath A, Fleming C, Pauker SG. Cost-effectiveness of streptokinase for acute myocardial infarction: a combined meta-analysis and decision analysis of the effects of infarct location and of likelihood of infarction. Med Decis Making 1994;14:108–117.

32. Herve C, Castiel D, Gaillard M, Boisvert R, Leroux V. Cost-benefit analysis of thrombolytic therapy. Eur Heart J 1990;11:1006–1010.

33. Mark DB, Hlatky MA, Califf RM, et al. Cost effectiveness of thrombolytic therapy with tissue plasminogen activator as compared with streptokinase for acute myocardial infarction. N Engl J Med 1995; 332:1418–1424.

34. Kalish SC, Gurwitz JH, Krumholz HM, Avorn J. A cost-effectiveness model of thrombolytic therapy for acute myocardial infarction. J Gen Intern Med 1995;10:321–330.

35. Lange RA, Hillis LD. Should thrombolysis or primary angioplasty be the treatment of choice for acute myocardial infarction? Thrombolysis—the preferred treatment. N Engl J Med 1996;335:1311–1317.

36. Grines CL. Should thrombolysis or primary angioplasty be the treatment of choice for acute myocardial infarction? Primary angioplasty—the strategy of choice. N Engl J Med 1996;335:1313–1317.

37. Berger AK, Schulman KA, Gersh BJ, et al. Primary coronary angioplasty vs thrombolysis for the management of acute myocardial infarction in elderly patients. JAMA 1999;282:341–348.

38. Grines CL, Browne KF, Marco J, et al. A comparison of immediate angioplasty with thrombolytic therapy for acute myocardial infarction. The Primary Angioplasty in Myocardial Infarction Study Group. N Engl J Med 1993;328:673–679.

39. Gibbons RJ, Holmes DR, Reeder GS, Bailey KR, Hopfenspirger MR, Gersh BJ. Immediate angioplasty compared with the administration of a thrombolytic agent followed by conservative treatment for myocardial infarction. The Mayo Coronary Care Unit and Catheterization Laboratory Groups. N Engl J Med 1993;328:685–691.

40. Zijlstra F, de Boer MJ, Hoorntje JC, Reiffers S, Reiber JH, Suryapranata H. A comparison of immediate coronary angioplasty with intravenous streptokinase in acute myocardial infarction. N Engl J Med 1993;328:680–684.

41. Reeder GS, Bailey KR, Gersh BJ, Holmes DR Jr, Christianson J, Gibbons RJ. Cost comparison of immediate angioplasty versus thrombolysis followed by conservative therapy for acute myocardial infarction: a randomized prospective trial. Mayo Coronary Care Unit and Catheterization Laboratory Groups. Mayo Clin Proc 1994;69:5–12.

42. Stone GW, Grines CL, Rothbaum D, et al. Analysis of the relative costs and effectiveness of primary angioplasty versus tissue-type plasminogen activator: the Primary Angioplasty in Myocardial Infarction (PAMI) trial. The PAMI Trial Investigators. J Am Coll Cardiol 1997;29:901–907.

43. Every NR, Parsons LS, Hlatky M, Martin JS, Weaver WD. A comparison of thrombolytic therapy with primary coronary angioplasty for acute myocardial infarction. Myocardial Infarction Triage and Intervention Investigators. N Engl J Med 1996;335:1253–1260.

44. Grines CL, Cox DA, Stone GW, et al. Coronary angioplasty with or without stent implantation for acute myocardial infarction. N Engl J Med 1999;341:1949–1956.

45. Grines CL, Marsalese DL, Brodie B, et al. Safety and cost-effectiveness of early discharge after primary angioplasty in low risk patients with acute myocardial infarction. PAMI-II Investigators. Primary Angioplasty in Myocardial Infarction. J Am Coll Cardiol 1998;31:967–972.

46. Randomised trial of intravenous streptokinase, oral aspirin, both, or neither among 17,187 cases of suspected acute myocardial infarction: ISIS-2. ISIS-2 (Second International Study of Infarct Survival) Collaborative Group. Lancet 1988;2:349–360.

47. Collins R, Peto R, Baigent C, Sleight P. Aspirin, heparin, and fibrinolytic therapy in suspected acute myocardial infarction. N Engl J Med 1997;336:847–860.
48. Oler A, Whooley MA, Oler J, Grady D. Adding heparin to aspirin reduces the incidence of myocardial infarction and death in patients with unstable angina. JAMA 1996;276:811–815.
49. Cohen M, Demers C, Gurfinkel EP, et al. A comparison of low-molecular-weight heparin with unfractionated heparin for unstable coronary artery disease. Efficacy and Safety of Subcutaneous Enoxaparin in Non-Q-Wave Coronary Events Study Group (ESSENCE). N Engl J Med 1997;337:447–452.
50. Mark DB, Cowper PA, Berkowitz SD, et al. Economic assessment of low-molecular-weight heparin (enoxaparin) versus unfractionated heparin in acute coronary syndrome patients: results from the ESSENCE randomized trial. Efficacy and Safety of Subcutaneous Enoxaparin in Non-Q wave Coronary Events [unstable angina or non-Q-wave myocardial infarction]. Circulation 1998;97:1702–1707.
51. Topol EJ, Califf RM, Weisman HF, et al. Randomised trial of coronary intervention with antibody against platelet IIb/IIIa integrin for reduction of clinical restenosis: results at six months. The EPIC Investigators. Lancet 1994;343:881–886.
52. Mark DB, Talley JD, Topol EJ, et al. Economic assessment of platelet glycoprotein IIb/IIIa inhibition for prevention of ischemic complications of high-risk coronary angioplasty. EPIC Investigators. Circulation 1996;94:629–635.
53. Topol EJ, Ferguson JF, Weisman HF, et al. Long-term protection from myocardial ischemic events in a randomized trial of brief integrin beta 3 blockade with percutaneous coronary intervention. JAMA 1997;278:479–484.
54. Weintraub WS, Culler S, Boccuzzi SJ, et al. Economic impact of GPIIB/IIIA blockade after high-risk angioplasty: results from the RESTORE trial. Randomized Efficacy Study of Tirofiban for Outcomes and Restenosis. J Am Coll Cardiol 1999;34:1061–1066.
55. Weintraub WS, Culler SD, Kosinski A, et al. Economics, health-related quality of life, and cost-effectiveness methods for the TACTICS (Treat Angina With Aggrastat [tirofiban]] and Determine Cost of Therapy with Invasive or Conservative Strategy)-TIMI 18 trial. Am J Cardiol 1999;83:317–322.
56. Braunwald E, McCabe CH, Cannon CP, et al. Effects of tissue plasminogen activator and a comparison of early invasive and conservative strategies in unstable angina and non-Q-wave myocardial infarction: Results of the TIMI IIIB trial. Circulation 1994;89:1545–1556.
57. Boden WE, O'Rourke RA, Crawford MH, et al. Outcomes in patients with acute non-Q-wave myocardial infarction randomly assigned to an invasive as compared with a conservative management strategy. N Engl J Med 1998;338:1785–1792.
58. Ragmin F, Wallentin L, Swahn E, et al. Invasive compared with non-invasive treatment in unstable coronary-artery disease: FRISC II prospective randomised multicentre study. Lancet 1999;354:708–715.
59. Cannon CP, Weintraub WS, Demopoulos LA, et al. Invasive versus conservative strategies in unstable angina and non-Q wave myocardial infarction following treatment with tirofiban: rationale and study design of the international TACTICS-TIMI 18 trial. Am J Cardiol 1998;82:731–736.
60. Cannon CP, Weintraub WS, Demopoulos LA, et al. Comparison of early invasive versus conservative strategies in patients with unstable coronary syndromes treated with the glycoprotein IIb/IIIa inhibitor tirofiban. N Engl J Med 2001;344:1879–1887.
61. Weintraub WS. Plenary session. American College of Cardiology 50th Annual Scientific Session. Orlando, Florida. March 2001.
62. Yusuf S, Peto R, Lewis J, Collins R, Sleight P. Beta blockade during and after myocardial infarction: an overview of the randomized trials. Prog Cardiovasc Dis 1985;27:335–371.
63. Goldman L, Sia ST, Cook EF, Rutherford JD, Weinstein MC. Costs and effectiveness of routine therapy with long-term beta-adrenergic antagonists after acute myocardial infarction. N Engl J Med 1988; 319:152–157.
64. Brown NJ, Vaughan DE. Angiotensin-converting enzyme inhibitors. Circulation 1998;97:1411–1420.
65. Tsevat J, Duke D, Goldman L, et al. Cost-effectiveness of captopril therapy after myocardial infarction. J Am Coll Cardiol 1995;26:914–919.
66. McMurray JJ, McGuire A, Davie AP, Hughes D. Cost-effectiveness of different ACE inhibitor treatment scenarios post-myocardial infarction. Eur Heart J 1997;18:1411–1415.
67. Ades PA, Pashkow FJ, Nestor JR. Cost-effectiveness of cardiac rehabilitation after myocardial infarction. J Cardiopulm Rehabil 1997;17:222–231.

26

Smoking Cessation

Beth C. Bock, PhD and
Bruce Becker, MD, MPH

CONTENTS

OVERVIEW
TREATMENT APPROACHES
SPECIFIC TREATMENT PLANS
SUMMARY AND CONCLUSIONS
REFERENCES

OVERVIEW

Effects of Smoking on Health

Cigarette smoking continues to be one of the most prevalent causes of preventable morbidity and mortality in the United States *(1,2)*. In the United States, an estimated 47 million adults smoke, and over 400,000 deaths/yr are attributable to smoking *(3,4)*. Tobacco use is causally linked to diseases such as cancer, heart disease, stroke, and chronic obstructive pulmonary disease *(5)* and is responsible for over $50 billion in annual healthcare expenditures *(6)*. Moreover, Environmental Tobacco Smoke (ETS) or "second hand smoke" has been strongly associated with respiratory illness in children and with both cancer and heart disease in adults living with smokers *(7)*. The prevalence of smoking decreased dramatically in the United States between 1950 and 1980 *(8)*, coinciding with the release of a series of reports from the U.S. Surgeon General regarding the effects of tobacco smoking on health. However, this trend has not continued. Today, one quarter of all adults living in this country smoke *(9)*, and the rate of smoking among high school students increased throughout the 1990s *(10)*.

Smoking Cessation in Cardiac Patients

Each year, over 600,000 people are newly diagnosed with coronary heart disease (CHD), presenting with events such as myocardial infarction (MI) or chronic conditions such as angina pectoris, congestive heart failure, or arrhythmias *(11)*. CHD is the leading cause of mortality in the U.S., accounting for almost half of all deaths in the United States annually *(12,13)*. Cigarette smoking greatly increases the risk of death from heart disease. Specifically, mainstream smoke (MSS), which is smoke that is directly inhaled by the smoker, has pathophysiologic effects on the heart, blood vessels, coagulation

From: *Contemporary Cardiology: Management of Acute Coronary Syndromes, Second Edition*
Edited by: C. P. Cannon © Humana Press Inc., Totowa, NJ

system and lipoprotein metabolism *(14–16)*. MSS exposure leads to an increase in white blood cell count and an increase in blood neutrophils, producing chronic elevations in oxygen-derived free radicals, fostering the development of atherosclerosis. MSS exposure also reduces the number of circulating lymphocytes, suppresses T and B cell function, and increases the concentration of free fatty acids (FFAs) in the blood, which results in increased levels of low-density lipoproteins *(15)*. MSS exposure also reduces levels of high-density lipoprotens (HDL) and produces pathogenic changes in myocardial vasculature, resulting in vasoconstriction and reduced blood flow and oxygen and nutrient delivery to the myocardium. These pathological changes occur in non-smokers exposed to ETS as well and follow a dose-response relationship when ETS exposure is quantified in these subjects and compared to morbid cardiac outcomes.

While both mainstream smoking and ETS exposure significantly increase the individual's risk of CHD, smoking cessation produces marked reductions in cardiovascular risk *(5)*. The experience of hospitalization, particularly for cardiovascular disease, can result in smoking cessation even without intervention *(17–19)*. However, cessation rates vary greatly depending upon reason for hospitalization, length of stay, and the presence of depressive symptoms *(20)*. For example, Rigotti and colleagues *(21)* found high cessation rates (58%) 1 yr after hospitalization among coronary bypass patients, while other studies have shown very low cessation among smokers immediately after hospitalization (13.7%) and at 1-yr follow-up (9.2%) *(22)*. While the majority of individuals who quit smoking without intervention will relapse within 3 mo, individuals provided with professional intervention had lower rates of relapse *(23)*.

Physician Interventions for Smoking Cessation

While 70% of smokers visit a physician each year, very few of their doctors use this opportunity to address the patient's smoking *(24)*. Physicians practicing in specialties such as cardiology or emergency medicine are less likely to provide smoking cessation interventions than primary care physicians *(25)*. Possible explanations cited for low physician intervention rates include lack of time, deficient training in counseling skills, and an absence of organizational support *(26–29)*. This low prevalence is especially unfortunate as multiple studies have shown that even brief interventions, lasting less than 3 min, will significantly increase the probability that the smoker will quit *(30)*. Formal physician training, the use of cues or reminders, pharmacological aids, follow-up visits, and supplemental educational materials all increase the effectiveness of physician-delivered interventions *(31)*.

Cardiologists seeing smokers with coronary artery disease, hypertension, or histories of recurrent chest pain, can be especially effective because the patient's illness can be linked directly to smoking. The clinical encounter is a great teachable moment *(32)* which should be seized. Many physicians do not feel that they have the counseling skills or training to address smoking cessation effectively. This chapter will provide a well-studied, effective, and simple approach that cardiologists can use with their smoking patients.

TREATMENT APPROACHES

Recently, clinical guidelines have been developed through a joint collaboration between the Centers for Disease Control (CDC) and the Agency for Healthcare Research and Quality (AHRQ) together with the National Cancer Institute, the National Heart

Lung and Blood Institute, the National Institute on Drug Abuse, the Robert Wood Johnson Foundation, and the University of Wisconsin Medical School Center for Tobacco Research and Intervention *(30)*. The recommendations made as a result of this extensive systematic review and analysis of the extant peer-reviewed scientific literature form the basis of the approach taken in this chapter.

The key principles underlying these recommendations are:

1. Physicians should identify all of their patients who smoke.
2. Physicians should be conversant with all of the current effective treatments available for tobacco dependence.
3. Physicians should offer treatment to all of their smoking patients who are ready to quit.
4. Even smoking patients who are not yet ready or willing to quit should be offered treatment because intervention by a physician demonstrably increases the smoker's readiness and motivation to quit.
5. The physician should understand that tobacco dependence is a chronic condition that typically requires repeated intervention before long-term success is achieved.

The best practice model of brief intervention for smoking cessation is easily summarized by the mnemonic device of the "Five A's".

The Five A's are:

ASK: The physician should ask all patients if they smoke or have recently quit.

ADVISE: The physician should give every tobacco user clear, strong, and personalized advice to quit.

ASSESS: The physician should assess the patient's level of nicotine dependence and readiness to quit.

ASSIST: The physician should assist the patient in obtaining one or more of the effective treatments that exist for smoking cessation.

ARRANGE FOLLOW-UP: The physician should arrange follow-up to reinforce successful efforts and to identify slips early, so that barriers can be identified and motivation to try again can be renewed.

Each of the Five A's are summarized in Fig. 1, with links (in parentheses) to checklists and resources throughout the remainder of this chapter.

(1) ASK

National guidelines recommend that physicians systematically determine the smoking status of all patients at every visit. One simple method of accomplishing this goal incorporated a routine vital sign chart containing a smoking section. This small change

VITAL SIGNS:	Date of visit _____
Blood Pressure_____	Heart rate_____
Weight_____ Temperature_____	Respiration_____
Smoking Status: ☐ Current _____ rate (cigarettes/day)	
☐ Former _____ Quit date/date last smoked	
☐ Never	

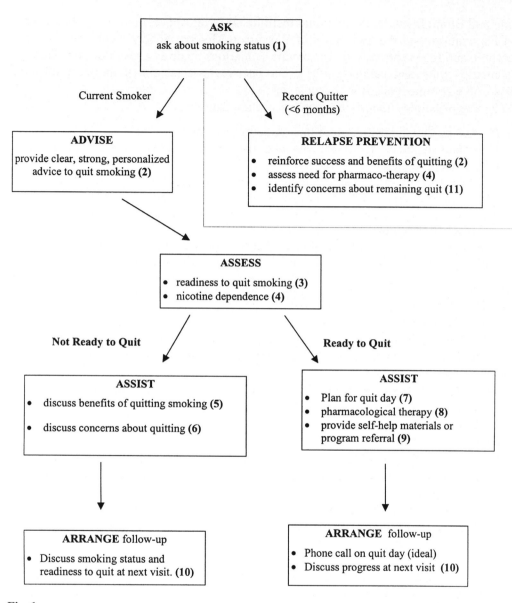

Fig. 1.

substantially increased the likelihood that smoking intervention was addressed during the patient visit *(33)*.

(2) ADVISE

EVERY TOBACCO USER SHOULD BE GIVEN ADVICE TO QUIT THAT IS CLEAR, STRONG, AND PERSONALIZED

Smoking cessation counseling is one of the most cost-effective healthcare interventions that can be made. Unfortunately research has repeatedly shown that smoking counseling is not provided at most physician visits *(27)*. Counseling does not need to be extensive to be effective. Advice which is clear, direct, and tailored to the individual patient's medical history or physical symptoms is more effective than generalized generic advice *(30)*. Brief, clear advice from a physician has been shown to double quit rates. For example, advice to a patient who is currently enrolled in cardiac rehabilitation might sound like this:

- Clear: "It is important for you to quit smoking."
- Strong: "Since you've already experienced heart disease (or specify condition), the most important thing you can do to avoid repeating this experience is to quit smoking."
- Personal: "Your risk of having a second MI will be a lot lower is you quit smoking."

Other phrases which work are: "As your physician, I want you to know that the most important thing you can do, to protect or improve your health, is to quit smoking." "Quitting smoking is important for everyone who smokes, but for you it's especially important because of (specify current health problem)."

ASSESS

ASSESS THE PATIENT'S READINESS TO QUIT SMOKING AND LEVEL OF NICOTINE DEPENDENCE

(3) Readiness to Quit Smoking. Readiness to quit smoking is a key determinant of treatment approach. Treatment for smokers who are ready to make a serious quit attempt should be focused on behavioral strategies, including selecting a Target Quit Date (TQD), reviewing and arranging appropriate pharmacological therapies, and referral to self-help or professional programs. Treatment for smokers who are not ready to quit should focus on increasing the patient's motivation to quit. Treatment for these smokers should focus on the psychological issues surrounding cessation, including reasons for quitting vs reasons for continuing smoking, concerns about the cessation process, the patient's self-confidence, and family and/or social supports and barriers to quitting (Fig. 2).

Motivation or readiness to quit smoking has most often been measured using Prochaska and DiClemente's Stages of Change model *(35)*, which was developed for use in outpatient populations. As most hospitals impose smoking restrictions in the inpatient setting, and hospitalization itself encourages serious thought about smoking habits, employing this algorithm in the inpatient setting introduces a bias misclassifying smokers into higher motivation to quit categories. Recent research has shown that a single question, "How likely it is that you will remain abstinent after hospital discharge?" has a higher predictive value for predicting sustained quits in hospital inpatients *(36)*.

(4) Nicotine Dependence. The most widely used and validated measure of nicotine dependence is the Fagerstrom Test for Nicotine Dependence (FTND). Patients scoring ≥ 6 are considered highly nicotine dependent. While research shows that most smokers benefit from nicotine replacement therapy (NRT) and that providing NRT is especially important for highly dependent smokers. Smokers who use nicotine replacement show double the success rates as those who do not *(30,37)*, but this effect is most pronounced among highly nicotine-dependent smokers. Highly nicotine-dependent smokers are $3\times$ more likely to be successful if they use nicotine replacement than if they do not. Moreover, the physician should choose the initial dose of NRT after considering the patient's level of nicotine dependence (see Table 1) and the patient's current smoking rate.

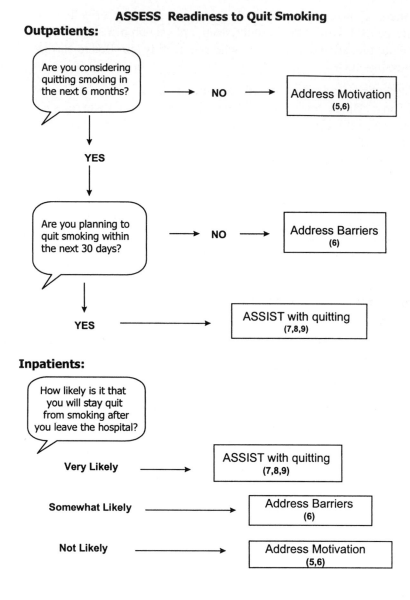

Fig. 2

SPECIFIC TREATMENT PLANS
ASSIST

A MOTIVATIONAL APPROACH

There are as many different types of smokers as there are people. For the sake of simplicity however, the physician can consider smokers as one of two groups: those who are ready to quit, and those who are not. Research studies have repeatedly shown that physicians who identify the two categories of smokers and take the appropriate motivational approach to addressing smoking with these groups are more successful in helping them to quit. Motivational approaches, including the "Transtheoretical" or

Table 1
Fagerstrom Test for Nicotine Dependence (FTND)

Points	0	1	2	3
How many cigarettes do you smoke per day				
	≤10	11–20	21–30	≥30
Do you smoke more in the morning (or when you first wake up) compared to the rest of the day ?				
	No	Yes		
Do you find it difficult to not smoke in places where smoking is not allowed, like church or the movies?				
	No	Yes		
How soon after waking do you smoke your first cigarette ?				
	>60 min	31–60 min	6–30 min	<5 min
Do you smoke when you are so ill that you must stay in bed?				
	No	Yes		
Which cigarette of the day would you most hate to give up?				
	any other	the first		

From ref. 38.

"Stages of Change" model and Motivational Interviewing, are widely used theoretical models of how people change health behaviors (6,35). Developed for use in outpatient populations, the basic tenet of these models is that individuals who are not yet ready to change behavior need to be approached differently than those who are ready to change. In practical terms, this means that treatment goals for smokers who are not yet ready to quit should focus on identifying reasons to quit, thus enhancing motivation for quitting, and identifying perceived barriers. Treatment for these smokers should avoid immediate behavioral goal-setting, such as discussing quit dates or selecting pharmacological treatments. Conversely, interventions for smokers who are ready to quit should focus on behavioral goals (e.g., choosing a TQD and pharmacotherapy) and coping strategies.

Not Ready to Quit

Patients who are not yet ready to quit need help identifying reasons to quit, improving their motivation and confidence in their ability to quit, and identifying barriers to smoking cessation. These patients may lack, or believe they lack, the needed financial resources to afford NRT or pharmacologic aids to quitting, or information about how smoking is affecting their health. They may have concerns about quitting—possibly related to prior failed attempts (39). The physician can intervene with these patients by providing information that is relevant and helping them identify barriers to quitting and the resources that are necessary to support cessation. Motivational interventions are most successful when the physician is empathic, promotes patient autonomy (provides choices among options), supports the patient's sense of self-confidence, and avoids argumentation (40,41).

(5) The "Good Reasons to Stop Smoking Now" and the "Benefits of Quitting Smoking" lists may be helpful.

GOOD REASONS TO STOP SMOKING NOW

Its never too late to quit. The body begins to repair itself within minutes of the last cigarette.

Within 20 min of your last cigarette:
- Blood pressure begins to decrease.
- Pulse slows to a more normal rate.
- The temperature of hands and feet increases to normal.

8 h:
- Carbon monoxide level in the blood returns to normal.
- Oxygen level in blood increases.

24 h:
- Chance of heart attack decreases.

48 h:
- Nerve endings start regrowing.
- Ability to smell and taste things is improved.

72 h:
- Bronchial tubes relax, making breathing easier.

2 wk to 3 mo:
- Circulation improves and walking becomes easier.
- Lung function increases up to 30%.

1 mo to 9 mo:
- Coughing, sinus congestion, fatigue, and shortness of breath all decrease.
- Cilia regrow in the lungs, increasing your ability to handle mucus, clean the lungs, and reduce infection.
- Body's overall energy level increases.

5 yr:
- The lung cancer death rate for the average smoker is cut in half.

10 yr:
- Risk of lung cancer is almost as low as for those who never smoked.
- Risk of other cancers (mouth, larynx, kidney, bladder, pancreas) all decrease.

Taken from the American Cancer Society's FreshStart program.

BENEFITS OF QUITTING SMOKING

- Fresher breath.
- Cleaner smelling hair and clothes.
- Whiter teeth.
- Saving money (a pack-a-day smoker will save almost $1000/yr).
- Freedom from social restrictions and the demands of addiction.
  - → no need to ensure continual cigarette supply.
- Improved circulation.
- Improved ability to exercise.
- Longer and better life.
- Less chance of having a heart attack, stroke, and cancer.
- Reduced risk of lung disease, fewer problems with existing respiratory disease.
- Improved health for the people you live with, especially your children.

Concerns about Quitting   (decisional balance worksheet)

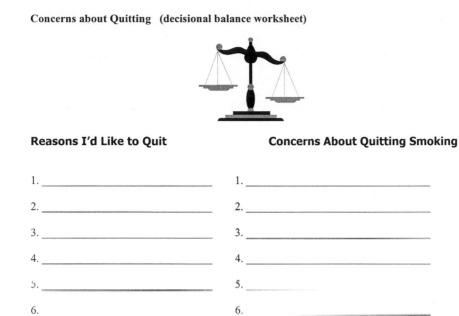

Reasons I'd Like to Quit   **Concerns About Quitting Smoking**

1. _____   1. _____

2. _____   2. _____

3. _____   3. _____

4. _____   4. _____

5. _____   5. _____

6.   6. _____

Fig. 3

- Better health: exsmokers have fewer days of illness, fewer health complaints, better self-reported health status.
- After 10 yr, the risk of lung cancer for exsmokers is cut in half.
- After 10 yr, the risk of stroke for exsmokers is the same as for people who never smoked.
- For people with heart disease, quitting smoking reduces the risk of repeat heart attacks and death from heart disease by over 50%.

(6) CONCERNS ABOUT QUITTING

Many patients are aware that they should quit smoking, but have concerns about the process of quitting or are discouraged from prior failed attempts. These patients may benefits by exploring their concerns about quitting. The Decisional Balance worksheet (Fig. 3) has been used in numerous smoking cessation trials to help smokers identify both their reasons for wanting to quit and perceived barriers to quitting.

READY TO QUIT

Effective treatments exist for smoking cessation and should be provided to all smokers who are ready to quit. Effective treatment components include:

- Selecting a TQD.
- Reviewing pharmacological therapies with the patient and selecting appropriate options.
- Anticipating challenges (work schedules, stressors, social supports, and saboteurs).
- Offering referral to self-help materials or specialized programs and resources.

(7) Planning to Quit

- Select a TQD.
  Usually this is within 2 wk of the office visit. Total abstinence on this date is essential.
- Prepare environment.
  If possible, eliminate ashtrays, smoking paraphernalia, and cigarette supply.
- Past experience.
  Review what worked in prior quit attempts and what caused relapses.
- Plan the day.
  Patients need to consider how they will alter their usual routine to avoid smoking. Avoid alcohol. For a few days, patients may need to avoid people and places associated with smoking. Patients should anticipate triggers and have a coping plan.
- Practice and preparation.
  Patients can begin to change their normal routine around smoking in the days before quitting. For example, if the patient always has a cigarette with coffee in the morning, he or she could begin drinking coffee without smoking in the days leading up to quit day. This gives the patient some practice in breaking up the behavioral cues associated with smoking.
- Recommend pharmacotherapy.
  Consider using medications if not contraindicated. Explain how these medications can reduce withdrawal symptoms and increase chances of success.
- Suggest social support.
  Have the patient identify family, friends, or coworkers who will be helpful. Arrange for other household smokers to restrict their smoking near the patient.
- Schedule follow-up visit.
  Follow-up contact should occur 1 wk after the Quit Day.

Short-Term Coping Strategies

- Remove all smoking-related paraphernalia (ashtrays, lighters, etc.) from the home, office, and car.
- Keep cigarettes out of easy reach (in an out-of-the-way kitchen cupboard, in the garage, in the trunk of the car).
- Be prepared to ask others to modify their behavior for a short while.
- Avoid alcohol.
- Exercise: taking brief walks during the day reduces stress and gets the smoker out of the environment where they were triggered to smoke.
- Reward positive change.

(8) Pharmacological Therapy for Smoking Cessation

All smokers who are ready to make a serious quit attempt should be strongly encouraged to use pharmacotherapy to aid their quitting efforts, except where contraindicated. As with other chronic disease conditions, nicotine dependence is best treated using multiple modalities including behavioral and pharmacotherapies. Physicians are advised to discourage patients from trying a single method and then switching to another single method only if the first approach fails. That strategy is likely to weaken the patient's resolve to quit before achieving success.

There are two first-line medications that are effective for smoking cessation; bupropion and NRT. NRT is currently available in four different delivery formats: transdermal patch, gum, nasal spray, and inhaler. The efficacy of nicotine replacement products is similar, with each agent leading to a doubling of the cessation rate, so the choice of product depends on patient factors such as smoking patterns, rate, and preference. Tailoring of NRT to the individual's ambient nicotine levels and smoking patterns appears to substantially increase treatment efficacy (Table 2). For example, a study by Sachs et al. *(42)* found that short-term cessation rates were over 75% when nicotine replacement was increased until blood nicotine levels matched those found when the patient was smoking. Higher-dose patches appear to be safe for the heavy smoker *(43)* and those who achieve a higher level of replacement of their smoking nicotine level may do better. However, there does not appear to be a general benefit to starting smokers at higher dose levels. While multiple patches are appropriate for the individual who is heavily nicotine-dependent, cost can become a prohibitive factor. In some heavily dependent smokers, it may be beneficial to combine nicotine replacement products such as gum plus a patch *(44)*. Using either NRT or bupropion increases the odds of successful cessation by 50–150% *(45–47)*. NRT and bupropion can be used simultaneously, since they have different mechanisms of action. They are synergistic: using both entities together is more effective than using either alone.

Beyond nicotine replacement and antidepressants such as bupropion, other agents such as clonidine, anti-anxiety agents, and nicotine antagonists have shown promise *(48,49)*, but have yet to demonstrate their efficacy in large-scale clinical trials *(50)*, thus they are not recommended for first-line treatment at present.

Key Points

- Pharmacotherapy doubles quit rates and is safe for most patients.
- Pharmacotherapy is effective for a broad range of patients and should NOT be reserved for "hard core" smokers or heavy smokers only.
- Different medication types (e.g., bupropion and NRT) can be combined to enhance chances of success.
- Combining the nicotine patch with self-administered forms of NRT (e.g., patch plus gum) may be more effective than using a single form of NRT.
- Long-term pharmacotherapy can reduce the risk of relapse.

NICOTINE REPLACEMENT IN CARDIAC PATIENTS

When used in medical settings, NRT plus a physician's advice can produce impressive abstinence rates *(51)*. Soon after the nicotine patch was approved for use, the media reported a possible link between patch use and cardiovascular incidents. The use of NRT in cardiac patients has been of concern, because some of the cardiotoxic effects of smoking are attributable to nicotine. While nicotine does have sympathomimetic effects that increase heart rate, blood pressure, and stimulate vasoconstriction *(52)*, the use of NRT generally leads to significantly lower blood nicotine levels compared to smoking *(53)* even in patients who smoke during NRT treatment *(54,55)*. Use of NRT is likely to result in fewer adverse cardiovascular effects than continued smoking. Anecdotal reports of adverse cardiac events *(56,57)* have made physician's hesitant to prescribe NRT for cardiac patients *(58)*. Systematic research over the past decade has documented that there is no reliable association between acute cardiovascular events and use of the nicotine

Table 2
First-Line Pharmacological Therapies

Medication	Bupropion (Zyban)	Nicotine patch	Nicotine polacrilex (gum)	Nicotine Inhaler	Nicotine nasal spray
Contraindications	Seizure disorder, current bupropion use (e.g., Wellbutrin) or MAO inhibitors, anorexia or bulimia, allergy to bupropion.	Severe eczema, allergy to adhesives or other skin disease.	Severe temporomandibular joint disease, jaw problems, dentures.	None.	Presence of asthma, rhinitis, nasal polyps, or sinusitis.
Precautions	Is usually well-tolerated by patients with cardiovascular disease—infrequent reports of hypertension.	Recent (2 wk) MI, severe arrhythmia, severe angina pectoris.	Same as nicotine patch.	Same as nicotine patch. Use caution with patients who have asthma, wheezing, or other pulmonary disease.	Same as nicotine inhaler.
Dosage/ use instructions	150 mg 1× /d for 3 d, 150 mg 2× /d for 7–12 wk. Start 7–10 d prior to quit date.	Available in 7–21 mg doses. Treatment usually lasts 4–12 wk with dosage tapering.	2 mg and 4 mg. One piece every 1–2 h (24/d maximum).	4 mg cartridge (80 inhalations/cartridge). 6–16 cartridges/d for 3–6 mo.	1 to 2 doses/h (5/h and 40/d maximum).3–6 mo.
Availability	Prescription.	OTC.	OTC.	Prescription.	Prescription.
Adverse reactions (possible remedy)	Dry mouth, insomnia.	Skin irritation (hydrocortisone cream/ rotate patch sites); vivid dreams (avoid wearing during sleep)	Mouth soreness, hiccups, dyspepsia, jaw ache (review correct chewing technique).	Irritation of mouth, throat, coughing, rhinitis.	Irritation in nose and throat, watering eyes, sneezing and cough.
Comments	May be used concurrently with NRT. Treatment can be maintained for 6 mo.	Vary initial dose with smoking rate (e.g., <15 cigarettes/d should start at lower-dosage; >35/d may need higher dose). May work best for regular-interval smokers.	May work especially well for light or irregular smokers. May help with oral substitution. Requires proper chewing technique.	May work especially well for light or irregular smokers. May help with oral substitution.	

MAO, monoamine oxidase; OTC, over-the-counter medications.

Table 3
Efficacy and Estimated Abstinence Rates for Intervention Types and Intensities

Level of Contact	Number studies	Estimated odds ratio (range)	Average abstinence rates
No intervention	39	1.0	10.9
Physician advice: (3 min)	10	1.3 (1.1–1.6)	13.4
Self-help	93	1.2 (1.1–1.4)	12.3
Telephone counseling	26	1.2 (1.1–1.4)	13.1
Group counseling	52	1.3 (1.1–1.6)	13.9
Individual counseling	67	1.7 (1.4–2.0)	16.8

From ref. 30.

patch, even among patients who continue to smoke while using the patch (59–62). Because cigarette smoking, in general, and nicotine ingestion, in particular, have cardiovascular effects, some caution is warranted regarding the safety of NRT among certain cardiac patients. These are:

- Patients with immediate (within 2 wk) history of MI.
- Patients with serious arrhythmias.
- Patients with severe or worsening angina pectoris.

Note that these are cautions, not contraindications. The physician must weigh the benefits of smoking cessation against any possible risk from nicotine replacement. Bupropion is generally well-tolerated in cardiac patients, although there have been rare reports of exacerbation of hypertension.

(9) Program Referral

Most smoking cessation efforts are enhanced by behavioral supports. These can include self-help materials, telephone calls, support groups, and individual therapy for smoking cessation. Intervention intensity is positively associated with cessation success: essentially "more is better". Minimal interventions, such as brief advice from a physician lasting less than 3 min increases the chance of successful cessation by approx 30%, while high-intensity interventions, such as individual counseling can more than double quit rates. Therefore, the more intervention resources the physician provides to the patient, the more likely it will be that he or she will quit smoking (Table 3).

Books and Other Self-Help Resources

Numerous books and tapes are available as self-help aids for smokers who are attempting to quit. Most recently, a number of Internet Web sites have sprung up offering assistance to smokers who are trying to quit. Internet sites may be especially helpful to some smokers since chats and other supports are available 24 h/d. There are many good books available to patients who want to quit smoking. A few of these are listed below.

1. **The Stop Smoking Workbook: Your Guide to Healthy Quitting** (Anita Maximin & Lori Stevio-Rust; New Harbinger Publications, 1995). This stop-smoking guide stands out because of its comprehensive content and its interactive workbook format. The practical exercises take smokers through a structured process that enables them to under-

stand the realities of addiction and the different phases of quitting, and helps them to make the changes in their lives that are necessary to quit for good.

2. **If Only I Could Quit : Recovering from Nicotine Addiction** (Karen Casey Hazelden. Information Education publishers, 1996). A motivational book based describing the experiences of 24 individuals while trying to quit smoking. Based on a Twelve Step philosophy, this book outlines a three-month, one-day-at-a-time program to begin recovery from nicotine addiction.

3. **No-Nag, No-Guilt: Do-It-Your-Own Way Guide to Quitting Smoking** (Tom Ferguson, Random House, Inc. publishers, 1998). Dr. Ferguson is an experienced medical writer who avoids anti-smoking rhetoric. Instead, he offers a reasonable, practical program for smokers who want to quit.

4. **American Cancer Society's "Fresh Start"** A 21-day gradual smoking reduction program that is helpful for smokers who wish to quit without using NRT. This book addresses coping with cigarette cravings, withdrawal symptoms and the benefits of quitting smoking.

5. **Quit Smoking for Good: A Supportive Program for Permanent Smoking Cessation** (Andrea Baer, Crossing Press, 1998). This book focuses on making emotional and behavioral changes needed to prepare for permanent smoke-free living.

6. **American Lung Association 7 Steps to a Smoke-Free Life** (Edwin Fisher, Jr. & C. Everett Koop, John Wiley & Sons, 1998). This book is based on the American Lung Association's "Freedom from Smoking" program. Helps smokers identify smoking triggers and develop coping strategies. Contains worksheets, checklists and "quick quit tips" .

7. **The Complete Idiot's Guide to Quitting Smoking** (Lowell Kleinman, MD. Deborah Messina-Kleinman & Mitchell Nides, Macmillan publishing, 2000). A solid, comprehensive guide to smoking cessation and pharmacotherapy.

8. **When It Hurts Too Much to Quit: Smoking and Depression** (Gerald Mayer, Desert City Press, 1997). This book presents information about the special challenges facing smokers who are trying to quit while experiencing clinical depression. This book addresses the relationship between smoking and depression, the basics of brain chemistry, the essentials of effective treatment and making choices about getting help.

9. **Out of the Ashes: Help for People Who Have Stopped Smoking** (Peter Holmes & Peggy Holmes, Fairview Press, 1992). This book offers ex-smokers new ways to cope with the challenges of remaining smoke-free.

Web sites. Many patients are familiar with computers and may have access at home or work to the Internet. This form of support can be particularly helpful to smokers who are having difficulty. They can access help and support on a 24-h basis using the Internet. The following is a list of smoking cessation support sites with a brief review of their contents. All site address (**in bold)** begin with *http://www* except for the Nicotine Anonymous site.

1. **Clever.net/chrisco/nosmoke/cafe.html** A long, convoluted Web address with high quality Web site at the other end: the "No Smoke Cafe". The site content includes "Counselor Larry": pages containing a wealth of information about making psychological and behavioral changes needed to quit. This site also features chat rooms, message boards, and inspirational information about tobacco use and quitting.

2. **Quitsmoking.about.com** This site is part of the "About.com" network of health-related Web sites. The site contains lots of information about smoking cessation methods, the "Ash Kickers" discussion forum and links to many other resources.

3. **Lungusa.com** American Lung Association Web site featuring *Freedom from Smoking* and *7-Steps to a Smoke-Free Life* programs. This site offers help in English and Spanish.

4. **Nicorette.com** This SmithKline Beecham Web site features nicorette gum and the "Committed quitters" program—a sound self-help cessation program for NRT gum users. Available in English and Spanish.

5. **Zyban.com** This is the Glaxo Wellcome site dedicated to providing information about Zyban and the "Zyban Advantage" smoking cessation support program.

6. **Smokehelp.org** The "Smokers Helpline" Web site. This site has general information about quitting smoking, the dangers of tobacco and so on. **Caution:** This site states that quitting cold turkey is the "best way" for most people to quit and discourages NRT use.

7. **Cancer.org** American Cancer Society Web site. This site is difficult to navigate and has only generalized informational pages about smoking related issues, without providing much hands-on help. For example, clicking on their "Fresh Start" program brings up a single page telling you that Fresh Start is a program to help people quit smoking—with no content about the program or information/links to any actual program.

8. **http://nicotine-anonymous.org** The Nicotine Anonymous (NA) Web site has contacts for local chapters and instructions on setting up an NA group. NA follows a traditional 12-step model of addiction recovery. **Caution:** This site states that "Nicotine Anonymous accepts that nicotine is a toxic addictive substance that endangers our quality of life.", but goes on to say "We neither endorse nor oppose such devices as nicotine gum or patches". This resource might be helpful to smokers who need group support, but the apparent bias against NRT and confusion between tobacco vs nicotine as toxic substances warrants caution.

(10) Arrange Follow Up

Follow-Up Visits

- Ideally the first follow-up should occur within 1 wk of the Quit Date.
- A phone contact on the quit day is helpful to most smokers.
- Congratulate and reinforce success.

If smoking has occurred,

- Identify circumstances surrounding slips.
- Reframe slips as learning experiences—not as signs of failure.
- Identify new target quit day.
- Reassess need for pharmacotherapy.
- Consider referral to a more intensive program.

A second follow-up visit is recommended within 1 mo.

(11) Discuss Concerns about Remaining Quit

Nicotine dependence is a chronic and recurring condition, often requiring several serious quit attempts before permanent success is achieved. Therefore, physicians should be prepared to address relapse prevention with any patient who has recently quit smoking (less than 6 mo abstinence). Physicians should reinforce success, underline the benefits of quitting smoking, and help patients identify any problems or concerns they may have about remaining quit. Even recently quit patients experiencing difficulties staying quit or verging on relapse may be helped with pharmacotherapy or behavioral therapy and referrals *(63,64)*.

Problem/Concern	Possible Solution
Strong, continued withdrawal symptoms or cravings.	Nicotine replacement therapy. If quit >1 wk, start at lower dose (e.g., 7-mg patch). Consider therapy with bupropion.
Depressive symptoms or negative mood.	Provide counseling. If significant, prescribe medication. Refer to specialist.
Weight gain.	Emphasize healthy diet (no strict dieting). Suggest increasing physical activity. Most people gain <10 lbs and is self-limiting. Consider medications known to delay/reduce weight gain (e.g., nicotine gum, bupropion).
Lack of support for cessation.	Schedule follow-up visit. Identify social or family supports. Refer to organization for support.
Low motivation.	Assess for cravings/withdrawal symptoms. Recommend rewarding activities. Emphasize benefits of quitting smoking.

OR

SUMMARY AND CONCLUSIONS

Because three quarters of all smokers will visit a physician at least once each year *(1)*, smoking cessation interventions delivered in medical settings can reach a wide range of smokers who otherwise might not present for treatment *(24)*. Medical settings may also provide a unique, teachable moment in which to influence patients' perception of risk from smoking related illness, and to enhance their motivation to quit *(65,66)*.

Tobacco use is unique in that it constitutes a highly significant public health threat, for which clinicians tend not to intervene consistently despite the presence of effective treatments. Smoking is the single, leading cause of preventable death in the U.S. today, killing more than 450,000 Americans each yr and causing uncounted morbidity and suffering. The annual cost of smoking and smoking related illness and death in the U.S. exceeds 130 billion dollars *(67)*.

Specialists are even less likely to provide smoking counseling than primary care physicians *(25,68)*. This is particularly unfortunate, since smokers are more likely to quit when counseling is provided within the context of a sick visit *(32)*. The reluctance of physicians to provide counseling can be traced to many factors including lack of counseling skills, inadequate training, time pressures (patients/h), and absent organizational support. Large, multilayered hospital systems, third-party insurers, and administrative structures often create barriers to physicians trying to provide preventive health counseling. Physicians should not bear the entire blame for this unfortunate deficit in proactive preventive health intervention. However, physicians can and should always strive to address smoking with their patients with the same vigor with which they address hypertension. The guidelines for physician intervention presented in this chapter reflect recommendations for clinician intervention produced by the AHRQ and US Public Health Service *(30)*. These recommendations should become the standard of care for the millennium embraced by physicians, mid-level providers, and healthcare systems as they strive together to free their patients once and for all from the addiction to nicotine and the morbidity and mortality that inevitably surround tobacco use.

REFERENCES

1. US Dept of Health and Human Services. Cigarette smoking among adults—United States 1994. *MMWR* 1996;45:588–590.
2. Peto R, Lopez AD, Boreham J, Thumn M, Heath C. Mortality from smoking in developing countries: 1950–2000. Oxford University Press, Oxford, 1994.
3. CDC. Smoking-attributable mortality and years of potential life lost—United States 1984. MMWR 1997;46:444–451.
4. Thun MJ, Apicella LF, Henley SJ. Smoking vs other risk factors as the cause of smoking-attributable deaths: confounding in the courtroom. *JAMA* 2000;284:706–712.
5. US Dept of Health and Human Services. Health Benefits of Smoking Cessation. Report of the US Surgeon General. Washington, DC: US GPO DHHS Pub. No. (CDC) 90–8416. 1990.
6. Miller LS, Zhang X, Rice DP, Max W. State estimates of total medical expenditures attributable to cigarette smoking, 1993. *Public Health Rep* 1998;113:447–458.
7. Ducatman AM, McLellan RK. Epidemiologic basis for an occupational and environmental policy on environmental tobacco smoke. *J Occup Environ Med* 2000;42:1137–1141.
8. Giovino GA, Henningfield JE, Tomar SL, Escobedo LG, Slade J. Epidemiology of tobacco use and dependence. *Epidemiol Rev* 1995;17:48–65.
9. CDC. Health objectives for the nation. Cigarette smoking among adults—United States, 1997. *MMWR* 1999;48:993–996.
10. CDC. Reducing tobacco use: A report of the Surgeon General Executive Summary. *MMWR* 2000;49:706–712.
11. Anderson RN, Kochanek KD, Murphy SL. Report of final mortality statistics, 1995. Monthly Vital Statistics Report 1997;45(Suppl. 2):1–80.
12. CDC. Mortality patterns—United States, 1997. *MMWR* 1999;48:664–668.
13. Kochanek KD, Smith BL, Anderson RN. Deaths: preliminary data for 1999. Natl Vital Statistics Reports 2001;49:1–48.
14. USDHHS. Office of the Assistant Secretary for Health and Surgeon General, Office on smoking and Health: The health consequences of involuntary smoking: A report of the Surgeon General, 1986. Rockville, MD. US Department of Health and Human Services, Public Health Service Centers for Disease Control, Center for Health Promotion and Education Office on Smoking and Health. For sale by the Superintendent of Documents, US Government Printing Office, 1986.
15. Taylor BV, Oudit GY, Kalman PG, et al. Clinical and pathophysiological effects of active and passive smoking on the cardiovascular system. *Can J Cardiol* 1998;13:1129.
16. Villablanca, AC, McDonald JM, Rutledge JC. Smoking and cardiovascular disease. Clin Chest Med 2000;21:159–172.
17. Houston-Miller N, Smith PM, DeBusk RF, Sobel DS, Taylor CB. Smoking cessation in hospitalized patients: results of a randomized trial. *Arch Intern Med* 1997;157:409–415.
18. Orleans CT, Ockene JK. Routine hospital-based quit-smoking treatment for the post myocardial infarction patient: an idea whose time has come. *J Am Coll Cardiol* 1993;22:1703–1705.
19. Rigotti N, Arnsten JH, McKool KM, Wood-Reid KM, Pasternak RC, Singer DE. Efficacy of a smoking cessation program for hospital patients. *Arch Intern Med* 1997;157:2653–2660.
20. Glasgow RE, Stevens VJ, Vogt TM, Mullooly JP, Lichtenstein E. Changes in smoking associated with hospitalization: quit rates, predictive variables, and intervention implications. *Am J Health Promo* 1991;6:24–29.
21. Rigotti N, McKool KM, Shiffman S. Predictors of smoking cessation after coronary artery bypass graft surgery. *Ann Intern Med* 1994;120:287–293.
22. Stevens VJ, Glasgow RE, Hollis JF, Lichtenstein E, Vogt TM. A smoking-cessation intervention for hospital patients. *Med Care* 1993;31:65–72.
23. Ockene JK, Emmons KM, Mermelstein RJ, et al. Relapse and maintenance issues for smoking cessation. *Health Psychol* 2000;19(Suppl. 1):17–31.

24. Goldstein MG, Niaura R, Willey-Lessne C, et al. Physicians counseling smokers: a population-based survey of patients' perceptions of health care provider delivered smoking cessation interventions. *Arch Intern Med* 1997;157:1313–1319.

25. Thorndike AN, Rigotti NA, Stafford RS, Singer DE. National patterns in the treatment of smokers by physicians. *JAMA* 1998;279:604–608.

26. Cohen SJ, Katz BP, Drook CA, Smith DM. Encouraging primary care physicians to help smokers quit. A randomized, controlled trial. *Ann Intern Med* 1989;110:648–652.

27. Cummings SR, Stein MJ, Hansen B, et al. Smoking counseling and preventive medicine. A survey of internists in private practices and health maintenance organizations. *Arch Intern Med* 1989;149:345–349.

28. Lewis CE, Clancy C, Leake B, Schwartz JS. The counseling practices of internists. *Ann Intern Med* 1991;114:54–58.

29. Strecher VJ, O'Malley MS, Villagra VG, et al. Can residents be trained to counsel patients about quitting smoking? Results from a randomized trial. *J Gen Intern Med* 1991;6:9–17.

30. Fiore MC, Bailey WC, Cohen SJ, et al. Treating Tobacco Use and Dependence. Clinical practice guideline. US Department of Health and Human Services, Public Health Service, Rockville, MD, June 2000.

31. Ockene JK, Kristeller J, Pbert L, et al. The physician-delivered smoking intervention projects: can short-term interventions produce long-term effects for a general outpatient population? *Health Psychol* 1994;13:278–281.

32. Daughton D, Susman J, Sitorius M, et al. Transdermal nicotine therapy and primary care: importance of counseling demographic and participant selection factors on 1-year quit rates. *Arch Fam Med* 1998;7:425–430.

33. Ellerbeck EF, Ahluwalia JS, Jolicoeur DG, Gladden J, Mosier MC. Direct observation of smoking cessation activities in primary care practice. *J Fam Pract* 2000;50:688–693.

34. Jackson G, Bobak A, Chorlton I, et al. Smoking cessation: a consensus statement with special reference to primary care. *Int J Clin Pract* 2001;55:385–392.

35. Prochaska JO, DiClemente CC. Stages and processes of self-change of smoking: toward an integrative model of change. *J Consult Clin Psychol* 1983;51:390–395.

36. Sciamanna CN, Hoch JS, Duke GC, Fogie MN, Ford DE. Comparison of five measures of motivation to quit smoking among a sample of hospitalized smokers. *J Gen Intern Med* 2000;15:16–23.

37. Leischow S, Muramoto ML, Cook G, Merikle E, Castellini S, Otte PS. OTC nicotine patches: effectiveness alone and with brief physician intervention. *Am J Health Behavior* 1999;23:61–69.

38. Heatherton TF, Kozlowski LT, Frecker RC, Fagerstrom KO. The Fagerstrom test for nicotine dependence: A revision of the Fagerstrom Tolerance Questionnaire. *Br J Addiction* 1991;86:1119–1127.

39. Rundmo T, Smedslund G, Gotestam KG. Motivation for smoking cessation among the Norwegian public. *Addict Behav* 1997;22:377–386.

40. Colby SM, Barnett NP, Monti PM, et al. Brief motivational interviewing in a hospital setting for adolescent smoking: a preliminary study. *J Consult Clin Psychol* 1998;66:574–578.

41. Prochaska JO, Goldstein MG. Process of smoking cessation. Implications for clinicians. *Clin Chest Med* 1991:12:727–735.

42. Sachs DPL, Benowitz NL, Bostron AG, et al. Percent serum replacement and success of nicotine patch therapy. Am Rev Respir Crit Care Med 1995;151:A688

43. Dale LC, Hurt RD, Offord KP, et al. High dose nicotine patch therapy: percentage of replacement and smoking cessation. JAMA 1995;274:1353–1358.

44. Kornitzer M, Boutsen M, Drammaix M, et al. Combined use of nicotine patch and gum in smoking cessation: a placebo-controlled clinical trial. Prev Med 1995;24:41–47.

45. Cepeda-Benito, A. Meta-analytical review of the efficacy of nicotine chewing gum in smoking treatment programs. *J Consult Clin Psychol* 1993;61:822–830.

46. Henningfield JE. Nicotine medications for smoking cessation. *N Engl J Med* 1995;333:1196–1203.

47. Jorenby DE, Leischow S, Nides M, et al. A controlled trial so sustained-release bupropion, a nicotine patch or both for smoking cessation. *N Engl J Med* 1999;340:685–691.

48. Hall SM, Reus VI, Munoz RF, et al. Nortriptyline and cognitive-behavioral therapy in the treatment of cigarette smoking. *Arch Gen Psychiatry* 1998;55:683–690.

49. Hughes J, Goldstein MG. Recent advances in the pharmacotherapy of smoking. *JAMA* 1999;281;72–76.

50. Prochazka AV. New developments in smoking cessation. *Chest* 2000;117(Suppl. 1):169S–175S.

51. Sachs DPL, Sawe U, Leischow SJ. Effectiveness of a 16-hour transdermal nicotine patch in a medical practice setting, without intensive group counseling. *Arch Intern Med* 1993;153:1881–1890.

52. Benowitz NL. Pharmacologic aspects of cigarette smoking and nicotine addiction. *N Engl J Med* 1984; 319:1318–1330.

53. Benowitz NL, Fitzgerald GA, Wilson M, Zhang Q. Nicotine effects on eicosanoid formation and hemostatic function: comparison of transdermal nicotine and cigarette smoking. *J Am Coll Cardiol* 1993;22:1159–1167.

54. Joseph AM, Westman EC. Transdermal nicotine therapy for older medically ill patients: a pilot study. *J Gen Intern Med* 1995;10(Suppl.):101.

55. Transdermal Nicotine Study Group. Transdermal nicotine for smoking cessation: six month results from two multicenter controlled clinical trials. *JAMA* 1991;266:3133–3138.

56. Jackson, M. Cerebral arterial narrowing with nicotine patch. *Lancet.* 1993;342:236–237.

57. Warner JG Jr, Little WC. Myocardial infarction in a patient who smoked while wearing a nicotine patch. *Ann Intern Med* 1994;120:695.

58. Arnaot MR. Treating heart disease: nicotine patches may not be safe. *Br Med J* 1995;310:663–664.

59. Benowitz NL, Gourlay SG. Cardiovascular toxicity of nicotine: implications for nicotine replacement therapy. *J Am Coll Cardiol* 1997;29:1422–1431.

60. Joseph AM, Norman SM, Ferry LH, et al. The safety of transdermal nicotine as an aid to smoking cessation in patients with cardiac disease. *N Engl J Med* 1996;335:1792–1798.

61. Mahmarian JJ, Moye LA, Nasser GA et al. Nicotine patch therapy in smoking cessation reduces the extent of exercise-induced myocardial ischemia *J Am Coll Cardiol* 1997;30:125–130

62. Working Group for the Study of Transdermal Nicotine in Patients with Coronary Artery Disease. Nicotine replacement therapy for patients with coronary artery disease. Arch Intern Med 1994;154:989–995.

63. Brandon TH, Tiffany ST, Obremski K, Baker TB. Postcessation cigarette use: the process of relapse. *Addictive Behaviors* 1990;15:105–114.

64. Carroll KM. Relapse prevention as a psychosocial treatment: a review of controlled clinical trials. Exp Clin Psychopharmacol 1996;4:46–54.

65. Bock BC, Becker B, Partridge R, Fisher S, Monteiro R, Spencer J. Physician intervention and patient attitudes among smokers with acute respiratory illness in the emergency department. Prev Med 2001; 32:175–181.

66. Emmons K, Goldstein MG. Smokers who are hospitalized: a window of opportunity for cessation interventions. *Prev Med* 1992;21:262–269.

67. Leistikow BN. The human and financial costs of smoking. Clin Chest Med 2000;21:189–197.

68. Jaen CR, Stange KC, Tumiel LM, Tumiel LM, Nutting P. Missed opportunities for prevention: smoking cessation counseling and the competing demands of practice. *J Fam Pract* 1997;45:348–354.

69. Bartecchi CE, MacKenzie MD, Schrier RW. The human costs of tobacco use. *N Engl J Med* 1994; 330:907–912.

70. Gourlay SG, Forbes A, Marriner T, et al. Double blind trial of repeated treatment with transdermal nicotine for relapsed smokers. BMJ 1995;311:363–366.

71. Miller W, Rollnick S. Motivational Interviewing: Preparing People to Change Addictive Behavior. New York, 1991.

72. Perkins K. Maintaining smoking abstinence after myocardial infarction. *J Subst Abuse* 1988;1:91–107.

73. Wei H, Young D. Effect of clonidine on cigarette cessation and in the alleviation of withdrawal symptoms. *Br J Addic* 1988;83:1221–1226.

27 Critical Pathways for Acute Coronary Syndromes

Christopher P. Cannon, MD and
Patrick T. O'Gara, MD

INTRODUCTION

Critical pathways are standardized protocols for the management of specific diseases that aim to optimize and streamline patient care *(1,2)*. Other names used for such programs are "clinical pathways" or simply "protocols" such as acute myocardial infarction (AMI) protocols used in the emergency department (ED) to reduce time to treatment with thrombolysis *(3)*. "True" critical pathways list in great detail all processes of care and potential inefficiencies for medical procedures such as coronary artery bypass surgery *(2)*. Some pathways are treatment recommendations and algorithms focusing on improving compliance with evidence-based medicine and have more relevance in the ambulatory setting (e.g., hypertension or hyperlipidemia) *(4)*. Critical pathways were first developed for business and industry as a tool to streamline production processes *(5)*. When applied to medicine, critical pathways initially were seen as a means to reduce length of hospitalization, but soon were recognized as an important tool for improving quality of care.

Goals of Critical Pathways

Use of "critical pathways" is currently growing rapidly primarily as a means of reducing hospital length of stay. However, several other components can be added to critical pathways, with the overall goal of improving patient care. These other goals focus on improving the use of appropriate treatments and on facilitating patient triage to the appropriate level of care (Table 1). In addition, limiting unnecessary tests can reduce costs and allow money to be spent on other treatments that have been shown to be beneficial.

NEED FOR CRITICAL PATHWAYS

For patients with acute coronary syndromes (ACS), critical pathways are needed because many patients do not receive evidence-based therapies. In addition, there is a wide variation in using procedures as well. Aspirin, heparin, and beta-blockers have been shown to improve outcomes in ACS, and their use was recommended in national guidelines released in 1994 and 2000 *(6,7)*. However, the National Registry of Myocardial Infarction (NRMI) showed that among 240,989 MI patients receiving thrombolytic

From: *Contemporary Cardiology: Management of Acute Coronary Syndromes, Second Edition*
Edited by: C. P. Cannon © Humana Press Inc., Totowa, NJ

Table 1
Goals of ACS Critical Pathways

1. Reducing time-to-treatment with reperfusion therapy.
2. Increase use of recommended medications (e.g., aspirin).
3. Decrease use of unnecessary tests/procedures.
4. Provide guidance on timing of cardiac procedures.
5. Reduce hospital, intensive care unit, and emergency department length of stay.
6. Increase participation in clinical research protocols.
7. Provide a framework for collecting information and feeding it back to clinicians and others (Continuous Quality Improvement).
8. Improve patient care and decrease costs.

therapy, only 87% received aspirin, and only 63% of patients with non-ST-segment elevation MI received aspirin (8). Similarly, in the Cooperative Cardiovascular Project, among patients fully eligible to receive aspirin (i.e., no contraindications to aspirin such as bleeding ulcer), only 80% of patients received aspirin (9). In the Thrombolysis In Myocardial Infarction (TIMI) III and Global Unstable Angina Registry And Treatment Evaluation (GUARANTEE) registries of unstable angina and non-ST-segment elevation MI, only 80% of patients received aspirin (10,11).

Another example of underutilization of medications concerns fibrinolysis. It has been suggested that only 25–30% of patients with acute MI receive thrombolysis. However, thrombolytic therapy is only beneficial in patients with STEMI (12). In the TIMI 9 Registry of patients with STEMI, 69% of patients received either thrombolysis (60%) or primary percutaneous coronary intervention (PCI) (9%) (13). Of those who presented to the hospital within 12 h of the onset of pain, 75% received reperfusion therapy (13). Similar findings have been reported in NRMI (14). Thus, despite a reasonable percentage of patients receiving reperfusion therapy for STEMI, opportunities for improvement exist, with the ultimate goal of extending the benefits of reperfusion therapy to all patients with STEMI.

Underutilization of most other guideline-recommended medications also has been observed. In the TIMI 9 Registry of STEMI, 91% of patients received heparin, and beta-blockers were given to 61% (13). In patients who developed congestive heart failure or had documented left ventricular (LV) dysfunction post MI, only 39% were treated with angiotensin-converting enzyme (ACE) inhibitors at hospital discharge. In the TIMI III and GUARANTEE registries of UA/NSTEMI, intravenous heparin was used in 60% of patients and beta-blocker therapy was also underused (10,11).

HOSPITAL AND ICU LENGTH OF STAY

Other opportunities for improvement in ACS are hospital length of stay and utilization of intensive care (ICU) and coronary care units (CCU). Hospital length of stay for ACS have ranged from 8 to 9 d in registries in the mid 1990s (10). Among patients treated with thrombolysis for STEMI, similar observations have been made. In GUSTO-I, the median length of stay was 9 d (15). In a follow-up analysis, which divided patients into those who had an uncomplicated course (no recurrent ischemia, congestive heart failure, or any other complication) vs any one of these complications, the median length of stay for both groups was 9 d (16). In the TIMI 9 Registry conducted in 1995, for uncomplicated patients with STEMI the median length of stay was 8 d *(17)*. Thus, it appears that length of stay has been long in all patients with acute coronary syndromes, and opportunities exist to safely reduce this length of stay, especially in low-risk patients.

A decade ago, admission to the CCU was standard for patients with unstable angina and MI. In the GUARANTEE registry, 40% of patients with unstable angina and non-ST-segment elevation MI were admitted to the CCU *(11)*. Current recommendations are to restrict CCU admissions to patients at higher risk (STEMI, hemodynamic compromise, or other complications) *(7,18)*.

Under- and Overutilization of Cardiac Procedures

Another area for potential improvement is in the use of cardiac procedures following admission for acute MI and unstable angina. Wide variation has been observed, especially between the United States and other countries. In acute STEMI, numerous studies have found wide differences in the use of cardiac procedures but no difference in mortality *(19,20)*. These data suggest that there may be unnecessary procedures performed in some patients; however, more contemporary trials are warranted to define this issue better.

On the other hand, in UA/STEMI, the recent FRISC II and TACTICS-TIMI 18 trials have shown a benefit of an early invasive strategy in intermediate- and high-risk patients *(21,22)*. In patients with positive troponin at admission, there is a 40-50% reduction in death or MI through 6–12 mo follow-up *(23)*. Because approx 60% of patients have positive cardiac markers *(23)*, this would mean that these patients should undergo procedures. In addition, for the remaining troponin-negative patients, a conservative strategy does involve catheterization and revascularization in patients who have recurrent ischemia. Thus, nearly three-quarters of patients with UA/NSTEMI are appropriate candidates for an early invasive strategy. Because current rates of catheterization are lower (approx 30% in Europe and Canada and 55 60% in the United States), in this population, based on current evidence of benefit in higher-risk patients, more patients should be undergoing cardiac catheterization procedures.

Thus, based on variations in care and the need to improve quality while reducing unnecessary use of resources, a strong rationale exists for using critical pathways in the management of ACS.

Emerging Evidence that Critical Pathway can improve care

Performance data on critical pathways in cardiology are beginning to emerge showing that these pathways can lead to improved outcomes. Several studies that have evaluated critical pathways in cardiac surgery demonstrated that they reduce length of stay and costs *(24)*. Studies of chest pain protocols have shown that they reduce length of stay, the number of patients with missed MIs, the number of hospital admissions, and, importantly, overall costs *(25–28)*.

For STEMI, several studies have reported that a standardized pathway or protocol can significantly decrease door-to-drug time by up to 50% *(29,30)*. Two studies have similarly show that quality improvement efforts and implementation of critical pathways can significantly reduce door-to-balloon time *(31,32)*. In one study, this reduction in door-to-balloon time was accompanied by a reduction in mortality *(31)*.

The Guidelines Applied in Practice (GAP) Project of the ACC was implemented in 10 hospitals in Michigan and led to improvements in several performance measures. The GAP Investigators put together materials designed to make it easier for hospitals to implement the ACC/AHA AMI guidelines in clinical practice. These materials included a critical pathway, standard orders, pocket cards, chart stickers, and patient handouts. Implementation of the protocols and pathways led to improvements in utilization of appropriate medications: beta-blocker use rose from 65% of patients to 77%, aspirin use in the hospital from 76% to 87%, and the use of aspirin at discharge from 81% to 93% *(33)*.

Another hospital-based quality improvement program, the Cardiac Hospital Atherosclerosis Management Program (CHAMP), used a treatment algorithm to increase utilization of aspirin, beta blockers, ACE inhibitors, and statins for secondary prevention *(4)*. These investigators were able to dramatically improve compliance with secondary prevention measures, and were able to show improve achievement of cholesterol lowering to a goal of low density lipoprotein (LDL) cholesterol <100 mg/dL. Importantly, these improvements in the quality of care were associated with a lower rate of death or MI *(4)*.

Improving the Cost-Effectiveness of Care

Several randomized studies have shown that one means of improving the cost-effectiveness of care is to reduce hospital length of stay. In STEMI, identification of low-risk patients has led to the possibility of early hospital discharge for patients with an uncomplicated course. A pilot trial of such a strategy in 80 patients suggested that hospital stay and costs could be significantly reduced without an increase in complications *(34)*. In the Primary Angioplasty in Myocardial Infarction (PAMI) - 2 trial, 471 low-risk patients were randomized to a strategy of early discharge or to conventional hospital discharge *(35)*. Clinical outcomes at 6 mo were similar in both groups: 0.8 vs 0.4% mortality for early discharge vs standard care ($p = 1.0$), unstable angina 10.1 vs 12.0% ($p = $ NS), recurrent MI 0.8 vs 0.4% ($p = $ NS), or the combination of death, unstable angina, MI, congestive heart failure or stroke, 15.2 vs 17.5% $p = 0.49$) *(35)*. On the other hand, hospital length of stay was 3 d shorter (4.2 d vs 7.1 d, $p = 0.0001$) and hospital costs were lower ($9,658 \pm $5,287 vs $11,604 \pm 6,125, p = 0.002$) *(35)*. Thus, a strategy of acute catheterization and primary PCI allowed identification of low risk patients. Early discharge was safe and resulted in substantial reduction in hospital length of stay and cost savings.

BRIGHAM AND WOMEN'S HOSPITAL ACUTE CORONARY SYNDROME PATHWAYS

An overview of our critical pathways for acute coronary syndromes is shown in Fig. 1. There are two pathways for the different types of syndromes: two for acute STEMI patients (one for fibrinolysis and one for primary angioplasty), two for UA/NSTEMI (one for high-risk and one for low-risk patients), and two for patients with chest pain of unclear etiology (ED-based rule out MI pathways).

STEMI Critical Pathway

The critical pathway for all acute coronary syndromes begins immediately with the triage nurse who brings patients with chest pain into an "acute" room of the ED. A brief

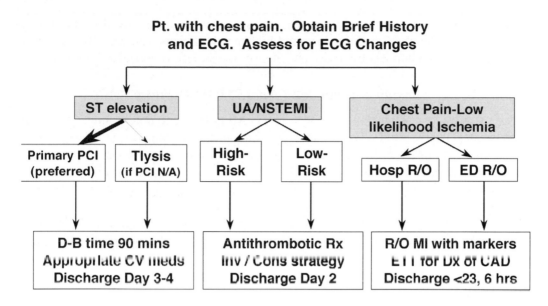

Fig. 1. Critical pathways for acute coronary syndromes at Brigham and Women's Hospital.

history is obtained and electrocardiogram performed. If ST segment elevation is present, the patient is immediately evaluated for reperfusion therapy. Based on the wealth of data showing superiority of primary PCI over thrombolysis *(36–39)*, primary PCI is the preferred strategy. Because of the importance of door-to-balloon time *(40)*, if there are extenuating circumstances (e.g., severe snow storm) and the time for the cardiac catheterization team to be available and perform the procedure is long, immediate thrombolysis would be carried out, so as to achieve more rapid reperfusion.

For the primary PCI pathway, the transfer of the patient to the cardiac catheterization laboratory has been found in two studies to be the longest part of the overall door-to-balloon time *(31,32)*, and thus we have focused on reducing this transfer time by having a single pager to call the cath lab personnel. Low-risk patients are admitted to the step-down unit after PCI in accord with the PAMI-II trial *(35)*. Primary stenting is common, as is the use of IIb/IIIa inhibition, usually with eptifibatide. No additional stress testing is performed except if patients have evidence of significant coronary stenoses in the non-infarct-related arteries. Discharge is targeted for hospital day 3 or 4 depending on the extent of infarction.

For the thrombolysis pathway, the goal is to start the thrombolytic drug in <30 min from arrival in the ED *(3)*. The second goal of the pathway (begun in the ED but continued in the CCU) is to treat the patient with all other appropriate medications, such as aspirin, an antithrombin (which is now specified as the low-molecular-weight heparin enoxaparin) *(41,42)*, anti-ischemic, and cholesterol-lowering medications. Patients are treated in the ED and admitted to the CCU. Low-risk patients are transferred out of the CCU after 24 h, whereas other are transferred after 2 d. Risk stratification is the next goal of the pathway. Rescue angioplasty is performed for patients who have evidence of ongoing symptoms and ST segment elevation. Otherwise, patients are treated according to the TIMI IIB conservative strategy *(43)*, with cardiac catheterization performed for ischemia or a positive stress test, the latter being performed on hospital d 3 or 5 for low- and higher-risk patients, respectively. Echocardiography is recommended for most patients to assess left ventricular function.

Unstable Angina and Non-STEMI Pathway

The pathway for unstable angina and non-STEMI at Brigham and Women's Hospital emphasizes (1) early relief of ischemic pain, which has been found to be a determinant of development of myocardial infarction (44); (2) administration of antithrombotic and anti-ischemic therapy; (3) reminders of eligibility criteria of ongoing clinical trials; (4) suggested list of blood tests in an effort to reduce unnecessary studies; (5) a recommendation for an early invasive or conservative strategy.

Patient eligibility for our pathway is based on clinical criteria for UA/NSTEMI, i.e., patients who present with typical angina at rest or with minimal exertion. It is felt that broad entry criteria are warranted to allow the pathway to benefit potentially as many patients as possible.

RISK STRATIFICATION

The presence of ST segment deviation (either depression or transient ST elevation) is a strong marker of high risk for adverse outcomes. Of note, ST change of 0.5 mm appears to have equal significance to ST depression of 1 mm or more (45,46). Because only a third of patients presenting with unstable angina have ECG changes (45), the admission diagnosis relies predominantly on the history. Similarly, benefit of more aggressive therapies is greatest in patients with ST segment changes (22,47).

CARDIAC MARKERS

The pathway includes three CK-MB and Troponin I determinations drawn at baseline, 8 and 16 h. Because serial troponin values have been found to improve the sensitivity of detecting high risk patients (without ST elevation) (48), we have included these in the pathway. As noted below, this is helpful in determining a high-risk group in whom IIb/IIIa inhibitors would have the greatest benefit (49,50).

TIMI RISK SCORE

The TIMI risk score was developed using multivariate analysis to predict the occurrence of death, MI, or recurrent ischemia leading to urgent revascularization in the TIMI 11B trial (51). Seven independent risk factors emerged: age $\geq$65 years, $\geq$3 risk factors for CAD, documented coronary artery disease at catheterization, prior ASA, $\geq$2 episodes of angina in last 24 h, ST deviation $\geq$0.5 mm, and elevated cardiac markers (Fig. 2). Use of this scoring system was able to risk stratify patients across a 10-fold gradient of risk, from 4.7 to 40.9% (p $<$ 0.001) (51). More important, the relative benefit of the newer therapies (enoxaparin vs unfractionated heparin, tirofiban vs heparin, and an invasive vs conservative strategy) were all seen to increase as the risk increased (22,51,52). Thus, these findings emphasize the importance of risk stratification as the first task in evaluating patients who present with UA/NSTEMI (7).

In our Emergency Department order set, we have incorporated all these three markers of risk, ST segment changes, positive troponin or CK-MB, and the TIMI Risk score to determine two pathways: a high-risk and a low-risk pathway.

1. **Age ≥ 65 years**

2. **≥ 3 CAD Risk Factors
    (↑ chol, FHx, HTN, DM, smoking)**

3. **Prior CAD (cath stenosis >50%)**

4. **ASA in last 7 days**

5. **≥ 2 Anginal events ≤ 24 hours**

6. **ST deviation**

7. **Elevated Cardiac Markers (CK-MB or Troponin)**

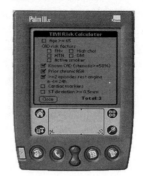

Fig. 2. Risk stratification with the TIMI Risk Score.

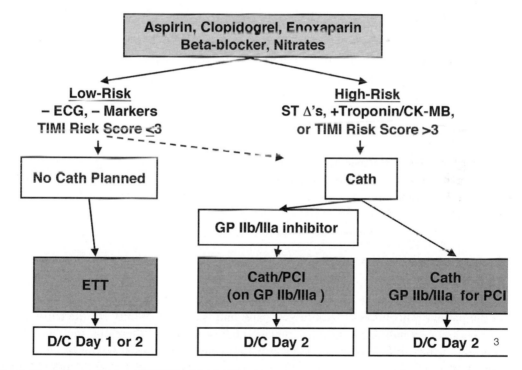

Fig. 3. Unstable angina/non-STEMI critical pathway.

MEDICAL MANAGEMENT

As shown in Fig. 3, initial management in both pathways is with aspirin, beta-blockers, and nitrates to control ischemic pain. Intravenous nitroglycerin is used if pain persists despite three sublingual nitroglycerin tablets. Calcium antagonists are used if needed to control ischemia after these agents are at optimal therapeutic doses.

Most recently, we have added clopidogrel and enoxaparin to the initial treatment of all patients, and have added glycoprotein IIb/IIIa inhibitors for patients in the high-risk pathway *(53)*. Clopidogrel plus aspirin was found to reduce cardiovascular death, MI, or stroke by 20% compared with aspirin alone *(54)*, a reduction that was seen in all subgroups, including patients with or without ST segment changes, and in those with positive or negative markers. A benefit of pretreatment with clopidogrel was seen in patients who went on to PCI, with a significant 30% reduction in death or MI at both 30 d, and through follow-up *(55)*.

Our pathway recommends glycoprotein llb/IIIa inhibitors to be used for high-risk patients, especially those with positive troponin *(49,50,56,57)*. Four studies have each shown a 50–70% reduction in death or MI in troponin-positive patients receiving glycoprotein IIb/IIIa inhibition compared with aspirin and heparin alone *(49,50,56,57)*. In contrast, those with a negative troponin have no benefit of GP IIb/IIIa inhibition compared with aspirin and heparin. Similar findings have been found with the TIMI Risk Score *(52)*. Diabetics also are a high-risk group who appear to have a mortality benefit fro IIb/IIIa inhibition *(58)*.

For enoxaparin, it has similarly been found that it is beneficial over unfractionated heparin in only high-risk patients *(51,59)*, but its ease of use, and the simplicity for the ED to have one standard antithrombin regimen for all ACS patients have enabled this to become the standard antithrombin in our new 2002 pathway.

The choice of an invasive vs conservative strategy is based also on risk: with an early invasive strategy in the high-risk pathway and the choice of a conservative or invasive strategy for the low-risk pathway *(22)*. In the high-risk pathway, catheterization is carried out immediately from the ED if the patient is having ongoing pain despite medical therapy, or later the same day if scheduling permits. Otherwise, it is carried out the following day. Based on the anatomic findings, revascularization is carried out as appropriate.

In the low-risk pathways, an early conservative strategy involves aggressive medical management, clinical monitoring, and non-invasive testing. In addition, if a patient is admitted with chest pain, but has an unclear diagnosis of coronary artery disease, a *diagnostic* stress test is done.

SECONDARY PREVENTION AND FOLLOW-UP

Because follow-up is critical, we ensure that both a phone call and a letter summarizing the hospital events are sent to the primary care physician and cardiologist caring for the patient. This allows continuity of care, and is an opportunity for the cardiologist to provide a rationale for long-term management with key medications such as aspirin, clopidogrel, beta-blockers, and cholesterol-lowering medications. Given the long-term benefit of aspirin in secondary prevention as well as that of clopidogrel in both CAPRIE and CURE *(60,61)*, the combination of aspirin and clopidogrel is recommended for most patients, with treatment for at least 1 y based on CURE.

Similarly beta-blockers are recommended for long-term management in all patients without contraindications. Given the results of the Heart Outcomes Prevention Evaluation (HOPE) trial *(62)*, ACE inhibitors should be considered at discharge. Cholesterol-lowering therapy is a key component of a long-term secondary prevention program and is recommended *(63–65)*. Follow-up care with the primary care physician to achieve an LDL less than 100 mg/dL is recommended by the National Cholesterol Education Program (NCEP-3) *(66)*.

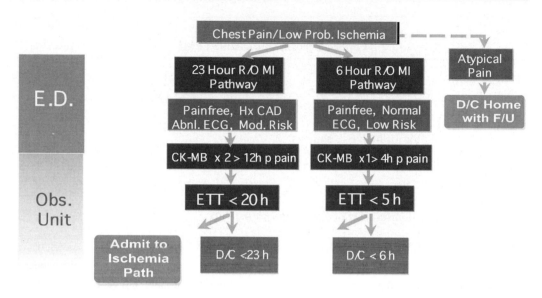

Fig. 4. "Rule-out MI" critical pathways.

Smoking cessation is a critical point of emphasis during hospitalization and at the time of discharge. Currently all cardiac patients are screened for current smoking, and are educated by trained nurses and given follow-up information about our smoking cessation classes and program. Finally cardiac rehabilitation is a key component following acute coronary syndromes. For patients with severe limitation of exercise capacity such as the very elderly, transfer to a rehabilitation facility is arranged, especially following CABG when needed. Patients are approached for participation in a cardiac rehabilitation program, either at our hospital or one near to their home. All patients receive a booklet outlining an exercise program and its outline is briefly reviewed by the cardiologist and the nurse.

"Rule-Out MI Pathways"

For the large population of patients without ECG changes, patients are risk stratified: Patients, with clearly atypical pain, not suggestive of ischemia, are discharged home with follow-up to their primary physicians (Fig. 4). The remaining patients with pain possibly suggestive of ischemia are observed in the ED. If stable, these patients undergo early exercise testing to determine the burden of ischemia. If positive, the patients are admitted for further evaluation and treatment. If negative, they are discharged home (ideally within 6 h of ED arrival) with follow-up by their physicians *(25)*.

FORMAT

The format of the pathways has evolved from a several page pathway listing all the indications, contraindications, and doses for each medicine (e.g. fibrinolytic therapy, heparin, beta-blockers) *(29,67–69)*, to a one-page document with all five pathways, each in a simple "checklist" format (Table 2) *(68)*. This checklist format was developed in order to simply the pathway and increase its usability—and use. The design is such that it serves as a quick reminder of the key medications to consider and tests to perform. In

Table 2
Cardiac Checklist for UA/NSTEMI

Medications:	
1. Aspirin	–
2. Clopidogrel	–
3. Heparin (or LMWH)	–
4. GP IIb/IIIa inhibitor for high risk patients	–
5. Beta-blocker	–
6. Nitrate	–
7. ACE inhibitor	–
Interventions:	
8. Cath/revascularization for intermediate high-risk patients	–
Secondary prevention:	
9. Cholesterol: check + treat as needed	–
10. Treat other risk factors (smoking)	–

From Cannon CP. Critical pathway for unstable angina and non-ST elevation myocardial infarction. February 2002. Crit Path Cardiol 2002;1:12–21, with permission

this way, a busy ED physician could use the pathway rapidly to improve care, but the pathway would not be a burden of paperwork for the physician. We have similarly developed a checklist for use at the time of hospital discharge. This "cardiac checklist" could be used in two ways: physicians could keep a copy on a small index card in their pocket, and run down the list when writing admission orders for patients, or it could be used in developing standard orders for an MI patient, either printed order sheets or computerized orders, which the physician can choose from when admitting a patient to the hospital.

We have recently developed a Palm Pilot program for these cardiac checklists to make them even more accessible at the bedside (70). The newest type of tool is the TIMI Risk Calculator developed for the Palm handheld device (Fig. 2). This tool is interactive and allows physicians to calculate the TIMI Risk Score for an individual patient. It then provides outcomes for the patient from several large trials and shows the benefits of new therapies, notably clopidogrel, enoxaparin, GP IIb/IIIa inhibition, and an early invasive strategy, all tailored to the patient's risk. The Palm Pilot program also provides the recommendation from the ACC/AHA UA/NSTEMI Guideline for management of the patient based on his/her risk score. The newest version includes the STEMI risk scores in addition to the UA/NSTEMI risk score (see www.timi.org).

We have also created standardized order sets for the ED physician and nurse to use utilizing much the same format (Fig. 5). Because all medications and other orders are now entered electronically—having a template with the critical pathway ensures that the physician sees the checklist of orders. The physician simply chooses a pathway based on the clinical diagnosis and clicks on the medications he or she wishes. It is hoped that this system, which guarantees that physicians will see the critical pathway for every patient, will further increase the use of evidence-based medications. A complete set of hospital admission orders also exists.

HOW TO DEVELOP A CRITICAL PATHWAY

In order to develop or update a pathway at your hospital, it is worthwile to consider the three phases of a critical pathway: pathway development, implementation, and

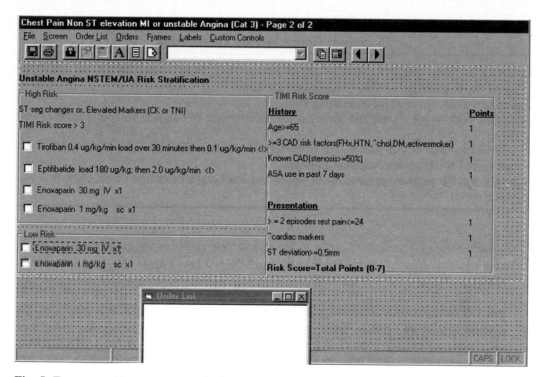

Fig. 5. Emergency Department standard orderset for unstable angina (page 2 is shown with some components of antithrombotic therapy).

Table 3
Approach to Critical Pathways

1. Pathway development
2. Implementation
3. Maintenance
   Collect and monitor data on pathway performance
   Periodically modify or update pathway as needed

maintenance (continuous quality improvement) (Table 3). Developing a pathway is itself a five-step process (Table 4): to first identify the problem, then assemble the team, assess the existing process, review the data, disseminate a draft pathway for input and revision to final pathway. The details of each step are outlined below:

1. **Identify the problem**. Development of a pathway begins with identifying the problem, such as underuse of newly available effective therapies (clopidogrel, GP IIb/IIIa inhibitors, and LMWH) and underutilization of existing therapies (aspirin, heparin, and beta blockers) for ACS patients. Another problem to be considered in STEMI patients is the timeliness of repefusion therapy. This measure will now be monitored by the Joint Commission of Accredidation of Hospital Organization, beginning in July 2002.
2. **Assemble the team**. The team should be multidisciplinary and include representatives from all groups that would be affected by the pathways and whose buy-in would be

Table 4
The Steps in Critical Pathway Development

1. Define problems (practice variation, excess resource use, failure to provide known evidence-based therapies,delays in time to reperfusion therapy).
2. Create a pathway (or adapt an existing one).
3. Form a working committee/task force for the development of optimal guidelines for medical care.
4. Distribute a draft critical pathway to all personnel and departments involved. Revise the pathway to reach a best consensus approach.
5. Implement the pathway, preferably via a pilot test involving a prominent, local clinical champion(s).

needed for implementation. This would include representatives from cardiology (interventional and noninterventional), emergency medicine, nursing, cardiac surgery, noninvasive laboratory, pharmacy, cardiac rehabilitation, social service, case management, and dietary service (71). A smaller group can be useful to do the initial draft. At Virginia Commonwealth University/Medical College of Virginia, organization of a multidisciplinary Acute Cardiac Team (ACT) was one of the key elements in the success of chest pain critical pathways (27). This was a multidisciplinary team of emergency physicians, cardiologists, and laboratory and nursing staff who participated in the decision making.

3. **Assess the existing process**. This step first involves an assessment of current ED and cardiology practice for ACS. The committee should undertake an inventory of procedures, protocols, and pathways currently in place. Some committees may want to undertake a more detailed analysis, consisting of a review of medical records to identify critical intermediate outcomes, rate-limiting steps, and high-cost areas on which to focus their efforts (2).

4. **Review the data**. The committee should review the literature to identify best practices and optimal processes of care. For ACS, new guidelines from the ACC/AHA and new studies define the optimal therapies and approach to risk stratification and management strategies (72). In brief, the ACC/AHA guidelines provide specific recommendations for early risk stratification, immediate medical management, and hospital care of patients with ACS. These guidelines provide a clinical risk stratification algorithm, review the role of the ECG, serum markers such as troponins, and functional testing, and outline an Acute Ischemia Pathway. Recommendations for anti-ischemic therapy and antithrombotic therapy are spelled out, as are the indications for early invasive or early conservative management strategies.

5. **Determine the pathway format and disseminate a draft pathway**. Although the format of a critical pathway may vary, an important feature is a time task matrix in which specific tasks are organized along a timeline (2). There is a spectrum of pathways ranging from a form that takes the place of the medical record to a simple checklist. Critical pathways may help reduce charting in more complicated situations. If the pathway format is too difficult to follow, it will not be used.

Reviewing the draft pathway with the committee and getting buy-in from all parties is an important step. With the many constituencies, it is important to have respect for everyone's perspective. Consensus meetings obtain buy-in from all parties involved with acceptance of the pathway components. To maximize the impact of the first announce-ment, the rollout should take a "Big Bang" approach.

PATHWAY IMPLEMENTATION

Implementing the pathway can be challenging and, if not handled well, can lead to barriers to utilization. All staff involved in any component of the pathway must be edu-cated about it; this includes non-participants who may be affected by the pathway. Mis-conceptions need to be dispelled. Questions about repercussions from failure to follow the pathway should be addressed. Roles and responsibilities must be clearly defined for all staff involved in implementation of the pathway *(2)*.

Pathways may be implemented in several ways. The pathway may be sent to physi-cians and nurses and presented at appropriate staff meetings, with implementation depending on voluntary participation. Another means of encouraging pathway use would be e-mail reminders triggered by admission diagnosis or monthly reminders to physicians and nurses. Or there could be independent screening of all admissions with copies of the pathway placed in the chart. Some hospitals have used designated case managers to evaluate each patient and ensure that the pathway is carried out. This obvi-ously has the drawback of requiring additional resources from the hospital.

An effective method of implementing a pathway is to release it in the form of a set of standard orders. Standard orders may be printed for use in the ED or in an electronic format. Tools such as wall chart, pocket cards, and simple checklists appear to be the key to successful implementation of critical pathways *(73)*.

PATHWAY MAINTENANCE

Along with putting the pathway in place, a continuous quality improvement (CQI) process should be instituted to monitor the pathway's use and effectiveness. Data must be collected and analyzed and processes refined to achieve the improvement in outcomes and resource utilization *(2)*. The continuous quality improvement team could present data at monthly multidisciplinary continuous quality improvement case conferences; CCU morning rounds; monthly ED cardiac case reviews; and Grand Rounds presentations. The frequency of such meetings should be tailored to the institution.

The monitoring of data can be through established registries such as the National Registry of Myocardial Infarction (NRMI) or newer initiatives such as the AHA's Get With the Guidelines program or the Can Rapid Risk Stratification of Unstable Angina Patients Suppress Adverse Outcomes with Early Implementation of the ACC/AHA Guidelines (CRUSADE) program. Alternatively, a more streamlined registry form can be a helpful tool to assist with a regular review process. As part of the maintenance process, the team should be reviewing new therapies and treatments and considering modification or updating of the pathway to improve it and keep it current.

CONCLUSION

Use of critical pathways is currently growing rapidly. They offer great potential for both reducing hospital length of stay and costs and improving patient care. A growing number of well conducted randomized trials and other studies have shown that they are effective in improving the quality of care in ACS. Having standardized approaches with simple "checklists" to ensure appropriate care is given appears to lead to a significant improvement in the outcomes of ACS patients. After development of pathways, it is important to monitor their performance to ensure that they meet the overall goal of reducing costs while improving quality of patient care. It is our belief that this goal can be achieved.

REFERENCES

1. Cannon CP, O'Gara PT. Critical pathways in acute coronary syndromes. In Cannon CP, ed. Management of Acute Coronary Syndromes. Totowa: Humana Press, 1999:611–627.
2. Every NR, Hochman J, Becker R, Kopecky S, Cannon CP, for the Committee on Acute Cardiac Care; Council of Clinical Cardiology; American Heart Association. Critical pathways : A review. An AHA Scientific Statement. Circulation 2000;101:461–465.
3. National Heart Attack Alert Program Coordinating Committee—60 Minutes to Treatment Working Group. Emergency department: rapid identification and treatment of patients with acute myocardial infarction. Ann Emerg Med 1994;23:311–329.
4. Fonarow GC, Gawlinski A, Moughrabi S, Tillisch JH. Improved treatment of coronary heart disease by implementation of a Cardiac Hospitalization Atherosclerosis Management Program (CHAMP). Am J Cardiol 2001;87:819–822.
5. Pearson SD, Goulart-Fisher D, Lee TH. Critical pathways as a strategy for improving care: problems and potential. Ann Intern Med 1995;123:941–948.
6. Braunwald E, Mark DB, Jones RH, et al. Unstable Angina: Diagnosis and Management. Clinical Practice Guideline Number 10. Rockville, MD: Agency for Health Care Policy and Research and the National Heart, Lung, and Blood Institute, Public Health Service, U.S. Department of Health and Human Services, 1994.
7. Braunwald E, Antman EM, Beasley JW, et al. ACC/AHA guidelines for the management of patients with unstable angina and non-ST segment elevation myocardial infarction: a report of the American College of Cardiology/American Heart Association Task Force on Practice Guidelines (Committee on the Management of Unstable Angina and Non-ST Segment Elevation Myocardial Infarction). J Am Coll Cardiol 2000;36:970–1056.
8. Rogers WJ, Bowlby LJ, Chandra NC, et al. Treatment of myocardial infarction in the United States (1990 to 1993). Observations from the National Registry of Myocardial Infarction. Circulation 1994; 90:2103–2114.
9. Ellerbeck EF, Jencks SF, Radford MJ, et al. Quality of care for medicare patients with acute myocardial infarction. A four-state pilot study from the Cooperative Cardiovascular Project. JAMA 1995;273: 1509–1514.
10. Stone PH, Thompson B, Anderson HV, et al. Influence of race, sex, and age on management of unstable angina and non-Q-wave myocardial infarction: The TIMI III Registry. JAMA 1996;275:1104–1112.
11. Scirica BM, Moliterno DJ, Every NR, et al. Differences between men and women in the management of unstable angina pectoris (The GUARANTEE Registry). Am J Cardiol 1999;84:1145–1150.
12. Fibrinolytic Therapy Trialists' (FTT) Collaborative Group. Indications for fibrinolytic therapy in suspected acute myocardial infarction: collaborative overview of early mortality and major morbidity results from all randomised trials of more than 1000 patients. Lancet 1994;343:311–322.
13. Cannon CP, Bahit MC, Haugland JM, et al. Underutilization of evidence-based medications in acute ST elevation myocardial infarction: Results of the Thrombolysis in Myocardial Infarction (TIMI) 9 Registry. Crit Path Cardiol 2002;1:44–52.
14. Barron HV, Bowlby LJ, Breen T, et al. Use of reperfusion therapy for acute myocardial infarction in the United States: data from the National Registry of Myocardial Infarction 2. Circulation 1998;97: 1150–1156.
15. The GUSTO Investigators. An international randomized trial comparing four thrombolytic strategies for acute myocardial infarction. N Engl J Med 1993;329:673–682.
16. Newby LK, Califf RM, Guerci A, et al. Early discharge in the thrombolytic era: an analysis of criteria for uncomplicated infarction from the Global Utilization of Streptokinase and t-PA for Occluded Coronary Arteries (GUSTO) trial. J Am Coll Cardiol 1996;27:625–632.

17. Bahit MC, Cannon CP, Antman EM, et al. Critical pathway for acute ST-segment elevation myocardial infarction: evaluation of the potential impact in the TIMI 9 Registry. Crit Path Cardiol 2002;1:107–112.

18. Ryan KA, Rizzo M, Kelley MB, et al. Relationship between the presence and duration of chest pain and blood flow at 90 minutes following thrombolytic administration. J Am Coll Cardiol 1999;33 (Suppl. A):375A.

19. Rouleau JL, Moye LA, Pfeffer MA, et al. A comparison of management patterns after acute myocardial infarction in Canada and the United States. N Engl J Med 1993;328:779–784.

20. Every NR, Larson EB, Litwin PE, et al. The association between on-site cardiac catheterization facilities and the use of coronary angiography after acute myocardial infarction. N Engl J Med 1993;329: 546–551.

21. FRagmin and Fast Revascularisation during InStability in Coronary artery disease Investigators. Invasive compared with non-invasive treatment in unstable coronary-artery disease: FRISC II prospective randomised multicentre study. Lancet 1999;354:708–715.

22. Cannon CP, Weintraub WS, Demopoulos LA, et al. Comparison of early invasive and conservative strategies in patients with unstable coronary syndromes treated with the glycoprotein IIb/IIIa inhibitor tirofiban. N Engl J Med 2001;344:1879–1887.

23. Morrow DA, Cannon CP, Rifai N, et al. Ability of minor elevations of troponin I and T to predict benefit from an early invasive strategy in patients with unstable angina and non-ST elevation myocardial infarction: Results from a randomized trial. JAMA 2001;286:2405–2412.

24. Velasco FT, Ko W, Rosengart T, et al. Cost containment in cardiac surgery: results with a critical path way for coronary bypass surgery at the New York hospital-Cornell Medical Center. Best Pract Benchmarking Healthc 1996,1.21 28.

25. Nichol G, Walls R, Goldman L, et al. A critical pathway for management of patient with acute chest pain at low risk for myocardial ischemia: Recommendations and potential impact. Ann Intern Med 1997;127:996–1005.

26. Graff LG, Dallara J, Ross MA, et al. Impact on the care of the emergency department chest pain patient from the Chest Pain Evaluation Registry (CHEPER) Study. Am J Cardiol 1997;80:563–568.

27. Tatum JL, Jesse RL, Kontos MC, et al. Comprehensive strategy for the evaluation and triage of the chest pain patient. Ann Emerg Med 1997;29:116–125.

28. Farkouh ME, Smars PA, Reeder GS, et al. A clinical trial of a chest-pain observation unit for patients with unstable angina. Chest Pain Evaluation in the Emergency Room (CHEER) Investigators. N Engl J Med 1998;339:1882–1888.

29. Cannon CP, Johnson EB, Cermignani M, Scirica BM, Sagarin MJ, Walls RM. Emergency department thrombolysis critical pathway reduces door-to-drug times in acute myocardial infarction. Clin Cardiol 1999;22:17–22.

30. Pell ACH, Miller HC, Robertson CE, Fox KAA. Effect of "fast track" admission for acute myocardial infarction on delay to thrombolysis. BMJ 1992;304:83–87.

31. Caputo RP, Ho KK, Stoler RC, et al. Effect of continuous quality improvement analysis on the delivery of primary percutaneous transluminal coronary angioplasty for acute myocardial infarction. Am J Cardiol 1997;79:1159–1164.

32. Ward MR, Lo ST, Herity NA, Lee DP, Yeung AC. Effect of audit on door-to-inflation times in primary angioplasty/stenting for acute myocardial infarction. Am J Cardiol 2001;87:336–338.

33. Mehta RH, Montoye CK, Gallogly M, et al. Improving quality of care of acute myocardial infarction: The Guideline Applied in Practice (GAP) Initiative in Southeast Michigan. JAMA 2002;287:1269–1276.

34. Topol EJ, Bure K, O'Neill WW, et al. A randomized controlled trial of hospital discharge three days after myocardial infarciton in the era of reperfusion. N Engl J Med 1988;318.1083–1088.

35. Grines CL, Marsalese DL, Brodie B, et al. Safety and cost-effectiveness of early discharge after primary angioplasty in low risk patients with acute myocardial infarction. J Am Coll Cardiol 1998;31:967–972.

36. Weaver WD, Simes RJ, Betriu A, et al. Comparison of primary coronary angioplasty and intravenous thrombolytic therapy of acute myocardial infarction. A quantitative review. JAMA 1997;278: 2093–2098.

37. Andersen HR. Danish Trial in Acute Myocardial Infarction (DANAMI) -2. American College of Cardiology Scientific Sessions. Atlanta, 2002.

38. Aversano T, Aversano LT, Passamani ER, et al. Thrombolytic therapy vs primary percutaneous coronary intervention for myocardial infarction in patients presenting to hospitals without on-site cardiac surgery: a randomized controlled trial. JAMA 2002;287:1943–51.

39. Cannon CP. Primary percutaneous coronary intervention for all? JAMA 2002;287:1987–1989.

40. Cannon CP, Gibson CM, Lambrew CT, et al. Relationship of symptom-onset-to-balloon time and door-to-balloon time with mortality in patients undergoing angioplasty for acute myocardial infarction. JAMA 2000;283:2941–2947.

41. The Assessment of the Safety and Efficacy of a New Thrombolytic Regimen (ASSENT)-3 Investigators. Efficacy and safety of tenecteplase in combination with enoxaparin, abciximab, or unfractionated heparin: the ASSENT-3 randomised trial in acute myocardial infarction. Lancet 2001;358:605–613.

42. Antman EM, Louwerenburg HW, Baars HF, et al. Enoxaparin as adjunctive antithrombin therapy for ST-elevation myocardial infarction: Results of the ENTIRE-Thrombolysis in Myocardial Infarction (TIMI) 23 Trial. Circulation 2002;105:1642–1649.

43. TIMI Study Group. Comparison of invasive and conservative strategies after treatment with intravenous tissue plasminogen activator in acute myocardial infarction. Results of the Thrombolysis in Myocardial Infarction (TIMI) Phase II Trial. N Engl J Med 1989;320:618–627.

44. Cannon CP, Thompson B, McCabe CH, et al. Predictors of non-Q-wave acute myocardial infarction in patients with acute ischemic syndromes: An analysis from the Thrombolysis in Myocardial Ischemia (TIMI) III Trials. Am J Cardiol 1995;75:977–981.

45. Cannon CP, McCabe CH, Stone PH, et al. The electrocardiogram predicts one-year outcome of patients with unstable angina and non-Q wave myocardial infarction: Results of the TIMI III Registry ECG Ancillary Study. J Am Coll Cardiol 1997;30:133–140.

46. Hyde TA, French JK, Wong CK, Straznicky IT, Whitlock RM, White HD. Four-year survival of patients with acute coronary syndromes without ST-segment elevation and prognostic significance of 0.5-mm ST-segment depression. Am J Cardiol 1999;84:379–385.

47. Antman EM, McCabe CH, Gurfinkel EP, et al. Enoxaparin prevents death and cardiac ischemic events in unstable Angina/Non-Q-wave myocardial infarction: results of the Thrombolysis In Myocardial Infarction (TIMI) 11B trial. Circulation 1999;100:1593–1601.

48. Newby LK, Christenson RH, Ohman EM, et al. Value of serial troponin T measures for early and late risk stratification in patients with acute coronary syndromes. The GUSTO-IIa Investigators. Circulation 1998;98:1853–1859.

49. Hamm CW, Heeschen C, Goldmann B, et al. Benefit of abciximab in patients with refractory unstable angina in relation to serum troponin T levels. N Engl J Med 1999;340:1623–1629.

50. Heeschen C, Hamm CW, Goldmann B, et al. Troponin concentrations for stratification of patients with acute coronary syndromes in relation to therapeutic efficacy of tirofiban. Lancet 1999;354:1757–1762.

51. Antman EM, Cohen M, Bernink PJ, et al. The TIMI risk score for unstable Angina/Non-ST elevation MI: A method for prognostication and therapeutic decision making. JAMA 2000;284:835–842.

52. Morrow DA, Antman EM, Snapinn SM, McCabe CH, Theroux P, Braunwald E. An integrated clinical approach to predicting the benefit of tirofiban in non-st elevation acute coronary syndromes: Application of the TIMI risk score for UA/NSTEMI in PRISM-PLUS. Eur Heart J 2002;23:223–229.

53. Cannon CP. Critical pathway for unstable angina and non-ST elevation myocardial infarction. February 2002. Crit Path Cardiol 2002;1:12–21.

54. CURE Study Investigators. The Clopidogrel in Unstable angina to prevent Recurrent Events (CURE) trial program; rationale, design and baseline characteristics including a meta-analysis of the effects of thienopyridnes in vascular disease. Eur Heart J 2000;21:2033–2041.

55. Mehta SR, Yusuf S, Peters RJ, et al. Effects of pretreatment with clopidogrel and aspirin followed by long-term therapy in patients undergoing percutaneous coronary intervention: The PCI-CURE study. Lancet 2001;358:527–533.

56. Newby LK, Ohman EM, Christenson RH, et al. Benefit of glycoprotein IIb/IIIa inhibition in patients with acute coronary syndromes and troponin t-positive status: the paragon-B troponin T substudy. Circulation 2001;103:2891–2896.

57. Januzzi JL, Chai CU, Sabatine MS, Jang IK. Elevation in serum troponin I predicts the benefit of tirofiban. J Thromb Thrombolysis 2001;11:211–215.

58. Roffi M, Chew DP, Mukherjee D, et al. Platelet glycoprotein IIb/IIa inhibitors reduce mortality in diabetic patients with non-ST-segment-elevation acute coronary syndromes. Circulation 2001;104:2767–2771.

59. Morrow DA, Antman EM, Tanasijevic M, et al. Cardiac troponin I for stratification of early outcomes and the efficacy of enoxaparin in unstable angina: a TIMI 11B substudy. J Am Coll Cardiol 2000;36:1812–1817.

60. CAPRIE Steering Committee. A randomised, blinded, trial of clopidogrel versus aspirin in patients at risk of ischaemic events (CAPRIE). Lancet 1996;348:1329–1339.

61. Clopidogrel in Unstable Angina to Prevent Recurrent Events Trial Investigators. Effects of clopidogrel in addition to aspirin in patients with acute coronary syndromes without ST-segment elevation. N Engl J Med 2001;345:494–502.

62. Heart Outcomes Prevention Evaluation Study Investigators. Effects of ramipril on cardiovascular and microvascular outcomes in people with diabetes mellitus: results of the HOPE study and MICRO-HOPE substudY. Lancet 2000;355:253–359.

63. Scandinavian Simvastatin Survival Study Group. Randomised trial of cholesterol lowering in 4444 patients with coronary heart disease: the Scandinavian Simvastatin Survival Study (4S). Lancet 1994;344:1383–1389.

64. Sacks RM, Pfeffer MA, Moye LA, et al. The effect of pravastatin on coronary events after myocardial infarction in patients with average cholesterol levels. N Engl J Med 1996;335:1001–1009.

65. The Long-Term Intervention with Pravastatin in Ischaemic Disease (LIPID) Study Group. Prevention of cardiovascular events and death with pravastatin in patients with coronary heart disease and a broad range of initial cholesterol levels. N Engl J Med 1998;339:1349–1357.

66. Executive Summary of The Third Report of The National Cholesterol Education Program (NCEP) Expert Panel on Detection, Evaluation, And Treatment of High Blood Cholesterol In Adults (Adult Treatment Panel III). JAMA 2001;285:2486–2497.

67. Cannon CP, Antman EM, Walls R, Braunwald E. Time as an adjunctive agent to thrombolytic therapy. J Thromb Thrombolysis 1994;1:27–34.

68. Cannon CP. Optimizing the treatment of unstable angina. J Thromb Thrombolysis 1995;2:205–218.

69. Sagarin MJ, Cannon CP, Cermignani MS, Scirica BM, Walls RM. Delay in thrombolysis administration: Causes of extended door-to-drug times and the asymptote effect. J Emerg Med 1998;16:557–565.

70. Cannon CP. Palm Pilot programs to improve the quality of care for patients with acute coronary syndromes. Crit Path Cardiol 1;113–115.

71. Cannon CP, O'Gara PT. Goals, design and implementation of critical pathways In cardiology. In: Cannon CP, O'Gara PT, eds. Critical Pathways in Cardiology. Philadelphia: Lippincott, Williams and Wilkins, 2001:3–6.

72. Braunwald E, Antman EM, Beasley JW, et al. ACC/AHA guideline update for the management of patients with unstable angina and non-ST segment elevation myocardial infarction: a report of the American College of Cardiology/American Heart Association Task Force on Practice Guidelines (Committee on the Management of Unstable Angina). www.acc.org 2002;accessed 3/15/2002.

73. Eagle KA, Goodman SG, Avezum A, et al. Practice variation and missed opportunities for reperfusion in ST-segment-elevation myocardial infarction: findings from the Global Registry of Acute Coronary Events (GRACE). Lancet 2002;359:373–377.

INDEX

763

About the Editor

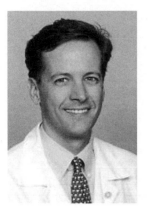

Christopher P. Cannon, MD, is Associate Physician in the Cardiovascular Division at Brigham and Women's Hospital in Boston, and Associate Professor of Medicine at Harvard Medical School. He earned his medical degree from Columbia University College of Physicians and Surgeons in New York and, after completing his residency in internal medicine, was a cardiovascular fellow in medicine at Brigham and Women's Hospital.

In addition to being a frequent lecturer, Dr. Cannon has published more than 300 original articles, reviews, editorials, book chapters and electronic publications in his areas of expertise. His research is published in numerous journals including *Circulation, Journal of the American College of Cardiology, American Journal of Cardiology, American Heart Journal, Journal of the American Medical Association* and the *New England Journal of Medicine.*

Dr. Cannon has received several awards including the Alfred Steiner Research Award, Upjohn Achievement in Research Award, and Robert F. Loeb Award for Excellence in Clinical Medicine. He is a member of a number of professional organizations and committees and serves as Chairman of the Acute Cardiac Care Committee of the Council of Clinical Cardiology of the American Heart Association and a fellow of the American College of Cardiology.

Dr. Cannon has been the principal investigator of several of the Thrombolysis in Myocardial Infarction (TIMI) trials, including most recently the TACTICS-TIMI 18 trial, which demonstrated the superiority of an early invasive strategy as compared with a conservative strategy in patients with unstable angina or non-ST elevation MI treated with a GPIIb/IIIa inhibitor. Dr. Cannon is currently principal investigator of the ongoing PROVE IT (TIMI 22) trial that will evaluate both the relative efficacy of pravastatin versus atorvastatin and the efficacy of an anti-chlamydial antibiotic in patients with acute coronary syndromes.